MOSBY'S
COMPREHENSIVE REVIEW OF
DENTAL HYGIENE

Edited by

MICHELE LEONARDI DARBY, BSDH, MS

Eminent Scholar and Graduate Program Director
School of Dental Hygiene and Dental Assisting
Old Dominion University
Norfolk, Virginia

FOURTH EDITION
Illustrated

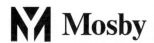 Mosby

St. Louis Baltimore Boston Carlsbad Chicago Minneapolis New York Philadelphia Portland
London Milan Sydney Tokyo Toronto

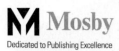
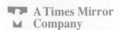

Publisher: John Schrefer
Acquisitions Editor: Penny Rudolph
Associate Developmental Editor: Angela Reiner
Project Manager: Mark Spann
Production Editor: Holly Roseman
Designer: Judi Lang
Manufacturing Manager: Karen Boehme
Editing and Production: Graphic World Publishing Services

Printed in the United States of America
Composition by Graphic World, Inc.
Lithography/color film by Graphic World, Inc.
Printing/binding by Maple-Vail Book Mfg.

Mosby, Inc.
11830 Westline Industrial Drive
St. Louis, Missouri 63146

Library of Congress Cataloging in Publication Data

Mosby's comprehensive review of dental hygiene / edited by Michele
    Leonardi Darby. — 4th ed.
        p.   cm.
    Includes bibliographical references and index.
    ISBN 0-8151-2267-5
    1. Dental hygiene—Outline, syllabi, etc.   2. Dental hygiene—Case
studies.   3. Dental hygiene—Examinations, questions, etc.
I. Darby, Michele Leonardi, 1949-   .
    [DNLM: 1. Dental Prophylaxis—examination questions.   2. Dental
Prophylaxis–outlines.   WU 18.2 M894 1998]
RK60.7.M67   1998
617.6'01'076–dc21
DNLM/DLC
for Library of Congress   97-34800
                                                                  CIP

98 99 00 01 / 9 8 7 6 5 4 3 2 1

Contributors

Stephen C. Bayne, M.S., Ph.D.

Professor and Section Head of Biomaterials
Department of Operative Dentistry
University of North Carolina
Chapel Hill, North Carolina

Marilyn Beck, R.D.H., B.S.D.H., M.Ed.

Associate Professor
Department of Dental Hygiene
Marquette University
Milwaukee, Wisconsin

Denise M. Bowen, R.D.H., M.S.

Professor
Department of Dental Hygiene
Idaho State University
Pocatello, Idaho

Patricia Regener Campbell, R.D.H., M.S.

Assistant Professor and Clinic Coordinator
Caruth School of Dental Hygiene
Baylor College of Dentistry
The Texas A&M University System
Dallas, Texas

Catherine C. Davis, Ph.D.

Associate Clinical Professor
Department of Basic Science and Oral Research
University of Colorado
Denver, Colorado

Mary Catherine Dean, R.D.H., M.S.

Assistant Professor and Clinic Coordinator
Department of Dental Hygiene
University of Maryland at Baltimore
Baltimore, Maryland

Linda Rubinstein DeVore, R.D.H., M.A.

Associate Professor and Chair
Department of Dental Hygiene
University of Maryland at Baltimore
Baltimore, Maryland

Dianne M. Frazier, Ph.D., M.P.H., R.D.

Assistant Professor
Department of Pediatrics and Biochemistry
School of Medicine
University of North Carolina
Chapel Hill, North Carolina

Kara T. Hansen, Ph.D., R.D.H.

Dental Hygiene Practitioner
Phoenix, Arizona

Barbara Heckman, R.D.H., M.S.

Program Coordinator
Department of Dental Hygiene
Diablo Valley College
Pleasant Hill, California

Olga A.C. Ibsen, R.D.H., M.S.

Adjunct Professor
Department of Dental Hygiene
University of New Haven
West Haven, Connecticut

Beverly Entwistle Isman, R.D.H., M.P.H.

Oral Health Consultant
Davis, California

Sandra Kramer, R.D.H., M.A.

Dental Hygiene Practitioner and Consultant
Berkeley, California

Sally Mauriello, R.D.H., M.Ed.

Associate Professor
Division of Dental Hygiene
University of North Carolina
Chapel Hill, North Carolina

Jill Nield-Gehrig, R.D.H., M.A.

Division of Allied Health and Public Service Education
Asheville-Buncombe Technical Community College
Asheville, North Carolina

Lynn Markley Ray, R.D.H., B.S.

Director of Test Development and Analysis
Central Regional Dental Testing Service, Inc.
Tulsa, Oklahoma

Barbara Requa-Clark, Pharm.D.

Professor of Dentistry (Pharmacology)
University of Missouri at Kansas City
School of Dentistry
Kansas City, Missouri

Maureen Dotzel Savner, R.D.H., M.S.

Assistant Professor and Clinic Coordinator
Department of Dental Health
Luzerne County Community College
Nanticoke, Pennsylvania

Edward J. Swift, Jr., D.M.D., M.S.

Associate Professor
Department of Operative Dentistry
University of North Carolina
Chapel Hill, North Carolina

Jeffrey Y. Thompson, Ph.D.

Assistant Professor and Biomaterials Laboratory Director
Department of Operative Dentistry
University of North Carolina
Chapel Hill, North Carolina

Lynn Utecht, M.D., M.A., R.D.H.

Head, Dermatology
Naval Medical Center Portsmouth
Portsmouth, Virginia

Esther M. Wilkins, R.D.H., D.M.D.

Associate Clinical Professor
Department of Periodontology
Tufts University School of Dental Medicine
Boston, Massachusetts

Pamela Zarkowski, J.D., M.P.H., B.S.D.H.

Professor and Associate Dean of Academic Administration
University of Detroit Mercy
School of Dentistry
Detroit, Michigan

Susan Zimmer, R.D.H., M.Ed.

Curriculum Specialist
Salish Kootenai College
Pablo, Montana

To my husband, Dennis, and our children, Devan and Blake,
for the joy and peace they bring me
M.L.D.

Preface

The success of earlier editions of *Mosby's Comprehensive Review of Dental Hygiene* and the plethora of new research discoveries that are expanding the education, practice, and future of dental hygiene serve as the prime forces directing the development of the fourth edition. Educational trends, changing societal needs, and new healthcare systems require today's dental hygienist to possess a breadth and depth of knowledge in the biological, social, behavioral, and dental hygiene sciences and in general education.

Publishing a book that selectively reviews the current body of dental hygiene knowledge is a challenge. This book meets that challenge with several key purposes in mind: first, to assist the dental hygiene student in reviewing the theory, skills, and judgments required on national, regional, and state dental hygiene board examinations; second, to prepare the individual for reentry into the field by updating knowledge for contemporary dental hygiene roles—clinician, educator/health promotor, change agent, consumer advocate, researcher, and manager; and third, to provide dental hygiene educators with salient information that can be used for course development and evaluation.

The reader will notice some major changes from the previous edition. A special effort was made to design case-based questions that include client health and dental history information, dental charts, radiographs and photographs, and some photographs are in color. Throughout the book, the term "client" is used instead of "patient" because the term is congruent with dental hygiene's disease prevention and health promotion and wellness focus. Most important, "client" conveys dental hygiene's partnership with consumers who take responsibility for their own health. Last, the term "client" encompasses individuals, families, groups and communities who may be the focus of dental hygiene services. Both the American Dental Hygienists' Association and the Canadian Dental Hygienists' Association have embraced the term "client" in their policies and actions.

The fourth edition of *Mosby's Comprehensive Review of Dental Hygiene* is divided into 18 independent yet interrelated chapters. Fifteen of the chapters cover the subject areas traditionally found on the National Board Dental Hygiene Examination. The remaining three chapters focus on board examinations; practice management and career development strategies; and historical, professional, ethical, and legal issues facing dental hygienists.

Chapter 1 provides guidance and practical suggestions for anyone preparing for a board examination. Also included is basic information on licensure/practice requirements for dental hygienists interested in international employment in select countries. Chapters 2 through 18 contain theoretical and practical information in an outline format and review questions with rationales explaining why the correct answer is appropriate and why each incorrect choice is wrong. The rationales for the correct and incorrect answers provide an additional strategy for board preparation. This information should enable the reviewer to assess both decision-making and judgment in using professional knowledge and facilitate mastery of each chapter's content.

This edition includes a Simulated National Board Dental Hygiene Examination also with rationales for right and wrong answers. Paralleling the National Board Dental Hygiene Examination in content and question format, this test permits students to experience the reality of a board examination. To achieve the maximum benefit of this test, students should record their responses, and score the test using the answers provided. The Simulated National Board Dental Hygiene Examination assists persons who are attempting to improve their objective test-taking ability and enables the individual to make the most effective use of study time by identifying areas of weakness. Having first identified specific areas for study and then reviewing the comprehensive information provided in the text, the individual should feel prepared and confident about board examinations.

A comprehensive index enables the user to locate information quickly and easily. Illustrations throughout the text and the Appendixes minimize the need to search alternate sources; however, reference lists are provided for those who desire a more in-depth study.

I would like to express my sincere appreciation to those who helped make this edition of *Mosby's Comprehensive Review of Dental Hygiene* a reality. The outlined materials, multiple-choice and case-based questions, and rationales were developed by educators and practitioners who are recognized experts. Comments and suggestions from students, faculty, and returning dental hygienists who have used the book are embodied in this fourth edition. The exemplary work of these contributors has made *Mosby's Comprehensive Review of Dental Hygiene* a classic in the field.

My special thanks go to Penny Rudolph, Acquisitions Editor, and Angela Reiner, Associate Developmental Editor, from Mosby–Year Book, who facilitated the many steps of the publication process.

Recognition and appreciation go to Deborah L. Miller, graphic design supervisor, Susan T. Cooke, graphic designer, and Donald K. Emminger, graphic designer, from Old Dominion University Academic Television Services Graphics Unit, and B. Yvonne Wilson, freelance illustrator, for some of the illustrations provided. Appreciation is extended to Karen Caspers, Director of Administration and Special Projects from the American Dental Hygienists' Association, for providing current information on association activities. Also acknowledged are the authors and publishers who granted permission to use quotes, concepts, photographs, figures, and tables.

Since the work of those who contributed to the earlier editions remains central to this revision, I want to gratefully acknowledge their efforts, particularly the work of Dr. Eleanor Bushee, whose competence and good humor as an oral health professional, editor, teacher, administrator, colleague, and friend will forever be missed, and Dr. Marcia Brand, Jan Shaner Greenlee, Charlotte Hangorsky, Dr. Donald E. Isselhard, Patricia Damon-Johnson, Mary M. Lee, Susan Schwartz Miller, Cara Miyasaki, Dr. Marlene Moss-Klyvert, Dr. John Powers, Dr. Peggy Reep, Dr. Lindsay Rettie, Nancy Webb and K. Cy Whaley. Without all these generous and talented people, the fourth edition of *Mosby's Comprehensive Review of Dental Hygiene*, would not have been possible.

Michele Leonardi Darby

Contents

Preparing for National, Regional, and State Dental Hygiene Board Examinations

Lynn Ray

Preparing for board examinations requires careful planning, study and review, time management, organization of information and schedules for applications, and a positive attitude. Conscientious dental hygienists will organize a plan for success well in advance and be prepared to satisfy board requirements with confidence in their professional knowledge and skills. This book is a guide through a comprehensive body of knowledge that constitutes the basis of dental hygiene practice. Systematic use of this book can enable one to reinforce professional education, benefit from exposure to concepts and ideas from a variety of dental hygiene educators, and identify those areas where additional study is needed.

This introductory chapter outlines suggestions on how a dental hygienist—whether a new graduate, a practicing dental hygienist who is moving to another licensing jurisdiction, or a dental hygienist who wishes to begin practicing again after an extended period of inactivity—can prepare for board examinations. The chapter takes into consideration preparation for both theoretic and clinical examinations. A dental hygienist must master the basic

subject matter and skills necessary for practice; therefore, each chapter of this book focuses on different aspects of such knowledge and skills. However, there have been instances where highly knowledgeable and skillful dental hygienists have failed to successfully complete board examinations. It is just as essential that the dental hygienist be psychologically, emotionally, and physically prepared to demonstrate competence and be thoroughly familiar with the format, logistics, and requirements of any examination preparatory to licensure.

This chapter provides basic information about how the credentialing system is organized and how it functions with the interaction of many different agencies and organizations. A more detailed discussion is included on the Joint Commission on National Dental Examinations, its testing program, and the development of test items. Further discussion is devoted to regional testing services and clinical board examinations in general. The chapter concludes with an overview of this review book, including its purposes and organization, as well as instructions on how to use it effectively.

Structure of Credentialing Agencies

In preparing for board examinations, one should understand the credentialing system. Many dental hygienists, particularly new graduates who have never been licensed, often have only a vague understanding of the system with which they are interacting. Such lack of awareness has even resulted in a few dental hygienists assuming that receiving a certificate for successful completion of an examination is authorization to practice, and they have begun practicing illegally without a license. Passing board examinations satisfies the major requirements for licensure, but there are usually other prerequisites as well. There is often a complex interrelationship of agencies involved in the board examination process. It behooves the examination candidate to have a clear understanding of which agency is administering an examination, how that agency functions, and by what authority the agency administers examinations and issues credentials.

State Boards of Dentistry/Dental Hygiene

The basic authority to recognize any credential for licensure lies with the state board of dentistry. Each state or licensing jurisdiction has a *state practice act* or some statutes that regulate the practice of dentistry/dental hygiene within that jurisdiction. Such statutes also establish a regulatory agency to enforce the law, conduct examinations for competence, and regulate the practice of dentistry/dental hygiene. There are features that virtually all state practice acts have in common; however, even a cursory review of state practice acts will alert one to the fact that they are inconsistent in defining the legal practice of dentistry/dental hygiene. Great variations exist from state to state in the way regulatory boards are organized, in the power or authority they have, and even in the names with which they are entitled. For the purpose of clarity in this text, the term *state board or state board of dentistry* is used to refer to the regulatory agency in a respective state that is empowered to determine prerequisites for licensure and issue licenses to practice dental hygiene. One of the first things a candidate for licensure should know is the correct title of the state board for the state(s) in which licensure is sought.

It is far too common for licensure candidates, and even licensed practitioners in a state, to have a fuzzy conception of what the state board actually is. Many professionals confuse the board with the local state dental association. Although strong ties usually exist between a state board and the state dental association, legally there are distinct differences in their organization and purpose. The state board of dentistry is a *government agency,* established by law, that functions as an arm of the state legislature to regulate the practice of dentistry. Its sole purpose is to protect the public from incompetent or unethical practi-

tioners. In contrast, a state dental or dental hygiene association is a *voluntary organization* of practitioners who join together to promote the oral health of the public and advance the profession. As one studies the credentialing system, it becomes evident that dental/dental hygiene associations are integrally involved in activities that affect the legal requirements for licensure. However, it is important to understand the distinction between state boards and professional associations. Professional associations *do not* determine requirements for licensure or regulate practice; that is determined by law and implemented through state boards. Professional associations *do,* however, initiate programs and research projects, studies, and legislative changes that are ultimately incorporated into the legal requirements for practice. Specific examples of the interrelationship between state boards and professional associations are provided with further explanation of the credentialing system.

Because state boards of dentistry are charged with the responsibility of conducting examinations for competence to practice, the candidate for licensure should be aware of how board members are identified. It is of particular interest to candidates for clinical examinations because state board members are very likely to be the clinical examiners. In the vast majority of states, state board members are appointed by the governor; in only two states (North Carolina and Oklahoma) are board members selected by an elective process within the profession. Despite the fact that gubernatorial appointments are the prevailing method, professional associations have an effect on this process as well. It is general practice in most states for the state association to submit a list of nominees from which the governor appoints. Although the governor is often not limited to such a list, in most instances appointments are made from the nominees designated by the association. Most states have few if any formal criteria for qualifications of board members.

Dental hygienists may be interested in activities of their professional associations that have changed the face of the credentialing system. In the early 1970s, state boards consisted almost universally of dentists, with a few boards having public members. As a result of the legislative initiatives of many state dental hygiene associations, within 10 years about 40 state boards included one or more dental hygienists in their membership, and by the early 1990s, all states had some form of dental hygiene representation on the board. The 1980s brought a thrust in some states to establish separate dental hygiene state boards and/or examining committees. Since the 1960s, another area of activity in many states has been to expand the functions that constitute the legal practice of dental hygiene. Changes in these functions and in the structure of state boards have had and will continue to have an impact on the content and format of board examinations. One should understand that the legislative and political arenas in health professions are fluid and constantly changing, as are technologic advancements. This dictates an ongoing necessity for the dental hygienist to continually update professional skills and knowledge, and it requires constant revision of examinations and redefining of standards of competence. Although this places demands on the individual practitioner, on the educational system, and on those agencies that are responsible for evaluating competence, it is the means by which the profession is able to advance its standards of care.

Having briefly reviewed the structure and nature of state boards and how they may interact with professional associations, it is appropriate to refocus attention on the responsibilities of the state boards with respect to board examinations. Typically, state practice acts charge the state board with conducting both theoretic and practical examinations to determine competence to practice. Some state laws even define the content of such examinations and specify the passing score. Most practice acts authorize the state board to recognize other examinations equivalent to their own. The act may even specify recognition of certain examinations, such as national or regional boards. This is the basis on which other agencies become a part of the credentialing process, but it must be recognized that the fundamental authorization to recognize credentials for licensure lies with the state board of dentistry.

Dental/Dental Hygiene Professional Associations

Any review of the credentialing system would be incomplete without reference to an essential licensure requirement (i.e., graduation from a program accredited by the Commission on Dental Accreditation of the American Dental Association [ADA]). Because it is implied that dental hygienists preparing for board examinations will have satisfied this requirement, it is not relevant to dwell on a lengthy discussion of accreditation standards. Suffice it to say that accreditation for dental hygiene education programs was instituted in 1951 with the encouragement and extensive involvement of the American Dental Hygienists' Association (ADHA). Graduation from an accredited school has become a basic licensure requirement in most state practice acts. Those states that provide for licensure of a dentist or dental hygienist from a nonaccredited school generally require evidence of an educational program that is equivalent to an accredited program. It should be noted that recognition of an accrediting agency is a governmental function. In most healthcare fields with a specialized educational system, accreditation is conducted by a specialized agency within the profession. In dentistry, the US Department of Education Council on Post-Secondary Accreditation (COPA) has recognized the ADA Commission on Dental Accreditation (CODA) as the official accrediting body for schools of dentistry, dental hygiene, dental assisting, and dental laboratory technology. The diploma or certificate of graduation is an essential credential for licensure for dental hygienists that is based on the accreditation program carried out under the auspices of the ADA.

Joint Commission on National Dental Examinations

The National Board Examination Program is another prime example of how the concerns of dental practitioners and educators, expressed through their professional associations, influence the legal requirements for licensure. In the early part of this century, each individual state board prepared and administered its own theoretic and clinical examinations. Obviously, there were extreme variations in the difficulty, content, and format of such examinations. Any practitioner wishing to move from one state to another had to take more examinations. Although it is reasonably feasible for a practitioner to remain current in clinical procedures and be able to demonstrate competence at any point professionally, it is much more difficult to remain current in all the didactic material included in theoretic examinations. It was equally difficult for state boards to keep their examinations up-to-date and secure the resources to ensure the comprehensiveness and reliability of the examinations. Interest grew in developing a national, comprehensive, theoretic examination that would satisfy state board requirements for licensure and reduce barriers to the mobility of dental practitioners. The logical source for organizing such a collaborative effort was the ADA.

In 1928 the ADA established the Council of National Board of Dental Examiners, composed of three ADA members, three members of the American Association of Dental Schools (AADS), and three members of the American Association of Dental Examiners (AADE). The first National Board Dental Examination was administered in 1933. The program gradually gained acceptance, and over a period of years most state practice acts were revised to recognize successful completion of National Board Dental Examinations as satisfying the theoretic examination requirement.

Interest in a dental hygiene national board examination program emerged in the 1950s during the period when national accreditation standards were established for dental hygiene educational programs. In 1959 the ADHA instituted an achievement testing program and also formed a liaison committee with the American Association of Dental Examiners. Working with this liaison committee and also through its involvement with the ADA's Council on Dental Education accreditation program, the ADHA gained support for a dental hygiene national board examination. In 1960 the ADHA requested that the ADA Board of Trustees consider assigning the development of a dental hygiene national board to an appropriate ADA agency. In 1961 the ADA Council of National Board of Dental Examiners was charged with this responsibility; the ADA agreed to underwrite the developmental costs for the examination, and the ADHA agreed to provide the test-item files and information from the ADHA achievement testing program. This brief history is the basis for the ADA and ADHA involvement in the National Board Dental Hygiene Examination, which was first administered in the spring of 1962.

The original ADA Council of National Board of Dental Examiners has evolved through its own history of structural and political changes up until 1980 when it became the Joint Commission on National Dental Examinations. Its membership is composed of three ADA members, three AADS members, six AADE members, one ADHA member, one public member, and one member from the American Student Dental Association. Dental hygiene involvement has historically been broadened by the Committee on Dental Hygiene, which was established in 1962. This committee has five dental hygienists—two educators and two practitioners appointed by the ADHA (one of whom is the ADHA Commissioner) and a dental hygiene student representative—plus one commissioner from each of the respective parent organizations: the ADA, AADE, and AADS. The Committee on Dental Hygiene assumes fundamental responsibility for guiding the development and administrative policies of the dental hygiene examinations. The committee reviews examinations, considers problems that arise, and recommends policy and regulations for the examination program. The commission has final authority to act on all recommendations of the committee, but historically the Committee on Dental Hygiene has been the guiding force of the dental hygiene examination program.

Having reviewed the basic structure of the credentialing system and how it is influenced by other professional organizations, it is appropriate to review the actual National Board Dental Hygiene Examination Program in more detail.

National Board Dental Hygiene Examination Program

Examination Format

When the National Board Dental Hygiene Examination was first administered in 1962, the test was organized according to subject matter. That is, 12 subjects were organized into groups of 3 to make a 4-part examination. Special test construction committees were formed to develop test items related to community dental health, dental health education, and clinical dental hygiene. Other subjects, such as microbiology, pathology, and histology, were assigned to appropriate dental test construction committees. The subject-oriented examination format was used from 1962 through 1972.

In 1969 the Committee on Dental Hygiene recommended the development of a comprehensive, function-oriented examination that would be organized according to the services that a dental hygienist may be expected to provide in practice. The purposes were to emphasize the more practical application of knowledge to clinical situations and to eliminate some of the overlapping of test items between subjects. The Committee on Dental Hygiene, in conjunction with the ADHA Education Committee, spent almost 2 years developing a function-oriented examination outline, which was widely circulated throughout the profession for input. The first function-oriented examination was developed and administered in March 1973, and its basic format remained in effect through 1986. The most notable problem with the function-oriented examination was that the outline did not clearly reflect the basic science foundation of the test. Although the technical skills essential to the practice of dental hygiene were evident, the scientific knowledge that is the basis of competent practice was less clearly defined. Therefore, the outline was revised for the 1987 examination to include a basic science section.

In the mid 1990s, the Committee on Dental Hygiene explored the feasibility of a case-based examination format that would focus on a candidate's ability to use and apply knowledge in a client-oriented, clinical simulation. Such a format was field-tested in 1995 and targeted for full-scale administration in 1998. Each case should contain a client's medical and dental history; a dental chart, including periodontal information; radiographs; extra/intra-oral photographs, as appropriate; and laboratory reports, as needed. The case material is followed by 10 to 15 related questions. The Committee has specified that each examination should contain at least one case for such client types as: geriatric, adult-periodontal, pediatric, special needs and medically-compromised.

Introduction of the case-based items does not substantially change the *content* of the examination outline; however, it does change the examination *format*. The examination lasts one day and includes approximately 350 questions. The morning session presents 200 items covering the three basic sections of the traditional examination outline—(1) scientific basis for dental hygiene practice, (2) provision of clinical dental hygiene services, (3) community health activities. The afternoon session presents 150 case-based items, which focus primarily on the provision of dental hygiene services and test the candidate's knowledge of assessing client characteristics, obtaining and interpreting radiographs, planning and managing dental hygiene care, performing periodontal procedures, using preventive agents, and providing supportive treatment services. Some basic science items are integrated into case problems, along with a few questions that assess knowledge of professional responsibility and occupational safety.

Examination Outline

The examination outline should be carefully reviewed by all examination candidates; it is the blueprint from which all editions of the test are constructed. The outline defines the specific topics or functions that are included in the examination content, with an itemization of the number of questions devoted to each area. The examination outline is circulated constantly for review and comment and is routinely refined and modified by the Committee on Dental Hygiene in order to keep the examination current. The examination content includes only those functions that are legal in the majority of states. Functions such as the administration of local anesthesia are covered only to the extent of background information that a dental hygienist is expected to know in relation to such basic sciences as pharmacology or anatomy. Questions regarding functions such as the technique for injection of anaesthetic agents are not included unless that function is legal in the majority of states.

It is not appropriate to print the examination outline within this text since ongoing revisions may render such a duplication inaccurate or misleading. Any dental hygienist preparing for the examination should secure a current copy of the examination outline and use it as a guide for study and review.

Test Construction Committees

National Board Dental Hygiene Examinations are developed through an extensive structure of test construction committees. Test constructors are selected by the Joint Commission on National Dental Examinations from applications solicited from schools, state boards, and professional associations and generally serve a term of 5 years. The membership of test construction committees is balanced according to the content of the examinations being developed and the disciplines that are covered. The commission maintains criteria for the selection of test constructors, and in addition to the qualifications of experience and expertise, geographic distribution is an important consideration.

The emphasis on dental hygiene functions necessitates the use of interdisciplinary committees to construct the examination. Each interdisciplinary committee is composed of a dentist or dental hygienist with an advanced degree in one of the basic sciences, a dentist or dental hygienist with expertise in radiography, a periodontist, a clinical dental hygienist, a dental hygienist with a strong curriculum background, and a dentist or dental hygienist with expertise in community oral health. Each edition of the examination is reviewed by at least two interdisciplinary committees: the first committee drafts the examination, and the second committee reviews and finalizes it. In addition, every examination edition is reviewed after it has been administered and statistics have been generated for each question. Items that are statistically unsatisfactory are reviewed, revised, or discarded. Therefore test construction committees have three routine responsibilities: drafting new examinations, reviewing examination drafts prepared by another committee, and reviewing unsatisfactory test items after an examination has been administered. The test construction committees work with test-item files containing thousands of questions that are classified according to the content area of the examination outline. The committees also develop new items, and questions are constantly solicited from throughout the profession.

Examination Scoring System

A norm-referenced scoring system is used for all National Board Dental Hygiene Examinations to ensure uniform meaning of scores from edition to edition of the tests. The converted score that is reported is known as a standard score, which indicates how an individual's score relates to the average. Standard scores can be averaged and correlated, and the results are generally proportional to differences in raw scores. The examinations maintain a degree of difficulty high enough to spread candidates out over a broad range of performance. Therefore there tend to be distinct differences in the performances of those who pass and those who fail, and guessing correctly on a few test items has minimal effect on an individual's score in relation to the other candidates. The average raw score on an examination is usually around 65%, which would convert to a standard score of approximately 85.

A candidate's examination score depends on two factors. The first, of course, is the raw score or number of correct answers the candidate selects. The second is the distribution of raw scores of the norming group. The norming group used for National Board Dental Hygiene Examinations consists of all candidates taking the examination for the first time who are students in fully accredited dental hygiene programs. The mean raw score of the norming group is always assigned the standard score of 85. Next, the raw score 1.5 standard deviations below the mean raw score is assigned the standard score of 75. All other standard scores are computed by using the relationship between these two. There is no fixed failure rate, but the results have remained stable for many years, and the failure rate is typically less than 10% for first-time candidates. A standard score of 75 is required to pass. It is obvious that as new editions of the examination are drafted, some may be more difficult than others; it is impossible to predict the difficulty level of new questions that are introduced. The norm-referenced scoring system eliminates inconsistencies in the results that may be caused by differences in difficulty between editions of the examination. Another potential inconsistency exists, however, in the possible differences among norming groups. If there is any possibility that the overall performance of new graduates in 1 year was less than that of graduates 5 years previously, then a norm-referenced score would not mean the same thing from year to year. To measure any significant differences in norming groups from year to year, the commission uses anchor items. Anchor items are selected questions that are used in repeated editions of the examination. The statistics on these anchor items are monitored and compared to see if there is any difference in the performance of the norming groups.

Examination Irregularities

The commission maintains a program to identify any irregularities or cheating on the examinations. For many years this has been done during the scoring process by computer comparison of answers to detect improbable similarities. The commission began implementing a plan in 1984 to use alternate forms of the examination so that different test booklets have the same questions in scrambled order. The commission is committed to maintaining the integrity of each candidate's individual results and can be expected to use as effective a system as possible to control irregularities.

Released Examinations

The commission has traditionally released examinations almost every year and has maintained that policy with the dental examinations. Since the implementation of the function-oriented examination in 1973, National Board Dental Hygiene Examinations have been released far less frequently, at intervals of 3 to 5 years. This is primarily because it is much more difficult to develop questions that require the application of knowledge to specific clinical functions. Test constructors must not only have knowledge in their area of expertise but must also understand how that knowledge is relevant to the practice of dental hygiene. The bank of test items must be large enough that the release of questions does not jeopardize the integrity and security of the examination program. The commission recognizes the desirability of releasing examinations frequently and circulating ample information so that misconceptions do not develop about the testing program. They are guided in their decisions by both the need to provide information and the necessity of maintaining a secure bank of reliable test items. Certainly, released examinations are an invaluable study guide for dental hygienists preparing for the National Board Dental Hygiene Examination. However, their greatest value is simply as a study guide; it is not constructive for a candidate to attempt to memorize questions. Changing one or two words in a question can alter the entire item, and the candidate who has memorized questions by rote will be utterly confused. It is far more constructive to invest one's energy in building a solid knowledge base that allows one to respond to many questions.

Release of Examination Results

It takes approximately 7 weeks to process and report examination scores. The candidate receives an individual score report, the school of graduation receives a report, and scores are sent to those state boards that have been specified by the candidate to receive a report. There is no limit on the number of times a candidate may retake the examination; however, a dental hygienist who fails the examination twice within a 25-month period must wait 1 year to retake the examination. Some jurisdictions require successful completion of the National Board Dental Hygiene Examination before a candidate is eligible for a clinical examination. The prerequisites of each jurisdiction in which a candidate is interested in obtaining licensure should be researched well in advance so that the necessary preparations to satisfy such requirements can be effectively scheduled.

Examination Availability

The National Board Dental Hygiene Examination is offered three times a year: usually in March, July, and December. Any graduate of an accredited dental hygiene program is eligible to take the examination; students who are certified by their program director as being within 4 months of graduation are also eligible. The results are accepted in all states, the District of Columbia, Puerto Rico, and the Virgin Islands. Some states, such as Florida and Hawaii, as well as Puerto Rico and the Virgin Islands, have time restrictions for accepting examination results. These jurisdictions require that examination scores be current within a certain number of years for licensure to be granted.

Characteristics of Multiple-Choice Test Items

National Board Dental Hygiene Examinations are composed of approximately 350 questions, all of which are multiple-choice items. There are several different approved formats for the structure of these items. A multiple-choice item consists of a stem, which poses a problem, and a set of possible answers or options. All of the questions in this examination must have at least three and not more than five possible answers. Only one choice should be correct or clearly the best answer. Other possible options are termed "distractors" because they are designed to distract the candidate from the correct answer.

Item Stems

The stem of an item either poses a question or forms an incomplete statement. The candidate should be able to determine what is being asked on the basis of the stem alone. The stem should contain all the information necessary to present the question, but there should be no extraneous information. The purpose of the stem is to test, not to teach. Key words in the stem such as *best, most, first,* or *least* are usually highlighted or italicized.

Distractors

The quality of the distractors determines the effectiveness of a question. A good distractor is plausible enough to attract the attention of candidates who lack the knowledge or skill being tested. Common misconceptions are frequently included as distractors, as well as responses that meet some but not all of the conditions posed in the stem. Possible answers are usually ordered according to length, and good distractors are of relatively uniform length. A well-constructed question also has distractors that are grammatically consistent with the stem (i.e., all options are nouns or verbs or whatever is appropriate grammar to complete the stem).

Correct Answer

Each test item should have only one option that is correct or clearly the best answer. Every effort is made to use only those items for which a correct or best answer is nationally agreed upon. Answers that reflect regional philosophies are avoided.

Formats of National Board Multiple-Choice Items

A variety of item formats are approved for use in National Board Dental Hygiene Examinations. Familiarity with these formats and knowing how to respond to each of them will help the candidate avoid confusion. A description of the types of approved formats follows, along with examples of questions.

Completion-Type Items

The stem of a completion-type item contains a statement that is completed by the addition of the selected answer. These items are generally easy to read and understand. For example:

The term used to describe the radiographic appearance of the trabecular (cancellous) bone is
A. Honeycomb
B. Herringbone
C. Sunburst
D. Webbed
It should be noted that the options in the above question all contain a verbal phrase that completes the statement in the stem in the proper grammatical context. The options are ordered according to length.

Question-Type Items

The stem of a question-type item contains a complete question. These items are generally simple, straightforward, and easily understood. This is probably the most frequently used type of item in National Board examinations. An example follows:
Which primary tooth usually erupts after the primary maxillary lateral incisors?
A. Mandibular canine
B. Maxillary canine
C. Mandibular first molar
D. Mandibular second molar

Negative Items

A negative test item is characterized by a word such as *except, not,* or *least* in the stem of the question. The key negative word is always capitalized or italicized to call the candidates' attention to it. Negative items can be either completion-type or question-type items. All the options for a negative item are generally stated in the positive form. Negative items are useful for testing exceptions to general principles. Examples are shown below:
The side effects of antineoplastic agents include all of the following EXCEPT
A. Anemia
B. Thrombocytopenia
C. Addison's syndrome
D. Leukopenia

Paired True-False Items

In a paired true-false item, the stem is the only portion of the question that varies. The stem consists of two statements on the same topic. The options always provide all possible true-false combinations. For example:
Disclosing solution is an important adjunct for teaching individuals their strengths and weaknesses in bacterial plaque removal. It is especially important for assessing subgingival plaque removal techniques.
A. Both statements are *TRUE.*
B. Both statements are *FALSE.*
C. The first statement is *TRUE;* the second is *FALSE.*
D. The first statement is *FALSE,* the second is *TRUE.*

Paired true-false items do not occur frequently in National Board Dental Hygiene Examinations.

Cause-and-Effect Items

A cause-and-effect item is very similar to a paired true-false item in that the only portion of the question that varies is the stem. The stem contains a statement and a reason that are written as a single sentence and connected by *because*. The possible answers are always the same, as in the example below:

Questionable or incipient carious lesions are an indication for sealant placement, because the sealant will interrupt or eliminate the progress of the decay process.

A. Both statement and reason are correct and related.
B. Both statement and reason are correct but *NOT* related.
C. The statement is correct, but the reason is *NOT.*
D. The statement is *NOT* correct, but the reason is accurate.
E. *NEITHER* the statement *NOR* the reason is correct.

This type of item requires the candidate to judge both the accuracy and the relationship of two statements. Such items should be read very carefully to avoid confusion. Cause-and-effect items generally appear with limited frequency in National Board Dental Hygiene Examinations.

Case Problems

For many years, National Board Dental Hygiene Examinations have typically contained several case problems. These items describe a client's condition or clinical situation and are followed by several test items related to the case problem. The case problem may include only written material or may be supplemented with charts, line drawings, or radiographs.

This concept was being expanded in the late 1990s. The case-based portion of the examination presents the candidate with brief histories containing medical, dental, and social histories along with the chief complaint; a complete periodontal chart; a complete mouth radiographic survey and panographic survey and high-quality, colored clinical photographs. The candidate must answer questions based on observations and judgments of the client's clinical condition as documented in the case material. Questions that relate to the case problem may be presented in any of the test-item formats that have been described.

Tips for Taking Multiple-Choice Tests

Alert candidates will use some general strategies in taking any multiple-choice examination. A poorly constructed examination will contain many clues for a test-wise candidate. The careful construction process and editing to which National Board Dental Hygiene Examination items

are subjected minimizes many of these typical clues. However, developing a system for reading and responding to questions will facilitate a candidate's performance.

1. Read the stem of the question carefully and completely before looking at the answers.
   a. Clearly determine what the question is asking, identify key words, and try to formulate the answer in your mind before looking at the answers.
   b. Reach each answer carefully, and determine whether it is an appropriate response to the question and gives as complete an answer as possible.
   c. Immediately eliminate any answers that are obviously incorrect, and attempt to narrow the choices to not more than two.
   d. For combination multiple-choice items, narrow the choices by eliminating any answer that contains an incorrect response, and consider only those answers that contain responses that you confidently know are correct.
   e. When the choices have been narrowed as much as possible and the correct answer is still not clear, make an educated guess. There is no penalty for guessing.
2. Avoid selecting any answer that contains such words as *always, never, none, all,* or *every.* There are seldom any conditions that are absolute in the health field, and unconditional responses are usually incorrect answers.
3. Look for the answer that *best* applies to the conditions presented in the question. An option may be partially true or may apply under certain conditions. Select the *best* answer that will generally apply under most conditions and is specifically applicable to the question. If several options might be true but one option would incorporate all possibilities, that option should clearly be the *best* answer.
   a. Avoid selecting answers that are based on isolated rules, are applicable only to certain locales or regions, or refer to procedures and techniques that are not broadly practiced.
   b. If the question asks for an immediate action, such as what is the *first* thing one would do, all of the options may be correct. The *best* answer would have to be based on identified priorities and on the conditions stipulated in the question.
4. Be alert for grammatical clues. A well-edited question will offer options that are all grammatically correct with the stem. If the question indicates a plural response, all the options should be in plural form. Any response that is inconsistent with the flow of the question may be an indication of an incorrect answer.
5. Watch for the words *not, least,* or *except* in the stem of the question. If an item does not make sense, re-

read it carefully to be sure a key word has not been overlooked.

6. Carefully review questions that include as a response "all of the above" or "none of the above." These responses impose broadly inclusive and exclusive conditions. "None of the above" has limited usefulness as a response because it entirely negates the premise of the question.

7. The pattern of numbers for correct answers should be fairly random. Do not be overly concerned if the same-numbered answer is selected repeatedly, and it is not advisable to base answer selections on a pattern of numbers.

8. Be careful to mark the correct space on the answer sheet that relates to the item. Periodically review the answer sheet to make sure you have not inadvertently marked in the wrong space.

9. The spaces on the answer sheet should be completely marked with a dark line, but no marks should extend outside the lines. Listen carefully when instructions are given for marking the answer sheet. Do not assume it is just like others you may have used.

Guidelines for Preparing for National Board Dental Hygiene Examinations

1. Organize a study plan 4 to 6 months in advance that will allow an orderly, progressive review without undue pressure.

2. Obtain an examination outline and application materials, including a brochure or any information about the examination provided by the Joint Commission on National Dental Examinations. Study the information carefully to clearly understand the format and design of the examination and the protocol for its administration.

3. Obtain a copy of the most recently released National Board Dental Hygiene Examination. Released examinations are usually available through a dental or dental hygiene school library or from the Commission itself. Set aside a day without interruptions; take the examination without advance preparation but with the same time limitations that are prescribed in the examination. As you take the test, mark all questions about which you are unsure.

4. Grade yourself with the key that is included in the released examination.

5. Prepare an outline of the areas in which you have identified weaknesses. Be guided by your experience in school as indicated by grades or difficulty in certain subjects and by the items from the released examination that you missed or marked as questionable. Dental hygienists who have been out of school or practice

for some period of time should focus on basic science material and any developments in dental technology or services that may have expanded the knowledge base since their graduation.

6. Gather a personal resource library for ready reference throughout the review process. Properly used, this book should be the mainstay of your study guides; directions for its use are included further on in this chapter. This book is designed to direct you through a comprehensive review of dental hygiene, provide questions by which you can assess your mastery of the subject material, and offer documentation for correct and incorrect answers. This review book should be supplemented with textbooks and appropriate reference material from a professional library when further study is needed in particular areas. Dental hygienists whose textbooks and reference material may be substantially outdated should make it an immediate priority to obtain adequate resources. They might contact recent graduates to request an extended loan of textbooks and visit the nearest dental library to review current publications. Those references that are particularly helpful should be ordered and purchased.

7. If possible, organize a study club of several candidates who are preparing for the examination. The group should be small, perhaps three to five colleagues. It is best to collaborate only with those individuals whose study habits, personal habits, and self-discipline will contribute to the group's efforts; otherwise, it would be better to study alone. Never rely on someone else to do your preparation; however, several heads can be better than one if the group is intentional in its purpose.

8. If a study group is formed, organize a schedule and procedures for it to operate. Content areas can be assigned to individuals for specific study and research; then the members of the group can pool their information and notes to be shared by all. Open discussion of questions or content areas that are confusing can contribute to the review process of each candidate.

9. Outline an orderly system to guide your review, and establish target dates to complete each area. It would be logical to set deadlines for the review of each chapter in this book. You may wish to organize your review around the functions specified in the examination outline, although you should be aware that each function will probably require the review of several different disciplines. Another option would be to assess and prioritize your own needs as you perceive them and be guided by the priorities you have established. The important point is to plan a system for your

review, with goals and deadlines to monitor your process.

10. When you have formulated a plan, get going and stick with it. If the plan bogs down, reassess the obstacles and modify your goals so you can continue through a comprehensive review.

11. Plan to complete your review at least 3 to 5 days before the examination date. Having prepared yourself intellectually, you should prepare yourself physically. As an educated health professional, you would be wise to adhere to principles of good health. Eat well-balanced meals, get plenty of sleep, avoid any chemical stimulants, and set aside time for exercise, such as brisk daily walks or any form of physical activity to which you are routinely accustomed. Last-minute cramming all night before the examination is not advisable. A good night's sleep is far more likely to enable you to assess your knowledge during the test.

12. Prepare yourself psychologically to set aside all distractions or immediate concerns on the day of the test. Focus on whatever enhances your powers of concentration. Above all, read the instructions for the examination thoroughly, and read each question carefully so that you are sure you understand exactly what is being asked.

13. Take a watch or accurate timepiece, and keep it in front of you during the examination. The time allowed for each section of the examination should be clearly stated, and you should pace yourself accordingly. Do not dwell on difficult items about which you are unsure. Move along and come back to those items as time permits. If time is available when you have completed all items, briefly review all your answers; be sure you have recorded the answer you intended.

14. As breaks are available during the day of the examination, seek out brief activities that are refreshing and help to restore your energy and concentration for the remaining portions of the test.

Future Trends in the National Board Testing Program

The ADA Department of Testing Services has computerized the application process for National Board examinations. They are also proposing to computerize the examination itself. This would eliminate printed test booklets, answer sheets, and pencils. By the end of the 1990s, candidates may be reading and answering test questions on the computer screen. Computerization will not necessarily change the content of the examination. It should make the examination more readily available and expedite the scoring, norming, and analysis process.

Regional Testing Agencies

Having reviewed some of the structural intricacies of the credentialing system and the National Board Dental Hygiene Examination program in particular, it is appropriate to devote some discussion to regional testing agencies. The thrust toward regional board examinations began in the late 1960s and gained momentum throughout the 1970s. Because of the barriers to mobility that are created by having to take repeated state board examinations to qualify for licensure in another state, interest grew in consolidating standards so that one examination might qualify a practitioner for licensure in several states. There was some impetus for a national clinical examination and licensure at the federal level. However, because of the historical advantages of licensure at the state level, regional examinations were perceived as a viable alternative to usurping those state rights and imposing national requirements. The basic rationale for the formation of regional testing services has been the standardization of requirements among states and the pooling of resources to develop and administer reliable clinical examinations.

The development of each of the regional boards has followed a similar pattern. Typically, each region began with a core group of states that initiated discussions about joining forces with one another. Usually this was followed by the states giving simultaneous examinations at a common testing site and then working to consolidate their respective state examinations into one test that they could all accept. As the regions have matured, more states have joined, and the combined examinations have gradually been revised and replaced with a regional test developed with the consensus of the member states. The important feature to be remembered about regional boards, which is often misunderstood by members of the profession, is that they are voluntary organizations made up of individual state boards of dentistry. The regional boards have no authority to supersede state boards or implement policy that goes beyond the statutory authorization of the member state boards. Only the individual state boards can make the determination to accept the results of the regional board as satisfying its requirements for licensure. It is typical to find numerous inconsistencies in the policies and procedures of states within the same region. A regional board only standardizes the examination offered by member states; it does not standardize other aspects of state board responsibilities.

The membership of regional boards may fluctuate from time to time as states join or withdraw. The Northeast Regional Board (NERB) was the first of all the regions and has remained the largest, with 15 member states. The NERB began in the late 1960s. The Central Regional Dental Testing Service (CRDTS) followed in 1972 and took in 11

Table 1-1

Membership in the Four Regional Testing Agencies in the United States

NERB	CRDTS
Connecticut	Colorado
D.C.	Illinois
Illinois	Iowa
Maine	Kansas
Maryland	Minnesota
Massachusetts	Missouri
Michigan	Nebraska
New Hampshire	North Dakota
New Jersey	South Dakota
New York	Wisconsin
Ohio	Wyoming
Pennsylvania	
Rhode Island	**WREB**
Vermont	Alaska
West Virginia	Arizona
	Idaho
SRTA	Montana
Arkansas	New Mexico
Georgia	Oklahoma
Kentucky	Oregon
South Carolina*	Texas
Tennessee	Utah
Virginia	Washington

*Regional Testing for Dentists Only

states between the Rocky Mountains and the Mississippi River. In the mid-1970s the Southern Regional Testing Agency (SRTA) was formed and now includes six of the middle southern states. In the late 1970s the Western Regional Examining Board (WREB) was established; it began with 3 member states and has grown to 10 (Table 1-1).

The concept of regional board examinations has been supported by both the ADA and the ADHA, although these associations have no actual involvement in any of the regional testing services. The political environment of the 1980s, which deemphasized federal involvement in health services and returned control to the states, diminished the momentum for growth of regional testing services. Nevertheless, the advent of regional testing agencies has had notable impact on the content and format of clinical board examinations in both dentistry and dental hygiene.

The four regional testing agencies, comprising a total of 40 member state boards, are very similar in their organization and structure. Typically, a steering committee or board of directors is responsible for determining policies of the agency and financial management. Generally, each member state board is represented on the steering committee. A second key part of the organizations is usually the examination committee, on which each member state board is also represented. In addition, the examination committee generally has several faculty members representing regional educational institutions. The examination committee is charged with reviewing and revising the examinations and developing new examinations. Most regions have some sort of mechanism to review complaints or appeals of results, and they all maintain their own office and staff separate from that of the member state boards.

Whereas national boards satisfy the state requirements for theoretic examinations, the regional boards' emphasis is on evaluating clinical knowledge and skills. The methodology for testing clinical competence generally involves clinical treatment of clients, but it should not be assumed that hands-on client procedures are the only mechanisms for assessing clinical ability. It is quite common for clinical examinations to include some written exercises and some clinical simulations using typodonts, radiographs, photographs, models, and so on. No general statement can be made about the distinctions between regional board examinations and state board examinations. Their content and format often appear quite similar on the surface. Obviously, regional board examinations have the advantage of qualifying a candidate for licensure in more than one state and are often offered more frequently than individual state board examinations. They also offer the advantage of bringing collective resources to bear on developing and maintaining reliable examinations. Examiners and educators have a forum in which they can cooperatively determine appropriate standards of competence and concentrate on technical aspects of testing without the distractions of the many other responsibilities that burden state boards. Some candidates believe that regional boards are better organized and present more specific documentation of candidate requirements, scoring systems, and performance criteria. Certainly, the circumstances will vary depending on which jurisdictions and examinations are being compared.

Examiner Selection and Training

The pool of examiners for regional agencies comes from the member state boards. Usually each state has the right to be represented at any or all regional examinations. All active board members of each state board are eligible to serve as examiners. In addition, many states are authorized to designate deputy examiners to represent them; such deputy examiners are generally practitioners who are not board members but are certified to serve as examiners for their state and help carry out the board's examining responsibilities. Testing dates and sites are scheduled well in advance by the region and the schools. The number of candidates at each test determines the number of examiners that is necessary, and each state is asked to assign examiners to represent them. From the pool of examiners assigned to a particular test, further assignments are made to administer the dental hygiene examination or different portions of the dental examination.

Training programs for the examiners vary according to the region, but it is becoming increasingly common for the regions to place heavy emphasis on standardization and grading exercises and train examiners to apply the examination criteria. The result of this is a more thorough and specific evaluation for dental hygienists, in comparison with a cursory inspection and flash of the mirror around the mouth, as may have been the practice in some jurisdictions in the past.

State and Regional Clinical Examinations

Only general statements can be made about the content of clinical dental hygiene board examinations because it varies from jurisdiction to jurisdiction and is continually being revised. Three basic categories of clinical skills are commonly included in regional and state clinical examinations. These are data-gathering/client assessment skills, oral prophylaxis, and radiographic skills. Client assessment may include such functions as dental and periodontal charting, head and neck examination, health history taking, and charting the location of subgingival deposits. An oral prophylaxis on at least one client is a universal requirement. However, requirements for the difficulty of the case may vary, and some jurisdictions demand a complete prophylaxis, whereas others may require a more difficult client and assign only a portion of the mouth for the purposes of the examination. Some jurisdictions may require treatment of more than one client as well.

The radiographic evaluation may include an assessment of the ability to interpret or recognize radiographic features and/or an assessment of technical ability. Some jurisdictions require a full-mouth survey of radiographs; others require only selected films. In some instances radiographs may be exposed in advance, whereas other agencies require all radiographic exercises to be completed during the examination.

The time schedule is another factor that may vary considerably in different jurisdictions. Some board examinations place specific time limits for the completion of assignments, whereas others allow such an ample amount of time that it is not a matter of concern for most candidates. It is essential for a candidate to be thoroughly familiar with examination requirements, not only concerning *what* one is expected to do but also *how* and *when* it must be done.

Anonymous Examinations

In recent years there has been a growing trend toward administering clinical board examinations anonymously. This means that the candidates are identified only by number and the examiners are usually segregated from the candidates. Clients are brought to a clinical area reserved for the examiners, and the candidates are not present while the examiners conduct their evaluations. Candidates often have mixed responses to this arrangement. Some candidates feel it is extremely stressful to be present during the examiners' evaluation and are relieved to avoid it. Others are enormously curious to perceive any clue from the examiners about their performance. Many candidates interrogate their clients about every comment or facial expression they observed among the examiners. Making assumptions based on the reports of clients, who generally understand little about the examination process, invites misinformation and erroneous conclusions. In any case, anonymous evaluations have a definite impact on the logistics of the examination process. The purpose, of course, is to eliminate any potential examiner bias based on personality, race, gender, or personal background so that the candidate's clinical performance is the only basis for the evaluation.

Examination Scoring

There is no uniform scoring system for regional or state board clinical examinations. Such scoring tends to be highly specific to the content, design, and format of each individual examination. However, some generalities can be reviewed. Clinical examinations are ordinarily criterion-referenced as opposed to the norm-referenced scoring system described for National Board Dental Hygiene Examinations. That is, a candidate's clinical performance is measured against a specific standard of competence rather than against the performance of another candidate or group of candidates. The best and most objective clinical examinations are generally considered to be those that set forth specific performance criteria and define the cutoff point that separates acceptable from unacceptable performance.

The emphasis on determining acceptable versus unacceptable performance is a distinctive feature of clinical board examinations. It is not relevant to the purposes of board examinations to rank candidates as good, better, or best, nor is it important whether a candidate scores 85 or 95 on an examination. The essential question is whether or not the candidate has demonstrated adequate competence to be licensed to practice. The critical decisions, then, in clinical board examinations lend themselves to pass/fail or acceptable/unacceptable determinations. Numerical values are almost always assigned to the examiners' determinations of acceptability, but such numerical scores often do not have the same meaning as test scores in school or on other standardized tests. For example, a test score of 100 on a 100-item pathology final would very likely mean that a student answered every question correctly. In contrast, a score of 100 on a criterion-referenced, pass/fail examination would not necessarily indicate that a candidate performed perfectly; it could mean only that the candidate consistently demonstrated minimal competence in all aspects of the examination.

Clinical board examinations generally use raw scores without any kind of conversion system; even written sections of the examination are scored strictly on the basis of the number of correct answers. However, it is common in board examinations to use a system of weighting. Weighting in examinations is simply a method of emphasizing the importance or recognizing the difficulty of certain skills and treatment procedures. For instance, most dental hygienists would acknowledge that root debridement is a more difficult task, and more important to the practice of dental hygiene, than the charting of restorations. Consequently, one would expect to see root debridement weighted with more point value in an examination than dental charting. If dental charting is included in the examination, examiners will carefully evaluate the candidate's ability to chart correctly; however, acceptable performance in dental charting may be worth only 10 points in the overall test as opposed to a weight of 30 points assigned to root debridement. A candidate should strive to demonstrate competence in all skills that are evaluated in an examination. The candidate should study the weighting system before the examination and may wish to concentrate time and attention on each skill in proportion to the weighted importance that is built into the examination.

There undoubtedly is much variation in the amount of information that different testing agencies release about their scoring systems. An examination scoring system is of concern to the candidate to the extent that it appears to be fair and reasonable, and it may offer guidance in preparing the candidate to take the examination. It is unwise, however, for a candidate to become too absorbed in analyzing the grading system. Indeed, some candidates have tended to become more interested in how to *give* the examination than in how to *take* it. The grading system is the testing agency's concern, and demonstrating competence in performing dental hygiene procedures is the candidate's concern. Successful candidates are those who do not allow themselves to be distracted from their primary task.

Clinical Facilities

Most jurisdictions today have access to modern clinical facilities in which to administer board examinations. Fortunately, it is a thing of the past to hear stories of board examinations given in poorly equipped prison clinics or with portable equipment set up in the basement of a courthouse. Today most candidates have the benefit of adequate lighting, water, evacuation systems, and functional equipment. For many states without any educational institutions, gaining access to adequate clinical facilities was a primary reason for joining a regional testing service. No state or regional board owns or operates its own clinical facility. Boards must elicit the cooperation of schools or large clinics to make their facilities available for board examinations. It is no small concession on the part of schools to release their facilities for several days for board examinations. It requires scheduling adjustments and substantial loss of clinic income, and it places heavy demands on faculty and staff to accommodate examination requirements and personnel.

Candidates are often oblivious to clinical facilities as long as they have equipment that is functional, reasonably comfortable, and efficient and they are able to find what they need when they need it. This poses no problem to candidates who take an examination at their school of graduation or at a familiar site. Problems may arise, however, for those who are operating in an unfamiliar facility. Candidates should be aware that the clinical facility is *not* under the management and control of the board examiners. In fact, the examiners may be scarcely more familiar with the facilities and equipment than are the candidates. The testing site may charge a separate fee to candidates for the use of the facilities and supplies and may have its own institutional requirements or record keeping for which the candidate is responsible. Rental of equipment or instruments is typically handled through the testing site, as well as obtaining information about the compatibility of handpieces and so on. An equipment breakdown during the examination can create stress for the candidate and result in the loss of time. Maintenance is also usually managed by the testing site, and many schools are accommodating enough to keep maintenance personnel on call during the examination.

The purpose of this discussion is simply to point out that candidates should not assume that all aspects of the examination process are totally under the control of the testing agency. The candidate will be involved with the testing site, the testing agency, and the state board(s) of the jurisdiction(s) in which licensure is sought. When problems or questions arise, the candidate should be aware of which agency can respond to his or her concerns. The testing site addresses concerns about the facilities, the testing agency addresses questions about the test itself, and the state board deals with actually issuing a license to practice. For those jurisdictions that are not part of a regional testing service, the state board and the testing agency are one and the same.

Client Selection and Classification

All dental hygiene clinical board examinations place the greatest weight on client treatment procedures, particularly scaling and extrinsic stain removal. Therefore selection of a board client is undoubtedly the single most important factor in preparation for an examination. Most testing agencies provide some criteria for client acceptability. Some agencies may be quite specific, to the point of defining exactly how many teeth and surfaces must have subgingival calculus and acceptable ranges of sulcular probing depths. Other agencies set forth more general descriptions. Experience has shown that no matter how detailed the criteria may be, candidates still worry desperately about whether their client is acceptable.

One of the difficulties in defining client criteria is that there is no standardized definition of client classification that is universally accepted and, of course, judgments differ among individuals when it comes to placing a client in a particular category. Most jurisdictions require a client with moderate to heavy subgingival deposits. Clients exhibiting only plaque or soft deposits are probably not difficult enough to present a valid test of the candidate's skills. A person with grossly heavy calculus or significant periodontal involvement is too difficult for the purposes of a board examination. Many experienced board examiners have observed that educators tend to classify clients as being more difficult than examiners would. Perhaps this is because for most board examinations the baseline for minimally acceptable clients begins with moderate deposits of calculus, and the degree of difficulty escalates from that point.

Many testing agencies classify the difficulty of clients and vary the examination criteria according to such classification. The most common factors that determine the client's classification are the amounts of subgingival calculus and supragingival stain. The classification of difficulty may be used to determine how well the candidate is expected to perform and/or how much work the candidate is assigned. For example, a candidate who presents a client with minimal deposits of subgingival calculus and light stain obviously has a much easier task than the candidate whose client is a pipe smoker and has heavy deposits of subgingival and supragingival calculus. One method of compensating for such variabilities in client conditions is to assign the first candidate three or four quadrants for treatment and expect at least 85% of the deposits to be completely removed. In contrast, the second candidate may be assigned to treat only one quadrant and be expected

to remove at least 75% of the deposits. Such compensation designed into the examination criteria tends to equalize the difficulty of the candidates' tasks and make the examination more equitable for all.

Recruitment of Clients

Most testing agencies cannot and do not provide clients for candidates. The burden of that responsibility falls on the candidate. Candidates frequently turn to the testing site for assistance in recruiting clients, but there is considerable variation in the amount of assistance that may be provided. Schools often assist their students in client recruitment and selection but are unable to provide clients to other candidates. Some schools will make operatories available for client screening shortly before a board examination or may screen and make lists of potential board clients through the oral diagnosis department. Ultimately, however, it is the responsibility of the candidate to present a suitable client, and the examiners make the final decision regarding acceptability. It is not helpful for a candidate to challenge an examiner's decision by pointing out that an instructor or family dentist said the client would be acceptable. It is the candidate's responsibility to know how a client may or may not satisfy the examination criteria. It is not advisable to present a marginally acceptable client and hope to "squeak by" the criteria. Having a client dismissed places enormous stress on the candidate, may penalize the grade or reduce the operating time, and delays the entire examination process.

Candidates often exhibit incredible resourcefulness in recruiting clients. Family and friends are a primary source. One's school, family dentist, or dental hygienist may also be sources for contacts. Students or staff at hospitals or health science centers are frequently recruited. Many candidates have contacted local police and fire stations, studied the shift schedule to determine who would be off duty on the day of the examination, and then visited the station when that shift was on duty in order to screen and recruit clients. Sometimes graduating classes develop plans of action and organize themselves to recruit clients for the entire class. Candidates have been known to advertise in local newspapers or post notices on bulletin boards to obtain clients; some candidates have even accosted people on the streets. Bizarre and unprofessional methods of client recruitment are obviously directly proportional to the desperation of the candidate. Such desperation can be avoided if the candidate begins a search for clients well in advance and maintains an attitude of professionalism in all contacts with potential clients. The pressure of board examinations can often influence candidates to perceive clients as walking typodonts instead of relating to them as human beings whose oral health needs certainly extend beyond the day of the examination.

Client selection is primarily dictated by the criteria defined by the testing agency. Such criteria may stipulate requirements for systemic health conditions, calculus deposits, stain, gingival conditions, a minimal number of teeth and items to be charted, and periodontal pockets. There also may be requirements for legal consent from the client for treatment and requirements for radiation hygiene. Candidates should carefully review all prerequisites before recruiting clients. The wise candidate will also take into consideration the attitude and cooperativeness of the client and ascertain the client's pain threshold or tolerance of the treatment. Part of the candidate's preparation for the examination should include careful preparation of the client.

Clinical examinations usually require long treatment sessions and periods of waiting for examiners. It is a difficult day for the clients, who are subjected not only to the necessary treatment by the candidate but also to inspection and instrumentation by the examiners. Examiners usually do not have the time or opportunity to build rapport with the client or provide the same kind of support that they would in a practice setting. Moreover, clients frequently ask examiners questions about the candidate's performance that the examiners are not at liberty to answer. The examiners' lack of response to clients and/or candidates may make them appear abrupt, when in actuality they are only doing their jobs. Candidates are in a stressful situation during the examination, which often makes it more difficult for them to maintain good client rapport. If clients are poorly prepared for the demands of the examination setting or if they have not been informed of the amount of time they will be detained, they can cause great difficulty for the candidate by refusing to cooperate, threatening to leave, or actually leaving the examination. Therefore the candidate should advise the client of the purposes of the examination, its importance to the candidate's career, the treatment that will be provided, what the examiners will be doing, the time schedule, and delays that may be encountered. Certainly, the client should be made aware of additional treatment that may be necessary but will not be provided during the examination. Some clients are so eager for the candidate to succeed that they may regard the examiners as adversaries. However, when they are made to understand the purpose and format of board examinations, most clients are supportive and appreciative of the efforts of the dental profession to ensure the competence of practitioners.

It is obvious that not all candidates will be fortunate enough to find the perfect client who satisfies all criteria. However, some candidates are able to secure several clients who are potentially suitable. It is highly advisable to recruit more than one client and have a backup client available. These clients should be informed that they may not be needed for the examination; however, it is often likely that if the candidate who recruited them does not need them, another candidate will. The candidate should stay in contact with any clients who have been recruited, confirm the time and date, and make sure that transportation is arranged and that the client has clear directions about where to appear, how to get there, and where to park.

Instrument Requirements

In recent years there has been an increasing tendency for testing agencies to specify certain instruments that are required for the examination. Some testing agencies supply or sell them, and others merely specify what the candidate is responsible for providing. While such requirements may impose some inconvenience on the candidate, it tends to serve the best interests of the candidate by standardizing the examination process. Ordinarily, it is only the examining instruments that are standardized, such as the mirror, explorer, and periodontal probe. Handpieces, scalers, and curets are usually selected at the candidate's discretion.

Every clinician has certain instruments that are most effective for that individual. Certainly, the candidate should use those instruments that are familiar and provide the best tactile sensitivity. If the examination requires instruments with which the candidate is not familiar, it is advisable to begin practicing with those instruments well in advance. For instance, it may be that a testing agency requires the candidate to have a No. 11/12 explorer, which the examiners use for detection of calculus. Perhaps the candidate has the greatest tactile sensitivity with a No. 13/14 curet. In preparing for the examination, the candidate should practice with both instruments, double-checking first with the curet and then with the explorer, until the explorer becomes as familiar as an extension of the candidate's operating hand. During the examination the same procedure should be followed, with the candidate exploring delicately and thoroughly for any remaining deposits before the client is presented for evaluation.

Candidates should be sure that their instruments are in excellent condition and *very sharp*. It would be poor strategy to provide examiners with a dull curet or scaler with the hope that they could not find or remove any calculus. Very likely, this would serve only to convince examiners that anyone who operates with such dull instruments is a poor practitioner and has only burnished calculus instead of removing it. It is advisable to have extra sterile sets of instruments on hand in case a client is not acceptable or an instrument is dropped.

The air syringe is an examining instrument that is often overlooked or forgotten by candidates. Careful candidates will take the time to thoroughly inspect their work with good light and a dry field before presenting the client for evaluation.

Examination Forms

For whatever charting, record keeping, or documentation that is necessary during the examination, forms are an important consideration. There are innumerable systems for charting and for taking client histories, and most individuals are familiar with only those few they have used. If it is possible to obtain examination forms or facsimiles thereof in advance, candidates should study them carefully and practice using them. If examination forms are not available before the test, time should be taken to read and review them at the examination site; candidates should be sure they understand and are properly oriented to the use of the forms before beginning any charting procedures. Most testing agencies will provide adequate orientation to their forms before any clinical exercises begin; however, candidates should not expect the testing agency to tell them how to record every specific oral condition that may occur with a client. The purpose of a charting examination is to measure a candidate's ability to recognize and record oral conditions; it is not intended to be a copying exercise. Therefore familiarity with the examination forms will allow the candidate to avoid confusion and exercise good clinical judgment in the gathering of data.

Release of Examination Results

Regional board examination results are often reported more slowly than those of state boards; some are released within a few days. Generally speaking, the larger the testing agency, the longer it takes to receive results, and in some instances it may be 8 weeks. Candidates should investigate when they might anticipate receiving results and schedule their practice plans accordingly.

How to Prepare for State or Regional Clinical Board Examinations

1. Obtain application forms, a candidate's guide or brochure, and any information pertaining to the examination that is published by the testing agency. This should be done several months before the examination.
2. Carefully review the application materials and highlight or make a list of all the requirements for the examination, including forms or documentation you must provide, client requirements, instruments, supplies, etc.
3. Make a note of the application deadline, and schedule on your calendar all pertinent dates for completing examination and licensure requirements.
4. If you are taking a regional examination, contact the individual state board offices for the states in which you are seeking licensure. Obtain licensure applications from each state, along with all pertinent information and deadlines for fulfilling licensure prerequisites. It is also advisable to obtain copies of the state dental practice act and rules and regulations for any jurisdiction in which licensure is sought.
5. If you are taking a regional examination, ascertain what additional requirements the state board may have for the jurisdiction(s) in which you are applying for licensure. On successful completion of the regional examination, it is common for a state board to require an examination over its state practice act—perhaps an oral interview or other forms of examination. You should plan your preparation and schedule deadlines for these requirements as well.
6. Begin gathering whatever credentials are necessary to complete the examination and licensure applications. These credentials may include such items as your school transcript, National Board Dental Hygiene Examination score, a copy of your diploma, current CPR certification, evidence of malpractice/liability insurance, and a passport-type photograph.
7. It may be helpful to talk with several dental hygienists who have taken the same examination within the past year and ask them for helpful hints in preparing for the examination. Keep the conversation constructive to your concerns. Board examinations create stress for virtually all candidates, and everyone has "war stories" about difficulties they may have encountered or how nervous they were. It is in your best interest to manage such stress constructively, pursue factual information, and employ a positive attitude in your preparations.
8. With the client-selection criteria firmly in mind, begin searching for suitable clients. Be prepared to present a prospective client with a clear and professional explanation of both the client's and your role in the examination. Refer to the section on "Recruitment of Clients" for a more comprehensive discussion of client selection.
9. Candidates who are enrolled in school should attempt to arrange clinical sessions that duplicate board requirements as much as possible. Many schools conduct "mock boards" for just this purpose; however, additional practice sessions can also be helpful. Seek out those instructors who provide critical, constructive feedback on clinical skills. Make an effort to obtain additional experience with clients whose difficulty level is commensurate with board requirements. Try to sharpen your clinical skills in any area in which you perceive weaknesses.

10. Dental hygienists who are in practice should also set up clinical simulations of board requirements. Begin a period of critical self-assessment; allow time to carefully evaluate your treatment before releasing a client. Make arrangements with your employer-dentist or with a fellow dental hygienist to occasionally evaluate your performance and give you specific feedback. Many testing agencies do not permit the use of ultrasonic instruments on board examinations. If it is your practice to use ultrasonic scalers routinely for clients with substantial deposits, make a point to limit yourself to hand scalers and curets until you are sure the strength of your hand and tactile sensitivity with these instruments is at its peak.

11. It is particularly important for dental hygienists who have been out of practice for some period of time to arrange to sharpen their clinical skills. A number of dental and dental hygiene schools periodically offer refresher and update courses for dental hygienists. Such courses should be investigated and pursued well before the examination date; particularly those courses that emphasize clinical skills. A hygienist who is not employed but who is licensed in the jurisdiction might seek the cooperation of a local dentist and/or dental hygienist to treat selected clients in the office and obtain feedback. A nonpracticing hygienist who is not licensed in the jurisdiction might contact a few local hygienists and request assistance through a few practical sessions in the evening—not involving any client treatment.

12. Ascertain whether any specific instruments are required for the examination. If so, obtain such instruments and practice using them until they are completely comfortable and familiar. Refer to the previous discussion in this chapter on standardized instruments.

13. If it is possible to obtain examination forms before the test, practice using them. If not, carefully study the examination manual for information about forms and materials to be used during the test.

14. Some examinations require the use of a particular tooth numbering system for the purposes of the test. If a standardized numbering system is used, be sure you are familiar with it and can apply it accurately. Confusion with an unfamiliar system can cause unnecessary charting errors or result in a candidate's failing to comprehend which teeth are assigned by examiners.

15. In addition to your attention to clinical skills, preparation should be ongoing for any written sections of the board examination. The examination manual or guide should contain some information about written portions of the test. Many clinical board examinations include written slide examinations covering radio-graphic recognition or interpretation. In such instances a review of Chapter 5 of this book and a radiographic textbook would be appropriate. Projected slides of common pathologic conditions are also frequently included in board examinations. Your study should be guided by the content of the examination for which you are preparing.

16. A few days before the test, prepare clinic attire and organize your instruments and supplies. Be *sure* your instruments are *sharp* and in excellent condition. Confirm arrangements with your client(s) and make sure the time, date, location, and relevant directions are clearly understood. For safety's sake, it is advisable to check with the client again the night before the examination.

17. If you are taking the examination at an unfamiliar testing site, try to arrange a brief tour of the clinical facilities before taking the test. Sometimes such a tour is provided in conjunction with a candidate's orientation session that is conducted at the beginning of the examination. Check among your fellow candidates to identify those who are familiar with the facility and request any assistance you may need in locating supplies or in operating equipment.

18. Maintian especially good health habits during the final days before the examination so you will be at your best physically, emotionally, and psychologically. This includes a nutritious diet, plenty of rest, and mild, routine exercise. Plan your arrival at the testing site to allow plenty of time for mishaps, traffic, parking problems, locating your operatory, setting up, and orienting yourself. Avoid starting the day feeling rushed, harried, and distracted.

19. At the examination, *listen* carefully to instructions and *read* thoroughly all material that is provided. Above all, follow instructions. Failure to read and follow instructions is undoubtedly the single most important factor in problems encountered by candidates.

20. *Relax* and concentrate on providing the dental hygiene care that your entire professional education and experience has prepared you to skillfully deliver. Try to plan appropriate breaks and rest periods during the examination for both yourself and your client. Eat and drink sensibly during the day to maintain your physical well-being.

Future Trends in Clinical Examinations and Regional Boards

In the 1990s, there has been a groundswell of demand for greater portability of credentials in dentistry and dental hygiene. This includes broader implementation of licensure by credentials for active practitioners who wish to move to another state and a variety of proposals to create a standardized national clinical examination that would be recognized by most if not all states. Federal legislation has been introduced that, if enacted, would have a substantial impact on examination and licensure responsibilities at the state level. As a result of this activity, one may expect to see movement throughout the 1990s toward more uniformity in board examination requirements across the country. Studies have already been conducted by both the ADHA and the ADA to compare clinical board examination requirements across the country in both dental hygiene and dentistry. A common core content has been proposed for a dental clinical examination. More individual states are exploring membership in one of the existing regional boards. Regional boards are proposing the development of joint examinations based on uniform standards of competence for both dental hygiene and dentistry. Although the outcome of this evolutionary process cannot be precisely predicted, the trend is definitely toward more uniformity in examinations, reduction of licensure barriers to mobility, and greater portability of credentials.

International Requirements

With our increasingly global society, recognition of credentials throughout the United States becomes a more pertinent concern. International licensure requirements vary more radically than those among the States. Maintaining *current* information about foreign licensure requirements is a process fraught with cumbersome obstacles. A dental hygienist contemplating employment in a foreign country should contact the ADHA and the ADA for all pertinent information and potential contacts and utilize whatever individual resources or personal contacts within the country of destination are available.

At the very least, the dental hygienist must gather documentation for all credentials—from passports or visas to transcripts, licenses, diplomas, employment history, etc. Some countries require language proficiency before credentials are granted. Others require the hygienist to secure employment *before* receiving a work permit. Several countries require only graduation from an accredited school and successful completion of a clinical board examination. Others require written and clinical examinations very similar to American requirements.

Special mention is warranted of the Canadian National Dental Hygiene Certification Board which was established in 1994. The Canadian National Dental Hygiene Certification Examination (NDHCE) is now accepted in 7 of the 10 Canadian provinces, as indicated in Table 1-2. Some of these provinces have other licensure requirements, but the portability of credentials has been greatly facilitated with the establishment of the Canadian National Board. An application guide and examination blueprint may be obtained by contacting the Certification Board at PO Box 58006, Orleans, ON K1C 7H4.

The rigor of a country's requirements appears to be strongly correlated to the number of dental hygienists in the country, how long dental hygiene has been established there, and the size and strength of its educational system. A dental hygienist who has followed the suggestions outlined in this book to prepare for board examinations should be well prepared to successfully fulfill foreign licensure requirements.

The information displayed in Table 1-1 summarizes data available through the International Federation of Dental Hygienists.

Content and Organization of This Review Book

This text presents a review in outline form of basic, dental, and clinical sciences. Each review outline is followed by related questions that test the candidate's knowledge of concepts, principles, and theories underlying the practice of dental hygiene.

Following the review questions covering the subject matter, each chapter contains a section that provides justification for the correct answer and every distractor. The rationale supporting the correct answer is specified, as well as an explanation of why each distractor is inappropriate as a response to the question. By reviewing these rationales, the candidate should be able to confirm facts and reinforce knowledge.

How to Use This Book in Studying

1. Review one section of content material at a time. Study the material outlined in the section. Refer to other textbooks and references to research additional details if you encounter any areas that are unclear to you.
2. When you have reviewed the content material, answer the review questions that immediately follow. As you answer each question, write a few words about why you think that answer is correct; in other words, simply justify why you selected that answer. If you guess at an answer to a question, you should make a special mark to identify the answer you selected as a guess. This will enable you to readily identify areas that need further review and clarification of facts. It will also provide a measure of how correct your guessing may be. Remember that analyzing a question, narrowing the choices, and then making an educated guess, if necessary, can

Table 1-2

Requirements for Licensure/Work Eligibility as a Dental Hygienist in Some Foreign Countries

Country/province	Clinical exam	Written/oral exam	Accredited school	Currently licensed in USA	Language proficiency	Employment commitment	Practice experience
Australia:							
S. Australia	Yes	Yes	Yes				
New S. Wales	Yes	Yes	Yes				
Queensland	Yes	Yes	Yes				
Canada:							
Ontario	Yes	NDHCE	Yes				
British Columbia	Yes	NDHCE	Yes	Yes			
New Brunswick			Yes				
Saskatchewan		NDHCE	Yes				
Quebec			Yes		Yes		
Manitoba			Yes	Yes			
Nova Scotia		NDHCE	Yes				
Newfoundland		NDHCE	Yes				
Prince Edward		NDHCE	Yes				
Alberta		NDHCE	Yes				
Other Countries:							
Bahrain	No specific regulations						
Denmark	Yes	Yes	Yes	Yes	Yes	Yes	
Germany		Yes	Yes	Yes	Preferred	Yes	Preferable
Italy			Yes			Yes	
Japan	Yes	Yes	Yes				
Korea	No specific regulations						
Netherlands	Yes	Yes	Yes	Yes		Yes	
Nigeria	Yes	Yes	Yes				
Norway			Yes	Yes	Yes		
South Africa	Varies by case						
Sweden	Yes	Yes	Yes	Yes	Yes		
Switzerland			Yes	Yes	Yes	Yes	1 yr
United Kingdom	Yes	Yes	Yes				

improve your performance. On board examinations, guessing is preferable to leaving any blank spaces.

3. Compare your answers with the answers at the end of each chapter. If you answered the item correctly, check the reason you noted for selecting the answer with the rationale that is presented. If you answered the item incorrectly, read the rationale to determine why the distractor you selected is incorrect. In addition, for each item you answered incorrectly, you should review the correct answer and its rationale. If your mistake on that item is still not clear to you, review the theory in the chapter pertaining to that question and research information in your reference material. You should carefully review all questions and rationales for items you identified as guesses since you did not have mastery of the material covered by the questions.

4. After an interval of several days or weeks, review the chapter again and reanswer the review questions. If you miss the same questions, it should be a clear sign that further study of the material is necessary.

Completion of the Review Processes

When a candidate has completed the comprehensive review presented in this book, assessed areas of strength and weaknesses with the aid of the chapter review questions, reinforced concentrated study of particular material pinpointed by the review, become familiar with the board examination process, protocol, and purpose, and followed instructions for preparation, board examinations can be successfully completed with confidence and composure. Preparation for board examinations actually begins with the first class in dental hygiene school and continues throughout the educational process. This book is designed to present a cohesive, comprehensive review of that professional educational base, reinforce existing knowledge, and guide the candidate toward areas requiring concentrated study.

Histology and Embryology

Maureen Dotzel Savner*

The dental hygienist plays a key role in the assessment phase of client treatment. In the process of evaluating a client's health, it is important to distinguish normal, a variant of normal, or a developmental abnormality from pathology. A clear sense of the developmental process and the histologic make-up of tissues provides the background for this assessment.

The knowledge of tissue components and embryologic tissue origin supports an understanding of the physiologic changes that take place during the course of disease progression. It also gives insight into the tissue capability of responding to this pathologic condition. Based on these scientific principles, a clinician can formulate a feasible dental hygiene care plan and accurately assess the success of the interventions taken.

This chapter contains basic general histology information with a focus on oral tissue components and oral and facial development.

General Histology

Cells (Fig. 2-1)

A. Smallest structures and functionally self-contained units in the body; vary in size, shape, and surface, depending on functional specialization

---

*Revision based in part on original material by Marlene Moss-Klyvert.

B. Possess similar common physiologic properties that permit
   1. Growth and reproduction
   2. Response to external stimuli
   3. Assimilation and synthesizing of materials
C. The building blocks of tissues in the body are attached to each other and noncellular surfaces via cell junctions; there are various types of cell junctions whose structure is dependent on location and function; types of junctions are
   1. Desmosomes
   2. Tight junctions
   3. Gap junctions
   4. Hemidesmosomes
D. Are surrounded by a cell membrane that separates them from the extracellular environment; cell membrane encloses all components of the cell
   1. Cytoplasm
   2. Organelles
   3. Inclusions
   4. Nucleus

Cell Membrane

A. Referred to as plasma membrane or plasmalemma; usually too thin to be seen with a light microscope; average width is approximately 7 nm; is considered selectively permeable because it controls passage of materials in and out of the cell

B. Trilaminar structure composed of two layers of lipid molecules facing each other into which large globular proteins are inserted (Fig. 2-2)
   1. Lipid bilayers consist mainly of phospholipid molecules; are oriented with hydrophilic ends facing outer and inner surfaces of the cell; hydrophobic ends attract and face each other
   2. Globular proteins are of two types
      a. Integral proteins that extend through the full width of the cell membrane and protrude; may have carbohydrate units attached to them
      b. Peripheral proteins linked or attached to the cell membrane surface

Cytoplasm

A. Translucent homogeneous gel enclosed in the cell by the cell membrane; organelles and inclusions are suspended in the cytoplasmic gel
B. All metabolic activities of the cell occur in the cytoplasm
   1. Assimilation (digestion)
   2. Synthesizing of substances such as proteins, proteoglycans, and glycoproteins

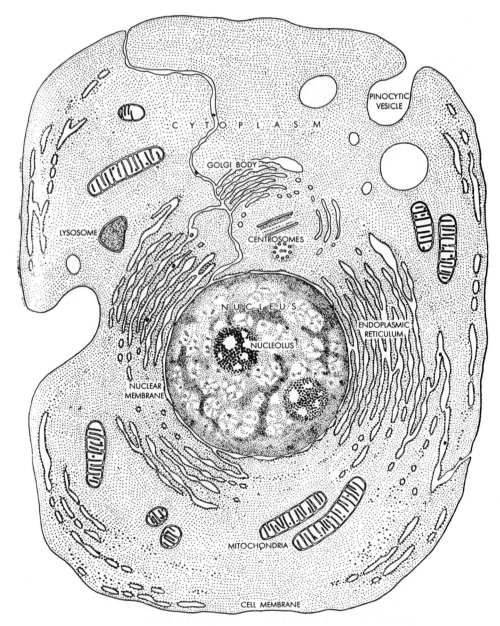

Fig. 2-1 Typical cell. (From Brachet J: The living cell, *Sci Am* 205:50, 1961. Copyright 1969 by Scientific American, Inc. All rights reserved.)

Nucleus

A. Controls the two major functions of the cell
  1. Chemical reactions of the cell; synthetic activities
  2. Stores genetic information of the cell
B. Genetic information is stored in chromosomes—chromosomal deoxyribonucleic acid (DNA); human nucleus contains 46 chromosomes
C. Chromosomes are visible only during cell division when they become long, coiled strands; other times chromosomal material is dispersed in granular clumps of material called chromatin
D. Each nucleus contains one or more round dense structures referred to as nucleoli; these produce ribosomal ribonucleic acid (RNA) (protein plus RNA)

Synthetic Activities

A. Three types of RNA are necessary for protein synthesis
  1. Messenger RNA—copies of short segments of DNA, the genetic code
    a. Messenger RNA can be compared to a tape that contains all the genetic information of proteins but must pass through the ribosomes attached to the endoplasmic reticulum

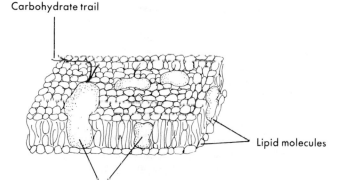

Carbohydrate trail

Lipid molecules

Proteins

Fig. 2-2 Proposed model for structure of cell membrane—two layers of lipid molecules facing each other, into which large globular proteins are inserted (trilaminar membrane).

  b. As the tape passes through the ribosomes, transfer RNA adds the exact amino acid to the newly forming proteins (Fig. 2-3)
  2. Transfer RNA—carriers of specific amino acids (building blocks of proteins)
  3. Ribosomal RNA—found floating free in the cytoplasm (polyribosomes) or attached to the endoplasmic reticulum
B. Protein synthesis can also occur on polyribosomes floating free in the cytoplasm; proteins synthesized on the free polyribosomes are used by the cell; proteins synthesized on the ribosomes attached to the endoplasmic reticulum are transported out of the cell

Inclusions

A. Transitory, nonliving metabolic by-products found in the cytoplasm of the cell
B. May appear as lipid droplets, carbohydrate accumulations, or engulfed foreign substances

Lysosomes

A. Membrane-bound organelles responsible for the breakdown of foreign substances engulfed by the cell by the process of phagocytosis or pinocytosis
B. Produced by the Golgi complex; they bud off as spherical vesicles containing digestive enzymes; enzymes are first produced by endoplasmic reticulum and then transported to the Golgi complex
C. Fuse with engulfed substances to form a secondary vesicle; vesicle with digestive materials may remain in the cell as a residual body or be discharged outside of the cell

Golgi Complex

A. Stacks of closely spaced membranous sacs where newly formed proteins are concentrated and prepared for export out of the cell (Fig. 2-4)
  1. Small membrane-bound vesicles pinch off from the Golgi complex and form secretory granules (newly formed proteins)

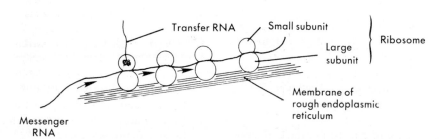

Transfer RNA

Small subunit

Large subunit

Ribosome

Membrane of rough endoplasmic reticulum

Messenger RNA

Fig. 2-3 Ribosomes showing protein synthesis on rough endoplasmic reticulum; messenger RNA is being passed through ribosomes on endoplasmic reticulum where transfer RNA becomes incorporated in protein (being formed) that is assembled in ribosome.

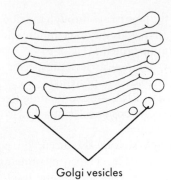

Fig. 2-4 Golgi complex, which consists of a series of flat membranous sacs filled with newly formed proteins; small vesicles pinch off and form secretory granules.

2. Granules attach to the inside of the cell membrane and are then discharged outside of the cell
C. Also involved in production of large carbohydrate molecules and lysosomes

Mitochondria (Fig. 2-5)

A. Membranous structures bounded by a double, inner and outer cell membrane; inner part is thrown into folds (cristae) that extend like shelves inside the mitochondria to provide an additional work surface for the organelle; usually more than one mitochondrion is present in a cell; number tends to be dependent on amount of energy required by the cell
B. Provide the chief source of energy for the cell— "powerhouse of the cell" (oxidation of nutrients)— by enzymatic breakdown of fats, amino acids, and carbohydrates

Endoplasmic Reticulum

A. Extensive membranous system found throughout the cytoplasm of the cell; composed of lipoprotein membranes existing in the form of connecting tubules and broad, flattened sacs (cisternae); outer membrane may or may not be covered with ribosomes
  1. Rough-surfaced endoplasmic reticulum (RER) or
  2. Smooth-surfaced endoplasmic reticulum (SER), which is minus the ribosomes; agranular
B. Proteins are synthesized on ribosomes attached to the endoplasmic reticulum and are transported to the Golgi complex for packaging
C. Smooth endoplasmic reticulum has a number of diverse roles and is found in a variety of cell types

Filaments and Tubules

A. Threadlike structures about 7 to 10 nm thick; thicker filaments are the same as those seen in muscle (protein myosin strands) and have been associated with contractility in cells

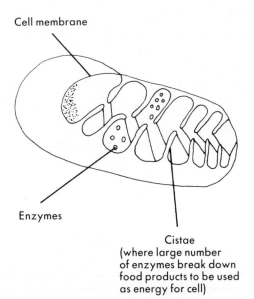

Fig. 2-5 Mitochondria.

B. Microfilaments act as a support system for the cell cytoskeleton
C. Bundles of microfilaments form tonofibrils and become part of the attachment apparatus (desmosomes) between cells

Microtubules

A. Delicate tubes 20 to 27 nm wide found in cells that are undergoing mitosis and alterations in cell shape (cell morphology)
B. Have an internal support function, particularly in long cellular processes such as neurites or odontoblastic processes
C. Capacity for directing intracellular transport through the cytoplasm of cell

Centrioles

A. Cylindrical structures composed of microtubule-like components
B. Function in self-duplication and the formation of cellular extensions

Concepts Relating to Dental Tissues

A. All calcified dental tissues are produced by secretory cells that require a great amount of energy in producing their organic matrix, which becomes calcified; organelles such as mitochondria play an important role in helping to provide energy
B. Mitochondria have been associated with the calcification (mineralization) process that occurs in dental tissues

C. Cell organelles help maintain tissues after initial formation by the cell

Basic Tissues

A. At the beginning of human development, individual cells multiply and differentiate to perform specialized functions; groups of cells with similar morphologic characteristics and functions come together and form tissues
B. Tissue components
   1. Cells
   2. Intercellular substance—a product of living cells; a medium for passage of nutrients and waste within the tissue; amount varies with different tissues
   3. Tissue fluid—blood plasma that diffuses through capillary walls; carries nutrients to intercellular substance and waste materials to capillaries
C. Tissues in the human body can be classified into four types
   1. Epithelial tissue
   2. Connective tissue
   3. Nerve tissue
   4. Muscle tissue
D. Each of the four basic tissues may be further subdivided into several variations

Epithelial Tissue

A. Main categories
   1. Surface epithelia
   2. Glandular tissue
B. Consists exclusively of cells held together by specialized cell junctions (very little intercellular material between the cells); cells rest on an underlying connective tissue, the basement membrane
C. Epithelial cells (keratinocytes) form continuous sheets (tissues) and perform the following functions
   1. Protection—covers all outer surfaces of the body (e.g., skin)
   2. Absorption—lines all inner surfaces of the body (e.g., digestive tract)
   3. Secretion—forms glands (glandular tissue)
D. Epithelial tissue varies depending on its function—may have surface specializations on its free surfaces
   1. Microvilli—for absorption
   2. Cilia—for surface transportation

Surface Epithelia

A. Epithelium is classified according to
   1. Shape of the most superficial cells
      a. Squamous (flat)
      b. Cuboidal
      c. Columnar
   2. Number of cell layers present
      a. One cell layer—simple
      b. Several cell layers—stratified
B. Combination characteristics allow for six different types of epithelium (Fig. 2-6)
   1. Simple squamous
   2. Simple cuboidal
   3. Simple columnar
   4. Stratified squamous
   5. Stratified cuboidal
   6. Stratified columnar
C. Other intermediate forms of epithelium
   1. Pseudostratified columnar (e.g., trachea)
   2. Transitional (e.g., urinary tract)
D. Other cell types found in epithelium
   1. Melanocytes—produce melanin (pigmentation); intensity of brown skin color is not due to difference in the number of melanocytes present but is due to difference in the *rate* of melanin production, the *size* of pigment granules, and the *length of time* of their preservation
   2. Inflammatory cells—transient cells usually associated with inflammation
   3. Langerhans cells—antigen presenting cells
   4. Merkel's cells—mechanoreceptors
E. Epithelium lining the oral cavity (oral mucosa) and the skin (dermis) are examples of stratified squamous epithelium

Glandular Tissue

A. Most glands develop from epithelium; the epithelial basal cell grows downward into the underlying connective tissue
B. Types
   1. Exocrine
      a. Serous; mucous or seromucous secretions
      b. Ducts carry secretions
   2. Endocrine
      a. Hormone secretions
      b. Bloodstream carries secretions; no ducts

Connective Tissue

Connective Tissue Proper

A. All connective tissue proper develops from embryonic mesenchyme; has two main functions
   1. Provides mechanical and biologic support
   2. Provides pathways for metabolic substances
B. Types of connective tissue
   1. Loose connective tissue
   2. Bone
   3. Cartilage

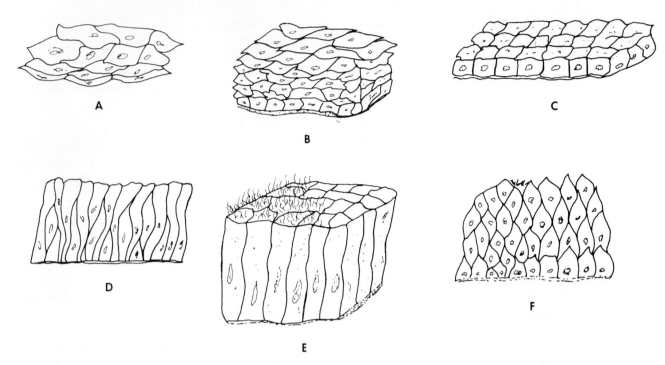

Fig. 2-6 Classification of epithelia according to morphologic shape and number of cell layers. **A,** Simple squamous. **B,** Stratified squamous. **C,** Simple cuboidal. **D,** Pseudostratified columnar. **E,** Simple columnar. **F,** Stratified columnar.

4. Bone marrow
5. Lymphoid tissue (tonsils and lymph nodes)
6. Fat (special type of connective tissue—composed of fat cells)
7. Dental tissues
   a. Pulp
   b. Dentin
   c. Cementum
C. Types of connective tissues differ in composition of cell products and proportions of products present
   1. Dense connective tissue—consists predominantly of heavy, tightly packed collagen fibers; main function is to resist tension
   2. Loose connective tissue—collagen and reticulin fibers extending in all directions; main function is to provide biologic support and fill spaces between organs and tissues

Connective Tissue Components

A. Cells
   1. Types of cells normally present
      a. Fibroblasts—produce the fibrous matrix and ground substance of connective tissue
      b. Macrophages—capable of digestive activity
      c. Mast cells—contain vesicles filled with heparin and histamine
      d. Mesenchymal cells—primitive cells that have the capability to differentiate into various con-
nective tissue cells; play a key role in the replacement of connective tissue lost as a result of injury or disease
   2. Cells that are normally in the bloodstream but move in and out of the blood vessels into surrounding connective tissue when needed (wandering cells) are
      a. Monocytes
      b. Polymorphonuclear leukocytes
      c. Lymphocytes
      d. Plasma cells
B. Fibrous matrix
   1. Matrix of connective tissue composed of some or all of the following fibers
      a. Collagen fibers—consist of three long polypeptide chains coiled in a left-handed helix to form a tropocollagen unit, which is assembled in a "quarter-stagger" model outside of the cell; are highly resistant to tension; most abundant fibers found in connective tissue (Fig. 2-7)
      b. Reticulin fibers—comparable to collagen fibers in their protein composition; usually found in border areas between connective tissue and other tissues
      c. Elastic fibers—consist of long fibrous proteins different in composition from collagen; are the branching fibers responsible for recoil in tissues when stretched

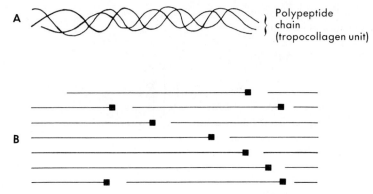

A   Polypeptide chain (tropocollagen unit)

B

Fig. 2-7 Structural arrangement of polypeptide units forming collagen molecule, **A,** and orderly arrangement of tropocollagen forming collagen fiber—quarter-stagger model, **B.**

    d. Oxytalan fibers—resemble elastic fibers in morphology and chemical composition; are thought to be immature elastic fibers

C. Ground substance

    1. Amorphous substance that consists of many large, highly organized carbohydrate chains attached to long protein cores—proteoglycans

    2. Molecular structure and the composition are responsible for the ground substance's resistance to compression—compressive loading from any direction

Types (Cartilage and Bone)

Cartilage

A. Cartilage and bone are sister tissues, both highly specialized forms of connective tissues whose intercellular substances have assumed particular properties that allow them to perform support functions

    1. Very "bouncy" resilient tissue that is specialized to resist compression; has a gel-like matrix where the ground substance predominates over the intercellular matrix

    2. Relatively avascular tissue

    3. In humans most of the embryonic skeleton is preformed as hyaline cartilage but is eventually replaced by bone (endochondral ossification); depending on the location and loading pattern imposed on the cartilage, it may specialize and form fibrous or elastic cartilage

    4. All mature cartilage is surrounded by a fibrous connective tissue, perichondrium, which serves a biomechanical function; it acts as an attachment site for muscles and tendons

B. Cartilage, like all connective tissues, has three components

    1. Cells—chondroblasts and chondrocytes

    2. Fibrous matrix—type II collagen fibers and in some cases elastic fibers

    3. Ground substance—proteoglycans, which have a protein core with side chains of chondroitin sulfate and keratin sulfate (glycosaminoglycans); because of the chemical nature and organization of the proteoglycans, the ground substance can readily bind and hold water, which allows the tissue to assume a gelatinous nature that can resist compression and also permit some degree of diffusion through the matrix

C. Types

    1. Hyaline cartilage

      a. Found in the adult human

        (1) Covering articular surfaces of movable long bones

        (2) Forming skeletal support parts of

          (a) Trachea

          (b) Larynx

          (c) External ear

          (d) Nasal septum

          (e) Ends of ribs

      b. Most abundant type of cartilage; forms the embryonic skeleton in humans; is best suited to resist compression; appears as a homogenous, translucent tissue because its intercellular matrix dominates its collagenous fibers; major type of fiber in collagen

    2. Fibrous cartilage (fibrocartilage)

      a. Has a very sparse amount of intercellular substance dominated by collagen fibers, which are in such proportions that they are visible with a light microscope and are seen running between the chondrocytic cells in the cartilage

      b. Resembles tendons except for the presence of the chondrocytes enclosed in lacunae

   c. Usually found in areas that are subjected to both compression and tension, as in
      (1) Intervertebral disk
      (2) Temporomandibular joint of older adults
      (3) Pubic symphysis
3. Elastic cartilage
   a. In areas that are in need of elastic recoil, hyaline cartilage becomes highly specialized and elastic fibers are added to its intercellular matrix, as in
      (1) External ear
      (2) Epiglottis
   b. Elastic fibers are highly branched and form a delicate fibrous matrix, often obscuring the intercellular substance; fibers can be seen only with a light microscope when stained with a specific elastic stain

Bone

A. Very rigid tissue; calcified connective tissue capable of resisting tension; has a calcified matrix that contains the mineral salt hydroxyapatite; very vascular tissue
B. Two main functions
   1. Provides skeletal support and protection of soft tissues
   2. Acts as a reservoir for calcium and phosphorus ions—when these two ions drop below a critical level in the blood (100 mg Ca/100 ml blood and 600 mg P/100 ml blood), they can be withdrawn from the bone
C. Can be identified on two levels
   1. Macroscopic (gross) level—compact (dense) and spongy (cancellous)
      a. Compact (dense) bone appears as a continuous solid mass
      b. Spongy (cancellous) bone appears as branching bony spicules (trabeculae with large intervening marrow spaces between them)
   2. Microscopic level—woven, spongy (cancellous), and lamellar bone
D. Bone morphology
   1. Woven bone—earliest formed embryonic bone; fibers in the matrix have no distinct preferential orientation
   2. Lamellar bone—mature bone has become functionally loaded and can withstand a variety of loading patterns (Fig. 2-8)
      a. Concentric lamellae—form around blood vessels to form osteons (primary or secondary)
      b. Circumferential lamellae—form on the outer and inner layers of compact bone
      c. Trabecular bone—reflects loading patterns; tra-

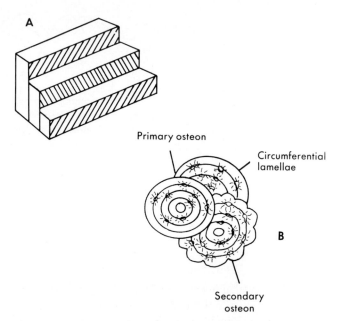

Fig. 2-8 Microscopic morphology of bone tissue. **A,** Compact lamellar bone where collagen fibers in each lamella run in opposite direction from adjacent lamella. **B,** Osteons, primary and secondary, that form as a result of bone resorption and remodeling; note scalloped edge of secondary osteon. (Modified from Salentijin-Moss L, Klyvert M: *Dental and oral tissues: an introduction for paraprofessionals in dentistry,* ed 3, Philadelphia, 1990, Lea & Febiger.)

   beculae are oriented in two main directions: one parallel with the principal loading direction, the other at right angles with the first; if the loading pattern changes, bone remodeling follows, with the size/shape and direction of the trabeculae adjusted to new conditions
      d. Primary osteons—form initially around blood vessels in embryonic woven bone and when bone is remodeled and resorbed; are replaced by mature secondary osteons; secondary osteons differ from primary osteons in that their outer surfaces have a scalloped border rather than a smooth one as with primary osteons; scalloping reflects the areas of resorbed lacunae by the osteoclasts before the secondary osteon was built
      e. Thickness of any bone (compact lamellar, spongy lamellar) is limited by the nutritional needs of its cells (osteocytes); furthest distance any osteocyte can be from any blood vessel is about 200 μm
E. Bone tissue
   1. Bone, like all connective tissues, has three main components
      a. Cells

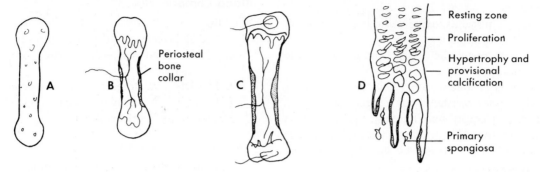

Fig. 2-9   Stages of endochondral bone formation in long bone growth. **A,** Preformed cartilage model of bone. **B,** Primary centers of ossification in epiphysis and periosteal collar. **C,** Secondary center of ossification starting in diaphysis. **D,** Growth plate with four zones.

    (1) Osteoblasts—bone-forming cells
    (2) Osteoclasts—bone-resorbing cells
    (3) Osteocytes—osteoblasts that are embedded in lacunae of bone matrix and that maintain the bone tissue
  b. Fibrous matrix—collagen fibers (type I) are the dominant component of the bone matrix
  c. Ground substance—proteoglycans containing chondroitin sulfates and seeded with the mineral salt hydroxyapatite
2. Bone is formed by osteoblasts developed in one of two ways
  a. Intramembranous ossification—mesenchymal cells move closer together (condensation); differentiate into osteoblasts and begin to deposit bone matrix; this is how the maxilla and mandible are formed
  b. Endochondral ossification—future bone is preformed in a cartilage model that is eventually resorbed and replaced by new bone formed by osteoblasts (Fig. 2-9)
    (1) Cartilage must undergo two important changes before being resorbed and replaced by new bone
      (a) Chondrocytic hypertrophy
      (b) Calcification of the cartilage model
    (2) Endochondral ossification is the process by which all long bones in the human body are formed
      (a) Bone growth in length—occurs in the cartilaginous epiphyseal growth plate
      (b) Bone growth in diameter—occurs in the cellular layer of the fibrous covering of connective tissue periosteum, which produces a periosteal bone collar on the outer bone surface
E. Structure of long bones (macroscopic)
  1. Typical long bone is composed of

  a. Diaphysis (shaft)—thick compact bone forming a hollow cylinder with a central marrow cavity; is the primary center of ossification in a long bone
  b. Epiphyses (ends)—spongy bone covered by a thin layer of compact bone; is the secondary growth center
  c. Metaphysis—transitional region between the epiphyses and the diaphysis where the cartilage growth plate is located
  d. All articular surfaces of long bones are covered by articular cartilage
2. While active, the epiphyseal growth plate usually has four zones, proceeding from first to last
  a. Primary spongiosa with resorption
  b. Hypertrophy and provisional calcification
  c. Proliferation
  d. Resting zone (Fig. 2-9)

Blood and Lymph

A. Vascular system
  1. Develops embryonically from mesenchymal cells that come together and form delicate tubular structures composed of endothelial cells
  2. Consists of the heart, blood vessels, and lymphatics
  a. Is a closed system that runs from the heart to the organs of the body and back to the heart
  b. Between the heart and the organs, the blood vessels branch progressively into finer and finer vessels and finally enter organs
    (1) Here a delicate network of capillaries form, called the capillary bed—the most essential part of the vascular system
    (2) Exchanges of gases and substances occur in this capillary bed
  c. Blood is then carried back to the heart via larger vessels, the veins

3. Functions
   a. Carries nutrients, oxygen, and hormones to all parts of the body
   b. Carries metabolic waste products to the kidneys
   c. Transports inflammatory cells and antibodies
   d. Maintains a constant body temperature
B. Lymph vessels empty into filtering organs (nodes); generally flow toward larger lymph vessels, the thoracic duct, and the right lymphatic duct; lymph enters venous branches of the circulatory system

Blood Vessels

A. Arteries—the largest of the blood vessels; walls are composed of
   1. Thick layer of smooth muscle cells
   2. Elastic tissue—the largest amount found in large arteries close to the heart
B. Veins—usually accompany arteries but carry blood in the opposite direction
   1. Walls are composed of
      a. Layer of endothelial cells
      b. Connective tissue layer
      c. Occasionally a few smooth muscle cells
   2. Veins contain about 70% of the total blood volume of the body at any given time
C. Capillaries—the simplest of the blood vessels in their structure
   1. Walls consist of a simple layer of endothelial cells and a basal lamina
   2. Usually the diameter of a capillary lumen is so small that only one blood cell at a time can pass through the vessel
   3. Form a barrier between the blood and the tissues
   4. Transport of substances occurs at the capillary level via
      a. Pores in the endothelial wall of the capillary
      b. Openings between adjacent endothelial cells
      c. Pinocytotic vesicles formed by the wall of the capillary

Microvasculature

A. Composed of the smallest arteries and veins located in the capillary bed
   1. At the end of the arterioles is a preferential channel that has several side branches entering into the capillary bed
   2. Blood passes through the capillary bed from the arterial side to the venous side
B. Selective openings and closings of the capillary bed occur in the microvasculature to ensure regulation of the amount of blood throughout the body at any given time

Blood Components

A. Cells
   1. Red blood cells—erythrocytes; most numerous
   2. White blood cells—leukocytes (granular and nongranular)
   3. Platelets—cell fragments of a specific cell type found in red bone marrow; have no nuclei
B. Plasma—liquid portion of blood

Functions of Blood Cells

A. Red blood cells—contain hemoglobin, which carries oxygen from the lungs to the tissues
B. Granular leukocytes
   1. Neutrophils—first line of defense against bacterial invasion
   2. Eosinophils—involvement in allergy reactions
   3. Basophils—antigen involvement
C. Nongranular leukocytes
   1. Monocytes—can become macrophages in connective tissue
   2. Lymphocytes—produce antibodies
D. Platelets—promote blood clotting

Lymphatic System

A. Made up of a series of vessels that carry excess tissue fluid from the capillaries to filtering organs such as lymph nodes on the way back to the bloodstream
B. Lymph nodes are found along the lymphatic pathway
   1. Consist of masses of lymph tissue that serve as a filtering system for the body
   2. Tonsils and the spleen are both filtering organs for the body
   3. Swollen and palpable lymph nodes can indicate that there may be an infection somewhere in the body
C. Function of lymph is to help protect and maintain the internal fluid environment of the body

Nerve Tissue

A. Main functions of the nervous system
   1. Directs and helps maintain the complex internal environment of the body
   2. Integrates and interprets incoming stimuli and directs appropriate responses at a conscious or unconscious level
B. Nervous system can be classified accordingly
   1. Central nervous system (CNS)
   2. Peripheral nervous system (PNS)
   3. Autonomic nervous system (ANS)
C. Afferent nerves transmit impulses (sensations) from the periphery to the CNS (sensory input); effer-

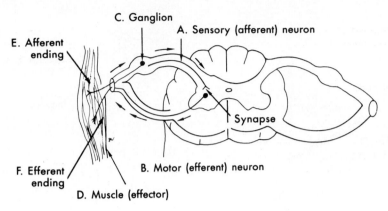

Fig. 2-10 Cross section of spinal cord and pathways used to transmit nerve impulses from periphery to central nervous system (see also Figs. 3-13 to 3-15). *A,* Sensory neuron sending impulses from periphery to central nervous system; *B,* motor neuron leaving spinal cord, transmitting commands to effector; *C,* nerve cell bodies located in dorsal root ganglia; *D,* effector; *E,* afferent ending; *F,* efferent ending.

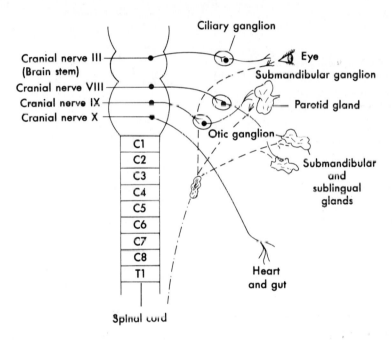

Fig. 2-11 Autonomic pathways for cranial nerves and synapses in their respective ganglia outside central nervous system (see also Fig. 3-17).

ent nerves transmit impulses (commands) from the CNS to muscles and other organs (motor output) (Fig. 2-10)

D. Divisions of the nervous system
　1. Central nervous system
　　a. Includes the brain and the spinal cord
　　b. Main functions
　　　(1) Receives incoming information at a conscious or unconscious level (sensory)
　　　(2) Integrates outgoing responses (motor) that are transmitted to various parts of the brain and the spinal cord

　2. Peripheral nervous system
　　a. Composed of 31 pairs of spinal nerves and 12 pairs of cranial nerves
　　b. All nerves transmit information to and from the CNS
　　c. Contains both sensory and motor nerves (neurons)
　3. Autonomic nervous system (Fig. 2-11)
　　a. Controls, regulates, and coordinates visceral activities (digestion, body temperature, blood pressure, and glandular secretions) on an unconscious level

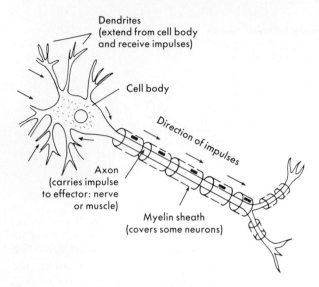

Fig. 2-12 Basic neuron.

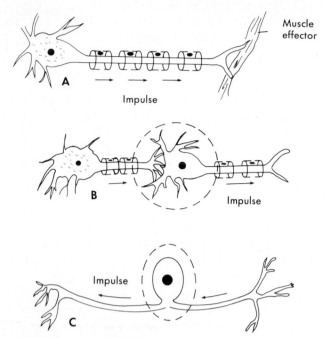

Fig. 2-13 Classification of neurons based on number of cell processes on neuron. **A,** Multipolar motor neuron with one of its axons going to effector (skeletal muscle). **B,** Two autonomic multipolar neurons; axon of one neuron in central nervous system communicates with cell body of neuron outside central nervous system (in ganglion). **C,** Sensory (afferent) neuron; cell process leaves cell body and divides into two processes; one process goes toward central nervous system; and one goes to periphery (e.g., skin, oral mucosa). (Modified from Salentijn-Moss L, Klyvert M: *Dental and oral tissues: an introduction for paraprofessionals in dentistry,* ed 3, Philadelphia, 1990, Lea & Febiger.)

b. Is further subdivided into
  (1) Sympathetic division—acts to regulate and mobilize activities during emergency and/or stress (flight activities); activities that require large outputs of energy produce an accelerated heart rate and increase in blood pressure
  (2) Parasympathetic division—works the opposite of the sympathetic division; stimulates those activities that restore or conserve energy
  (3) These two divisions are seen as acting reciprocally rather than antagonistically

Structural Components

A. Neurons (Fig. 2-12)
  1. Structural components of nerve tissue
  2. Receive and transmit information
  3. Highly specialized cells consisting of
    a. Cell body—contains the nucleus and the organelles; located in the ganglia in the CNS and PNS
    b. One or more cytoplasmic extensions
      (1) Dendrites—conduct impulses toward the cell body
      (2) Axons—conduct impulses away from the cell body
  4. Classified according to the number of cell processes (Fig. 2-13)
    a. Multipolar neurons—located in the CNS and autonomic ganglia; usually one process is the axon, and the other processes are the dendrites
    b. Unipolar neurons—have a short cell process that leaves the cell body and divides into two long

branches; one branch goes to the CNS, and the other goes toward the PNS (sensory neurons)
  5. Interneurons—lie within the CNS; receive and link sensory and motor impulses to bring about appropriate responses in the body
B. Glial cells—provide structural support and nourishment for the neurons; Schwann cells in the PNS and satellite cells in the ganglia

Definitions

A. Synapse—area that occurs between two neurons or between a neuron and its effector (muscle or gland); between the cell surfaces are
  1. Synaptic cleft—intercellular space separating a presynaptic and postsynaptic membrane
  2. Presynaptic membrane—situated before the synapse
  3. Postsynaptic membrane—situated after the synapse
B. Neurotransmitters—chemicals released from the neuron as electrical impulses travel along the axon and reach the terminal end

1. They increase the permeability of the cell membranes; impulses are relayed to the effector (impulses can be excitatory or inhibitory)
   2. Two membrane junctions
   3. Kinds of neurotransmitters
      a. Acetylcholine—secreted by cholinergic fibers
      b. Norepinephrine—secreted by adrenergic fibers
C. Myelin sheath—fatty layer surrounding the axon of the nerve
   1. Myelinated—contains a fatty sheath
   2. Unmyelinated—no fatty sheath is present
D. Neurilemma—a continuous sheath that encloses the segmented myelin sheath of some nerves
E. Neuroglia—extremely soft tissue that supports the nervous tissue of the brain and spinal cord
F. Free nerve endings—end portions of afferent (sensory) axons that are no longer covered by a supportive Schwann cells; are found in
   1. Dental pulp
   2. Oral epithelium
G. Encapsulated nerve endings—are composed of several portions of afferent axons surrounded by a capsule of several Schwann cells without a myelin sheath and some connective tissue; are associated with
   1. Touch perception (Meissner's corpuscles) found in the lamina propria of the oral mucosa
   2. Periodontal ligament

Cranial Nerves

A. Twelve pairs of cranial nerves originate from the brain
   1. Transmit information to the brain from the special sensory receptors and regulate the functions of
      a. Smell
      b. Sight
      c. Hearing
      d. Taste
   2. Bring impulses from the CNS to voluntary muscles of
      a. Eyes
      b. Mouth (masticatory muscles)
      c. Face (facial expression)
      d. Tongue (swallowing and speech)
      e. Larynx
B. Local anesthetic used in the dental profession is injected into a sensory peripheral nerve; it diffuses through the nerve fibers and blocks transmission of impulses to the brain in an area of several teeth or in a localized area of soft tissue

Muscle Tissue

A. Composed mainly of cells called muscle fibers that have differentiated from embryonic mesenchyme and become highly specialized in contracting (shortening)
B. Contracting ability of muscle fibers is a result of large amounts of intracellular, contractile protein filaments: actin and myosin
C. Three muscle tissue types
   1. Skeletal (striated) muscle
      a. Under conscious control; referred to as voluntary muscle
      b. Has rapid, short, strong contractions; requires a great deal of energy
      c. Innervated by motor nerves
      d. Skeletal muscles of the head region
         (1) Muscles of mastication
         (2) Muscles of facial expression
      e. Muscle attachments are made possible because of the connective tissues surrounding the muscle, bone, or cartilage; connecting tissues of the muscle run directly into the periosteum, cover the bone or perichondrium, cover the cartilage or perimysium, or cover the muscle. The exact nature of the attachment will depend on the site and function of the muscle. There may be intermediate structures such as
         (1) Tendons
         (2) Ligaments
         (3) Aponeuroses
      f. Muscles that change the shape of the tongue by their contractions are attached on both sides to the lamina propria of the oral mucosa of the tongue
   2. Smooth muscle
      a. Under the control of the ANS and not under conscious control
      b. Contractions are slow and can be maintained over a long period of time without the use of much energy
   3. Cardiac muscle
      a. Has some of both skeletal and smooth muscle characteristics
      b. Is involuntary; has fast, powerful contractions
      c. Purkinje's fibers—specialized cells that are present in the heart muscle; they act like nerves to conduct messages through the heart
      d. Bundle of His—a band of specialized cardiac muscle fibers; the heartbeat originates at this site

Muscle Contraction

A. Muscle can be stimulated to contract by one or many nerves
B. Each striated muscle contains bundles of highly organized contractile proteins called myofibrils; each myofibril consists of regularly arranged protein filaments: actin and myosin (Fig. 2-14)

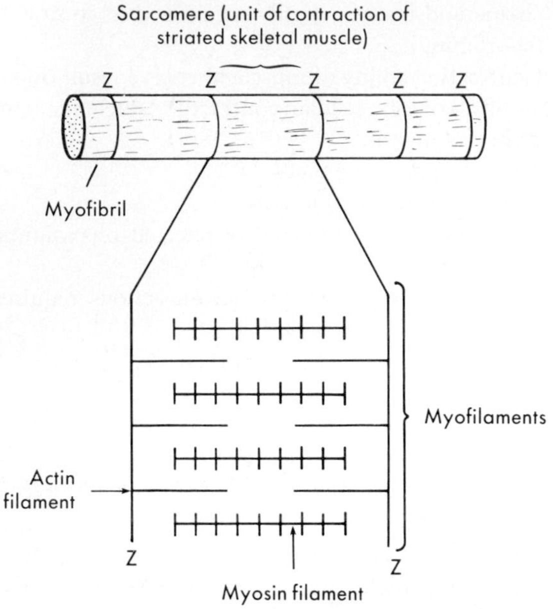

Sarcomere (unit of contraction of striated skeletal muscle)

Myofibril

Myofilaments

Actin filament

Myosin filament

Fig. 2-14 Enlarged segment of myofibril showing arrangement of actin and myosin filaments and their attachment to Z bands (see also Fig. 3-10).

C. Protein filaments are attached to a Z band; section of a myofibril between two Z bands is called a sarcomere, which is the contractile unit
D. As a muscle unit contracts, the actin and myosin filaments slide past each other, shorten the length of the individual sarcomere (sliding mechanism), and cause total shortening of the muscle fiber

Embryology

General Embryology

A. All human development begins by the uniting of a female germ cell (ovum) with a male germ cell (sperm), called fertilization
B. Each germ cell contains 23 chromosomes (haploid number); during the process of fertilization the number of chromosomes is restored to 46 (diploid number)
C. The developing organism, called the zygote, goes through a series of mitotic divisions producing
   1. Morula—16 to 32 cells having the appearance of a mulberry
   2. Blastocele—central cavity develops with an embryonic pole
   3. Blastocyst—becomes attached to and embedded in the uterine wall
      a. Two distinct layers become visible
         (1) Epiblast (ectoderm) layer
         (2) Hypoblast (endoderm) layer

      b. These two layers constitute the embryonic disk, which will give rise to the future embryo
D. Three distinct periods in human development
   1. Period of the ovum (first week)—fertilized ovum develops an embryonic disk
   2. Embryonic period (second through eighth week)—most of the organs and organ systems develop
      a. Period of differentiation
      b. At the end of this period a recognizable individual has developed
      c. Most congenital malformations occur during this time
   3. Fetal period (third through ninth month)—growth of the existing structures takes place
E. Development of some facial and oral structures is dependent on a group of cells (neural crest cells) derived from ectoderm as the neural tube is forming; these cells migrate cephalically and interact with the cephalic ectoderm and mesoderm to result in development of
   1. Facial skeleton—Meckel's cartilage
   2. Neck skeleton—hyoid bone
   3. Connective tissue components
   4. Tooth development
F. Neural crest cells migrate into each of the branchial arches and surround the existing mesoderm; in each arch the following components develop
   1. Cartilage rod (skeleton of each arch)—first branchial arch, Meckel's cartilage
   2. Muscular component—second branchial arch, facial musculature
   3. Vasculature component
   4. Nerve component—first branchial arch, trigeminal nerve
G. On the internal aspect of the branchial arches are corresponding pharyngeal pouches that give rise to
   1. External auditory meatus
   2. Pharyngotympanic tube
   3. Palatine tonsils
   4. Parathyroid glands

Facial Development

A. Begins in the fourth week of prenatal life (embryonic period) and is complete in the twelfth week
B. Future facial region is located between the bulging forebrain, frontal nasal process, and developing heart
C. At the beginning of the fourth week, five facial swellings appear on the embryo, called branchial arches
   1. Located between the first branchial arch and the frontal process (forebrain) is the oral stomadeum (primitive oral cavity) (Fig. 2-15, *A* and *B*); the stomodeum is the first sign of facial development

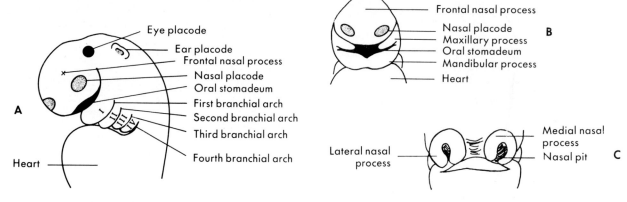

Fig. 2-15   Facial development in fourth week of embryo. **A**, and **B**, Facial development beginning with outgrowth of branchial arches; note relationship of oral stomadeum to heart and developing face. **C**, Nasal placodes develop from frontal nasal process and grow to become nostrils and form bridge of nose and philtrum.

2. The stomodeal ectoderm invaginates until it comes in contact with the primitive foregut; the stomodeum and foregut are initially separated by the buccopharyngeal membrane, which is composed of ectoderm and endoderm
3. Rathke's pouch—small invagination in roof of stomodeum; deepens into brain and forms anterior lobe of pituitary gland
4. Maxilla and mandible develop from the first branchial arch
5. Second through fifth branchial arches are involved with development of the neck
D. Frontal nasal process develops the forehead and nose
   1. On the surface of the frontal nasal process two bilateral thickened areas of specialized ectoderm arise—nasal placodes (Fig. 2-15, *C*); the nasal placodes become the nostrils which separate this area into
      a. Two lateral nasal processes—will form the sides of the nose
      b. Two medial and nasal processes—will form the bridge of the nose, the nostrils, and the globular process; the globular process will form the philtrum of the upper lip and the primary palate
   2. Face grows downward and forward around the developing nasal and oral cavities
E. Midface is formed by the bilateral processes of the maxillary process, which grow forward and make contact with the mandibular processes and the globular process
F. Lower face is formed by the bilateral swellings (mandibular processes) of the mandibular arch
G. Several facial or oral processes merge or fuse together during development; incomplete merging or fusing can result in cleft formation—cleft lip or cleft palate

Palatal Development

A. The globular process develops as medial nasal processes grow downward and gives rise to
   1. Philtrum of upper lip
   2. Primary palate (premaxillary process), which carries the incisor teeth
B. During the sixth week of embryonic life, two palatal shelves develop from each side of the maxilla and lie vertically on each side of the tongue (secondary palate)
C. During the seventh week of embryonic life, the developing tongue drops down, the vertical palatal shelves flip up, assume a horizontal position, and fuse with the primary palate
D. Where the two palatal processes (shelves) fuse in the midline, trapped epithelium between the two processes may result in epithelium remnants, which may result in cysts

Tongue Development

During the fourth week of embryonic life, the tongue develops from several swellings arising on the internal aspect of branchial arches 1 through 4 (pouches); these swellings eventually merge and form the body and root of the tongue
A. Branchial arch 1—two lateral swellings and one medial swelling merge to form body of the tongue
B. Branchial arches 2, 3, and part of 4—corpula merge to form tongue base
C. Branchial arch 4—epiglottis
D. Thyroid gland—develops from an invagination of ectoderm in the area of the foramen ceacum of the tongue; the thyroid gland eventually migrates down to its position in the neck; thyroid tissue that remains entrapped in the tissue of the tongue may result in a

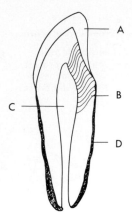

Fig. 2-16   Longitudinal cross section showing tissues of tooth. *A,* Enamel covering crown of tooth; *B,* dentin forming bulk of tooth in crown and root; *C,* pulp tissue centrally located in crown and root; *D,* cementum covering root.

developmental abnormality known as a lingual thyroid nodule

Oral Histology

Tooth Development

A. Begins in the seventh week of embryonic life with the 20 primary teeth; continues until the late teens with sequential exfoliation of the primary teeth and development and eruption of the secondary dentition—the 32 permanent teeth
B. Tissues of the tooth
  1. Each tooth consists of four tissues (Fig. 2-16)
    a. Enamel—calcified
    b. Cementum—calcified
    c. Dentin—calcified
    d. Pulp—uncalcified
  2. All tissues of the tooth are specialized forms of connective tissue, except enamel
  3. Each tooth is the product of two tissues that interact during tooth development
    a. Mesenchyme (ectomesenchyme)—derived from neural crest cells
    b. Epithelium—oral epithelium derived from ectoderm
C. Involves two major events
  1. Morphodifferentiation—shaping of the tooth
  2. Cytodifferentiation—cells differentiate into specific tissue-forming cells
    a. Ameloblasts—enamel-forming cells
    b. Cementoblasts—cementum-forming cells
    c. Odontoblasts—dentin-forming cells
    d. Fibroblasts—pulp-forming cells

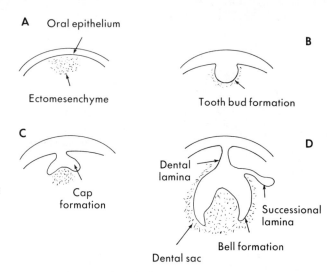

Fig. 2-17   Sequential stages of tooth development. **A,** Initial interaction between oral epithelium and ectomesenchyme. **B,** Bud stage. **C,** Cap stage. **D,** Bell stage.

Morphodifferentiation

A. Oral epithelium and underlying ectomesenchyme are responsible for shaping the tooth
  1. Both primary and permanent tooth germs go through the same stages of development
  2. Oral epithelium grows down into underlying ectomesenchyme; small areas of condensed mesenchyme will form future tooth germs
B. Stages (Fig. 2-17)
  1. Bud stage—condensed areas of ectomesenchymal cells that are continuous with oral epithelium; connection between the two is referred to as the dental lamina
  2. Cap stage—future shape of the tooth becomes evident; cells specialize to form the enamel organ
  3. Bell stage—final stage of morphodifferentiation; in the later part of this stage, cytodifferentiation begins in the enamel organ
  4. Apposition stage—cells have differentiated into tissue-forming cells; begin to deposit the dental tissues

Cytodifferentiation

A. Stages of cytodifferentiation and morphodifferentiation overlap; both the epithelial and mesenchymal components of the tooth germ become organized
  1. Epithelial components become the enamel organ, which is organized into four distinct cell layers
    a. Outer enamel epithelium (OEE)—outlines the shape of the future developing enamel organ on the outer surface; composed of small cuboidal cells, one cell layer thick

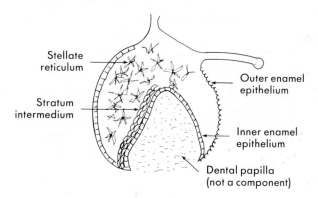

Stellate reticulum

Stratum intermedium

Outer enamel epithelium

Inner enamel epithelium

Dental papilla (not a component)

Fig. 2-18　Four distinct components of enamel organ.

　　b. Inner enamel epithelium (IEE)—innermost layer of enamel organ on the concave side of developing tooth germ; will become the future enamel-producing cells, the ameloblasts; composed of cuboidal-type cells, one cell layer thick

　　c. Stratum intermedium (STI)—flat, supporting squamous-type cells; two to three cell layers thick, lying on top of the inner enamel epithelial cells

　　d. Stellate reticulum (STR)—mechanically and nutritionally supporting cells that fill the bulk of the developing enamel organ; are star shaped with large amounts of intercellular space between them (Fig. 2-18)

　2. Mesenchymal components—become subdivided into

　　a. Dental sac (follicle)—surrounds the developing tooth germ and provides cells that will form the cementum, periodontal ligament, and the alveolar bone proper

　　b. Dental papilla—condensed ectomesenchyme located on the concavity side of the enamel organ; peripheral cells facing the IEE will differentiate into dentin-forming cells, the odontoblasts

　　c. Center of the dental papilla will become the dental pulp

B. Tooth development is dependent on a series of sequential cellular interactions between epithelial and mesenchymal components of the tooth germ

　1. First interaction—between oral epithelium and the mesenchyme; ectomesenchyme instructs the epithelium to grow down into the ectomesenchyme and shape the tooth

　2. Second interaction—given by cells of inner enamel epithelium (preameloblasts) to mesenchymal cells on the periphery of the dental papilla to differentiate into odontoblasts and begin deposition of dentin

　3. Third interaction—as soon as odontoblasts begin to deposit dentin, preameloblasts become true secreting ameloblasts and begin deposition of enamel

　4. Fourth interaction—occurs with development of root dentin and cementum

Dentin and Enamel Formation

A. Both enamel- and dentin-forming cells are polarized, tall, columnar secreting cells; just before ameloblasts and odontoblasts begin to deposit enamel and dentin, there is an increase in the number of organelles, especially the mitochondria; organelles move to the basal nonsecretory end of the cell; both cells require tremendous amounts of energy for production of their calcified tissues

B. All dentin and enamel formation begins at the dentoenamel junction of the cup or incisal edge of the tooth and continues in an apical direction

C. Permanent tooth germ grows off the primary (deciduous) tooth germ via an epithelial attachment similar to dental lamina, called successional lamina; true for all of the developing permanent teeth except first, second, and third molars; these develop from the dental lamina, which continues to grow back in oral arches

D. Dentin formation

　1. Odontoblasts produce Karff's fibers that unravel to produce a fibrous connective tissue matrix (fibrillar matrix) of predominantly collagen fibers with a rich proteoglycan ground substance; dentinal tissue is calcified by deposition of crystals of the calcium salt hydroxyapatite into the matrix

　2. Each odontoblast has a long cell extension, odontoblastic process, left behind in the calcified dentin and enclosed in a dentinal tubule (Fig. 2-19, A)

　3. Dentin remains a vital tissue throughout the life of the tooth; cells continue to produce dentin when needed

E. Enamel formation

　1. Ameloblasts produce an enamel matrix with protein components called amelogenins and enamelins; matrix is calcified immediately by deposition of crystals of the calcium salt hydroxyapatite

　2. Ameloblasts deposit enamel; each ameloblast has a secretory process, Tomes' process; Tomes' process has a six-sided pyrimidal and it is responsible for prism-shaped microscopic patterns of enamel rods; unlike the odontoblastic process, Tomes' process is not left behind embedded in the calcified tissue (Fig. 2-19, B)

　3. When the tooth emerges into the oral cavity, the enamel has no vital cells associated with the tissue; enamel is not a true tissue as the other dental tissues are and is incapable of tissue growth or repair; once

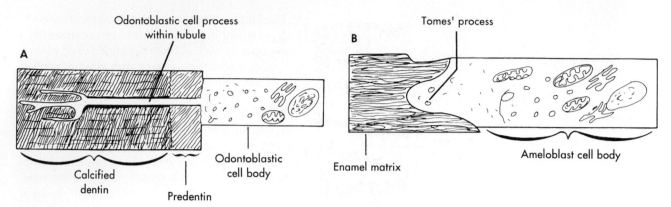

Fig. 2-19 Odontoblast and ameloblast with their cell extensions. **A,** Tall secretory odontoblast with its cell extension (odontoblastic process). **B,** Tall secretory ameloblast with its cell extension (Tomes' process).

formed the mineral substance cannot be physiologically withdrawn from the tooth

4. A final product of the ameloblasts is the primary enamel cuticle, a calcified coating on the enamel surface
5. Secondary cuticle—a noncalcified coating; product of the reduced enamel organ

F. Dentogingival junction formation
1. After enamel formation is completed, remains of the enamel organ (OEE, IEE, STI, and STR) come together
2. These form the reduced enamel epithelium, which plays an important role in formation of the dentogingival junction as the tooth emerges into the oral cavity

G. Cementum formation
1. Formation of root dentin and cementum follows after the crown of the tooth is completed
2. Hertwig's root sheath is formed by the joining of the outer enamel epithelium and the inner enamel epithelium; the sheath continues to grow down, shapes the root of the tooth and formation of root dentin, and is followed by differentiation of cells from the dental sac, which produce
   a. Cementum
   b. Periodontal ligament
   c. Alveolar bone proper

Soft Tissue of the Oral Cavity

Oral Mucosa

A. Oral epithelium (Fig. 2-20)
1. Covered by a layer of stratified squamous epithelium, which
   a. Acts as a mechanical barrier
   b. Protects the underlying tissues

2. Three types of stratified squamous epithelium are found in the oral cavity
   a. Orthokeratinized
      (1) Effective as a mechanical protector and barrier against fluids
      (2) Least common of the three types
      (3) Layers
         (a) Basal cell layer—deepest layer
         (b) Prickle cell layer
         (c) Granular layer—contains the keratohyaline granules, the precursor to keratin
         (d) Keratinized layer—contains degenerative cells with no nuclei or organelles; cells are filled with keratin, become hard (cornified), and are eventually lost from the surface epithelium
   b. Nonkeratinized
      (1) Functions as a selective barrier acting as a cushion and as protection against mechanical stress and wear
      (2) Layers
         (a) Basal cell layer
         (b) Prickle cell layer
         (c) Outer surface of nonkeratinized cells (squamae); no distinctly recognizable layer above the prickle cell layer; superficial cells in the outermost layer undergo a gradual increase in size; look empty but are filled with fluid sacs; cells act as a cushion and are firmly attached to each other
   c. Parakeratinized
      (1) Intermediate form of epithelium located between the orthokeratinized and nonkeratinized oral mucosa
      (2) Layers
         (a) Basal cell layer

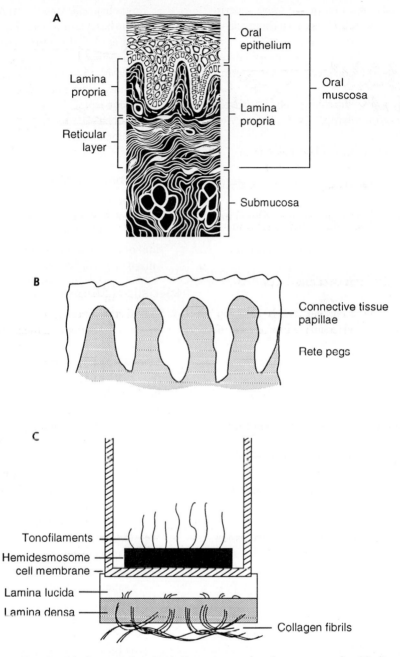

Fig. 2-20 Basic structure of oral epithelium. **A,** Two basic tissue types of oral mucosa: oral epithelium and connective tissue; connective tissue is composed of papillary layer and reticular layer; submucosal layer may or may not be present, depending on location of oral mucosa. **B,** Arrangements of rete pegs and connective tissue. **C,** Basal lamina interface between oral epithelium and connective tissue; hemidesmosome attachments between epithelial cells and basal lamina.

(b) Prickle cell layer

(c) Keratinized layer—no distinct granular layer present; gradually becomes filled with keratin; nuclei and other cell organelles remain present until the cell becomes cornified and are eventually lost

3. Stratified squamous epithelium is constantly being renewed by mitosis at the basal cell layer; turnover time ranges from 5 to 16 days

4. Other cell types in the oral epithelium—nonepithelial cells; these cells are normally found in oral epithelium and perpetuate themselves

   a. Melanocytes—usually found in the basal cell layer; responsible for the production of pigment (melanin)

b. Langerhans cells—located in the more superficial cell layers; they are antigen presenting cells—part of the body's immune system
c. Merkel cells—usually found in the basal cell layer, cells that are associated with nerve terminals (endings)
d. Inflammatory cells—transient cells associated with inflammation: lymphocytes, monocytes, neutrophils

B. Connective tissue—referred to as lamina propria
  1. Subdivided into two layers
    a. Papillary layer—directly under the epithelial layer
    b. Reticular layer—dense fibrous layer located under the papillary layer
  2. Forms a mechanical support system and carries
    a. Blood vessels
    b. Nerves

C. Submucosa
  1. Layer of loosely organized connective tissue
  2. Present only in areas that require a high degree of compressibility and flexibility (e.g., cheeks, soft palate)
  3. When present, is located between the lamina propria and areas where muscle tissue is present

D. Interface
  1. Area of interdigitation between oral epithelium and the connective tissue
  2. Epithelial extensions into the connective tissue (lamina propria) are called rete pegs
  3. Connective tissue extensions into overlying epithelium are called connective tissue papillae
  4. Corrugated arrangement
    a. Increases the surface area between the two tissues
    b. Increases the strength of the junction between the two tissues
    c. Decreases the distance between the blood supply and epithelium, which does not have its own blood supply; blood vessels are carried to epithelium in connective tissue via the connective tissue papillae

E. Basement membrane
  1. Located between oral epithelium and the connective tissue
  2. Noncellular
  3. Produced in part by epithelial cells and connective tissue cells
  4. Composed of two layers (lamina)
    a. Basal lamina (densa)—20 to 70 nm thick, seen as a thin dark line; produced by the epithelial cells
    b. Reticular lamina (lucida)—much thicker than basal lamina; produced by the connective tissue cells

5. Epithelial cells form hemidesmosome attachments to the basal lamina (see Fig. 2-20)

F. Clinical epithelial tumors—three types may occur in the oral cavity
  a. Papilloma—derived from the squamous epithelium of the oral mucosa
  b. Mucoepidermoid carcinoma—derived from salivary gland epithelium
  c. Ameloblastoma—derived from odontogenic (dental) epithelium

Classifications of Mucosa

A. Masticatory—gingiva, hard palate (orthokeratinized epithelial covering)
B. Lining—lips, cheeks, floor of mouth, ventral (underside) of tongue, soft palate, alveolar mucosa (nonkeratinized epithelial covering)

Specialized Mucosa of the Tongue

A. Specialized covering found only on the top of the tongue; covered with *lingual papillae*
B. Epithelial layer—stratified squamous epithelium that varies in thickness and degree of keratinization
C. Taste buds are epithelial organs of special sense (taste); most of these taste buds are found on the lingual papilla; isolated ones may be found on the soft palate and walls of the pharynx
D. Connective tissue papillae form specialized *lingual papillae*
  1. Fungiform papillae—located on the dorsal aspect of the tongue; mushroom shaped; a single taste bud may be present on the top surface
  2. Filiform papillae—most abundant of the papillae; found covering the entire top surface of the tongue; have no taste buds
  3. Vallate papillae—large papillae located in a V-shaped groove at the base of the tongue; encircled by a deep groove; mushroom shaped; taste buds are located on their sides; small salivary glands (von Ebner's glands) empty into surrounding grooves of taste buds
  4. Foliate papillae—located along the sides of the tongue, near the base of the tongue; taste buds may be located on only one of the sides
E. No submucosa is present

Tissues of the Tooth

Dentin

A. Mature dentin composition
  1. Chemical composition
    a. Organic matter, 18%

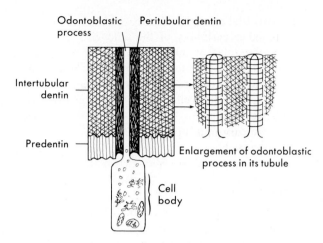

Odontoblastic process   Peritubular dentin

Intertubular dentin

Predentin

Enlargement of odontoblastic process in its tubule

Cell body

Fig. 2-21   Odontoblastic process with its cell process enclosed in dentinal tubule.

    b. Inorganic materials, 70%
    c. Water, 12%
  2. Tissue composition
    a. Cells—odontoblasts
    b. Fibrous material—collagen fibers (type I)
    c. Ground substance—proteoglycans and glyco proteins
  3. Calcification—deposition of crystals of the calcium salt hydroxyapatite in the dentin, fibrous matrix, and ground substance
B. Process of dentogenesis
  1. Dentin begins to form in the late bell state of the developing tooth germ
  2. Newly differentiated odontoblasts deposit the dentin matrix; odontoblastic processes become surrounded by predentin (a newly deposited uncalcified dentin matrix); predentin becomes calcified as cells deposit more dentin; predentin is adjacent to the pulp in young teeth
  3. Each cell process in mature calcified dentin is enclosed in a dentinal tubule (Fig. 2-21)
    a. Dentinal tubules can run from the dentoenamel junction to the periphery of the dental pulp, where cell bodies of odontoblasts are located
    b. Tubules follow a primary S-shaped curve (pathway) and secondary S-shaped curves along the length of the tubules
      (1) Primary S-shaped curves are caused by movement of odontoblasts from a wider area to a narrower area, which produces crowding of the odontoblasts; S-shaped curved movement is how odontoblasts adjust to the new crowding while moving back toward the dental pulp

      (2) Secondary S-shaped curves are seen along the length of the dentinal tubule as small waves in the tubules, about 4 μm apart; may possibly be reflecting changes in the movement of the odontoblasts during the night and day
    c. Tubules tend to have more branching at their terminal ends in the crown of the tooth than in the root dentin; root dentin has more lateral branching, with fewer primary S-shaped curves
    d. Higher tubular density in the peripheral dentin makes teeth particularly sensitive when exposed; almost as sensitive as the dentin near the pulp
    e. Diameter of tubules changes during the process of dentin formation; widest dentinal tubules are found in children and are about 4 μm wide
  4. First layer of dentin immediately adjacent to the dentoenamel junction (DEJ) is called mantle dentin; remainder of the deposited dentin is called circumpupal dentin (around the pulp)
    a. Mantle dentin
      (1) Layer of dentin about 10 to 30 μm thick
      (2) Differs from circumpulpal dentin because in addition to collagen fibers normally found in dentin, it contains a second group of thicker and heavier collagen fibers
        (a) These fibers are deposited perpendicular to the dentoenamel junction
        (b) Are referred to as von Korff's fibers
      (3) Is less calcified than circumpulpal dentin
    b. Circumpulpal dentin
      (1) Contains finer collagen fibers than mantle dentin
      (2) Fibers are deposited parallel to the dentoenamel junction
  5. Dentin that forms immediately around the odontoblastic process is called *peritubular dentin*
    a. Forms a sheath around each odontoblastic process about 1 μm thick
    b. Consists of a matrix of delicate collagen fibers
    c. Is highly calcified
    d. First dentin to be decalcified by the bacterial enzymes when exposed to caries is the peritubular dentin
  6. Remainder of dentin is called *intertubular dentin*
    a. Consists of large, coarse collagen fibers
    b. Matrix is less calcified than that of the peritubular dentin
    c. Produced first by the odontoblast; then the odontoblast produces its peritubular dentin

7. Once the dentin is deposited, it does not undergo any remodeling

C. Types
1. Primary dentin—refers to dentin deposited *before* completion of the apical foramen
2. Secondary dentin—refers to dentin formed *after* completion of the apical foramen; tends to be more calcified than the primary dentin; forms at a slower rate
3. Reactive dentin—forms rapidly in localized areas where dental tubules have been exposed to external traumas such as
   a. Caries preparation
   b. Attrition or bruxism (enamel has been worn away)
   c. Thermal water sprays
4. Sclerotic dentin occurs when the dentinal fibers have degenerated and the tubules become filled with calcium salts
5. Dead tracts are dentinal tubules that remain unfilled after dentinal fiber degeneration
6. Interglobular dentin—small areas of unmineralized dentin near DEJ
7. Tome's granular layer is composed of small unmineralized areas of dentin beneath the cementum (may play role in root sensitivity)

D. Sensory conduction
1. Nerves associated with dentin are located in the dental pulp, but it is believed that they monitor changes in the environment of odontoblasts, which allows for perceptions of pain
2. When dentinal tubules become exposed to the outside environment, a direct contact is made with pulp; fluid in open, exposed tubules begins to evaporate, and the movement of fluid caused by evaporation may stimulate nerves nearest odontoblasts to produce pain (dentinal hypersensitivity)

Pulp Tissue

A. Structure
1. Most centrally located tissue in the tooth
2. Loose connective tissue
3. Cells
   a. Fibroblasts—undifferentiated mesenchymal cells
   b. Histiocytes—found along blood vessels; sometimes referred to as macrophages when filled with ingested materials
   c. Lymphocytes—when present, tend to be near the odontoblastic layer
   d. Cells present in diseased pulp include monocytes, polymorphonuclear leukocytes, eosinophils, and plasma cells
   e. No fat cells are present

4. Structural arrangement
   a. Outer periphery of the pulp gives rise to the odontoblastic cell layer
   b. Subjacent layer to the odontoblastic layer is called the cell-free zone or zone of Weil
   c. Next to the cell-free zone is a relatively cell-rich zone
   d. Core of the pulp is centrally located

B. Functions
1. Nutritive functions—very rich blood supply that forms a capillary plexus that surrounds the odontoblasts
2. Formative function—peripheral layer of pulp cells gives rise to the odontoblasts
3. Sensory function—naked nerve fibers travel as free nerve endings and make contact with odontoblasts
4. Protective function—pulp can respond to stimuli that occur outside of the tooth; response may trigger the formation of reactive dentin

C. Blood supply and nerves
1. Blood vessels enter pulp via the apical foramen; one or more small arterioles form a rich capillary plexus under the odontoblastic layer; exchange of nutrients occurs across the capillary wall
2. Two types of nerve fibers enter the pulp
   a. Autonomic nerve fibers—only the sympathetic autonomic nerve fibers are found; regulate the flow of blood in the vessels
   b. Afferent nerve fibers—come from the second and third branches of the trigeminal nerve; lose their myelin sheath and terminate as free nerve endings in close association with odontoblasts; the presence of *free nerve* endings is thought to be responsible for the perception of pain by the dental pulp

D. Pulp changes
1. Changes resulting from age
   a. As the tooth ages, there is an increase in the amount of collagen fibers and a decrease in the number of reticulin fibers; ground substance loses considerable water
   b. Pulp becomes less cellular and more fibrous
   c. Size of the pulp decreases because of the continued deposition of dentin
2. Small calcified bodies called denticles may be present
   a. Three types of denticles
      (1) True denticles—form during tooth development in the root; have dentinal tubules present in their structure; odontoblasts are present on their periphery
      (2) False denticles—form when components of the pulp start to degenerate; calcify and grow

into irregular calcified bodies; dentinal tubules are not usually present

(3) Diffuse calcifications—occur in sick pulps in many locations; are likely to grow and cause problems

b. Both true and false denticles may be loose in the dental pulp, attached to the dentin wall, or embedded in the dentin tissue

c. Calcified structures in pulp appear radiopaque on radiographs

Comparison of Pulp and Dentin

A. Dentin and pulp are closely related functionally and developmentally; both are products of the dental papilla (derived from neural crest cells)

B. Two major differences between the tissues
1. Pulp is a loose, noncalcified connective tissue; dentin is a highly specialized calcified connective tissue
2. Pulp is a very vascular tissue; dentin is avascular

C. Dentin and pulp form the bulk of the fully developed tooth

D. During tooth development the peripheral cells of the dental papilla differentiate into odontoblasts and form dentin, while the core of the dental papilla becomes the pulp

Enamel

A. Composition
1. Most highly calcified of the dental tissues
2. Composed mainly of inorganic calcium salt, hydroxyapatite, with a small amount of protein material and water in the matrix
   a. Inorganic component, 95%
   b. Organic component, 1%
   c. Water, 4%

B. Process of amelogenesis
1. Enamel formation, like dentin formation, begins in the late bell stage of tooth development
2. Shortly after the deposition of dentin, the inner enamel epithelial cells of enamel organ become secretory ameloblasts
   a. Begin to deposit enamel matrix, which is mineralized almost immediately
   b. Have tall columnar cell bodies that are hexagonal in cross section
   c. Secretory process is shovel shaped and called Tomes' process; shape of the process is closely related to the form of the structural units that make up the fully developed enamel tissue
3. Ameloblasts pass through two main stages while depositing enamel
   a. Secretory stage—ameloblasts deposit enamel matrix, which contains both organic and inorganic components

b. Resorbing stage—ameloblasts remove most of the water and organic components from the matrix

4. Enamel maturation begins before completion of enamel formation
   a. First, hydroxyapatite crystals deposited in matrix are very thin and needlelike
   b. During process of enamel maturation, crystals increase in all dimensions, which is made possible by continual removal of water and organic components from the matrix
   c. Hydroxyapatite crystals in enamel are four times larger than those in bone, dentin, and cementum

C. Enamel rods—structural units of enamel
1. Enamel is composed of tightly packed masses of hydroxyapatite crystals called enamel rods or prisms
2. Rod formation is related to the shape of Tomes' process and orientation of crystals as they are deposited by ameloblasts
3. Are rod-shaped structures that run from the dentoenamel junction to the outer edge of the enamel surface
4. Are stacked in interlocking rows, one row on top of the other; stacking arrangement causes rods to appear as keyhole shaped prisms when viewed in cross section, with the top of the keyhole facing the occlusal or incisal edge of the tooth and the tail facing the cervical portion; four ameloblasts contribute to form one keyhole (Fig. 2-22)
5. Average width of an enamel rod is approximately 4 μm; rods are narrower near the dentoenamel junction and wider near the outer surface of the enamel
6. Crystals in the rod head region are oriented with their long axis parallel to the long axis of the rod; in the tail region crystals are perpendicular to the long axis of the rod
7. Adjacent rods are separated from each other by a rod sheath approximately 0.1 to 2.0 μm wide; can be observed in the head region of the rod but are not so clearly defined in the tail region; are produced by an abrupt change in angulation (orientation) of the crystals as they are deposited by the moving ameloblast (Fig. 2-23)
8. Rodless enamel may be found near the dentoenamel junction and outer surface of enamel
9. Are perpendicular to the outer surface of enamel; near the cervix of the tooth they tend to be oriented apically; toward the inner third of the enamel, groups of rods curve but then straighten out to form right angles with the enamel surface

D. Microscopic structures
1. Bands of Hunter-Schreger—alternating light and

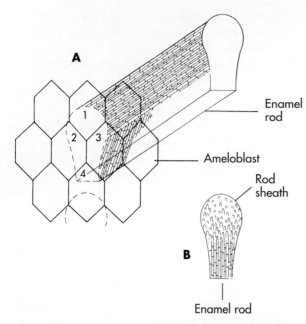

Fig. 2-22 Formation of enamel rod. **A,** Cross-sectional, hexagonal outline of ameloblast is superimposed over cross-sectional, keyhole outline of enamel rod; note that it takes four ameloblasts to form one enamel rod. **B,** Outline of rod with rod sheath surrounding rod head. (Modified from Salentijn-Moss L, Klyvert M: *Dental and oral tissues; an introduction for paraprofessionals in dentistry,* ed 3, Philadelphia, 1990, Lea & Febiger.)

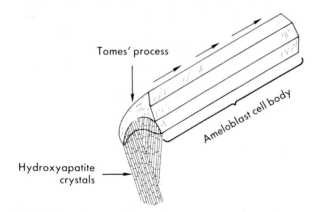

Fig. 2-23 Ameloblast depositing hydroxyapatite crystals from Tomes' process; note angular change in orientation of crystals being deposited, which accounts for rod sheath around head of rod.

    dark bands; perpendicular to the DEJ; manifest result of enamel rod curvature
2. Stripes of Retzius—narrow brown lines, extend diagonally from enamel rods, on tooth surface end in shallow furrows known as perikymata
3. Enamel lamellae—cracks occurring during enamel crystallization

4. Enamel tufts—hypomineralized inner ends of some enamel rods; DEJ area
5. Enamel spindles—terminal portions of dentinal fibers that extend across DEJ into the enamel

E. Clinical importance
  1. Dental procedures performed on enamel
    a. Application of fluoride—because enamel is semipermeable, fluoride ions are absorbed on the hydroxyapatite crystals; tooth becomes more resistant to bacteria-produced acids
    b. Acid etching of enamel—structure of enamel (rods and rod sheaths) allows acid to penetrate enamel for a limited distance (30 μm) and attacks the mineral at the periphery of the sheaths; leaves a rough enamel surface so bonding materials adhere more readily; acid may attack the rod core and produce the same effect
    c. Cavity preparations—all rods are supported by dentin; margins of cavity will fail if enamel is left unsupported
  2. Tetracycline stains
    a. Appear clinically as dark bands through the enamel, especially near the cervix of the tooth where enamel is thin
    b. Caused by the administration of tetracycline (antibiotic) while teeth were forming
    c. Tetracycline binds chemically to organic and inorganic components of bone and dentin
    d. Resulting darkened area shows through enamel with fully developed tooth becoming aesthetically unattractive
    e. Are difficult to bleach out; affected teeth may need crowns for aesthetic purposes only
  3. Pits and fissures in enamel
    a. Are often less-calcified areas
    b. Form where ameloblasts become crowded between adjacent areas (cusps), causing incomplete maturation of enamel

Cementum

A. General properties and functions
  1. Calcified connective tissue that covers the roots of the teeth; in conjunction with the alveolar bone proper and the periodonal ligament forms the attachment apparatus of the teeth, allowing the teeth to become suspended in the jaw
  2. Derived from the dental sac (dental follicle)
  3. Resembles bone in structure and composition; major differences are
    a. Bone is a vascularized tissue
    b. Cementum is avascular
  4. Least mineralized of the calcified tissues of the tooth
B. Mature cementum composition

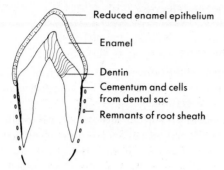

Fig. 2-24 Relationship of epithelial root sheath to the forming root and formation of cementum.

1. Chemical composition
   a. Organic components, 23%
   b. Inorganic components, 65%
   c. Water, 12%
2. Tissue composition
   a. Cells—cementoblasts, cementocytes
   b. Fibrous matrix—collagen fibers (type I); dominant component of the tissue, 90%
   c. Ground substance—proteoglycans
C. Process of cementogenesis (Fig. 2-24)
   1. After crown formation is complete, the epithelial root sheath (Hertwig's root sheath) begins to grow down
      a. Shapes the root of the tooth
      b. Induces formation of root dentin
   2. After the first root dentin is deposited, the root sheath breaks down; cells from the dental sac migrate onto newly deposited dentin; differentiate into cementoblasts
D. Mature cementum (fibrous matrix)
   1. Very little cementum is deposited on the developing root until the tooth reaches functional occlusion (only about two thirds of the root has been formed when the tooth erupts)
   2. Two groups of fibers found in cementum
      a. Group I
         (1) Collagen fibers produced by the cementoblasts
         (2) Form in the fibrous component of cementum
         (3) Run parallel to the long axis of the root (internal fibers)
      b. Group II
         (1) Fibers produced by cells from the dental sac
         (2) Form fibers of the periodontal ligament (external fibers)
         (3) Insert into cementum at right angles to the dentoenamel junction or at right angles to the internal fibers of cementum

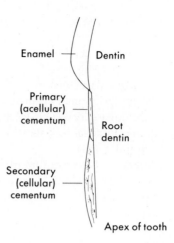

Fig. 2-25 Relationship of primary acellular cementum to secondary (cellular) cementum or root of tooth; note thickness of cellular cementum near tooth apex.

   3. Group II fibers (external fibers) are coarser than internal fibers; cores of fibers remain uncalcified in the calcified cementum; referred to as Sharpey's fibers
E. Cellular and acellular cementum (Fig. 2-25)
   1. Acellular cementum
      a. Cervical half of the tooth is covered with a thin layer of cementum, approximately 10 μm thick
      b. Does not contain any embedded cementocytes (cementoblasts) in the lacunae
      c. Forms at a slower rate than cellular cementum
      d. Does not increase during the life of the tooth
      e. Appears to be involved more in maintenance of the tissue than in production
      f. Contains less inorganic matrix than cellular cementum
      g. Better calcified than cellular cementum
   2. Cellular cementum
      a. Apical portion of the tooth is covered with cellular cementum reaching a thickness of 100 to 150 μm
      b. Contains cementocytes trapped in the lacunae of the tissue
      c. Deposited throughout the life of the tooth
      d. Deposited at intervals (pauses), producing arrest lines—highly calcified lines similar to those seen in bone tissue
F. Abnormalities
   1. Reversal lines
      a. May be present in cementum as in bone tissue
      b. Reflect resorption of the tissue (remodeling)
      c. Resorption of cementum does not occur as frequently as in bone tissue; when it does occur, is usually associated with

(1) Extreme orthodontic movement of the teeth

(2) Trauma to the teeth

2. Cementicles

a. Small abnormal calcified bodies occasionally found in the periodontal ligament

b. Result of cellular debris (i.e., degenerating remnants of the epithelial root sheath)

c. May be found

(1) Attached to the cementum surface

(2) Free in the periodontal ligament

(3) Embedded in the cementum of the root

3. Hypercementosis

a. Local abnormal thickening of parts of the cementum

b. Usually found in the apical region, occurring on one or all of the teeth

c. May be seen in cases of

(1) Chronic inflammation of the tooth

(2) Loss of an antagonist tooth (no opposing tooth in the jaw)

(3) Additional eruption; compensatory cementosis takes place

(4) Tooth may become fused to surrounding alveolar bone proper

Cementoenamel Junction

A. Three types of cementoenamel relationships can occur during the development of the tooth

1. Cementum *meets* the enamel edge to edge—occurs in approximately 30% of all teeth

2. Cementum *overlaps* a small part of the enamel—occurs in approximately 60% of all teeth

3. Cementum and enamel *do not meet* and expose dentin—occurs in approximately 10% of all teeth

B. Cementoenamel relationships occur when root-cementum development begins; related to the timing of the disruption (breakdown) of the epithelial root sheath; allow cells from the dental sac to differentiate and begin depositing cementum

C. Differentiation of root dental papilla into odontoblasts is mediated by a cell-to-matrix type of inductive interaction (between the basal lamina of Hertwig's root sheath and undifferentiated root dental papilla)

D. Differentiation of dental sac cells into cementoblasts is mediated by a cell-substrate type of inductive interaction between sac cells and newly deposited dentin

E. Practicing dental hygienists should use caution during instrumentation in areas where cementum is thin or absent

F. Recession of gingiva may also leave exposed cementum or dentin and create root sensitivity or root caries

Supporting Tissues

Alveolar Bone

A. That part of the bony maxilla and mandible, the alveolar process, in which teeth are suspended in alveoli (bony sockets)

B. Existence or presence of alveolar bone is totally dependent on the presence of dental roots; when teeth do not develop and erupt, alveolar bone will not develop; when teeth are extracted, alveolar bone resorbs

C. Formed during development and eruption of teeth; developing teeth, primary or permanent, are located in bony crypts in bone of the maxilla or mandible

D. Has the same biophysical and chemical properties as other bone tissue in the body; has the same basic components as other connective tissues

1. Cells—osteoblasts, osteocytes, osteoclasts

2. Fibrous matrix—collagen fibers dominant component; calcified by deposition of calcium salt, hydroxyapatite, into the matrix

3. Ground substance—proteoglycans

E. Gross anatomy of a mature bone socket

1. Each tooth is suspended in its own alveolus (socket), with each alveolus having the same structure and anatomy (Fig. 2-26)

a. Outer cortical (compact lamellar) plate bone—faces the cheek and lips (buccal)

b. Inner cortical (compact lamellar) plate of bone—faces the tongue and palate (lingual)

c. Spongiosa—cancellous bone sandwiched between cortical plates of bone

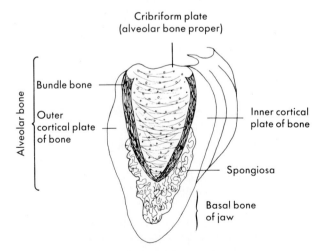

Fig. 2-26 Components of alveolar bone proper. (Modified from Schroeder HE: *Oral structural biology: embryology, structure, and function of normal hard and soft tissues of the oral cavity and temporomandibular joints,* Stuttgart, 1991, Georg Thieme Verlag.)

2. Alveolar bone proper—that part of the alveolus directly facing the root of the tooth; follows the general outline of the root; sometimes referred to as the cribriform plate or lamina dura
   a. Cribiform plate
      (1) Contains numerous small openings; allows blood vessels and nerves in the periodontal ligament and bone to communicate
      (2) Consists of two layers of bone
         (a) Compact lamellar bone
         (b) Layer of bundle bone into which the periodontal fibers insert; cores of the fibers remain uncalcified in the calcified tissues of bone or cementum—called Sharpey's fibers
   b. *Lamina dura* is purely a radiographic term based on the fact that this area appears more radiopaque on radiographs; is not more calcified than the rest of the bone socket; rather, opaqueness is caused by geometry in the area
   c. Alveolar bone proper that forms sockets around multirooted teeth consists of the cribriform plates of both roots and some spongy bone, called interradicular alveolar bone
   d. Alveolar bone proper between teeth consists of the cribriform plates of both teeth and some spongy bone, called interdental alveolar bone
   e. Spongiosa is composed of small trabeculae of bone with large narrow spaces between the trabeculae
3. Alveolar bone proper/cribriform plate is the only essential part of the bone socket; spongiosa and outer and inner cortical plates of bone are not always present; spongiosa may be absent, and outer and inner cortical plates may be fused together
4. Trabeculae of the spongiosa reflect functional forces or loading patterns imposed on teeth; pattern will change when forces are altered; two principal directions of the trabeculae are parallel and perpendicular to the direction of the imposed forces; trabecular bone orientation can be observed on radiographs; the number of trabeculae increases with increased function
5. Orthodontic movement of teeth always causes remodeling of the alveolar bone proper to accommodate movement of the teeth; affects the insertion of periodontal ligament fibers in the bundle bone, but is a localized type of resorption; when the bundle bone is redeposited, fibers become firmly attached again; with pressure bone is resorbed; when tension is applied there is bone formation

6. Radiographs of teeth may be used to show the height and/or slope of the interdental bone septum, which may reflect periodontal or other disease

Periodontal Ligament

A. Specialized form of connective tissue derived from the dental sac that contributes to attachment of the tooth
B. Made up of groups of fiber bundles called gingival fibers and principal fiber bundles; between the principal fiber bundles are areas of loose connective tissue, blood vessels, and nerves; areas of loose connective tissue are called interstitial spaces
C. Tissue components
   1. Fibroblasts of the periodontal ligament (PDL) are responsible for production of fibrous matrix and ground substance; are continually engaged in synthetic activities rebuilding and producing new fibers to be incorporated into existing fibers, which are constantly being remodeled; PDL has a very fast turnover rate
   2. Ground substance—proteoglycans
   3. Fibrous matrix is dominant component of the PDL
      a. Fibers are collagen and oxytalan with a few elastic fibers associated with blood vessels
      b. Fibers are arranged in dense bundles inserted into the alveolar bone proper and the cementum
      c. Fibers are arranged into two groups
         (1) Gingival fiber groups (Figs. 2-27 and 2-28; see also Chapter 11, Fig. 11-2)
            (a) Dentogingival fibers extend from the cervical cementum to the free gingiva and from the cervical cementum to the lamina propria of the gingiva, over the alveolar crest

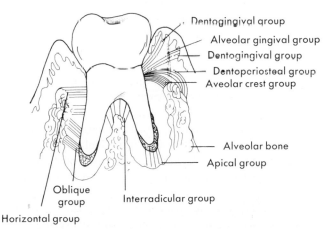

Fig. 2-27 Connective tissue fibers of gingiva and principal fiber groups of periodontal ligament (transseptal and circular fibers shown in Fig. 2-28; see also Figs. 11-2 and 11-3).

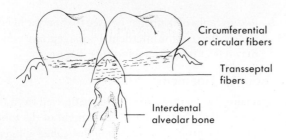

Fig. 2-28 Transseptal fibers are shown between two teeth passing over alveolar crest; circumferential fibers are around teeth within free gingiva.

(b) Dentoperiosteal fibers—extend from the cervical cementum over the alveolar crest to the periosteum of the cortical plates of bone

(c) Transseptal fibers—extend from the cementum of the tooth to the adjacent tooth, over the alveolar crest

(d) Circumferential fibers—extend horizontally around the most cervical part of the root and insert into the cementum and lamina propria of the gingiva and the alveolar crest

(2) Principal fiber groups (Fig. 2-27; see also Chapter 11, Fig. 11-3)

(a) Alveolar crest fibers—extend from the cervical cementum and insert into the alveolar crest

(b) Horizontal fibers—extend at right angles to the long axis of the root of the tooth in a horizontal plane from the alveolar bone to the cementum; found in the cervical third of the root

(c) Oblique fibers—slant occlusally from the cementum to the alveolar bone; most abundant of the fiber bundles; start at the apical two thirds of the root

(d) Apical fibers—radiate from the apical cementum into the alveolar bone

(e) Interradicular fibers (seen only in multirooted teeth)—extend from the cementum in the furcation area of the tooth to the interradicular alveolar bone

d. Sharpey's fibers—the terminal portion of a PDL fiber that is embedded in bone and cementum

e. Fiber groups are oriented to give the tooth optimal resistance to all kinds of functional loading patterns

(1) Circumferential fibers resist rotational movements of the tooth (Fig. 2-28)

(2) Alveolar crest and apical fibers resist pull of the tooth from its socket

(3) Transseptal fibers connect all teeth and maintain integrity of the dental arches

f. Elastic fibers in the PDL do not contribute to support of the tooth; role of the oxytalan fibers is not clear

D. Blood vessels

1. Blood supply of the PDL is very rich and highly developed, more than in any other connective tissues; vessels are found in the interstitial spaces of the ligament

2. Each tooth, with its PDL and alveolar bone, has a common blood supply; a small artery will branch off of the main artery that supplies the jaw and enter

a. Apical foramen of the tooth—supplies pulp of the tooth

b. Periodontal ligament—supplies areas all around the tooth

c. Alveolar bone of the tooth

3. Once blood vessels enter pulp chambers, they are isolated from surrounding tissues, but vessels supplying the PDL and alveolar bone are richly interconnected via openings in the cribiform plate

E. Nerves

1. PDL contains two types of nerves

a. Autonomic—sympathetic fibers that travel with blood vessels; regulate flow of blood to the tissues

b. Afferent sensory fibers—mostly myelinated nerves from branches of the second and third divisions of the trigeminal nerve (cranial nerve V)

2. Two types of nerve endings are found in the PDL

a. Free, unmyelinated nerve endings—responsible for pain sensation

b. Encapsulated nerve endings—responsible for registering pressure changes

F. Width of the PDL varies with functional forces placed on the tooth and at different levels of the root (apex and cervix)

1. Width is greater in young adults (0.21 mm) than in older adults (0.15 mm)

2. Width is greater near cervical and apical areas than in the middle of the root

3. Minimal movements (rotations) of any tooth occur around the axis in the middle of the root; greatest movements occur near the apex and cervix, accounting for difference in width of the PDL along the root

4. Width is related to the amount of function; actively functioning tooth will have a slightly wider PDL than a nonfunctioning tooth

G. Abnormalities

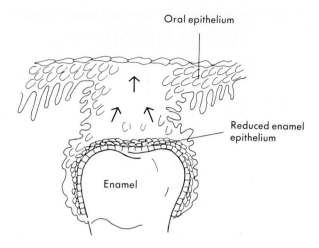

Fig. 2-29 Tooth emerging into oral cavity; note reduced enamel epithelium covering tooth and joining of oral epithelium and reduced enamel epithelium, which will form initial junctional epithelium.

1. Cementicles
2. Epithelial rests (cell rests of Malassez)
   a. Remnants of epithelium from the root sheath that did not disintegrate; formed from a cluster of epithelial cells surrounded by a basement membrane
   b. In most cases are harmless, but they have the potential to become cystic
3. Untreated periodontal disease can result in damage to the supporting apparatus of the tooth and cause eventual loss of the tooth

Dentogingival Junction

A. Area on the tooth where enamel and epithelium form a junction; with age, the junction is displaced more apically between cementum and epithelium
B. First established as the tooth emerges into the oral cavity (Fig. 2-29)
   1. Developing tooth is covered with reduced enamel epithelium (REE), consisting of
      a. Layer of outer enamel epithelial cells
      b. Remnants of the stratum intermedium cell layers
      c. Stellate reticulum
      d. Postsecretory ameloblasts
   2. Basal cells of oral epithelium covering the emerging tooth and outer layer of cells of the REE begin to proliferate; soon grow together and form one continuous unit; as tooth emerges through the combined epithelia, it forms the initial dentogingival junction on the enamel of the tooth
C. Dentojunctional epithelium
   1. Gingival epithelium that faces the tooth

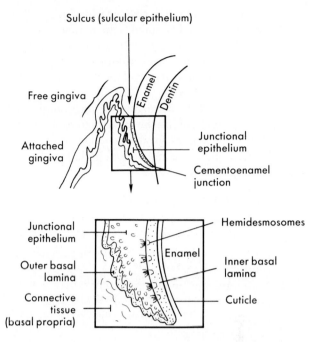

Fig. 2-30 Junctional epithelium and its relationship to clinical and histologic structures; note enlarged section of junctional epithelium showing outer and inner basal lamina that is continuous around junctional epithelium and cuticle that is seen intervening between junctional epithelium and tooth surface.

2. Composed of nonkeratinized stratified squamous epithelium and divided into
   a. Sulcular epithelium
      (1) Found occlusally at the same height as the free gingiva
      (2) Sulcus forms a shallow pocket around the tooth, about 0.5 mm deep
   b. Junctional epithelium
      (1) Begins at the base of the sulcus
      (2) Is firmly attached to the tooth, enamel, and/or cementum by hemidesmosomes
      (3) Located between two basal laminae
         (a) One basal lamina faces the enamel surface
         (b) Second basal lamina faces the connective tissue of the gingiva
         (c) Basal laminae are continuous at the base of the junctional epithelium (Fig. 2-30)
3. A membrane intervenes between the basal lamina of the junctional epithelium and tooth surface, called the primary cuticle
   a. Formed during the late states of eruption of the tooth
   b. Composition of the cuticle is not known but thickens with age

4. Newly erupted tooth is covered with a thin, delicate membrane called Nasmyth's membrane
   a. Will float off of the tooth surface if placed in a 10% solution of hydrochloric acid
   b. Contains some of cells of the REE and the dental cuticle
5. In the area of the dentogingival junction the junctional epithelium has the capacity to repair itself
6. Site of the dentogingival junction is easily invaded by microorganisms and is where periodontal disease often begins

Gingiva—Masticatory Oral Mucosa

A. Histologic structure
   1. Keratinized stratified squamous epithelium; rete pegs—projections of epithelium into underlying connective tissue
   2. No submucosa; no salivary glands
   3. Fibrous connective tissue; gingival fibers (pp. 47-48) (Figs. 2-27 and 2-28; see also Chapter 11, Fig. 11-2)
B. Clinical appearance
   1. Color—coral pink; influenced by vascularity and pigmentation cells
   2. Texture—stippled result of rete peg arrangement
   3. Consistency—firm because of fibrous underlying tissue

SUGGESTED READINGS

Avery JK: *Essentials of oral histology: a clinical approach,* St. Louis, 1992, Mosby.

Bath-Balogh M, Fehrenbach MJ: *Dental embryology, histology and anatomy,* Philadelphia, 1987, WB Saunders.

Brand RW, Isselhard DE: *Anatomy of orofacial structures,* St. Louis, 1993, Mosby.

Ibsen OA, Phelan JA: *Oral pathology for the dental hygienist,* ed 2, Philadelphia, 1996, WB Saunders.

Melfi RC: *Permar's oral embryology and microscopic anatomy,* ed 9, Philadelphia, 1994, Lea & Febiger.

Neville BW, Douglas DD, Allen CM, Bouquot JC: *Oral and maxillofacial pathology,* Philadelphia, 1995, WB Saunders.

Perry DA, Beemsterboer PL, Taggart EJ: *Periodontology for the dental hygienist,* Philadelphia, 1996, WB Saunders.

Ten Cate AR: *Oral histology: development, structure, and function,* ed 4, St. Louis, 1994, Mosby.

Trowbridge HO, Emling RC: *Inflammation: a review of the process,* ed 4, Chicago, 1993, Quintessence.

Review Questions

1 The cellular organelle that contains digestive enzymes is the:
   A. Mitochondria
   B. Ribosome
   C. Chromosome
   D. Lysosome
   E. Centriole

2 The medium that carries nutrients and waste materials between the tissue and the capillaries is the:
   A. Formed elements
   B. Ground substance
   C. Tissue fluid
   D. Endoplasmic reticulum
   E. Cytoplasm

3 An attached plaque between a cell and noncellular surface is called a
   A. Desmosome
   B. Hemidesmosome
   C. Tight junction
   D. Gap junction

4 The tissue component that is derived from the blood is the
   A. Cells
   B. Fibrous intercellular substance
   C. Amorphous intercellular substance
   D. Tissue fluid

5 The blood supply of the periodontal ligament and the alveolar bone proper anastomose and communicate because of the
   A. Compact structure of the alveolar bone proper
   B. Structure of the cribriform plate of the alveolar bone proper
   C. Lamina dura of the alveolar bone proper
   D. Bundle bone of the alveolar bone proper
   E. Arrangement of Sharpey's fibers in the alveolar bone proper

6 The embryonic origin of all connective tissue is:
   A. Mesenchyme
   B. Endoderm
   C. Fascia
   D. Ectoderm
   E. Epithelium

7 Cells that devour debris within connective tissue of a client with periodontitis are called
   A. Lysosomes
   B. Melanocytes
   C. Fibroblasts
   D. Macrophages
   E. Mast cells

8 With the exception of the _____, the oral and nasal cavities develop from the first branchial arch and the frontal process.
   A. Lower lip
   B. Lower border of the cheeks
   C. Anterior portion of the hard palate
   D. Base of the tongue
   E. Base of the nasal septum

9 Rathke's pouch is the embryonic origin of the
A. Thyroid gland
B. Globular process
C. Palate
D. Pituitary gland
E. Nasal septum

10 The lateral palatine process initially grows downward toward the future floor of the mouth. It does not grow medially at this time of initial development because of the presence of the
A. Nasal septum
B. Maxillary process
C. Premaxilla
D. Tongue
E. Mandibular process

11 An infant born without a primary palate is presented for consultation. What teeth will never be present, even after a surgical repair of the existing condition?
A. Both the primary and the permanent incisors in the maxilla
B. Both the first primary and the permanent premolars in the maxilla
C. Both 6-year molars in the maxilla
D. Both the primary and the permanent canines in the maxilla
E. Only the primary incisors in the maxilla

12 The buccopharyngeal membrane is composed of:
A. Mesoderm and endoderm
B. Ectoderm and mesoderm
C. Ectoderm, mesoderm, and endoderm
D. Ectoderm and endoderm

13 In the area of the foramen cecum, epithelium invaginates deep into the tissues and will eventually become the
A. Pituitary gland
B. Lingual salivary gland
C. Submandibular salivary gland
D. Trachea
E. Thyroid gland

14 What anatomic feature separates the root and the body of the tongue?
A. The lingual frenum
B. The fungiform papillae
C. The median groove
D. The third branchial arch
E. The circumvallate papillae

15 The olfactory (nasal) pits appear on the lateral sides of the
A. Maxillary process
B. Olfactory process
C. Mandibular process
D. Frontal process
E. Globular process

16 During palatal fusion, epithelial cells may become entrapped in the line of fusion. These cells may later contribute to the formation of
A. Teeth
B. Cleft lips
C. A cleft palate
D. Cysts
E. Ectopic teeth

17 The earliest signs of development of the human face occurs during the third week in utero with the formation of the
A. Stomodeum
B. Maxillary process
C. Olfactory pits
D. Globular process

18 A cleft lip occurs when the maxillary process fails to fuse with the
A. Palatine process
B. Globular process
C. Lateral nasal process
D. Mandibular process
E. Opposing maxillary process

19 The three types of muscle tissue are:
A. Skeletal, smooth, and striated voluntary
B. Cardiac, striated involuntary, and smooth
C. Nonstriated involuntary, cardiac, and skeletal
D. Striated involuntary, smooth, and cardiac

20 The site of muscle contraction is called
A. Sarcomere
B. Sarcolemma
C. Actin
D. Myosin
E. Z line

21 The part of the neuron that conducts impulses toward the cell body is called the
A. Dendrite
B. Axon
C. Neurilemma
D. Myelin sheath
E. Neuroglia

22 Dentin, cementum, and pulp are derived from
A. Ectoderm
B. Mesoderm
C. Endoderm
D. Epithelium
E. Endothelium

23 In what area of enamel is rodless enamel most often found?
A. At the base of pits and fissures
B. In the outermost enamel
C. In the central region of enamel

24 The relationship between enamel and cementum at the CEJ that cannot occur is
A. Enamel overlaps cementum
B. Enamel and cementum just meet
C. Enamel and cementum do not meet
D. Cementum overlaps enamel

25 Which of the following microscopic structures show evidence of the curvature of the enamel rods?
A. Bands of Hunter-Schreger
B. Stripes of Retzius
C. Enamel lamellae
D. Enamel tufts
E. Enamel spindles

26 In a person born without teeth, what part of the bone of the maxilla and the mandible would be absent?
   A. The cribriform plate of the alveolar bone proper
   B. The alveolar bone
   C. The basal bone of the maxilla and the mandible
   D. The bundle bone of the alveolar bone proper
   E. The interradicular bone of the alveolar process

27 The reduced enamel epithelium will ultimately produce all of the following except
   A. Junctional epithelium
   B. Hertwig's epithelial root sheath
   C. Primary enamel cuticle
   D. Secondary enamel cuticle

28 Which statement *BEST* describes the status of tooth enamel?
   A. Calcium is lost from enamel during pregnancy.
   B. Calcium is withdrawn during periods of malnutrition.
   C. Low blood calcium causes demineralization.
   D. Calcium loss is similar to that of bone.
   E. none of the above

29 The layer of dentin found adjacent to the pulp in young teeth is called
   A. Tome's granular layer
   B. Predentin
   C. Interglobular dentin
   D. Dead tracts
   E. Sclerotic dentin

30 The stippled texture of the gingiva may be attributed to
   A. Keratinization
   B. Rete pegs
   C. Presence of submucosa
   D. Optimal blood supply
   E. Pigmentation

31 The dentinal fibers that occupy the dentinal tubules are part of the
   A. Korff's fibers of the pulp
   B. Fibrillar dentin matrix
   C. Odontoblasts of the pulp
   D. Sclerotic dentin
   E. Interrod substance

32 Caries in the dentin of the tooth progresses through the
   A. Interglobular dentin
   B. Dentinal tubule
   C. Secondary dentin
   D. Predentin
   E. Sclerotic dentin

33 The outer, less calcified layer of cementum is called
   A. Cellular cementum
   B. Acellular cementum
   C. Cementoid
   D. Cementicles
   E. Sharpey's fibers

34 The connective tissue that underlies the epithelium of the gingiva is
   A. Reticular
   B. Elastic
   C. Fibrous
   D. Submucosa
   E. Oxytalan

35 The periodontal fibers that are located in the root furcation area are the
   A. Sensory fibers
   B. Apical fibers
   C. Septum fibers
   D. Interradicular fibers
   E. Transseptal fibers

36 The ends of the periodontal ligament fibers that are embedded in the cementum and bone are called
   A. Principal fibers
   B. Korff's fibers
   C. Sharpey's fibers
   D. Dentinal fibers
   E. Gingival fibers

37 Remnants of Hertwig's epithelial root sheath found in the periodontal ligament of a functional tooth are called:
   A. Enamel pearls
   B. Denticles
   C. Rests of Malassez
   D. Cementicles
   E. Intermediate plexus

38 Bone trabeculation increases as functional activity decreases; the periodontal ligament increases in width as functional activity decreases.
   A. The first statement is true; the second is false.
   B. The first statement is false; the second is true.
   C. Both statements are true.
   D. Both statements are false.

39 In the oral cavity, one way in which lining mucosa differs from masticatory mucosa is that
   A. Lining mucosa contains more muscle fibers
   B. Masticatory mucosa contains glands
   C. Lining mucosa has no submucosa
   D. Lining mucosa is not keratinized

40 The first permanent molar develops from
   A. Primary dental lamina
   B. Secondary dental lamina
   C. Enamel pearls

41 The first cell to reach an injured area is the
   A. Neutrophil
   B. Monocyte
   C. Macrophage
   D. Lymphocyte
   E. Plasma cell

42 The last visible layer in nonkeratinized stratified squamous epithelium is the
   A. Basal cell layer
   B. Prickle cell layer
   C. Granular layer
   D. Corneum layer

43 Dentin is the product of
   A. Dental lamina
   B. Dental organ
   C. Dental papilla
   D. Dental cuticle
   E. Dental sac

44 The cellular component that provides the internal support for the long odontoblastic processes is the
A. Microtubule
B. Microfilament
C. Tonofibrils
D. Cilia

45 The cellular organelle that provides the vast amount of energy required for the organic matrix deposition is the
A. Endoplasmic reticulum
B. Golgi complex
C. Nucleus
D. Mitochondria

46 The mandible and maxilla are formed through _____ bone formation
A. Endochondral
B. Circumferential
C. Intermembranous
D. Lamellar
E. Haversian

47 Bone and cementum are similar in all of the following aspects except for the presence of
A. Canaliculi
B. Approximately the same amount of inorganic components
C. Lacuna
D. Volkmann's canals

48 Fibrous cartilage is found in all of the following locations except
A. Intervertebral disk
B. Temporomandibular joint
C. Pubic symphysis
D. Epiglottis

49 What type of attachment is present between the epithelial cells and the basal lamina of the basement membrane?
A. Desmosome
B. Heimdesmosome
C. Tight junction
D. Gap junction

50 The color of the gingiva is influenced by:
A. Rete pegs
B. Pigment cells
C. Vascularity
D. 2 & 3
E. All of the above

Answers and Rationales

1. (D) The lysosome is a cellular organelle that contains digestive enzymes.
   (A) The mitochondria is responsible for cellular metabolism.
   (B) Ribosomes are the site of messenger RNA attachment and amino acid assembly.
   (C) Chromosomes store genetic information.
   (E) Centriole is involved in self-duplication and in the formation of cellular extensions.

2. (C) Tissue fluid carries nutrients to the intercellular substance and waste to the capillaries.
   (A) Formed elements are fibrous intercellular substances that function as a medium between cells.
   (B) Ground substance is an amorphous intercellular substance that functions as a medium between cells.
   (D) Endoplasmic reticulum functions in transportation within the cell.
   (E) Cytoplasm is the fluid medium within the cell.

3. (B) Hemidesmosome is the attachment plaque or cellular junction between a cell and the noncellular surface. This is the form of attachment in the area of the junctional epithelium.
   (A) Desmosome is a round attachment plaque between two cells.
   (C) Tight junction is an attachment plaque between two cells in which their membranes are fused.
   (D) Gap junction is an attachment plaque between two cells that contains a channel for free transport.

4. (D) Tissue fluid is blood plasma that diffuses through the capillary walls.
   (A) Cells are the basic building block of the human body.
   (B) Fibrous intercellular substance lies between cells and is derived from cells.
   (C) Amorphous intercellular substance lies between cells and is derived from cells

5. (B) The cribriform plate of the alveolar bone proper has minute small openings in it to allow for the passage of blood vessels, which communicate with the blood vessels in the periodontal ligament.
   (A) The compact bone of the alveolar bone proper does not have the morphology to permit the blood vessels to pass through and communicate with those in the periodontal ligament.
   (C) *Lamina dura* is a radiographic term used to describe an opaque line seen on radiographs outlining the alveolar bone proper.
   (D) The bundle bone proper is that part of the bone into which the periodontal ligament is inserted.
   (E) Sharpey's fibers are not related to the blood supply of the periodontal ligament or alveolar bone; they are uncalcified cores of the ligament found in cementum and alveolar bone.

6. (A) Mesenchyme is the middle embryonic layer from which all connective and muscle tissue is derived.
   (B) Endoderm is the inner embryonic layer from which the gastrointestinal tract and related glands are derived.
   (C) Fascia is composed of connective tissue.
   (D) Ectoderm is the outer embryonic layer from which epithelial and nervous tissue is derived.
   (E) Epithelium along with connective, nervous, and muscle tissue is one of the four basic types of tissue found in the human body. It is derived from ectoderm and it covers surfaces and cavities of the body and has secretory functions.

7. (C) Macrophages function in the removal of dead and dying cells and in the debridement of damaged tissue.
   (A) Lysosome is a cellular organelle that contains digestive enzymes.
   (B) Melanocyte is a pigment cell found in the epithelium.
   (C) Fibroblasts produce proteins such as collagen, elastin, and proteoglycans and function in wound repair.
   (E) Mast cells contain vesicles of heparin and histamine and are involved in inflammatory and immediate hypersensitivity reactions.

8. (D) The base of the tongue is derived from a swelling that develops from the inner aspect of the 2nd, 3rd, and 4th branchial arches.
   (A) (B) (C) (E) Lower lip, lower border of the cheeks, anterior portion of the hard palate, and the base of the nasal septum are all formed from derivatives of the first branchial arch.

9. (D) The pituitary gland develops from an invagination of stomadeal ectoderm known as Rathke's pouch.
   (A) The thyroid gland forms from an invagination of lingual epithelium in the area of the foramen ceacum.
   (B) The globular process is the down-growth of the median nasal process.
   (C) The palate develops from the fusion of the premaxillary and lateral palatine processes.
   (E) The nasal septum develops from the inner aspect of the median nasal process.

10. (D) When the tongue initially develops it extends upward and forward; as a result, the growing lateral palatine processes grow downward. Between 8 and 12 weeks the tongue drops down and the lateral palatine processes begin to grow medially and fuse.
    (A) The nasal septum develops from the inner aspect of the median nasal process; its inferior border will fuse with the formed palate.
    (B) The lateral palatine processes are derived from the maxillary processes
    (C) The premaxilla will fuse with the anterior border of the lateral palatine processes to form the palate.
    (E) The mandibular process is below the stomadeum and does not affect palatal development.

11. (A) Incisors develop in the primary palate; if the primary palate is absent, neither primary nor permanent incisors will ever be present.
    (B) Premolars would not be affected because they do not develop in the primary palate.
    (C) First permanent molars do not develop in the primary palate.
    (D) Primary and permanent canines do not develop in the primary palate.
    (E) Both the primary and the permanent incisors would be affected because the permanent incisors develop from the successional lamina.

12. (D) The buccopharyngeal membrane marks the separation of the stomadeum which is composed of ectoderm and the primitive foregut which is composed of ectoderm. There is no intervening mesoderm in this membrane.

13. (E) The lingual epithelial tissue invaginates in the area of the foramen ceacum to form the thyroid gland.
    (A) The pituitary gland develops from an investigation of stomadeal ectoderm known as Rathke's pouch.
    (B) (C) The lingual and submandibular glands form in the sublingual area.
    (D) The trachea forms in the area below the larynx.

14. (E) The circumvalate papillae are at the boundary of the base of the tongue and the body of the tongue.
    (A) The lingual frenum is the sublingual soft tissue attachment.
    (B) The fungiform papillae are the mushroom shaped papillae that cover the dorsum of the tongue.
    (C) The median groove runs anterior to posterior in the middle of the dorsal tongue surface.
    (D) The 2nd, 3rd, and part of the 4th branchial arch form the base of the tongue.

15. (D) The olfactory pits appear on the lateral sides of the lower border of the frontal process. With the appearance of the nasal pits, this area is then separated into the median, and left and right lateral nasal processes.
    (A) The maxillary processes develop from two buds that grow from the 1st branchial arch. They grow medially to form sides of the cheeks.
    (B) There is no olfactory process, the lower border of the frontal process is usually referred to as nasal processes once the pits appear.
    (C) The mandibular process is below the stomadeum.
    (E) The globular process is the down-growth of the median nasal process.

16. (D) Epithelial rest cells that become entrapped in the lines of fusion are the source of cyst formation. They do not play a role in cleft or tooth formation.

17. (A) The stomadeum marks the earliest sign of human face development around 3 weeks in utero.

18. (B) The maxillary processes grow medially and fuse with the globular process to form the upper lip. A cleft lip can occur on one side or both sides of the globular process.
    (A) The maxillary processes' inner aspects give rise to the lateral palatine processes. The palatine processes (palatine shelves) form the inferior aspects of the bilateral maxillary processes.
    (C) The lateral nasal process forms the sides of the nose.
    (D) Failure of the maxillary process to fuse with the mandibular process results in macrostomia (large mouth).
    (E) The maxillary processes grow medially and fuse with the globular process to form the upper lip.

19. (C) The three types of muscle tissue are skeletal (voluntary striated), cardiac (striated involuntary), and smooth (nonstriated involuntary).

20. (A) The site of a muscle contraction is called a sarcomere. It is the segment of the myofibril that is found between the two Z lines.
    (B) Sarcolemma is the cell membrane of the muscle fiber.
    (C) (D) Actin and myosin are myofilaments present in the muscle fiber.
    (E) Z line is the line that bisects the I Band.

21. (A) The dendrite conducts impulses toward the cell body.
    (B) The axon conducts the impulse away from the cell body.
    (C) The neurilemma is a continuous sheath that encloses the segmented myelin sheath of peripheral nerve fibers.
    (D) Myelin sheath is a fatty layer surrounding the axon of the nerve.
    (E) Neuroglia is the soft tissue that supports the central nervous system.

22. (B) Mesoderm gives rise to the dental papilla portion of the tooth germ from which the dentin and pulp are derived. The dental sac portion of the tooth germ is also derived from mesoderm; the dental sac gives rise to the periodontal ligament which produces the cementum and alveolar bone.
    (A) (D) Epithelium and enamel are derived from ectoderm.
    (C) (E) The teeth are not derived from the endodermal layer or its derivatives.

23. (B) Rodless enamel is most often found around the DEJ, in the outermost surface of most primary teeth, and the outermost surface of the gingival one third of permanent teeth.

24. (A) Enamel forms before cementum so that it is not possible for it to overlap cementum.
    (B) Enamel and cementum just meet in approximately 30% of all teeth.
    (C) Enamel and cementum do not meet in 10% of all teeth.
    (D) Cementum overlaps a small part of enamel in approximately 60% of all teeth.

25. (A) The bands of Hunter-Schreger are the alternating light and dark bands that are perpendicular to the DEJ and extend to the tooth surface. They manifest the result of curvature of the enamel rods.
    (B) The Stripes of Retzius are narrow brown lines extending diagonally from the enamel rods.
    (C) Enamel lamellae are cracks occurring during enamel crystallization.
    (D) Enamel tufts are the small hypomineralized inner ends of some enamel rods that are found in the enamel near the DEJ.
    (E) Enamel spindles are the terminal portions of the cytoplasmic extensions of the odontoblasts (dentinal fibers) which extend across the DEJ into the enamel.

26. (B) Alveolar bone will develop in the oral cavity only if teeth develop and erupt into the mouth.
    (A) The cribriform plate could not be present because it is part of the alveolar bone proper.
    (C) Basal bone would be present because it is that part of the maxilla and mandible below the alveolar bone and is unrelated to tooth formation.
    (D) Bundle bone is part of the alveolar bone proper and would not be present; it houses Sharpey's fibers of the periodontal ligament.
    (E) The interradicular alveolar bone is that part of the alveolar bone located between the roots of multirooted teeth and would not be present.

27. (C) The primary enamel cuticle is formed by the ameloblasts. It is a calcified coating on the tooth surface.
    (A) The reduced enamel epithelium plays an important role in the attachment of the gingiva to the tooth as it erupts.
    (B) Hertwig's root sheath is formed by the joining of the outer and inner enamel epithelium. It moves downward and plays a role in root formation.
    (D) The secondary enamel cuticle is formed by the reduced enamel epithelium. It is an uncalcified coating on the crown surface.

28. (E) Once enamel is formed the mineral substance cannot be physiologically withdrawn from the tooth.

29. (B) Predentin is found adjacent to the pulp. It is actually the organic matrix which has not yet mineralized.
    (A) Tome's granular layer is the unmineralized areas of dentin found beneath the cementum.
    (C) Interglobular dentin is unmineralized dentin in the area near the DEJ.
    (D) Dead tracts are unfilled dentinal tubules, the dentinal fibers have degenerated and the tubules remain unfilled.
    (E) Sclerotic dentin occurs when the dentinal fibers have degenerated and the tubules become filled with calcium salts.

30. (B) The epithelial extensions (rete pegs) into the connective tissue and the connective tissue papilla, which extend into the epithelium enhance tissue strength and bring the blood supply to the epithelium. This corrugated arrangement at the histologic level creates the stippled appearance of the gingiva at the clinical level.
    (A) (D) (E) The keratinization, the blood supply, and the pigmentation affect the color of the gingiva.
    (C) The gingiva has no submucosa.

31. (C) The cytoplasmic extensions of the odontoblasts occupy the dentinal tubules of the dentin. The odontoblastic cell bodies move inward during the dentin formation and eventually reside in the pulp.
    (A) (B) Korff's fibers are the corkscrew-shaped collagen fibers located between the bodies of the odontoblasts. They unwind to form the fibrillar dentin matrix of the dentin. These fibers are found in the pulp tissue.
    (D) Sclerotic dentin occurs when the dentinal fibers have degenerated and the tubules become filled with calcium salts.
    (E) The interrod substances are found between the encased rods of the enamel.

32. (B) Once a carious lesion reaches the dentin it progresses through the dentinal tubule.
    (A) Interglobular dentin is unmineralized dentin in the area near the DEJ.
    (C) Secondary dentin is dentin produced after the completion of the apical foramen.
    (D) Predentin is found adjacent to the pulp. It is actually the organic matrix which has not yet mineralized.
    (E) Sclerotic dentin occurs when the dentinal fibers have degenerated and the tubules become filled with calcium salts.

33. (C) Cementoid is the outer, less calcified layer of the cementum. It is believed that this less calcified layer prevents cemental resorption under normal pressure.
    (A) Cellular cementum is cementum that is found in the apical portion of the root. It contains cementocytes and is capable of remodeling.
    (B) Acellular cementium is cementum that is found in the cervical portion of the root. It does not contain cementocytes and is not capable of remodeling.
    (D) Cementicles are small calcified bodies of cementum found in the periodontal ligament.
    (E) Sharpey's fibers are the terminal ends of the periodontal ligament fibers that are embedded in the cementum and bone.

34. (C) Fibrous connective tissue underlies the epithelium of the gingiva. Approximately 60% of the connective tissue of the gingiva is composed of collagen fibrils.
    (A) Reticular is not a type of connective tissue, but connective tissue fibers that resemble collagen fibers and are usually found in border tissues between connective tissue and other tissues.
    (B) Elastic is not a type of connective tissue, but a fiber of the connective tissue that causes the tissue to recoil when stretched. It is found in the alveolar and buccal mucosa.
    (D) Submucosa is not present in the gingival tissue.
    (E) Oxytalan resemble elastic fibers and are thought to be immature elastic fibers.

35. (D) Interradicular fibers are located in the furcation of multirooted teeth. They are thought to reduce tooth tipping.
    (A) The periodontal ligament has a sensory capability. There are no principal periodontal fibers named sensory fibers.
    (B) Apical fibers are at the apex of the root. They reduce tooth tipping.
    (C) There are no principal periodontal fibers named septum fibers. The bone between the roots of multirooted teeth is referred to as a septum.
    (E) Transseptal fibers are located at the proximal surfaces of the teeth. They run from the cementum of one tooth to the cementum of the adjacent tooth. They work to maintain teeth in their proper relationship with one another.

36. (C) Sharpey's fibers are the terminal ends of the periodontal ligament fibers that are embedded in the cementum and bone.
    (A) The principle fibers of the periodontal ligament are the fiber groups that run from the cementum to the bone.
    (B) Korff's fibers are the corkscrew-shaped collagen fibers located between the bodies of the odontoblasts. They unwind to form the fibrillar dentin matrix of the dentin. These fibers are found in the pulp tissue.
    (D) Dentinal fibers are the odontoblast's cytoplasmic extension that reside in the dentinal tubules of the dentin.
    (E) Gingival fibers are collagen fibers that maintain gingival tone.

37. (C) Rests of Malassez are the remnants of Hertwig's epithelial root sheath that are present in the periodontal ligament after eruption.
    (A) Enamel pearls are spherical enamel formations on the root surface that are thought to be the result of the differentiation of the Hertwig's epithelial root sheath cells into ameloblasts.
    (B) Denticles are calcified bodies found in the pulp. True denticles have dentinal tubules. False denticles are calcified bodies in which the dentinal tubules are not present and necrotic cells may be found.
    (D) Cementicles are small calcified bodies of cementum found in the periodontal ligament.
    (E) Intermediate plexus is an area of apparently interwoven fibers in the central region of the periodontal ligament.

38. (D) Bone trabeculation increases with increased functional activity. The width of the periodontal ligament increases with excessive functional activity.

39. (D) Lining mucosa is nonkeratinized.
    (A) Lining mucosa does contain more muscle fibers than masticatory mucosa.
    (B) Masticatory mucosa does not contain glands; lining mucosa does.
    (C) Lining mucosa does have submucosa.

40. (A) The first, second & third permanent molars develop from primary dental lamina.
    (B) Only those permanent teeth that succeed a primary tooth grow from secondary (successional) lamina which grows off the primary tooth bud.
    (C) Enamel pearls are calcified bodies of enamel that appear on the root surface. They are thought to be the result of the differentiation of Hertwig's epithelial root sheath cells.

41. (A) The neutrophil is the first cell in the line of defense against bacterial invasion and it reaches the site of injury first.
    (B) The monocyte is a nongranular leukocyte that travels through the bloodstream and becomes a macrophage as it enters the connective tissue.
    (C) Although the macrophage does not arrive to the site of injury first, it is capable of staying for a longer period of time than the neutrophils.
    (D) The lymphocyte plays a key role in the immune system. It differentiates into plasma cells which secrete antibodies.

42. (B) The prickle cell layer is the last visible layer in nonkeratinized stratified squamous epithelium.
    (A) The basal layer is the deepest layer in all stratified squamous epithelium.
    (C) The granular layer is the last visible layer in parakeratinized stratified squamous epithelium. Eventually, it becomes filled with keratin, but the nuclei remains visible in this layer.
    (D) The corneum of keratinized layer is the last visible layer in orthokeratinized stratified squamous epithelium. It contains degenerative cells with no nuclei.

43. (C) Dentin is the product of the dental papilla.
    (A) (B) The dental lamina produces the enamel (dental organ), which produces enamel.
    (D) The dental cuticle covers the completed tooth crown.
    (E) The dental sac produces the periodontal ligament which in turn gives rise to alveolar bone and cementum.

44. (A) The microtubule provides the internal support function for the long cellular process of the odontoblasts.
    (B) Microfilaments have a support function for the cell cytoskeleton.
    (C) Tonofibrils are the intercellular filaments that attach to desmosomes.
    (D) Cilia are fine minute hair-like structures of an epithelial cell that contains microtubules.

45. (D) The cellular organelle that is responsible for cellular metabolism or producing energy is the mitrochondria.
    (A) Endoplasmic reticulum functions in transportation within the cell.
    (B) The Golgi apparatus or complex is involved in the production of large carbohydrate molecules and lysosomes.
    (C) The nucleus controls synthetic activities and stores genetic information.

46. (C) The maxilla and the mandible are formed from intermembranous bone formation which is bone formation that is not preceded by cartilage formation.
    (A) Endochondral bone formation is bone formation that occurs after cartilage has formed and provided a pattern. The bone forms replacing the cartilage.
    (B) Circumferential bone describes a particular type of bone, not a method of bone formation. It is that bone that covers the periphery or outer portion of lamellar bone.
    (D) Lamellar describes a particular type of bone, not a method of formation. It is bone that is formed in thin layers and is not arranged in small concentric circles.
    (E) The haversian describes a particular type of bone, not a method of bone formation. In haversian system bone, the lamellae are arranged in small concentric circles around a central haversian canal.

47. (D) Only bone contains Volkmann's canals. Volkmann's canals are the areas where blood vessels enter the bone. Cementum is not vascular.
    (A) (B) (C) Both bone and cementum have a similar amount of inorganic components, contain lacuna and canaliculi.

48. (D) Elastic cartilage is found in the epiglottis.
    (A) (B) (C) Fibrous cartilage is usually found in areas that are subject to compression and tension such as the intervertebral disc, temporomandibular joint, and pubic symphysis.

49. (B) Hemidesmosome is the attachment plaque or cellular junction between the epithelial cell and the noncellular surface of the basal lamina.
    (A) Desmosome is a round attachment plaque between two cells.
    (C) Tight junction is an attachment plaque between two cells in which their membranes are fused.
    (D) Gap junction is an attachment plaque between two cells that contains a channel for free transport.

50. (D) The color of gingiva is influenced by the vascularity and the presence of pigment cells.
    (A) The rete pegs (epithelial projections into the underlying connective tissue) influence the clinical appearance of stippling.

Human Anatomy and Physiology

Catherine C. Davis

Anatomy and physiology are sciences that describe the organization, structure, and function of the human body. The dental hygienist uses concepts of anatomy and physiology most often during client assessment and evaluation. Knowledge of these concepts allows the dental hygienist to determine the location of normal structures and to determine if structures are within normal limits, deviate from normal, or are ectopic. Anatomic landmarks also are important in oral radiologic and pathologic examinations and for the administration of a local anesthetic agent. The anatomic and physiologic review covers basic concepts, definitions of terms, cell structure and function, and the systems of the body, including the skeletal, muscular, nervous, circulatory, digestive, endocrine, and reproductive systems.

Sciences of Anatomy and Physiology

Basic Concepts

Anatomy

A. Definition—the science that describes the structure of the body; word is derived from the Greek roots that translate into "the act of cutting up" (i.e., dissection)

B. Branches of anatomy
  1. Gross anatomy—study of structures that can be identified with the naked eye; usually involves the use of cadavers (corpses)
  2. Microscopic anatomy (histology)—study of cells that compose tissues and organs; involves the use of a microscope to study the details of the specimens
  3. Developmental anatomy (embryology)—study of an individual from beginning as a single cell to birth
  4. Comparative anatomy—comparative study of the animal structure in regard to similar organs or regions

Descriptive Terms

A. Anatomic position—erect body position with the arms at the sides and the palms upward
B. Plane or section
  1. Definition—imaginary flat surface formed by an extension through an axis
  2. Median plane—a vertical plane that divides a body into right and left halves (Fig. 3-1)
  3. Sagittal plane
    a. Any plane parallel to the median plane
    b. Divides the body into right and left portions
  4. Frontal plane
    a. Vertical plane that forms at right angles to the sagittal plane

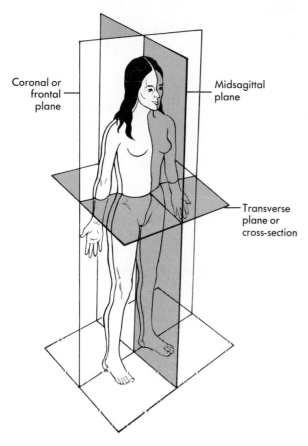

Fig. 3-1   Directions and planes of section. (From McClintic JR: *Human anatomy,* St Louis, 1983, Mosby.)

  b. Divides the body into anterior and posterior sections
  c. Synonymous with the term *coronal plane*
 5. Transverse plane
  a. Horizontal plane that forms at right angles to the sagittal and frontal planes
  b. Divides the body into upper and lower portions
  c. Synonymous with the term *horizontal plane*
C. Relative positions
 1. Anterior
  a. Nearest the abdominal surface and the front of the body
  b. Synonymous with the term *ventral*
  c. In referring to hands and forearms, the terms *palmar* and *volar* are used
 2. Posterior
  a. Back of the body
  b. Synonymous with the term *dorsal*
 3. Superior
  a. Upper or higher
  b. Synonymous with the term *cranial* (head)

 4. Inferior
  a. Below or lower
  b. Synonymous with the term *caudal* (tail)
  c. In referring to the top of the foot and the sole of the foot, the terms *dorsal* and *plantar* are used, respectively
 5. Medial—near to the median plane
 6. Lateral—farther away from the median plane
 7. Proximal—near the source or attachment
 8. Distal—away from the source or attachment
 9. Superficial—near the surface
 10. Deep—away from the surface
 11. Afferent—conducting toward a structure
 12. Efferent—conducting away from a structure

Physiology

A. Definition—study of mechanisms by which the body performs various functions; attempts to explain vital processes by using principles outlined in the biologic, chemical, and physical sciences; roots of the word are derived from the Greek words that translate into "the study of nature"
B. Branches of physiology
 1. Comparative physiology—study of comparing and contrasting the vital processes in different organisms
 2. Developmental physiology—study of the vital processes related to embryonic development
 3. General physiology—study of the functions of the vital processes
 4. Human physiology—study of the functions within the human body
 5. Pathologic physiology—study of disease that relates to an imbalance in function

Body Cavities—Formation and Contents (Fig. 3-2)

A. Dorsal cavity—contains the brain and spinal cord
 1. Cranial cavity—formed by bones of the skull
 2. Vertebral cavity—formed by the vertebrae
B. Ventral cavity
 1. Thoracic cavity
  a. Pericardial cavity contains the heart
  b. Pleural cavity contains the lungs
  c. Trachea, bronchi, esophagus, and thymus lie between these subdivisions
 2. Abdominopelvic cavity
  a. Upper cavity contains the liver, small and large intestines, stomach, spleen, pancreas, and gallbladder
  b. Lower cavity contains the bladder, rectum, sigmoid colon, and reproductive organs

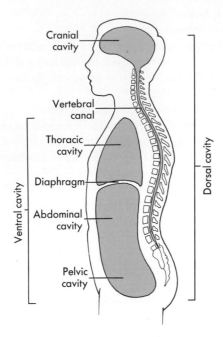

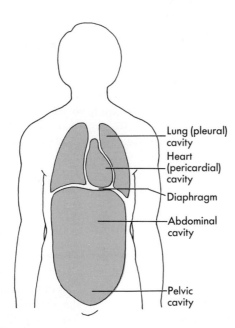

Fig. 3-2 Lateral and anterior views of human figure identifying body cavities. (From McClintic JR: *Human anatomy*, St Louis, 1983, Mosby.)

Cells

Common Functions

See also Chapter 2, section on general histology, and Fig. 2-1.

A. Excitability
1. Change in the environment stimulates the cell to bring about a response to adapt to the change in the environment
2. Example—nerve cells conduct impulses
B. Synthesis
1. Cells must be able to form substances to produce products that aid in the body's function
2. Example—glands synthesize and secrete products to aid body function
C. Membrane transport
1. Fluids, chemical elements, and compounds must be able to move both in and out of the cells
2. Example—nutrients are transported across the epithelial lining of the gastrointestinal tract
D. Reproduction
1. Cells must be able to preserve the species by giving rise to offspring
2. Example—union of a sperm and an ovum can lead to the formation of an offspring

Specialization

A. Differentiation
1. Cells that recognize one another will group together
2. Cancer cells do not recognize each other
B. Organize chemicals
1. Chemicals appear early in the development of the embryo
2. Endocrine substances are produced by one type of cell and can affect other types of cells
C. Cells → tissues → organs → organ systems

Cellular Structures—Organelles

See also Chapter 2, section on general histology, and Chapter 7, sections on prokaryotic (bacterial) cell structure and function and on eukaryotic cell structure and function.

A. Cell membrane
1. Surrounds the cell; is semipermeable, allowing some substances to pass through it and others to be excluded
2. Its permeability may be varied
3. Selective permeability characteristics
   a. Protects cell from external environment
   b. Permits entrance and exit of selected substrates
   c. Uses active transport, passive transport, or facilitated diffusion
4. Has a 3:2 ratio of proteins to lipids; lipids and proteins are the major components
5. Consists of a bipolar membrane with a central core of lipids between two layers of protein
6. The 8 Å pores in the surface allow diffusion of small lipid-insoluble substances

B. Endoplasmic reticulum
1. A complex series of tubules in the cytoplasm of the cell
2. Membranous system of channels that can permeate the entire cytoplasm, sometimes leading from the plasma membrane to the nuclear membrane
3. Synthesizes, circulates, and packages intracellular and extracellular materials
4. Contains enzymes and is involved in a variety of metabolic activities (e.g., lipogenesis and glycogenesis)
5. Granular
   a. Contains ribosomes, which are attached to the cytoplasmic side of the membrane
   b. Site of protein synthesis
6. Agranular
   a. No ribosomes present
   b. Site of steroid synthesis
C. Golgi apparatus or body
1. Network of flattened smooth membrane and vesicles
2. Responsible for secreting to the external environment a variety of proteins synthesized on the endoplasmic reticulum
3. Major site of membrane formation and recycling
4. Storage site for newly synthesized proteins
5. Site for packaging and transporting many cell products (e.g., polysaccharides, proteins, and lipids)
6. Synthesis site for lysosomes
D. Mitochondria
1. Ellipsoid bodies that consist of an outer and inner membrane that contain enzyme complexes in a particular array (e.g., tricarboxylic acid cycle enzymes)
2. Function as the powerhouse of the cell by transforming the chemical energy bond of nutrients into the high-energy phosphate bonds of adenosine triphosphate (ATP)
3. A single cell may contain 50 to 2500 of these organelles, depending on the cell's energy needs
E. Lysosomes
1. Tiny closed vesicles with a single limiting membrane containing powerful degradative or hydrolytic enzymes
2. Involved in the normal degradation of both intracellular and extracellular substances that must be removed by the cell
3. Vitamins A and E and zinc are important stabilizers for the membrane
F. Cytoplasm
1. Aqueous environment that surrounds and supports all of the organelles within a cell

2. Transport medium in which all nutrients and metabolites are carried from one organelle to another
3. Contains enzyme and electrolytes in which specific metabolic reactions take place (e.g., glycolysis)
G. Ribosomes
1. Ribonucleoprotein particles usually attached to the endoplasmic reticulum
2. Synthesis site for protein molecules
H. Nucleus
1. Consists of a nuclear membrane, nucleolus, and nuclear matrix with chromosomes
2. Ultimately controls cellular function; determines cellular nutrient needs
3. Genetic code for cell duplication and construction of the cell's proteins is found in the deoxyribonucleic acid (DNA) portion of the chromosome
4. Mitosis—process of cell replication (Fig. 3-3)
   a. Interphase
      (1) Genetic material of each chromosome replicates
      (2) Chromosomes are dispersed as chromatin material in the nucleus
   b. Prophase
      (1) Nuclear envelope disappears
      (2) Two centrioles separate and move to opposite poles of the cell
      (3) Spindle fibers develop
   c. Metaphase
      (1) Chromatids line up at the center
      (2) Spindle fibers attach at the centromere
      (3) Centromere replicates, allowing separation of the chromatids
   d. Anaphase
      (1) Spindle fibers pull the new chromosomes to opposite poles of the cell
   e. Telophase
      (1) Nuclear membrane forms around each set of chromosomes
      (2) Centrioles replicate in each cell

Internal Environment and Homeostasis

A. Extracellular fluid
1. The mass of fluid that circulates on the outside of the cells and in between them
2. Composition must be regulated exactly

$$[Na^+] = 142 \text{ mEq/L}$$
$$[K^+] = 5 \text{ mEq/L}$$
$$[Cl^-] = 103 \text{ mEq/L}$$
$$[Ca^{+2}] = 5 \text{ mEqL}$$
$$pH = 7.4$$

3. Claude Bernarde called it the "milieu interne"
B. Intracellular fluid
1. The fluid located inside the cells of the body

2. Composition must be regulated exactly

$$[Na^+] = 10 \text{ mEq/L}$$
$$[K^+] = 141 \text{ mEq/L}$$
$$[Cl^-] = 4 \text{ mEq/L}$$
$$[Ca^{+2}] = <1 \text{ mEq/L}$$
$$pH = 7.0$$

C. Homeostasis
   1. The delicate balance that must be maintained between the two fluid compositions
   2. Phrase coined by William Cannon

Transport Through the Cell Membrane

A. Diffusion
   1. Definition—continuous movement of molecules among one another in liquids or in gases
   2. Molecules may move across a membrane
   3. Direction of diffusion of a substance is from a region of high concentration to a region of low concentration, which is the diffusion gradient
   4. If equal amounts of a substance are placed at either end of the chamber, they diffuse toward each other and the net rate of diffusion equals zero
   5. Factors that affect the rate of diffusion

a. The higher the concentration difference, the greater the rate of diffusion
b. The greater the cross-sectional area of the chamber, the greater the rate of diffusion
c. The greater the temperature, the greater the rate of reaction
d. The lesser the square root of the molecular weight, the greater the rate of reaction
e. The shorter the distance, the greater the rate of reaction

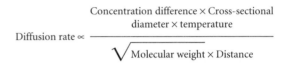

$$\text{Diffusion rate} \propto \cfrac{\text{Concentration difference} \times \text{Cross-sectional diameter} \times \text{temperature}}{\sqrt{\text{Molecular weight} \times \text{Distance}}}$$

6. How rapidly a substance can diffuse through the lipid matrix of the cell membrane is determined by its solubility in lipids
   a. Oxygen, carbon dioxide, and alcohol can diffuse through the membrane rapidly because they are lipid-soluble
   b. Water is not lipid-soluble and therefore must

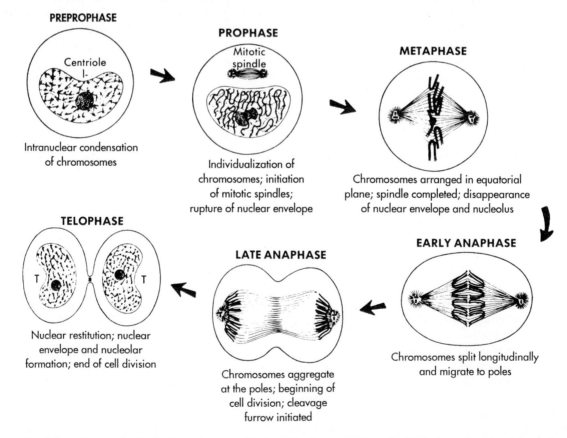

PREPROPHASE

Centriole

Intranuclear condensation of chromosomes

PROPHASE

Mitotic spindle

Individualization of chromosomes; initiation of mitotic spindles; rupture of nuclear envelope

METAPHASE

Chromosomes arranged in equatorial plane; spindle completed; disappearance of nuclear envelope and nucleolus

EARLY ANAPHASE

Chromosomes split longitudinally and migrate to poles

LATE ANAPHASE

Chromosomes aggregate at the poles; beginning of cell division; cleavage furrow initiated

TELOPHASE

Nuclear restitution; nuclear envelope and nucleolar formation; end of cell division

Fig. 3-3 Phases of mitosis. (From Junqueira LC: *Basic histology,* ed 7, Norwalk, 1992, Conn, Appleton & Lange.)

depend on another mechanism to diffuse through the cell membrane

7. Facilitated diffusion involves the use of a carrier substance to transport a non–lipid-soluble substance across the cell membrane
   a. Once the substance reaches the opposite side of the membrane, it breaks away from the carrier
   b. This system does not involve the use of energy
8. Diffusion through pores
   a. Substance must be less than 8 Å in diameter to move through the pore
   b. Calcium ions line the pores; therefore positive elements such as potassium are repelled
   c. Antidiuretic hormone (ADH) from the hypothalamus can cause the pores in kidney tubule cells to decrease in diameter

B. Osmosis
1. Definition—process of net diffusion of water through a semipermeable membrane caused by a concentration difference
2. Osmotic pressure—pressure that develops in a solution as a result of net osmosis into that solution; is affected by the number of dissolved particles per unit volume of fluid
3. Isotonic solution—when placed on the outside of a cell, will not cause osmosis (e.g., 0.9% sodium chloride)
4. Hypertonic solution—when placed on the outside of a cell, will cause osmosis out of the cell (e.g., greater than 0.9% sodium chloride) and lead to crenation of the cell
5. Hypotonic solution—when placed on the outside of a cell, will cause osmosis into the cell (e.g., less than 0.9% sodium chloride) and lead to lysis of the cell)

C. Active transport
1. Used by a cell when large quantities of a substance are needed inside of the cell and only a small amount is present in the extracellular fluid
2. Involves pumping the substance against its concentration gradient
3. Uses a carrier system and energy (ATP)
4. Keeps sodium extracellularly (sodium pump) and potassium intracellularly; important for transmission of impulses
5. Almost all monosaccharides are actively transported into the body

D. Phagocytosis—movement of a solid particle into the cell
1. Cell wall invaginates around the particle
2. Pinches off from the rest of the membrane and floats inward

E. Pinocytosis—movement of fluid into a cell; similar to phagocytosis, except cell invaginates around fluid

Tissues

A. Definition—an aggregate of cells that have nonliving intracellular substances between the cells
1. Classification
   a. Epithelial
   b. Connective
   c. Nerve
   d. Muscle
2. Differ in structure because each tissue can differ in function
B. Types
1. Epithelial tissue
   a. Contains little intercellular substance; therefore is composed mainly of cells
   b. Does not contain blood vessels
   c. Cells composing this tissue undergo mitosis
   d. Subtypes
      (1) Simple squamous
         (a) One layer of flat cells
         (b) Example—lining of blood vessels
      (2) Stratified squamous
         (a) Several layers thick
         (b) Example—mucous membranes
      (3) Simple columnar
         (a) Two types of cells—columnar and goblet
         (b) Example—lining of the intestines
2. Connective tissue
   a. Contains large amounts and various types of intercellular material and few cells
   b. Is usually highly vascular
   c. Functions
      (1) Supports structures
      (2) Aids in distribution of nutrients
   d. Classifications
      (1) Reticular—network of branching fibers; acts as a filter; loose and stretchable; serves as a connection between structures
      (2) Adipose—located under the skin; insulates
      (3) Dense fibrous—flexible; serves as a connection between structures
      (4) Bone—hard and calcified; serves a supportive, protective function
      (5) Cartilage—firm but flexible; serves a supportive function
      (6) Blood—large amount of fluid within the various cells; carries on vital functions of the body

3. Nervous tissue
   a. Neurons—nerve cells that are irritable and are the conducting units
   b. Neuroglia—supporting framework
4. Muscle tissue
   a. Function—contraction
   b. Types
      (1) Skeletal—voluntary, striated
      (2) Cardiac—involuntary, striated
      (3) Visceral—involuntary, smooth

Membranes and Glands

Membranes

A. Function—to cover or line parts of the body
B. Types
   1. Mucous
      a. Line cavities of the body that communicate with the exterior
      b. Protect, secrete, and absorb
   2. Serous
      a. Line cavities that do not communicate with the exterior
      b. Visceral layer covers organs
      c. Parietal layer lines cavities
      d. Synovial membranes line joint cavities
   3. Cutaneous
      a. Skin functions in protection, excretion, and sensation
      b. Skin consists of epidermis and dermis
      c. Skin contains hair follicles and glands

Glands

A. Function—synthesizes compounds
B. Types
   1. Endocrine—secrete product directly into the blood system
   2. Exocrine—secrete product directly into ducts
      a. Simple—nonbranching duct
      b. Compound—branching duct

Systems of the Body and Their Components

Skeletal System

A. Functions
   1. Provides a rigid support system
   2. Protects delicate structures (e.g., the protection pro-

vided by the bones of the vertebral column to the spinal cord)
   3. Bones supply calcium to the blood; are involved in the formation of blood cells (hemopoiesis)
   4. Bones serve as the basis of attachment of muscles; form levers in the joint areas, allowing movement
B. Formation
   1. Bones begin to form during the eighth week of embryonic life in the fibrous membranes (intramembranous ossification) and hyaline cartilage (endochondral ossification)
   2. Ossification
      a. Intramembranous—found in the flat bones of the face
         (1) Mesenchymal cells cluster and form strands
         (2) Strands are cemented in a uniform network, which is known as osteoid
         (3) Calcium salts are deposited; osteoid is converted to bone
         (4) Trabeculae are formed and make cancellous bone with open spaces known as marrow cavities
         (5) Periosteum forms on the inner and outer surfaces of the ossification centers
         (6) Surface bone becomes compact bone
      b. Endochondral—primary type of ossification in the human
         (1) Cartilage model is covered with perichondrium that is converted to periosteum
            (a) Diaphysis—central shaft
            (b) Epiphysis—located at either end of the diaphysis
            (c) Growth in length of the bone is provided by the metaphyseal plate located between the epiphyseal cartilage and the diaphysis
         (2) Blood capillaries and the mesenchymal cells infiltrate the spaces left by the destroyed chondrocytes
            (a) Osteoblasts are derived from the undifferentiated cells; form an osseous matrix in the cartilage
            (b) Bone appears at the site where there was cartilage
         (3) Ossification is completed as the proximal epiphysis joins with the diaphysis between the twentieth and twenty-fifth year
C. Microscopic structure
   1. Compact bone is found on the exterior of all bones; cancellous bone is found in the interior
   2. Surface of compact bone is covered by periosteum that is attached by Sharpey's fibers

3. Blood vessels enter the periosteum via Volkmann's canals and then enter the haversian canals that are formed by the canaliculi and lacunae
4. Marrow
   a. Fills spaces of spongy bone
   b. Contains blood vessels and blood cells in various stages of development
   c. Types
      (1) Red bone marrow
         (a) Formation of red blood cells (RBCs) and some white blood cells (WBCs) in this location
         (b) Predominant type of marrow in the newborn
         (c) Found in spongy bone of adults (sternum, ribs, vertebrae, and proximal epiphyses of long bones)
      (2) Yellow bone marrow
         (a) Fatty marrow
         (b) Generally replaces red bone marrow in the adult, except in areas mentioned above

D. Types
   1. Long bones (e.g., femur and humerus)
   2. Short bones (e.g., wrist and ankle bones)
   3. Flat bones (e.g., ribs)
   4. Irregular bones (e.g., vertebrae)
E. Descriptive terminology
   1. Projections
      a. Process—prominence
      b. Spine—sharp prominence
      c. Tubercle—rounded projection
      d. Tuberosity—larger rounded projection
      e. Trochanter—very large bony prominence
      f. Crest—ridge
      g. Condyle—round process for articulation
      h. Head—enlargement at end of a bone
   2. Depression
      a. Fossa—pit
      b. Groove—furrow
      c. Sulcus—synonymous with groove
      d. Sinus—cavity within a bone
      e. Foramen—opening
      f. Meatus—tubelike
F. Divisions of the skeleton (Figs. 3-4 and 3-5)
   1. Axial skeleton (74 bones total)
      a. Upright axis of the skeleton
      b. Consists of the skull, hyoid, vertebral column, sternum, and ribs
   2. Appendicular skeleton (126 bones total)
      a. Bones attached to the axial skeleton
      b. Upper and lower extremities

3. Auditory ossicles (six total)
G. Articulations
   1. Classified according to their structure, composition, and movability
      a. Fibrous joints—surfaces of bones almost in direct contact with limited movement
         (1) Syndesmosis—two bones united by interosseous ligaments
         (2) Sutures—serrated margins of bones united by a thin layer of fibrous tissue
         (3) Gomphosis—insertion of a cone-shaped process into a socket
      b. Cartilaginous joints—no joint cavity and contiguous bones united by cartilage
         (1) Synchondrosis—ends of two bones approximated by hyaline cartilage
         (2) Symphyses—approximating bone surfaces connected by fibrocartilage
      c. Synovial joints—approximating bone surfaces covered with cartilage; may be separated by a disk; attached by ligaments
         (1) Hinge—permits motion in one plane only
         (2) Pivot—permits rotary movement in which a ring rotates around a central axis
         (3) Saddle—opposing surfaces are convex-concave, allowing great freedom of motion
         (4) Ball and socket—capable of movement in an infinite number of axes; rounded head of one bone moves in a cuplike cavity of the approximating bone
   2. Bursae
      a. Sacs filled with synovial fluid that are present where tendons rub against bone or where skin rubs across bone
      b. Some bursae communicate with a joint cavity
      c. Prominent bursae found at the elbow, hip, and knee
   3. Movements
      a. Gliding
         (1) Simplest kind of motion in a joint
         (2) Movement on a joint that does *not* involve any angular or rotary motions
      b. Flexion—decreases the angle formed by the union of two bones
      c. Extension—increases the angle formed by the union of two bones
      d. Abduction—occurs by moving part of the appendicular skeleton away from the median plane of the body
      e. Adduction—occurs by moving part of the appendicular skeleton toward the median plane of the body

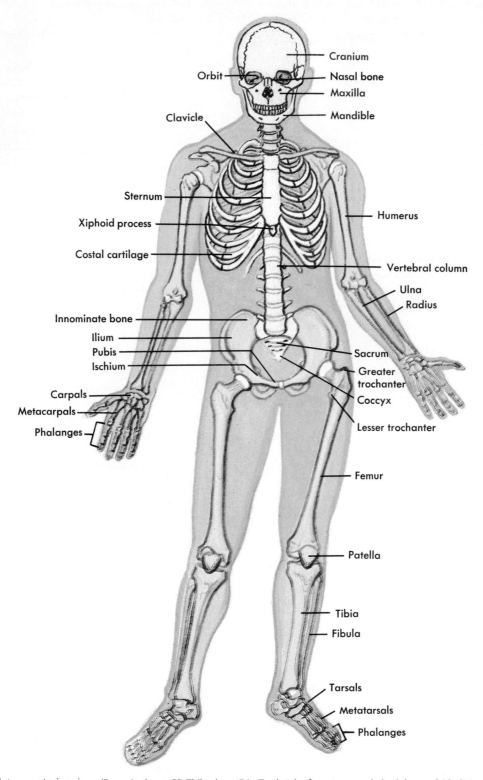

Fig. 3-4 Skeleton, anterior view. (From Anthony CP, Thibodeau GA: *Textbook of anatomy and physiology,* ed 12, St Louis, 1987, Mosby.)

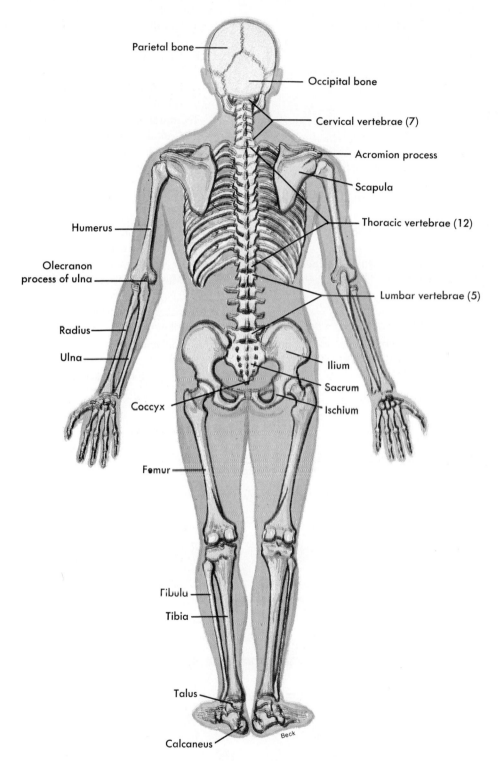

Fig. 3-5   Skeleton, posterior view. (From Anthony CP, Thibodeau GA: *Textbook of anatomy and physiology,* ed 12, St Louis, 1987, Mosby.)

f. Circumduction
   (1) Occurs in ball-and-socket joints
   (2) Circumscribes the conic space of one bone by the other bone
g. Rotation—turning on an axis without being displaced from that axis

Axial Skeleton

A. Skull (Figs. 3-6 and 3-7 and Table 3-1)
   1. Cranium
      a. Superior portion formed by the frontal, parietal, and occipital bones
      b. Lateral portions formed by the temporal and sphenoid bones
      c. Cranial base formed by the temporal, sphenoid, and ethmoid bones
      d. Fontanels—soft spots in which ossification is incomplete at birth
   2. Frontal bone
      a. Forms the forehead
      b. Contains the frontal sinuses
      c. Forms the roof of the orbits
      d. Union with the parietal bones forms the coronal suture
   3. Parietal bones
      a. Union with the occipital bone forms the lambdoid suture
      b. Union with the temporal bone forms the squamous suture
      c. Union with the sphenoid bone forms the coronal suture
   4. Temporal bones
      a. Contains the external auditory meatus and middle and inner ear structures
      b. Squamous portion—above the meatus; zygomatic process—articulates with the zygoma to form the zygomatic arch
      c. Petrous portion
         (1) Contains organs of hearing and equilibrium
         (2) Prominent elevation on the floor of the cranium
      d. Mastoid portion
         (1) Protuberance behind the ear
         (2) Mastoid process
      e. Glenoid fossa—articulates with the condyle on the mandible
      f. Styloid process—anterior to the mastoid process; several neck muscles attach here

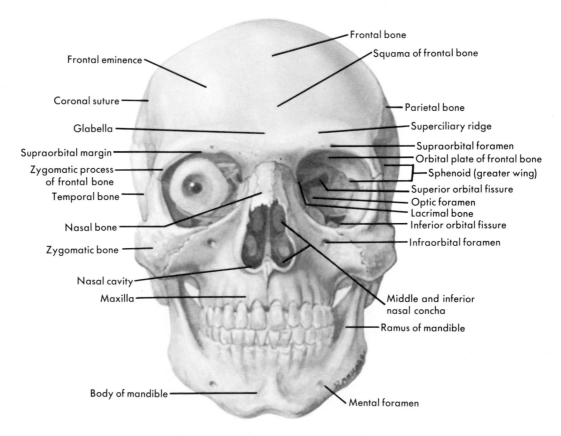

Fig. 3-6   Skull viewed from front. (From McClintic JR: *Human anatomy,* St Louis, 1983, Mosby.)

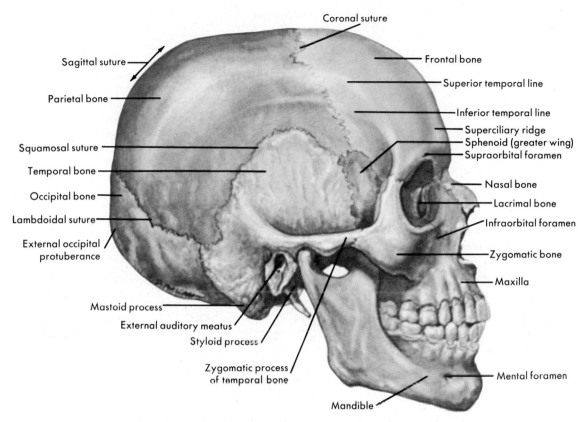

Fig. 3-7   Skull viewed from right side. (From McClintic JR. *Human anatomy*, St Louis, 1983, Mosby.)

Table 3-1	
Bones of the Skull	
Bones	**No.**
BONES OF THE CRANIUM	
Occipital	1
Frontal	1
Sphenoid	1
Ethmoid	1
Parietal	2
Temporal	2
BONES OF THE FACE	
Mandible	1
Vomer	1
Maxillae	2
Zygomae	2
Lacrimal	2
Nasal	2
Inferior nasal conchae	2
Palatine	2

g. Stylomastoid foramen—located between the styloid and mastoid processes; facial nerve emerges through this opening

h. Jugular foramen—located between the petrous portion and the occipital bone; cranial nerves IX, X, and XI exit

5. Sphenoid bone (Fig. 3-8)

a. Bounded by the ethmoid and frontal bones anteriorly and the temporal and occipital bones posteriorly

b. Greater wings—lateral projections

(1) Form outer wall and floor of the orbits

(2) Foramen rotundum—maxillary division of cranial nerve V exits

(3) Foramen ovale—mandibular division of cranial nerve V exits

(4) Foramen spinosum—transmits an artery to the meninges

(5) Foramen lacerum—contains the internal carotid artery

(6) Superior orbital fissure—transmits cranial nerves III and IV and part of cranial nerve V

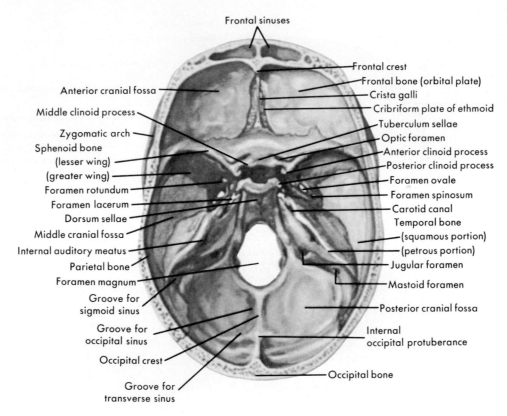

Fig. 3-8 Floor of cranial cavity. (From McClintic JR: *Human anatomy,* St Louis, 1983, Mosby.)

c. Lesser wings
   (1) Posterior part of the root of the orbits
   (2) Optic foramen—cranial nerve II exits
d. Body
   (1) Sella turcica—holds the pituitary gland
   (2) Contains the sphenoid sinuses
   (3) Medial and lateral pterygoid processes located here
6. Ethmoid bone
   a. Contributes to the formation of the base of the cranium, the orbits, and the roof of the nose
   b. Perpendicular plate—forms the superior part of the nasal septum
   c. Horizontal plate (cribriform plate)
      (1) Located at right angles to the perpendicular plate
      (2) Olfactory nerves pass through
      (3) Contains the crista galli—meninges of the brain attach to this process
   d. Lateral masses
      (1) Form the orbital plates
      (2) Contain the superior and middle conchae (lateral walls of the nose)
      (3) Contain the ethmoid sinuses
7. Occipital bone (Fig. 3-9)
   a. Forms the posterior part of the cranium

b. Foramen magnum—spinal cord enters to attach to the brainstem
c. Condyles (two) on either side of the foramen magnum—articulate with depression on the C1 vertebra
d. External occipital protuberance—located on the posterior surface
   (1) Superior nuchal lines—curved ridges extending laterally
   (2) Inferior nuchal lines—parallel superior nuchal lines
e. Transverse sinuses—located on the inner surface
B. Facial bones
   1. Appear suspended from the middle and anterior parts of the cranium
   2. Ethmoid and frontal bones also contribute to the framework of the face
   3. All the facial bones except the mandible touch the maxilla
      a. Alveolar process—forms the upper jaw containing the maxillary teeth
      b. Forms the floor of the orbit; infraorbital foramen is inferior from the orbit
      c. Forms the walls of the nasal cavities and the hard palate (palatine process)
      d. Maxillary sinus—large air space

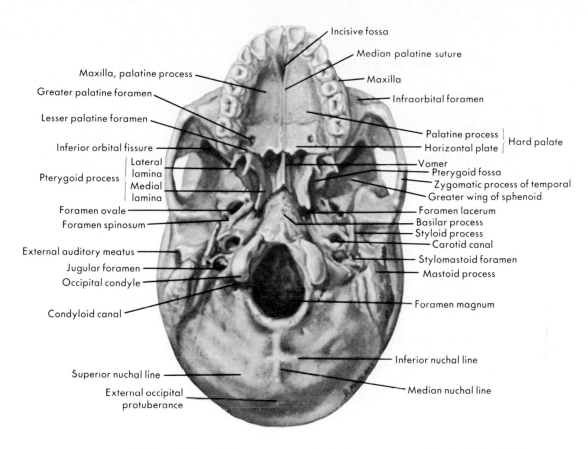

Fig. 3-9   Skull viewed from below. (From McClintic JR. *Human anatomy*, St Louis, 1983, Mosby.)

4. Mandible
   a. Body—central horizontal portion
     (1) Chin—symphysis in midline
     (2) Alveolar process—contains the mandibular teeth
     (3) Mental foramen
       (a) Below the first bicuspid on the outer surface
       (b) Transmits nerves and blood vessels; frequent site of injections of local anesthetics
   b. Ramus—upward process on either side of the posterior body of the mandible
     (1) Condyle—articulates with the glenoid fossa (neck—constriction located inferior to the condyle)
     (2) Coronoid process—attachment site for the temporalis muscle
     (3) Mandibular foramen—located on the inner surface
5. Zygomatic bone
   a. Prominence of cheek—attaches to the zygomatic process of the temporal bone to form the zygomatic arch
   b. Other margin of the orbit

6. Lacrimal—medial part of the wall of the orbit
7. Nasal bones—upper bridge of the nose
8. Inferior nasal concha
   a. Horizontally placed along the lateral wall of the nasal fossa
   b. Inferior to the middle and superior conchae of the ethmoid
9. Palatine bones
   a. Horizontal plates—form the posterior part of the hard palate
   b. Perpendicular plates—form the sphenopalatine foramen
10. Vomer
   a. Plowshare shaped
   b. Forms the lower part of the nasal septum
C. Hyoid
   1. U-shaped bone
     a. Body
     b. Greater horn
     c. Lesser horn
   2. Suspended by ligaments from the styloid process
D. Vertebral column
   1. Part of the axial skeleton; strong, flexible rod
     a. Supports the head
     b. Gives base to the ribs

c. Encloses the spinal cord
2. Vertebrae
   a. Consists of 34 bones composing the spinal column
      (1) Cervical—7 bones
      (2) Thoracic—12 bones
      (3) Lumbar—5 bones
      (4) Sacral—5 bones
      (5) Coccygeal—4 to 5 bones
   b. In the adult the vertebrae of the sacral and coccygeal regions are united into two bones, the sacrum and the coccyx
3. Curvatures—from a lateral view there are four curves, alternately convex and concave ventrally
   a. Two convex curves are the cervical and lumbar
   b. Two concave curves are the thoracic and sacral
4. Vertebral morphology
   a. Each vertebra differs in size and shape but has similar components
   b. Body—central mass of bone
      (1) Weight bearing
      (2) Forms anterior part of the vertebra
      (3) Encloses the vertebral foramen
   c. Pedicles of the arch—two thick columns that extend backward from the body to meet with the laminae of the neural arch
   d. Processes (7)
      (1) One spinous, two transverse, two superior articular, and two inferior articular
         (a) Spinous process extends backward from the point of the union of the two laminae
         (b) Transverse processes project laterally at either side from the junction of the lamina and the pedicle
         (c) Articular processes arise near the junction of the pedicle and the lamina— superior processes project upward; inferior processes project downward
      (2) Surfaces of the processes are smooth
         (a) Inferior articular processes of the vertebra fit into the superior articular processes below
         (b) Form true joints, but the contacts established serve to restrict movement
5. Distinguishing features
   a. Cervical region—triangular shape
      (1) All have foramina in the transverse process (upper six transmit the vertebral artery)
      (2) Spinous processes are short
         (a) C3 to C5 are bifurcated
         (b) C7 is long—prominence felt at the back of the neck
      (3) Have small bodies (except for C1 vertebra)
      (4) C1 vertebra (atlas)
         (a) No body
         (b) Anterior and posterior arch and two lateral masses
         (c) Superior articular processes articulate with the condyles of the occipital bone
      (5) C2 vertebra (axis)—process on the upper surface of the body (dens) forms a pivot about which the axis rotates
   b. Thoracic region
      (1) Presence of facets for articulation with the ribs (distinguishing feature)
      (2) Processes are larger and heavier than those of the cervical region
      (3) Spinous process is directed downward at a sharp angle
      (4) Circular vertebral foramen
   c. Lumbar region
      (1) Large and heavy bodies
      (2) Four transverse lines separate the bodies of the vertebrae on the pelvic surface
      (3) Triangular shape—fitted between the halves of the pelvis
      (4) Four pairs of dorsal sacral foramina communicate with four pairs of pelvic sacral foramina
   d. Sacral vertebrae
   e. Coccygeal vertebrae
      (1) Four to five modular pieces fused together
      (2) Triangular shape with the base above and the apex below
   f. Defects
      (1) Lordosis—exaggerated lumbar concavity
      (2) Scoliosis—lateral curvature of any region
      (3) Kyphosis—exaggerated convexity in the thoracic region
E. Bones of the thorax
   1. Sternum
      a. Forms the medial part of the anterior chest wall
      b. Manubrium (upper part)—clavicle and first rib articulate with the manubrium
      c. Body (middle blade)—second and tenth ribs articulate with the body via the costal cartilages
      d. Xiphoid (blunt cartilaginous tip)
   2. Ribs (12 pairs)
      a. Each rib articulates with both the body and the transverse process of its corresponding thoracic vertebra
      b. The second to ninth ribs articulate with the body of the vertebra above
      c. Ribs curve outward, forward, and then downward

d. Anteriorly, each of the first seven ribs joins a costal cartilage that attaches to the sternum

e. Next three ribs (eighth to tenth) join the cartilage of the rib above

f. Eleventh and twelfth ribs do not attach to the sternum; are called "floating ribs"

Appendicular Skeleton (Table 3-2)

A. Upper extremity

1. Shoulder—clavicle and scapula

   a. Clavicle

      (1) Articulates with the manubrium at the sternal end

      (2) Articulates with the scapula at the lateral end

      (3) Slender S-shaped bone that extends horizontally across the upper part of the thorax

   b. Scapula

      (1) Triangular bone with the base upward and the apex downward

      (2) Lateral aspect contains the glenoid cavity that articulates with the head of the humerus

      (3) Spine extends across the upper part of the posterior surface; expands laterally and forms the acromion (forms point of shoulder)

      (4) Coracoid process projects anteriorly from the upper part of the neck of the scapula

2. Arm (humerus)

   a. Consists of a shaft (diaphysis) and two ends (epiphyses)

   b. Proximal end has a head that articulates with the glenoid fossa of the scapula

   c. Greater and lesser tubercles lie below the head

      (1) Intertubercular groove is located between them; long tendon of the biceps attaches here

      (2) Surgical neck is located below the tubercles

   d. Radial groove runs obliquely on the posterior surface; radial nerve is located here

   e. Deltoid muscles attaches in a V-shaped area in the middle of the shaft, called the deltoid tuberosity

   f. Distal end has two projections, the medial and lateral epicondyles

      (1) Capitulum—articulates with the radius

      (2) Trochlea—articulates with the ulna

3. Forearm

   a. Radius

      (1) Lateral bone of the forearm

      (2) Radial tuberosity is located below the head on the medial side

      (3) Distal end is broad for articulation with the wrist; has a styloid process on its lateral side

   b. Ulna

      (1) Medial side of the forearm

      (2) Conspicuous part of the elbow joint (olecranon)

      (3) Curved surface that articulates with the trochlea of the humerus is the trochlear notch

      (4) Lateral side is concave (radial notch); articulates with the head of the radius

      (5) Distal end contains the styloid process

4. Hand

   a. Carpal bones (8)

      (1) Arranged in two rows of four

      (2) Scaphoid, lunate, triquetral, and pisiform (proximal row); trapezium, trapezoid, capitate, and hamate (distal row)

   b. Metacarpal bones (5)

      (1) Framework of the hand

      (2) Numbered 1 to 5 beginning on the lateral side

   c. Phalanges (14)

      (1) Fingers

      (2) Three phalanges in each finger; two phalanges in the thumb

B. Lower extremity

1. Hip

   a. Constitutes the pelvic girdle

   b. United with the vertebral column

   c. Union of three parts that is marked by a cup-shaped cavity (acetabulum)

   d. Ilium

      (1) Prominence of the hip

      (2) Superior border is the crest

Table 3-2

Appendicular Skeleton

Upper extremity		Lower extremity
Shoulder	Shoulder girdle	Hip
Scapula		Pelvic girdle
Clavicle		Thigh
Arm		Femur
Humerus		Kneecap
Forearm		Patella
Ulna, radius, carpals (wrist) (8 bones)		Leg
		Tibia, fibula, tarsals (ankle) (7 bones)
Hand		Foot
Metacarpals (5 bones), phalanges (fingers) (14 bones)		Metatarsals (5 bones), phlanges (toes) (14 bones)

(3) Anterosuperior spine—projection at the anterior tip of the crest

(4) Corresponding projections on the posterior part are the posterosuperior and posteroinferior iliac spines

(5) Greater sciatic notch—located beneath the posterior part

(6) Most is a smooth concavity (iliac fossa)

(7) Posteriorly it is rough and articulates with the sacrum in the formation of the sacroiliac joint

e. Pubic bone

(1) Anterior part of the innominate bone

(2) Symphysis pubis—joining of the two pubic bones at the midline

(3) Body and two rami

(a) Body forms one fifth of the acetabulum

(b) Superior ramis extends from the body to the median plane; superior border forms the pubic crest

(c) Inferior ramus extends downward and meets with the ischium

(d) Pubic arch is formed by the inferior rami of both pubic bones

f. Ischium

(1) Forms the lower and back part of the innominate bone

(2) Body

(a) Forms two fifths of the acetabulum

(b) Ischial tuberosity—supports the body in a sitting position

(3) Ramus—passes upward to join the inferior ramus of the pubis; known as the obturator foramen

2. Pelvis

a. Formed by the right and left hip bones, sacrum, and coccyx

b. Greater pelvis

(1) Bounded by the ilia and lower lumbar vertebrae

(2) Gives support to the abdominal viscera

c. Lesser pelvis

(1) Brim of the pelvis corresponds to the sacral promontory

(2) Inferior outlet is bounded by the tip of the coccyx, ischial tuberosities, and inferior rami of the pubic bones

d. Female pelvis

(1) Shows adaptations related to functions as a birth canal

(2) Wide outlet

(3) Angle of the pubic arch is obtuse

e. Male pelvis

(1) Shows adaptations that contribute to power and speed

(2) Heart-shaped outlet

(3) Angle of the pubic arch is acute

3. Thigh

a. Femur—longest and strongest bone of the body

b. Proximal end has a rounded head that articulates with the acetabulum

c. Constricted portion—the neck

d. Greater and lesser trochanters

e. Slightly arched shaft; is concave posteriorly

(1) Linea aspera—strengthened by this prominent ridge

(2) Site of attachment for several muscles

f. Distal end has two condyles separated on the posterior side by the intercondyloid notch

4. Kneecap

a. Patella—sesamoid bone

b. Embedded in the tendon of the quadriceps muscle

c. Articulates with the femur

5. Leg

a. Tibia—medial bone

(1) Proximal end has two condyles that articulate with the femur

(2) Triangular shaft

(a) Anterior—shin

(b) Posterior—soleal line

(c) Distal—medial malleolus that articulates with the latus to form the ankle joint

b. Fibula—lateral bone

(1) Articulates with the lateral condyle of the tibia but does not enter the knee joint

(2) Distal end projects as the lateral malleolus

6. Ankle, foot, and toes

a. Adapted for supporting weight but similar in structure to the hand

b. Talus

(1) Occupies the uppermost and central position in the tarsus

(2) Distributes the body weight from the tibia above to the other tarsal bones

c. Calcaneus (heel)—located beneath the talus

d. Navicular—located in front of the talus on the medial side; articulates with three cuneiform bones distally

e. Cuboid—lies along the lateral border of the navicular bone

f. Metatarsals

(1) First, second, and third metatarsals lie in front of the three cuneiform bones

(2) Fourth and fifth metatarsals lie in front of the cuboid bone

g. Phalanges
    (1) Distal to the metatarsals
    (2) Two in the great toe; three in each of the other four toes

h. Longitudinal arches in the foot (2)
    (1) Lateral—formed by the calcaneus, talus, cuboid, and fourth and fifth metatarsal bones
    (2) Medial—formed by the calcaneus, talus, navicular, cuneiform, and first, second, and third metatarsal bones

i. Transverse arches—formed by the tarsal and metatarsal bones

Skeletal Muscular Tissue

A. Organization (Fig. 3-10; see also Fig. 2-14)
    1. Muscles as a whole are composed of various numbers of the fascicles
        a. Muscle fascicles are formed from grouping the skeletal muscle fibers (long, multinucleated cells and surrounded by endomysium) together and surrounding the muscle fibers with perimysium
        b. Muscle is formed by groups of the muscle fascicles bound together and surrounded with epimysium
        c. Epimysium and perimysium fuse together; form the junction between the muscle and the tendon
        d. Tendons fuse together with the periosteum of the bone; allow the muscles to produce traction of the bone
    2. Subcellular system of the muscle fibers consists of the tubules and fibrils
        a. Skeletal muscle fibers are composed of many longitudinally arranged myofibrils
            (1) Sarcoplasmic reticulum is analogous to the endoplasmic reticulum of other cells; contains Ca^{+2}
            (2) T tubules communicate with the extracellular fluid of the fiber
            (3) These systems provide a pathway for exchange of chemical material, which is important in muscle contraction

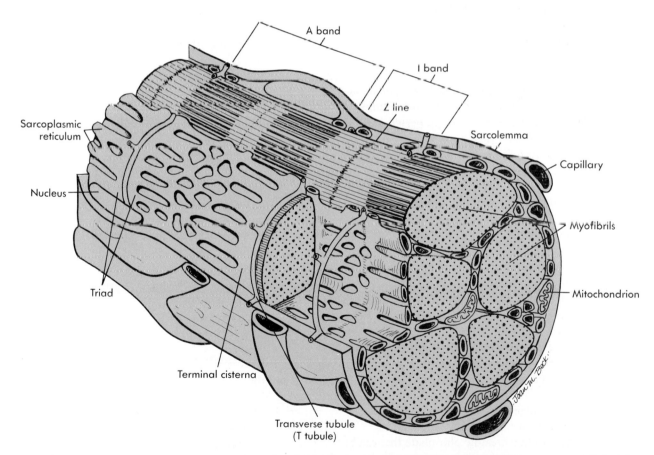

Fig. 3-10   T tubules and sarcoplasmic reticulum of skeletal muscle. (From Seeley R, Stephens T, Tape P: *Anatomy and physiology,* St Louis, 1989, Mosby.)

b. Myofibrils are formed by myofilaments
   (1) Thin—actin
   (2) Thick—myosin
c. Functional unit of the muscle is designated the sarcomere
   (1) Relationship of the myofilaments forms several unique patterns
      (a) Z line → Z line forms the sarcomere; distance between two Z lines contains the sarcomere unit; consists of only actin and is in the middle of the I band
      (b) M line consists of only myosin; is in the middle of the A band
      (c) I band contains actin that is lined up; shortens during contraction
      (d) A band consists of actin and myosin that interdigitate; is bisected by the M line
      (e) H zone appears in the A band when the muscle is relaxed
B. Muscular contraction
   1. Myoneural junction
      a. Unmyelinated end of a motor nerve almost touches a skeletal muscle fiber with its terminal buttons (end feet)
         (1) Terminal buttons contain the transmitter substance acetylcholine
         (2) Space between the nerve and muscle is the synaptic cleft
      b. Nerve impulse that reaches the myoneural junction causes acetylcholine to be released into the synaptic cleft, causing increased permeability in the muscle and creating an action potential
      c. Effect of acetylcholine is catabolized by the enzyme acetylcholinesterase to form choline and acetate
      d. Action potential is sent to the deeper myofibrils via the T tubules
   2. Muscle contraction
      a. Calcium is released from the cisterns of the sarcoplasmic reticulum; combines with the protein myosin to activate it
      b. Cross-linkages are developed by projections from the myosin filament touching the actin filament
      c. ATP, located on the myosin, is split so that energy can be released
      d. Contraction mechanism is known as the ratchet theory since the myosin filaments pull the actin filaments, thereby shortening the sarcomere
   3. Energy for contraction
      a. Muscles contain creatine phosphate that can be broken down by enzymatic activity to creatine, phosphate, and energy

b. Muscles also use glucose to form energy and pyruvic acid
c. Oxygen debt occurs in muscles when oxygen is not provided in sufficient amounts; pyruvic acid is changed to lactic acid if there is not enough oxygen
   4. Muscle relaxation
      a. Ca^{+2} is pumped into the sarcoplasmic reticulum
      b. Myosin projections are released from the actin filaments

Forms

A. Arrangement of muscle fibers may vary
   1. Fusiform fibers consist of two tendons with a belly between the fibers parallel to the long axis
   2. Pennate oblique fibers attach to a central tendon
      a. Unipennate—approach central tendon from one side
      b. Bipennate—approach central tendon from both sides
      c. Circumpennate—cylindric muscle mass
B. Muscle power is proportional to the cross-sectional area; is measured at right angles to the long axis of the muscle fascicles
C. Attachments
   1. Origin—attachment to a relatively immovable structure
   2. Insertion—attachment to a relatively movable structure
   3. Bones serve as levers and their joints as fulcrums; contraction of a muscle pulls the insertion end toward the origin of a muscle
   4. Muscles generally act in groups
      a. Agonists (prime movers)—give power for flexion
      b. Synergists—assist the agonists and reduce unnecessary movement
      c. Antagonists—are at rest while the agonists are contracting
D. Types of contraction
   1. Isometric—muscle length is unchanged, but tension is developed
   2. Isotonic—muscle length is shortened, and work is done

Physiologic Activities

A. Conditions of contraction
   1. Electrical, chemical, or mechanical stimulant must be applied to a muscle for contraction to occur
   2. If a stimulus is strong enough to cause a muscle fiber to contract, the entire muscle fiber (not just part of it) will contract (all-or-none law); strength of the stimulus will not change the response

3. Summation—muscles need to contract with varying amounts of force; therefore the number of muscle fibers that are stimulated and contract are in direct proportion to the force of the contraction
   a. Wave summations occur when a muscle fiber(s) contracts in rapid succession
   b. Strength of contraction will increase as the rate of stimulation increases
   c. Tetanization—muscle twitches eventually fuse into a single contraction; has a shortened refractory period

4. Treppe—a muscle contracts more forcefully after it has been stimulated a few times (staircase phenomenon)
5. Fibrillation—muscle fibers contract randomly, producing an ineffective fluttering action

Description (Origin, Insertion, Function, and Innervation)

A. Muscles of facial expression (Table 3-3)
B. Muscles of mastication (Table 3-4)
C. Muscles that move the head (Table 3-5)
D. Muscles that move the shoulder (Table 3-6)

Table 3-3

Muscles of Facial Expression

Muscle	Origin	Insertion	Function	Innervation
Epicranius (occipitofrontalis)	Occipital bone	Tissues of eyebrows	Raises eyebrows, wrinkles forehead horizontally	Cranial nerve VII
Corrugator supercilii	Frontal bone (superciliary ridge)	Skin of eyebrow	Wrinkles forehead vertically	Cranial nerve VII
Orbicularis oculi	Encircles eyelid		Closes eye	Cranial nerve VII
Procerus	Bridge of nose	Skin over epicranius	Narrows eye opening	Cranial nerve VII
Inferior labial depressor	Mandible	Skin of lower lip	Draws lower lip downward	Cranial nerve VII
Mentalis	Incisive fossa of mandible	Skin of chin	Raises and protrudes lower lip	Cranial nerve VII
Nasalis	Maxilla	Ala of nose	Compresses nasal aperture	Cranial nerve VII
Zygomaticus major	Zygomatic bone	Angle of mouth	Laughing (elevates angle of mouth)	Cranial nerve VII
Zygomaticus minor	Zygomatic bone	Upper lip	Elevates upper lip	Cranial nerve VII
Orbicularis oris	Encircles mouth		Draws lips together	Cranial nerve VII
Platysma	Fascia of upper part of deltoid and pectoralis major	Mandible (lower border) Skin around corners of mouth	Draws corners of mouth down—pouting	Cranial nerve VII
Buccinator	Maxillae	Skin of sides of mouth	Permits smiling Blowing, as in playing a trumpet	Cranial nerve VII

From Anthony CP, Thibodeau GA: *Textbook of anatomy and physiology,* ed 12, St Louis, 1987, Mosby.

Table 3-4

Muscles of Mastication

Muscle	Origin	Insertion	Function	Innervation
Masseter	Zygomatic arch	Mandible (external surface)	Closes jaw	Cranial nerve V
Temporal	Temporal bone	Mandible	Closes jaw	Cranial nerve V
Pterygoids (internal and external)	Undersurface of skull	Mandible (mesial surface)	Grates teeth	Cranial nerve V

From Anthony CP, Thibodeau GA: *Textbook of anatomy and physiology,* ed 12, St Louis, 1987, Mosby.

Table 3-5

Muscles that Move the Head

Muscle	Origin	Insertion	Function	Innervation
Sternocleidomastoid	Sternum Clavicle	Temporal bone (mastoid process)	Flexes head (prayer muscle) One muscle alone, rotates head toward opposite side; spasm of this muscle alone or associated with trapezius called torticollis or wryneck	Accessory nerve
Semispinalis capitis	Vertebrae (transverse processes of upper six thoracic, articular processes of lower four cervical)	Occipital bone (between superior and inferior nuchal lines)	Extends head; bends it laterally	First five cervical nerves
Splenius capitis	Ligamentum nuchae Vertebrae (spinous processes of upper three or four thoracic)	Temporal bone (mastoid process) Occipital bone	Extends head Bends and rotates head toward same side as contracting muscle	Second, third, and fourth cervical nerves
Longissimus capitis	Vertebrae (transverse processes of upper six thoracic, articular processes of lower four cervical)	Temporal bone (mastoid process)	Extends head Bends and rotates head toward contracting side	

From Anthony CP, Thibodeau GA: *Textbook of anatomy and physiology,* ed 12, St Louis, 1987, Mosby.

Table 3-6

Muscles that Move the Shoulder

Muscle	Origin	Insertion	Function	Innervation
Trapezius	Occipital bone (protuberance)	Clavicle	Raises or lowers shoulders and shrugs them	Spinal accessory, second, third, and fourth cervical nerves
	Vertebrae (cervical and thoracic)	Scapula (spine and acromion)	Extends head when occiput acts as insertion	
Pectoralis minor	Ribs (second to fifth)	Scapula (coracoid)	Pulls shoulder down and forward	Medial and lateral anterior thoracic nerves
Serratus anterior	Ribs (upper eight or nine)	Scapula (anterior surface, vertebral border)	Pulls shoulder forward; abducts and rotates it upward	Long thoracic nerve

From Anthony CP, Thibodeau GA: *Textbook of anatomy and physiology,* ed 12, St Louis, 1987, Mosby.

E. Muscles that move the chest wall (Table 3-7)
F. Muscles that move the upper arm (Table 3-8)
G. Muscles that move the lower arm (Table 3-9)
H. Muscles that move the hand (Table 3-10)
I. Muscles that move the trunk (Table 3-11)

J. Muscles that move the pelvic floor (Table 3-12)
K. Muscles that move the abdominal wall (Table 3-13)
L. Muscles that move the thigh (Table 3-14)
M. Muscles that move the lower leg (Table 3-15)
N. Muscles that move the foot (Table 3-16)

Table 3-7

Muscles that Move the Chest Wall

Muscle	Origin	Insertion	Function	Innervation
External intercostals	Rib (lower border; forward fibers)	Rib (upper border of rib below origin)	Elevate ribs	Intercostal nerves
Internal intercostals	Rib (inner surface, lower border; backward fibers)	Rib (upper border of rib below origin)	Probably depress ribs	Intercostal nerves
Diaphragm	Lower circumference of thorax (of rib cage)	Central tendon of diaphragm	Enlarges thorax, causing inspiration	Phrenic nerves

From Anthony CP, Thibodeau GA: *Textbook of anatomy and physiology,* ed 12, St Louis, 1987, Mosby.

Table 3-8

Muscles that Move the Upper Arm

Muscle	Origin	Insertion	Function	Innervation
Pectoralis major	Clavicle (medial half) Sternum Costal cartilages of true ribs	Humerus (greater tubercle)	Flexes upper arm Adducts upper arm anteriorly; draws it across chest	Medial and lateral anterior thoracic nerves
Latissimus dorsi	Vertebrae (spines of lower thoracic, lumbar, and sacral) Ilium (crest) Lumbodorsal fascia	Humerus (intertubercular groove)	Extends upper arm Adducts upper arm posteriorly	Thoracodorsal nerve
Deltoid	Clavicle Scapula (spine and acromion)	Humerus (lateal side about halfway down—deltoid tubercle)	Abducts upper arm Assists in flexion and extension of upper arm	Axillary nerve
Coracobrachialis	Scapula (coracoid process)	Humerus (middle third, medial surface)	Adduction; assists in flexion and medial rotation of arm	Musculocutaneous nerve
Supraspinatus	Scapula (supraspinous fossa)	Humerus (greater tubercle)	Assists in abducting arm	Suprascapular nerve
Teres major	Scapula (lower part, axillary border)	Humerus (upper part, anterior surface)	Assists in extension, adduction, and medial rotation of arm	Lower subscapular nerve
Teres minor	Scapula (axillary border)	Humerus (greater tubercle)	Rotates arm outward	Axillary nerve
Infraspinatus	Scapula (infraspinatus border)	Humerus (greater tubercle)	Rotates arm outward	Suprascapular nerve

From Anthony CP, Thibodeau GA: *Textbook of anatomy and physiology,* ed 12, St Louis, 1987, Mosby.

Nervous System

A. Adapts to environmental influences by stimulating skeletal, cardiac, and smooth muscle; adaptation by the muscle system is almost immediate
1. Responds to various stimuli (chemical, electrical, mechanical, and thermal)
2. Stimulus must be at least at the threshold or liminal level; that is the weakest stimulus that will cause a response (Fig. 3-11, p. 85)
   a. Subthreshold stimulus is below the threshold level and will not produce an effect
   b. Maximal stimulus causes the maximum re-

Table 3-9

Muscles that Move the Lower Arm

Muscle	Origin	Insertion	Function	Innervation
Biceps brachii	Scapula (supraglenoid tuberosity) Scapula (coracoid)	Radius (tubercle at proximal end)	Flexes supinated forearm Supinates forearm and hand	Musculocutaneous nerve
Brachialis	Humerus (distal half, anterior surface)	Ulna (front of coronoid process)	Flexes pronated forearm	Musculocutaneous nerve
Brachioradialis	Humerus (above lateral epicondyle)	Radius (styloid process)	Flexes semipronated or semisupinated forearm; supinates forearm and hand	Radial nerve
Triceps brachii	Scapula (infraglenoid tuberosity) Humerus (posterior surface—lateral head above radial groove; medial head, below)	Ulna (olecranon process)	Extends lower arm	Radial nerve
Pronator teres	Humerus (medial epicondyle) Ulna (coronoid process)	Radius (middle third of lateral surface)	Pronates and flexes forearm	Median nerve
Pronator quadratus	Ulna (distal fourth, anterior surface)	Radius (distal fourth, anterior surface)	Pronates forearm	Median nerve
Supinator	Humerus (lateral epicondyle) Ulna (proximal fifth)	Radius (proximal third)	Supinates forearm	Radial nerve

From Anthony CP, Thibodeau GA: *Textbook of anatomy and physiology,* ed 12, St Louis, 1987, Mosby.

Table 3-10

Muscles that Move the Hand

Muscle	Origin	Insertion	Function	Innervation
Flexor carpi radialis	Humerus (medial epicondyle)	Second metacarpal (base of)	Flexes hand Flexes forearm	Median nerve
Palmaris longus	Humerus (medial epicondyle)	Fascia of palm	Flexes hand	Median nerve
Flexor carpi ulnaris	Humerus (medial epicondyle) Ulna (proximal two thirds)	Psiform bone Third, fourth, and fifth metacarpals	Flexes hand Adducts hand	Ulnar nerve
Extensor carpi radialis longus	Humerus (ridge above lateral epicondyle)	Second metacarpal (base of)	Extends hand Abducts hand (moves toward thumb side when hands supinated)	Radial nerve
Extensor carpi radialis brevis	Humerus (lateral epicondyle)	Second, third metacarpals (bases of)	Extends hand	Radial nerve
Extensor carpi ulnaris	Humerus (lateral epicondyle) Ulna (proximal three fourths)	Fifth metacarpal (base of)	Extends hand Adducts hand (move toward little finger side when hand supinated)	Radial nerve

From Anthony CP, Thibodeau GA: *Textbook of anatomy and physiology,* ed 12, St Louis, 1987, Mosby.

Table 3-11

Muscles that Move the Trunk

Muscle	Origin	Insertion	Function	Innervation
Sacrospinalis (erector spinae)			Extend spine; maintain erect posture of trunk Acting singly, abduct and rotate trunk	Posterior rami of first cervical to fifth lumbar spinal nerves
Lateral portion: Iliocostalis lumborum	Iliac crest, sacrum (posterior surface), and lumbar vertebrae (spinous processes)	Ribs, lower six		
Iliocostalis dorsi	Ribs, lower six	Ribs, upper six		
Iliocostalis cervicis	Ribs, upper six	Vertebrae, fourth to sixth cervical		
Medial portion: Longissimus dorsi	Same as iliocostalis lumborum	Vertebrae, thoracic ribs		
Longissimus cervicis	Vertebrae, upper six thoracic	Vertebrae, second to sixth cervical		
Longissimus capitis	Vertebrae, upper six thoracic and last four cervical	Temporal bone, mastoid process		
Quadratus lumborum (forms part of posterior abdominal wall)	Ilium (posterior part of crest) Vertebrae (lower three lumbar)	Ribs (twelfth) Vertebrae (transverse processes of first four lumbar)	Both muscles together extend spine One muscle alone abducts trunk toward side of contracting muscle	First three or four lumbar nerves
Iliopsoas	See muscles that move thigh		Flexes trunk	

From Anthony CP, Thibodeau GA: *Textbook of anatomy and physiology*, ed 12, St Louis, 1987, Mosby.

Table 3-12

Muscles of the Pelvic Floor

Muscle	Origin	Insertion	Function	Innervation
Levator ani	Pubic (posterior surface) Ischium (spine)	Coccyx	Together form floor of pelvic cavity; support pelvic organs; if these muscles are badly torn at childbirth or become too relaxed, uterus or bladder may prolapse, that is, drop out	Pudendal nerve
Coccygeus (posterior continuation of levator ani)	Ischium (spine)	Coccyx Sacrum	Same as levator ani	Pudendal nerve

From Anthony CP, Thibodeau GA: *Textbook of anatomy and physiology*, ed 12, St Louis, 1987, Mosby.

Table 3-13

Muscles that Move the Abdominal Wall

Muscle	Origin	Insertion	Function	Innervation
External oblique	Ribs (lower eight)	Ossa coxae (iliac and pubis by way of inguinal ligament) Linea alba by way of an aponeurosis	Compresses abdomen Important postural function of all abdominal muscles is to pull front of pelvis upward, thereby flattening lumbar curve of spine; when these muscles lose their tone, common figure faults of protruding abdomen and lordosis develop	Lower seven intercostal nerves and iliohypogastric nerves
Internal oblique	Ossa coxae (iliac crest and inguinal ligament) Lumbodorsal fascia	Ribs (lower three) Pubic bone Linea alba	Same as external oblique	Last three intercostal nerves; iliohypogastric and ilioinguinal nerves
Tranversalis	Ribs (lower six) Ossa coxae (iliac crest, inguinal ligament) Lumbodorsal fascia	Pubic bone Linea alba	Same as external oblique	Last five intercostal nerves; iliohypogastric and ilioinguinal nerves
Rectus abdominis	Ossa coxae (pubic bone and symphysis pubis)	Ribs (costal cartilage of fifth, sixth, and seventh ribs) Sternum (xiphoid process)	Same as external oblique; because abdominal muscles compress abdominal cavity, they aid in straining, defecation, forced expiration, childbirth, etc.; abdominal muscles are antagonists of diaphragm, relaxing as it contracts and vice versa Flexes trunk	Last six intercostal nerves

From Anthony CP, Thibodeau GA: *Textbook of anatomy and physiology,* ed 12, St Louis, 1987, Mosby.

sponse; if a higher stimulus is given, the same response will be produced
  c. Submaximal threshold is less than a maximal stimulus but greater than a threshold stimulus
 3. Basic requirements for a stimulus to be effective
  a. It must be sufficient strength
  b. It must be applied for a minimal duration of time
  c. It must produce a rapid rate of change in the environment
B. Organized into various systems
 1. Central nervous system (CNS) consists of the brain and spinal cord

2. Peripheral nervous system (PNS) contains the nerves to and from the body wall, which connect to the CNS; also known as the somatic division since it is under voluntary control
3. Autonomic nervous system (ANS) is not under conscious control (involuntary); provides stimulus for the viscera and smooth and cardiac muscle
  a. Sympathetic division (thoracolumbar) involves motor (afferent) nerves from the ANS
  b. Parasympathetic division (craniosacral) involves motor (efferent) nerves from the ANS
4. Nerve cell is called a neuron
  a. Structure
   (1) Cell body or soma contains a nucleus

Table 3-14

Muscles that Move the Thigh

Muscle	Origin	Insertion	Function	Innervation
Iliopsoas (iliacus and psoas major)	Ilium (iliac fossa) Vertebrae (bodies of twelfth thoracic to fifth lumbar)	Femur (small trochanter)	Flexes thigh Flexes trunk (when femur acts as origin)	Femoral and second to fourth lumbar nerves
Rectus femoris	Ilium (anterior, inferior spine)	Tibia (by way of patellar tendon)	Flexes thigh Extends lower leg	Femoral nerve
Gluteal group				
Maximus	Ilium (crest and posterior surface) Sacrum and coccyx (posterior surface) Sacrotuberous ligament	Femur (gluteal tuberosity) Iliotibial tract	Extends thigh—rotates outward	Inferior gluteal nerve
Medius	Ilium (lateral surface)	Femur (greater trochanter)	Abducts thigh—rotates outward; stabilizes pelvis on femur	Superior gluteal nerve
Minimus	Ilium (lateral surface)	Femur (greater trochanter)	Abducts thigh; stabilizes pelvis on femur Rotates thigh medially	Superior gluteal nerve
Tensor fasciae latae	Ilium (anterior part of crest)	Tibia (by way of iliotibial tract)	Abducts thigh Tightens iliotibial tract	Superior gluteal nerve
Piriformis	Vertebrae (front of sacrum)	Femur (medial aspect of greater trochanter)	Rotates thigh outward Abducts thigh Extends thigh	First or second sacral nerves
Adductor group				
Brevis	Pubic bone	Femur (linea aspera)	Adducts thigh	Obturator nerve
Longus	Pubic bone	Femur (linea aspera)	Adducts thigh	Obturator nerve
Magnus	Pubic bone	Femur (linea aspera)	Adducts thigh	Obturator nerve
Gracilis	Pubic bone (just below symphysis)	Tibia (medial surface behind sartorius)	Adducts thigh and flexes and adducts leg	Obturator nerve

From Anthony CP, Thibodeau GA: *Textbook of anatomy and physiology,* ed 12, St Louis, 1987, Mosby.

(which has a distinct nucleal pattern); is not capable of reproducing nerve cells

(2) Neurofibrils are threadlike fibers in the interior of the nerve cells; contain typical cytoplasm structures plus Nissl granules (clusters of ribonucleic acid [RNA])

(3) Dendrite carries impulse toward the cell body under normal conditions

(4) Axon carries impulse away from the cell body and makes contact with the next cell at the button that contains chemicals in vesicles; release of chemicals starts impulse in the next neuron

(5) Myelin sheath is a fatty substance around some cell axons; provides insulation

    (a) Myelin is laid down by Schwann cells in layers

    (b) Neuron must have a neurilemma to regenerate

    (c) Nodes of Ranvier are between myelin segments and are unmyelinated

b. Neurons can carry impulses in different directions

(1) Afferent neurons carry the sensory information to the CNS

(2) Efferent neurons carry the motor information away from the CNS

(3) Central or internuncial neurons are found entirely within the CNS; relay information within the system

c. Neurons have various numbers of processes

(1) Unipolar—one process from the cell body

(2) Bipolar—two distinct processes arising from opposite poles of the cell body

Table 3-15

Muscles that Move the Lower Leg

Muscle	Origin	Insertion	Function	Innervation
Quadriceps femoris group				
Rectus femoris	Ilium (anterior, inferior spine)	Tibia (by way of patellar tendon)	Flexes thigh Extends leg	Femoral nerve
Vastus lateralis	Femur (linea aspera)	Tibia (by way of patellar tendon)	Extends leg	Femoral nerve
Vastus medialis	Femur	Tibia (by way of patellar tendon)	Extends leg	Femoral nerve
Vastus intermedius	Femur (anterior surface)	Tibia (by way of patellar tendon)	Extends leg	Femoral nerve
Sartorius	Os innominatum (anterior, superior iliac spines)	Tibia (medial surface of upper end of shaft)	Adducts and flexes leg Permits crossing of legs tailor fashion	Femoral nerve
Hamstring group				
Biceps femoris	Ischium (tuberosity)	Fibula (head of)	Flexes leg	Hamstring nerve (branch of sciatic nerve)
	Femur (linea aspera)	Tibia (lateral condyle)	Extends thigh	Hamstring nerve
Semitendinosus	Ischium (tuberosity)	Tibia (proximal end, medial surface)	Extends thigh	Hamstring nerve
Semimembranosus	Ischium (tuberosity)	Tibia (medial condyle)	Extends thigh	Hamstring nerve

From Anthony CP, Thibodeau GA: *Textbook of anatomy and physiology,* ed 12, St Louis, 1987, Mosby.

Table 3-16

Muscles that Move the Foot

Muscle	Origin	Insertion	Function	Innervation
Tibialis anterior	Tibia (lateral condyle of upper body)	Tarsal (first cuneiform) Metatarsal (bone of first)	Flexes foot Inverts foot	Common and deep peroneal nerves
Gastrocnemius	Femur (condyles)	Tarsal (calcaneus by way of Achilles tendon)	Extends foot Flexes lower leg	Tibial nerves (branch of sciatic nerve)
Soleus	Tibia (underneath gastrocnemius)	Tarsal (calcaneus by way of Achilles tendon)	Extends foot (plantar flexion)	Tibial nerve
Peroneus longus	Tibia (lateral condyle) Fibula (head and shaft)	First cuneiform Base of first metatarsal	Extends foot (plantar flexion) Everts foot	Common peroneal nerve
Peroneus brevis	Fibula (lower two thirds of lateral surface of shaft)	Fifth metatarsal (tubercle, dorsal surface)	Everts foot Flexes foot	Superficial peroneal nerve
Tibialis posterior	Tibia (posterior surface) Fibula (posterior surface)	Navicular bone Cuboid bone All three cuneiforms Second and fourth metatarsals	Extends foot (plantar flexion) Inverts foot	Tibial nerve
Peroneus tertius	Fibula (distal third)	Fourth and fifth metatarsals (base of)	Flexes foot Everts foot	Deep peroneal nerve

From Anthony CP, Thibodeau GA: *Textbook of anatomy and physiology,* ed 12, St Louis, 1987, Mosby.

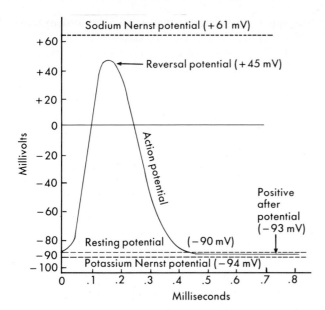

Fig. 3-11 Action potential. (From Guyton AC: *Textbook of medical physiology,* ed 8, Philadelphia, 1990, WB Saunders.)

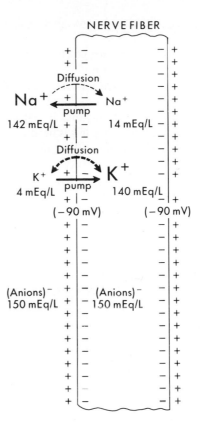

Fig. 3-12 Membrane potential. (From Guyton AC: *Textbook of medical physiology,* ed 8, Philadelphia, 1990, WB Saunders.)

(3) Multipolar—contain several processes, usually an axon and three or more dendrites

C. Nerve impulse results from a change in the membrane potential (Fig. 3-12)

1. Membrane potential results from the concentration difference of two ions on the inside and outside of the nerve

2. Inside the axon membrane

$$[K^+] = 141mEq/L$$
$$[Na^+] = 10mEq/L$$ at rest

3. Outside the axon membrane

$$[K^+] = 4mEq/L$$
$$[Na^+] = 137mEq/L$$ at rest

4. Balance is mostly maintained by the sodium pump; potassium pump is not very important in this phenomenon because the membrane is extremely permeable to potassium

5. A void of positive electrons is created on the inside; leads to a state of electronegativity that gives a reading of −65 mV to −85 mV on the voltmeter
   a. Creates the depolarization wave or nerve impulse (+35 mV)
   b. Law of forward conduction—impulse can leave in only one direction

6. Vesicles in the buttons are ruptured; various chemicals are released to carry the impulse to the next neuron
   a. Acetylcholine is released at all preganglionic fibers of the ANS, at all postganglionic fibers of the parasympathetic division, at some of the sympathetic fibers of the parasympathetic division, and at all of the motor neurons at the myoneural junction (cholinergic fibers)
   b. Acetylcholine is destroyed by acetylcholinesterase, so nerve stimulation will be for a definite amount of time
   c. Norepinephrine is released by the adrenergic fibers (most of the sympathetic postganglionic nerve fibers)
   d. Norepinephrine is destroyed by monoamine oxidase

7. Immediately after the depolarization wave the nerve is repolarized because the membrane becomes impermeable to sodium ions but potassium can diffuse back in the membrane; this high potassium concentration causes the positive electrons to migrate outward, creating electronegativity inside the membrane

8. Refractory period—nerve will not react to another stimulus
   a. Absolute refractory period—will not react to any stimulus no matter how strong the stimu-

lus; will extend through the depolarization stage

    b. Relative refractory phase—can produce a response if the stimulus is stronger than the original; starts at repolarization and prevents nerve impulses from piling up

  9. Once an impulse begins, it remains constant throughout the nerve if it is healthy

    a. Greatest velocity will be over a coarse, myelinated nerve

    b. Least velocity will be over a fine, nonmyelinated nerve

    c. All-or-none principle in effect

    d. Graded response; the stronger the stimulus, the more impulses per second

 10. Nerve impulses can be blocked by pressure, chemicals, or cold

    a. Sensory nerves are usually blocked before motor nerves

    b. Strychnine reduces resistance at the synapse; leads to convulsions

    c. Curare causes increased resistance at the synapse; produces paralysis

 11. Nerves cannot store glycogen; need a constant supply of glycogen; can also function without oxygen for short periods

D. Spinal cord is approximately 45.8 cm long; occupies the upper two thirds of the vertebral canal

  1. Conus medullaris—pointed up where the spinal cord terminates between the L1 and L2 vertebrae

  2. Filum terminale—thin threadlike fiber from the coccyx to the spinal cord; acts as an anchor; has no nervous function

  3. Cauda equina—bundle of spinal nerve roots located below the L1 vertebra

  4. Has a unique structure in cross section (Fig. 3-13)

E. There are 31 pairs of spinal nerves; each has a dorsal (afferent) root and a ventral (efferent) root

  1. Spinal nerves come out of the spinal cord to form plexuses along the spinal cord except in the thoracic region

    a. Cervical plexus—first four cervical nerves innervate the muscles and skin of the upper chest; phrenic nerve originates here and innervates the diaphragm

    b. Brachial plexus—base of the neck; fifth to eighth cervical nerves and first thoracic nerve provide nerves to the shoulders and arms

      (1) Radial—lateral side of the arm

      (2) Medial—middle portion of the arm

      (3) Ulnar—medial side of the arm

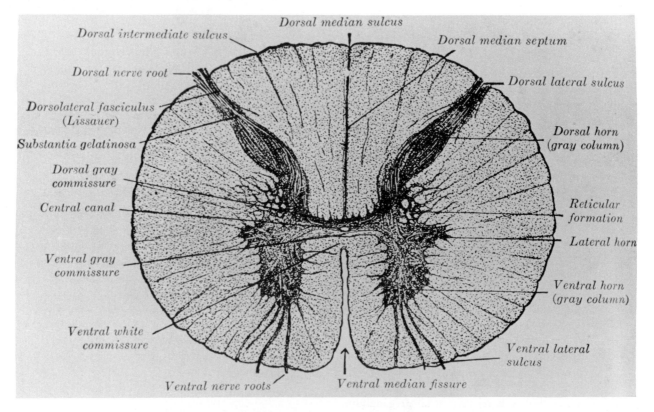

Fig. 3-13 Cross section of spinal cord. (From Clement CD: *Gray's anatomy,* American ed 30, Philadelphia, 1985, Lea & Febiger.)

c. T2 to T12 compose the intercostal nerves; do not form a plexus

d. Lumbrosacral plexus—includes L1 to S4

   (1) Lumbar portion—first four lumbar nerves contribute to the femoral nerve

   (2) Sacral portion—sacral nerves, last lumbar nerve, and coccygeal nerve supply the pelvis and legs; contribute to the sciatic nerve (largest nerve in the body)

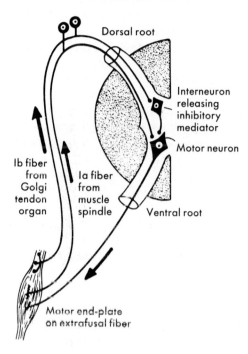

Fig. 3-14 Pathways responsible for stretch reflex. (From Ganong WF: *Review of medical physiology,* ed 15, Norwalk, Conn, 1991, Appleton & Lange.)

F. Spinal cord acts as a relay and reflex center

1. Reflex—unconscious response
2. Reflex arc—structures over which the reflex impulses pass (Fig. 3-14)
3. Conditioned reflex—becomes unconscious after repeated reinforcement (e.g., walking)
4. Simple reflex—involves only one set of muscles
5. Coordinated reflex—several reflexes performed in an orderly manner
6. Convulsive reflex—several reflexes performed in a random order
7. First-level spinal reflex—impulse enters the spinal cord and passes out of the same nerve
   a. Involves three neurons
     (1) Impulse picked up by the receptor and passed over to the afferent neuron (afferent neuron enters the spinal cord via the dorsal root)
     (2) In the posterior horn of the gray matter the afferent neuron synapses with the central or association neuron
     (3) Central neuron passes to the anterior horn and synapses with the efferent neuron
     (4) Efferent neuron leaves the spinal cord via the ventral root; passes to a muscle or gland and produces action
8. Second-level spinal reflex—impulse goes up or down the spinal cord; may involve the cerebellum or medulla
9. Third-level reflex—involves the cerebrum; most complex reflex arc

G. Fiber tracts are bundles of white fibers with the same origin (cell body location) and termination (axon button location) (Fig. 3-15)

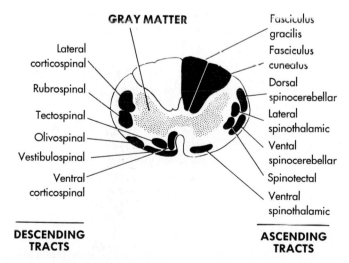

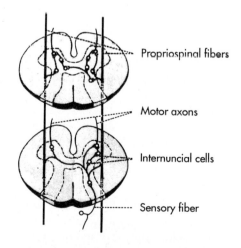

Fig. 3-15 Motor and sensory tracts in spinal cord. (From Guyton AC: *Physiology of the human body,* ed 8, Philadelphia, 1990, WB Saunders.)

1. All ascending fibers are afferent
   a. First-order neuron—associated with receptors; cell body located in the dorsal root ganglion
   b. Second-order neuron—passes up the spinal cord
   c. Third-order neuron—located in the brain; terminates in the outside layer of the cortex
2. All descending fibers are efferent
   a. Upper motor neurons—extend down the brain from the spinal cord and end in the ventral gray matter
   b. Lower motor neurons—cell body located in the ventral gray matter and goes out to muscles or glands
3. Ascending tracts
   a. Fasciculus gracilis—fibers from pressure and touch receptors; provides proprioception; involves first-order neurons
   b. Fasciculus cuneatus—first-order neurons pick up impulses from the skin; nerves travel up either side of the spinal cord to the medulla; make a synapse with a second-order neuron; this neuron crosses to the opposite side to the thalamus, synapses with a third-order neuron, and finally reaches the cerebral cortex
   c. Spinothalamic tract—second-order neurons cross over to the opposite side and can pass up the spinal cord
      (1) Ventral (nerves associated with touch)—synapses with the third-order neuron and ends in the cortex
      (2) Lateral (nerves associated with pain and temperature)—involves the second-order neurons that end in the thalamus
4. Descending tracts
   a. Lateral corticospinal—originates in the motor cortex; crosses over in the medulla and continues down the spinal cord on the opposite side (main motor tract)
   b. Ventral corticospinal—crosses over (decussates) in the spinal cord; provides voluntary responses
   c. Rubrospinal—originates in the midbrain; decussates immediately and comes down on the opposite side of the brain (coordinates muscles to maintain balance)
H. Brain consists of four regions (Fig. 3-16)
   1. Cerebrum—seat of conscious activities; largest portion of brain; located most superiorly
      a. Cerebral cortex—thin, outside layer; gray color; consists of several layers of cells; convoluted surface
      b. Longitudinal fissure—divides into two hemispheres
      c. Corpus callosum—heavy band of white fibers; forms the floor of the longitudinal fissure
      d. Central fissure—posterior to the midline
      e. Frontal lobe—anterior to the central fissure
      f. Parietal lobe—posterior to the central fissure
      g. Temporal lobe—below the lateral fissure
      h. Occipital lobe—posterior part of the brain
      i. Broca's area—controls the muscular part of speech
      j. Somasthetic area—interprets body sensations
      k. Visual area—fibers from the medial part of the retina cross to opposite sides in the brain; fibers from the lateral portion do not cross
      l. Auditory area—superior central portion of the temporal lobe
      m. Prefrontal area—personality characteristics
      n. Aphasia—results from damage to the cerebral cortex
   2. Cerebellum—coordinates balance and equilibrium
      a. Cortex—consists of gray matter
      b. Vermis—bridgelike connection between the two hemispheres
      c. Arbor vitae—white matter in the cerebellum; similar to leaf veins
      d. Ataxia—results from damage to the cortex of the cerebellum
   3. Medulla oblongata—bulb of the spinal cord located inside the foramen magnum
      a. White on the outside; gray on the inside
      b. Controls three vital functions: cardiac, respiratory, and vasomotor
      c. Also controls mastication, salivation, swallowing, emesis, lacrimation, blinking, coughing, and sneezing
      d. Pons—ropelike mass of white fibers; connects the halves of the cerebellum
   4. Mesencephalon—short part of the brainstem above the pons—mostly white matter
      a. Tectum—four large ropelike masses
      b. Cerebral aqueduct—connects the third and fourth ventricles of the brain
      c. Corpora quadrigemina
         (1) Colliculus superior—inferior pair; synapse cranial nerves II and III
         (2) Colliculus inferior—inferior pair; relay point of cranial nerve VIII
      d. Cerebral peduncles—make up the ventral columns of white fibers
      e. Reticular formation—acts as a clearing station for information; is associated with muscular movement; damage to this area results in coma
I. Meninges are the membranous coverings of the brain and spinal cord

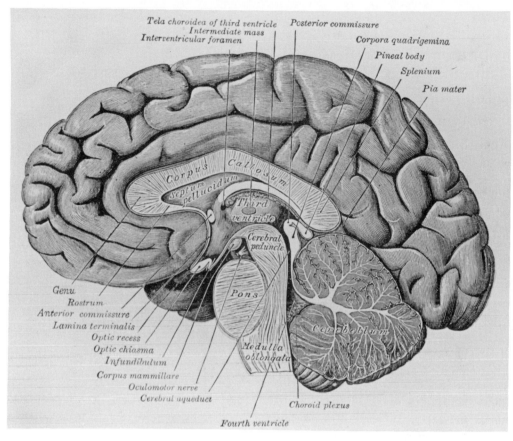

Fig. 3-16   Brain. (From Clemente CD. *Gray's anatomy*, American ed 30, Philadelphia, 1985, Lea & Febiger.)

1. Dura mater—double layers around the brain; single layer around the spinal cord including the cauda equina
2. Arachnoid—membrane just inside the dura mater; relatively thin; is attached via the arachnoid of cranial nerve VIII
3. Pia mater—soft covering that fits against the brain and spinal cord; contains an enormous amount of blood
   a. Leptomeninges—soft, delicate membrane; consists of the arachnoid and pia mater
   b. Subarachnoid space—threadlike structure where cerebrospinal fluid circulates; located between the pia mater and arachnoid
J. Cranial nerves are part of the PNS and originate at the base of the brain (Fig. 3-17); there are 12 pairs of cranial nerves, which can be referred to by name or by Roman numerals; can provide motor impulses, sensory impulses, or mixed impulses
   1. Olfactory nerve (cranial nerve I)—provides the sensation of smell by innervating the olfactory epithelium of the nasal cavity
      a. Does not provide motor function
      b. Originates in the olfactory bulb of the brain;

passes through the cribriform plate of the ethmoid bone
2. Optic nerve (cranial nerve II)—innervates the retina of the eye with sensory neurons; provides the sensation of vision
   a. Does not provide motor function
   b. Originates from the base of the brain; forms two optic tracts that converge at the optic chiasma; passes through the optic canal (foramen)
3. Oculomotor nerve (cranial nerve III)—provides motor fiber for the ocular muscles and parasympathetic fibers for the ciliary ganglion
   a. Primarily a motor nerve but contains some proprioceptive fibers from the brain
   b. Originates near the pons and enters the superior orbital fissure; has two divisions: superior and inferior
4. Trochlear nerve (cranial nerve IV)—smallest cranial nerve; supplies the superior oblique muscle of the eyeball
   a. Does not provide sensory function
   b. Originates near the optic tract; passes through the superior orbital fissure

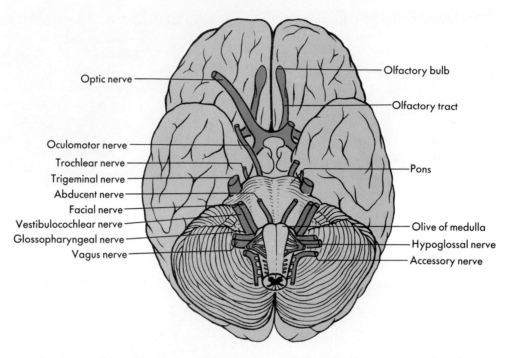

Fig. 3-17 Basal view of brain showing cranial nerves. (From McClintic JR: *Human anatomy,* St Louis, 1983, Mosby.)

5. Trigeminal nerve (cranial nerve V)—provides motor and sensory neurons
   a. Originates from two roots from the pons: a large sensory root and a small motor root
   b. Fibers are mixed in the trigeminal ganglion; produce three branches
      (1) Ophthalmic branch (cranial nerve V_1)—provides sensory fibers only; produces three nerves; passes through the superior orbital fissure
         (a) Lacrimal nerve
         (b) Nasociliary nerve
         (c) Frontal nerve
      (2) Maxillary branch (cranial nerve V_2)—provides sensory fibers only; produces several nerves; passes through the foramen rotundum to the pterygopalatine fossa (Table 3-17)
      (3) Mandibular branch (cranial nerve V_3)—provides motor and sensory fibers; produces several nerves; passes through the foramen ovale to the infratemporal fossa (Table 3-18)
6. Abducens nerve (cranial nerve VI)—provides motor fibers to the rectus lateralis muscle of the eyeball; passes through the superior orbital fissure
   a. Does not provide sensory fibers
   b. Originates at the inferior border of the pons

7. Facial nerve (cranial nerve VIII)—has two roots of unequal size; provides motor and sensory fibers
   a. Originates at the base of the pons; emerges from the stylomastoid foramen
   b. Innervates the muscles of facial expression: the buccinator, platysma, stapedius, stylohyoid, and the posterior belly of the digastric muscles
   c. Provides fibers to the submandibular and sublingual salivary gland
   d. Provides the taste sensation in the anterior two thirds of the tongue (gives all sensations except bitter)
   e. Branches from the geniculate ganglion; greater petrosal nerve provides sensory fibers to the soft palate
   f. Branches from the pterygopalatine plexus; innervates the lacrimal glands and the mucous membrane of the nose and palate
   g. Branch of the facial nerve within the facial canal is the chorda tympani—unites with the lingual nerve (cranial nerve V_3) to provide taste to the anterior two thirds of the tongue
   h. Branches from the submandibular ganglion; innervates the submandibular and sublingual glands
   i. Branches of the facial nerve in the face and neck

Table 3-17

Maxillary Branch (V$_2$) of the Trigeminal Nerve

Location	Comments	Branch
Cranium		Middle meningeal
	Foramen rotundum	Zygomatic
		Pterygopalatine branches; distribution from ganglion
	Inferior orbital fissure	Orbital
Pterygopalatine fossa		Greater (anterior) palatine
	Pterygopalatine canal	Posterior inferior nasal
	Greater (anterior) palatine	Lesser (posterior) palatine
	Lesser (posterior) palatine foramen	
	Sphenopalatine foramen	Posterior superior nasal
	Incisive foramen	Nasopalatine
	Pharyngeal foramen	Pharyngeal
	Posterior superior alveolar foramen	Posterior superior alveolar
Infraorbital groove and canal	Infraorbital fissure	Middle superior alveolar
	Infraorbital nerve	Anterior superior alveolar
Face	Infraorbital foramen	Inferior palpebral
		External nasal
		Superior labial

Table 3-18

Mandibular Branch (V$_3$) of the Trigeminal Nerve

Location	Comments	Branch
Main trunk	Foramen ovale	Nervus spinosus (ramus meningeus)
	Foramen spinosum	Medial pterygoid (M)
		Tensor veli palatini
	Auditory tube	Tensor tympani (M)
Anterior division		Masseteric (M)
	Mandibular notch	Deep temporal (M)
		Lateral pterygoid (M)
		Long buccal (buccinator)
		Auriculotemporal
		Otic ganglion—6 branches
Posterior division		Lingual nerve
		Chorda tympani (cranial nerve VII)
		Submandibular ganglion
		Hypoglossal (cranial nerve XII)
	Mandibular foramen	Inferior alveolar
	Mandibular canal	Mylohyoid (M)
		Dental branches
	Mental foramen	Mental and incisive (4)

M, Muscle.

(1) Posterior auricular nerve supplies the occipital muscle

(2) Digastric branch supplies the posterior belly of the digastric muscle

(3) Stylohyoid branch supplies the stylohyoid muscle

(4) Temporal branch supplies the frontalis, orbicularis oculi, and corrugator muscles

(5) Zygomatic branches innervate the orbicularis oculi

(6) Buccal branches supply the procerus, zygomaticus, levator labii superioris, buccinator, and orbicularis oris muscles

(7) Mandibular branch supplies the muscles of the lower lip and chin

8. Acoustic nerve (cranial nerve VIII)—originates in the middle peduncle by the pons; passes through the internal auditory meatus

   a. Provides sensory nerve fibers only

   b. Vestibular nerve division innervates the semicircular canals of the ear; controls equilibrium

   c. Cochlear nerve innervates the cochlea; provides the sensation of sound

9. Glossopharyngeal nerve (cranial nerve IX)—originates in the superior aspect of the medulla oblongata; passes through the jugular foramen

   a. Mixed nerve that provides taste to the posterior one third of the tongue, motor function to the muscles of the throat, and secretory fibers to the parotid salivary gland

   b. Tympanic nerve supplies of the parotid gland and the mucous membrane covering of the middle ear; its continuation through the tensor tympani is known as the lesser petrosal nerve

   c. Carotid sinus nerve provides sensory fibers for the carotid sinus; main function is to monitor blood pressure

   d. Pharyngeal branches supply the muscular pharynx

   e. Tonsillar branch supplies the palatine tonsils

   f. Lingual branches innervate the circumvallate papillae

10. Vagus nerve (cranial nerve X)—has the widest distribution of any nerve in the body; is the dominant nerve to the heart; originates in the medulla oblongata; leaves the cranial cavity through the jugular foramen

    a. Provides sensory fibers to the larynx, lungs, arch of the aorta, and stomach; provides motor fibers to the heart, stomach, small intestine, larynx, esophagus, and gastric glands

    b. Right vagus nerve crosses the subclavian artery; forms the posterior pulmonary plexus by following the dorsal aspect of the lung; continues on to form the posterior vagus nerve

    c. Left vagus nerve passes between the left carotid and subclavian arteries; also forms a posterior pulmonary plexus on the dorsal surface of the lung; joins the right vagus nerve above the diaphragm to form the anterior vagus nerve

    d. Superior laryngeal nerve contributes motor and sensory fibers to the larynx

    e. Recurrent nerves—the right one loops under the subclavian artery and innervates the muscles of the larynx; the left one loops under the arch of the aorta and innervates all muscles of the larynx except one

    f. Inferior cardiac branches innervate the cardiac muscle and great vessels

    g. Esophageal branches innervate the esophagus

    h. Branches continue through the abdominal cavity; form gastric, hepatic, and celiac branches

11. Accessory nerve (cranial nerve XI)—provides motor fibers to the muscles of the upper trunk region; consists of a cranial and spinal part

    a. Provides motor fibers to the muscles of the shoulder

    b. Cranial portion originates in the medulla oblongata and exits the cranial cavity through the jugular foramen; its fibers are distributed to the soft palate, pharynx, larynx, and esophagus

    c. Spinal part originates from the first five cervical segments of the spinal cord; pass up through the foramen magnum to join the cranial portion of cranial nerve XI; gives motor innervation to the sternocleidomastoid and trapezius muscles

12. Hypoglossal nerve (cranial nerve XII)—originates from the medulla oblongata and runs through the hypoglossal canal

    a. Provides motor fibers for the tongue muscles

    b. Forms the ansa cervicalis near the cricoid cartilage

K. ANS is the coordinator of internal actions; used to regulate (not initiate) the rate of internal action

   1. Sympathetic division (thoracolumbar) is located on either side of the spine

      a. Actions involve a great expenditure of energy

      b. Cell bodies of the preganglionic neurons are found in the gray matter of the spinal columns; are cholinergic in nature

      c. Cell bodies of the postganglionic neurons are found in the ganglia near the spinal cord; release norepinephrine as neurotransmitter substance fibers

	Table 3-19	

Autonomic Nervous System

Visceral effector	Effect of sympathetic stimulation (neurotransmitter, norepinephrine unless otherwise stated)	Effect of parasympathetic stimulation (neurotransmitter, acetylcholine)
Heart	Increased rate and strength of heartbeat (beta receptors)	Decreased rate and strength of heartbeat
SMOOTH MUSCLE OF BLOOD VESSELS		
Skin blood vessels	Constriction (alpha receptors)	No parasympathetic fibers
Skeletal muscle blood vessels	Dilation (beta receptors)	No parasympathetic fibers
Coronary blood vessels	Dilation (beta receptors)	No parasympathetic fibers
Abdominal blood vessels	Constriction (alpha receptors)	No parasympathetic fibers
Blood vessels of external genitals	Ejaculation (contraction of smooth muscle in male ducts, e.g., epididymis and vas deferens)	Dilation of blood vessels causing erection in male
SMOOTH MUSCLE OF HOLLOW ORGANS AND SPHINCTERS		
Bronchi	Dilation (beta receptors)	Constriction
Digestive tract, except sphincters	Decreased peristalsis (beta receptors)	Increased peristalsis
Sphincters of digestive tract	Contraction (alpha receptors)	Relaxation
Urinary bladder	Relaxation (beta receptors)	Contraction
Urinary sphincters	Contraction (alpha receptors)	Relaxation
Eye		
Iris	Contraction of radial muscle; dilated pupil	Contraction of circular muscle; constricted pupil
Ciliary	Relaxation; accommodates for far vision	Contraction; accommodates for near vision
Hairs (pilomotor muscles)	Contraction produces goose pimples, or piloerection (alpha receptors)	No parasympathetic fibers
GLANDS		
Sweat	Increased sweat (neurotransmitter, acetylcholine)	No parasympathetic fibers
Digestive (salivary, gastric, etc.)	Decreased secretion of saliva; not known for others	Increased secretion of saliva
Pancreas, including islets	Decreased secretion	Increased secretion of pancreatic juice and insulin
Liver	Increased glycogenolysis (beta receptors); increases blood sugar level	No parasympathetic fibers
Adrenal medulla	Increased epinephrine secretion	No parasympathetic fibers

From Anthony CP, Thibodeau GA: *Textbook of anatomy and physiology,* ed 12, St Louis, 1987, Mosby.

2. Parasympathetic division (craniosacral) is formed by nerves from the brain and sacrum
   a. This system is active except under stress
   b. Cell bodies of the preganglionic neurons are found in various nuclei of the brain and sacral segments of the spinal cord; use acetylcholine at the neurotransmitter junctions
   c. Cell bodies of the postganglionic neurons are usually located near the organs that they innervate; release acetylcholine
3. Fight-or-flight mechanism prepares the body to deal with stresses; sympathetic and parasympathetic systems tend to produce opposite effects (Table 3-19)

Special Senses

A. Eyeball is located in the orbital fossa for protection; is surrounded by fat
   1. Eyelids—keep the eyes moist and clear; blinking reflex is controlled by the medulla
   2. Eyelashes—shade the eyeball and protect it

3. Conjunctiva—thin mucous membrane that covers the front of the eye and lines the eyelid
4. Lacrimal glands—located bilaterally on the outer border of the orbital cavity; secrete about 1 ml of fluid per day; contain lysozyme to destroy bacteria
5. Nasolacrimal duct—carries fluid away from the gland
6. Contains intrinsic and extrinsic muscles of the eye
7. Parts of the eyeball
   a. Iris—colored part of the eye that is a circular diaphragm; regulates the amount of light that enters the eye
   b. Pupil—where light enters the eye; black in color
   c. Lens—biconvex disk without blood
   d. Sclera—white covering on the anterior aspect of the eye
   e. Vitreous body—colloid inside of the eyeball; maintains the shape
   f. Optic disk—located on the posterior surface of the eyeball; contains no rods or cones, only optic nerves
   g. Retina—contains cones in its center (fovea) and rods on the outer periphery
8. Physical process of forming an image on the retina is much like that used by a camera to produce a picture
   a. Light rays are bent as they enter the eye
   b. Lens adjusts to the amount of light
   c. Light rays are converged on the fovea
   d. Rays cause changes in the chemistry of the rods and cones
   e. Optic nerve sends impulses to the occipital lobes of the brain
B. Ear controls the sense of hearing
   1. External ear consists of an ear flap
   2. Middle ear is separated by the tympanic membrane (eardrum); contains the ossicles (malleus, incus, and stapes) and eustachian tube (to equalize pressure)
   3. Inner ear contains a vestibule, cochlea, and the semicircular canals
      a. Cranial nerve VIII innervates this structure
      b. Small hairs detect various frequencies and pitches; impulses are sent to the temporal lobes of the brain
      c. Semicircular canals maintain equilibrium
C. Tongue provides the sensation of taste
   1. Cranial nerve VIII provides sensory fibers to the anterior two thirds of the tongue, including the fungiform and foliate papillae; sensations of sweet, sour, and salt are detected
   2. Cranial nerve IX provides sensations of taste to the posterior one third of the tongue's circumvallate papillae; taste sensation of bitter is noted here

3. Food must be in solution in the mouth before the tastebuds can transfer the information to the brain
4. Most taste sensations are made up of various combinations of the four basic tastes
5. Olfactory system also provides sensory input to taste detection (cranial nerve I)
D. Olfactory sense is provided through the cranial nerve I
   1. Stimulates hairs (upper nasal cavity)
   2. Sensitive to slight odors
E. Sensation of touch is modulated by various nerve endings
   1. Meissner's corpuscles control the sensation of touch
   2. Pacinian corpuscles control the sensation of pressure
   3. Ruffini's corpuscles control the sensation of heat
   4. Krause's end bulbs control the sensation of cold
   5. Naked nerve fibers produce pain when stimulated

Blood

Blood is a connective tissue that originates from embryonic mesoderm
A. Serves the following body functions: nutrition, respiration, fluid balance, acid-base balance, excretion, protection, temperature regulation, and as an endocrine adjunct
   1. Whole blood has a specific gravity of 1.055 and a viscosity three to five times greater than that of water; makes up 9% of the total body; an adult has approximately 5 L of blood; pH remains fairly constant
   2. If whole blood is centrifuged in a test tube, various components can be separated out
      a. Plasma—clear straw color; at top (55%)
      b. White blood cells (WBCs)—white line in the center (less than 1%)
      c. Red blood cells (RBCs)—red color (45%)
   3. Hematocrit measures the volume of RBCs in blood by percent
      a. Women—less than 45%
      b. Men—greater than or equal to 45%
B. Consists of plasma and three cellular elements
   1. Erythrocytes (RBCs) transfer oxygen to the body and remove carbon dioxide
   2. Leukocytes (WBCs) are involved in the body's immune and protective function
   3. Thrombocytes (platelets) are involved in blood coagulation
   4. Plasma composes the fluid portion of the blood: 90% water plus 10% proteins and solids
      a. Serum albumin—important in maintaining osmotic pressure

b. Globulins—important in maintaining osmotic pressure

c. Fibrinogen—important for coagulation of blood; converted to fibrin to form the blood clot

d. Nonprotein nitrogenous material (NPN)—amino acids and urea

e. Nonnitrogenous materials—carbohydrates and fats

f. Others—inorganic salts and bicarbonate buffers

C. Three types of cells (RBCs, WBCs, and platelets) in blood are unique in both their structure and functions

1. Erythrocytes are biconcave disks that do not contain a nucleus; the advantages of a disk shape are that it allows for greater surface area for absorption and diffusion and allows for greater flexibility

   a. Cells stack up like coins (rouleaux formation) when they are out of circulation

   b. Hematocrit is measured by a hemocytometer; is reported in millimeters cubed
      (1) Women—4.7 mm^3
      (2) Men—5.4 mm^3

   c. Elevation in the hematocrit is known as polycythemia; polycythemia vera is a serious pathologic condition that is often caused by a malignant tumor in the bone marrow and leads to sluggish blood, which damages the heart and other vessels

   d. Hemoglobin (Hb) is a functional part of the RBC and is a protein-pigment compound; a combination of acetic acid and glycine forms protoporphyrin; protoporphyrin plus one atom of iron produce the heme molecule; four heme molecules plus one globin form hemoglobin; each iron atom combines loosely with one molecule of oxygen to form oxyhemoglobin (HbO$_2$); this compound is very quick at combining and breaking down
      (1) Blood will appear bright scarlet if the tissue has less oxygen than the blood
      (2) Oxyhemoglobin breaks up and gives up the oxygen; becomes reduced hemoglobin (HHb), which looks blue through the tissue
      (3) Fetal hemoglobin (HbF) will pick up oxygen faster than adult hemoglobin (HbA)

   e. Formation of blood, erythropoiesis, occurs in the red bone marrow of the adult in the ribs, sternum, vertebrae, and angle of the mandible

   f. Effete RBCs are removed from circulation by the liver and spleen

2. WBCs (leukocytes) average 7500/mm^3 in number

   a. An increase in WBCs is known as leukocytosis; a decrease is called leukopenia

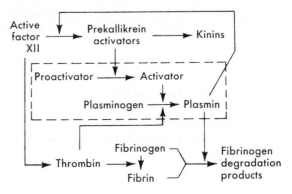

Fig. 3-18   Clotting scheme. (From Ganong WF: *Review of medical physiology*, ed 15, Norwalk, Conn, 1991, Appleton & Lange.)

   b. All WBCs have nuclei that aid in their identification

   c. Granulocytes are the most numerous
      (1) Neutrophils—most common with a polynuclear pattern; have an ameboid movement
      (2) Eosinophils—double-lobed nucleus with red granules; function in detoxification
      (3) Basophils—S-shaped nucleus with blue granules; produce heparin

   d. Agranulocytes
      (1) Lymphocytes—large nucleus with a small amount of cytoplasm; involved in the immune system
      (2) Monocytes—C-shaped nucleus; function is to destroy necrotic tissue

3. Thrombocytes (platelets) function in coagulation

   a. Fragments of megakaryocyte

   b. Average of 150,000 in the blood circulation

D. Blood clotting occurs when the platelets encounter rough, injured tissue (Fig. 3-18)

E. Erythrocytes carry antigens on their surfaces that make blood typing important; serum carries antibodies

1. Type A blood carries the A agglutinogen; plasma carries the anti-B agglutinins

2. Type B blood carries the B agglutinogen; plasma carries the anti-A agglutinins

3. Type AB blood has the A and B agglutinogens; plasma does not carry any agglutinins

4. Type O blood does not carry any agglutinogen; serum carries both the anti-A and anti-B agglutinins

Heart

The heart is composed of cardiac muscle and serves to pump the blood through the circulatory system

A. Located behind the sternum; is the size of a human fist; the apex of the heart points down and to the left (Fig. 3-19)
  1. Located in a space between the lungs in the thoracic cavity known as the *mediastinum*
  2. Consists of four chambers: two atria and two ventricles
     a. Blood from the superior and inferior venae cavae fills the right atrium and passes into the right ventricle through the tricuspid valve (three flaps)
     b. From the right ventricle, the unoxygenated blood is sent to the lungs by passing through the semilunar valve and pulmonary artery
     c. Oxygenated blood is sent from the lungs to the left atria through the pulmonary veins; the left semilunar valve separates the left atria from the pulmonary veins
     d. From the left atrium, blood flows through the mitral valve (two flaps) into the left ventricle
     e. Blood enters circulation by passing through the left semilunar valve into the aorta
  3. Heart wall consists of three layers
     a. Visceral pericardium or epicardium
     b. Myocardium—heaviest covering
     c. Endocardium—smooth continuous covering
     d. All valves and chambers are lined by endothelium
  4. Valves of the heart are unique
     a. Atrioventricular (AV) valves—tough, fibrous tissue; open except when ventricles contract; hang into the ventricle like a leaf; held in place by chordae tendineae at the edge of the valves
        (1) Tricuspid AV valve—three flaps form it
        (2) Bicuspid AV valve (mitral valve)—two parts form it
     b. Semilunar (SL) valves—pressure opens them, and reverse pressure closes them; remain closed until the ventricles contract
        (1) Pulmonary SL valve—located on the right
        (2) Aortic SL valve—located on the left
  5. Heartbeat averages 70 to 72 beats per minute and cannot contract without nerve impulses; nerves regulate the rate of the beat
     a. Sinoatrial (SA) node—located in the wall of the right atrium near the superior vena cava; heartbeat begins here (Fig. 3-19)
        (1) From here, the action current spreads out and passes down to the fibrous layer and stops
        (2) Current goes through the AV node at the upper end of the interventricular septum
        (3) Modified cardiac muscle (bundle of His) divides into right and left branches
        (4) Along the AV bundle, fibers pass out into the cardiac muscle (Purkinje's fibers)
     b. Action current consists of the impulse starting at the SA node, spreads to the atria, passes to the AV node, is picked up and sent down through all the cardiac fibers from the Purkinje's fibers, and ends by spreading up over the ventricles; muscle contracts after the impulse spreads over the heart
        (1) Purkinje's fibers provide for uniform contraction
        (2) If the AV node is blocked, ventricles will set up their own rhythm
  6. Cardiac cycle consists of a relaxation-contraction cycle; lasts for approximately 0.8 seconds
     a. SA node discharge begins the cycle
     b. First isometric period—beginning of the atrial systole (contraction, very short in length); atria build up enough pressure to get the blood moving
     c. Second isometric period—beginning of the atrial diastole (relaxation) and beginning of ventricular systole; AV valve is closed, and SL valve is open
     d. At the beginning of ventricular systole the AV valve opens and the SL valve is closed
  7. The heart sound is a "lubb-dubb" noise
     a. First sound—AV valves close (louder, longer sound)
     b. Second sound—SL valves close

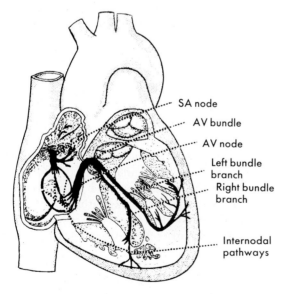

Fig. 3-19   Transmission of cardiac impulse. (From Guyton AC: *Physiology of the human body,* ed 6, Philadelphia, 1984, WB Saunders.)

SA node
AV bundle
AV node
Left bundle branch
Right bundle branch
Internodal pathways

c. Damage to the valves may yield stenosis (scarred), prolapse (limpness), or weakness (murmurs); dental hygienist may need to pre-medicate clients with antibiotics before starting any procedure that may produce a bacteremia; check with the guidelines established by the American Heart Association

8. Electrocardiogram is a record of the action current as it travels across the heart (Fig. 3-20)
   a. P wave—depolarization of the atria
   b. QRS complex—depolarization of the ventricles
   c. T wave—repolarization of the ventricles

9. Starling's law—force of contraction is directly proportional to the initial tension of the muscle; allows for a more powerful contraction when blood piles up
   a. Medulla—houses the cardiac control center
   b. Right vagus nerve—most important nerve to the heart (goes to the SA node); left vagus nerve goes to the AV node
      (1) Releases acetylcholine
      (2) If the vagus nerve is injured, the heart rate increases
      (3) Rapid vagus stimulation will stop the heart, but after a while, vagal escape takes over and the heart begins to beat on its own
   c. Sympathetic nervous system—first four thoracic spinal nerves (accessory nerves) contribute adrenergic fibers to the heart; affect the heart's irritability
      (1) Stimulation leads to increased discharge from the SA node
      (2) Produces more rapid, forceful contractions

10. Bainbridge's reflex—increase in the heart rate is initiated by an excess amount of blood returning to the right atrium; receptor cells in the right atrium are sensitive to pressure and stretch
    a. Message is sent to the medulla via afferent fibers in the vagus nerve
    b. This in turn causes efferent signals to be transmitted back through the vagus nerve
    c. Final outcome will be to increase the heart rate and strength of the contractions

Circulatory System

The circulatory system involves the connection of the heart to the arteries, arterioles, capillaries, venules, and veins; the lymphatic system also interacts with this circulatory system

A. Arteries are thick-walled, elastic vessels; end in arterioles
   1. Tunica adventitia is the outside layer; thicker in the large arteries; allows for stretch and recoil of the arteries
   2. Tunica media contains the smooth muscle; circular pattern
   3. Tunica intima is the innermost covering; continuous with the endocardium
   4. Vasa vasorum are tiny capillaries that pass into the walls of the arteries and provide nourishment

B. Arteriole is the smallest branch of an artery; connected to venules by capillaries

C. Venules are connected to veins that carry blood toward the heart and carry unoxygenated blood (exception is the pulmonary vein)

D. Lymphatic system carries lymph; is involved in the maintenance of fluid pressure; contains lymph glands that filter out foreign particles
   1. Tissue fluid is located in the intracellular spaces and is derived from the blood; is constantly moving; similar to plasma without large proteins
   2. Lymph is tissue fluid that has been reabsorbed into the lymphatic vessels; these vessels begin blindly in the tissues; similar to capillaries except that they are much more permeable; lacteals are lymphatic capillaries in the intestines that are important for digestion
   3. Valves are necessary in the lymphatic system to keep fluid flowing in the right direction; most valves are located in the arms and legs where gravity is a problem
      a. If a person does not move around, lymph fluid will collect in the feet and hands
      b. Hydrostatic pressure forces fluid out
      c. Protein osmotic pressure tends to pick up fluid from the tissues

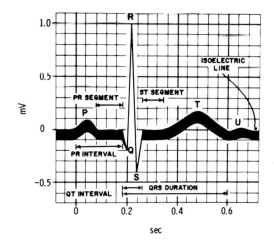

Fig. 3-20 QRS-T-P complex. (From Ganong WF: *Review of medical physiology,* ed 15, Norwalk, Conn, 1991, Appleton & Lange.)

4. Lymph nodes are spongy masses of tissue through which lymph filters; macrophages engulf foreign substances
5. Lymphocytes are small WBCs that originate from stem cells
   a. T lymphocytes are involved in cell-mediated immunity
   b. B lymphocytes are involved in the humoral immune system
6. Lymph nodes have more afferent vessels coming to the node than efferent vessels leaving the node
7. An aggregate is a large number of lymph nodes in an area; usually named after a gland or organ
   a. Posterior auricular lymph nodes—located behind the ears
   b. Deep cervical lymph nodes—located around the sternocleidomastoid muscle
   c. Axillary lymph nodes—drain the chest and arm
   d. Inguinal lymph nodes—drain the legs
   e. Popliteal lymph nodes—located behind the knee
8. Right lymphatic duct drains the upper right quadrant, right arm, and right side of the head and empties into the right subclavian vein
9. Thoracic duct drains the rest of the body; begins at the cisterna chyli (bulblike enlargement at the L2 vertebra) and passes up the left side of the vertebral column through the aortic hiatus of the diaphragm into the left subclavian vein
10. Lymphoidal tissue contains a spongelike network; found in various anatomic structures
    a. Spleen—contains the largest concentration of macrophages; the graveyard of RBCs
    b. Thymus—atrophies after puberty but is involved in the cell-mediated immune system
    c. Tonsils—located in the oral cavity
       (1) Palatine tonsils—located between the anterior and posterior pillars
       (2) Lingual tonsils—located on the posterior part of the tongue
       (3) Pharyngeal tonsils—located in the nasopharynx
       (4) Waldeyer's ring—formed by these structures; guards the opening to the digestive and respiratory systems

E. Veins have the same layers as arteries, except they are thinner
   1. Veins will collapse without blood
   2. Valves in the veins help to resist the forces of gravity
F. Capillaries connect small veins and small arteries; are lined by a thin layer of endothelium
   1. Metarterioles are the main pathways between the arterioles and venules; give rise to smaller capillary networks
   2. Networks have an average thickness of 1 μm
      a. Permeable to water but not RBCs or large proteins
      b. Functional part of circulatory system; exchange center
   3. Capillaries can dilate or constrict, depending on the tissues' needs
   4. RBCs go through capillaries one cell at a time
   5. More active tissue has a greater number of capillaries
   6. Sinusoids are modified capillaries that are important in the liver, lymph nodes, and spleen
G. Arteriovenous shunt (anastomosis) is a large blood vessel that connects an arteriole and venule directly; thick walled; smooth muscle that surrounds it is controlled by a nerve
   1. Skin color is caused by blood in the capillaries and anastomoses; important for heat distribution
      a. Warm and red skin—capillaries constricted and anastomoses open
      b. Warm and pale skin—capillaries constricted and anastomoses open
      c. Cool and red skin—capillaries open and anastomoses closed
   2. Found only in the hands, face, and toes where the body is exposed to weather
H. Arterial systemic circulation
   1. Aorta arises from the left ventricle of the heart; first 5 cm is called the ascending aorta; two left and right coronary arteries branch off it directly above the left semilunar valve and supply blood to the cardiac muscle
   2. Aortic arch loops back over the top of the heart and left of the trachea; continues down in back of the heart; three arteries come off of the arch
      a. Brachiocephalic artery—only a few centimeters in length
         (1) Right subclavian artery (first branch) supplies blood to the right shoulder
         (2) Right common carotid artery supplies blood to the right side of the head
      b. Left common carotid artery supplies blood to the left side of the head
      c. Left subclavian artery supplies branches to the upper chest and scapula
   3. Descending aorta consists of the thoracic and abdominal sections of the aorta
      a. Thoracic aorta starts after the left subclavian artery branches off the aortic arch and extends to the T4 vertebra; passes down and in front of the vertebral column and through the diaphragm

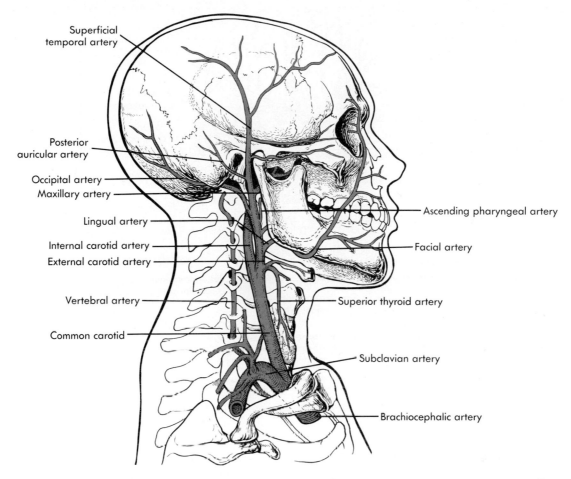

Fig. 3-21   Arteries of the head and neck. The brachiocephalic artery, the right common carotid artery, the right subclavian artery, and their branches. The major arteries to the head are the common carotid and vertebral arteries. (From Seeley R, Stephens T, Tate P: *Anatomy and physiology*, St Louis, 1989, Mosby.)

b. After it passes through the diaphragm, it is called the abdominal aorta; extends to the L4 vertebra; bifurcates into the left and right common iliac arteries

4. Carotid arteries supply the head; right carotid artery originates from the brachiocephalic artery; left carotid artery originates from the aortic arch (Fig. 3-21)

a. External carotid artery
   (1) Lingual artery—located from the branch of the tongue
   (2) Facial artery—comes out at an angle; serves the face
   (3) Occipital artery—located behind the scalp
   (4) Superficial temporal artery—main branch of the external carotid artery; moves into the scalp and toward the eye
   (5) External maxillary artery—branches off just below the ear; serves the face and part

of the jaw; located in the mandibular canal and exits through the mental foramen

b. Internal carotid artery—supplies most of the blood for the brain and eye
   (1) Cervical part comes up the neck without branching; goes through the carotid foramen in the temporal bone
   (2) Ophthalmic artery supplies the eyeball, eye muscles, and lacrimal glands; middle cerebral artery provides blood for the temporal and lateral parietal lobes
   (3) Anterior cerebral artery passes forward through the longitudinal fissure where it joins other arteries to form the circle of Willis (Fig. 3-22)

5. Subclavian arteries provide blood to the shoulder and arms; left one comes from the aortic arch, right one from the brachiocephalic artery
a. Pass over the first rib and under the clavicle

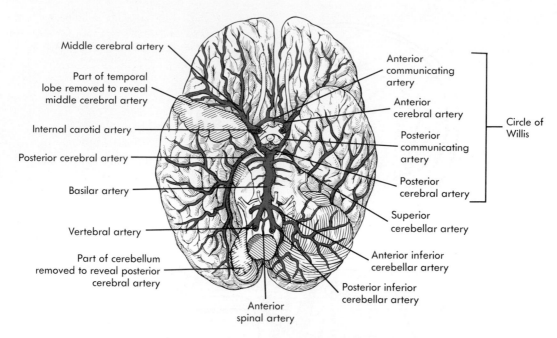

Fig. 3-22 Inferior view of the brain showing the vertebral, basilar, and internal carotid arteries and their branches. (From Seeley R, Stephens T, Tate P: *Anatomy and physiology,* St Louis, 1989, Mosby.)

b. Become the axillary arteries as they pass through the shoulder region

c. First branch off the subclavian artery is the vertebral artery, which passes up the neck through the transverse foramen of the cervical vertebrae and enters the skull through the foramen magnum; the two paired arteries join on the ventral side of the medulla and become the basilar artery (this artery joins branches from the internal carotid artery to form the circle of Willis) (Fig. 3-22)

d. Axillary artery becomes the brachial artery at the humerus; moves along the medial surface across the elbow region and then divides
   (1) Radial artery moves along the radius and crosses it at the distal end (one can feel a pulse here); moves across the metacarpals and deep into the palm; forms a loop that connects with the ulnar artery
   (2) Ulnar artery travels down the medial surface of the forearm; becomes the superficial palmar artery that joins with the radial artery
   (3) Digital arteries supply the fingers and branch off from the palmar loop

6. Thoracic aorta gives off several branches
   a. Nine pairs of intercostal arteries serve the last nine ribs (subclavian artery serves the first three ribs)

   b. Two bronchial arteries supply the lungs
   c. One esophageal artery comes off the front part of the thoracic aorta and spreads into a network
   d. One or two superior phrenic arteries serve the upper surface of the diaphragm

7. Abdominal aorta gives rise to the visceral and parietal arteries
   a. Celiac artery—visceral artery that is 1.5 cm long and then divides
      (1) Left gastric artery—smallest branch to the stomach
      (2) Hepatic artery—supplies most of the blood to the liver; divides at the liver
         (a) Cystic artery—serves the gallbladder
         (b) Gastroduodenal artery—divides into the gastroepiploic artery (serves the stomach and pancreas) and the pancreaticoduodenal artery (serves the pancreas and duodenum)
      (3) Splenic artery—largest branch to the spleen
   b. Superior mesenteric artery—supplies all of the small intestine (except the duodenum) and superior ascending and transverse portions of the large intestine; comes off the front of the aorta below the celiac artery
   c. Inferior mesenteric artery—supplies blood for part of the transverse colon and all of the

descending and sigmoid colon, rectum, and bladder

d. Renal artery—supplies the kidneys; located below the superior mesenteric artery
   (1) Right renal artery slightly longer and lower because the aorta is slightly left of the midline
   (2) Enters the kidney at the hilus

e. Suprarenal artery—branches off the aorta above the renal artery (may be branches of the renal arteries)

f. Spermatic arteries—located below the renal arteries; pass through the inguinal canal

g. Ovarian arteries do not leave the abdominal cavity

h. Parietal artery branches off the thoracic aorta
   (1) Inferior phrenic artery—supplies the undersurface of the diaphragm
   (2) Lumbar arteries (four pairs)—opposite L1 to L4 vertebrae
   (3) Spinal arteries—serve the vertebral canal

i. Aorta terminates at the L4 vertebra

8. Aorta then divides and becomes the common iliac artery and then bifurcates again
   a. Internal iliac artery supplies the pelvic wall and viscera
   b. External iliac artery goes on to the leg

9. External iliac artery then passes over the pelvic brim and under the inguinal ligament; becomes the femoral artery

10. Just above the knee it becomes the popliteal artery and goes behind the knee to bifurcate
    a. Anterior tibial artery
    b. Posterior tibial artery

11. Anterior and posterior tibial arteries spread out at the ankle; become the dorsal artery of the foot

I. Venous systemic circulation

1. Consists of one set of superficial veins and one set of deep veins

2. Veins have a higher blood capacity than the arteries but have lower blood pressure and velocity than do the arteries

3. Three sets of veins that connect to the heart
   a. Vena cava—serves the body; returns unoxygenated blood
   b. Coronary sinus—serves the heart; returns unoxygenated blood
   c. Pulmonary veins—serve as the lung (two per lung); return oxygenated oxygenation blood to the left atrium

4. Superior vena cava begins at the level of the first rib; formed by two veins
   a. Left and right brachiocephalic veins (return blood from the head, shoulders, and arms)

b. Each brachiocephalic vein is a union of the internal jugular vein with the subclavian vein

5. Jugular veins drain blood from the head
   a. External jugular vein drains the face and the scalp; is the union of three main veins (unite just below the ear and empty into the subclavian vein)
      (1) Superficial temporal vein
      (2) Posterior auricular vein
      (3) Posterior facial vein
   b. Internal jugular vein returns from the internal carotid vein; originates in the skull
      (1) Begins as cerebral veins (drains cortex)
      (2) Superior sagittal sinus (center of falx cerebri)
      (3) Confluence of sinuses (just inside the external occipital protuberance)
      (4) Straight sinus (short vessel from the inferior sagittal sinus)—confluence of sinuses and passes laterally
      (5) Left and right transverse sinuses flow around the occipital bone to the temporal bone; become the sigmoid sinus, which eventually passes out the jugular foramen to become the internal jugular vein

6. Vertebral veins arise outside of the skull at the level of the atlas and pass through the transverse foramen to the subclavian artery

7. Arms and shoulders are drained by the deep veins that run alongside the arteries
   a. Palmar vein drains into the radial and ulnar veins, which drain into the brachial vein, which drains into the axillary vein, which drains into the subclavian vein
   b. Superficial veins—cephalic vein along the lateral forearm and arm drains into the axillary vein; basilic vein along the medial surface of the forearm drains into the brachial vein, which drains into the axillary vein

8. Inferior vena cava is formed by two common iliac veins at the L5 vertebra in front of the vertebral column; goes through the diaphragm via the caval opening
   a. Azygous vein branches off of the inferior vena cava at the level of the renal veins; goes through the aortic hiatus of the diaphragm just above the heart and empties into the superior vena cava; picks up veins from the esophagus and bronchi
      (1) Esophageal vein
      (2) Bronchial vein
      (3) Intercostal vein
   b. Parietal veins—four pairs of lumbar veins, one sacral vein, and two inferior phrenic veins that empty into the inferior vena cava

c. Renal veins (visceral) return blood from the kidneys; right renal vein is shorter than the left renal vein

d. Ovarian or spermatic veins—located just below the renal veins
   (1) Paired veins
   (2) One set appears only in females, the other only in males

e. Suprarenal veins—located from the adrenal glands to the inferior vena cava

f. Hepatic vein returns blood from the liver to the inferior vena cava; part of the hepatic portal system

g. Veins of the lower extremities
   (1) Deep veins have same names as the arteries; plantar vein drains into the anterior and posterior tibial veins, which drain into the popliteal veins, which drain into the femoral veins, which drain into the external iliac vein, which drains into the common iliac vein
   (2) Superficial veins
      (a) Great saphenous vein drains the dorsalis pedis area of the foot
      (b) Small saphenous vein drains the lateral side of the foot
      (c) Popliteal vein drains the lateral side of the leg
   (3) Connections exist between the path and superficial veins along their paths

Blood Pressure

A. Pressure created by the force of the blood against the vessel walls in a closed system
   1. Highest in the arteries and lowest in the capillaries
   2. Pressure created in the veins is between the valves of the arteries and capillaries

B. Velocity of the blood flow is inversely related to the total cross-sectional area of the blood vessels

C. Five factors essential for maintaining the blood pressure
   1. An increase in cardiac output, especially ventricular systole, will lead to an increase in blood pressure
   2. The greater the peripheral resistance inside the blood vessels, the higher the blood pressure
   3. An increase in the volume of blood will cause an increase in blood pressure
   4. A decrease in the elasticity of the arterial walls will lead to an increase in blood pressure
   5. An increase in the viscosity of blood will cause an increase in blood pressure

D. Methods for measuring the pressure inside the vessel wall
   1. Direct method (uses a cannula)
      a. Cannula is inserted into a blood vessel
      b. When the pressure rises, a thin membrane inside of the cannula bulges outward; electric sensor detects the movement
      c. Information regarding the rate and frequency of the movement produced on the membrane is recorded on a moving sheet of paper
   2. Indirect method (involves the auscultatory method)
      a. Cuff with an inflatable bladder is placed around the upper arm
      b. Cuff is attached to either a mercury or aneroid monometer so the pressures can be measured
      c. Cuff is inflated until sounds can no longer be heard through a stethoscope that has been placed over the brachial artery
      d. Air is gradually released until the pressure in the cuff is great enough to close the artery during part of the arterial pressure cycle; Korotkoff sounds are heard
      e. Systolic pressure is noted when the Korotkoff sounds are first noted
      f. Diastolic pressure is noted when the Korotkoff sounds become muffled
      g. Blood pressure is reported with the systolic reading over the diastolic reading in millimeters of mercury (average 120 mm Hg/80 mm Hg)
      h. Pulse pressure is the difference between the systolic pressure and the diastolic pressure
   3. Factors affecting the blood pressure
      a. Age (newborn 40 mm Hg/20 mm Hg)
         (1) Onset of puberty leads to a sharp increase in blood pressure
         (2) Continued increase in blood pressure as age increases; increase is greater in systolic reading
      b. Exercise can increase the blood pressure; rest can decrease the blood pressure
      c. Weight gain can cause an increase in the blood pressure because the extra fat around the blood vessels will not allow them to expand; will also be more capillaries to serve the adipose tissue, leading to an increased amount of resistance created
      d. Disturbing emotions can cause a drop in blood pressure, leading to a decreased blood and oxygen supply to the brain and producing syncope (fainting)
      e. Pathologic changes can lead to hypertension
         (1) Primary or essential hypertension is seen with an increase in age; usually resulting

from a loss of elasticity in the arteries or atherosclerosis.

(2) Secondary or renal hypertension is more serious; usually associated with damaged kidneys

(3) Essential hypertension has an unknown cause; exhibits a very strong hereditary tendency

(4) As the blood passes through the various vessels, blood pressure changes

    (a) Average systolic pressure in the arteries—100 to 120 mm Hg

    (b) Average systolic pressure in the arterioles—30 to 70 mm Hg

    (c) Average systolic pressure in the capillaries—17 to 30 mm Hg

    (d) Average systolic pressure in the veins—0 to 17 mm Hg

E. Factors affecting pressure in the veins

1. Force produced during ventricular contraction

2. Vacuum created through the dilation of the ventricles

3. Gravity and massaging action created by the contraction of the muscles

4. Respiratory pump created during inhalation that causes a drop in pressure in the lungs and allows the blood to flow into the lungs

5. Pressure almost at zero in the veins connected to the heart (therefore the blood flows through the veins toward the heart)

F. Blood pressure is controlled by the vasomotor center in the medulla; consists of two parts

1. Vasoconstrictor system has a dominant role unless another stimulus overcomes it

2. Vasodilator system is less dominant; even when it is in control, some vessels in the body remain constricted

G. Carotid sinus reflex also controls the blood pressure

1. Carotid sinus is located where the internal and external carotid arteries branch

2. Carotid sinus is composed of nerve endings that are sensitive to pressure; impulses are sent to the vasomotor system via the glossopharyngeal nerve (cranial nerve IX)

3. Pressure on the sinus will result in vasodilation and a slowing of the heart rate

H. Marey's law states that there is an inverse relationship between the heart rate and the blood pressure

I. Chemical and hormonal regulators of blood pressure

1. If body tissues are not receiving enough oxygen, the capillaries will automatically dilate

2. Levels of carbon dioxide control both the rate of respiration and blood pressure

3. Carbon dioxide acts to dilate the vessels and leads to a decrease in blood pressure

4. Angiotensin II is a very active enzyme that works on the arterioles to cause a rise in the blood pressure

    a. Stimulates the sympathetic nervous system

    b. Causes aldosterone to be released, which causes the kidneys to retain salt and water, thus causing an increase in blood pressure

    c. If the kidney becomes ischemic, this will lead to an increased production of renin that will intensify the effects of angiotensin II and aldosterone

5. Oxytocin, antidiuretic hormone, and epinephrine also raise the blood pressure

Respiratory System

The respiratory system performs two functions for the body: supplies oxygen to the tissues and removes carbon dioxide from the tissues

A. Respiration is the sum of the processes concerned with gaseous reception, distribution, and elimination; involves gaseous oxygen, carbon dioxide, and nitrogen

1. External respiration—exchange of gases between the air sacs of the lungs and the bloodstream

2. Internal respiration—exchange of gases between the bloodstream and tissue cells of the body

3. Cellular respiration—use of oxygen within the cell

B. Respiratory quotient (RQ) is the ratio of the volume of carbon dioxide liberated to the volume of oxygen used

1. RQ in the use of carbohydrates is 1

2. RQ in the use of fats is 0.7

3. RQ in the use of proteins is approximately 0.8

C. Respiratory tract begins at the nostril opening and extends to the alveoli of the lungs (Fig. 3-23)

1. Air is drawn in through the nose, where it is warmed, humidified, and cleansed

2. Nasal cavity is lined with olfactory epithelium in the sphenoethmoidal recess and by respiratory epithelium in the lower part

3. Superior, middle, and inferior turbinates are located on the lateral surface of the nasal cavity

4. Frontal, ethmoidal, maxillary, and sphenoidal paranasal sinuses empty into the nasal cavity

5. Pharynx is the second part of the respiratory tract; starts at the base of the skull and extends to the esophagus; divided into three parts

    a. Nasopharynx—located behind the nasal cavity

    (1) Eustachian tube connects the middle ear with the pharynx; open only during swallowing; functions to equalize the pressure

    (2) Pharyngeal tonsils (adenoids)—located on the upper back wall of the nasopharynx; are masses of lymphoid tissue

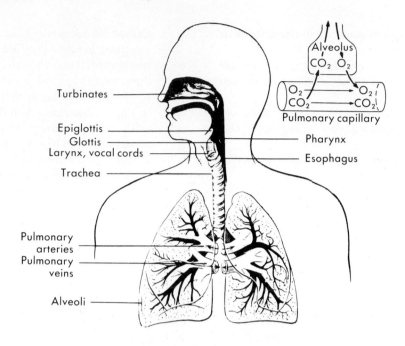

Fig. 3-23 Respiratory system. (From Guyton AC: *Physiology of the human body,* ed 6, Philadelphia, 1984, WB Saunders.)

b. Oropharynx extends from the soft palate to the base of the tongue; separated from the oral cavity by the palatine arches

c. Laryngopharynx extends from the hyoid bone to the larynx

6. Larynx is located at the base of the tongue; made up of nine cartilages: three single cartilages and three pairs of cartilage that are held together by membranes and ligaments

   a. Thyroid cartilage—largest cartilage; one on each side—fuse at the anterior surface to form one continuous cartilage; thyroid gland rests on the lower part of the cartilage

   b. Cricoid cartilage forms a signet-ring shape; attached by membranes to the upper part of the trachea

   c. Arytenoid cartilages—small, paired cartilages that are shaped like pyramids and located on the back of the larynx; serve as points of attachment for the vocal cords

   d. Other cartilages are the corniculate and cuneiform cartilages

   e. Epiglottis—large leaf-shaped cartilage that attaches to the thyroid cartilage and extends toward the base of the tongue; during swallowing the larynx comes up and the epiglottis folds over it to protect it

7. Vocal cords are folds of mucous membranes with elastic connective tissue at the edges

   a. Connective tissue tightens via the arytenoid cartilage; air passes through the glottis; vibrations for sounds are made from the true vocal cords

   b. False vocal cords protect against the entrance of food and water into the trachea

8. Trachea is approximately 12 cm long; located in front of the esophagus; composed of several C-shaped rings that prevent its collapse; lined with ciliated epithelium that beats upward

9. At the level of the T4 vertebra the trachea divides into left and right branches known as the primary bronchi

   a. Left primary bronchus is longer than the right; forms a sharp angle

   b. Right primary bronchus has a larger diameter than the left; comes off almost forming a straight line

10. Secondary bronchi branch off the primary bronchi

    a. Three secondary bronchi for the right lung (one per lobe)

    b. Two secondary bronchi for the left lung (one per lobe)

11. Tertiary bronchi branch off the secondary bronchi; 10 tertiary bronchi per lung because there are ten segments per lung

12. Bronchioles are smaller branches of the tertiary bronchi; surrounded by smooth muscle

    a. Terminal bronchioles—1 mm in diameter; do

not contain cartilage for support; not involved in gaseous exchange

b. Respiratory bronchioles—branch off the terminal bronchioles; first site of diffusion of oxygen into the blood

13. Alveolar ducts branch off the respiratory bronchioles; alveolar sacs attach to the alveolar ducts

14. Surfactant is produced by pneumocytes
   a. Lipoprotein that is formed along the alveolar wall
   b. Acts to decrease surface tension and allows the lungs to expand

D. Two cone-shaped lungs in the thoracic cavity; base rests on the diaphragm, and the apex is located at the level of the clavicle

1. Right lung has three lobes: superior, middle, and inferior; is larger than the left lung

2. Left lung is smaller than the right lung since two thirds of the heart is located on the left side and it contains only two lobes

3. Ten bronchopulmonary segments per lung
   a. Each one has a branch from the tertiary bronchi
   b. Used as points of reference for surgery

4. Cardiac notch is a depression on the medial surface of the lungs

5. Point of attachment to a lung is designated as the hilus
   a. Blood vessels, bronchiole tree, and nerves enter at the hilus
   b. Hilus is located in the cardiac notch

6. Pleura is the serous membrane surrounding the visceral and parietal layers of each lung
   a. Space between the two layers is the pleural cavity
   b. Lungs are not located in the pleural cavity

E. Mechanics of respiration involve changing the pressure in the lungs to cause inspiration or expiration (Fig. 3-24)

1. Inspiration occurs when the air pressure in the lungs is decreased; causes the volume of the lungs to increase
   a. External intercostal muscles cause the ribs to elevate; increase the size of the chest cavity
   b. Dome-shaped diaphragm (between the thoracic and abdominal cavity) pulls downward when contracted; will also increase the size of the chest cavity

2. Expiration is basically a passive movement; ribs fall down, and the diaphragm is pushed up by the abdominal viscera
   a. Abdominal muscles force the abdominal contents upward
   b. Internal intercostal muscles pull the ribs downward

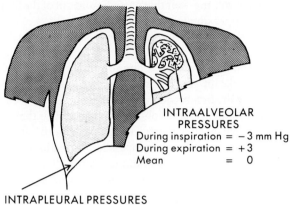

INTRAALVEOLAR
PRESSURES
During inspiration = −3 mm Hg
During expiration = +3
Mean   = 0

INTRAPLEURAL PRESSURES
During inspiration   = −8 mm Hg
During expiration   = −2
At end of expiration = −4
At end of inspiration = −6
Mean   = −5

Fig. 3-24   Alveolar and intraalveolar pressures in lung. (From Guyton AC: *Physiology of the human body*, ed 6, Philadelphia, 1984, WB Saunders.)

3. During inspiration the enlargement of the thoracic cavity decreases the pressure in the alveoli to −3 mm Hg; therefore pulls air inside the lung; during expiration the opposite effects occur—the pressure in the alveoli increases to +3 mm Hg, pushing the air outside of the lung

4. Intrapleural pressure is always negative
   a. During inspiration the pressure is equal to −8 mm Hg
   b. During expiration the pressure is equal to −2 mm Hg

5. Differences in the alveolar and intrapleural pressures cause the lungs to pull away from the thoracic cage and cause a negative pressure

6. Malfunctions that can occur in the respiratory system
   a. Pneumothorax—when the chest wall is punctured, air enters the pleural cavity, causing the lung(s) to collapse
   b. Dyspnea—difficult or labored breathing
   c. Apnea—cessation of breathing
   d. Hyperpnea—increased respiration
   e. Orthopnea—person can breathe better in one position than another
   f. Cheyne-Stokes respiration—abnormal periodic respiration that consists of a long period of apnea followed by a short burst of hyperpnea followed by apnea

F. Normal lungs always contain air during breathing; amount of air can be measured with a spirometer

1. Tidal volume—air that passes in and out of the lungs
   a. Approximately 500 ml of air
   b. Normal rate of respiration is about 12 times per minute
2. Inspiratory capacity—amount of air that a person can take into the lungs beyond the amount brought in by the first breath; about 3000 ml
3. Expiratory reserve volume—amount of air that one can exhale after normal expiration; about 1100 ml
4. Residual volume—air that is left in the lungs after the most forceful expiration; about 1200 ml
5. Vital capacity—greatest amount of air that one can exchange in a forced respiration; approximately 4500 ml
6. Hering-Breuer reflex prevents overinflation of the lungs
   a. Pressure receptors located in the lungs are stimulated with inhalation and expansion
   b. Stimuli are sent over the afferent vagus nerve to the respiratory control centers
   c. When stimuli reach the critical level, inspiration ceases and expiration ceases (unless one holds his breath)
7. Carbon dioxide concentration in the blood is the most important stimulus; respiratory control center
   a. Direct—blood passes through the respiratory center
   b. Indirect—chemoreceptors in the aortic arch and carotid sinuses are stimulated by an increase in the carbon dioxide content, causing a nerve reflex to stimulate the respiratory center
   c. Four percent carbon dioxide in inhaled air leads to doubled respiratory rate; 20% carbon dioxide in inhaled air leads to loss of consciousness; 40% carbon dioxide in inhaled air leads to death
8. Cyanosis occurs when there is an excess amount of reduced hemoglobin (HHb) in the capillary circulation; causes the skin to turn blue
9. Hypoxia—decreased oxygen supply to tissue below physiologic levels despite adequate perfusion of blood
   a. Hypoxic hypoxia—decreased pressure in the lungs
   b. Anemic hypoxia—blood has decreased oxygen-carrying power
   c. Stagnant hypoxia—poor circulation
   d. Histiocytic anoxia—tissue cells are poisoned, making them incapable of picking up oxygen
G. Air that we breathe consists of several different gases and some water (Table 3-20)
   1. Each gas exerts pressure against the walls surrounding it (known as the partial pressure of a gaseous mixture); the greater the partial pressure of a gas, the greater the rate of diffusion of the gas through the pulmonary membrane
   2. Alveolar air constantly loses oxygen to the blood; blood allows diffusion of carbon dioxide into the alveolar air space
   3. Pulmonary membrane is thin; composed of surfactant and epithelial cells; allows for rapid diffusion of gases
   4. Gases pass through the membrane; follow the law of diffusion
   5. Oxygen is picked up in the blood (from the lungs) and forms oxyhemoglobin (HbO_2); blood leaving the lungs is saturated with oxygen and carries oxygen (20 ml oxygen/100 ml blood) to the tissues with decreased oxygen pressure; oxygen splits away from the hemoglobin and creates reduced hemoglobin; blood returning to the lungs has 15 ml oxygen/100 ml blood (Fig. 3-25)

Table 3-20

Gaseous Composition of Air Involved in Respiration

	Inspired (%)	Alveolar (%)	Expired (%)
Oxygen	20.84	13.6	16.3
Carbon dioxide	0.15	5.3	4.0
Nitrogen	79.0	75.0	79.7

Modified from Guyton AC: *Physiology of the human body,* ed 6, Philadelphia, 1984, WB Saunders.

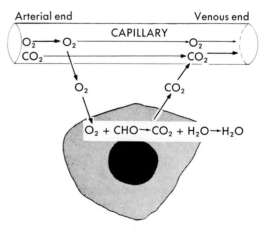

Fig. 3-25 Diffusion of oxygen from capillary to tissues. (From Guyton AC: *Physiology of the human body,* ed 6, Philadelphia, 1984, WB Saunders.)

6. Oxygen is loaded and unloaded with the use of hemoglobin
   a. Loading tension (t_L)—oxygen tension in lungs will produce 97% saturation of blood; same as normal pressure in the lungs; 97 mm Hg
   b. Unloading tensions (t_U)—blood has given up 50% oxygen—oxygen pressure in tissues is approximately equal to 30 mm Hg; venous blood unloads faster than arterial blood (part of hemoglobin molecule)
7. When iron is in the ferric state, it is unable to carry and release oxygen normally (methemoglobin)
8. Carbon dioxide is carried away from the tissues to the lungs to be expired; most carbon dioxide is carried in the form of the bicarbonate ion (HCO_3^-); chloride shift uses carbonic anhydrase (c-a) to form carbonic acid

$$(CO_2 + H_2) \overset{\text{c-a}}{\rightleftarrows} (H_2CO_3)$$

9. Small amounts of carbon dioxide are dissolved in the blood or carried away in carbaminohemoglobin

Digestive System

A. Digestive or alimentary tract consists of a tube 6 m long from the mouth to the anus; selectively absorbs nutrients and water for the body (Fig. 3-26)
B. Mouth—location where food processing and digestion commences
   1. Secondary teeth (32 in the adult) tear and grind the food
   2. Tongue—fibromuscular organ that contains the taste buds; transmits the sensation of taste to the brain; rolls the food into a bolus for swallowing
   3. For the food to be rolled into a bolus, saliva must be added; saliva contains glycoproteins that enable the bolus to slip down the esophagus with greater ease; produced by three major paired glands and many minor glands (Fig. 3-27)
      a. Parotid glands are located in the preauricular region; saliva contains ptyalin, which initiates digestion of starches; saliva travels down Stensen's duct, which opens opposite the second maxillary molar (serous secretion)
      b. Sublingual glands lie under the tongue and rest against the mandible in the sublingual fossa; saliva travels down Bartholin's duct and enters the oral cavity through Rivinus' ducts on the sublingual fold
      c. Submandibular glands lie on the medial surface of the mandible; saliva travels down the tortuous Wharton's duct and is released into the

mouth at the sublingual caruncles (seromucous secretion)
   4. Bolus of food is conducted from the mouth and pharynx to the esophagus, a muscular tube located posterior to the trachea and connected to the stomach
      a. During swallowing the soft palate is pushed back against the posterior pharyngeal wall, closing the passage to the nasopharynx
      b. Larynx is elevated; superior opening is protected by the epiglottis
C. Stomach is a dilated portion of the alimentary canal lying in the upper abdomen just under the diaphragm
   1. Several functions
      a. Stores food
      b. Digests—secretes pepsin, rennin, and gastric lipase
      c. Produces hydrochloric acid (parietal cells)
   2. Shaped like a J; internal surface is wrinkled (rugae)
      a. Cardiac portion—esophagus enters
      b. Body—main part
      c. Fundus—bulge at the upper end, left of the esophageal area
      d. Pyloric portion—narrows and connects with the small intestine
D. Small intestine—thin-walled muscular tube
   1. Three portions
      a. Duodenum—bile and pancreatic secretions are added to the small intestine; horseshoe shaped
      b. Jejunum—greatest amount of absorption occurs here; 1.5 m long
      c. Ileum—connects with the large intestine; 2.4 m long
   2. Secretes several enzymes and substances
      a. Brunner's glands—located only in duodenum; secrete alkaline mucus
      b. Sucrase—acts on sucrose; end product is one molecule of glucose and one of fructose
      c. Maltase—acts on maltose; produces two molecules of glucose
      d. Lactase—acts on lactose; produces one molecule of glucose and one molecule of galactose
      e. Aminopeptidase—acts on the amino end of the protein chain; produces one amino acid and simpler proteins
      f. Dipeptidase—acts on dipeptides to produce two amino acids
      g. Enterokinase (coenzyme)—acts on trypsinogen to produce trypsin
      h. Secretin—hormone carried to the pancreas; stimulates the pancreas to produce watery pancreatic juice

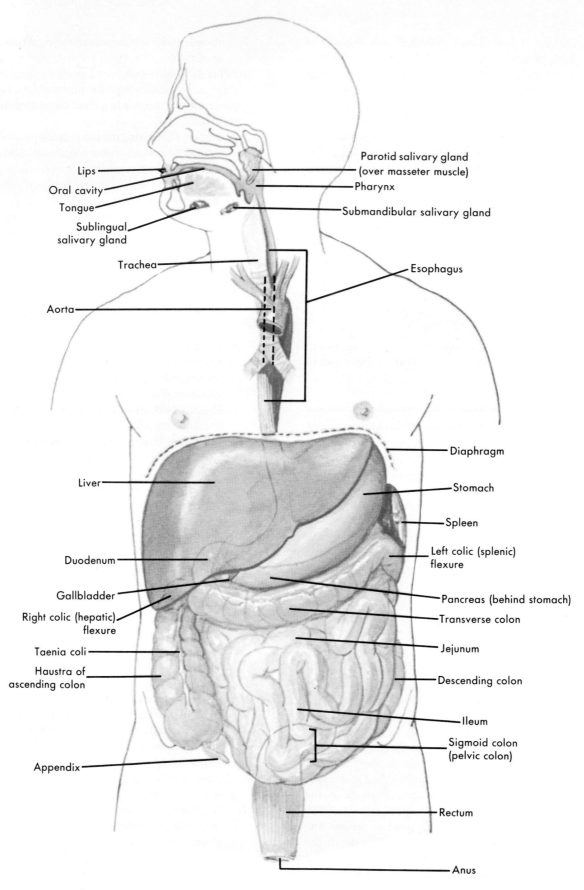

Fig. 3-26 Digestive system. (From McClintic JR: *Human anatomy,* St Louis, 1983, Mosby.)

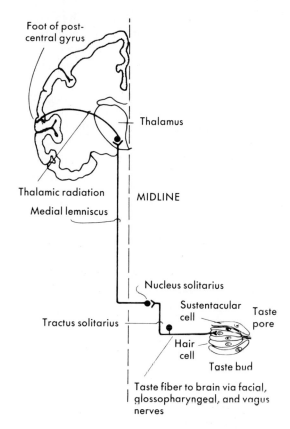

Foot of post-
central gyrus

Thalamus

Thalamic radiation

MIDLINE

Medial lemniscus

Nucleus solitarius

Sustentacular
cell

Taste
pore

Tractus solitarius

Hair
cell

Taste bud

Taste fiber to brain via facial,
glossopharyngeal, and vagus
nerves

Fig. 3-27 Taste pathways. (From Ganong WF: *Review of medical physiology*, ed 15, Norwalk, Conn, 1991, Appleton & Lange.)

i. Enterogastron—hormone carried to the stomach; produced when fatty foods are in the intestine; reduces gastric motility

E. Large intestine—approximately 1.5 m long; divided into several parts

1. Cecum—blind pouch in the lower right quadrant; appendix attaches to the cecum; ileocecal sphincter separates the ileum from the cecum
2. Colon
   a. Ascending—from the cecum to the hepatic flexure
   b. Transverse—from the hepatic flexure to the splenic flexure
   c. Descending—to the level of the pelvic bone, on the left side of the body
   d. Sigmoid—S-shaped curve
3. Rectum—from the sigmoid colon down to the pelvic diaphragm
4. Anus—3 cm in length (internal and external sphincters)

F. Pancreas—endocrine and exocrine gland
1. Exocrine—acinar cells produce pancreatic juice

that is collected by the pancreatic duct (Wirsung's duct) and carried away; joins the common bile duct to form Vater's ampulla, which penetrates the walls of the duodenum
2. Endocrine—releases insulin that controls the blood glucose levels

G. Liver—largest and most active gland in the body
1. Two main lobes and several lobules; lobules produce bile that is carried away and stored in the gallbladder
2. Other functions
   a. Acts as a storehouse for glycogen
   b. Produces fibrinogen for blood clotting
   c. Synthesizes prothrombin with the aid of vitamin K
   d. Synthesizes some amino acids from simpler compounds
   e. Produces erythrocytes in the embryo and fetus
   f. Detoxifies nitrogenous waste
   g. Deaminates 50% to 60% of the absorbed amino acids
   h. Stores some cyanocobalamin (vitamin B_{12})
   i. Removes old erythrocytes and foreign substances by the action of the phagocytic Kupffer's cells
   j. Stores iron, copper, and vitamins A and D
   k. Synthesizes and destroys uric acid
   l. Acts as a center for fat and carbohydrate metabolism

H. Digestion starts in the mouth; absorption of molecules occurs in the small intestine
1. Functions of saliva in the oral cavity
   a. Lubricating—reduces friction
   b. Solvent—important for stimulation of taste buds
   c. Moistening—important for speech
   d. Cleansing—decreases bacterial population
   e. Buffering—helps to protect teeth from acid insults
   f. Minor digestion of starches
2. Elevating the tongue causes the tongue to push the bolus of food toward the pharynx
3. Wavelike contraction (peristalsis) keeps the bolus moving down the rest of the digestive system
4. Food that is converted to a semifluid mass in the stomach is known as chyme
5. Three phases of gastric digestion
   a. Cephalic—taste, smell, and sight of food stimulate the cerebral cortex; cause the salivary glands to produce saliva
   b. Gastric—food reaches the stomach, causing a copious flow of juices to form chyme
   c. Intestinal—chyme is in small intestines; causes

enterogastrone to be released, which will inhibit gastric movement and secretion

6. Davenport's theory of hydrochloric acid secretions in the stomach
   a. Parietal cells contain more carbonic anhydrase than the blood, which will form

   $$H_2CO_3 \rightarrow H^+ + HCO_3$$

   b. Carbonate ion moves out into the blood and causes the chloride ions to shift back out of the blood into the interstitial spaces
   c. Chloride ion attaches to the free hydrogen ion to form hydrochloric acid (HCl)
7. Mucus is also secreted in the stomach to protect against self-digestion
8. Hydrochloric acid acts on pepsinogen to produce pepsin; converts milk protein and collagen to proteases and peptones
9. Pancreas produces several enzymes that act on the chyme in the small intestine
   a. Lipase—acts on emulsified fats to form fatty acids and glycerol
   b. Amylase—acts on carbohydrates to form disaccharides
   c. Carboxypeptidase—works on the —COOH end of the protein chain to produce one amino acid and simpler proteins
   d. Trypsinogen—inactive enzyme until the coenzyme enterokinase activates it to trypsin; splits large protein chains
   e. Chymotrypsinogen—inactive enzyme until the coenzyme enterokinase activates it to chymotrypsin; acts on amino acids
10. After the enzymes have broken up the molecules (catabolism), they are selectively absorbed through the small intestine
    a. Amino acids are used to build new tissue or repair tissue; those not used are deamidized in the liver; ammonia formed is converted to urea and eliminated by the kidneys; nonnitrogenous portion may be oxidized to supply energy or synthesized to glucose (1 g of protein equals 4 calories); passes into the body via the blood capillaries in the villi
    b. Fats are oxidized to carbon dioxide and water with the release of energy; fat not used can be stored in the liver or body and passed into the body via the lacteals of the lymphatic system (1 g of fat equals 9 calories)
    c. Carbohydrates may be oxidized in the tissue cells to supply energy or may be stored in the liver or muscles as glycogen; passes into the body via the blood capillaries in the villi
       (1) Glycogenesis—synthesis of glucose to glycogen
       (2) Glycogenolysis—hydrolysis of glycogen to glucose
       (3) One gram of carbohydrates equals 4 calories
11. Large intestine holds the fecal material that is not absorbed; reabsorbs water to maintain the internal environment

I. Kidneys
1. Important because they also excrete waste products from metabolism and maintain the water and acid-base balance in the body
2. Paired bean-shaped organs on either side of the vertebral column
   a. Renal artery and vein and the ureter (which attaches to the bladder) attach to the center of the kidney at the hilus
   b. Outer part of the kidney is designated the cortex and the inner part the medulla
      (1) Medulla consists of several pyramids
      (2) Apices of the pyramids project into the calyces
   c. Nephron is the functional unit of the kidney (Fig. 3-28)
   d. Renal circulation is renal arteries to interlobar artery to arcuate artery to glomerulus to efferent arterioles to secondary capillary network to interlobular vein to arcuate vein to interlobar vein to renal vein
3. Kidney connected to the bladder by the ureters
   a. Are approximately 27 cm long
   b. Urine flows down the ureters via peristalsis
4. Bladder lies behind the symphysis pubis; serves as a reservoir for the urine
   a. Smooth muscle (detrusor muscle) readjusts constantly to the amount of urine entering
   b. Three orifices form a trigone
5. Urethra connects the bladder to the exterior
   a. Female urethra is approximately 4 cm long
   b. Male urethra is approximately 20 cm long
6. Urine is a liquid with unique properties
   a. Colored by bile pigments
   b. pH varies from 4.5 to 9
   c. Specific gravity varies from 1.015 to 1.025
   d. Amount excreted daily is approximately 1400 ml
   e. Consists of 95% water and solids
      (1) Urea, uric acid, creatinine, and urea
      (2) Sodium chloride and various phosphates and sulfates

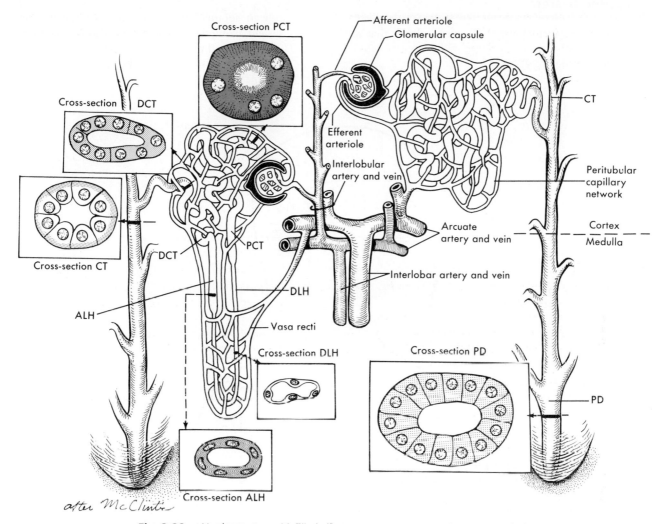

Fig. 3-28   Nephron. (From McClintic JR: *Human anatomy,* St Louis, 1983, Mosby.)

7. Blood is filtered first in the glomeruli
   a. Ultrafiltrate of water and nonprotein solutes pass through the glomerular membranes into Bowman's capsule and then into the proximal tubules
   b. Filtration rate is determined by the filtration pressure, which is equal to the blood pressure in the glomerulus minus the sum of the protein osmotic pressure plus the intercapsular pressure
      (1) Approximately 75 L of blood flow through the kidney per hour
      (2) Most of the filtrate is reabsorbed before reaching the collecting tubules
   c. Ultrafiltrate is modified as it passes through the tubules via reabsorption and secretion
      (1) Proximal convoluted tubule—all glucose and some sodium, chloride, potassium, bi-carbonate, and hydrogen ions are reabsorbed in the blood
      (2) Loop of Henle—more precise adjustment of the sodium concentration is made
      (3) Distal collecting tubule—final adjustment is made in the levels of the sodium ions, acids, bases, and water
   d. Waste products are not reabsorbed
   e. Adjustments of the sodium/potassium and calcium/phosphorus ratios are done in the distal convoluted tubules under the influence of aldosterone and the parathyroid gland
   f. Hydrogen ions are exchanged in the distal convoluted tubules so that the pH levels are controlled
   g. Water levels are also regulated in the distal convoluted tubules, depending on the amount of antidiuretic hormone in the body

Endocrine System

The endocrine system consists of several glands that secrete hormones

A. Functions (Fig. 3-29)
   1. Composed of a number of glands that play a major role in supplementing the effect of the nervous system, in regulating the rate of various physiologic processes, and in maintaining the constancy of the internal environment of the body
   2. Glands

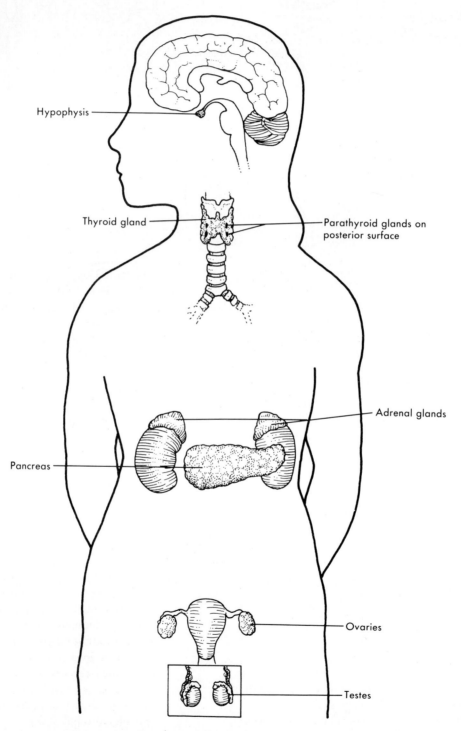

Hypophysis

Thyroid gland

Parathyroid glands on posterior surface

Adrenal glands

Pancreas

Ovaries

Testes

Fig. 3-29 Location of endocrine glands. (From McClintic JR: *Human anatomy,* St Louis, 1983, Mosby.)

    a. Do not secrete their products into ducts; instead are secreted into the system

    b. Product of an endocrine gland is called a hormone

        (1) Ectodermally derived endocrines secrete amine hormones

        (2) Mesodermally derived endocrines secrete steroid hormones

        (3) Endodermally derived endocrines secrete protein hormones

   3. Hormones secreted by the endocrine system

    a. Main regulators of metabolism, reproduction, and maintenance of fluid and electrolyte balance and acid-base balance

    b. Produce slow and long-lasting responses in target cells

B. Control of endocrine secretion

   1. Blood levels of specific inorganic substances

   2. Total osmolarity of blood

   3. Blood levels of organic substances

   4. Positive and negative feedback

   5. Chemicals produced by nerve cells

   6. Nervous stimulation

C. Pituitary gland (Table 3-21)

   1. Located in the sella turcica of the sphenoid bone

   2. Composed of a portion derived from the roof of the oral cavity (adenohypophysis) and a portion from the hypothalamus (neurohypophysis)

   3. Arterial blood supply is derived mainly from the superior and inferior hypophyseal arteries

   4. Hypophyseal portal veins arise from the capillaries of the median eminence of the hypothalamus

   5. Veins empty into the sinusoid in the pars distalis

   6. Hypophysis receives its nerve supply from the sympathetic plexus around the carotid artery

   7. Adenohypophysis

    a. Contains three types of cells (pars distalis)

        (1) Acidophils—stain red-orange from an orange G or purplish red from an azocarmine stain

        (2) Basophils—stain blue from a periodic acid–Schiff's stain

        (3) Chromophobes—stain little if at all

    b. Growth hormone (somatotropin)

        (1) Produced by acidophils

        (2) Stimulates growth of both bone and soft tissues

        (3) Causes cells to shift from using carbohydrate to using fat for energy

        (4) Excess production of growth hormone

            (a) Pituitary gigantism—before epiphysial closure; large size but proportionally balanced

            (b) Acromegaly—full-grown adult; characterized by enlarged hands, feet, and jaws

        (5) Deficient secretion of growth hormone

            (a) Pituitary dwarfism—develops during skeletal development; diminuitive size but proportionally balanced

            (b) Simmond's disease—develops during adult years; presents with premature aging and cachexia

    c. Prolactin (lactogenic hormone)

        (1) Produced by acidophils

        (2) Stimulates milk production by the mammary glands

            (a) Secreted during pregnancy breast development

            (b) Secreted after delivery of child—lactation

        (3) Stimulates progesterone secretion by corpus luteum

    d. Adrenocorticotropic hormone (ACTH)

        (1) Secreted by basophils; also possibly secreted by chromophobes

        (2) Controls the synthetic and secretory activity of the two inner zones of the adrenal cortex

        (3) Atrophy of the adrenal cortex results in Addison's disease; can result in death because of a loss of sodium in the extracellular fluid

        (4) Hypertrophy of the adrenal cortex results in Cushing's syndrome; characterized by moon face, hirsutism, and possible hypertension

    e. Thyroid-stimulating hormone (TSH)

        (1) Secreted by basophils

        (2) Affects thyroid gland activity (accumulation of material, synthesis, and secretion)

        (3) Hypersecretion results in Grave's disease

        (4) Hyposecretion results in cretinism (young) or myxedema (adult)

Table 3-21

Divisions of the Hypophysis

Major divisions	Subdivisions
Adenohypophysis	Pars distalis
	Pars tuberalis
	Pars intermedia
Neurohypophysis	Infundibulum
	Neural lobe

   f. Luteinizing hormone (LH)
      (1) Secreted by basophils
      (2) Also classified as a gonadotropin
      (3) Female
         (a) Forms corpus luteum in the ovary
         (b) Causes corpus luteum to secrete progesterone
         (c) Necessary for ovulation and implantation of the zygote
      (4) Male
         (a) Interstitial cell–stimulating hormone
         (b) Stimulates the production of testosterone by the interstitial cells of the seminiferous tubules
   g. Follicle-stimulating hormone (FSH)
      (1) Female—controls maturation of primary follicles to vesicular fossicles
      (2) Male—controls spermatogenesis
   h. Pars intermedia has no proven function in mammals
   i. Pars tuberalis has no proven function in mammals
8. Neurohypophysis
   a. Contains pituicytes
      (1) Axons, with their cell bodies in the hypothalamus, terminate on or near the pituicytes
      (2) Hypothalamus produces the hormones and passes them over a nerve tract to be stored or released from the neurohypophysis
   b. Antidiuretic hormone (ADH)
      (1) Acts on the kidney to decrease urine formation
      (2) Acts on smooth muscle of arteries and arterioles; increases blood pressure
      (3) Hyposecretion of ADH results in diabetes insipidus
         (a) Polyuria
         (b) Polydipsia
         (c) Polyphagia
      (4) Release is controlled by osmosensitive cells in the hypothalamus
   c. Oxytocin
      (1) Secreted during parturition; affects the uterus
      (2) Aids milk ejection of the mammary glands
D. Thyroid gland
   1. Consists of two lobes that are interconnected by an isthmus; located on the ventral surface of the trachea; superior border is the thyroid cartilage; inferior border is the sixth tracheal ring
   2. Receives approximately 120 ml of blood per minute, which is supplied by the superior thyroid arteries (from the external carotid arteries) and by the inferior thyroid arteries (from the subclavian arteries); capillary system of the gland drains into the superior and middle thyroid veins to the internal jugular veins to the inferior thyroid veins to the left brachiocephalic vein
   3. Receives sympathetic fibers from the inferior and superior ganglia and parasympathetic fibers from branches of the vagus nerve
   4. Thyroxine (T_4) and triiodothyronine (T_3) are iodinated amino acids secreted by the follicles of the gland
      a. T_3 is more potent than T_4, but the thyroid contains more T_4 (under normal conditions)
      b. T_3 and T_4 must attach to a plasma protein in the circulating blood
      c. If T_3 and T_4 are to be stored, thin thyroglobulin is formed in the follicular colloid
      d. Effects of T_4
         (1) Accelerates catabolic reactions of glycolysis
         (2) Necessary for proper development of the brain
         (3) Controls metabolism by affecting glycogen levels; can control urine production
         (4) Influences cardiac metabolism
   5. Secretes calcitonin in response to high plasma concentrations of calcium and phosphate; can cause increased absorption of minerals by the kidneys; can increase mineralization of bones
   6. Effects of thyroid hormones on oral structures
      a. Injection of T_4 in newborn rats causes marked acceleration in the rate of eruption of the incisor teeth; can also affect eruption of the molars[1]
      b. Large doses of thyroid hormone given to guinea pigs affects the odontoblasts; dentin formation is adversely affected[1]
      c. Children with cretinism may exhibit a small dental arch; exfoliation patterns of the teeth are delayed
E. Parathyroid gland
   1. Variable number of parathyroid glands in the human; most people have two pairs, but the range varies from one to three pairs
   2. Small in size (approximately 5 mm); usually located on the posterior side of the thyroid gland
   3. Composed of two types of cells
      a. Chief cells—produce parathyroid hormone (PTH)
      b. Oxyphil cells—reserve cells capable of producing PTH
   4. Parathyroid hormone
      a. Controls serum calcium, magnesium, and phosphate levels
      b. Decreased calcium concentration in the blood stimulates secretion
      c. Affects the gut, bone, and kidneys

(1) Gut—causes increased absorption of calcium, magnesium, and phosphate

(2) Bone—stimulates osteoclasts; causes calcium and phosphate to be released into the blood

(3) Kidney—causes increased calcium and phosphate reabsorption and increased phosphate excretion

d. Disorders caused by unregulated PTH levels

(1) Hyperparathyroidism (von Recklinghausen's disease)

(a) Extremely high blood calcium levels leading to muscular weakness

(b) Cysts in the bones may develop (osteitis fibrosa cystica)

(2) Hypoparathyroidism (tetany)—extremely low blood calcium levels leading to muscular rigidity and convulsion

e. Effects of PTH on oral structures

(1) Hypoparathyroidism during tooth development produces defects in the matrix, mineralization in the enamel and dentin, and delays in eruption

(2) Hyperparathyroidism, seen radiographically, shows loss of the lamina dura; alveolar bone can become osteoporotic with no change in density of the teeth

F. Pancreas gland

1. Single gland that extends horizontally across the posterior abdominal wall on the left side

2. Consists of three parts

a. Head—duodenal portion

b. Body—between the head and tail

c. Tail—splenic portion

3. Has an exocrine and endocrine function

a. Exocrine—trypsin and trypsinogen (digestive functions)

b. Endocrine—α-cells, glucagon (controls blood glucose; β-cells (control insulin levels)

4. Insulin

a. Complex protein hormone that is secreted in response to a rise in the blood glucose level

b. Effects

(1) Causes glycogenesis in the liver (conversion of glucose to glycogen)

(2) Stimulates cells to take up glucose

(3) Increase in blood glucose levels (caused by a lack of insulin) can lead to infection and bacteremias when bacteria are introduced into the blood system

5. Glucagon—secreted by α-cells in response to a decrease in the blood glucose level; causes glycogenolysis (conversion of glycogen to glucose) in the liver

6. Diabetes mellitus can be caused by an insulin deficiency

a. Signs and symptoms

(1) Hyperglycemia—high blood glucose level

(2) Glucosuria—kidney tubules cannot reabsorb all of the glucose, and the excess appears in the urine

(3) Ketoacidosis—body uses fats as the main source of energy; ketone levels increase; acidosis can result from overtaxed buffering systems

(4) Polyuria—excess water is lost with glucose in urine

(5) Polydipsia—loss of water triggers thirst

(6) Polyphagia—glucose loss triggers a desire to eat

b. If the β-cells are destroyed, the patient must receive insulin and control diet

c. If some β-cells survive, oral sulfonylurea compounds may be prescribed to stimulate the β-cells

7. Hypoglycemia can develop from low blood glucose levels; can result from insulin shock, islet tumors, and starvation

a. Mainly affects the brain

b. Can also lower the body temperature, disturb respiration, and depress the reflexes

G. Adrenal glands

1. These paired glands are located on the top of each kidney; adrenal cortex develops from the embryologic mesoderm; adrenal medulla develops from the neural ectoderm

2. Adrenal cortex secretes several hormones that can be classified as steroids

a. Cells located in the zona glomerulosa secrete mineralocorticoids (aldosterone and corticosterone) that regulate electrolytes in the extracellular fluids

(1) Sodium is reabsorbed into the blood from the glomerular filtrate

(2) Potassium (a positive ion) is lost in the urine because of the electronegativity created by the reabsorption of sodium in the kidney tubules

(3) Chloride (a negative ion) is reabsorbed from the glomerular filtrate because of the electronegativity created by the reabsorption of sodium in the kidney tubules

b. Secretion of aldosterone is regulated in response to changes in the extracellular fluid; decreased sodium concentration produces a weak effect on the cortex to increase secretion, causes the kidneys to secrete renin, which stimulates the release of angiotensin in the cortex, and causes the pituitary gland to release ACTH

   c. Addison's disease is caused by the hyposecretion of aldosterone and cortisol

     (1) Causes brown pigmentation of the skin

     (2) Causes hypotension

   d. Cells located in the zona fasiculata secrete glucocorticoids (cortisol) that affect the body's metabolic system

     (1) Glucocorticoid secretion causes an increased concentration of the blood glucose

     (2) Cortisol causes a decrease in the quantity of protein in most tissues and an increase in protein in the liver

     (3) Cortisol can stabilize lysozymes and therefore inhibit cell death

     (4) Cushing's syndrome can be manifested from an increase in glucocorticoids

       (a) Moon face

       (b) Buffalo hump on shoulders

       (c) Fat abdomen

   e. Cells located in the zona reticularis secrete androgens and produce masculine features; excess production in women can lead to masculine features

Reproductive System

Male

A. Testes
1. Two ovoid bodies that lie in the scrotum
2. Suspended in the inguinal region by the spermatic cord
3. Sperm is formed and stored in the seminiferous tubules of the testes
4. Testosterone is produced in the testes
5. Epididymis is adjacent to the testes in the scrotum
   a. Acts as a storage reservoir for sperm along with the seminiferous tubules
   b. Sperm may live for as long as a month in both the epididymis and tubules
6. If the testes have failed to descend in an infant, the condition is referred to as cryptorchidism

B. Vas deferens
1. Conducts sperm from the epididymis to the urethra
2. Acts as a storage site for sperm

C. Urethra
1. Passageway for semen from the vas deferens through the penis
2. Passage for urine from the bladder through the penis
3. Ends at the urinary meatus, which is the opening in the glans penis through which urine and semen are excreted

D. Seminal vesicles
1. Membranous pouches located posterior to the bladder
2. Produce a secretion that contains fructose, amino acids, and mucus
3. Secrete mucoid material into the upper end of the vas deferens

E. Prostate gland
1. Located inferior to the bladder
2. Secretes an alkaline fluid to activate the sperm
3. Secretes its milky fluid into the vas deferens

F. Bulbourethral glands (Cowper's glands)
1. Located inferior to the prostate gland
2. Secretes a mucous secretion into the urethra that precedes ejaculation; aids in lubrication

G. Penis
1. Organ of copulation that is divided into a shaft and glans penis
   a. Glans penis is the most sensitive portion of the penis
   b. Foreskin covers the glans penis (removed by circumcision)
2. Erective tissue (corpus cavernosum) surrounds the penile urethra; causes erection when engorged with blood

H. Sperm
1. Spermatozoa formed in the testes
2. Contains head, neck, body, and tail
   a. Head contains the genetic material of the male
   b. Tail provides motility through flagella movement
   c. Sperm move through the female genital tract to seek the ovum at a velocity of approximately 1 to 4 mm per minute
3. Spermatogenesis
   a. After a spermatogonium has been divided by mitosis for the last time, it increases in size and forms a primary spermatocyte
   b. Primary spermatocyte is divided by meiosis to form secondary spermatocyte with haploid number of chromosomes (23)
   c. Division of the secondary spermatocytes results in spermatoids being formed
   d. Spermatids are transformed into motile cells called spermatozoa

I. Physiology of ejaculation
1. Erection is the stiffening of a flaccid penis
2. Rhythmic peristalsis in the genital ducts during orgasm causes semen to be propelled through the epididymis, vas deferens, seminal ducts, and urethra

3. Semen is a thick, whitish fluid of high viscosity
  a. Between 2.5 and 5 ml are secreted at ejaculation
  b. Each milliliter contains 10 to 150 million sperm
  c. Sperm usually move at about 3 mm/min
C. Hormonal influences
  1. Hormones are essential to the mechanism of reproduction and to the development and maintenance of secondary sex characteristics
  2. Anterior pituitary gland secretes FSH and LH, which cause growth and function of the testes at puberty
  3. Secondary sex characteristics in the male that appear during adolescence
    a. Deepening of voice; widening of musculature of chest and shoulders
    b. Growth of facial and body hair

Female

A. Pelvis
  1. Contains the reproductive organs, bladder, and rectum
  2. Shaped like a funnel with a wide mouth
  3. Divided into true and false pelvis by the inlet or brim; sacral promontory and ileopectineal lines are dividing points between the true and false pelvis
  4. Forms part of the birth canal
  5. Perineum, vagina, muscles, and ligaments form the soft structures of the pelvis
    a. Retain pelvic organs in place
    b. During labor direct presenting part of the infant forward
B. Ovaries
  1. Flat, oval shaped bodies about 2.5 cm long
  2. Supported in the pelvis by the broad ligament and suspensory ligament
  3. Three types of follicles located in the ovaries
    a. Primordial follicles—contain a primary oocyte
      (1) Present at birth
      (2) Follicles finish first maturation under the influence of FSH
    b. Growing follicles—contain a mature ovum and spaces that contain fluid
    c. Mature follicles—seen bulging from the surface of the ovary
C. Fallopian tubes (oviducts)
  1. Lie in the folds of the broad ligaments
  2. Fimbriae (fingerlike projections) located at the ovarian ends; isthmus portion is connected to the uterus
  3. Important events occurring in the fallopian tube—fertilization of the ovum by a spermatozoa, segmentation, and formation of the blastocyst
D. Uterus

1. Hollow organ with thick muscular walls
2. Located behind the bladder and in front of the rectum
3. Pear-shaped; divided into three parts
  a. Fundus—rounded upper part
  b. Body—narrows from the fundus
  c. Cervix—tapering projection
4. Muscular layers
  a. Endometrium—one layer of ciliated columnar cells except for lower one third of the cervical canal where it changes to stratified squamous epithelium; contains glands and a good blood supply
  b. Myometrium—contains smooth muscle and large blood vessels
  c. Exometrium—contains the pelvic peritoneum
5. Serves as the womb for a developing fetus
E. External genitalia
  1. Vagina—female organ of copulation
    a. Muscular, membranous orifice; 7.6 to 12.7 cm long
    b. Connects the uterus to the external surface (vaginal orifice)
    c. Serves as the birth canal
  2. Mons pubis—rounded eminence in front of the pubic symphysis
  3. Labia majora—two longitudinal folds; protect the inner vulva
  4. Labia minora—two inner folds; smaller; protect the clitoris
  5. Clitoris
    a. Homologue of the penis in the male
    b. Can increase in size with sexual stimulation
F. Perineum contains the structures found between the pubic symphysis and the coccyx
G. Mammary glands
  1. Composed of compound alveolar glands
  2. Secrete milk to the nipples under the influence of lactogenic hormone from the pituitary gland
  3. Pigmented circular region (areolae surround the nipple)
  4. Active glandular growth occurs during pregnancy to prepare the mammary glands to produce milk (lactation)
H. Hormonal cycle (Fig. 3-30)
  1. Begins at puberty and ends at menopause
  2. FSH is secreted by the anterior pituitary gland; activates the primary graafian follicle
  3. Maturing follicle produces estrogen; causes the endometrium to become engorged with blood and prepares it to receive the fertilized ovum
  4. Both hormones (FSH and estrogen) allow the ova to mature

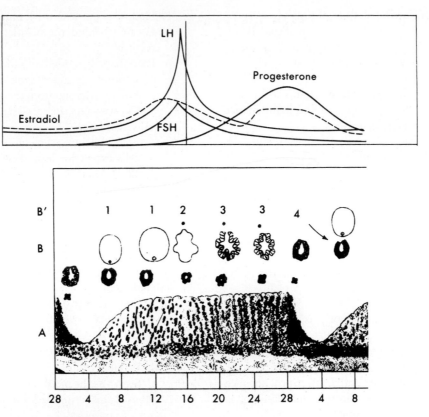

Fig. 3-30 Relationship of pituitary gonadotropins and ovarian hormones to follicular development and uterine changes. (From McClintic JR: *Human anatomy,* St Louis, 1983, Mosby.)

5. Mature ovum is released into the fallopian tube by a ruptured graafian follicle; LH assists ovulation; follicle forms the corpus luteum and secretes progesterone
6. Increased progestogen levels reduce FSH and increase LH; cause the corpus luteum to secrete progesterone
   a. Stimulate uterus to store glycogen and increase the uterine blood supply
   b. Corpus luteum begins to involute as a result of lowered FSH levels
7. Menstrual cycle lasts 21 to 35 days
   a. Menstruation begins if the ovum is not fertilized
   b. If fertilization occurs, the placenta will secrete chorionic gonadotropin, which will maintain the corpus luteum; estrogens and progesterone will also continue to be secreted and will maintain the rich vascular supply in the endometrium for the developing embryo
I. Secondary sex characteristics that develop in response to estrogen and progesterone secretion during puberty
   1. Widening of hips
   2. Breast and genital enlargement
   3. Growth of axillary and pubic hair

REFERENCE

1. Jenkins GN: *The physiology and biochemistry of the mouth,* ed 4, Oxford, 1978, Blackwell Scientific.

SUGGESTED READINGS

Anthony CP, Thibodeau GA: *Textbook of anatomy and physiology,* ed 12, St Louis, 1987, Mosby.

Clemente CD, ed: *Gray's anatomy,* American ed 30, Philadelphia, 1985, Lea & Febiger.

Ganong WF: *Review of medical physiology,* ed 15, Norwalk, Conn, 1991, Appleton & Lange.

Guyton AC: *Physiology of the human body,* ed 6, Philadelphia, 1984, WB Saunders.

Guyton AC: *Textbook of medical physiology,* ed 8, Philadelphia, 1990, WB Saunders.

Hoyle G: How is muscle turned on and off? *Sci Am* 22:84, April, 1970.

Jungueira LC, Carneiro J: *Basic histology,* ed 7, Los Altos, Calif, 1992, Appleton & Lange.

McClintic JR: *Human anatomy,* St Louis, 1983, Mosby.

McClintic JR: *Physiology and the human body,* ed 3, 1985, Wiley.

Seeley R, Stephens T, Tate P: *Anatomy and physiology,* St Louis, 1989, Mosby.

Schmidt RF, Thews G: *Human physiology,* ed 2, Berlin, 1989, Springer-Verlag.

Squier CA, Johnson NW, Hopps RA: *Human oral mucosa: development, structure and function,* Oxford, 1976, Blackwell Scientific.

Review Questions

Anatomy and Physiology

1 The pancreas is only an endocrine gland. It secretes parathormone.
   A. Statement one is *TRUE*. Statement two is *FALSE*.
   B. Statement one is *FALSE*. Statement two is *TRUE*.
   C. Both statements are *TRUE*.
   D. Both statements are *FALSE*.

2 Three sets of veins connect to the heart. Which one serves the heart?
   A. Vena cava
   B. Coronary sinus
   C. Pulmonary veins

3 Which group of lymph nodes drains the chest and arm?
   A. Posterior auricular
   B. Axillary
   C. Inguinal
   D. Popliteal

4 Erythrocytes carry antigens on their surfaces. Which of the following blood types will carry anti-A and anti-B agglutinins in their serum?
   A. A
   B. B
   C. A,B
   D. O

5 Sensation of pressure is modulated by
   A. Meissner's corpuscles
   B. Pacinian corpuscles
   C. Ruffini's corpuscles
   D. Krause's end bulbs

6 Which of the following phrases is *TRUE* about the middle ear?
   A. Maintains equilibrium
   B. Contains the eustachian tube
   C. Is innervated by cranial nerve VIII

7 Which of the following parts of the eye structure lines the eyelid?
   A. Iris
   B. Sclera
   C. Nasolacrimal duct
   D. Conjunctiva

8 The brain consists of four regions. Which one is the largest part and the center of conscious activities?
   A. Cerebrum
   B. Cerebellum
   C. Medulla oblongata
   D. Mesencephalon

9 There are a total of 12 pairs of spinal nerves. Each has a dorsal efferent root and a ventral afferent root.
   A. Statement one is *TRUE*. Statement two is *FALSE*.
   B. Statement one is *FALSE*. Statement two is *TRUE*.
   C. Both statements are *TRUE*.
   D. Both statements are *FALSE*.

10 Nerve impulses result from a change in membrane potential. Balance is mostly maintained by:
   A. The sodium pump
   B. The potassium pump
   C. A collection of positive electrons created internally
   D. A state of neutrality

11 The neuron has various components. Which component carries impulses toward the cell?
   A. Soma
   B. Dendrite
   C. Axon

12 The functional unit of a muscle is designated by the sarcomere. This space is from:
   A. Z line to Z line
   B. M line to A line
   C. I band
   D. H zone

13 All of the following blood cells have a nucleus *EXCEPT* one. Which one is that *EXCEPTION?*
   A. Macrophage
   B. Lymphocyte
   C. Erythrocyte
   D. Eosinophil

14 The mechanics of respiration involve several sets of muscles. What pulls the ribs downward during expiration?
   A. Abdominal muscles
   B. Internal intercostal muscles
   C. External intercostal muscles
   D. Pleura

15 Repolarization of the cardiac ventricles is represented by what part of the electrocardiogram?
   A. QRS complex
   B. P wave
   C. T wave

16 Which of the following descending spinal tracts is the main motor tract?
   A. Fasciculus gracilis
   B. Fasciculus cuneatus
   C. Spinothalamic
   D. Lateral corticospinal
   E. Rubrospinal

17 What is the name of the plowshare-shaped bone forming the lower part of the nasal septum?
   A. Calvarium
   B. Xiphoid
   C. Lacrimal
   D. Vomer
   E. Sphenoid

18 Which vertebra articulates with the condyles of the occipital bone?
   A. C1 (atlas)
   B. C2 vertebrae
   C. Thoracic vertebrae
   D. Coccygeal vertebrae

19 The following definition describes which of the following bones? "The bone is located beneath the talus and forms the heel"
   A. Femur
   B. Patella
   C. Tibia
   D. Fibula
   E. Calcaneus

20 A tooth is inserted into the jawbone and attached to it by the periodontal ligament. What type of articulations exist in this joint?
   A. Gomphosis
   B. Syndesmosis
   C. Synchondrosis
   D. Cartilaginous joint

21 The maxillary division of the trigeminal nerve exits through which of the following foramina?
   A. Rotundum
   B. Ovale
   C. Magnum
   D. Spinosum

22 Which of the following cranial nerves innervates the muscles of facial expression?
   A. I
   B. V
   C. VII
   D. XII

23 The levator anguli oris muscle is part of which of the following groups of muscles?
   A. Cranial
   B. Facial expression
   C. Extrinsic muscles of the tongue
   D. Mastication

24 From the paired information given below, identify the origin and insertion of the masseter muscle.

ORIGIN	INSERTION
A. Zygomatic process	coronoid process
B. Greater wing of the sphenoid	condyloid process of the mandible
C. Pterygoid fossa	posterior body of ramus
D. Hyoid bone	tongue

25 The heart is which type of muscle?
   A. Voluntary, striated
   B. Involuntary, striated
   C. Involuntary, smooth

CASE A. Mrs. Thompson is a 74-year-old female with a chief complaint of dry mouth after surgical removal of both parotid salivary glands 5 years ago. She reports taking 25 µg of Capoten (captopril) bid. Her blood pressure is 120/92 mm Hg. After the surgery to remove her salivary glands, she reported that she developed Bell palsy. Laboratory analysis of her blood indicates that her white blood cells are 7500/mm³. Questions 26 to 40 (and Figure 3-31) relate to Case A.

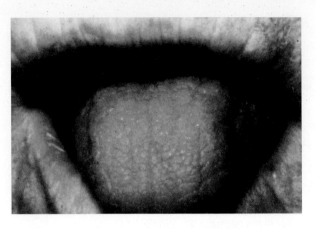

Fig. 3-31 Intraoral photograph of Case A showing a cobblestone appearance of tongue. (From Woodall IR: *Comprehensive dental hygiene care,* ed 4, St Louis, 1993, Mosby.)

26 What is captopril used to treat?
   A. Bacterial infections
   B. Viral infections
   C. Type II diabetes
   D. Hypertension

27 What is the target of the drug?
   A. Bacterial cell wall biosynthesis
   B. Microbial chromosomal replication
   C. Angiotensin converting enzyme
   D. Beta-lactamase

28 Captopril works on which of the following systems?
   A. Peptidoglycan wall
   B. DNA gyrase
   C. Renin-angiotensin-aldosterone system
   D. Pituitary gland

29 What does bid indicate?
   A. The client is taking the medication as needed.
   B. The client is taking the medication by mouth.
   C. The client is taking the medication twice daily.
   D. The client is taking the medication four times a day.

30 As the blood passes through the various vessels, blood pressure changes. What is the average systolic pressure in the capillaries?
   A. 100 to 120 mm Hg
   B. 30 to 70 mm Hg
   C. 17 to 30 mm Hg
   D. 1 to 17 mm Hg

31 Which of the following factors affects pressure in the veins?
   A. Force is produced during ventricular contraction.
   B. A vacuum is created through the dilation of the atria.
   C. A respiratory pump is created during inhalation that causes an increased pressure in the lungs.
   D. Pressure is at the highest in the veins connected to the heart.

32 What is the correct term for dry mouth?
   A. Xerophthalmia
   B. Keratoconjunctivitis sicca
   C. Polyuria
   D. Polydypsia
   E. Xerostomia

33 A white blood cell count of 7500 cells/mm³ is indicative of:
   A. An infection
   B. Leukemia
   C. Normal range

34 What is the most numerous white blood cell?
   A. Neutrophil
   B. Lymphocyte
   C. Monocyte
   D. Macrophage

35 Because the client reports Bell palsy, which nerve was most likely severed during her salivary gland surgery?
   A. Trigeminal
   B. Abducens
   C. Facial
   D. Glossopharyngeal

36 Where does the nerve in question 35 originate in the brain?
   A. Two equal roots from the pons
   B. Inferior border of the pons
   C. Base of the pons
   D. Superior aspect of the medulla oblongata

37 ACE inhibitors usually increase renal blood flow. Glomerular filtration rate is usually unchanged.
   A. Statement one is *TRUE*. Statement two is *FALSE*.
   B. Statement one is *FALSE*. Statement two is *TRUE*.
   C. Both statements are *FALSE*.
   D. Both statements are *TRUE*.

38 Synthesized by the kidneys, renin is released into the circulation where it acts on a plasma globulin substrate to produce _____.
   A. Angiotensin I
   B. Angiotensin II
   C. Aldosterone

39 Cranial nerve VII emerges from the _____ foramen.
   A. Stylomastoid
   B. Optic
   C. Jugular

40 Blood from the superior and inferior vena cava fills the right atrium and passes into the right ventricle. The blood will pass through the tricuspid valve.
   A. Statement one is *TRUE*. Statement two is *FALSE*.
   B. Statement one is *FALSE*. Statement two is *TRUE*.
   C. Both statements are *TRUE*.
   D. Both statements are *FALSE*.

Case B. A 17-year-old female is scheduled with the dental hygienist for an oral examination and periodontal maintenance care. Intraoral examination reveals loss of the enamel on the lingual surfaces of the maxillary anterior teeth. Questions 41 to 43 (and Figure 3-32) refer to this case.

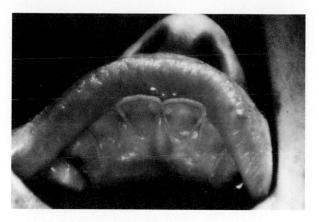

Fig. 3-32 Intraoral photograph of Case B showing the maxillary lingual view of the teeth of a young woman. (From Woodall IR: *Comprehensive dental hygiene care*, ed 4, St Louis, 1993, Mosby.)

41 The dental hygienist should suspect the client is suffering from:
   A. Decreased insulin
   B. Bulimia
   C. Taurodontism
   D. Extensive toothbrushing

42 The loss of tooth enamel is from:
   A. Erosion
   B. Abrasion
   C. Attrition

43 The pH of the stomach contents is usually:
   A. 0
   B. 1
   C. 7
   D. 14

Case C. Mrs. Otto, a 54-year-old female, was scheduled for a continued care appointment with the dental hygienist. During the extraoral examination, the clinician noticed lesions on the upper right part of the client's face, which the client reported to be quite painful. Questions 44 through 47 (and Figure 3-33) refer to this case.

44 The client is most likely suffering from:
   A. Herpes simplex
   B. Herpes zoster
   C. Hyperthyroidism
   D. Hypothyroidism

45 This client would be treated with:
   A. Acyclovir
   B. Penicillin
   C. Estrogen

46 This case is illustrative of a spread of a recurrent infection through which division of the trigeminal nerve?
   A. Ophthalmic (V_1)
   B. Maxillary (V_2)
   C. Mandibular (V_3)

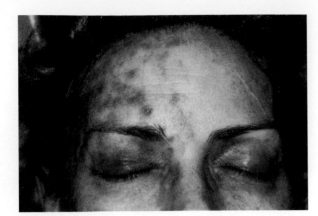

Fig. 3-33 Extraoral photograph of individual noted in Case C. Observe the unilateral distribution of painful vesicles along the V_1 of the trigeminal nerve. (From Smith, Turner, and Robbins: *Atlas of oral pathology*, St Louis, 1981, Mosby.)

47 The other *MOST* common site for signs of this disease to occur is:
A. On the fingers
B. On the trunk
C. On the legs
D. On the soles of the feet

48 There are several types of cells in the gastric glands that secrete different products. Which *ONE* of the following cells secretes hydrochloric acid?
A. Goblet
B. Parietal
C. Chief
D. Argentaffen

49 Intestinal motility—the movement of chyme through the intestine—is relatively fast. This is due to the fact that the pressure at the pyloric end of the small intestine is less than the distal end.
A. Both statements are *TRUE.*
B. The first statement is *TRUE;* the second statement is *FALSE.*
C. The first statement is *FALSE;* the second statement is *TRUE.*
D. Both statements are *FALSE.*

50 The products of digestion that are absorbed into the blood capillaries in the intestines are delivered first to the liver. The term portal system is used to describe the unique pattern of circulation in the liver. This pattern is:
A. Arteries → arterioles → capillaries → venules → veins
B. Veins → venules → capillaries → arterioles → arteries
C. Capillaries → vein → capillaries → vein
D. Vein → capillaries → arteries

Answers and Rationales

1. (D) The pancreas is both an endocrine and exocrine gland. The parathyroid gland secretes parathormone.
   (A) See statement (D)
   (B) See statement (D)
   (C) See statement (D)
2. (B) The coronary sinus serves the heart and returns unoxygenated blood.
   (A) The vena cava serves the body.
   (C) The pulmonary veins serve the lung.
3. (B) The axillary lymph nodes drain the chest.
   (A) The posterior auricular nodes are located behind the ears.
   (C) The inguinal nodes drain the legs.
   (D) The popliteal nodes are located behind the knees.
4. (D) Type O blood carries both anti-A and anti-B agglutinins.
   (A) Type A blood carries the A agglutinogen; plasma carries anti-B agglutinins.
   (B) Type B blood carries the B agglutinogen; plasma carries the anti-A agglutinins.
   (C) Type AB plasma does not carry any agglutinins.
5. (B) Pacinian corpuscles control the sensation of pressure.
   (A) Meissner's corpuscles control the sensation of touch.
   (C) Ruffini's corpuscles control the sensation of heat.
   (D) Krause's end bulbs control the sensation of cold.
6. (B) The eustachian tube equalizes pressure and is located in the middle ear.
   (A) Semicircular canals maintain equilibrium.
   (C) Cranial nerve VIII innervates the inner ear.
7. (D) The conjunctivae are the thin mucous membranes that cover the front of the eye and line the eyelid.
   (A) The iris is the colored part of the eyeball.
   (B) The sclera is the white covering on the anterior aspect of the eye.
   (C) This carries fluid away from the eye.
8. (A) This is the most superior part of the brain.
   (B) This portion coordinates balance and equilibrium.
   (C) This forms the bulb of the spinal cord located inside the foramen magnum.
   (D) This is the short part of the brainstem above the pons.
9. (D) Both statements are *FALSE.* There are 31 pairs of spinal nerves; each has a dorsal afferent and a ventral efferent root.
   (A) Statement one is *FALSE.*
   (B) Statement two is *FALSE.*
   (C) Both statements are *FALSE.*
10. (A) Balance is mostly maintained by the sodium pump.
    (B) The potassium pump is not very important in this phenomenon.
    (C) A void of positive electrons is created on the inside.
    (D) A state of electronegativity is created.

11. (B) Dendrites carry impulses toward the cell body under normal conditions.
    (A) The soma is the cell body.
    (C) Axons carry impulses away from the neuron.

12. (A) The Z line to Z line forms the sarcomere; it consists only of actin and is in the middle of the I band.
    (B) The M line consists only of myosin and is in the middle of the A band.
    (C) I band contains actin that is lined up; shortens during contraction.
    (D) The H zone appears in the A band when the muscle is relaxed.

13. (C) A mature erythrocyte, in the human bloodstream, does not have a nucleus.
    (A) The macrophage is a leukocyte with a nucleus.
    (B) The lymphocyte is a leukocyte with a nucleus.
    (D) The eosinophil is a leukocyte with a nucleus.

14. (B) The internal intercostal muscles pull the ribs downward during expiration.
    (A) The abdominal muscles force the abdominal contents upward during expiration.
    (C) The external intercostal muscles cause the ribs to elevate during inspiration.
    (D) The pleura are the serous membranes surrounding the visceral and parietal layers of the lung.

15. (C) Repolarization of the ventricles is represented by the T wave.
    (A) Depolarization of the ventricles is detected by the QRS complex.
    (B) Depolarization of the atria is represented by the P wave.

16. (D) The lateral corticospinal tract is a descending tract and is the main motor tract.
    (A) Fasciculus gracilis is an ascending fiber tract.
    (B) Fasciculus cuneatus is an ascending fiber tract.
    (C) The spinothalmic tract is an ascending fiber tract.
    (E) The rubrospinal tract originates in the midbrain, decussates immediately, and comes down on the opposite side of the brain.

17. (D) The vomer is the plowshare-shaped bone forming the lower part of the nasal septum.
    (A) Calvarium is the name given to the domelike superior portion of the skull.
    (B) The xyphoid is part of the sternum
    (C) The lacrimal bones form part of the medial surface of the orbital cavity.
    (E) The sphenoid is the butterfly-shaped bone of the skull.

18. (A) The atlas (C1 vertebra) articulates with the condyles of the occipital bone.
    (B) The C2 vertebra has a process on the upper surface of the body (dens) that forms a pivot about which the C1 vertebra rotates.
    (C) The thoracic vertebrae have articulations for the ribs.
    (D) The coccygeal vertebrae are fused together.

19. (E) The calcaneus is located beneath the talus and forms the heel of the foot.
    (A) The femur is located in the thigh and is the longest and strongest bone of the body.
    (B) The patella is a sesmoid bond and forms the kneecap.
    (C) The tibia is the medial bone of the leg and approximates with the femur.
    (D) The fibula is the lateral bone of the leg and articulates with the tibia.

20. (A) Gomphosis is a fibrous joint that is the insertion of a cone-shaped process into a socket.
    (B) Syndesmosis is a fibrous joint with two bones united by interosseous ligaments.
    (C) Synchondrosis is a cartilaginous joint with approximation.
    (D) A cartilaginous joint contains no joint cavity, and contiguous bones are united by cartilage.

21. (A) Cranial nerve V_2, exits through the foramen rotundum.
    (B) Cranial nerve V_3, exits through the foramen ovale.
    (C) The spinal column exits through the foramen magnum.
    (D) An artery to the meninges is transmitted to the foramen lacerum.

22. (C) The facial nerve (VII) innervates the muscles of facial expression.
    (A) The olfactory nerve (I) provides sensory innervation only.
    (B) The trigeminal nerve (V) innervates the muscles of mastication.
    (D) The hypoglossal nerve (XII) innervates the muscles of the tongue.

23. (B) This muscle elevates the corner of the mouth and is part of the muscles of facial expression.
    (A) This muscle is not a part of the scalp.
    (C) The muscle is not part of the fibromuscular tongue.
    (D) This muscle is not one of the muscles of mastication.

24. (A) The zygomatic process is the origin and the coronoid process is the insertion of the masseter muscle.
    (B) The greater wing of the sphenoid is the origin and the condyloid process of the mandible is the insertion of the lateral pterygoid.
    (C) The pterygoid fossa is the origin and the posterior body of the ramus is the insertion of the medial pterygoid muscle.
    (D) The hyoid bone is the origin and the tongue is the insertion of the hypoglossus muscle.

25. (B) Involuntary, striated muscle describes cardiac muscle.
    (A) Skeletal muscles are classified as voluntary, striated muscle.
    (C) Involuntary smooth muscle describes the uterus.
    (D) Voluntary, smooth muscle tissue does not fall into this classification.

26. (D) Captopril is used to treat high blood pressure.
    (A) This is not an antibiotic.
    (B) This is not an antiviral drug.
    (C) This drug does not treat diabetes.

27. (C) Captopril is an ACE inhibitor (angiotensin converting enzyme).
    (A) Penicillin would be an example of an antibiotic that is effective against formation of the bacterial cell wall.
    (B) Ciprofloxacin would be an example of an antibiotic that has a target of bacterial DNA gyrase.
    (D) Betalactamases are enzymes produced by bacteria in response to beta-lactam antibiotics.
28. (C) ACE inhibitors work on this system.
    (A) This is part of the bacterial cell wall.
    (B) This is part of the bacterial chromosome.
    (D) See answer C.
29. (C) b.i.d. = twice daily
    (A) p.r.n. = take as needed
    (B) p.o. = take by mouth
    (D) q.i.d. = four times daily
30. (C) The average systolic pressure in the capillaries is 17 to 30 mm Hg.
    (A) The average systolic pressure in the arteries is 100 to 120 mm Hg.
    (B) The average systolic pressure in the arterioles is 30 to 70 mm Hg.
    (D) The average systolic pressure in the veins is 0 to 17 mm Hg.
31. (A) Force is produced during ventricular contraction.
    (B) A vacuum is created through the dilation of the ventricles.
    (C) A respiratory pump is created during exhalation.
    (D) The pressure is almost zero in the veins connected to the heart.
32. (E) Xerostomia is the correct answer.
    (A) This term relates to dry eyes.
    (B) This term relates to the eyes.
    (C) This term implies frequent urination.
    (D) The term implies frequent thirst.
33. (C) This is the normal range for white blood cells.
    (A) This number would be increased, most likely with neutrophils.
    (B) This is a normal amount of cells.
34. (A) The neutrophil is the most numerous circulating white blood cell.
    (B) The lymphocyte is the second most numerous circulating white blood cell.
    (C) The monocyte is the third most numerous cell.
    (D) Macrophages are found in tissue.
35. (C) The facial nerve innervates the muscles of facial expression.
    (A) The trigeminal nerve provides motor and sensory neuron.
    (B) The abducens nerve provides motor fibers to the rectum lateralis muscle of the eyeball.
    (D) The glossopharyngeal nerve profices taste to the posterior one third of the throat.
36. (C) This describes the origin of the facial nerve.
    (A) This describes the origin of the trigeminal nerve.
    (B) This describes the origin of the abducens nerve.
    (D) This describes the origin of the hypoglossal nerve.
37. (D) Both statements are true.
    (A) See statement D.
    (B) See statement D.
    (C) See statement D.
38. (A) Renin is converted into angiotensin I.
    (B) See statement A.
    (C) See statement A.
39. (A) Cranial nerve VII emerges from the stylomastoid foramen.
    (B) The optic nerve emerges from the optic canal/foramen.
    (C) The glossopharyngeal nerve emerges from the jugular foramen.
40. (D) Both statements are *TRUE*.
    (A) Both statements are *TRUE*.
    (B) Both statements are *TRUE*.
    (C) Both statements are *TRUE*.
41. (B) One of the intraoral signs of bulimia is wearing away of the lingual surfaces of the anterior maxillary teeth.
    (A) Decreased insulin production is a sign of diabetes.
    (C) This is a condition where teeth are fused to bone.
    (D) There are no signs of abrasion in this client.
42. (A) Erosion is the loss of tooth structure from chemical effects on teeth.
    (B) Abrasion is the loss of tooth structure from mechanical effects on the teeth.
    (C) Attrition is the physiological wearing away of tooth structure.
43. (B) The pH is usually at one.
    (A) See answer B
    (C) It is not neutral.
    (D) The pH of the stomach is acidic, not basic.
44. (B) This is an example of herpes zoster (shingles). Notice the unilateral eruption of lesion.
    (A) Herpes simplex is a recurrent viral disease caused by HSV I and II.
    (C) See statement B.
    (D) See statement B.
45. (A) Acyclovir is the appropriate antiviral drug.
    (B) Penicillin is not effective against viral replication.
    (C) Estrogen therapy is not used to treat viral infections.
46. (A) This virus is spreading through VI.
    (B) See statement A.
    (C) See statement A.
47. (B) The trunk between vertebrae T3 and L2 is another common site for this latent viral disease.
    (A) Herpetic whitlow can be found on the fingers.
    (C) See statement B.
    (D) See statement B.
48. (B) Parietal cells secrete hydrochloric acid.
    (A) Goblet cells secrete mucus.
    (C) Chief cells secrete pepsinogen.
    (D) Argentaffen cells secrete serotonin and histamine.

49. (D) Both statements are *FALSE*. Normal intestinal motility is relatively slow and is due primarily to the fact that the pressure at the pyloric end of the small intestine is greater than that at the distal end.
    (A) See statement D in the rationales.
    (B) Intestinal motility is normally slow.
    (C) Pressure is greater at the pyloric end than the distal end of the intestine.

50. (C) In addition to receiving venous blood from the intestine, the liver also receives arterial blood via the hepatic artery.
    (A) This pattern of circulation is true for general circulation in the body, not the liver.
    (B) This pattern is capillaries → vein → capillaries → vein.
    (D) Capillaries in the digestive tract drain into the hepatic portal vein, which carries this blood to capillaries in the liver; it is not until the blood has passed through the second capillary bed that it enters the general circulation through the hepatic vein that drains the liver.

Clinical Oral Structures, Dental Anatomy, and Root Morphology

Marilyn Beck   Susan Zimmer

Oral anatomy is a fundamental dental science upon which the clinical practice of dental hygiene is based. A dental hygienist must be thoroughly familiar with the clinical appearance of normal oral structures throughout the process of care. A thorough knowledge of dental anatomy provides the basis for assessing, planning, implementing, and evaluating dental hygiene care. Specifically, a knowledge of *crown* anatomy gives the dental hygienist the background information needed to identify the teeth present in a dentition, educate clients in proper oral health, and make decisions about fluoride therapy and pit and fissure sealants. Dental morphology is integrally related to instrumentation theory. A thorough knowledge of *root* anatomy is necessary for periodontal assessment, instrumentation, and maintenance. The critical skills necessary for periodontal probing, exploring, scaling, root planing and debridement demand that the dental hygienist use mental imagery and tactile sensations in the adaptation and activation of instruments and the evaluation of care. The dental hygienist also observes and assesses the relationship a tooth has with adjacent teeth in the same and the opposing arch. The identification of alterations in the expected alignment and their cause is essential to individu-

alized plans for oral health, instrument selection, and referral to other healthcare specialists.

This chapter addresses the clinical appearance of oral structures, dental terminology, morphology of the permanent and primary teeth, eruption, and the relationship of the teeth within and between the dental arches.

Clinical Oral Structures

Oral tissues are indicators of oral and general health. Abnormal conditions can be recognized if the appearance of normal oral structures is known. The color and morphology of the structures may vary with genetic patterns and age.

A. Lips and cheeks
   1. Philtrum—midline vertical depression of the skin between the nose and the upper lip.
   2. Vermilion zone—transition area between the skin of the face and the oral mucosa of the lips
   3. Labial commissure—junction of the upper and lower lip at the corner of the mouth
   4. Vestibule—space between the cheeks, lips, and facial surfaces of the teeth and gingiva

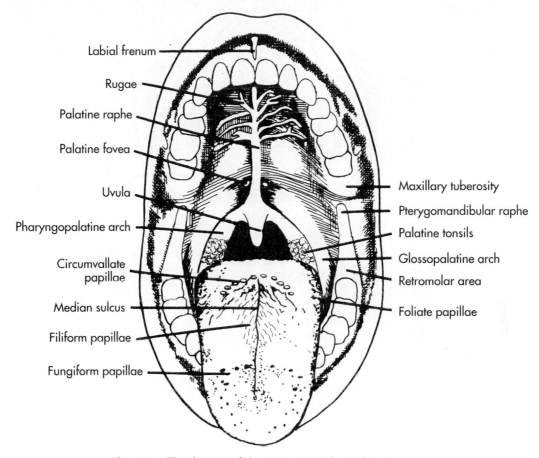

Fig. 4-1 The dorsum of the tongue and the oral cavity.

5. Labial mucosa—mucous membrane lining of the inner lip; its surface has small elevations that are the external manifestation of the minor labial salivary glands
6. Labial frenum—fold of tissue at the midline (maxillary and mandibular) between the inner surface of the lip and the alveolar mucosa (Figs. 4-1 and 4-2)
7. Buccal mucosa—mucous membrane lining of the inner cheek
8. Buccal frena—folds of tissue between the cheek and the attached gingiva (maxillary and mandibular) in the first premolar area
9. Parotid papilla—flap of tissue on the cheek opposite the maxillary first molar; contains the opening for Stenson's duct, which carries saliva from the parotid gland
10. Alveolar mucosa—thin, movable, lining-type mucosa covering the alveolar bone on the facial and mandibular lingual
11. Mucobuccal fold—fold or "gutter" area between the alveolar and buccal or labial mucosa

B. Tongue and floor of the mouth (Figs. 4-1 and 4-2)—the tongue is a flat muscular organ of speech and taste; numerous small elevations called papillae make the dorsum rough
1. Median sulcus—midline depression on the dorsum of the tongue; if additional grooves are present it is called a fissured tongue
2. Fungiform papillae—red to dark brown papillae scattered over the anterior third of the dorsum of the tongue; contain taste buds
3. Filiform papillae—small papillae with fringe-like keratinized projections; concentrated in the middle third of the dorsum of the tongue; readily collect plaque and stain
4. Circumvallate papillae—8 to 10 large papillae arranged in an inverted V-shaped row posterior to the filiform papillae; contain taste buds; ducts of von Ebner's salivary glands open around them
5. Foliate papillae—folds or "ruffles" of tissue on the posterior lateral border of the tongue; contain taste buds
6. Lingual tonsils—mass of lymphoid tissue on the

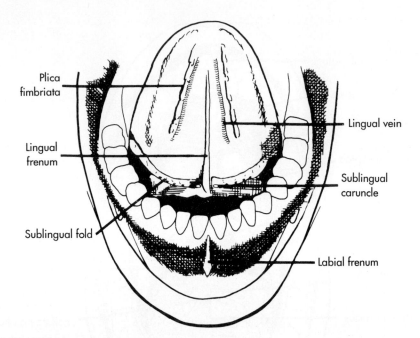

Fig. 4-2 The undersurface of the tongue and the floor of the mouth.

base of the dorsum of the tongue behind the circumvallate papillae

7. Lingual frenum—thin fold of epithelium between the undersurface of the tongue and the floor of the mouth; if short, tongue movement is limited (ankyloglossia)

8. Sublingual folds—two ridges of tissue on the floor of the mouth arranged in a V-shaped direction from the lingual frenum to the base of the tongue; contain duct openings from the sublingual salivary glands

9. Sublingual caruncle—round elevation at the anterior end of each sublingual fold on either side of the lingual frenum; contains the opening for Wharton's duct, which carries saliva from the submandibular (also called submaxillary) salivary gland and a major duct of the sublingual salivary gland

10. Lingual vein—vein visible on the undersurface of the tongue on either side of the lingual frenum

11. Plicae fimbriatae—fringelike projections lateral to the lingual vein

C. Palate (Fig. 4-1)—consists of two parts: the hard palate of attached masticatory mucosa and bone form the anterior two thirds of the roof of the mouth; the soft palate of loose lining-type mucosa forms the posterior third of the roof of the mouth

1. Incisive papilla—pad of tissue lingual to the maxillary central incisors; protects the nasopalatine

nerve, which enters through the underlying incisive foramen

2. Rugae—firm, irregular ridges of masticatory mucosa on the anterior half of the hard palate

3. Palatine fovea—small dimple on either side of the midline at the junction of the hard and soft palate

4. Palatal salivary gland duct openings—small red or dark spots scattered on the hard and soft palate; represent the duct openings from the minor palatal salivary glands

5. Palatine raphe—hard linear elevation along the midline of the hard palate; external manifestation of the palatine suture joining the right and left maxillary and palatine bones

6. Maxillary tuberosity—protuberance of the alveolar bone distal to the last maxillary molar

D. Tonsillar region (Fig. 4-1)

1. Retromolar area—triangular area of bone and pad of tissue distal to the last mandibular molar

2. Pterygomandibular raphe—fold of tissue extending from the retromolar area to an area near the maxillary tuberosity; separates the soft palate from the cheek

3. Anterior or glossopalatine arch—thin fold of tissue extending lateral and inferior from both sides of the soft palate to the base of the tongue; marks the entry to the pharynx

4. Posterior or pharyngopalatine arch—thin fold of tissue more posterior and narrower than the ante-

rior arch; with the anterior arch forms the boundary of the tonsillar recess

5. Palatine tonsils—globules of lymphoid tissue located in the tonsillar recess
6. Uvula—fleshy tissue suspended from the midline of the posterior border of the soft palate
7. Pharyngeal tonsils—globules of lymphoid tissue (adenoids) on the oropharyngeal wall
8. Fauces—isthmus (narrowing) of the space from the oral cavity into the pharynx

Dental Terminology

A. Parts of a tooth
   1. Crown
      a. Anatomic crown—part of the tooth covered by enamel
      b. Clinical crown—two definitions
         (1) Portion of the tooth visible in the oral cavity; determined by the location of the gingival margin; or
         (2) Unattached portion of the tooth; determined by the junction of the epithelium to the tooth surface; includes that portion of the tooth bounded by the marginal gingiva
   2. Root—part of the tooth covered by cementum
      a. Apex—rounded end of the root
      b. Foramen—opening at the apex through which blood vessels and nerves enter
      c. Furcation—area of a two- or three-rooted tooth where the root divides
         (1) Furcation entrance—area of opening into the furcation
         (2) Roof of the furcation—most coronal area of the furca; the "ceiling" of a mandibular furcation; the base of a maxillary furcation
         (3) Interfurcal area—area between the roots of a two- or three-rooted tooth
      d. Root trunk—area from the cementoenamel junction (CEJ) to the furcation
      e. Root concavity—broad, shallow vertical depression on the root; named by location; mesial, distal, and lingual; a concavity located on the furcation side of a root is called a furcal concavity
   3. Enamel—hardest calcified tissue covering the dentin in the crown of the tooth; 96% mineralized
   4. Cementum—bonelike calcified tissue covering the dentin in the root of the tooth; 50% mineralized
   5. Dentin—hard calcified tissue surrounding the pulp and underlying the enamel and cementum; makes up the bulk of the tooth; 70% mineralized
   6. Pulp—the innermost noncalcified tissue containing blood vessels, lymphatics, and nerves

   7. Pulp cavity—the space containing the pulp
      a. Pulp canal—portion of the pulp cavity in the root of the tooth
      b. Pulp chamber—portion of the pulp cavity in the crown of the tooth
      c. Pulp horns—crownward extensions of the pulp chamber
B. Junction of parts
   1. CEJ (cervical line)—junction of the cementum and enamel
   2. DEJ—junction of the dentin and enamel
   3. CDJ—junction of the cementum and dentin
C. Tooth surfaces
   1. Facial—surface toward the face
      a. Labial (toward the lips)—facial surfaces of anterior teeth
      b. Buccal (toward the cheeks)—facial surfaces of posterior teeth
   2. Lingual—surface toward the tongue; may also be called palatal for the maxillary teeth
   3. Proximal—surface toward the adjacent tooth
      a. Mesial—proximal surface toward the midline
      b. Distal—proximal surface farthest from the midline
   4. Contact area—area that touches the adjacent tooth in the same arch
   5. Incisal—surface of an incisor that is toward the opposite arch; the biting surface; newly erupted permanent incisors have *mamelons* (projections of enamel) on this surface
   6. Occlusal—surface of a posterior tooth that is toward the opposite arch; the chewing surface. This surface has elevations and depressions; the expression of these anatomic landmarks varies with the population from which they are derived
      a. Cusp—large, rounded, elevated area of enamel
      b. Ridge—rounded, linear elevation of enamel
         (1) Marginal ridge—forms the mesial and distal border of the lingual surface of anterior teeth and the occlusal surface of posterior teeth
         (2) Triangular ridge—ridge from the tip of the cusp to the central developmental groove; formed by the junction of two cuspal inclines
         (3) Oblique ridge—a collective term referring to two triangular ridges meeting in an oblique line; a characteristic of maxillary molars
         (4) Transverse ridge—a collective term referring to two triangular ridges meeting in a faciolingual line
         (5) Cingulum—large, rounded elevation of enamel on the linguocervical third of anterior teeth

c. Cuspal inclines—the two surfaces of a cusp that slant or slope down and away from the crests of the triangular ridge toward the developmental grooves

d. Groove—narrow linear depression

(1) Developmental groove—groove that divides cusps or lobes, which are primary anatomic divisions of a crown; referred to as a fissure, if deep

(2) Supplemental groove—a less distinct groove that branches from a developmental groove

e. Fossa—a shallow, broad depression

f. Pit—sharp depression where two or more grooves meet; deepest part of a fossa

D. Junction of surfaces—a tooth has curved surfaces; therefore, there is no "corner" where one surface begins and another ends. The transition area is called a *line angle area* and is named for the surfaces that are involved (e.g., MB—mesiobuccal, DL—distolingual, MO—mesioocclusal)

E. Embrasure—an interproximal space that begins at the contact area and widens toward the facial, lingual, occlusal/incisal, and cervical; functions as a spillway and escapement area by deflecting food and reducing forces placed upon the periodontum during chewing; also provides a self-cleaning area; interproximal gingiva fills the cervical embrasure

Dental Anatomy

A. Permanent dentition

1. Humans are diphyodonts, having two sets of teeth in a lifetime—a permanent and a primary dentition

2. The permanent dentition consists of 8 incisors, 4 canines, 8 premolars, and 12 molars

3. The Universal Numbering System uses Arabic numerals 1 to 32 to specify the permanent teeth, beginning with the maxillary right third molar and ending with the mandibular right third molar; the International Standards Organization (ISO) TC 106 designation system (also referred to as the International Numbering System) uses a two digit code; the first digit, 1 to 4, designates the quadrant in the dentition, clockwise from the upper right quadrant; the second digit, 1 to 8, designates the tooth, from the central incisor to the third molar

4. General characteristics of tooth form

a. All proximal surfaces converge toward the apex from the crests of curvature (height of contour) (Fig. 4-3)

(1) This convergence provides spacing for interproximal gingiva and bone

(2) In an ideal dentition the proximal crest of curvature is also the contact area, which functions to stabilize adjacent teeth and protect the interproximal gingiva

(3) Proximal crests are located in the incisal or middle third of the crown

(4) The general rule is the mesial crest is more incisal/occlusal than the distal crest and mesial cusp ridges are shorter than distal cusp ridges; mesial outlines are straighter than distal outlines (Fig. 4-4)

b. All facial and lingual surfaces converge toward the apex and toward the incisal/occlusal surface from the crests of curvature; this convergency facilitates mastication (Fig. 4-5)

c. All facial surfaces of the crown are convex, and the crest of the curvature is located in the cervical third; the lingual surfaces of posterior teeth are convex, and the crest of curvature is located in the middle third; the lingual surfaces of anterior teeth are concave in the middle third; these

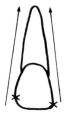

Fig. 4-3 The apical convergence of proximal surfaces.

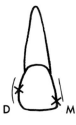

Fig. 4-4 Mesial and distal outlines compared.

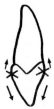

Fig. 4-5 The apical and incisal/occlusal convergence of facial and lingual surfaces.

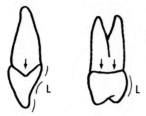

Fig. 4-8 The lingual convergence of proximal surfaces.

Fig. 4-6 Facial and lingual contours and the proximal curvature of the CEJ.

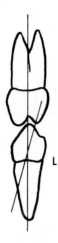

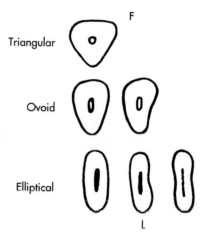

Fig. 4-9 Root shapes in cervical cross section: triangular, ovoid, and elliptical.

Fig. 4-7 The lingual inclination of the mandibular posterior crowns.

contours deflect food away from the gingiva and facilitate the function of the teeth (Fig. 4-6)

d. The CEJ on the proximal surface curves toward the incisal/occlusal surface and is more prominent on the anterior teeth than on the posterior teeth; the CEJ curves more on the mesial than on the distal surface (see Fig. 4-6)

e. From a proximal view, the long axis of the crown and root are in line except for the mandibular posterior teeth, which have the long axis of the crown tilting lingual to the long axis of the root; this lingual inclination enables the intercusping relationship of the posterior teeth and the distribution of forces along their long axes (Fig. 4-7)

f. Proximal surfaces converge to the lingual; this is most prominent on the maxillary incisors and canines (two exceptions are the mandibular second premolar and maxillary first molar) (Fig. 4-8)

5. General characteristics of roots

a. Root anatomy is not as complex as crown anatomy, but variations in size, shape, and number occur frequently

b. Teeth have one, two, or three roots:

(1) One root—incisors, canines, maxillary second premolar, mandibular premolars

(2) Two roots—maxillary first premolar (buccal and lingual) and mandibular molars (mesial and distal)

(3) Three roots—maxillary molars (mesiobuccal, distobuccal, and lingual)

c. Teeth with two or three roots have a root trunk with depressions that deepen until the trunk divides at the furcation

d. Some roots have longitudinal depressions called root concavities

e. Individual roots are basically cone shaped, being widest at the CEJ and converging to the apex

f. A cervical cross section of teeth with one root shows three basic shapes (Fig. 4-9) that may be slightly altered by the presence of root concavities

(1) Triangular—maxillary incisors

(2) Ovoid (egg shaped)—canines and some mandibular premolars

(3) Elliptical—maxillary premolars, mandibular incisors, and some mandibular premolars

g. Roots that are triangular or ovoid in cross section have narrower lingual surfaces

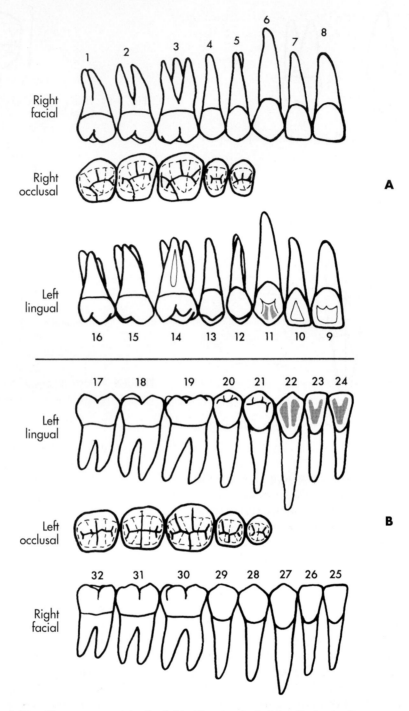

Fig. 4-10 The permanent teeth: **A,** Maxillary teeth; **B,** Mandibular teeth.

h. A cervical cross section of molars follows the form of the crown
i. From a facial or lingual view, roots have a distal inclination
j. Second and third molar roots are more likely to be closer together, fused, and distally inclined
6. The permanent incisors (Fig. 4-10)

a. General characteristics
    (1) There are eight incisors, two in each quadrant, named central and lateral incisors
    (2) Only teeth with an incisal ridge; newly erupted incisors have mamelons on the incisal ridge that are usually worn away shortly after eruption

(3) Only teeth with incisal angles; formed by the proximal surface and the incisal ridge; central incisal angles are sharper than lateral incisal angles; mesioincisal angles are sharper than distoincisal angles, which are more rounded

(4) Lingual anatomy consists of a lingual fossa bounded by a cingulum, mesial and distal marginal ridges, and a linguoincisal ridge

(5) Maxillary lateral incisors vary the most in size and shape; they may also be congenitally missing

b. Maxillary incisor crown anatomy

(1) Maxillary central incisor is the largest of the incisors; the lateral is next largest

(2) Mesiodistal width is greater than faciolingual

(3) Lingual anatomy is distinct

    (a) Central incisor cingulum is broad; grooves make it appear scalloped

    (b) Lateral incisor cingulum is narrow; a lingual pit is common

c. Maxillary incisor root anatomy

(1) Roots are short; sometimes no longer than the length of the crown; the lateral incisor crown/root ratio is larger than the central incisor

(2) Central incisor root is thicker than the lateral incisor root

(3) Maxillary incisors generally do not have root concavities; lateral incisors may have a deep lingual groove that starts on the distolingual marginal ridge and extends onto the root

(4) In cervical cross section, maxillary incisor roots are triangular with broad facial and proximal surfaces that converge toward a very small lingual surface; the mesial surface is quite flat

d. Mandibular incisor crown anatomy

(1) Mandibular central incisor is the smallest tooth in the dentition; the lateral is only slightly larger

(2) Faciolingual width is greater than mesiodistal width

(3) Incisal angles are sharp and the contact areas are often near the incisal ridge

(4) Lingual surface is concave; the lingual anatomy is not distinct and there are no pits

(5) Mandibular central, from a facial view, appears almost symmetric

(6) Mandibular lateral is characterized by the distal twist of the crown on the root; the

cingulum is displaced slightly toward the distal

e. Mandibular incisor root anatomy

(1) Roots are longer than the crown

(2) In cervical cross section the root is elliptical in shape with very small facial and lingual surfaces and broad proximal surfaces with root concavities

f. Clinical considerations of incisor form

(1) Maxillary lingual anatomy is more prominent than mandibular; however, plaque, calculus, and stain readily collect on the mandibular lingual surfaces

(2) Proximal surfaces of maxillary incisors are more accessible from the lingual because of the convergence of the proximal surfaces; the proximal surfaces of mandibular incisor roots are difficult to approach because of limited interproximal space and root concavities

(3) As people keep their teeth and live longer, repeated instrumentation on the roots of mandibular incisors place the crowns of these teeth in jeopardy; the very narrow facial and lingual root surfaces are more subject to loss of structure resulting in unsupported cervical enamel

7. The permanent canines

a. General characteristics

(1) One in each quadrant

(2) Only teeth with one cusp

(3) Considered the "cornerstone" teeth because of the long, large root externally manifested by the canine eminence of the alveolar bone

b. Maxillary canine crown anatomy

(1) Cusp ridges and tip occupy the incisal third of the crown

(2) Lingual anatomy includes a cingulum, mesial and distal marginal ridges, and a vertical lingual ridge between two lingual fossae; rarely has lingual pits

c. Mandibular canine crown anatomy

(1) Cusp ridges and tip occupy the incisal fourth of the crown, which appears longer and narrower than the maxillary canine

(2) Lingual anatomy same as maxillary canine but not as prominent

d. Canine root anatomy

(1) Root is the longest in the dentition, averaging one and one half times the length of the crown; the maxillary root is usually a little longer

(2) In cervical cross section the root is ovoid,

with broad facial and proximal surfaces that converge to the lingual; proximal root concavities are expected

(3) Rarely, a mandibular canine root is bifurcated into a facial and lingual root

e. Clinical considerations of canine form

(1) Crown length and bulk make these teeth very stable

(2) Proximal surfaces are more accessible from the lingual than the facial approach because of the convergence of the proximal surfaces

8. The premolars

a. General characteristics

(1) All posterior teeth have these characteristics

(a) Shorter crowns

(b) Less curvature of the CEJ

(c) Occlusal surfaces with marginal ridges, cusps, pits, and grooves

(2) Replace the primary molars

(3) Generally have two cusps; the mandibular second premolar frequently has a three-cusped or tricuspidate form

(4) Have one root except for the maxillary first premolar, which has two roots

(5) First premolars are sometimes extracted for orthodontic purposes

b. Maxillary premolar crown anatomy

(1) Faciolingual width is greater than mesiodistal width

(2) From an occlusal view the outline of the first premolar is hexagonal and angular; the second premolar is rounded

(3) Have two cusps of relatively equal size, one facial and one lingual

(4) Occlusal anatomy of the first premolar includes a long central developmental groove that crosses the mesial marginal ridge and two pits; the second premolar has a shorter central developmental groove, and numerous supplemental grooves

(5) First premolar has a prominent concavity in the cervical third of the mesial surface of the crown that becomes continuous with a root concavity that deepens to the furcation

c. Maxillary premolar root anatomy

(1) First premolar usually has two roots, one facial and one lingual; furcations are on the mesial and distal surfaces in the middle of the apical third midway between the facial and lingual surfaces; often has only one root with a prominent mesial root concavity; sometimes has three roots, two facial and one lingual

(2) Second premolar usually has one root

(3) In cervical cross section both maxillary premolar roots are elliptical with proximal root concavities

d. Mandibular premolar crown anatomy

(1) Faciolingual and mesiodistal widths are almost equal

(2) First premolar has two cusps (one large facial and one small lingual cusp form a transverse ridge), two pits, and a mesiolingual groove

(3) Second premolar is larger and has one facial and one (bicuspidate form) or two (tricuspidate) small lingual cusps

(a) Bicuspidate form has an H-shaped groove pattern and two pits

(b) Tricuspidate form has one facial and two lingual cusps; has a Y-shaped groove pattern and a central pit; proximal surfaces of this form do not converge toward the lingual

e. Mandibular premolar root anatomy

(1) One root with proximal root concavities, some of which are deeply grooved in the apical third

(2) In cervical cross section are ovoid or elliptical

f. Clinical considerations of premolars

(1) Distinctive pit and groove patterns facilitate the identification of premolars present

(2) Proximal root concavities, especially the mesial of the maxillary first premolar, make subgingival instrumentation difficult on proximal surfaces

(3) Mandibular premolar crowns, with their small lingual surfaces and lingual inclinations, make instrumentation difficult

9. The permanent molars

a. General characteristics

(1) Erupt distal to the second primary molars

(2) First molars are the largest teeth in the dentition; the maxillary first is the largest; the second and third molars are progressively smaller

(3) Mandibular first molars are the first permanent teeth to erupt

(4) Maxillary molars have pits and grooves on occlusal and lingual surfaces; mandibular molars have pits and grooves on occlusal and buccal surfaces

(5) Maxillary molars have three roots; mandibular molars have two

(6) Presence, size, and shape of third molars vary greatly

b. Maxillary molar crown anatomy
   (1) Appear rhomboidal in outline from occlusal view
   (2) A characteristic oblique ridge extends from the mesiolingual to the distobuccal cusp
   (3) A characteristic distolingual groove ends in a pit on the lingual surface
   (4) First molar has five cusps; four on the occlusal surface and one off the mesial half of the lingual surface called the cusp of Carabelli; the mesiolingual cusp is the largest and the distolingual is the smallest
   (5) Second molar has four occlusal cusps and resembles the first molar but is smaller; sometimes does not have a distolingual cusp
   (6) Occlusal pits are located in mesial, central, and distal fossae
c. Maxillary molar root anatomy
   (1) Roots are mesiobuccal, distobuccal, and lingual
   (2) First molar roots are larger and more divergent; the lingual root is the largest and longest and extends beyond the crown outline
   (3) Furcations are located on the mesial, facial, and distal surfaces and begin near the junction of the cervical and middle thirds of the root; the facial furcation is located midway between the mesial and distal surfaces; the mesial and distal furcations are located more to the lingual than the facial surface
   (4) Root concavities are found on the mesial surface of the mesiobuccal root, the lingual surface of the lingual root, and the furcal surfaces. In a study on furcal concavities in maxillary first molars, R.C. Bower found 94% of mesiobuccal, 31% of distobuccal, and 17% of lingual roots to have furcal concavities[1] (Fig. 4-11)
d. Mandibular molar crown anatomy
   (1) Mesiodistal wider than faciolingual; crown appears rectangular
   (2) First molar usually has five cusps, three buccal and two lingual; a Y-shaped groove pattern is formed by the mesiobuccal, distobuccal, and lingual grooves; the two buccal grooves on the facial surface are extensions of the occlusal grooves and end in a pit; the occlusal surface has mesial, central, and distal pits
   (3) Second molar has four cusps, two buccal and two lingual; a + shaped groove pattern is formed by the central, buccal, and lingual grooves; the buccal surface has one groove that ends in a pit; the occlusal surface has mesial, central, and distal pits
e. Mandibular molar root anatomy
   (1) Roots are mesial and distal
   (2) First molar roots are larger, longer, and more divergent
   (3) Furcations are located on the facial and lingual midway between the proximal surfaces, at a level of one-fourth root length; the root trunk of a second molar is longer
   (4) Root concavities are found on the mesial surface of the mesial root and on furcal surfaces of both mesial and distal roots. In a study on furcal concavities on mandibular first molars, R.C. Bower found 100% of the mesial and 99% of the distal roots to have furcal concavities.[1] The root concavities on the mesial root of the first molar are especially prominent because this root has two root canals (Fig. 4-11)
f. Clinical considerations of molars
   (1) Complex pit and groove patterns make them relatively susceptible to dental caries; they should be sealed shortly after eruption
   (2) Lingual inclination of mandibular molar

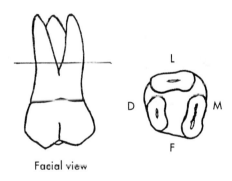

Facial view

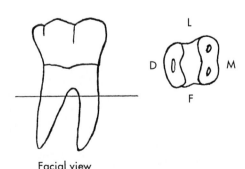

Facial view

Fig. 4-11 Furcal concavities of the maxillary and mandibular first permanent molars.

crowns makes the placement of instruments subgingivally more difficult on the lingual surface

(3) Proximal furcation areas of the maxillary molars should be approached from the lingual because the furcations are located closer to the lingual surface

(4) Roots with furcation involvement are especially difficult to manage; success of instrumentation is questionable without surgery

B. The primary dentition

1. The primary (deciduous) dentition consists of 20 teeth: 8 incisors, 4 canines, and 8 molars

2. The universal numbering system utilizes capital letters A through T for the primary teeth, beginning with the maxillary right second primary molar and ending with the mandibular right second primary molar; the International Standards Organization (ISO) TC 106 designation system uses a two digit code. The first digit, 5 to 8, designates the quadrant in the dentition, clockwise from the upper right quadrant; the second digit, 1 to 5, designates the tooth, from the central incisor to the second primary molar

3. The anatomy of the primary teeth is similar to that of permanent teeth except (Fig. 4-12)

a. Primary teeth are smaller in size than their permanent counterparts; the primary molars are wider than the premolars that replace them but are smaller than permanent molars

b. They are whiter

c. The crowns are shorter with pronounced labial and lingual cervical ridges and a constricted cervical area

d. The occlusal table is narrower faciolingually and the cuspal anatomy is not as pronounced

e. Enamel depth is more consistent and thinner (0.5 to 1 mm as compared with that of permanent teeth, which is 2.5 mm)

f. Pulp chambers (relative to the size of the tooth) are larger and the pulp horns extend more occlusally; the amount of dentin is proportionally less

g. Roots are slender and longer, about twice the crown length

h. Root trunks are shorter and the roots are more divergent in order to accommodate the developing premolar crown

i. Have fewer anomalies and variation in tooth form

4. Anatomy of primary teeth (Fig. 4-13)

a. Incisors—resemble the outline of their permanent counterpart except they may not have mamelons on the incisal ridge and no pits on the lingual surface

b. Canines—resemble the outline of their perma-

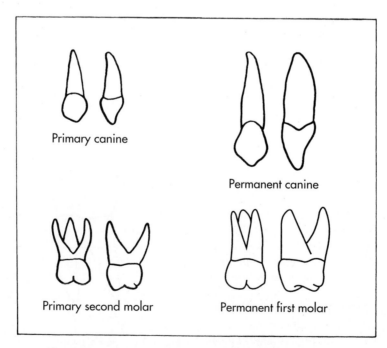

Primary canine

Permanent canine

Primary second molar

Permanent first molar

Fig. 4-12 The primary and permanent teeth compared.

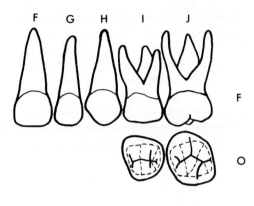

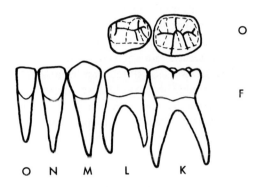

Fig. 4-13 The primary teeth.

nent counterpart; the maxillary canine has a sharp cusp and appears especially wide and short

c. Molars

(1) First primary molars

(a) They do not resemble any other teeth

(b) They have the same number and position of roots as the permanent molars

(c) CEJ on the mesial half of the buccal surface curves apically around a very prominent cervical ridge

(d) Maxillary first primary molar has an H-shaped groove pattern and usually three cusps; the mesial cusps are the largest

(e) Mandibular first primary molar has four or five cusps; the mesial cusps are larger and the ML cusp is long, pointed, and angled in on the occlusal surface

(2) Second primary molars are larger than the first primary molars and resemble the form of the *first permanent molar*

Eruption

A. General comments

1. Frequently defined as emergence of the tooth through the gingiva

2. More comprehensively defined as those movements a tooth makes to attain and maintain a relationship with the teeth in the same and the opposing arch

3. Developmental stages that relate to the broader definition are

a. Beginning of hard tissue formation

b. Enamel (crown) completion, after which actual tooth movement begins

c. Eruption

d. Root completion (approximately 50% of the root is formed when eruption begins)

4. Ages given in classical eruption tables are based on studies by Logan and Kronfeld (1933)

5. Sequential patterns are reflected throughout the developmental stages, and knowledge of these patterns can be used to predict and/or approximate the age of one stage, given another

6. Generally mandibular teeth erupt before maxillary teeth, and first of a type before the second

7. Clinically, eruption tables are helpful, but a better approach may be to correlate a given age with the teeth expected to be present

B. Primary teeth

1. A guide for the emergence into the oral cavity follows:

	Maxillary	Mandibular
Central incisor	7 ½ months	6 months
Lateral incisor	9 months	7 months
Canine	18 months	16 months
First molar	14 months	12 months
Second molar	24 months	20 months

2. The sequential pattern for primary tooth development is central incisor, lateral incisor, first molar, canine, second molar

3. Hard tissue formation begins between 4 and 6 months in utero

4. Crowns are completed between 1 ½ and 10 months of age

5. Roots are completed between 1 ½ and 3 years of age, 6 to 18 months after eruption

6. By age 3 years all of the primary and permanent teeth (except for the third molars) are in some stage of development

7. Root resorption of primary teeth is triggered by the pressure exerted by the developing permanent tooth; it is followed by primary tooth exfoliation in sequential patterns

8. The primary dentition ends when the first permanent tooth erupts

C. The mixed dentition

1. Transition dentition between 6 and 12 years of age with primary tooth exfoliation and permanent tooth eruption

2. Physiologic and psychologic effects may be noted for both parent and child
3. Its characteristic features have led to this being called the ugly duckling stage because of
   a. Edentulated areas
   b. Disproportionately sized teeth
   c. Various clinical crown heights
   d. Crowding
   e. Enlarged and edematous gingiva
   f. Different tooth colors

D. Permanent teeth
   1. Those that have primary predecessors are called *succedaneous;* they are the incisors, canines, and premolars
   2. The permanent teeth begin formation between birth and 3 years of age (except for the third molars)
   3. The crowns of permanent teeth are completed between 4 and 8 years of age, at approximately one-half the age of eruption
   4. The sequential pattern for permanent tooth development is

Maxillary	Mandibular
First molar	First molar
Central incisor	Central incisor
Lateral incisor	Lateral incisor
First premolar	Canine
Second Premolar	First premolar
Canine	Second premolar
Second molar	Second molar
Third molar	Third molar

   5. A guide for the emergence into the oral cavity follows:

	Maxillary	Mandibular
Central incisor	7-8 years	6-7 years
Lateral incisor	8-9 years	7-8 years
Canine	11-12 years	9-10 years
First premolar	10-11 years	10-12 years
Second premolar	10-12 years	11-12 years
*First molar	6-7 years	6-7 years
Second molar	12-13 years	11-13 years
Third molar	17-21 years	17-21 years

*First permanent tooth to erupt.
Based on studies by Logan and Kronfeld (1933)

   6. The roots of the permanent teeth are completed between 10 and 16 years of age, 2 to 3 years after eruption

E. Age changes in the dentition
   1. Biomarkers of aging are fluid; after the teeth have reached full occlusion, microscopic tooth movements occur to compensate for wear at the contact areas (by mesial drift) and occlusal surfaces (by deposition of cementum at the root apex)
   2. Attrition of incisal ridges and cusp tips may be so severe that dentin may become exposed and intrinsically stained
   3. Secondary dentin may be formed in response to dental caries, trauma, and aging and result in a decrease in size of the pulp cavity and tooth sensation

Intraarch and Interarch Relationships

Each tooth has a relationship with adjacent teeth in the same and the opposing arch. The relationships are influenced by a number of factors, including size and shape of the maxillae, mandible, and teeth and a wide variety of external factors such as oral habits and dental disease.

A. Intraarch relationship refers to the alignment of the teeth within an arch
   1. Position of the teeth in the jaw
      a. In an ideal alignment teeth contact at their proximal crests of curvature; a continuous arch form is observed from an occlusal view.
      b. Axial positioning—relationship of the long axis of individual teeth to an imaginary, horizontal or median plane. Ideally, each tooth "sits" at an angle that best withstands the forces placed on it
         (1) Incisors are placed with their axes at about 60° to the horizontal plane; the more posterior the tooth the less acute the angle. (Fig. 4-14)
         (2) Mandibular posterior teeth tip lingually, toward the median plane; the long axis of maxillary posterior teeth are more parallel to the median plane
      c. Curves of the occlusal plane (a line connecting the cusp tips of the canines, premolars, and molars) are observed from a buccal and a proximal view
         (1) Curve of Spee; anterior to posterior curve; for mandibular teeth the curve is concave and for maxillary teeth it is convex (Fig. 4-15, A)
         (2) Curve of Wilson; medial to lateral curve; for mandibular teeth the curve is also concave and for the maxillary teeth it is convex (Fig. 4-15, B)
   2. Contact does not always exist
      a. Some permanent dentitions have normal spacing
      b. Primary dentitions often have developmental spacing in the anterior area; some primary dentitions have a pattern of spacing called *primate spaces* between the primary maxillary lateral incisors and canine and between the mandibular canine and first molar (Fig. 4-16)
   3. Disturbances to the intraarch alignment are described as

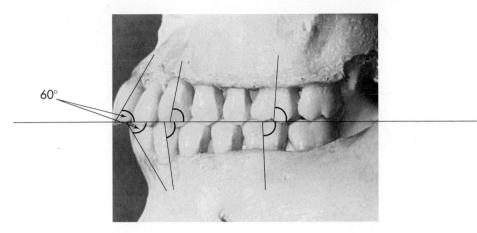

Fig. 4-14 Tooth positioning in relation to the horizontal plane. (Modified from Okeson JP. Management of temporomandibular disorders and occlusion, ed 4, St Louis, 1998, Mosby.)

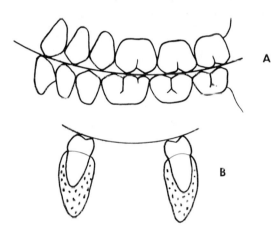

Fig. 4-15 The curves of occlusions. **A,** The curve of Spee; **B,** The curve of Wilson.

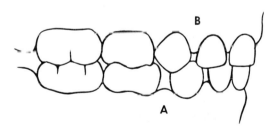

Fig. 4-16 Primary teeth showing primate spaces. **A,** Mandibular primate space between canine and first molar; **B,** Maxillary primate space between lateral incisor and canine. (From Wilkins E: *Clinical practice of the dental hygienist,* ed 7, Philadelphia, 1994, Lea & Febiger.)

 a. *Open contacts,* where interproximal space exists because of normal alignment, missing teeth, oral habits, dental disease, or overdeveloped frena
 b. *Versions,* where contact or position is at an unexpected area because of developmental disturbances, crowding, oral habits, dental caries or

periodontal disease; named for their misplaced position: facio-, linguo-, mesio-, disto-, supra (supererupted), infra (undererupted), and torso (rotated) version
B. Interarch relationships can be viewed from a stationary (fixed) and a dynamic (movable) perspective
 1. Stationary relationships
  a. *Centric relation* is the most superior relationship of the condyle of the mandible to the articular fossa of the temporal bone as determined by the bones, ligaments, and muscles of the temporomandibular joint; in an ideal dentition it is the same as centric occlusion
  b. *Centric occlusion* is habitual occlusion where maximum intercuspation occurs. (Note: a normal physiologic rest position of the mandible occurs during nonfunction when a freeway space with no interocclusal contact should occur.) The characteristics of centric occlusion are
   (1) *Overjet,* or that characteristic of maxillary teeth to overlap the mandibular teeth in a horizontal direction by 1 to 2 mm; the maxillary arch is slightly larger; functions to protect the narrow edge of the incisors and provide for an intercusping relationship of the posterior teeth (Fig. 4-17)
   (2) *Overbite,* or that characteristic of maxillary anterior teeth to overlap the mandibular anterior teeth in a vertical direction by a third of the lower crown height; facilitates the scissor-like function of incisors (Fig. 4-18)
   (3) *Intercuspation,* or that characteristic of posterior teeth to intermesh in a faciolingual direction; the mandibular facial and maxillary lingual cusps are centric cusps that con-

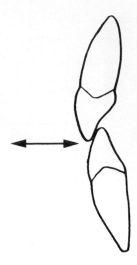

Fig. 4-17 Overjet, the horizontal overlap of the maxillary on the mandibular teeth.

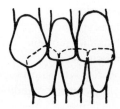

Fig. 4-18 Overbite, the vertical overlap of the maxillary anterior to the mandibular anterior teeth.

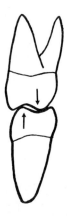

Fig. 4-19 Intercuspation of the posterior teeth. The centric cusps have interocclusal contact with the opposing teeth.

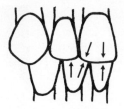

Fig. 4-20 Interdigitation of the teeth.

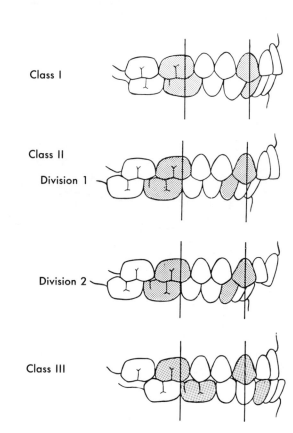

Class I

Class II

Division 1

Division 2

Class III

Fig. 4-21 Normal occlusion and classification of malocclusions. (From Wilkins E: *Clinical practice of the dental hygienist,* ed 7, Philadelphia, 1994, Lea & Febiger.)

tact interocclusally in the opposing arch (Fig. 4-19)

(4) *Interdigitation,* or that characteristic of each tooth to articulate with two opposing teeth (except for the mandibular central incisors and the maxillary last molars); a mandibular tooth occludes with the same tooth in the upper arch and the one mesial to it; a maxillary tooth occludes with the same tooth in the mandibular arch and the one distal to it (Fig. 4-20)

(a) Edward H. Angle classified these relationships using the first permanent molars (Fig. 4-21)

• Normal or neutral occlusion (ideal): mesiobuccal groove of the mandibular first permanent molar aligns with the mesiobuccal cusp of the maxillary first permanent molar

• Class I malocclusion: normal molar relationships with alterations to other

characteristics of the occlusion such as versions, crossbites, excessive overjets, or overbites
  - Class II malocclusion: a distal relation of the mesiobuccal groove of the mandibular first permanent molar to the mesiobuccal cusp of the maxillary first permanent molar
    Division I: protruded maxillary anterior teeth
    Division II: one or more maxillary anterior teeth retruded
  - Class III malocclusion: a mesial relation of the mesiobuccal groove of the mandibular first permanent molar to the mesiobuccal cusp of the maxillary first permanent molar
  (b) Canines may also be used to confirm the molar relationships or to classify occlusion when a molar is missing; a class I canine relationship shows the cusp tip of the maxillary canine facial to and aligned with the interproximal space between the mandibular canine and first premolar
  (c) Second primary molars are used to classify the occlusion in a primary dentition
  (d) In a mixed dentition the first permanent molars will erupt into a normal occlusion if there is a terminal step between the distal surfaces of the maxillary and mandibular second primary molars; if these surfaces are flush, a terminal plane exists and the first permanent molars will first erupt into an end-to-end relationship until there is a shifting of space or exfoliation of the second primary molar (Fig. 4-22)

2. Disturbances to interarch alignment are described as
  a. Excessive overbite where the incisal edges of the maxillary incisors extend to the cervical third of the mandibular incisors
  b. Excessive overjet where the maxillary teeth overjet the mandibular teeth by more than 3 mm
  c. End-to-end relationships: edge-to-edge bite where the anterior teeth meet at their incisal edges with no overjet or overbite; cusp-to-cusp bite where the posterior teeth meet cusp to cusp with no intercuspation
  d. Openbite where there is no incisal or occlusal contact between maxillary and mandibular

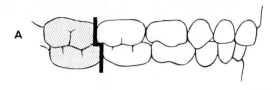
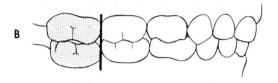

Fig. 4-22 Permanent first molar relationships in the mixed dentition. **A,** With a terminal step; **B,** With a terminal plane. (From Wilkins E: *Clinical practice of the dental hygienist,* ed 7, Philadelphia, 1994, Lea & Febiger.)

teeth; teeth cannot be brought together, a space is created
  e. Crossbites where the normal faciolingual relationship of the maxillary to the mandibular teeth is altered; for the anterior teeth, the mandibular tooth or teeth are facial rather than lingual to the maxillary teeth; for the posterior teeth, normal intercuspation is not observed; numerous alterations are possible and result in maxillary or mandibular, buccal or lingual, or partial or total crossbites

3. Dynamic interarch relationships are a result of functional mandibular movements that start and end with centric occlusion during mastication
  a. Mandibular movements are
    (1) Depression (opening)
    (2) Elevation (closing)
    (3) Protrusion (thrust forward)
    (4) Retrusion (bring back)
    (5) Lateral movements right and left; one side is always the working or chewing side and one the balancing or nonworking side
  b. Mandibular movements from centric occlusion are guided by the maxillary teeth
    (1) Protrusion is guided by the incisors; called incisal guidance
    (2) Lateral movements are guided by the canines on the working side in young, unworn dentitions (canine protected occlusion); and may be guided by incisors and posterior teeth in older, worn dentitions
  c. As mandibular movements commence from centric occlusion, the posterior teeth should disengage in protrusion; the posterior teeth on

the balancing side should disengage in lateral movement

d. If tooth contact occurs where teeth should be disengaged, occlusal interferences or premature contacts exist

REFERENCE

1. Bower RC: Furcation morphology relative to periodontal treatment, *J Periodontol* July 366-374, 1979.

SUGGESTED READINGS

Brand RW and Isselhard DE: *Anatomy of orofacial structures,* ed 5, St Louis, 1994, Mosby.

McKechnie LB: Root morphology in periodontal therapy. *Dental Hygienist News* 6:3-6, 1993.

Woelfel JB: *Dental anatomy,* Philadelphia, 1990, Lea & Febiger.

Wilkins E: *Clinical practice of the dental hygienist,* ed 7, Philadelphia, 1994, Lea & Febiger.

Wong MG: *Root morphology in dental hygiene theory and practice,* Darby ML, Walsh MM, eds, Philadelphia, 1995, WB Saunders.

Woodall I: *Comprehensive dental hygiene care,* ed 4, St Louis, 1993, Mosby.

Review Questions

1 Each of the following is descriptive of alveolar mucosa *EXCEPT* one. Which one is the *EXCEPTION*?
   A. Covers the facial and lingual alveolar bone
   B. Forms part of the mucco-buccal fold
   C. Movable, not attached to the alveolar bone
   D. Thin lining mucosa

2 Which of the following is *MOST* closely associated with the retromolar area?
   A. Last maxillary molar
   B. Lingual tonsils
   C. Pterygomandibular raphe
   D. Tonsillar recess

3 What type of tissue is located in the tonsillar recess?
   A. Connective tissue
   B. Lymphoid tissue
   C. Muscle tissue
   D. Nerve tissue

4 What structure is associated with the accumulation of stain on the dorsum of the tongue?
   A. Circumvallate papillae
   B. Filiform papillae
   C. Fungiform papillae
   D. Foliate papillae

5 The salivary gland associated with the accumulation of mineralized deposits on the facial surface of the maxillary first molars is the
   A. Parotid salivary gland
   B. Submandibular salivary gland
   C. Sublingual salivary gland
   D. von Ebner's salivary gland

6 When determining the cause of gingival recession on the facial surface of a first premolar, the clinician should observe the attachment of the
   A. Buccal frena
   B. Labial frenum
   C. Buccal mucosa
   D. Alveolar mucosa

7 Which of the following oral structures is associated with a torus palatinus?
   A. Incisive papilla
   B. Maxillary tuberosity
   C. Palatine fovea
   D. Palatine raphae

8 The following structures are associated with the hard palate *EXCEPT* one. Which one is the *EXCEPTION*?
   A. Incisive papilla
   B. Palatine fovea
   C. Rugae
   D. Uvula

9 What does ankyloglossia refer to?
   A. Blocked eruption
   B. Fused roots
   C. Impacted third molars
   D. Short lingual frenum

10 To examine the pharyngeal tonsillar area, the clinician should guide the person to
   A. Depress the tongue
   B. Elevate the tongue
   C. Hold the tongue in a normal position
   D. Move the tongue to both sides

11 What is the name of the area that forms the mesial and distal border of the occlusal surface?
   A. Fossae
   B. Marginal ridge
   C. Triangular ridge
   D. Transverse ridge

12 *EXCEPT* for one, all of the following surfaces normally have a groove(s) that extend(s) from the occlusal surface. Which one is the *EXCEPTION*?
   A. Facial surface of mandibular first molars
   B. Facial surface of maxillary second molars
   C. Lingual surface of maxillary first molars
   D. Mesial surface of maxillary first premolars

13 The apical limit of the clinical crown is determined by the location of the marginal gingiva *OR* the location of the
   A. Alveolar bone
   B. Cementoenamel junction
   C. Dentinoenamel junction
   D. Junctional epithelium

14 Which of the following arch relationships is associated with embrasures?
   A. Contact areas
   B. Curves of the occlusal plane
   C. Open contacts
   D. Open bites

15 In the Universal Tooth Numbering System, the mandibular left first molar is #19. What is the International Standards Organization TC 106 System's code (also known as the International Numbering System) for this tooth?
A. 19
B. 36
C. 46
D. L

16 What is the relationship between tooth #20 and tooth K?
A. Both are mandibular second premolars
B. Both are mandibular molars
C. It is the same tooth in different tooth identification systems
D. Tooth #20 replaces tooth K

17 What dental anatomy is common *ONLY* to multi-rooted teeth?
A. Apical foramen
B. Fossa
C. Furcal concavity
D. Pulp horns

18 Which of the following anatomical characteristics is similar in the primary and permanent molars?
A. Extension of the pulp horns
B. Location of the root trunk
C. Number of roots
D. Thickness of the enamel

19 Which furcal root surface of molars is *LEAST* likely to have a concavity?
A. Mesial root of the mandibular first molar
B. Distal root of the mandibular first molar
C. Mesiobuccal root of the maxillary first molar
D. Lingual root of the maxillary first molar

20 To determine if there is furcation involvement of a maxillary second molar, the clinician should probe the
A. Midfacial and midlingual areas
B. Both proximal surfaces
C. Both proximal surfaces and the midfacial area
D. Both proximal surfaces and midlingual area

21 What tooth anatomy is common *ONLY* to anterior teeth?
A. Cingulum
B. Fossa
C. Pits
D. Marginal ridges

22 The CEJ curves the greatest on the
A. Facial and lingual surfaces of anterior teeth
B. Facial and lingual surfaces of posterior teeth
C. Proximal surfaces of anterior teeth
D. Proximal surfaces of posterior teeth

23 Which tooth has a mesial furcation and the longest root trunk?
A. Mandibular first premolar
B. Maxillary first premolar
C. Mandibular first molar
D. Maxillary first molar

24 Each of the following is a normal anatomic change associated with aging *EXCEPT* one. Which one is the *EXCEPTION?*
A. Attrition of the occlusal/incisal surfaces
B. Decrease in the size of the pulp cavity
C. Formation of cementum at the root apex
D. Formation of mamelons

25 Which of the following teeth is the *LEAST* likely to have proximal root concavities?
A. Maxillary central incisor
B. Maxillary canine
C. Mandibular central incisor
D. Mandibular canine

26 An oblique ridge separates the central and distal occlusal fossae. Mandibular molars have an oblique ridge.
A. Both statements are *TRUE.*
B. Both statements are *FALSE.*
C. The first statement is *TRUE*, the second is *FALSE.*
D. The first statement is *FALSE*, the second statement is *TRUE.*

27 Which of the following proximal surfaces is more easily reached from the lingual?
A. Proximal surfaces of maxillary incisors and mandibular incisors
B. Proximal surfaces of maxillary incisors and mandibular premolars
C. Proximal surfaces of maxillary and mandibular premolars
D. Proximal surfaces of mandibular incisors and maxillary premolars

28 What are the last succedaneous teeth to erupt?
A. Maxillary second molars
B. Third molars
C. Maxillary first premolars
D. Maxillary canines

29 What permanent tooth replaces the first primary molar?
A. First premolar
B. Second premolar
C. First molar
D. Second molar

30 When do the primary teeth begin to develop?
A. 4 to 6 weeks in utero
B. 8 to 10 weeks in utero
C. 12 to 14 weeks in utero
D. 18 to 20 weeks in utero

31 Normally, a child has a mixed dentition between the ages of _____ and _____.
A. 24 months and 6 years
B. 6 years and 10 years
C. 6 years and 13 years
D. 8 years and 16 years

Questions 32-34: A mother of 3 children is concerned about the eruption of her children's teeth. Dick is almost 12, Susan is aged 10, and Marilyn is 14 months old

32 If Dick, aged 12, has followed the normal eruption pattern, what primary teeth would Dick still have?
A. Maxillary primary canines
B. Maxillary and mandibular primary canines
C. Maxillary first primary molars
D. Maxillary second primary molars

33 Susan, aged 10, is concerned about her appearance. The following are expected oral appearances *EXCEPT* one. Which one is the *EXCEPTION?*
A. Crowding
B. Darker color of the permanent teeth
C. Enlarged, edematous gingiva
D. Primate spacing

34 If Marilyn, aged 14 months, has followed the normal eruption pattern, what primary teeth are unerupted?
A. Central incisors
B. Lateral incisors
C. Canines
D. First molars

35 In addition to the central incisors, what permanent teeth would you expect to see in an 8-year-old child?
A. Canines and first molars
B. First premolars and first molars
C. Lateral incisors and canines
D. Lateral incisors and first molars

36 When are the roots of the permanent teeth fully formed?
A. At the time of eruption
B. Six months after eruption
C. One year after eruption
D. Two years after eruption

37 An edge-to-edge tooth relationship is correctly described as:
A. A disturbance in intraarch alignment
B. A normal tooth relationship
C. Insufficient intercuspation
D. Insufficient overbite

38 Which of the following teeth guide protrusive mandibular movement?
A. Canines
B. Incisors
C. Centric cusps of the molars
D. Non-centric cusps of the molars

39 What relationship of the primary molars guides the eruption of the first permanent molars in an end-to-end relationship?
A. Primate spaces
B. Terminal step between the distal surface of the maxillary and mandibular primary molars
C. Terminal plane between the distal surface of the maxillary and mandibular primary molars
D. Tooth versions

40 A maxillary first molar is approximately 12 mm in length. How many millimeters from the CEJ would a clinician feel a furcation?
A. 2 mm
B. 4 mm
C. 6 mm
D. 8 mm

41 Which is the largest and longest root of maxillary molars?
A. Mesiobuccal
B. Distobuccal
C. Lingual
D. All roots are equal in size and length

42 If the mandibular left molars are lost and not replaced, over time which of the following is the *MOST* probable effect on the position of the maxillary left molars?
A. Mesial drift
B. No change
C. Rotation
D. Supereruption

43 Tooth #3 is in a normal axial position; tooth #30 is in buccal version. What is the *MOST* likely relationship of tooth #3 and tooth #30?
A. Crossbite
B. Excessive overjet
C. Excessive overbite
D. Openbite

44 In centric occlusion, the mesiobuccal cusp of tooth #14 is in the facial embrasure of tooth #19 and #20. What is the classification of malocclusion?
A. Neutral
B. I
C. II
D. III

45 Which of the following occurs in lateral mandibular movements of a young adult?
A. Canines on the working side guide the movement
B. Incisors guide the movement
C. Molars on the balancing side guide the movement
D. There is contact of the maxillary and mandibular posterior teeth

46 During an assessment of interarch relationships the clinician notes enlarged, reddened gingiva on the lingual surface of teeth #7 through #10. What is the *MOST* likely cause?
A. Anterior crossbite
B. Anterior openbite
C. Excessive overbite
D. Excessive overjet

47 When a tooth is turned from its normal intraarch alignment, it is in
A. Facioversion
B. Infraversion
C. Supraversion
D. Torsoversion

48 Which of the following interarch relationships is associated with the axial positioning of anterior teeth?
A. Intercuspation
B. Interdigitation
C. Overbite
D. Overjet

49 The following facilitate the intercuspation of maxillary and mandibular posterior teeth, *EXCEPT* one. Which one is the *EXCEPTION?*
A. Axial position of the mandibular posterior teeth toward the median plane
B. Axial position of the maxillary posterior teeth parallel to the median plane
C. Axial position of the maxillary posterior teeth more parallel to the horizontal plane
D. Lingual inclination of the crowns of mandibular posterior teeth

50 Which of the following is characteristic of an openbite?
A. A disturbance in intraarch alignment
B. Deviation in the arch form
C. Lack of incisal or occlusal contact
D. Insufficient overjet

Answers and Rationales

1. (A) There is no alveolar mucosa on the maxillary lingual surface; attached, masticatory mucosa covers the palate
   (B) Alveolar and buccal or labial mucosa form the mucobuccal fold
   (C) Alveolar mucosa is unattached and movable
   (C) Alveolar mucosa is thin, lining type mucosa
2. (C) The pterygomandibular raphe is a fold of tissue extending from the retromolar area to the maxillary tuberosity area
   (A) The last maxillary molar is most closely associated with the maxillary tuberosity
   (B) The lingual tonsils are on the base of the dorsum of the tongue
   (D) The tonsillar recess is in the tonsillar area, posterior to the retromolar area
3. (B) Palatine tonsils are located in the tonsillar recess; tonsils are lymphoidal tissue
   (A) Connective tissue is associated with support of structures
   (C) Muscle tissue is associated with contraction/movement
   (D) Nerve tissue is associated with sensory functions
4. (B) Filiform papillae are on the dorsum of the tongue, their fringe-like shape easily collects stain
   (A) Circumvallate papillae, 8 to 10 in number, are posterior to the fungiform papillae; they are round and not easily seen
   (C) Fungiform papillae are singularly scattered anterior to the filliform papillae; their surface is smoother
   (D) Foliate papillae are on the lateral border of the tongue, they are smooth ridges

5. (A) The opening of the parotid gland is on the parotid papillae, opposite the maxillary first molars
   (B) The opening of the submandibular salivary gland is on the sublingual caruncle, lingual to the mandibular incisors
   (C) The openings of the sublingual salivary gland are on the sublingual fold, on the floor of the mouth
   (D) The openings of von Ebner's salivary gland surround the circumvalate papillae on the posterior dorsum of the tongue
6. (A) The buccal frena, folds of tissue between the cheek and attached gingiva in the premolar area; may be thick and tight contributing to gingival recession
   (B) Labial frenum located at the midline, may contribute to gingival recession on the buccal of the central incisors
   (C) Buccal mucosa, mucous membrane lining of the inner cheek, is not associated with recession
   (D) Alveolar mucosa, lining mucosa of the alveolar bone, is not a cause of gingival recession
7. (D) The palatine raphe is an external elevation along the midline of the hard palate; torus palatinus is an exostosis at the midline of the hard palate
   (A) The incisive papilla is a pad of tissue lingual to the maxillary central incisors
   (B) The maxillary tuberosity is a protuberance of the alveolar bone distal to the last maxillary molar
   (C) The palatine fovea is a small dimple on either side of the midline at the junction of the hard and soft palate
8. (D) The uvula is at the distal border of the soft palate
   (A) The incisive papilla is a pad of tissue at the anterior midline of the hard palate
   (B) The palatine fovea are two small depressions at the distal border of the hard palate
   (C) Rugae are ridges of mucosa on the hard palate
9. (D) Ankyloglossia is the more stable joining (ankylo) of the tongue (glossia) to the floor of the mouth. The lingual frenum is shorter than normal
   (A) Blocked tooth eruption may be caused by the joining of the cementum to the alveolar bone (ankylosis)
   (B) Fusion is the merging of singular parts of a tooth; it usually refers to the merging of the roots of a tooth
   (C) Same as A
10. (A) The pharyngeal tonsillar area is on the oropharyngeal wall; depressing the tongue allows a view of this area
    (B) Elevating the tongue would not help to view the oropharyngeal wall
    (C) In a normal position the base of the tongue is too high to view the pharyngeal tonsillar area
    (D) Moving the tongue to both sides is necessary to view the posterior lateral sides of the tongue
11. (B) The occlusal surface is bounded on the mesial and distal by ridges of enamel called marginal ridges
    (A) Fossae are depressions on the occlusal surface, at the base of the marginal ridges
    (C) A triangular ridge is the area of an occlusal cusp, from the tip of the cusp to the central developmental groove
    (D) A transverse ridge collectively refers to two triangular ridges that meet in a faciolingual line

12. (B) A buccal groove is not normally present on the facial surface of maxillary second molars
    (A) Two grooves extend from the occlusal surface onto the facial surface of mandibular first molars
    (C) A groove extends from the occlusal surface onto the lingual surface of maxillary first molars
    (D) A groove extends over the marginal ridge onto the mesial surface of maxillary first premolars
13. (D) The clinical crown is the portion of the tooth visible in the oral cavity OR the unattached portion of the tooth; the junctional epithelium is the apical limit of unattached gingiva.
    (A) The alveolar bone is apical to the clinical crown
    (B) The cementoenamel junction is the apical limit of the anatomic crown
    (C) The enamel forms a junction with the dentin in the anatomic crown; this junction is not visible
14. (A) Embrasures are interproximal spaces that begin at the contact area and widen toward the facial, lingual, occlusal/incisal, and cervical
    (B) Curves of the occlusal plane are associated with the anterior, posterior or medial lateral curve of the occlusal/incisal surfaces
    (C) Open contacts are a lack of contact area between adjacent teeth
    (D) Open bites are a lack of contact between opposing teeth
15. In the International Standards Organization TC 106 Dentition Identification System (also known as the International Numbering System)
    (B) The lower left quadrant is 3; the first molar is #6
    (A) The upper right quadrant is 1; there is no tooth #9
    (C) The lower right quadrant is 4; the first molar is #6
    (D) The system does not use letters
16. (D) The mandibular left second premolar (#20) replaces the second primary molar (K)
    (A) There are no premolars in the primary dentition
    (B) Tooth #20 is a premolar
    (C) The Universal Tooth Numbering System uses numbers to identify the permanent teeth and letters to identify the primary teeth
17. (C) Furcal concavities are located on the furcation side of a root; only multi-rooted teeth have furcations
    (A) An apical foramen is the opening at the apex of a root; all roots have an apical foramen
    (B) A fossa is a shallow depression; fossae are present on the lingual surface of anterior teeth and the occlusal surface of posterior teeth
    (D) Pulp horns are the crownward extensions of the pulp chamber; they are present on all teeth
18. (C) Primary molars have the same number of roots as permanent molars; maxillary molars have three roots, mandibular molars have two roots
    (A) The pulp horns of primary molars extend more occlusally
    (B) The root trunks of primary molars are shorter, located in the cervical third
    (D) The enamel depth of primary molars is more consistent and thinner

19. (D) Study of furcal concavities found only 17% of the lingual roots of maxillary first molars have a furcal concavity
    (A) 100% of the mesial roots of mandibular first molars have a furcal concavity
    (B) 99% of the distal roots of mandibular first molars have a furcal concavity
    (C) 94% of the mesiobuccal roots of maxillary first molars have a furcal concavity
20. (C) The maxillary second molar has three furcations: facial, mesial, and distal
    (A) Mandibular molars have furcation areas on the facial and lingual surfaces
    (B) The facial furcation area would be missed if the clinician probed only the proximal surfaces
    (D) There is no furcation area on the lingual of maxillary molars
21. (A) A cingulum is a smooth, broad elevation of enamel present only on the lingual, cervical third of anterior teeth
    (B) Fossae are present on the lingual surface of anterior teeth and the occlusal surface of posterior teeth
    (C) Pits are normally present on the lingual surface of maxillary anterior teeth and the occlusal surface of posterior teeth
    (D) Marginal ridges are present on the lingual surface of anterior teeth and the occlusal surface of posterior teeth
22. (C) On the proximal surfaces of anterior teeth the CEJ curves apically in a V shape
    (A) On the facial and lingual surfaces of anterior teeth the CEJ is a gradual convex curve
    (B) The CEJ curves less on the facial and lingual surfaces of posterior teeth
    (D) The CEJ curves slightly on the proximal surfaces of posterior teeth
23. (B) The maxillary first premolar has a mesial (and distal) furcation in the middle to apical third of the root
    (A) The mandibular first premolar has one root
    (C) The mandibular first molar has a deep mesial concavity but no mesial furcation
    (D) The maxillary first molar has a mesial (distal and facial) furcation near the junction of the cervical and middle thirds of the root
24. (D) Mamelons are developmental scallops on the incisal edge of newly erupted permanent incisors; they are worn away shortly after eruption
    (A) Attrition of the incisal ridges and cusp tips occurs; if severe, dentin is exposed
    (B) Formation of secondary dentin decreases the size of the pulp cavity
    (C) Cementum deposits at the root apex; it compensates for wear on incisal and occlusal surfaces

25. (A) The root of a maxillary central incisor is convex, with no root concavities
    (B) Proximal root concavities are expected on a maxillary canine
    (C) The root of a mandibular central incisor has prominent proximal root concavities
    (D) Proximal root concavities are expected on a mandibular canine
26. (C) A ridge of enamel, the oblique ridge, separates the central and distal occlusal fossae; only maxillary molars have an oblique ridge
    (A) Only maxillary molars have an oblique ridge
    (B) A ridge of enamel, the oblique ridge, separates the central and distal occlusal fossae
    (D) A ridge of enamel, the oblique ridge, separates the central and distal occlusal fossae; only maxillary molars have an oblique ridge
27. (B) Maxillary incisor and mandibular premolar roots are triangular ovoid in shape; the lingual surface is smaller than the facial creating a wider lingual embrasure area
    (A) Maxillary incisor roots are more easily approached from the lingual; mandibular incisor roots are elliptical in shape, proximal surfaces are broad; facial and lingual embrasures are approximately the same size
    (C) Mandibular premolar roots are more easily approached from the lingual; maxillary premolar roots are elliptical in shape, proximal surfaces are broad; facial and lingual embrasures are approximately the same size
    (D) Mandibular incisor and maxillary premolar roots are elliptical in shape; proximal surfaces are broad; facial and lingual embrasures are approximately the same size
28. (D) Although maxillary canines are anterior teeth, they are usually the last permanent teeth to replace primary teeth at age 11-12
    (A) Although maxillary second molars erupt later, age 12-13; they are not succedaneous, they do not replace primary teeth
    (B) Although third molars are the last teeth to erupt, about age 17 or above, they are not succedaneous, they do not replace primary teeth
    (C) Maxillary first premolars usually erupt earlier, at age 10-11; they are succedaneous, they replace the first primary molar
29. (A) The first premolar replaces the first primary molar
    (B) The second premolar replaces the second primary molar
    (C) The first molar is not succedaneous, it erupts distal to the second primary molar
    (D) The second molar is not succedaneous, it erupts distal to the first permanent molar
30. (A) Primary teeth begin to develop 4 to 6 weeks in utero
    (B) Primary teeth begin to develop several weeks before this
    (C) Primary teeth begin to develop 6 to 8 weeks before this
    (D) Primary teeth begin to develop 12 to 14 weeks before this

31. (C) The first permanent tooth erupts about age 6; the last succedaneous tooth erupts about age 13; between these years, primary and permanent teeth are present
    (A) During this time only primary teeth are present
    (B) The mixed dentition continues for several years past age 10
    (C) The first permanent teeth erupt before age 8, and the last primary tooth is exfoliated several years before age 16
32. (A) The permanent maxillary canines are usually the last succedaneous teeth to erupt; they replace the primary canines at about 11-12 years of age
    (B) The mandibular primary canine would be exfoliated when the permanent canine erupted at about 9-10 years of age
    (C) The maxillary first premolars replace the maxillary first primary molars at about 10-11 years of age
    (D) It is more probable that the maxillary second premolars have erupted by 10-12 years of age and replaced the maxillary second primary molars
33. (D) Primate spacing is a characteristic of primary teeth; this spacing is usually closed when the larger permanent teeth erupt
    (A) The larger permanent teeth are often crowded until the mandible grows
    (B) Permanent teeth are darker in color than primary teeth
    (C) Enlarged, edematous gingiva occur with the process of exfoliation and eruption
34. (C) Primary canines do not erupt until 16-18 months
    (A) Primary central incisors erupted at 6-7 months
    (B) Primary lateral incisors erupted at 7-9 months
    (D) Primary first molars erupted at 12-14 months
35. (D) At 8 years of age the central incisors, lateral incisors, and first molars should be present
    (A) Central incisors and first molars will be present; mandibular canines erupt age 9 to 10; maxillary canines erupt 2 years later
    (B) Central incisors and first molars will be present; premolars begin to erupt about 10 years of age
    (C) Central and lateral incisors will be present; mandibular canines erupt at 9-10 years of age; maxillary canines erupt 2 years later
36. (D) Roots of permanent teeth are fully formed 2-3 years after eruption
    (A) The root of the tooth is not fully formed at the time of eruption
    (B) Complete formation of the root occurs 2-3 years after eruption
    (C) Complete formation of the root occurs 2-3 years after eruption
37. (D) An edge-to-edge bite occurs when anterior teeth meet at their incisal edges; the maxillary teeth do not overlap the mandibular teeth
    (A) This disturbance involves both arches; it is a disturbance in interarch alignment
    (B) It is normal for the maxillary teeth to overlap the mandibular teeth
    (C) Intercuspation involves posterior teeth; in a cusp-to-cusp bite there is insufficient intercuspation

38. (B) Protrusion is guided by the incisors, and is called incisal guidance
    (A) Canines guide lateral movements
    (C) Posterior teeth disengage in protrusive movements
    (D) Posterior teeth disengage in protrusive movements
39. (C) A flush, terminal plane relationship of the primary molars will guide the permanent first molars into an end-to-end relationship
    (A) Primate spaces is a spacing pattern between the maxillary lateral and canine and the mandibular canine and first primary molar
    (B) First permanent molars will erupt in a normal relationship if there is a terminal step relationship
    (D) Tooth versions are disturbances in intraarch alignment; versions involve individual tooth position
40. (B) Furcations of the maxillary molars begin near the junction of the cervical and middle thirds of the root, 3-5 mm from the CEJ
    (A) Root trunks of maxillary first molars are longer than 1-2 mm; furcations are further from the CEJ
    (C) Root trunks of maxillary first molars are shorter than 6 mm; furcations are closer to the CEJ
    (D) Same as C
41. (C) The lingual root is the longest and largest root of maxillary molars
    (A) The lingual root is larger and longer than the mesiobuccal root
    (B) The lingual root is larger and longer than the distobuccal root
    (D) All the roots are not the same size and length; the lingual root of maxillary molars is larger and longer
42. (D) Without opposing teeth, the maxillary teeth will supererupt
    (A) Contact with adjacent teeth will prevent an excessive mesial drift
    (B) Loss of teeth does have an effect on the opposing teeth, usually they supererupt
    (C) Contact with adjacent teeth will prevent rotation of the teeth
43. (A) Tooth #30 is in buccoversion; tooth #3 is lingual to tooth #30; this is a crossbite
    (B) Excessive overjet occurs when the maxillary tooth overlaps the opposing teeth more than 3 mm in a horizontal direction
    (C) Excessive overbite is a greater than normal vertical overlap of anterior teeth
    (D) An openbite occurs when teeth do not reach the line of occlusion
44. (C) The mesiobuccal cusp of tooth #14 should align with the mesiobuccal groove of tooth #19; in this case tooth #19 is distal to this relationship, this is a Class II malocclusion
    (A) In neutral occlusion, the mesiobuccal cusp of tooth #14 would align with the mesiobuccal groove of tooth #19
    (B) A neutral relationship and Class I molar relationship are the same
    (D) In a Class III malocclusion, the mesiobuccal groove of tooth #19 would be mesial to the mesiobuccal cusp of tooth #14

45. (A) Canines on the working side guide lateral movements
    (B) Incisors guide protrusion
    (C) Molars on the balancing side disengage in lateral movements
    (D) Molars on the balancing side disengage in lateral movements
46. (C) An excessive overbite may result in the mandibular incisors occluding in the lingual gingiva of the maxillary incisors
    (A) In an anterior crossbite the mandibular anterior teeth are facial to the maxillary anterior teeth
    (B) In an anterior openbite there is no vertical overlap of the maxillary and mandibular anterior teeth
    (D) In an excessive overjet the maxillary teeth are more than 3 mm facial to the mandibular teeth in a horizontal direction
47. (D) Torso version refers to the rotation of a tooth in the alveolus
    (A) Facial version refers to the facial position of a tooth in relation to the overall curvature of the arch
    (B) Infra version refers to the less than full eruption of a tooth into occlusion
    (C) Supra version refers to the eruption of a tooth past the occlusal plane
48. (D) Anterior teeth normally "sit" at a 60° angle to the horizontal plane; this places the crowns in a definite facial position. Overjet is the position of the maxillary teeth in a horizontal direction
    (A) Intercuspation is a characteristic of posterior teeth
    (B) Interdigitation is a characteristic of each tooth to articulate with two opposing teeth
    (C) Overbite is a characteristic of maxillary teeth to overlap the mandibular anterior teeth in a vertical direction
49. (C) The axial positioning in relation to the horizontal plane affects the amount of overjet of anterior teeth
    (A) The axial position of the mandibular posterior teeth toward the median plane brings the facial cusps into intercuspation in the occlusal surface of the maxillary posterior teeth
    (B) The axial position of the maxillary posterior teeth more parallel to the median plane brings the lingual cusps into intercuspation in the occlusal surface of the mandibular posterior teeth
    (D) The lingual inclination of the crowns of posterior teeth brings the facial cusps into intercuspation in the occlusal surface of the maxillary posterior teeth
50. (C) In an openbite there is no incisal or occlusal contact; there is a space between the maxillary and mandibular teeth
    (A) An openbite is a disturbance in alignment between the arches, interarch alignment
    (B) The arch form is usually maintained, with no teeth in buccal or lingual version
    (D) Teeth may have a normal horizontal relationship and normal overjet

Oral and Maxillofacial Radiology*

Evelyn M. Thomson-Lakey

An important aspect of the practice of dental hygiene essential for total client care is the utilization of comprehensive oral and maxillofacial imaging modalities that aid in the assessment, care planning, and evaluation of oral health.

Knowledge and skill in applying that information are critical for the safe use of radiant energy in the oral health-care setting. Therefore special emphasis is given to radiation physics, production, protection, and ethics; radiographic imaging techniques and receptor systems; radiographic film processing and quality assurance procedures; and radiographic anatomy and principles of interpretation.

General Considerations

Radiation Physics

A. Emission or propagation of energy in the form of waves or particles[1]
B. Types of radiation
  1. Particulate radiation

---

*Revisions based in part on original material by Nancy B. Webb and K. Cy Whaley.

  a. Particles that have both mass and energy
  b. Some particles may have a positive, negative, or neutral charge
  c. Cannot reach speed of light
  d. Examples—neutrons, protons, electrons, α-particles, and β-particles
2. Electromagnetic radiation
  a. Definitions
    (1) Wavelength—distance from one crest of a wave to the next; wavelength of electromagnetic radiation ranges from 10^6 to 10^{-16} m
    (2) Frequency—number of crests passing a particular point per unit of time and measured in hertz (Hz); 1 Hz is equal to 1 cycle/sec; frequency of electromagnetic radiation ranges from 10^2 to 10^{24} Hz
    (3) Photon and quantum—terms used to designate a single unit or bundle of energy
    (4) Energy—ability to do work; energy of electromagnetic radiation is measured in electron volts (eV); ranges from 10^{-12} to 10^{10} eV (1 keV is equal to 1000 eV)
  b. Characteristics
    (1) Bundles of energy that have neither mass nor charge

(2) Electric and magnetic fields are associated with the travel of the electromagnetic energy through space

(3) Electromagnetic energies exist over a wide range of magnitudes; are termed the electromagnetic spectrum

(4) Interaction of electromagnetic radiation with matter may be described in terms of wave and particle behavior

(5) Electromagnetic spectrum is measured according to frequency, energy, and wavelength

  c. Examples—radiowaves, microwaves, infrared light, visible light, ultraviolet light, x-rays, gamma rays, and cosmic rays

  3. Ionizing radiation

    a. Definitions

(1) Ion—charged particle; either positive or negative

(2) Ion pair—positive ion and negative ion

(3) Ionization—process by which radiant energy removes an orbital electron from an atom to yield an ion pair

(4) Ionizing radiation—particulate and electromagnetic radiation with sufficient energy to cause ionization of atoms; radiation must have energy greater than the electron-binding energy

    b. Biologic significance—damage of biologic systems results from the ionization process

    c. Examples—α-particles, β-particles, x-rays, and gamma rays

C. Sources of radiation

  1. Natural background radiation is the greatest contributor to population exposure from radiation

    a. Naturally occurring radionuclides in the soil (a radionuclide is an unstable atom that decays by emitting particles and energy from the nucleus to become electrically stable; deposited within the human body through the inhalation of air and the ingestion of food, and water)

    b. Cosmic radiation from outer space

  2. Healing arts

    a. Radiopharmaceutical agents

    b. X radiation

  3. Production and use of nuclear energy

    a. Atmospheric weapons tests

    b. Nuclear power reactors

  4. Research facilities

    a. High-voltage x-ray machines

    b. Particle accelerators

    c. Diffraction units

    d. Electron microscopes

  5. Consumer and industrial products may contain radioactive materials or use ionizing radiation

    a. Building materials

    b. Some smoke detectors

  6. Miscellaneous sources

    a. Transportation of radioactive materials

    b. Smoke from tobacco products

D. Average annual effective dose equivalent of ionizing radiation[2]

  1. The average annual effective dose equivalent of ionizing radiation to a member of the U.S. population is 3.63 mSv

  2. Natural sources (cosmic, terrestrial, and internal) account for 3.0 mSv, or 82%

  3. Man-made sources (medical, nuclear medicine, consumer products, occupational, etc.) account for 0.63 mSv, or 18%

    a. Of the man-made sources, medical/dental x-rays account for 0.39 mSv, or 11%

Discovery of X Radiation

A. Crookes tube

  1. Developed by Sir William Crookes

  2. Also known as a cathode ray tube

  3. Evacuated glass tube with two electrodes (cathode and anode) through which an electrical current is passed

B. Wilhelm Conrad Roentgen

  1. Discovered X rays on November 8, 1895

  2. Was investigating properties of the cathode ray with a Crookes tube

  3. Enclosed the Crookes tube with black paper; noticed glowing of fluorescent material on a workbench several feet away

  4. Because he knew that the cathode ray could only travel 6-8 cm, Roentgen knew he had discovered a new form of energy[3]

  5. Termed the unknown energy: X ray

Electricity

A. Definition

  1. The flow of electrons through a wire or other electrical conductor

B. Types

  1. Direct current (DC)—electrons flow in one direction only along an electrical conductor

  2. Alternating current (AC)—electrons flow in one direction and then reverse to flow in the opposite direction

    a. *Cycle* is used to refer to the flow of electrons in one direction and then the opposite direction

    b. One cycle is equal to $\frac{1}{60}$ second

c. Alternating current is designated as 60-Hz current (European countries use 50-Hz current)
C. Units of measurement
1. Ampere (A)—measurement of the number of electrons flowing in an electrical circuit; one milliampere (mA) is equal to $\frac{1}{1000}$ ampere; dental units usually operate between 7 mA and 15 mA
2. Volt (V)—measurement of the electrical potential or force that moves the electrons along an electrical conductor; one kilovolt (kV) is equal to 1000 volts; kilovolt peak (kVp) refers to the peak voltage of an alternating current
D. The power supply to dental x-ray machines is primarily 110-V, 60-Hz alternating current

X-Ray Machines

A. Types
1. Intraoral units are designed to provide sufficient radiation output for standard intraoral radiographs: bitewing, periapical, and occlusal
    a. X-ray beam is restricted to provide exposure of small anatomic sites
    b. Kilovolt peak (kVp) and milliamperage (mA) settings may be constant or variable, depending on the manufacturer
2. Extraoral units are designed to provide greater radiation output as required by the extraoral procedures; x-ray beam is larger to accommodate larger anatomic areas under study
B. Components of the x-ray unit
1. Generator—device that supplies electrical power to the x-ray tube
    a. Transformer[4]
        (1) Device that changes the potential difference of the incoming electrical energy to any desired level
        (2) Consists of two wire coils wound around opposite sides of an iron ring
        (3) Current flows through the primary coil; creates a magnetic field in the iron ring
        (4) Magnetic field then induces a current in the second coil
        (5) Voltage in the two circuits is proportional to the number of turns in the two coils
        (6) An increase in the voltage must be accompanied by a corresponding decrease in the current
    b. Types of transformers
        (1) Step-up transformer has more turns in the secondary coil than in the primary coil, which increases the voltage; used to supply voltage to the high-voltage (kVp) tube circuit
        (2) Step-down transformer has fewer turns in the secondary coil than in the primary coil, which decreases the voltage; used to supply voltage to the filament (mA) circuit
        (3) Autotransformer is a special type of transformer because the primary and secondary windings are incorporated into a single winding
            (a) Has a number of connections called electrical taps located along the length of the coil
            (b) Designed to supply voltage of varying magnitude to several different circuits of the x-ray machine (e.g., filament circuit and high-voltage tube circuit)
    c. Rectification
        (1) Definition—the process of changing an alternating current into a direct current
        (2) A *rectifier* is an electrical device that changes AC into DC
        (3) Dental x-ray units are considered to be *self-rectified* or *half-wave rectified*
            (a) In half-wave rectification, X rays are generated during the first half (positive half) of the electrical cycle; the filament is negative and the target is positive
            (b) X rays are *not* generated during the second half (negative half) of the electrical cycle
            (c) With a 60-cycle alternating current, 60 pulses of X rays are generated per second, each having a duration $\frac{1}{120}$ second[5]
        (4) In *full-wave rectification*, X rays are generated during both phases of the alternating current cycle
            (a) Solid-state diodes (or vacuum tube diodes) are employed to redirect the electrical current so that the filament remains negatively charged and the target remains positively charged for x-ray production
            (b) With a 60-cycle alternating current and full-wave rectification, 120 pulses of X rays are generated per second
2. X-ray tube (Fig. 5-1)
    a. Protective housing
        (1) Lead-lined metal casing for the x-ray tube designed to prevent excessive radiation exposure and electrical shock
        (2) Limits the amount of leakage radiation escaping from the unit

(3) Provides mechanical support for the x-ray tube and protection from handling

b. Cooling system
   (1) Oil is sealed in the protective housing and surrounds the x-ray tube
   (2) Serves as both a thermal cushion and an electrical insulator

c. Glass envelope
   (1) Usually made of Pyrex glass to withstand high heat produced
   (2) Surrounds the electrodes of the x-ray tube to provide a vacuum
   (3) Aperture, or window, is a thin segment of the glass that allows maximum emission of X rays and minimum absorption by the glass

d. Cathode
   (1) Electrically negative portion of the x-ray tube
   (2) Composed of:
       (a) Filament (tungsten wire)
       (b) Focusing cup
   (3) Milliamperage control regulates the:
       (a) Step-down transformer
       (b) Heating of the filament
       (c) Quantity of electrons "boiled off" during thermionic emission (when electrical current is passed through the coil of

tungsten wire, atoms of the wire absorb thermal energy and some of the outer-shell electrons acquire enough energy to move a small distance away, forming an electron cloud)
   (4) Because like charges repel, the electron beam is directed to a small area of the anode

e. Anode
   (1) Electrically positive portion of the x-ray tube
   (2) Composed of:
       (a) Tungsten target (tungsten is used as the target material because of its high atomic number, which yields higher efficiency in x-ray production plus higher-energy x-ray photons; conducts heat well; has a high melting point (3380°C)
       (b) Copper stem (which functions to conduct heat away from target)
   (3) Kilovoltage control regulates the:
       (a) Step-up transformer
       (b) Voltage between cathode and anode
       (c) Accelerating potential (speed) of the electrons
   (4) Portion of the target bombarded by the electrons is termed the focal spot

f. Filtration

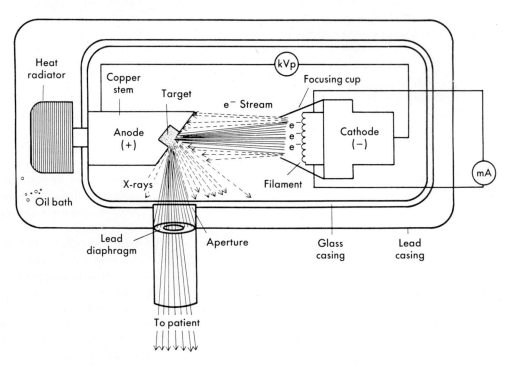

Fig. 5-1   X-ray tube. (From Matteson S, Whaley C, Crandell CE: *Dental assisting manual no 5: Dental radiology,* 1980, University of North Carolina Press, with permission.)

(1) Process of selectively removing X rays from the beam

(2) Total filtration is the result of inherent and added filtration

   (a) Inherent filtration is the filtering of the beam by the glass envelope

   (b) Added filtration occurs by placing metal disks (usually aluminum) within the path of the x-ray beam

(3) Low-energy, nonpenetrating X rays are removed from the beam

(4) Federal regulations require 1.5 mm of aluminum equivalent filtration for units operating below 70 kVp and 2.5 mm of aluminum equivalent filtration for units capable of operating above 70 kVp

  g. Collimation

   (1) Process of restricting the size and/or shape of the x-ray beam

   (2) Lead diaphragm disk with a circular or rectangular opening through which the beam is narrowed

3. Position indicating device (PID)

  a. Definition—"That part of the x-ray machine (cone, rectangle, or cylinder) that aligns the useful beam to the object and film."[1]

  b. Open-ended, lead-lined cylinders or rectangular devices are the only PIDs that should be used

  c. Federal regulations limit the size of the x-ray beam at the patient's face to 7 cm (2¾ inches) in diameter

  d. Rectangular PIDs have an exit size of 3.5 × 4.4 cm (1⅜ × 1¾ inches)

  e. Common lengths of PIDs are 20 cm (8 inches), 30 cm (12 inches), and 40 cm (16 inches)

  f. The longer PID

   (1) Decreases client radiation exposure because the x-ray beam is less divergent

   (2) Provides better image resolution

4. Console

  a. Description—exposure factors (milliamperage, kilovolt peak, and exposure time) are set and electrical circuits are activated by using the controls located on the x-ray machine console

  b. Function

   (1) May control up to three x-ray tube heads

   (2) Usually, settings of 7, 10 or 15 mA are available; kilovolt peak settings range from 50 to 100 kVp

   (3) Depending on the machine type, the automatic timer is adjusted in impulses (1/60th of a second) or seconds

(4) Exposure switch is depressed to initiate the emission of X radiation

(5) Emission of X radiation from the machine is noted by an audible "chirping" sound and the glowing of the exposure indicator light

(6) Console should be located adjacent to the x-ray cubicle so that continuous observation of the patient is possible; however, the operator should be protected from any radiation exposure

Production of X Radiation

A. X-ray machine preparation

1. Initial process for x-radiation production is achieved by the activation of the on-off switch located on the unit console; this process completes the filament circuit, and the filament is heated

2. Appropriate milliamperage, kilovolt peak, and exposure time are set by using controls located on the unit console

  a. Milliamperage control, which is connected to the milliamperage-filament circuit (step-down transformer), allows for the warming of the cathode filament and determines the number of electrons available for x-ray production; the higher the milliamperage, the hotter the filament becomes, resulting in a greater number of available electrons

  b. Kilovolt peak control, which is connected to the high-voltage circuit (step-up transformer), establishes the high voltage needed for x-ray production (65,000 to 100,000 volts); this also provides the condition in which the anode is positively charged and the cathode is negatively charged for the attraction and high-speed acceleration of electrons from the cathode to the anode; the higher the kilovolt peak setting, the greater the speed of acceleration of electrons from the cathode to the anode

  c. Exposure time establishes the time during which electrons are available for bombardment of the target material

B. Electronics of x-ray production

1. X rays are produced by the interactions that occur when high-speed electrons strike a target material

2. Phenomenon of x-ray production occurs only when the exposure switch on the console is depressed, thereby completing the high-voltage circuit

  a. Heated filament provides electrons for x-ray production by thermionic emission

  b. Thermionic emission occurs when electrons absorb sufficient thermal energy (from the milliamperage circuit) to allow for the electrons' short movement away from the filament; commonly referred to as a "boiling off" of electrons; electron cloud surrounding the filament is formed

   c. Closure of the high-voltage circuit creates an electrical potential difference whereby electrons are attracted from the negative cathode to the positive anode

   d. The one-directional flow of electrons (from the negative cathode to the positive anode) is influenced by the focusing cup of the cathode; electrons are repelled away from the negatively charged focusing cup because like charges repel; this mechanism controls the size and shape of the electron stream

C. Electron-target interactions

  1. Electron stream is directed at a small portion of the target, referred to as the focal spot

  2. Actual production of X radiation occurs by the interaction of the accelerating electrons and the target atoms

   a. Accelerating electrons have variable kinetic energy because the electrical power source for the x-ray unit is an alternating current

   b. Example—at 70 kVp the current begins at 0, rises to the peak (potential) of 70, then is fol-

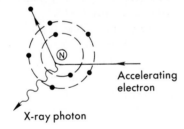

Fig. 5-2 Bremmstrahlung interaction. (Redrawn from Christensen EE, Curry TS III, Dowdy JE: *An introduction to the physics of diagnostic radiology,* ed 2, Philadelphia, 1978, Lea & Febiger.)

lowed by a return to 0; only a small number of electrons leaving the cathode will possess the peak energy; most electrons will be leaving the cathode when the current is rising from or returning to 0

   c. A range of x-ray photon energies will be emitted from the unit as a result of the alternating current

  3. Two types of interactions for x-ray production

   a. Bremsstrahlung radiation (Fig. 5-2)

    (1) Also known as general radiation or braking radiation

    (2) Accelerating electron passes near the nucleus of the target atom and is slowed down by the attraction of the nucleus

    (3) Slowing-down process results in a transference of the electron's kinetic energy into x-ray energy plus a change in the traveling direction of the electron

    (4) Energy of the photon produced depends on the amount of kinetic energy transferred

    (5) Electron may give up its energy in stages, yielding photons of various energy levels

    (6) The closer the accelerating electron passes by the nucleus, the greater the nuclear attraction, thereby yielding greater energy transference and higher photon energy

    (7) The primary source of x-ray photons from an x-ray tube is Bremsstrahlung radiation[5]

   b. Characteristic radiation (Fig. 5-3)

    (1) Also known as discrete radiation

    (2) Radiation is characteristic of the target material

    (3) Steps for characteristic radiation production involve ionization of the target atom by removing an orbital electron and restabilization of the atom by shifting orbital electrons

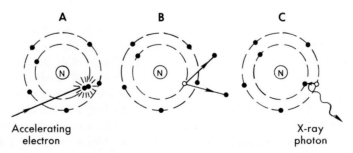

Fig. 5-3 Characteristic interaction. **A,** Collision of accelerating electron and orbital electron; **B,** Vacancy of inner shell; **C,** Shifting of outer-shell electron to inner vacancy with generation of x-ray photon. (Redrawn from Christensen EE, Curry TS III, Dowdy JE: *An introduction to the physics of diagnostic radiology,* ed 2, Philadelphia, 1978, Lea & Febiger.)

(4) During restabilization of the ionized atom the hole created by the ejected orbital electron is filled by an outer-shell electron; movement of the outer-shell electron results in the transference of electron-binding energy into x-ray energy

(5) Energy of the resulting characteristic x-ray photon is a result of the difference in the binding energies of the orbital electrons involved

(6) Characteristic radiation is a minor source of radiation[5]

D. Emanation of the x-ray beam from the tube
   1. X rays are isotropically emitted from a point source (focal spot); however, only a small portion is allowed to exit the machine and be used for image production
   2. X-ray beam emitted is described as polychromatic, meaning a range in the photon energies, as compared with a monochromatic beam, in which all photons have the same energy
   3. Long-wavelength, low-energy x-ray photons have less penetrating ability and are commonly referred to as soft rays; short-wavelength, high-energy x-ray photons have greater penetrating ability and are commonly referred to as hard rays
   4. Characteristics of the x-ray beam emitted from the tube are altered for various reasons
      a. Soft, nonpenetrating, non-radiographic image-producing X rays are removed by filtration
      b. Mean photon energy of the x-ray beam increases following filtration (removal of low-energy photons), yielding a "harder beam"
      c. Field size of the x-ray beam is restricted (collimated) to match the image receptor size
      d. Preceding factors provide a reduction in patient radiation exposure

E. Characteristics of X rays
   1. Portion of the electromagnetic spectrum
   2. Pure energy without mass or charge
   3. Travel at the speed of light (186,000 miles/sec)
   4. Affect photographic emulsion
   5. Cause fluorescence of certain chemicals
   6. Can adversely affect biologic tissues

Interactions of X Rays with Matter

A. Considerations[6]
   1. When x-ray photons interact with matter, they may be either absorbed or scattered
      a. If an incident (initial) photon is absorbed, it ceases to exist
      b. If an incident photon is scattered, its direction of travel is altered; does not aid in formation of the radiographic image and only increases film density; scattered radiation causes film fog (or noise) that destroys image quality
   2. Attenuation (removal) of x-ray photons from the beam as they travel through matter (tissue) is determined by the intensity (energy) of the radiation and the density, atomic number, and electrons per gram of the matter
      a. As the energy of the radiation increases, the number of photons passing through the matter increases
      b. As the density, atomic number, or electrons per gram of the material increase, the number of photons passing through the matter decreases
   3. Definitions[1]
      a. Primary radiation—photons coming directly from the target of the x-ray tube
      b. Secondary radiation—radiation resulting from the interaction of primary radiation and matter
      c. Scattered radiation—one form of secondary radiation in which the direction of travel was altered

B. Types of interactions
   1. No interaction
      a. Refers to the passing of x-ray photons through a material without any alteration of the photon or the material
      b. Photons proceed to expose the silver halide crystals of the film emulsion
   2. Thomson scattering
      a. Also termed unmodified or coherent scattering
      b. Refers to the interaction of an incident photon passing near an outer-shell electron and being scattered without losing energy
      c. Incident photon causes the electron to vibrate
      d. Incident photon ceases to exist, and a new photon of identical energy is released from the vibrating electron
      e. Direction of travel of the Thomson scattered photon is different from that of the incident photon
      f. In the diagnostic energy range Thomson scattering accounts for 5% of the total interactions
   3. Photoelectric effect
      a. Results from an incident photon colliding with a tightly bound inner-shell electron
      b. Incident photon ceases to exist; electron is ejected as a recoil electron (or photoelectron)
      c. Ionization of the atom occurs; ejected electron leaves a vacancy in the shell that must be filled
      d. Low-energy characteristic radiation is produced by the shifting of an outer-shell electron to the inner vacancy

e. In the diagnostic energy range the photoelectric effect accounts for 75% of the interactions

4. Compton effect
   a. Results from an incident photon colliding with a loosely bound outer-shell electron
   b. Incident photon gives up part of its energy in the ejection of the orbiting electron
   c. Ionization of the atom occurs
   d. Direction of travel of the incident photon is changed; its energy is reduced
   e. Energy of the Compton-scattered x-ray photon is equal to the difference between the energy of the incident photon and the energy imparted to the ejected electron
   f. Scattered photon and ejected electron may have sufficient energy to undergo many more ionizing interactions before losing their entire energy
   g. Compton-scattered X radiations may exit the patient's tissues and cause film fog
   h. In the diagnostic energy range Compton scattering accounts for 20% of the interactions

C. Image formation and differential attenuation
   1. Radiographic image formation depends on differential attenuation of x-ray photons from the primary beam by the patient's tissues
   2. If all photons exited the patient (no absorption), the film would be totally exposed; if all photons were attenuated (absorbed), the film would be unexposed
   3. X-ray photons in the primary beam are in a uniform distribution
   4. As a result of the Thomson, Compton, and photoelectric interactions, x-ray photons are removed from the beam
   5. Distribution of transmitted photons represents the patient's tissues
   6. Variances in attenuating ability of the tissues produce radiographic contrast
   7. As previously stated, attenuation is dependent on the intensity (energy) of the radiation plus the density, atomic number, and electrons per gram of the tissue
   8. Example—when the kilovolt peak setting is increased, more X rays are produced and the mean energy of the beam is increased; x-ray photons with higher energy have greater penetrating ability; at a 50-kVp setting many photons are unable to pass through the structures, and a high-contrast radiographic image is obtained; at a 90-kVp setting many photons are able to pass through the structures, and a low-contrast radiographic image is obtained (NOTE: As the kilovolt peak is increased, the exposure time must be decreased to prevent overexposure and thus provide a film of acceptable density)

   9. Generally as the density, atomic number, and electrons per gram of tissue increase, the number of attenuated photons increases; gold, amalgam, enamel, dentin, cementum, and bone attenuate photons to a great extent and are radiopaque structures; bone marrow spaces, sinuses, pulps, and periodontal ligament spaces do not attenuate photons and are radiolucent structures

Interactions of Ionizing Radiation with Cells, Tissues, and Organs

A. Definitions
   1. Whole-body exposure (total body)—each gram of tissue in the entire body absorbs equal amounts of radiation
   2. Specific-area exposure (localized)—each gram of tissue of the body in the specific area irradiated absorbs equal amounts of radiation (e.g., facial exposure from four bitewing radiographs)
   3. Direct effect—transfer of energy by the ionization mechanism from an x-ray photon to a biologically critical molecule such as deoxyribonucleic acid (DNA)
   4. Indirect effect—transfer of energy by the ionization mechanism from an x-ray photon to a noncritical molecule, which in turn delivers the energy to the biologically critical molecule
   5. Genetic effect—mutations in future generations; results from exposure of the reproductive cells, yielding alterations in the genetic code
   6. Somatic effect—refers to injury in the person being irradiated
   7. Latent period—time between the exposure and the development of the biologic effect
   8. Acute effects (short-term or early)—effects that may occur minutes, hours, or weeks after the exposure; usually result from high doses of whole-body exposure
   9. Chronic effects (long-term or late)—effects observed years after the original exposure

B. Units of radiation measurement
   1. Roentgen (R) is a unit of radiation exposure or intensity
      a. One roentgen is that amount of X radiation or gamma radiation that will produce 2.08×10^9 ion pairs in 1 cc of air
      b. International System of Units (SI) unit for exposure is defined as electrical charge per unit mass of air

$$1\ R = 2.58 \times 10^{-4}\ \text{coulomb (C)/kg}$$

2. Direct imaging refers to the exposure of the x-ray film by the interaction of the photographic emulsion and remnant x-ray beam
3. Indirect imaging refers to the exposure of the x-ray film primarily by the light emitted from an intensifying screen and, to a lesser extent, by the remnant x-ray beam

B. Radiographic film
   1. X-ray film used with direct and indirect imaging systems is similar in composition
   2. Quality control procedures are followed during the manufacture of film for standardization
   3. Film composition
      a. Base material must possess dimensional stability to withstand processing procedures; a polyester is used
      b. Adhesive is applied evenly to the base; used to provide for uniform attachment of the emulsion to the base
      c. Emulsion consists of the gelatin and silver halide crystals; records the information within the x-ray beam
      d. Protective coating is applied to protect the emulsion from scratching
   4. Film classifications
      a. Intraoral film and extraoral film refer to the designated use of the film
         (1) Intraoral means the film is placed within the oral cavity (e.g., bitewing or periapical)
         (2) Extraoral refers to film placed outside of the mouth for exposure of large areas (e.g., panoramic or cephalometric)
      b. Screen film is characteristically a much slower film with a thinner emulsion layer and must be used with an intensifying screen (e.g., panoramic film); nonscreen film is exposed by X rays alone and has a thicker emulsion to increase its sensitivity to radiation
      c. Speed refers to the film's responsiveness to X radiation and is directly related to image visibility
         (1) Fast film has larger silver halide crystals and decreased image resolution
         (2) Slow film has smaller silver halide crystals and increased image resolution
         (3) Traditionally, speed ranges have been designated from A to F, with A being the slowest
         (4) Radiation hygiene factors prevent A- to C-speed films from being commercially available for patient use; D- and E-speed films are available for use
         (5) E-speed intraoral film is twice as fast as D-speed intraoral film; E-speed film should

be used to reduce
radiation

d. Size—various sizes are a
film and nonscreen film
   (1) Nonscreen film
      (a) No. 0—22 × 35
      (b) No. 1—24 × 40
      (c) No. 2—31 × 41
      (d) No. 3—27 × 54
      (e) No. 4—57 × 76
   (2) Screen film
      (a) 5 × 7 in
      (b) 5 × 12 in
      (c) 8 × 10 in
e. Use
   (1) Nonscreen films
      cal, bitewing, and
      projections
   (2) Screen films are us
      tions such as the p
      metric projections
f. Intraoral nonscreen filr
   double film packets; do
   a duplicate radiograph

5. Packet construction of int
   a. Light-tight, leakproof
      film from light and the
   b. Black protective paper
      protection of the film f
   c. Lead foil is inserted bet
      the outer wrapping on
      packet; the purpose of
      backscatter from fogg
      help reduce exposure t
   d. Double or single films

6. Intensifying screens
   a. Housed inside a light-t
   b. Used as a component
      systems to reduce
      radiation for study of l
   c. Screen construction
      (1) Base material com
      (2) Reflective layer, c
         terial, may be e
         or titanium diox
         ward the film to
         the film
      (3) Phosphor layer
         (a) Composed o
            (e.g., calciun
            crystals); crys
            the remnant
            light; visible
            the film

2. Rad (rad) is the unit for absorbed dose; 1 rad is equal to 100 ergs of energy from any type of radiation per gram of absorbing material; SI unit for absorbed dose is the gray (Gy); 1 Gy is equal to 100 rad; 1 Gy is equal to 1 joule (J)/kg
3. Rem (rem) is the unit of dose equivalent and refers to the occupational dose received by radiation workers; SI unit for dose equivalent is the sievert (Sv); 1 sievert is equal to 100 rem
   a. Some radiations are more damaging than X rays; rem facilitates comparisons among the biologic effects of various radiations
   b. Rem is the product of the absorbed dose in rad times the quality factors (QF), indicating the relative biologic effectiveness
      (1) The relative biologic effectiveness is a function of the *linear energy transfer (LET)* of the radiant energy; LET is the amount of energy deposited per unit length of travel and is expressed in keV per micrometer[6]
      (2) In comparison of an electron and proton with equal energy, the proton will be attenuated faster than the electron; "the proton deposits more energy per unit length of travel, so it is a higher LET radiation"[6]
      (3) X rays have a qualifying factor of 1, protons have a qualifying factor of 5, and α-particles have a qualifying factor of 20
      (4) Absorption of 0.01 Gy of x-radiation would yield an occupational dose of 0.01 Sv (0.01 Gy × 1 QF = 0.01 Sv)
      (5) Absorption of 0.01 Gy of protons would yield an occupational dose of 0.05 Sv (0.01 Gy × 5 QF = 0.05 Sv)
      (6) Absorption of 0.01 Gy of α-particles would yield an occupational dose of 0.20 Sv (0.01 Gy × 20 QF = 0.20 Sv)
4. Curie (Ci) is the unit of radioactivity; refers to the quantity of radioactive material and *not* the radiation emitted by radioactive decay; 1 Ci is equal to that quantity of material in which 3.7×10^{10} atoms disintegrate per second; SI unit for radioactivity is the becquerel (Bq); 1 Ci is equal to 3.7×10^{10} Bq
5. The SI units are based on the metric system and were adopted for use in 1985; note that the traditional units may be used by various agencies until the SI units become commonplace

C. Radiation dose-response relationships
   1. Applications
      a. Design of radiation therapeutic treatment regimens for patients with malignant disease
      b. To provide information on low-dose radiation effects

2. Characteristics of dose-response relationships
   a. Linear—response is directly proportional to the dose
   b. Nonlinear—response is not directly proportional to the dose
   c. Nonthreshold—any dose, regardless of its size, is expected to produce a response
   d. Threshold—from zero to a particular point, no response would be expected; above the threshold point any dose will produce a response

D. Biologic responses to irradiation
   1. Considerations
      a. Radiation exposure is harmful to all living tissues and should be used cautiously
      b. Although the interaction between X rays and tissues occurs at the atomic level, it is theorized that observable human radiation injury results from molecular derangement of macromolecules and water
      c. Injury to cells, tissues, and organs occurs at the time of exposure but may require hours, days, or generations for manifestations
      d. Radiation injury is induced immediately following the interaction of X rays and tissues; caused by ionization
      e. Ionization
         (1) Refers to the excitation of orbital electrons in an atom and to the deposition of energy in the tissues
         (2) Occurs when the atoms of a molecule are separated into charged atomic particles (e.g., table salt; NaCl yields Na$^+$ + Cl$^-$ when mixed in H_2O)
         (3) May cause a breakage in the molecule or relocation of the atom in the molecule
         (4) Altered molecules may function improperly or cease to function altogether
   2. Radiation effects on cells
      a. Two types of cells in the human body
         (1) Genetic cells are the oogonium of the female and the spermatogonium of the male
         (2) Somatic cells comprise all other cells
      b. Nucleus of proliferating somatic and genetic cells is considered to be the most sensitive area of the cell to the ionizing effects
         (1) Exposure to the nucleus results in cell inhibition
         (2) Most sensitive sites within the cell's nucleus are the DNA and chromosomes
         (3) Chromosome aberrations in somatic cells are observed during the metaphase stage of mitosis (cell division); changes in genetic

material can occur during meiosis or reduction division

    (a) Chromosomes control the growth, development, and maintenance of the cell

    (b) Sufficient radiation damage to the DNA may yield visible or invisible chromosome aberrations that may lead to cell death or malfunction

    (c) Tissue or organ destruction occurs when several cells are damaged and not sufficiently repaired by the body's repair mechanism

    (d) DNA damage can result in an uncontrolled, rapid proliferation of cells, the principal characteristic of radiation-induced malignant disease

    (e) Genetic cell or germ cell injury may be observed only in future generations (ranging from increased susceptibility to disease to birth defects to cancer)

  c. Cells found to be the most sensitive to radiation exposure are young, rapidly dividing, nondifferentiated cells such as those of the developing fetus

  d. Cell responses to irradiation

    (1) Cell death refers to the immediate or delayed death of a cell following exposure to a lethal dose

    (2) Swelling of the cell results from interference of fluid exchange through the cell wall

    (3) Alterations in specific cell function, such as the production of a protein or enzyme of changed chemical composition, can also occur following excessive exposure

    (4) Cell aberration results from damage occurring during mitosis or meiosis

3. Radiolysis of water

  a. Yields radicals that combine to form hydrogen peroxide

  b. Hydrogen peroxide is a toxic agent to living tissues; its formation is an indirect damaging effect of ionizing radiation

4. Biologic effects on tissues and organs

  a. Bergonié-Tribondeau law of radiosensitivity

    (1) The more mature a cell is, the more resistant it is to radiation

    (2) The younger tissues and organs are, the greater the radiosensitivity

    (3) The higher the metabolic activity is, the higher the radiosensitivity

    (4) The greater the proliferation rate for cells and the growth rate for tissues, the greater the radiosensitivity

    (5) The more differenti... function) a cell is, th... is to biologic effects

  b. Degree of tissue sensitivi...

    (1) Reproductive (most...

    (2) Lymphatic

    (3) Circulatory

    (4) Endocrine

    (5) Respiratory

    (6) Digestive

    (7) Nervous

  c. Determinants of the organ[4]

    (1) Function of the org...

    (2) Rate at which cells... over in the organ

    (3) Inherent radiosensi...

  d. Organ tissues considere... sensitivity are skin, thy... etic and genetic tissue

  e. The most radiosensitiv... gans is the endothelial... capillary walls

  f. Repeated exposure to th... to functional impairme... in performance and red... infection

  g. Continued low-dose e... the repair mechanism; ... system by time or amou... in somatic or genetic d...

5. Repair and accumulation

  a. Most injury resulting ... exposure is repaired wi... organs (depending on ... aging ability of the rad...

  b. Repeated exposure ma... effects that accumula...

  c. Accumulated radiatio... crease the probability... normal aging process; ... rapid expression of th...

Image Receptors

A. Definition

1. Serve as a mechanism fo... contained in an attenua... into a visible image

2. For dental radiology, a... often either a piece of x-r... of film and an intensifyi...

B. Types

1. Classified as either di... systems

    (b) Phosphorescent crystals

      [1] Have a higher atomic number to increase the probability of their interaction with the x-ray photons

      [2] Should emit a large amount of light per interaction

      [3] Should emit light of proper wavelength to match sensitivity of the film to light

      [4] Should stop emitting light once the x-ray exposure has been terminated

    (4) Protective coating is applied to the phosphor layer to prevent abrasion of the phosphor and must be transparent to light

  d. Calcium tungstate phosphor

    (1) Emits blue light

    (2) Traditionally used in the phosphor layer of the intensifying screen

  e. Rare earth phosphors

    (1) Primarily emit green light

    (2) Represent recent research in indirect imaging systems

    (3) Use gadolinium oxysulfide or lanthanum oxysulfide

    (4) Respond more efficiently to X radiation; result in a significant decrease in patient exposure

7. Extraoral film identification methods

  a. Lead letter (R or L) is attached to the tube-side surface of the cassette but positioned away from the structures of interest; can be used to record the date and patient's name

  b. Radiopaque tape is also available for recording the patient's name and date

  c. Light flasher units are used to record the patient's name, date, and social security number or other identifying data onto the emulsion before processing

C. Film care storage methods

1. Must be stored away from heat, moisture, chemical vapors, and radiation

2. Should be stored by expiration date so that the oldest films are used first

D. Latent image formation

1. Film considerations

  a. Crystals within the emulsion are composed of positive silver ions (Ag^+) and negative bromine and iodine (I^-) ions

  b. Crystals contain imperfections

    (1) Free interstitial silver ions

    (2) Crystals are chemically sensitized by sulfur compounds bound to the surface

  c. Irregularities of crystals are termed latent image sites; trap recoil electrons to begin image-formation process

2. Silver halide crystals are irradiated

3. X-ray photons are absorbed by bromide ions; bromide ions are converted to bromine atoms; process produces high-speed recoil electrons and scattered photons

4. High-speed recoil electrons travel through crystal with the ability to dislodge other electrons

5. High-speed recoil electrons are trapped by latent image sites (crystal imperfections); impart a negative charge to the site

6. Free interstitial silver ions are attracted to the negatively charged latent image site

7. Atom of metallic silver is produced by the combination of the trapped electron and silver ion

8. When photons interact with bromide ions, the process occurs

9. Accumulation of silver atoms at the latent image sites (crystal imperfection sites) constitutes the latent (invisible) image

10. Crystals with metallic silver deposits are subject to chemical reduction by the developer solution during film processing

11. Individual crystals are completely reduced to metallic silver or not at all during film-processing procedures

12. Crystals not exposed to radiation are removed from the emulsion by the fixer solution

Darkroom Techniques—Radiographic Film Processing

A. Chemical solutions

1. Developer

  a. Reducing agent (a hydroquinone and elon combination)—functions to reduce the latent image-containing silver bromide crystals to black metallic silver

  b. Alkalizer (sodium carbonate)—provides the required alkaline medium for the reducer to work; softens and swells the gelatin of the emulsion to allow reducers to reach the silver bromide crystals

  c. Preservative (sodium sulfite)—slows the oxidation of the solution to prolong its life span

  d. Restrainer (potassium bromide)—slows down the action of the chemicals

2. Fixer

  a. Clearing or fixing agent (sodium or ammonium thiosulfate)—removes the unexposed or undeveloped crystals from the emulsion

Table 5-1	
Time-Temperature Processing	
Temperature of developer (°F)	**Time in developer (min)**
60	8
65	5½
68	4½ optimum
70	4
75	3
80	2¼

From Matteson S, Whaley C, Crandell CE: *Dental assisting manual no 5: Dental radiology,* 1980, University of North Carolina Press. Used with permission of the publisher.

b. Acidifier (acetic acid)—provides the required acidity so the fixing solutions can work; stops the action of the developer
c. Preservative (sodium sulfite)—slows the oxidation of the solution to prolong its life span
d. Hardener (potassium aluminum)—shrinks and hardens the emulsion
3. Vehicle (distilled water)—used to mix the chemicals
B. Processing methods
1. Basic procedure of film processing
a. Developing—reduces latent image-containing silver bromide crystals to black metallic silver
b. Rinsing—washes away excess developer solution to avoid contamination and neutralization of the fixer
c. Fixing—removes the unexposed or undeveloped crystals from the emulsion
d. Washing—removes the fixer solution to avoid staining the film
e. Drying—removes water from the emulsion; prepares the film for viewing
2. Time-temperature method
a. Recommended scientific method for film processing
b. Optimum amount of reduction of silver bromide crystals occurs
c. Developer activity is dependent on the temperature of the solution
d. Less activity occurs at lower temperatures; greater activity occurs at higher temperatures
e. Optimum results are obtained at 20° C (68° F) (Table 5-1)
3. Sight method*
a. Unscientific method of film processing

*Method is not recommended, but is described here only for completeness of the topic area.

b. Films are removed periodically from the developer solution, examined under a safelight to determine the presence of visible images
c. Disadvantages
(1) Lack of quality control
(2) Nonstandardized procedures
(3) Radiographic density of variable range
4. Manual method
a. Films are placed on racks and hand-dipped in solutions
b. Normally associated with the time-temperature method
5. Automatic method
a. Films are carried from solution to solution and through the dryer by a roller assembly
b. Completed in 5 to 7 minutes
c. Advantages over manual processing method
(1) Standardized procedure
(2) Solutions of proper strength provided
(3) Controlled-temperature solutions
(4) Processing time regulated
(5) Increased number of films can be processed
(6) Reduction in processing time
6. Rapid processing method
a. Sometimes referred to as "hot processing"
b. Accomplished by use of high-temperature solutions or concentrated solutions at room temperature
c. Completed in 1 minute or less
d. Film quality is less than that obtained with standard methods
e. Recommended for processing working films (i.e., endodontic or emergency procedures)
7. Wet reading
a. Immediate evaluation of radiographic technique and dental disease
b. Often used in manual processing
c. Minimum fixing time of 3 minutes required before viewing films
d. For archival quality films, normal time-temperature processing procedures must be resumed as soon as possible
C. Darkroom design and requirements[1,7]
1. Location and size
a. Located near rooms where x-ray units are placed
b. Minimum of 16 square feet for one person to work
c. Size-determining factors
(1) Number of radiographs to be processed
(2) Number of personnel using the darkroom
(3) Processing method(s) used (i.e., manual, automatic, or both)
(4) Space for duplicating, drying, and storage

d. Light-tight room
e. Revolving light-sealed door or door with inside lock to prevent accidental white light exposure of films during processing

2. Lighting
a. Illuminating safelight
(1) Any illumination that will not expose x-ray film
(2) Determining factors include x-ray film sensitivity to light, film position, and intensity of light
(3) Ideal safe lighting consists of a 15 watt bulb covered with a red filter placed 4 feet away from the working surface
(4) Panoramic and other extraoral films are more sensitive to light than intraoral films; therefore extraneous light (e.g., from equipment dials, indicator lights, luminous watch faces) should be eliminated
b. Overhead white light
(1) Provides adequate illumination for the room
(2) Because of fluorescent lighting's tendency for afterglow, incandescent lighting is preferred
(3) Locate light switches out of easy reach to prevent accidental exposure to white light
c. Viewing safelight—mounted on the wall behind the processing tanks for wet readings (after films have been in the fixer solution for 3 minutes)
d. X-ray viewbox—for wet readings
e. Outside warning light
(1) To prevent accidental entry of personnel during film-processing procedures
(2) Should be wired to the safelight so that both are on at the same time

3. Plumbing
a. Hot and cold water supply for time-temperature processing
b. Adequate drainage
c. Thermostatically controlled intake valve to maintain constant temperatures of solutions
d. Constant water flow for automatic processors must be considered
e. Noncorrosive pipes to withstand chemicals
f. Large sink with gooseneck faucet needed to accommodate cleaning procedures

4. Darkroom contents
a. Processing tanks
b. Processing solutions
c. Timer
d. Thermometer
e. Film hangers
f. Dryer
g. Stirring paddles for solutions
h. Cleaning supplies

5. Record keeping
a. Inventory of chemicals
b. Dates of solution changes
c. Film identification records
(1) Client's name
(2) Number of films
(3) Rack numbers
(4) Date of film exposure and processing

D. Film-processing errors
1. Fogged films
a. Causes
(1) Unsafe darkroom illumination
(2) Safelight too close to the working surface
(3) Overactive chemicals (freshly made)
(4) Exposure to scattered radiation
b. Corrective action
(1) Check safelight filter for cracks
(2) Check appropriate filter for film sensitivity
(3) Check wattage of the light bulb in the safelight
(4) Check distance of the safelight from the working surface

2. Underdeveloped films
a. Causes
(1) Temperature of developer solution too cool
(2) Insufficient developing time
(3) Developer solution exhausted
(4) Developer solution in automatic processor too low
b. Corrective action
(1) Check developer temperature with a thermometer
(2) Check developing time with an accurate timing device
(3) Replace old developer solution
(4) Replenish developer solution to appropriate level

3. Overdeveloped films
a. Causes
(1) Temperature of developer solution too high
(2) Excessive developing time used
(3) Overactive solutions (no restrainer chemical)
b. Corrective action
(1) Check developer temperature with a thermometer
(2) Check developing time with an accurate timing device
(3) Check chemistry of solutions and mixing procedures

4. Developer cut off
   a. Caused by film that is partially immersed in the developer solution
   b. Corrective actions
      (1) Check height of the developer solution in the tank
      (2) Replenish the developer solution if necessary
      (3) Do not attach films to the top clip of the developing rack
5. Clear films
   a. Causes
      (1) Film placed in the fixer solution first, which removed all silver bromide crystals
      (2) Excessive washing to cause removal of emulsion
   b. Corrective actions
      (1) Label solution tanks
      (2) Post appropriate processing procedures in the darkroom
      (3) Remove films from wash after appropriate time
6. Stained films
   a. Developer stains
      (1) Dark overdeveloped areas caused by contamination of the film with developer solution before the normal processing cycle
      (2) Corrected by keeping the darkroom work area clean, preventing dripping or splashing of the developer solution on the work counter, and washing hands if handling solutions
   b. Fixer stains
      (1) Clear or light spots on the film that result from contamination of the film by fixer solutions before the normal processing cycle; corrected by keeping the work area clean to avoid dripping and splashing of the fixer solution on the counter
      (2) Brown or yellow stains result from insufficient fixing time or insufficient washing time for removal of fixer chemicals from the film emulsion; corrected by employing appropriate film-processing procedures
   c. Dark stains
      (1) Fluoride artifacts
         (a) Dark areas on the film caused by contamination of the film with fluoride
         (b) Corrected by washing hands to remove fluoride before unwrapping film
      (2) Saliva stains
         (a) Dark areas on the film
         (b) Corrected by wiping saliva from the film packet after removal from the oral cavity and preventing the black protective paper from sticking to the emulsion
      (3) Glove powder artifacts
         (a) Contact of gloved hand or when gloves were removed, powder residue remained on hands and came in contact with the film
         (b) Corrected by removing latex gloves and washing hands, or placing vinyl/plastic overgloves over latex gloves before handling film
   d. Green film
      (1) Film emulsion not in contact with processing chemicals
      (2) Corrected by separating double film packets
7. Reticulation of emulsion
   a. Caused by transferring the film from one solution to another with extreme changes in temperature
   b. Corrected by monitoring solution temperatures
8. Torn or scratched films
   a. Caused by the emulsion coming into contact with rough objects or the sides of the tanks while wet
   b. Corrected by monitoring placement of the film in the processing tanks
9. Lost films
   a. Causes
      (1) Film not securely attached to the rack (manual processing)
      (2) Film did not proceed through the roller assembly properly (automatic processing)
   b. Corrective actions
      (1) Repair the manual rack, and securely fasten the film
      (2) Repair the roller assembly if defective, and review the method of film insertion
      (3) Replace processing solutions with fresh chemistry; exhausted developer solution in automatic processors can cause films to slide around on roller transports and fail to advance through the processing unit
10. Air bubbles
    a. Caused by air bubbles caught on the film emulsion when placed in the developer solution
    b. Corrected by agitating the film rack for 5 seconds to release air bubbles
11. Static electricity
    a. Caused by rapid removal of the film from the packet or cassette when humidity level is very low (e.g., during winter) which yields dark tree-like streaks, or smudge-like dots

b. Corrected by careful removal of the film from the packet or cassette

12. Light leaks
  a. Cause
    (1) Film packet covering is torn
    (2) Accidental opening of the packet under the white light
    (3) Failure to cover the film-processing tanks during the procedure
    (4) Failure to allow the film to be fully accepted by the rollers for automatic processing before turning on the white light
    (5) Cuffs of the daylight loader of the automatic processor not tight enough around the arms; light enters during the unwrapping of the film
  b. Corrective action
    (1) Follow proper procedures
    (2) Examine the daylight loader cuffs for secure fit

E. Film duplication
  1. Purpose
    a. Provide copies of radiographs for third party payment
    b. Forward the client's treatment records to a new oral healthcare practice
    c. For referrals to specialists
    d. Use in litigation
  2. Equipment
    a. Radiographic duplicating film
      (1) Base—blue-tinted polyester base
      (2) Solarized emulsion
        (a) Emulsion composed of gelatin and silver bromide crystals
        (b) Refers to the phenomenon in which more light exposure of the film yields a decrease in film density and less light exposure of the film yields an increase in film density
        (c) Often the term *direct positive* is used
      (3) Antihalation coating
        (a) Layer of gelatin containing a dye
        (b) Process of halation occurs when the light passing through the film and into the air is reflected back toward the emulsion, causing unsharp edges
        (c) Dye absorbs the reflected light to prevent image unsharpness
        (d) Dye is washed away during film processing
    b. Film-duplicating printer
      (1) Box-type device with a glass top, adjustable timer, and ultraviolet light source
      (2) Printing area of variable size; dependent on dealer and model type
  3. Procedure
    a. Original radiographs are positioned on the glass top
    b. Right and left sides are identified
    c. Under safelight conditions, remove the duplicating film from the box; place the solarized emulsion side down over the film
    d. Appropriate exposure time is selected; ultraviolet light passes through the original radiographs to expose the duplicating film
    e. Duplicating film is processed by either manual or automatic processing such as that used for normal dental radiographs
  4. Duplication errors
    a. Light duplicate film results from overexposure of the duplicating film
    b. Dark duplicate film results from underexposure of the duplicating film
    c. Poor definition of the film results from loss of intimate contact between the original and copy film

Oral Radiographic Procedures

Description of the Radiographic Image

A. Definitions
  1. Radiolucent—black to dark gray areas on the radiograph resulting from more exposure of the film by radiation passing through the less dense anatomic structures
  2. Radiopaque—white to light gray areas on the radiograph resulting from less exposure of the film by radiation being absorbed by the dense anatomic structures
  3. Radiographic density—overall blackening of a radiograph; density is read with a densitometer
  4. Radiographic contrast—differences in densities of adjacent areas of the radiograph
    a. Long-scale contrast (also called low contrast)—scale with many shades of gray resulting from the small differences in densities; obtained with a high kilovolt peak technique
    b. Short-scale contrast (also called high contrast)—scale with few shades of gray resulting from a large difference in densities; obtained with a low kilovolt peak technique
  5. Detail (definition)—degree of clarity on a radiograph
  6. Resolution—ability to record separate images of small objects that are placed close together

7. Sharpness—ability of the x-ray film to define an edge
8. Fog—overall gray appearance, yielding a lower film contrast; results from exposure of the film by scattered radiation or by unsafe illumination of the darkroom

B. Factors affecting visualized radiographic image
1. Exposure time
   a. Directly proportional to film density
   b. Increased exposure time provides more x-ray photons to interact with the emulsion
2. Milliamperage
   a. Directly proportional to film density
   b. Increased milliamperage yields more heat in the filament; produces more electrons by thermionic emission, which yields more x-ray photons
   c. With more X rays produced, more X rays interact with the film emulsion
3. Kilovolt potential
   a. Directly proportional to film density; a higher kilovolt peak technique yields a more penetrating x-ray beam, and a greater number of x-ray photons are produced; therefore more of the film emulsion is exposed
   b. Inversely proportional to film contrast; decreased kilovolt peak yields film with high contrast because the beam has less penetrating ability; increased kilovolt peak yields film with low contrast because the beam has more penetrating ability
4. Collimation
   a. Inversely proportional to film density; increased collimation of the x-ray beam decreases density because there is a reduction in the number of scattered photons that cause film fog
   b. Directly proportional to film contrast; with fewer scattered photons causing fog, the contrast is higher (short scale)
5. Filtration—inversely proportional to film density; the greater the filtration of the x-ray beam, the fewer photons available to penetrate the patient and interact with the film
6. Target-to-film distance
   a. Inversely proportional to film density
   b. Based on the phenomenon of the inverse square law

$$\frac{I_1}{I_2} = \frac{d_2^2}{d_1^2}$$

   where I_1 is the intensity at the first distance (d_1) from the source and I_2 is the intensity at the second distance (d_2) from the source

   (1) States that the intensity of the x-ray beam is inversely proportional to the square of the distance
   (2) Rapid decrease in intensity results from the spreading out of the x-ray photons over a larger area as they move farther from the source
   (3) Example—if the intensity of an x-ray beam is 400 milliroentgens (mR) at 36 inches, then at 72 inches (double the distance) the intensity is only one fourth as great and is 100 mR
   c. To maintain film density when switching from a short target-to-film distance to a long target-to-film distance, the milliamperage or exposure time must be increased
7. Client-object thickness—inversely proportional to film density; as thickness increases, more of the beam is attenuated, yielding a decrease in film density
8. Client-object density—inversely proportional to film density; more of the beam is attenuated by the patient, yielding a decrease in film density

Radiographic Techniques

A. Shadow-casting principles
1. Smallest focal spot (x-ray source) possible
   a. Yields more parallel x-ray photons
   b. Reduces penumbra
   c. Enhances image sharpness
2. Longest focal spot (x-ray source-to-object [tooth] distance) possible
   a. Results in use of more parallel x-ray photons
   b. Decreases image magnification
   c. Enhances image sharpness
3. Shortest object (tooth)-to-film distance possible
   a. Decreases image magnification
   b. Enhances image sharpness
4. Object (tooth) and film should be in a parallel relationship; reduces image distortion (e.g., elongation and foreshortening)
5. X-ray beam should be perpendicular to the tooth and film; reduces image distortion

B. Angulation of the x-ray beam
1. The position of the x-ray beam is described in relation to the client's teeth when the occlusal plane is parallel to the floor[8]
2. *Vertical angulation* indicates the position of the x-ray tube head (PID) in the vertical plane
   a. Positive vertical angulation means that the PID is pointing downward
   b. Negative vertical angulation means that the PID is pointing upward

c. Vertical angulation is noted in degrees (positive or negative) by the dial on the side of the tube head
3. *Horizontal angulation* indicates the position of the x-ray tube head (PID) in the horizontal plane
C. Intraoral procedures
  1. Paralleling technique
    a. Theory
      (1) Introduced by McCormack
      (2) Yields radiographs with a minimum of image distortion
      (3) Minimizes the superimposition of adjacent oral structures
      (4) Commonly referred to as the long-cone technique or right-angle technique
      (5) Applies shadow-casting principles Nos. 1, 2, 4, and 5
    b. Application (Fig. 5-4)
      (1) Film packet is placed parallel to the long axis of the tooth and perpendicular to the horizontal axis of the tooth
      (2) X-ray beam is directed perpendicular to the long axis of the tooth and image receptor (film)
      (3) X-ray beam is directed through the interproximal spaces
      (4) X-ray beam centered over the anatomic structures and image receptor
  2. Bisecting-the-angle technique
    a. Theory
      (1) Introduced by Cieszynski
      (2) Applies the rule of isometry (correct length of the tooth image obtained if the x-ray beam is perpendicular to the bisector of the angle formed by the plane of the film and the long axis of the tooth)
      (3) Commonly referred to as the short-cone technique
      (4) Does not use shadow-casting principles Nos. 4 and 5 as listed under A
    b. Application (Fig. 5-5)
      (1) Film packet is placed against the teeth
      (2) X-ray beam is directed perpendicular to the imaginary bisector of the angle formed by the plane of the film and the long axis of the tooth
      (3) X-ray beam is directed through the interproximal spaces
      (4) X-ray beam is centered over the anatomic structures and image receptor
  3. Intraoral radiographic techniques
    a. Periapical projection demonstrates the entire tooth and surrounding structures (Fig. 5-6); indications are[9]
      (1) Suspected periapical condition (e.g., fistula or sinus tract infection)
      (2) Evidence of periodontal involvement
      (3) Injury or trauma to teeth
      (4) Endodontic therapy
      (5) Deep or large caries
      (6) Suspected impaction
      (7) Unusual eruption, malposition or unexplained missing teeth
      (8) Unexplained sensitivity
      (9) Unexplained tooth mobility
      (10) Unusual tooth morphology or color
      (11) Evaluate implants
    b. Bitewing projection demonstrates anatomic

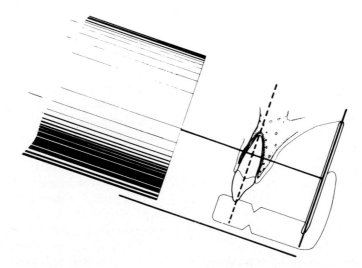

Fig. 5-4 Paralleling technique. (From Whaley KC: *Intraoral radiography: The paralleling technique,* Chapel Hill, NC, 1977, Learning Resource Center, School of Dentistry, University of North Carolina.)

crowns of the maxillary and mandibular teeth plus height of the alveolar bone (Fig. 5-7); indications are
  (1) Suspected interproximal caries
  (2) Defective restorations
  (3) Localized periodontal involvement
c. Occlusal projection demonstrates a large ana-

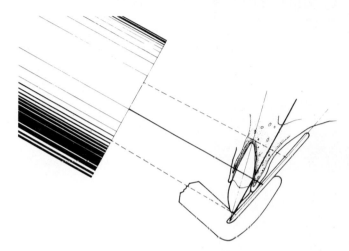

Fig. 5-5 Bisecting-the-angle technique. (From Whaley KC: *Intraoral radiography: The paralleling technique,* Chapel Hill, NC, 1977, Learning Resource Center, School of Dentistry, University of North Carolina.)

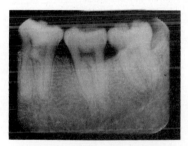

Fig. 5-6 Periapical radiograph.

tomic region or entire arch (Fig. 5-8); indications are[9]
  (1) Image margins of large pathological conditions
  (2) Localization of objects (foreign or impactions)
  (3) Injury or trauma to surrounding bone structure
  (4) Suspected supernumerary teeth
  (5) Unexplained swelling or growth abnormality
d. Complete radiographic survey is a combination of periapical and bitewing projections that image entire dentition, with the number of projections variable (Fig. 5-9)
4. Intraoral film holding devices are used to stabilize the film position, reduce film movement during exposure, and eliminate the need for the client to hold the film
D. Intraoral technique errors (Fig. 5-10)
  1. Typical packet placement errors involve improper positioning of the film behind the teeth of interest and failure to achieve shadow-casting principles
  2. Vertical angulation (Fig. 5-11)
    a. Typical vertical angulation errors with the paralleling technique are visualized as missing apical or coronal structures
    b. Typical vertical angulation errors with the bisecting-the-angle technique are visualized as foreshortened or elongated structures
  3. Horizontal overlap
    a. Visualized as the radiopaque density resulting from the superimposition of adjacent interproximal tooth surfaces
    b. Commonly occurs by directing the beam from an excessively mesial or distal horizontal position

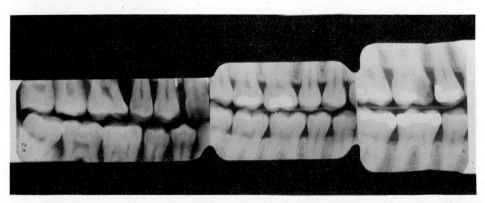

Fig. 5-7 Bitewing radiographs. *Left to right:* Long horizontal bitewing, standard horizontal bitewing, and vertical bitewing.

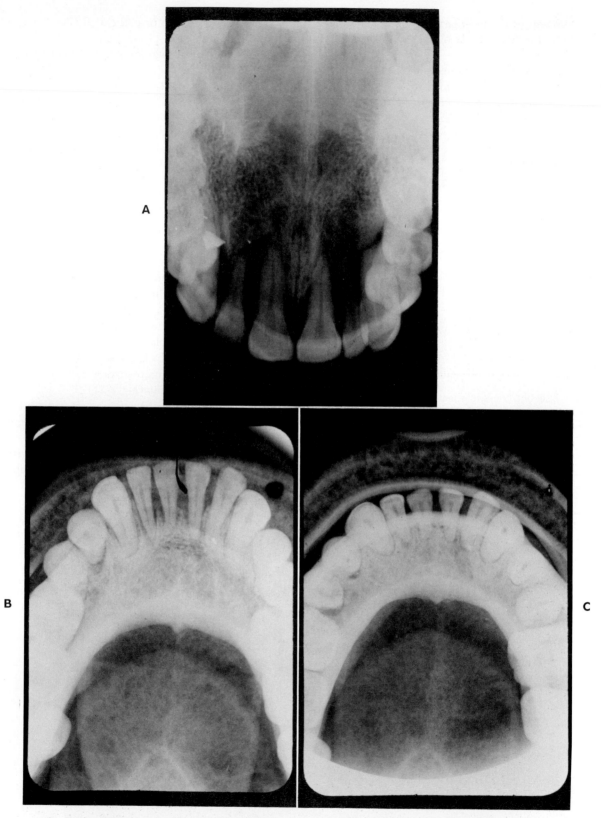

Fig. 5-8 Occlusal radiographs. **A,** Topographic occlusal radiograph of maxillary arch. **B,** Topographic occlusal radiograph of mandibular arch. **C,** Cross-sectional occlusal radiograph of mandibular arch.

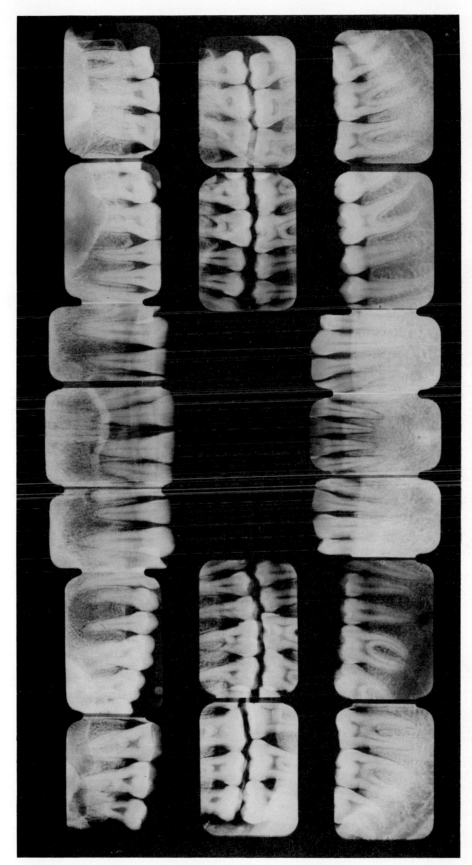

Fig. 5-9   Full-mouth radiographic survey. (From Mattesor S, Whaley C, Crandall CE: *Dental radiology*, 1980, University of North Carolina Press, with permission.)

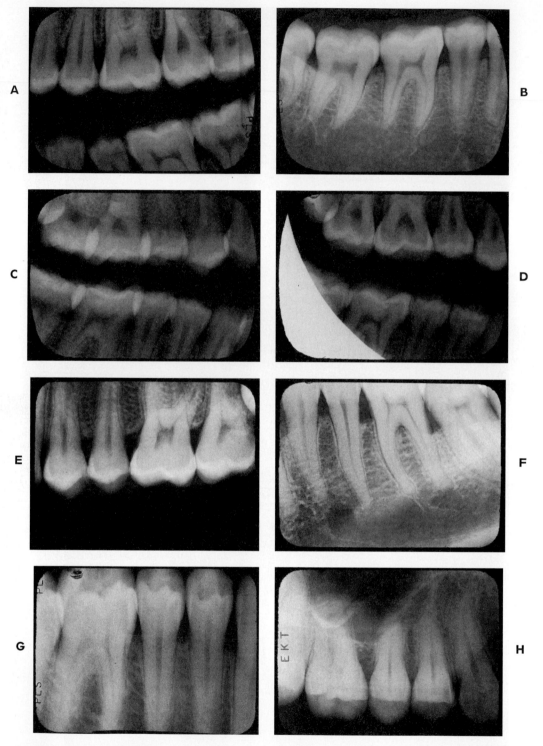

Fig. 5-10 Intraoral technique errors. **A,** Packet placement: packet tilted; **B,** Packet placement: third molar not fully recorded on film; **C,** Horizontal overlap; **D,** Cone cut; **E,** Insufficient vertical angulation (paralleling technique): apices not imaged; **F,** Excessive vertical angulation (paralleling technique): occlusal edges not imaged; **G,** Insufficient vertical angulation (bisecting the angle technique): image elongated; **H,** Excessive vertical angulation (bisecting the angle technique): image foreshortened.

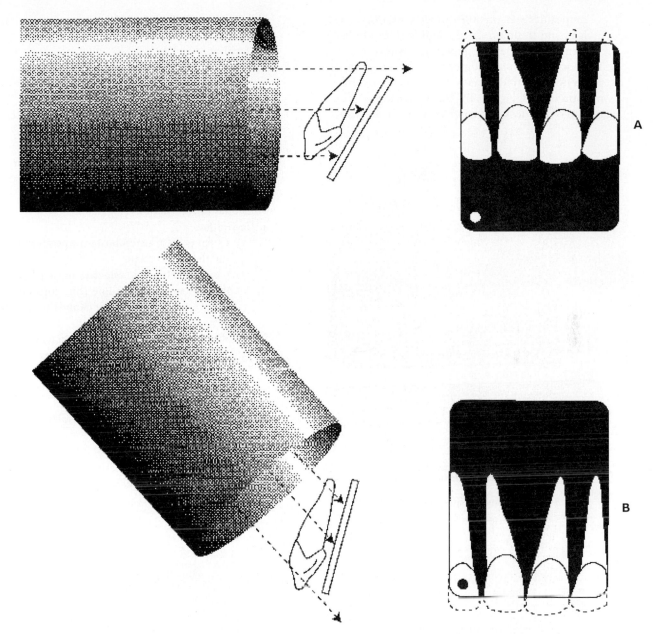

Fig. 5-11   Incorrect vertical angulation will result in incomplete recording of the entire tooth (crown edge to root tip) on the film when using the paralleling technique. **A,** Insufficient vertical angulation; vertical angulation that is too flat will cut off the root tips on the resultant radiograph. **B,** Excessive vertical angulation; vertical angulation that is too steep will cut off the crown edges on the resultant radiograph.

4. Centering
   a. Visualized as a clear area on the film (cone cut)
   b. Results from improper coverage of the image receptor by the x-ray beam
E. Extraoral procedures are considered supplemental projections and are used when evaluating a variety of maxillofacial conditions
   1. Lateral oblique mandible projection is used for visualizing the mandible from the canine region posteriorly to the mandibular body and ramus (Fig. 5-12)
      a. Technique
         (1) Occlusal plane is perpendicular to the plane of the film
         (2) X-ray beam is centered over the area of interest
         (3) PID is directed 25 degrees to the negative
      b. Indications—to evaluate radiolucencies and ra-

diopacities seen on other projections, third molars, and trauma-related conditions and to determine the extent of pathologic lesions
2. Temporomandibular joint (TMJ)—transcranial projection is traditionally the most preferred method of imaging the TMJ area; provides visualization of the neck and condylar head of the man-

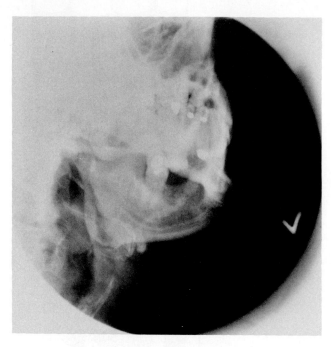

Fig. 5-12   Lateral oblique mandible.

dible and the TMJ space without superimposition of adjacent structures (Fig. 5-13)
  a. Technique
    (1) Midsagittal plane and film are parallel
    (2) X-ray beam is directed transcranially 25 to 30 degrees to the positive
    (3) X-ray beam exits at the joint space of interest, which is against the film
  b. Indication—TMJ dysfunction
3. Waters' projection is a supplemental extraoral projection used primarily for visualization of the maxillary sinuses with minimal superimposition of other anatomic structures (Fig. 5-14)
  a. Technique
    (1) Client is in an anteroposterior position facing the film cassette
    (2) Chin is extended, establishing a perpendicular mentomeatal line (line formed by the external auditory meatus and the mental region of the chin)
    (3) X-ray beam is directed perpendicular to the film and parallel to the mentomeatal line
    (4) Structures shown include the maxilla, maxillary sinuses, zygomatic arches, and orbital rims
  b. Indications include trauma and visualization of "cloudy" radiopaque sinuses
4. Cephalometric projection is used primarily during orthodontic treatment to measure changes in the cranial bones and by oral surgeons involved in maxillofacial reconstruction (Fig. 5-15)

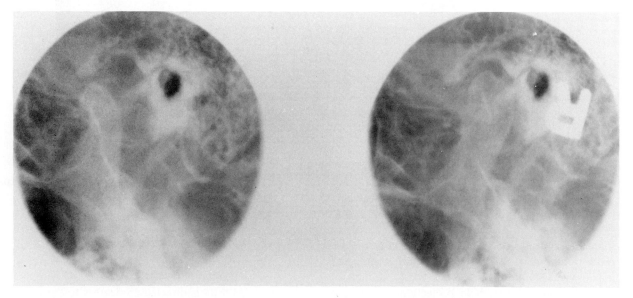

Fig. 5-13   Temporomandibular joint projections. Open *(left)*; closed *(right).*

a. Technique
  (1) Cephalostat with earpost is used to allow for reproduction of client position at subsequent examinations.

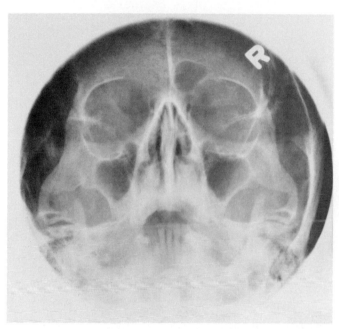

Fig. 5-14 Waters' projection for maxillary and frontal sinuses and orbital rims.

  (2) Client is instructed to look straight ahead in a natural position
  (3) Midsagittal plane-to-film distance of 11.5 cm is used
  (4) Target-to-film distance of 1.5 m is used
  (5) Placement of a wedge filter in the path of the x-ray beam provides a soft tissue outline
b. Indications
  (1) Orthodontic evaluations
  (2) Maxillofacial reconstructive procedures
  (3) Evaluation of growth and development
5. Panoramic radiography (Fig. 5-16)
  a. Single radiograph, usually 5 by 12 inches, which records both the maxillary and mandibular arches; all of the mandible (from condyle to condyle) and all of the maxillae (up to the middle third of the orbit) are imaged on a single film
  b. Types
    (1) Split image provides two lateral projections of the jaw; clear vertical strip of unexposed film is in the center of the radiograph; anterior structures, from approximately canine to canine, are imaged twice
    (2) Continuous image provides an uninterrupted view of the jaws without anterior redundancies

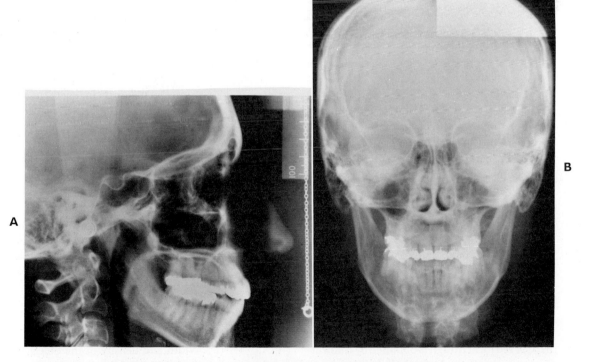

Fig. 5-15   **A,** Lateral cephalometric projection; **B,** Posteroanterior cephalometric projection.

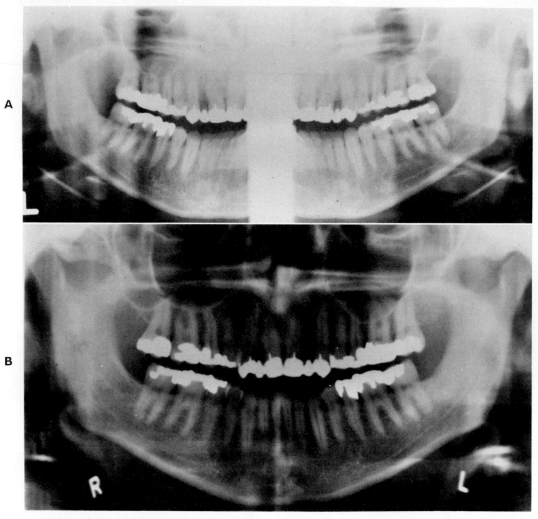

Fig. 5-16 Panoramic radiographs. **A,** Split image; **B,** Continuous image.

c. Image production
  (1) Based on the principle of tomography
  (2) Tomography is the radiographic technique that permits visualization of structures in a chosen plane or layer within an object while intentionally blurring out the images above and below the selected plane
  (3) Tomographic process is accomplished by moving the film and x-ray source parallel to each other and in opposite directions while the client remains stationary
  (4) Layer or plane of interest is termed the focal trough (the plane of acceptable focus)
  (5) Curved, horseshoe focal trough is needed to image the jaw; chin rest represents the focal trough
  (6) Curved focal trough is obtained by connecting the x-ray tube and the film carriage assembly and then circling them around the object such that the x-ray beam rotates around a pivot point
  (7) Depending on the machine design, the pivot points may be stationary or moving

d. Technique
  (1) Refer to the manufacturer's directions for specific operating procedures
  (2) Film cassette is loaded into the unit
  (3) Client is positioned in the unit so that the midsagittal plane is perpendicular to the floor and the occlusal plane is parallel to the floor
  (4) Dental arches are separated by a cotton roll or similar device (e.g., bite rod)
  (5) Client's head is stabilized
  (6) Width and density of the object is used to determine the kilovoltage setting

(7) Exposure is made, and film is processed by either the automatic or the manual method

e. Indications
   (1) As a survey film
   (2) Trauma to facial structures
   (3) Evaluation of growth and development
   (4) Evaluation of dental anomalies
   (5) To image extensive pathoses

6. Panoramic technique errors
   a. Client movement during the exposure cycle yields a blurred image that is not diagnostically useful
   b. Positioning errors
      (1) When the chin is positioned in front of the focal trough (closer to the film assembly), the anterior teeth will be blurred and diminished in size
      (2) When the chin is positioned behind the focal trough (farther from the film assembly), the anterior teeth will be blurred and magnified in size
      (3) When the chin is tilted upward, the resulting radiograph will appear to "frown"; additionally, the dense bony palatal structures will absorb much of the radiant beam, causing the maxillary anterior teeth to be obscured or faintly imaged
      (4) When the chin is tilted downward, the resulting radiograph will appear to "smile"; the condyles will tilt inward
      (5) When the midline is not centered and is turned too far to the right, more teeth will be imaged on the right and the teeth on the left will be magnified
      (6) When the midline is not centered and is turned too far to the left, more teeth will be imaged on the left and the teeth on the right will be magnified
      (7) If the tube head–film carriage assembly is positioned too low, the superior structures will not be imaged and the chin rest will be imaged excessively
      (8) If the tube head–film carriage assembly is positioned too high, the superior structures will be imaged excessively and the inferior border of the mandible will be absent
   c. Operator errors
      (1) Exposure errors
         (a) Double exposure of the film
         (b) Insufficient kilovolt peak producing less dense (light) radiographs
         (c) Failure to depress the exposure switch through the entire cycle

      (2) Processing errors—refer to the section on film processing
      (3) Lead apron and thyroid collar artifacts are radiopaque densities; if the protective device is positioned within the path of the x-ray beam, then the beam is absorbed and anatomic structures are obliterated
      (4) Metallic object artifacts are seen as radiopaque densities and result from failure to remove objects such as earrings, bobby pins, glasses, and partial dentures; often ghost images are present
   d. Equipment errors—failure of the equipment to function properly may yield no image, a partial image, or an extremely blurred image

F. Radiographic localization methods
   1. Purpose—periapical and bitewing projections image the teeth and bone in the superoinferior and anteroposterior dimensions; relative buccolingual position of structures is often required for diagnosis and treatment planning in a variety of clinical situations
   2. Indications
      a. Impacted teeth
      b. Supernumerary teeth
      c. Foreign objects
      d. Fractures or trauma
      e. Pathologic lesions
      f. Endodontic therapy
      g. Sialoliths
   3. Methods
      a. Definitive evaluation
         (1) Based on shadow-casting principle No. 3 (the shortest object to the film distance improves image sharpness)
         (2) Radiographic film is positioned lingually; therefore more lingually positioned objects have better radiographic sharpness
         (3) Additional radiographs are not necessary, which decreases the client's radiation exposure
      b. Clark's technique (Fig. 5-17)
         (1) Also referred to as the tube shift method or the buccal object rule
         (2) Requires a second periapical radiograph with an alteration of 20 degrees in either the vertical or the horizontal angulation
         (3) Key phrase is "same or olingual, opposite on buccal," the SLOB rule[8]
         (4) In a comparison of the initial and second radiographs, the buccal object will appear to have moved in the direction opposite to the tube shift

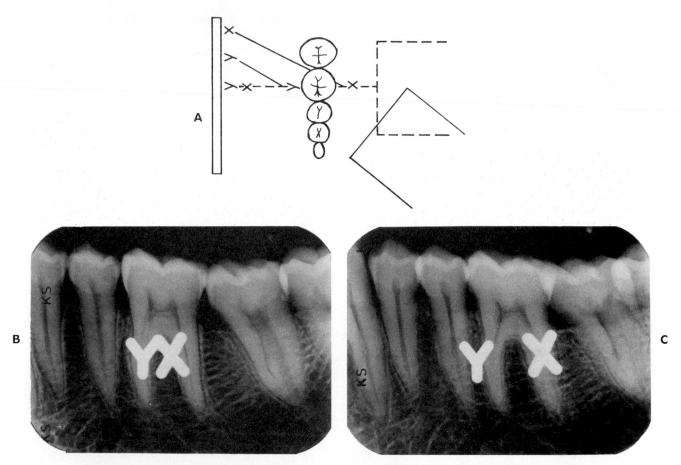

Fig. 5-17 Localization using Clark's technique. **A,** *Dotted-line* PID represents standard angulation; *solid line,* which superimposes first molar and objects, represents mesial cone shift to yield visual separation of first molar and objects; **B,** Radiograph taken with standard angulation yielding superimposition of first molar and lead letters *X* and *Y;* **C,** Radiograph taken with mesial PID yielding separation of first molar and lead letters *X* and *Y; X* is facially positioned and appears to move opposite tube shift (distally); *Y* is lingually positioned and appears to move with tube shift (mesially).

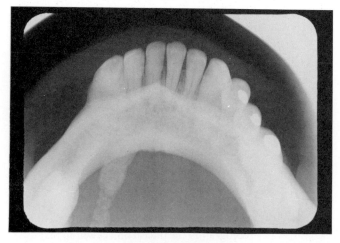

Fig. 5-18 Cross-sectional occlusal radiograph illustrating lingually positioned radiopacity.

(5) In a comparison of the initial and second radiographs, the lingual object will appear to have moved in the same direction as the tube shift

c. Miller's technique (Fig. 5-18)
   (1) Also referred to as the right-angle method
   (2) Requires a second radiograph taken at a right angle to the initial radiograph
   (3) Intraorally, the cross-sectional occlusal radiograph provides the buccolingual dimension

d. Panoramic
   (1) Requires use of a split-image panoramic radiograph in which the anterior regions are imaged twice
   (2) Anterior structures are imaged with two different horizontal angulations as a result of the split-image radiograph

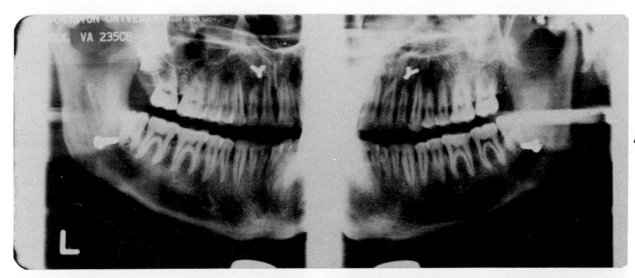

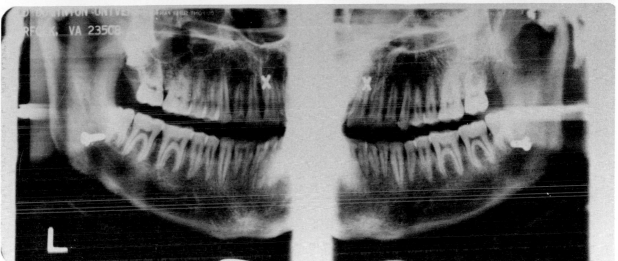

Fig. 5-19 Localization with split-image panoramic radiograph and SLOB rule. **A,** Lead letter *Y* is located lingually and appears to move in same direction as viewer's movement; **B,** Lead letter *X* is located facially and appears to move in direction opposite to viewer's movement

(3) Relative movement of the object is compared with the adjacent structures from one side of the film to the other

(4) Key phrase is "same or lingual, opposite on buccal," the SLOB rule[8]

(5) Buccal object will appear to have moved in the direction opposite to the clinician's viewing movement

(6) Lingual object will appear to have moved in the same direction as the clinician's viewing movement (Fig. 5-19)

Film Mounting

A. Purpose—provides a systematic approach for viewing and evaluating radiographs, with placement of the radiograph in a holding device according to anatomic considerations

B. Mount construction—made of either cardboard or plasticlike material; available with windows for placement of radiographs in various number and size combinations

C. Mounting procedures

  1. Intraoral radiographs

    a. Labial mounting

      (1) Raised portion of embossed dot is toward the viewer

      (2) Client's left side is the viewer's right side

      (3) Orientation is that the viewer is facing the client

    b. Lingual mounting

(1) Raised portion of embossed dot is away from the viewer
(2) Client's left side is the viewer's left side
(3) Orientation is that the viewer is on the client's tongue

2. Extraoral radiographs
   a. During film exposure the side(s) under examination should be identified with a lead letter (R or L) placed on the film cassette
   b. Radiographs may be placed on an illuminating viewbox with orientation so that the viewer is facing the client or that the viewer is on the client's tongue

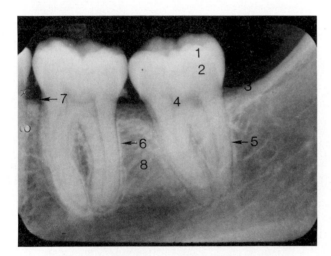

Fig. 5-20 Tooth anatomy. *1*, Enamel; *2*, dentin; *3*, cementum; *4*, pulp; *5*, periodontal membrane; *6*, lamina dura; *7*, alveolar crest; *8*, trabeculae.

Radiographic Anatomy

A. General considerations
   1. Radiographic examination is an essential component of the total assessment of the client's dental health
   2. When viewing dental radiographs, one must be able to distinguish between normal and abnormal appearances of radiographic anatomic conditions
   3. Occasionally, normal or a variation of a normal anatomic condition may be confused with dental disease; therefore the clinical examination is mandatory
   4. Radiographic evidence of dental disease is observed as an abnormal radiolucency or radiopacity in the radiographic image
   5. Most often evidence of caries, periodontal disease, and periapical inflammations are observed in dental radiographs; developmental disturbances, traumatic injuries, and neoplastic lesions are also observed
   6. Dental hygienists must be able to identify normal tooth and bony structure anatomic conditions to distinguish between signs of disease and variations of normal

B. Tooth anatomy
   1. Radiographic appearance is distinguished by the variations in radiographic densities
   2. Dense tooth structure (e.g., enamel) appears radiopaque; less dense tooth structure (e.g., pulp chamber) appears radiolucent
   3. Radiographic appearance of the tooth and supporting structures is seen in Fig. 5-20

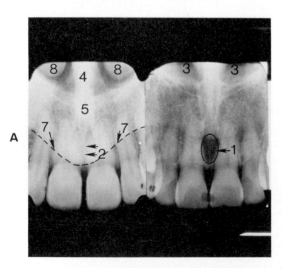

A

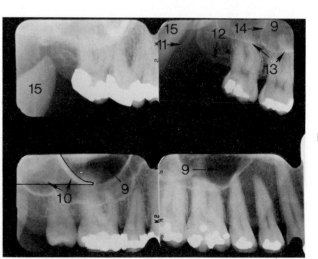

B

Fig. 5-21 Maxillary anatomy. **A,** *1,* Nasopalatine foramen; *2,* median palatine suture; *3,* nasal fossa; *4,* nasal septum; *5,* anterior nasal spine; *7,* soft tissue outline of nose *(dotted line)*; *8,* turbinates. **B,** *9,* Maxillary sinus; *10,* zygomatic process; *11,* hamular process; *12,* maxillary tuberosity; *13,* floor of sinus; *14,* sinus septum; *15,* coronoid process.

C. Radiographic anatomy of the maxilla (Fig. 5-21)
1. Nasopalatine foramen—oval radiolucency between the maxillary central incisors; provides passage for the nasopalatine nerve and artery; when superimposed over the apex of an incisor, it is often confused with periapical disease
2. Median palatine suture—radiolucent line extending vertically between the maxillary incisors; may be mistaken for a fracture line, nutrient canal, or fistula tract
3. Nasal fossae—two radiolucent densities observed superior to the central incisors outlining the nasal passages
4. Nasal septum—radiopaque density representing the bony division of the nasal cavities
5. Anterior nasal spine—increased radiopacity adjacent and superior to the incisive foramen
6. Typical Y formation—Y-shaped radiopacity created by the radiopaque lines that outline the nasal floor and anterior portion of the maxillary sinus
7. Maxillary sinus—bilateral radiolucency originating at the canine region and extending posteriorly; outlined by a radiopaque wall; represents the maxillary sinus air space
8. Nutrient canals—thin radiolucent lines often confused with fracture lines; generally seen in the maxillary sinus area
9. Zygomatic process (arch)—radiopaque structure observed superior to the maxillary posterior teeth that joins the maxilla and frontal and temporal bones
10. Maxillary tuberosity—most distal region of the maxilla; appears as a raised alveolar bony ridge
11. Hamular process—radiopaque spine located on the medial pterygoid plate
12. Lateral pterygoid plate—radiopaque extension of the sphenoid bone
13. Maxillary torus—radiopaque density superior to the apices; seen in some patients

D. Radiographic anatomy of the mandible (Fig. 5-22)
1. Genial tubercles—radiopaque spines (often seen as a circle) located inferior to the mandibular central incisors; serve as the attachment of the geniohyoid and genioglossus muscles
2. Lingual foramen—small radiolucency in the cen-

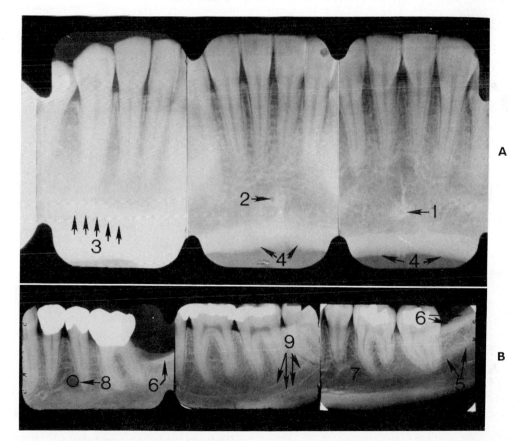

Fig. 5-22 Mandibular anatomy. **A,** *1,* Genial tubercules; *2,* lingual foramen; *3,* mental ridge; *4,* inferior border of mandible. **B,** *5,* Internal oblique ridge; *6,* external oblique ridge; *7,* submandibular fossa; *8,* mental foramen; *9,* mandibular canal.

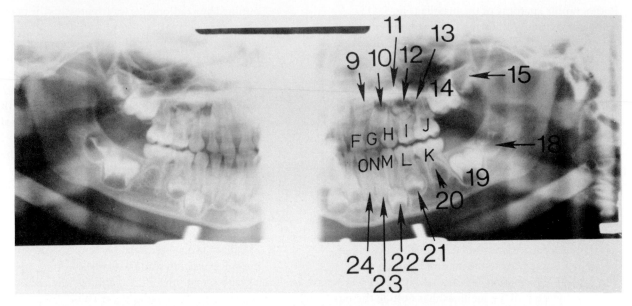

Fig. 5-23 Developing dentition. *9,* Permanent maxillary left central incisor; *10,* permanent maxillary left lateral incisor; *11,* permanent maxillary left canine; *12,* permanent maxillary left first premolar; *13,* permanent maxillary left second premolar; *14,* permanent maxillary left first molar; *15,* permanent maxillary left second molar; *18,* permanent mandibular left second molar; *19,* permanent mandibular premolar; *22,* permanent mandibular left canine; *23,* permanent mandibular left lateral incisor; *24,* permanent mandibular left central incisor; *F,* primary maxillary left central incisor; *G,* primary maxillary left lateral incisor; *H,* primary maxillary left canine; *I,* primary maxillary left first molar; *J,* primary maxillary left second molar; *K,* primary mandibular left second molar; *L,* primary mandibular left first molar; *M,* primary mandibular left canine; *N,* primary mandibular left lateral incisor; *O,* primary mandibular left central incisor. (Courtesy Dr. Henry Fields, Department of Pedodontics, University of North Carolina School of Dentistry, Chapel Hill, NC.)

ter of the genial tubercles for the passage of nerves and vessels

3. Nutrient canals—narrow radiolucent lines observed in the mandibular anterior regions
4. Mental ridge—radiopaque density (lines) corresponding to the raised bone level along the anterior aspect of the mandible
5. Inferior border of the mandible—radiopaque density representing the dense cortical bone
6. Internal oblique ridge (mylohyoid line)—radiopaque line representing a ridge of bone on the lingual surface of the mandible that serves as the attachment of the mylohyoid muscles
7. External oblique ridge—radiopaque ridge created by the raised bony surface on the facial side of the mandible for the attachment of the buccinator muscle; superior to the internal oblique ridge
8. Submandibular fossa—radiolucent area in the posterior body of the mandible that represents the lingual depression for the submandibular salivary gland
9. Mental foramen—circular radiolucency on the facial aspect of the mandible, near the apex of the second premolar, for the exit of the mental nerve;

often mistaken for a periapical pathologic condition of the premolars

10. Mandibular canal—radiolucent horizontal canal in the mandible through which the inferior alveolar nerve and artery pass; extends anteriorly from the mandibular foramen on the lingual aspect of the ramus through the body and terminates at the mental foramen
11. Mandibular torus—radiopacity below the apices; seen in some patients

E. Radiographic appearance of tooth development—radiography of the developing dentition normally includes most of the 20 primary or deciduous teeth and, depending on the age of the child, evidence of the development of the 32 permanent teeth (Fig. 5-23)

F. Panoramic anatomy (Fig. 5-24) and artifacts (Fig. 5-25)

G. Restorations (Fig. 5-26)
  1. Metallic (gold, amalgam)
  2. Nonmetallic (composite, gutta-percha, etc.)

Radiographic Interpretation

A. Systemic approach
  1. Mounting of radiographs

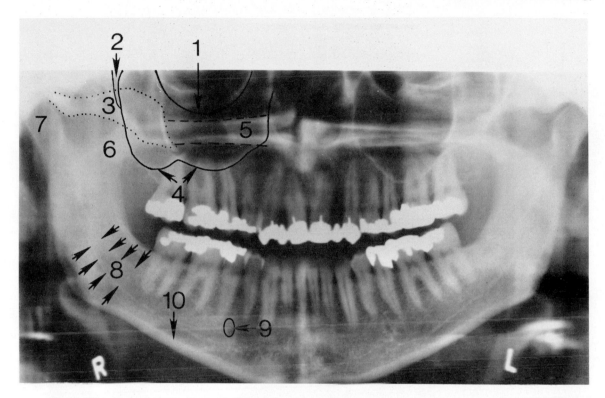

Fig. 5-24   Panoramic anatomy. *1*, Orbital floor; *2*, pterygoid maxillary fissure; *3*, zygomatic arch; *4*, walls of maxillary sinus; *5*, palate; *6*, coronoid process; *7*, mandibular condyle; *8*, mandibular canal; *9*, mental foramen; *10*, inferior border of mandible.

2. Placement of radiographs on the illuminating viewbox (labial mounting recommended)
3. Masking out of extraneous light around films and dimming of room light
4. Evaluation of technical quality of films
   a. Should be free of technical errors and artifacts
   b. Should adequately image anatomic regions of interest
5. Dentition evaluation
   a. Begin assessment at tooth No. 1 and proceed to tooth No. 32 (if present, continue with A through T)
   b. Order of evaluation
      (1) Presence or absence of teeth
      (2) Size of teeth
      (3) Shape of teeth
      (4) Eruption and location of teeth
      (5) Presence of restorative materials
      (6) Signs of pathoses (abnormal radiolucencies and radiopacities)
6. Supporting structure evaluation
   a. Periodontal membrane (ligament) space
   b. Lamina dura
   c. Bone trabecular pattern
   d. Cortical plates
   e. Alveolar bone height
   f. Sinuses (when present)
   g. Orbits (when present)
   h. Signs of pathoses (abnormal radiolucencies and radiopacities)
B. Developmental disturbances (Fig. 5-27, pp. 183-184)
C. Inflammatory responses (Fig. 5-28, p. 185)
D. Traumatic injuries (Fig. 5-29, p. 186)
E. Neoplastic conditions (Fig. 5-30, pp. 188-189)
F. Caries and bone loss (Fig. 5-31, p. 190)

Quality Assurance

A. Definition—"refers to the routine and special procedures developed to ensure that the final product is of consistently high quality"[4]
B. Components of a quality assurance program
   1. Practitioner competence
      a. Self-evaluation of radiographs for technique analysis
      b. Peer review of radiographs for technique analysis
      c. Continuing education courses
   2. Equipment inspections by state and local radiation regulatory agencies
      a. Timer accuracy; milliamperage accuracy
      b. Collimation and alignment of the x-ray beam
      c. Leakage radiation
      d. Mechanical support of unit

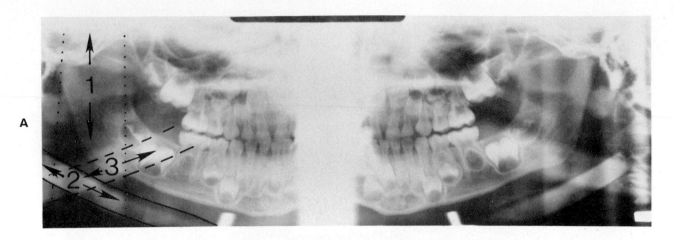

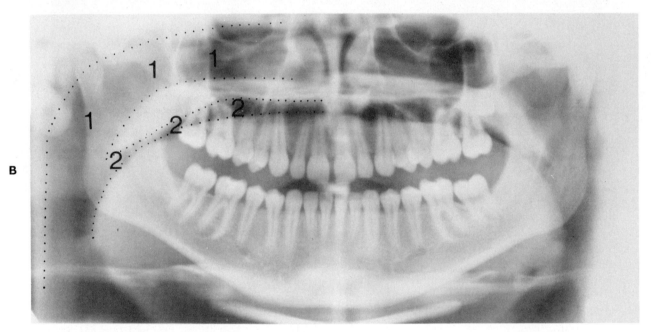

Fig. 5-25 Panoramic artifacts. **A,** *1,* Pancentric head positioner; *2,* chin rest of right side; *3,* shadow of chin rest of left side. **B,** *1,* Nasopharyngeal air space; *2,* palatal glossal air space. (Courtesy Dr. Henry Fields, Dean, The Ohio State University, College of Dentistry, Columbus, OH.)

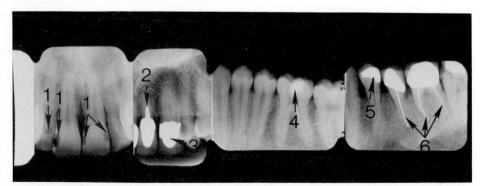

Fig. 5-26 Restorative materials. *1,* Radiolucent aesthetic restorations; *2,* post and core with porcelain-fused-to-metal crown; *3,* porcelain-fused-to-metal crown; *4,* temporary restoration; *5,* metallic restoration (amalgam); *6,* root canal filling material.

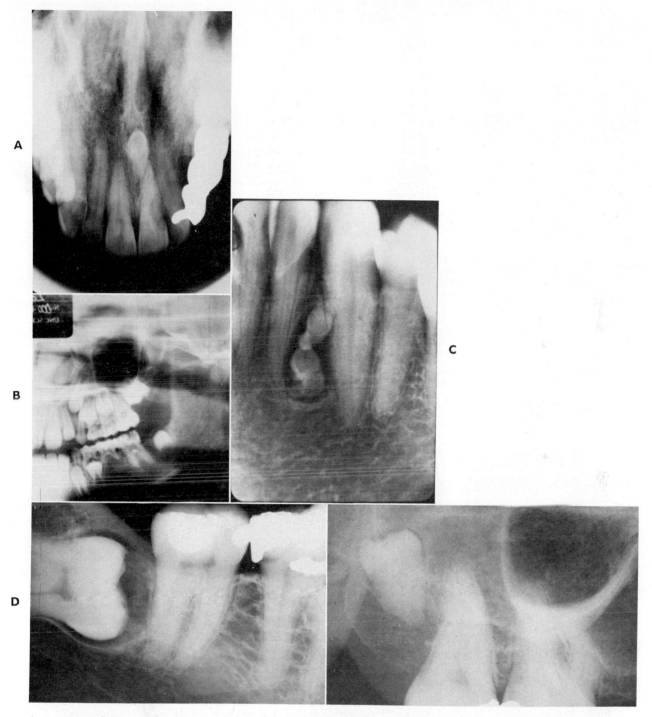

Fig. 5-27   Developmental disturbances. **A,** Supranumerary tooth (mesiodens); **B,** Tooth No. 20 is congenitally missing, and primary tooth K is retained; **C,** Compound odontoma; **D,** Dentigerous cyst; **E,** Impacted third molar.

Continued

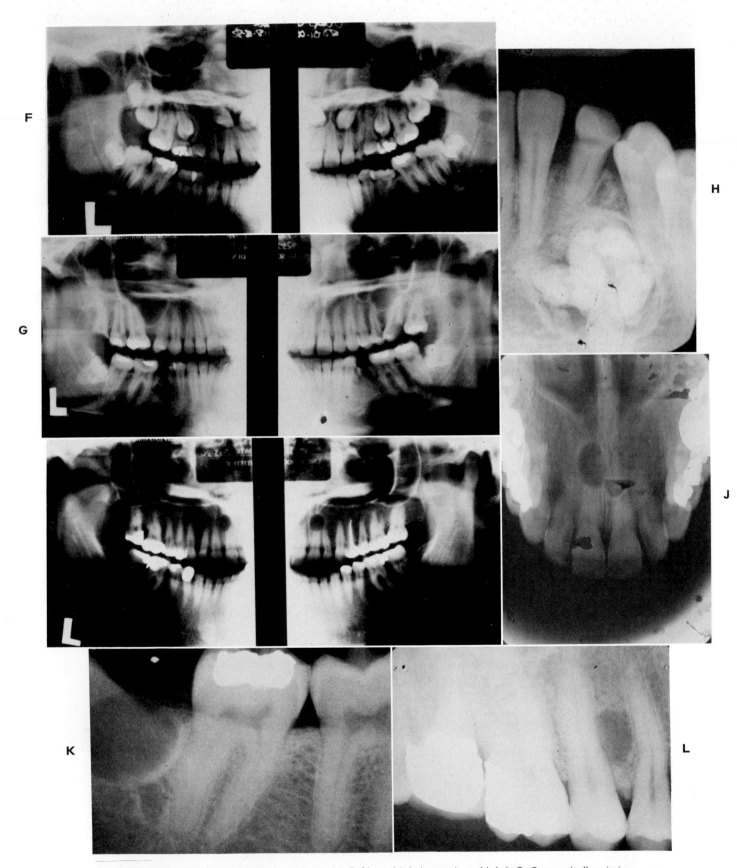

Fig. 5-27, cont'd   F, Missing tooth no. 20 *(left)*; multiple impactions *(right)*; G, Congenitally missing teeth Nos. 20 and 29 *(left)*; right and left maxillary sinus pneumatization *(right)*; H, Compound odontoma; I, Panoramic view of incisive canal cyst; J, Occlusal view of incisive canal cyst; K, Primordial cyst; L, Lateral periodontal cyst. (Courtesy Dr. Donald Tyndall and Dr. Stephen Matteson, Department of Oral Diagnosis, University of North Carolina School of Dentistry, Chapel Hill, NC.)

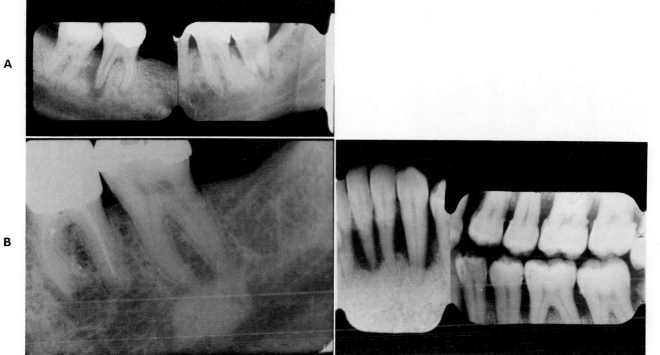

Fig. 5-28 Inflammatory response. **A,** Periapical radiolucencies; **B,** Condensing osteitis apical to tooth No. 18; **C,** Extensive bone loss resulting from periodontal disease.

e. Half-value layer (HVL) is the thickness of a material that when placed within the path of a beam of radiation, reduces the exposure by one half[4]
  (1) The HVL is measured by placing a series of aluminum filters (or other materials) within the path of the x-ray beam
  (2) The decrease in beam intensity is plotted as a function of the material thickness
  (3) Changes in the HVL may indicate a change in beam quality or the amount of added filtration
3. Quality assurance procedures for film processing
 a. Periodic evaluation of the darkroom
  (1) Check for light leaks
  (2) Check safelight illumination for cracks in the filter, bulb wattage, and safety (coin test)
  (3) Coin test for safelight evaluation involves the placement of a coin on an unwrapped, unexposed film under a safelight for 2 to 3 minutes; if the coin outline is present on the processed film, corrective action is necessary
 b. Periodic cleaning, maintenance, and daily monitoring of the processing equipment
  (1) Cleaning of the automatic roller assembly and manual racks is appropriate to prevent debris buildup and artifacts on films;

cleaning schedule should be based on usage
  (2) Records of unit cleaning should be kept
  (3) Scheduled maintenance and preventive maintenance are necessary for optimum equipment operation
  (4) Solution temperatures should be monitored daily
  (5) Solutions should be replenished in accordance with the volume of films processed
  (6) Sensitometric analysis for fog, speed, and contrast should be determined and recorded

Ethical Considerations Regarding the Use of Ionizing Radiation

A. Regulatory agencies
 1. International Commission on Radiological Protection (ICRP)
 2. National Council on Radiation Protection and Measurements (NCRP)
 3. Nuclear Regulatory Commission (NRC)
 4. Bureau of Radiological Health (BRH) of the Food and Drug Administration
 5. State and local agencies
 6. American Dental Association

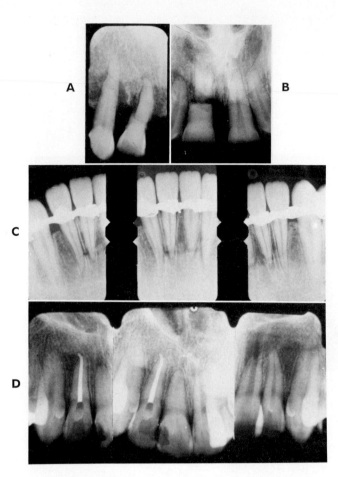

Fig. 5-29 Traumatic responses. **A,** Root fracture; **B,** Root fracture of tooth No. 8; **C,** Alveolar fracture; **D,** Pulp of tooth No. 8 is obliterated as a result of trauma; apical root resorption and widening of pulp of tooth No. 9 as a result of trauma. (Courtesy Dr. Donald Tyndall and Dr. Stephen Matteson, Department of Oral Diagnosis, University of North Carolina School of Dentistry, Chapel Hill, NC.)

Table 5-2

Guidelines for Prescribing Bitewing Radiographs for Clients with No Clinical Evidence of Caries and No High-Risk Factors for Caries[9]

Child
  (primary or transitional dentition)
    posterior bitewings every 12 to 24 months
Adolescent
  (permanent dentition before eruption of third molars)
    posterior bitewings every 18 to 36 months
Adult
    posterior bitewings every 24 to 36 months

---

7. American Academy of Oral and Maxillofacial Radiology (formerly the American Academy of Dental Radiology)

B. Assessment of need for radiographic procedures
  1. Only a licensed physician or dentist may prescribe radiographic services
  2. Dental hygiene assessment for recommendation of need for radiographs
    a. Must be based on a review of the client's medical/dental histories; clinical examinations; client signs/symptoms/complaints
    b. Radiographs are recommended only when there is reasonable expectation of benefit for the client[5]
    c. If no positive findings are noted in the clinical examination or the client's history, radiographs should not be exposed
      (1) The only exception to this rule may be the use of bitewing radiographs for caries detection when no clinical signs of early lesions exist[5]
      (2) Posterior bitewing radiographs may be exposed when there are no clinical signs present according to the guidelines developed by the FDA (Table 5-2)

C. Radiation protection
  1. Cardinal principles of radiation protection[4]
    a. "Keep the time of exposure to radiation short"
    b. "Maintain a large distance between the source of radiation and the exposed person"
    c. "Insert shielding material between the source and the exposed person"
  2. ALARA concept—those individuals working with radiation should attempt to keep all radiation exposure as low as reasonably achievable
  3. Maximum permissible dose (MPD) (Table 5-3)
    a. "The maximum dose of radiation that in light of present knowledge would *not* be expected to produce significant radiation effects"[4]
    b. Specified for the occupational exposure received by the radiation worker (e.g., dental personnel working with radiation)
    c. Assumes a linear, nonthreshold dose-response relationship
    d. Annual MPD for occupationally exposed workers is 5 rem or 5000 mrem (or 50 mSv)
    e. Cumulative MPD for occupationally exposed persons (whole-body exposure)
      (1) Formulas are

$$MPD = 5 \ (N - 18) \ \text{rem}$$
[in traditional units]

or

$$MPD = 50 \ (N - 18) \ \text{mSv}$$
[in SI units]

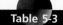

Table 5-3

Maximum Permissible Dose

Group	MPD
Radiation workers	
Combined whole-body occupational exposure	
Prospective annual limit	5 rem in any given year
Retrospective annual limit	10 to 15 rem in any given year
Long-term accumulation to age N years	$5(N-18)$ rem
Skin	15 rem in any given year
Hands	75 rem in any given year (25 rem per quarter)
Forearms	30 rem in any given year (10 rem per quarter)
Other organs, tissues, and organ systems	15 rem in any given year (5 rem per quarter)
Pregnant women (with respect to fetus)	0.5 rem in gestation period
Public or occasionally exposed individuals	0.5 rem in any given year
Students	0.1 rem in any given year
General population	
Genetic	0.17 rem average per year
Somatic	0.17 rem average per year

From Bushong SC: *Radiologic science for technologists: Physics, biology, and protection,* ed 6, St Louis, 1997, Mosby.

(2) Persons younger than age 18 should not be employed as radiation workers

(3) Older workers, not previously exposed may exceed the 5 rem/yr limit if the cumulative limit is not exceeded

(4) To convert rem to Sv, divide rem by 100; for example, 25 rem divided by 100 is equal to 0.25 Sv

  f. Nonoccupational exposure (whole body) is 10% of that for the radiation worker (500 mrem/yr or 5 mSv/yr)

4. Reduction of unnecessary client dose
   a. Eliminate unnecessary examinations
   b. Eliminate repeat examinations
   c. Use proper radiographic technique factors
   d. Use as fast an image receptor system as possible
   e. Position client and film properly
   f. Shield specific areas (gonads and thyroid)
5. Reduction of occupational exposure
   a. Protective shielding and apparel
   b. Distance from source
   c. Never hold client, film, or tube head during exposure
   d. Use of personnel monitoring devices and reports

D. Personnel monitoring devices
1. Film badge
   a. Description—small piece of film sandwiched between metal filters inside a plastic holder
   b. Film density is proportional to the exposure received

  c. Not accurate below 20 mR (read as minimal or "M"), but higher exposures are accurately reported

  d. Filters are usually made of copper and aluminum

  e. Advantages
    (1) Inexpensive
    (2) Easy to handle
    (3) Easy to process
    (4) Reasonably accurate

  f. Disadvantages
    (1) Cannot be worn for periods longer than 1 month
    (2) Film subject to fogging
    (3) Limited sensitivity

2. Thermoluminescent dosimeters (TLD)
   a. Lithium fluoride crystals absorb x-ray energy
   b. Ionizing radiation excites (raises the energy) of the outer-shell electrons of the crystal
   c. When the lithium fluoride crystals are heated, the excited electrons fall back to the normal orbital state and emit light
   d. Light emitted is proportional to the radiation exposure
   e. Advantages
      (1) More sensitive and accurate than film monitors
      (2) Not affected by humidity
      (3) Can be worn for 3 months
   f. Disadvantages—more costly than film monitors

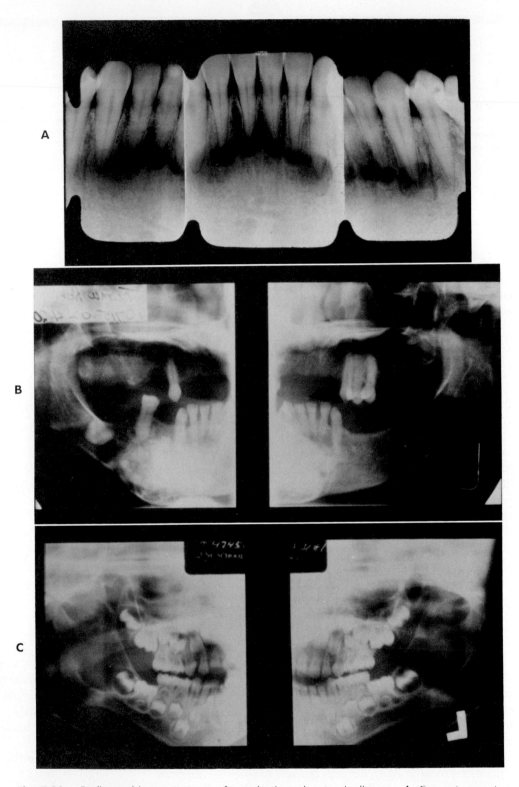

Fig. 5-30 Radiographic appearances of neoplastic and systemic diseases. **A,** Cementoma, stage I; **B,** Multiple cementoma, stage III; **C,** Cherubism; **D,** Ameloblastoma; **E,** Chondrosarcoma; **F,** Osteogenic sarcoma; **G,** Hyperparathyroidism; **H,** Histiocytosis X of left mandible. (Courtesy Dr. John R. Jacoway, Section of Oral Pathology, University of North Carolina School of Dentistry, Chapel Hill, NC.)

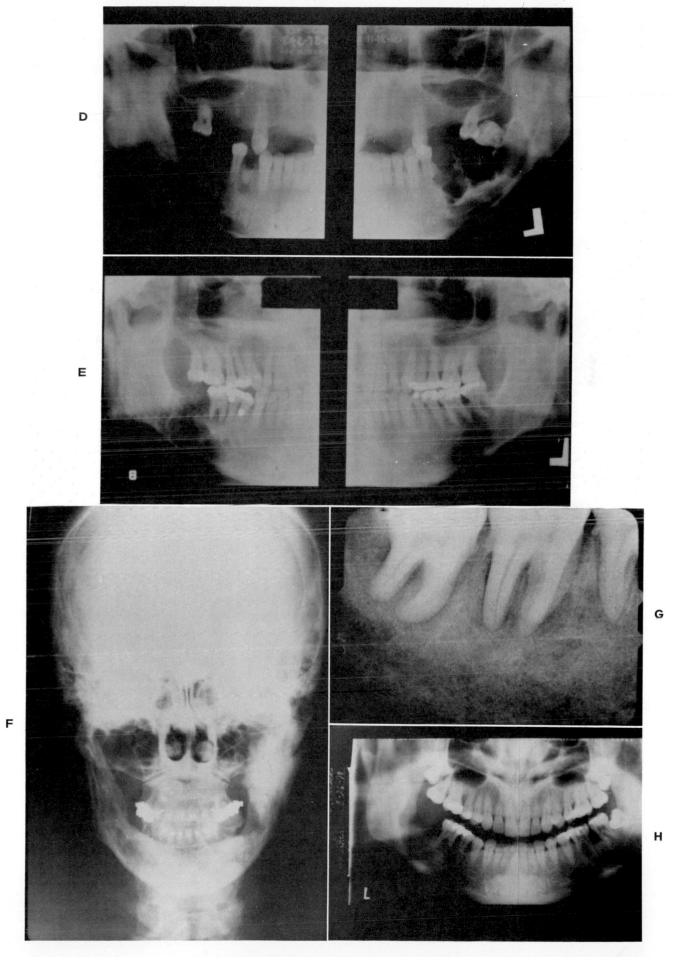

Fig. 5-30, cont'd See facing page for legend.

E. Documentation of client's radiographic exposure
1. Client's record should provide appropriate space for listing radiographic services
2. All radiographic exposures, both acceptable and unacceptable, should be entered sequentially and cumulatively
3. Essential information for radiographic services
   a. Date of radiographic examination
   b. Number of radiographs
   c. Type of radiographs

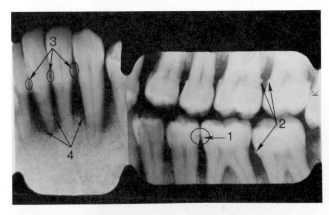

Fig. 5-31 Caries and bone loss. *1*, Interproximal caries; *2*, calculus deposits; *3*, heavy calculus deposits; *4*, height of alveolar bone following resorption.

d. Number and type of retake radiographs
e. Exposure factors used
   (1) Kilovoltage
   (2) Milliamperage
   (3) Exposure time
   (4) Target-to-film distance
   (5) Image receptor system and relative speed[10]
F. Documentation of client's refusal of radiographic services
1. Client must be informed of the possible diagnostic information and possible risks from the radiographic procedure
2. Client should be informed of all protection procedures employed (e.g., equipment standards, quality assurance, standard darkroom procedures, protective shielding, and operator competence)
3. For legal purposes client should sign refusal-for-radiographic-services form to release oral health provider of responsibility
4. Refusal form must be kept in client's dental record

Specialized Imaging Modalities

Although periapical, bitewing, and panoramic radiographs are the most often used images for the assessment and evaluation of oral disease, innovative oral and maxil-

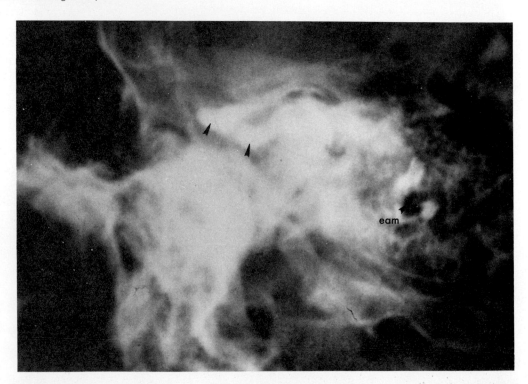

Fig. 5-32 Temporomandibular joint arthrography. *Arrows* indicate radiopaque contrast media in both anterior and posterior compartments as a result of ruptured disc. *eam,* External auditory meatus. (Courtesy Wesley Long Community Hospital, Department of Radiology, Greensboro, NC.)

lofacial imaging technologies are emerging and will have an influence on the scope of dental hygiene practice in the future.

A. Temporomandibular joint arthrography
  1. Definition—radiographic examination of the temporomandibular joint region using contrast medium to outline soft tissues in joint space (Fig. 5-32)
  2. Contrast medium—usually an iodine compound that appears radiopaque and serves to outline structures in the joint space
  3. Indications
    a. Subluxation of condyle
    b. Limited mobility or function
    c. Trauma
    d. Presence of degenerative disease
    e. Congenital deformities
    f. Pain
  4. Procedure used by radiologist
    a. Expose open/closed preliminary films in lateral projection
    b. Use sterile surgical technique
    c. Insert needle into joint spaces (separate insertions for anterior and posterior compartments)
    d. Inject contrast medium
    e. Take radiographs of joint in various positions periodically during procedure

B. Sialography
  1. Definition—radiographic examination of the major salivary glands (parotid and submandibular) using contrast agent to evaluate the ductal and acinar systems
  2. Indications
    a. Soft tissue swelling in submandibular region
    b. Soreness and pain
    c. Suspected salivary stone
  3. Procedure used by radiologist
    a. Expose anteroposterior (AP) and lateral oblique mandibular preliminary projections of salivary gland region
    b. Follow sterile surgical technique
    c. Place cannula into appropriate ductal orifice using fluoroscopy
    d. Secure cannula by taping to client's face
    e. Introduce contrast agent slowly into ductal system
    f. Monitor filling of ductal system with sequential radiographic exposures
    g. After removal of cannula, client receives sialagogue to stimulate glandular function and eliminate contrast agent
    h. Postclearing radiographs are exposed 5 minutes after cannula removal

C. Computerized tomography
  1. Definition—"tomographic process in which x-ray scanning produces digital data that measure the extent of the energy transmission through an object. This information is stored and transformed by a computer into a density scale that is used to generate an image"[1] (Fig. 5-33)
  2. Indications
    a. Trauma
    b. Pain
    c. Degenerative disease
    d. Enhanced imaging of soft tissues
    e. Evaluations done before dental implants
  3. Procedure used by radiologist
    a. Place client into gantry
    b. Position infraorbital meatal line perpendicular to horizon
    c. Establish condyle/fossa relationship
    d. Perform "cuts" using standard protocol (e.g., 0.5- to 1.0-mm section)

D. Nuclear medicine imaging
  1. Definition—the field of diagnostic imaging that uses injected isotopes to assess organ physiology by recording radiation emitted from the respective tissues (Fig. 5-33)
  2. Indications
    a. Suspected salivary gland disease
    b. Metastatic survey
    c. Supplement to previous diagnostic imaging procedures
  3. Procedure used by radiologist
    a. Technetium 99m isotope, which emits gamma rays, is injected approximately 1 hour before scanning
    b. Client is positioned in recumbent or seated position
    c. Gamma rays emitted by isotope from tissue are counted and recorded by a gamma counter
    d. Imaging time approximately 15 minutes

E. Magnetic resonance imaging
  1. Definition—"an imaging technique that utilizes magnetic fields and radio frequencies to produce computed tomographic sections of the body" (Fig. 5-34)[1]
  2. Indications
    a. Trauma
    b. Pain
    c. Degenerative disease
  3. Advantages
    a. Does not use ionizing radiation
    b. Sensitive to physiologic functions of organs
  4. Procedure used by radiologist
    a. Client positioned inside gantry
    b. Client in recumbent position

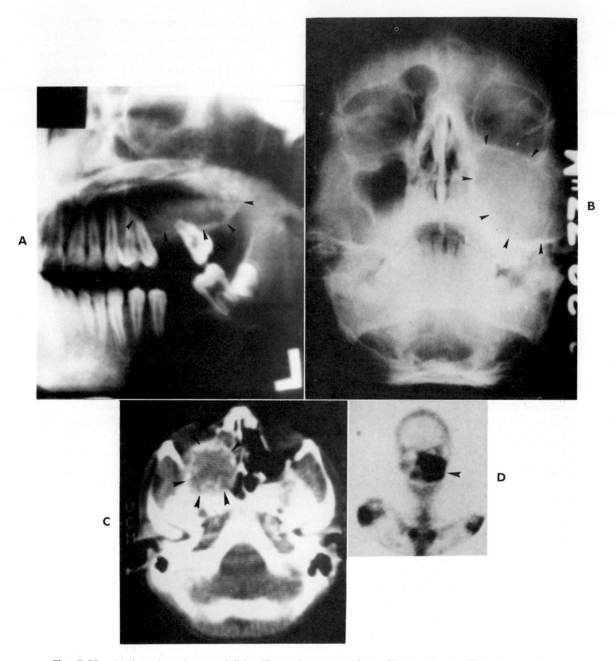

Fig. 5-33 Various imaging modalities illustrating an ossifying fibroma in maxillary sinus region. **A,** Panoramic radiograph demonstrating lesion in maxillary left sinus region. Note resorption of apices of maxillary molar. **B,** Waters' view showing radiopacity in maxillary sinus region. **C,** Computed tomographic image of lesion seen in **A** and **B**. **D,** Nuclear medicine bone scan reveals increased isotope uptake in maxillary left sinus region. (Courtesy Rick Platin, University of North Carolina School of Dentistry, Chapel Hill, NC.)

   c. Strong magnetic force is applied, causing disorientation of hydrogen atoms
   d. Radio frequency energy is emitted from tissues
   e. Computer interpretation provides static and paper images for diagnosis

   f. Examination time approximately 1 hour
5. Hazards
   a. Client with metallic prosthesis
   b. Client with pacemaker
   c. Loose metallic objects in examination suite

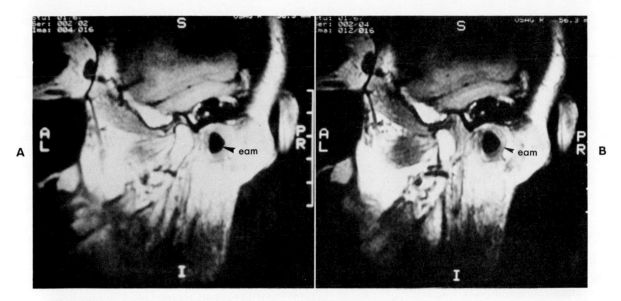

Fig. 5-34 Magnetic resonance images of right temporomandibular joint in open and closed positions. **A,** Closed. *eam,* External auditory meatus. **B,** Open. (Courtesy Moses H. Cane Memorial Hospital, Department of Radiology, Greensboro, NC.)

F. Digital imaging
1. Definition—use of computer-based devices and electronic x-ray detectors to produce an x-ray image on a monitor or video screen from a computer disk; the process is achieved by using sensors to record an exposure and having a computer interpret and convert the information into a numerical value for transmission into a digitized image[11]
2. Types of systems
    a. Intraoral detectors use charge-coupled devices (CCDs), which detect the X rays for conversion into a digitized image
    b. Panoramic detectors use photostimulable phosphor to produce "computed" panoramic radiographic images or a linear array of photodiodes with a scintillator to record exposure for image conversion[9]
3. Indications
    a. Detection of periodontal bone disease
    b. Assessment of temporomandibular joint and condylar changes
    c. Evaluation of all conditions typically seen on periapical and bitewing radiographs[12]
4. Advantages
    a. Generates an image for immediate evaluation on a screen or video monitor
    b. Eliminates the disruption associated with traditional imaging techniques that require film processing and produce variable standards in image quality

    c. Images can be preserved on computer disk for future reference
5. Digital subtraction radiography
    a. A technique used to compare two radiographic images taken over time
    b. Images are stored in computer memory and are electronically merged
    c. Changes in the anatomy of the two images are visibly demonstrated in the subtracted image
    d. Applications for assessing periodontal and TMJ disease[13]

Infection Control (See Chapter 7)

A. General considerations
1. Infection control procedures established for dental care setting must include guidelines for dental radiographic procedures
2. Client's health history must be reviewed before treatment
3. All clients should be considered potentially infectious
4. Infection control protocol, when followed, can reduce the risk of disease transmission during radiographic procedures[14]
B. Procedure
1. Unit preparation
    a. Disinfect equipment (control panel, exposure button, PID, lead apron, counter top, dental chair controls, etc.)

b. Use barrier technique and cover the following items with disposable plastic wrap: control panel, chair adjustments, tube head, PID, exposure button, and cord

c. Obtain radiographic supplies (film, film holders, cotton rolls, etc.) with aseptic technique

d. Disposable film wraps such as the Kodak Dental Barrier Envelope may be used to minimize the possibility of disease transmission during radiographic exposure and film processing[15]

2. Expose intraoral radiographs while wearing disposable latex gloves

a. After removal of film packet from client's mouth, wipe saliva from packet with accepted disinfectant

b. Moisture-proof film packets such as the Kodak Poly-Soft vinyl film packet may be immersed in disinfecting solutions

c. Paper packets should not be immersed in disinfecting solutions because the film may be damaged

3. Place exposed film packets in paper cup; *do not* place film packets in uniform or lab coat pockets

4. Process intraoral radiographs

a. Under safelight conditions, open all film packets and drop film onto a clean paper towel; avoid touching film with contaminated gloves

b. Dispose of all contaminated film wrappings and paper cup in appropriate biohazard container

c. Remove contaminated gloves and dispose in appropriate biohazard container

d. Wash hands thoroughly to remove any glove powder, which may cause film artifacts

e. Place overgloves (gloves as used in foodhandling services) on hands

f. Follow standard film processing procedures (e.g., for manual or automatic)

5. Retrieve processed radiographs and place in film mounts

6. Plastic barrier coverings should be removed and discarded, and radiographic unit and operatory should be disinfected; clean barriers should be placed for next client

7. Film holding devices should be sterilized

REFERENCES

1. Frommer HH: *Radiology for dental auxillaries,* ed 6, St Louis, Mosby, 1996.

2. Board on Radiation Effects Research, Commission on Life Sciences, National Research Council, Committee on the Biological Effects of Ionizing Radiations: Health effects of exposure to low levels of ionizing radiation-BEIR V, 1990, Washington, DC, 1990 National Academy Press.

3. Jacobsohn PH, Fedran RJ: Making darkness visible: The discovery of X-ray and its introduction to dentistry, *JADA* 126:1359-1366, 1995.

4. Bushong SC: *Radiologic science for technologists: Physics, biology, and protection,* ed 3, St Louis, 1984, Mosby.

5. Goaz PW, White SC: *Oral radiology: principles and interpretation,* ed 3, St Louis, 1994, Mosby.

6. Curry TS III, Dowdey JE, Murry RC: *Christensen's introduction to the physics of diagnostic radiology,* ed 3, Philadelphia, 1984, Lea & Febiger.

7. Thomson-Lakey EM: Designing the Ideal Darkroom, *Dent Hyg News* 7:22, 1994.

8. Langlais RP, Langland OE, Morris RR: Radiographic localization techniques, *Dent Radiogr Photogr* 52:67, 1979.

9. FDA: Guidelines for Prescribing Dental Radiographs. Kodak Publication No N-80A, Rochester, NY, 1995, Health Sciences Division, Eastman Kodak Co.

10. American Dental Association, Commission on Dental Accreditation: *Guidelines for evaluating radiograph curriculum and instruction,* Chicago, 1981, The Association.

11. McDavid WD, et al: Direct digital extraoral radiography of the head and neck with a solid-state linear x-ray detector, *Oral Surg, Oral Med, Oral Pathol* 74:811-817, 1992.

12. Nelvig P, et al: Sens-A-Ray, a new system for direct digital intraoral radiography, *Oral Surg, Oral Med, Oral Pathol* 74:818-823, 1992.

13. Kapa SF, et al: Assessing condylar changes with digital subtraction radiography, *Oral Surg, Oral Med, Oral Pathol* 75:247-252, 1993.

14. Infection control in the dental office, Kodak dental radiography series, Publication No N-415 P9742 10-89-AB, Rochester, NY, 1989, Health Sciences Division, Eastman Kodak Co.

15. Manson-Hing LR: *Fundamentals of dental radiography,* ed 3, Philadelphia, 1990, Lea & Febiger.

SUGGESTED READINGS

Haring JI, Lind LJ: Radiographic interpretation for the dental hygienist, Philadelphia, 1993, WB Saunders.

Miles DA, et al: Radiographic imaging for dental auxiliaries, ed 2, Philadelphia, 1993, WB Saunders.

Review Questions

1 Particulate and electromagnetic radiations with sufficient energy to remove orbital electrons from atoms are termed:
A. Electronic
B. Ionizing
C. Subatomic
D. Ultrasonic

2 Which of the following is affected by changing the mA on the dental x-ray unit?
A. Wavelengths
B. Speed of electron travel
C. Penetrating ability of the x-ray beam
D. Quantity of x-ray photons

3 Which of the following *BEST* describes the anode?
A. Negatively charged component
B. Composed of the focusing cup and filament
C. Contains the tungsten target
D. Is the source of electrons

4 Federal regulations limit the size of the intraoral x-ray beam at the client's skin to:
A. 1 ¾ inches
B. 2 ½ inches
C. 2 ¾ inches
D. 3 ½ inches
E. 3 ¾ inches

5 Because most dental x-ray units use alternating current, x-ray production is blocked during the negative half of the cycle. The term for this is:
A. Ionization
B. Self rectification
C. Thermionic emission
D. Transformation

6 What percentage of kinetic energy inside the vacuum tube is actually converted to X radiation?
A. 1%
B. 10%
C. 50%
D. 99%
E. 100%

7 The number of attenuated x-ray photons would be greatest with which of the following?
A. Bone marrow spaces
B. Dentin
C. Enamel
D. Periodontal ligament space
E. Pulp

8 Which of the following indicates radiation absorbed dose?
A. Curie
B. Gray
C. Rem
D. Roentgen
E. Sievert

9 Which of the following is the *MOST* radiosensitive?
A. Mature bone cells
B. Muscle cells
C. Nerve cells
D. White blood cells

10 The light and x-ray–sensitive component of the film is the:
A. Adhesive
B. Base
C. Gelatin
D. Protective coating
E. Silver halide crystals

11 Following irradiation, unexposed silver halide crystals are removed from the film emulsion by which of the following?
A. Elon
B. Hydroquinone
C. Potassium bromide
D. Sodium carbonate
E. Sodium thiosulfate

12 Which of the following temperatures produce optimal results when manually processing radiographs?
A. 58° F
B. 68° F
C. 78° F
D. 88° F
E. 98° F

13 Radiographic images that are too dark are the result of all of the following *EXCEPT*:
A. Overdevelopment
B. Film fog
C. Nonexposure to X rays
D. Hot temperature of solution
E. Over active chemicals

Questions 14 through 16 refer to Fig. 5-35

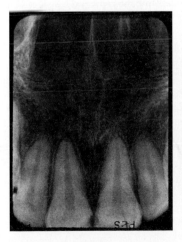

Film A

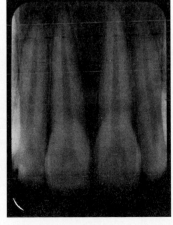

Film B

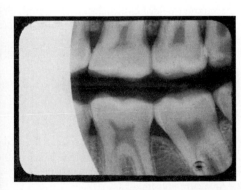

Film C

Fig. 5-35

14 To correct the technique error present in film A, you should do which of the following?
A. Increase vertical angulation
B. Decrease vertical angulation
C. Increase horizontal angulation
D. Decrease horizontal angulation

15 To correct the technique error present in film B, you should do which of the following?
A. Increase vertical angulation
B. Decrease vertical angulation
C. Increase horizontal angulation
D. Decrease horizontal angulation

16 To correct the technique error present in film C, you should move the PID in which of the following directions?
A. Apically
B. Distally
C. Mesially
D. Occlusally

17 With all other technique factors remaining constant, an increase in film speed will:
A. Increase image density
B. Decrease image density
C. Increase image contrast
D. Decrease image contrast
E. Have no effect on the image

18 Which of the following is the most likely reason that a dental hygienist recently removed an 8 inch PID (position indicating device or cone) and replaced it with a 16 inch PID prior to exposing a client's radiographs?
A. To decrease the exposure time
B. To enhance the film image sharpness
C. To reduce image distortion
D. To add more x-ray photons to the beam

19 Which of the following is the *most* important consideration prior to performing scaling procedures on a client with hypertension? (The client's current medications are nitroglycerine and Cardizem [diltiazem].)
A. Checking prothrombin time
B. Placing nitroglycerin on the counter
C. Monitoring blood pressure
D. Prescribing antibiotic premedication

20 When radiographs are mounted labially, which of the following accurately describes the labial mount method?
A. The embossed dot is up, and the viewer's orientation is facing the client.
B. The embossed dot is down, and the viewer's orientation is facing the client.
C. The embossed dot is up, and the viewer's orientation is from the client's tongue.
D. The embossed dot is down, and the viewer's orientation is from the client's tongue.

21 The prescribing of Cardizem (diltiazem) as a hypertension medication for a client may necessitate which of the following be added to the dental hygiene care plan?
A. Amalgam polishing
B. Impressions for study casts
C. Recommendation of saliva substitutes
D. Dietary counseling

22 Which of the following cannot be determined about a client's periodontal health from a full mouth survey?
A. Identification of predisposing factors
B. Location of bone loss
C. Pocket depths
D. Prognosis of affected teeth
E. Type of bone loss

23 Which of the following local irritating factors associated with periodontal disease may *not* be imaged on a radiograph?
A. Calculus
B. Bacterial plaque
C. Open contacts
D. Overhanging restorative margins

24 Which of the following is the *best* reason for exposing the panoramic survey on a client concerned with missing permanent teeth?
A. Deep pits and fissures present on permanent molars
B. Clinical evidence of moderate gingivitis
C. Mouth breathing
D. Suspected dental decay
E. Familial history of congenitally missing teeth

25 A radiograph produced by the movement of an electron from an outer shell to a vacancy in an inner shell is referred to as:
A. Thomson scatter
B. Bremsstrahlung radiation
C. Characteristic radiation
D. Particulate radiation

26 Which of the following is NOT a quality assurance procedure for film processing?
A. Daily replenishment of processing solutions
B. Assessment for light leaks
C. Milliamperage accuracy
D. Safelight evaluation

27 To correct the slender appearance of the anterior teeth on a radiograph, a dental hygienist should:
A. Position the client farther forward in the focal trough
B. Position the client farther back in the focal trough
C. Raise the client's chin up in the focal trough
D. Lower the client's chin down in the focal trough

28 Which of the following film identification methods could NOT be used to determine the right and left sides of a extra oral projection?
A. Lead letters
B. Flash printer unit
C. Radiopaque tape
D. Embossed dot

29 The client's earrings should be removed prior to exposure. Which of the following would a client be allowed to wear during a panoramic exposure?
A. Facial jewelry
B. Hearing aid
C. Necklace
D. Partial denture
E. Wrist watch

30 A duplicate of the panoramic radiograph may be needed for referral. If the duplicate radiograph is too dark, then a lighter duplicate could be obtained by:
A. Increasing duplication time
B. Decreasing duplication time
C. Placing the antihalation side against the original
D. Placing the solarized emulsion side against the original

Answers and Rationales

1. (B) This is the definition of ionizing radiations.
   (A,C,D) These are incorrect responses.
2. (D) Milliamperage controls the quantity of electrons.
   (A) Wavelength is controlled by the kilovoltage.
   (B) Speed of the electrons is controlled by the kilovoltage.
   (C) Penetrating ability of the x-ray beam is controlled by the kilovoltage.
3. (C) The anode contains the tungsten target
   (A) The cathode is the negatively charged component of the vacuum tube.
   (B) The cathode is composed of the focusing cup and filament.
   (D) The cathode is the source of electrons.
4. (C) 2¾ inches is correct.
   (A, B, D, E) These are incorrect responses.
5. (B) X rays are generated during the first half (positive half) of the electrical cycle and not generated during the negative half of the cycle.
   (A) Ionization is the process by which radiation with sufficient energy removes an orbital electron from an atom creating an ion pair.
   (C) Thermionic emission refers to the process by which electrons are "boiled" off, forming an electron cloud around the tungsten filament in the negatively charged (cathode) side of the vacuum tube.
   (D) Step-up and step-down transformers are used to supply voltage to the tube current and the filament circuit.
6. (A) Less than 1% of the kinetic energy is converted to X radiation
   (B) This is an incorrect response.
   (C) This is an incorrect response.
   (D) More than 99% of the kinetic energy is converted into heat energy.
   (E) This is an incorrect response.
7. (C) Dense structures attenuate more of the x-ray beam than less dense structures. Enamel is 92% mineralized.
   (A) Bone marrow spaces are less dense, attenuating little of the x-ray beam.
   (B) Dentin is 65% mineralized and attenuates less of the x-ray beam than enamel.
   (D) Periodontal ligament spaces contain soft tissue, which attenuates very little of the x-ray beam.
   (E) Pulp contains soft tissue, which attenuates very little of the x-ray beam.
8. (B) Gray is the International System of Units term for absorbed dose.
   (A) Curie measures radioactivity based on decay rate of a sample and is not used to measure electromagnetic radiation.
   (C) Rem is the traditional unit of measurement of dose equivalent used to calculate the effective absorbed dose for all types of ionizing radiation.
   (D) Roentgen is the traditional unit of measurement of radiation exposure or intensity.
   (E) Sievert is the International System of Units term of dose equivalent used to calculate the effective absorbed dose for all types of ionizing radiation.
9. (D) Based on the law of B and T that states cells' sensitivity to ionizing radiation is directly proportional to their reproductive activity and inversely proportional to their degree of differentiation, white blood cells are the most radiosensitive of this group.
   (A) Mature bone is relatively resistant to destruction by radiation.
   (B) Muscle cells are relatively resistant to destruction by radiation.
   (C) Nerve cells are relatively resistant to destruction by radiation.
10. (E) Silver halide crystals (bromide and iodide) are the light and x-ray sensitive material in the emulsion.
    (A) The adhesive is applied to the base to ensure union between the base and emulsion.
    (B) The base material (polyester) provides support for the emulsion.
    (C) Gelatin functions as a suspension medium for the silver halide crystals in the emulsion.
    (D) The protective coating keeps the emulsion from being scratched off.
11. (E) Sodium thiosulfate is the clearing agent in the fixer which removes the unexposed/undeveloped silver halide crystals from the emulsion.
    (A) Elon is a reducing agent, a component of the developing solution.
    (B) Hydroquinone is a reducing agent, a component of the developing solution.
    (C) Potassium bromide is a restrainer, a component of the developing solution.
    (D) Sodium carbonate is an activator, a component of the developing solution.
12. (B) 68° F produces archival radiographic images.
    (A) 58° F will not produce archival radiographic images.
    (C) 78° F will not produce archival radiographic images.
    (D) 88° F will not produce archival radiographic images.
    (E) 98° F will not produce archival radiographic images.
13. (C) Nonexposure to X rays results in an image that is clear.
    (A) Overdevelopment produces dark radiographic images.
    (B) Fogged film produces dark radiographic images.
    (D) Hot processing solution temperatures produce dark radiographic images.
    (E) Overactive chemicals produce dark radiographic images.

Oral Pathology

Olga A.C. Ibsen

O ne important skill of the dental hygienist is to be able to identify pathologic conditions and bring these findings to the attention of the dentist for dental diagnosis, treatment, or referral. A knowledge of pathology also is critical for infection control, background preparation in managing emergency situations, and formulation and implementation of dental hygiene care plans congruent with the health status and needs of the client.

The dental hygienist must be able to differentiate between normal and abnormal findings and to relate significant health history information to clinical, histologic, ethnocultural, and radiographic findings. Although the dental hygienist is not responsible for the dental diagnosis, skill in the use of the diagnostic process is essential for collaborative practice.

In this chapter the review of pathologic conditions and anomalies is outlined according to etiology, age and gender considerations, location, clinical features, radiographic appearance, laboratory tests/findings, histologic characteristics, and treatment/prognosis.

Benign Lesions of Soft Tissue Origin

General Characteristics

A. Etiology—unknown
B. Age and gender vary with the type of lesion
C. Clinical features
    1. Sharp line of demarcation outlines the lesion

    2. Sessile or pedunculated base
    3. Lesion is easily palpable
D. Histologic characteristics depend on the lesion (e.g., a lipoma is composed of fat cells)
E. Lesion grows slowly, which contributes to an evaluation of a benign state
F. Lesion is removed surgically and usually does not recur

Fibroma

A. Etiology—unknown
B. Age and gender affected—all ages affected (30 to 50 years most common age); males and females equally affected
C. Location
    1. Buccal mucosa, gingiva, floor of the mouth, palate, tongue, lips
    2. When on the gingiva or hard palate, the lesion lacks mobility and ease of palpation
D. Clinical features
    1. Smooth surface; round, ovoid, or elliptic shape
    2. Well-defined pale pink projection
    3. Size varies from the common size of a few millimeters to several centimeters
    4. Consistency varies from firm and resilient to soft, spongy, and easily palpable
E. Histologic characteristics
    1. Bundles of interlacing collagenous fibers are interspersed with fibroblasts, fibrocytes, and small blood vessels

2. Outer portion of the lesion is covered by a layer of stratified squamous epithelium

F. Treatment/prognosis
  1. Conservative surgical excision
  2. Seldom recurs

Irritative Fibroma

A. Etiology—mild irritant causes a pyogenic granuloma, which scars down to an irritative fibroma
B. Age and gender affected—50% between 20 and 50 years; males and females equally affected
C. Location—anywhere on the soft tissues; buccal mucosa, fauces, tongue, gingiva, floor of the mouth, or lips
D. Clinical features
  1. Pink to red color
  2. Round or semicircular shape
  3. Up to 2 cm in size
  4. Sessile or pedunculated base
E. Histologic characteristics
  1. Chronic hyperkeratosis; dense collagen and scar tissue covered with normal epithelium
  2. Contains fewer fibroblasts than a fibroma; inflammatory cells
F. Treatment—complete excision

Papilloma

A. Etiology—unknown; long duration; slow development
B. Age and gender affected—50% between 20 and 50 years; males and females equally affected
C. Location—usually on the soft palate or lips but can be found on the labial or buccal mucosa or tongue
D. Clinical features
  1. Cauliflower-like or wartlike surface
  2. Usually grayish or white color, can also be pink; color depends on amount of keratin
  3. Well-delineated, pedunculate growth; fingerlike projections
E. Histologic characteristics
  1. Composed primarily of long, fingerlike projections of squamous epithelium with a core of fibrous connective tissue
  2. "Acanthosis" of epithelium—increase in thickness of cells covered by a keratin layer
F. Treatment/prognosis
  1. Excision including the base
  2. Does not recur

Wart (Verruca Vulgaris)

A. Etiology—papillomavirus
B. Age and gender affected—all ages; males and females equally affected
C. Location—most common on skin (hands); also occurs on buccal mucosa, lips, tongue
D. Clinical features
  1. Differs from a papilloma in that warts grow faster, are more often a multiple lesion, are smaller, and develop in a shorter time
  2. Heals alone because it is of viral origin
  3. Self-inoculated (finger to mouth)
  4. Often sessile
E. Histologic characteristics
  1. Contains large clear squamous cells with large dark intranuclear inclusions
  2. Church-spiral effect
  3. Papillary acanthosis
F. Treatment—excision if necessary; lateral lipping of the epithelium undermines it, and the wart falls off

Hemangioma

A. Etiology—congenital or developmental during healing; proliferation of blood capillaries
B. Age and gender affected—present at birth or by the end of the first year; more common in females (2 : 1)
C. Location—most common on the tongue; also found on buccal mucosa, labial mucosa, vermilion of the lip
D. Clinical features
  1. Flat or raised, well-circumscribed lesion of mucosa
  2. Deep red or bluish purple color
  3. Pressure imparts a pallor to the lesion; when released, the lesion again appears bluish red
  4. Two types
    a. Venous or capillary—small to moderate size; soft
    b. Cavernous—located on the tongue and buccal mucosa; 2 or more cm in diameter; exhibits an impressive protrusion of tissue; deep purple; soft or semifirm
E. Histologic characteristics
  1. Venous or capillary—many small capillaries lined by a single layer of endothelial cells supported by a connective tissue stroma of varying density; endothelial cell proliferation
  2. Cavernous—large dilated blood sinuses with thin walls, each having an endothelial lining; sinusoidal spaces filled with blood and lymphatic vessels
F. Treatment/prognosis
  1. Treatment depends on the size and/or location
    a. Nonintervention in cases in which remission has occurred
    b. Surgical removal
    c. Radiation in infants or young children
    d. Sclerosing agents (sodium morrhuate or psylliate) injected into the lesion
    e. Electrocauterization

f. Carbon dioxide snow (cryotherapy)

g. Compression

2. Prognosis excellent; does not become malignant; does not recur

Lipoma

A. Etiology—unknown; rare; benign tumor of mature fat cells

B. Age and gender affected—all ages; males and females equally affected

C. Location—tongue, buccal mucosa, mucobuccal folds, gingiva

D. Clinical features

1. Single or lobulated, well defined, painless

2. Sessile or pedunculated base

3. Soft to palpation

4. Yellowish color

E. Histologic characteristics

1. Circumscribed mass of mature fat cells with collagen strands and a few blood vessels

2. Thin epithelium covers lesion

3. If fibrous connective tissue forms a more significant part of the lesion, it is called a fibrolipoma

F. Treatment/prognosis

1. Surgical excision

2. Recurrence is rare

Inflammatory Tumors (Granulomas)

General Characteristics

A. Growth or enlargement of tissue composed mainly of inflammatory cells

B. Account for the major portion of all mouth tumors

C. Benign tumors

Pyogenic Granuloma

A. Etiology—chronic irritants (calculus, poor restorative margins); response to injury

B. Age and gender affected—more common in age range of 15 to 45; more common in females (3:1), perhaps related to increased estrogen levels

C. Location—anterior maxillary labial gingiva; buccal mucosa, tongue, lips

D. Clinical features

1. Protrusive mass growing outward; pedunculated, sessile, or lobulate base

2. Deep red rather than pink surface

3. Soft and spongy; freely movable; bleeds easily

4. Sixty-five percent are ulcerated

5. Can scar down to an irritative fibroma—fibrogranuloma

6. When pyogenic granuloma occurs in a pregnant woman, it is called a pregnancy tumor

E. Histologic characteristics

1. Epithelium, if present, is thin

2. Rich in capillaries with proliferation of endothelial cells, which form blood vessels

3. Contains polymorphonuclear leukocytes, acute and chronic inflammatory cells, plasma cells, and lymphocytes

4. Has histologic characteristics similar to those of a pregnancy tumor

F. Treatment/prognosis

1. Removal of the irritant

2. Excision of the lesion

3. If cells infiltrate the underlying tissue, 5% to 10% of these lesions can recur

Papillary Hyperplasia of the Palate (Palatal Papillomatosis)

A. Etiology—chronic irritation to the palate caused by the suction chamber of a denture; excessive pressure of an ill-fitting denture; poor denture hygiene; can also be associated with an orthodontic appliance

B. Age and gender affected—denture wearers usually over 40 years of age; males and females equally affected

C. Location—vault of the palate

D. Clinical features

1. Closely clustered projections (papillary processes) 1 to 4 mm in diameter

2. Round, smooth glistening red surface; granular

3. Varying degrees of inflammation present

E. Histologic characteristics

1. Small vertical projections, each composed of parakeratotic or orthokeratotic stratified squamous epithelium and a central core of connective tissue

2. Epithelial proliferation

3. Infiltrated with inflammatory cells

F. Treatment/prognosis

1. Surgical excision via curettage

2. Electrosurgery preceding new denture construction

3. Denture removal at night to rest tissues

4. Prognosis good

Denture-Induced Fibrous Hyperplasia (Epulis Fissurata, Redundant Tissue)

A. Etiology—irritation caused by a denture flange producing a proliferation of tissue

B. Age and sex affected—age range of 40 to 50; males and females equally affected

C. Location—mucobuccal folds; alveolar ridge in anterior regions along the denture flange line

D. Clinical features in vestibular mucosa

1. Exophytic or elongated protrusion of tissue under or around the denture flange—linear irritative fibroma

2. Pink to reddish color
3. Firm to palpation
E. Histologic characteristics
1. Excessive bulk of dense fibrous connective tissue covered by stratified squamous epithelium
2. Connective tissue composed of coarse bundles of collagen fibers with a few fibroblasts or blood vessels (unless inflammation is present)
F. Treatment/prognosis
1. Surgical excision of the lesion is essential
2. Correction of the denture flange, irritant
3. Prognosis excellent if the cause is corrected

Peripheral Giant Cell Granuloma

A. Etiology—local irritant or trauma
B. Age and gender affected—either very young, 20 to 35 years, or elderly (edentulous); more common in females (2:1)
C. Location
1. Gingiva or alveolar process, anterior to the molars
2. Fifty-five percent occur in the mandible, 45% in the maxilla
3. In edentulous persons, the lesion occurs on the crest of the ridge
D. Clinical features
1. Outwardly growing lesion 0.5 to 1.5 cm in diameter
2. Red or pink color
3. Pedunculated or sessile base
4. Arises from a deeper area in the tissue than does a pyogenic granuloma or fibroma
E. Radiographic appearance—radiolucent "cuffing" or erosion of bone
F. Histologic characteristics
1. Composed of a delicate reticular and fibrillar connective tissue stroma containing a large number of ovoid or spindle-shaped young connective tissue cells
2. Multinucleated giant cells
3. Proliferation of collagen and blood vessels
4. Can infiltrate bone, but does not metastasize
5. Appears to originate from the periodontal ligament or mucoperiosteum
G. Treatment/prognosis
1. Surgical removal of the entire base to eliminate recurrence
2. Five to ten percent recur

Central Giant Cell Reparative Granuloma

A. Etiology—trauma caused by a fall or blow or even tooth extraction
B. Age and gender affected—children and young adults; more common in females (2:1)
C. Location

1. Sixty-six percent occur in the mandible, 33% in the maxilla
2. Anterior segment of the arch crossing the midline
D. Clinical features
1. Appears as a swelling or bulge resulting from expansion of cortical plates
2. No symptoms, so may be discovered accidentally
E. Radiographic appearance
1. Large or small radiolucent area with diffuse margins that are sometimes smooth, with faint trabeculae
2. Displacement of teeth
3. Root resorption
F. Histologic characteristics
1. Loose fibrillar connective tissue with many fibroblasts
2. Rich vascularity
3. Foreign-body multinucleated giant cells
G. Treatment/prognosis
1. Surgical excision or curettage; no radiation therapy
2. Invariably fills with new bone and heals

Chronic Hyperplastic Pulpitis (Pulpal Granuloma, Pulp Polyp)

A. Etiology—large, open, carious lesion
B. Age and gender affected—children and young adults; males and females equally affected
C. Location
1. Usually in primary molars or permanent first molars
2. Can occur in any tooth with a large carious lesion
D. Clinical features
1. Red to pink outgrowth of pulp tissue protruding from the crown of a large open carious lesion
2. Lesion is not painful
E. Histologic characteristics
1. Originates from pulpal tissue
2. Contains acute and chronic inflammatory cells, plasma cells, and lymphocytes
F. Treatment/prognosis
1. Extraction of the tooth involved or root canal therapy plus full restorative coverage, depending on the extent of the lesion
2. Prognosis good; no complications

Internal Resorption

A. Etiology—not clear; theories include
1. Trauma
2. Irritative factors
3. Chronic pulpal inflammation
B. Age and gender affected—any age; males and females equally affected
C. Location—usually found in permanent dentition within the tooth

D. Clinical features
   1. Dentin immediately surrounding the pulp in the area of resorption is destroyed
   2. Crown appears pink ("pink tooth") because of the vascularity of the lesion within
E. Radiographic appearance—well-defined radiolucent lesion in close proximity to the pulp canal
F. Histologic characteristics—highly vascularized chronic inflammatory tissue
G. Treatment—endodontic therapy if perforation of the root has not occurred; otherwise, extraction of the tooth

Periapical Granuloma

A. Etiology—dental caries or deep restorations
B. Age and gender affected—any age; males and females equally affected
C. Location—apex of a nonvital tooth
D. Clinical features
   1. Nonvital tooth
   2. Fistula or parulis may be present if the condition has been chronic
E. Radiographic appearance—varies from a well-defined circular radiolucent lesion at the apex of the tooth involved to a diffuse radiolucency or thickening of the periodontal ligament space
F. Histologic characteristics—contains proliferating endothelial cells, young fibroblasts, and epithelial rests of Malassez
G. Treatment—endodontic therapy or extraction of the tooth

Benign Intraosseous Neoplasms

General Characteristics

A. Etiology—generally unknown
B. Onset—gradual with slow development or enlargement
C. Early stages—asymptomatic
D. With expansion of the lesion, malocclusion may occur; bone tenderness on palpation; cortical bone may become thin

Osteoma

A. Etiology—generally unknown, but may be caused by irritation or inflammation
B. Age and gender affected—more common in young adults, but can be found at any age; males and females equally affected
C. Location—endosteal or periosteal; rarely found in the maxilla or mandible
D. Clinical features—individual may be unaware of the

lesion because it grows slowly; considerable growth must occur before cortical plates expand
E. Radiographic appearance—well-circumscribed radiopaque mass that is indistinguishable from scar bone; panoramic or lateral plate radiograph may be needed to view the lesion in its entirety
F. Histologic characteristics—extremely dense, compact bone or coarse, cancellous bone
G. Treatment/prognosis
   1. If it interferes with normal physiologic speech or eating, the lesion should be removed surgically
   2. Does not recur after surgical removal

Chondroma

A. Etiology—unknown
B. Age and gender affected—any age; males and females equally affected
C. Location
   1. Maxilla—anterior area
   2. Mandible—posterior to the canines
   3. May involve the body of the mandible or the coronoid or condylar process
D. Clinical features
   1. Painless
   2. Slow, progressive swelling of the jaw may loosen or malposition teeth
   3. Tendency toward malignancy
E. Radiographic appearance—irregular radiolucent or mottled area in bone; may displace surrounding teeth or cause root resorption
F. Histologic characteristics
   1. Mass of hyaline cartilage with areas of calcification or necrosis
   2. Cartilage cells are small and have one nucleus
   3. Large biopsy sample must be made because the lesion is similar to a malignant chondrosarcoma
G. Treatment/prognosis
   1. Nonconservative surgical removal; tumor resistant to radiation therapy
   2. Periodic evaluation necessary to detect recurrence or possible malignant transformation

Myxoma

A. Etiology—unknown; originates from mesenchymal tissue of the tooth germ
B. Age and gender affected—any age; males and females equally affected
C. Location—maxilla or mandible only (because of lesion's origin)
D. Clinical features—deep-situated lesion
E. Radiographic appearance
   1. Numerous small radiolucencies occurring in groups, giving a "honeycomb" appearance

2. May be large and multilocular
3. May show displaced teeth, mandibular canal, and antrum (may also invade the antrum)
4. Peripheral borders are irregular, diffuse, and not well defined

F. Histologic characteristics
1. Loose-textured tissue containing delicate reticulin fibers and mucoid material
2. Contains stellate, spindle- shaped cells
3. Tumor is not encapsulated and may invade surrounding tissues
4. Does not metastasize

G. Treatment/prognosis
1. Surgical removal
2. Recurrence is common

Exostosis

Torus Palatinus

A. Etiology—inherited, autosomal dominance
B. Age and gender affected—usually seen by puberty; rarely observed in children, but peak incidence is before 30 years; more common in females (2:1)
C. Location—midline of the hard palate
D. Clinical features
1. Bony hard protuberance in the midline in a variety of shapes—nodular, lobular, smooth
2. Occurs in 20% to 25% of the U.S. population
3. Ulcerated if traumatized by coarse foods or a toothbrush
E. Radiographic appearance—dense radiopaque area
F. Histologic characteristics—dense, compact bone
G. Treatment—surgical removal if it interferes with a prosthodontic appliance

Torus Mandibularis

A. Etiology—inherited, autosomal dominant
B. Age and gender affected—first observed in persons over 15 years of age
C. Location—lingual surface of the mandible above the mylohyoid line in the area of the premolars
D. Clinical features
1. Bony hard protuberance varying in size and shape
2. Slow growing—usually unnoticed
3. Bilateral incidence more common (80%)
E. Radiographic appearance—dense radiopaque area
F. Histologic characteristics—dense, compact bone
G. Treatment—surgical excision if it interferes with a prosthodontic appliance

Odontoma

A. Etiology—unknown; theories include
1. Infection

2. Local trauma
3. Inherited trait
4. Mutant gene
5. Postnatal interference with genetic control of tooth development

B. Age and gender affected—any age; males and females equally affected
C. Location—maxilla or mandible, usually between the roots of teeth
D. Clinical features
1. Usually small; asymptomatic
2. Two types
   a. Compound—tooth structures identified
   b. Complex—mass of radiopacity
3. Cyst involvement may occur
E. Radiographic appearance—irregular mass of calcified material ("toothlike structures") surrounded by a narrow radiolucent band with a smooth outer periphery; ranges from radiolucency to radiopacity
F. Histologic characteristics—tumor in which epithelial and mesenchymal cells show differentiation, resulting in abnormal enamel and dentin formation
G. Treatment/prognosis
1. Surgical removal
2. Prognosis good; rare recurrence

Gingival Fibromatosis

General Characteristics

A. Enlargement of gingival tissue, sometimes covering the teeth
B. Contains a proliferation of dense fibrous connective tissue
C. Classification includes
1. Irritative fibromatosis—localized areas associated with extraneous irritants
2. Hereditary fibromatosis—generalized enlargement of gingival tissue
3. Chemical fibromatosis—caused by certain drugs or medications

Irritative Fibromatosis

A. Etiology—irritant such as mouth breathing, orthodontic appliances, heavy bacterial plaque, calculus, debris, overhanging restorations, or ill-fitting prosthodontic appliances
B. Age and gender affected—any age; males and females equally affected
C. Location—localized areas on interproximal papillae; in mouth breathers, on maxillary and mandibular anterior labial gingivae

D. Clinical features—solitary round, smooth-surfaced, pink enlargement of papillae, well attached to surrounding structures
E. Histologic characteristics—proliferation of dense fibrous connective tissue, with an increase in the number of fibroblasts
F. Treatment/prognosis
   1. Removal of the irritant
   2. Improved oral hygiene
   3. Gingivectomy in severe cases
   4. Prognosis excellent

Hereditary Fibromatosis

A. Etiology
   1. Hereditary; believed to have genetic or developmental involvement or be related to hormonal imbalances
   2. Contributing factors include poor oral hygiene, food impaction, calculus, malocclusion, and mental deficiency
B. Age and gender affected—within the first 5 years of life; at the eruption of permanent teeth; slightly more common in females
C. Location—excessive enlargement of interproximal gingival tissues throughout the mouth
D. Clinical features
   1. Two varieties
      a. Symmetric type—diffuse smooth-surfaced, pink, firm tissue in interproximal papillae
      b. Nodular type—multiple protruding pink, stippled firm masses; labial and buccal areas most affected; teeth may be displaced; occurs after eruption of permanent teeth
   2. Primary teeth especially are affected; often mistaken for "unerupted teeth" because teeth may be completely covered by tissue overgrowth
E. Histologic characteristics—bundles of fibrous connective tissue with fibroblasts and fibrocytes (depending on the formative stage)
F. Treatment/prognosis
   1. Excision
   2. Rigid home care
   3. Recurrence is common

Chemical Fibromatosis

A. Etiology—reaction to drugs, specifically Dilantin and calcium channel blockers, especially Procardia
B. Age and gender equally affected
C. Location—papillae and gingivae
D. Clinical features—smooth, pink, firm enlargement of the papillae
E. Histologic characteristics—extensive proliferation of connective tissue

F. Treatment
   1. Change in the prescribed medication if possible
   2. Gingivectomy
   3. Improved oral hygiene

Ulcerative Diseases

General Characteristics

A. Ulcer—formed by destruction of epithelium and some underlying tissue
B. Factors aiding in the diagnosis of ulcers occurring in the oral cavity
   1. Number and size
   2. Location
   3. Depth
   4. Borders
   5. Personal, medical, and drug histories
C. Etiology—not always known
D. Can be classified as acute or chronic conditions
   1. Acute ulcerative conditions include traumatic ulcers, acute necrotizing ulcerative gingivitis (ANUG), recurrent ulcerative stomatitis (RUS), allergic reactions, and viral ulcerations
   2. Chronic ulcerative conditions include those caused by or associated with systemic diseases such as leukemia, colitis, malnutrition, tuberculosis, syphilis, sickle cell anemia, and drug toxicity

Traumatic Ulcer

A. Etiology—various types of trauma
   1. Physical—biting the mucosa, denture irritation, toothbrush injury, sharp tooth, fractured filling
   2. Chemical—mouth rinse, phenol, topical medication used to treat a "toothache"
   3. Thermal—hot foods ("pizza burn")
   4. Electrical
B. Age and gender affected—any age; males and females equally affected
C. Location—lateral border of the tongue, buccal mucosa, lips, palate (especially tori)
D. Clinical features
   1. Small, single, oval, round or irregular shape
   2. Flat or slightly depressed
   3. Covered by necrotic membrane and surrounded by an inflammatory halo
   4. Painful for 2 to 5 days
   5. Heals within 10 days
E. Histologic characteristics
   1. Loss of continuity of surface epithelium
   2. Fibrinous exudate covering exposed connective tissue

3. Infiltration of polymorphonuclear leukocytes in connective tissue
4. Fibroblastic activity can be prominent

F. Treatment/prognosis
1. Removal of the irritant
2. Orabase with benzocaine to relieve symptoms (or Kenalog in Orabase)
3. Denture adhesive to protect the area
4. Anesthetic-type mouth rinse to relieve discomfort
5. Antibacterial mouth rinse to reduce or eliminate secondary infection
6. Hydrogen peroxide rinses
7. Tetracycline suspension (120 ml/1 tsp/4 hr)
8. Tincture of benzoin compound
9. Prognosis good

Acute Necrotizing Ulcerative Gingivitis (ANUG, Vincent's Infection, Trenchmouth)

A. Etiology
1. Anaerobic bacteria, fusiform bacilli
2. *Borrelia vincentii*, a spirochete
3. Contributory factors
   a. Systemic—fatigue, poor hygiene, stress, malnutrition, suppressed immune system
   b. Local—poor restorations, gingivitis, poor oral hygiene, heavy smoking
B. Age and gender affected—any age, usually 17 to 35 years; males and females equally affected
C. Location—free gingival margin, crest of gingiva, interdental papillae
D. Clinical features
1. Acute gingivitis with extensive necrosis
2. Craters form with punched-out interdental papillae
3. Fetid mouth odor, pain, bleeding, bad taste
4. Headaches, low-grade fever
5. Regional lymphadenopathy
E. Histologic characteristics
1. Ulcerated stratified squamous epithelium
2. Thick fibrinous exudate containing polymorphonuclear leukocytes
3. Lack of keratinization
4. Connective tissue infiltrated by dense numbers of polymorphonuclear leukocytes
F. Treatment/prognosis
1. Therapeutic scaling and debridement with ultrasonic instruments and topical anesthetics; will need to be repeated in a few days once pain subsides
2. Use of an oxygenating rinse 4 or more times daily
3. Use of antibiotics such as penicillin if client has fever and lymphadenopathy
4. Home care to improve oral hygiene status (toothbrushing, interdental cleaning, antimicrobial rinse)

5. One month follow-up evaluation to reinforce home care; repeat therapeutic scaling if necessary and encourage regular professional care
6. Can recur if individual lacks good bacterial plaque control or has risk factors

Minor Aphthous Ulcers

Recurrent Ulcerative Stomatitis (RUS); Recurrent Aphthous Stomatitis

A. Etiology
1. Theories
   a. Autoimmune response of oral epithelium
   b. L-form *Streptococcus sanguis*
   c. Nutritional deficiencies
   d. Inherited predisposition
2. Contributory factors
   a. Hormonal imbalance
   b. Endocrine conditions—premenstrual (incidence increases), pregnancy (eruptions occur after delivery)
   c. Psychologic—anxiety, depression, acute emotional problems, stress
   d. Allergic—asthma, hay fever, food, drug, gluten
B. Age and gender affected—first episode occurs in the 20s; more common in females
C. Location—buccal and labial mucosa, soft palate, pharynx, tongue; more common in anterior regions
D. Clinical features
1. Oval or round shape with a red halo having a distinct border
2. Range from 1 to 100 in number (3 to 10 most common)
3. Size—0.5 to 1 cm
4. Pain, tenderness, discomfort
5. Interference with function—speech, eating
6. Prodromal period 1 to 2 days characterized by burning in the area where ulcer will appear
7. Contributory factors include low-grade fever and localized lymphadenopathy
E. Laboratory tests/findings—blood tests and cultures for exclusion of other conditions
F. Histologic characteristics—superficial erosion of soft tissue covered by a membrane
G. Treatment/prognosis—self-limiting, healing in 10 to 12 days; recurrence is common
1. Topical application of nonprescription corticosteroids, chlorhexidine gluconate mouth rinse, topical tetracyclines
2. Nonprescription products for relief of pain, e.g., tannic acid, benzoin, benzocaine

Major Aphthous Ulcers

Recurrent Scarifying Ulcerative Stomatitis (RSUS); Periadentis Mucosa Necrotica Recurrens; Mikulicz' Aphthae; Sutton's Disease

A. Etiology
   1. Autoimmune response of oral epithelium
   2. L-form *Streptococcus sanguis*
B. Age and gender affected—usually adults; more common in females
C. Location—oral cavity, buccal mucosa, tongue, soft palate, lips, posterior fauces
D. Clinical features
   1. Multiple large ulcers, 1 to 10 in number, 2 cm in diameter
   2. Craterlike formations with irregular shapes
   3. Lesions last 5 to 6 weeks, producing scars at healing that are firm and grayish or pale pink
   4. Very painful
   5. Occur at frequent intervals
E. Histologic characteristics
   1. Fibrinopurulent membrane covering the ulcerated area
   2. Necrotic epithelium
   3. Intense inflammatory cell infiltration in connective tissue
   4. Neutrophils and lymphocytes present
   5. Granulation tissue at the base of the lesion
   6. Microscopic picture is nonspecific; conclusive diagnosis cannot be made without thorough clinical and historical data
F. Treatment/prognosis
   1. Tetracycline mouthwash (250 mg) used in doses of 5 ml four times a day for 5 to 7 days
   2. Topical application of corticosteroids
   3. Orabase
   4. Recurrence is common; patient seldom without an ulcer; remission periods of 2 to 3 months; long-term problem

Chronic Benign Mucosal Pemphigoid (Benign Mucous Membrane Pemphigoid, Ocular Pemphigus)

A. Etiology—chronic autoimmune disease
B. Age and gender affected—40 to 55 years; more common in females (2:1)
C. Location
   1. Mucous membranes—nose, larynx, vulva, mouth, eye tissues, vagina, anus (ocular most severe)
   2. Only 30% are skin lesions
D. Clinical features
   1. Bullous lesion appears; thick-walled; takes 24 to 48 hours to rupture
   2. After rupture, the surface is eroded, raw
   3. Lesions heal by scar formation
   4. Gingiva exhibits persistent erythema long after the lesion heals
E. Histologic characteristics
   1. Vesicles and bullae are subepithelial
   2. No evidence of acantholysis—degeneration of cohesive elements of cells (bridges)
F. Treatment/prognosis
   1. Mild forms—no treatment
   2. With bullous eruptions or conjunctival involvement, use systemic corticosteroids
   3. Long duration of lesions, extending many years; few remissions

Herpes

See Chapter 7, section on herpes

Primary Herpes

A. Etiology
   1. Virus—herpes simplex
   2. Transmission—droplet infection; direct contact; highly contagious
B. Age and gender affected—2 to 11 years (85%), not younger than 6 months; males and females equally affected
C. Location—lips, gingiva, tongue, pharynx, floor of the mouth, buccal mucosa
D. Clinical features
   1. Systemic symptoms
      a. Abrupt onset of fever
      b. Headache, irritability
      c. Pain on swallowing—pharyngitis
      d. Regional lymphadenopathy
   2. Oral symptoms
      a. Hypertrophic gingivitis
      b. Painful ulcers 1 to 3 mm in size; filled with yellowish fluid
      c. Shallow craters covered by white or yellow plaque; bright red margins—"halo"
      d. Third to seventh day most acute
E. Laboratory tests/findings
   1. Rabbit eye test—virus injected into a rabbit eye; keratoconjunctivitis results; results take several days
   2. Embryonated egg—"pock" formation occurs; results take several days; expensive
   3. Cytologic smear—ulcer scraped and stained; multinucleated cells observed; not dependable
   4. Serologic—first sample taken before fourth day; second sample taken within 7 to 21 days to see if antibodies are present
F. Histologic characteristics
   1. Vesicle is an intraepithelial blister filled with fluid
   2. Degenerating cells show "ballooning" or intranuclear inclusions (Lipschütz' bodies)

3. Displacement of chromatin
4. When the vesicle ruptures, the surface of the tissue is covered by exudate composed of fibrin, polymorphonuclear leukocytes, and degenerated cells

G. Treatment/prognosis
1. Symptomatic therapy—bed rest, fluids, mouthwash; antibiotics on the third day to prevent secondary infections (especially in persons with rheumatic fever)
2. Self-limiting, healing in 7 to 14 days (21 at most)

Herpes Labialis (Cold Sore)

A. Etiology
1. Residual form of primary herpesvirus infection
2. Contributory factors
   a. Exposure to sunlight
   b. Trauma
   c. Menstruation, pregnancy
   d. Upper respiratory tract infection
   e. Emotional stress, anxiety, fatigue
   f. Allergic reactions
   g. Systemic diseases, gastrointestinal upset

B. Age and gender affected—adults; males and females equally affected

C. Location
1. Lips—most common
2. Intraorally—hard palate, attached gingiva, alveolar ridge

D. Clinical features
1. Burning sensation, feeling of tightness, swelling, and soreness where the vesicle eventually appears
2. Small lesion or several in clusters
3. Gray to white vesicles rupture, leaving a red "halo"
4. Lip vesicles covered with a brownish crust when dried
5. Pain and discomfort varies

E. Histologic characteristics
1. Ballooning degeneration; chromatin margination
2. Lipschütz' bodies; multinucleated giant cells
3. Isolation of herpes simplex virus

F. Treatment/prognosis
1. Topical remedies—camphor, calamine lotions, *Lactobacillus* tablets
2. Acyclovir
3. Vitamin supplements
4. Self-limiting, healing in 7 to 10 days

Herpes Zoster (Shingles)

A. Etiology
1. Varicella virus, which causes chickenpox; injury to the dorsal nerve root
2. Contributory factors
   a. Systemic disease
   b. Drug toxicity
   c. Malnutrition
   d. Trauma to cranial nerve V (oral)
   e. Extreme fatigue
   f. Immunosuppressed patient

B. Age and gender affected—adults, usually over 50 years; males and females equally affected

C. Location—skin or mucosa supplied by the affected sensory nerve

D. Clinical features
1. Clusters of vesicles along the pathway of a sensory nerve
2. Inflammation with severe pain, itching, and burning preceding vesicle eruption
3. Unilateral distribution

E. Treatment/prognosis
1. Propoxyphene (Darvon), meperidine (Demerol), or morphine to control pain
2. Topical anesthetics; Orabase
3. Antibacterial mouth rinses
4. Radiation—three treatments of 150 rad to involved dorsal root ganglia to reduce pain
5. Prognosis good if cranial nerve V involvement (healing in 2 to 3 weeks); involvement of other nerve ganglia may be long lasting

Herpangina (Aphthous Pharyngitis)

A. Etiology—coxsackievirus

B. Age and gender affected—children 6 months to 8 years; males and females equally affected

C. Location—posterior hard or soft palate, tongue, fauces (pillars), uvula, tonsils

D. Clinical features
1. Systemic symptoms
   a. Comparatively mild and short duration
   b. Sore throat
   c. Fever—101° to 105° F, peaks in 2 days
   d. Headache
   e. Vomiting; dysphagia
   f. No lymphadenopathy—differs from primary herpes
2. Oral symptoms
   a. Eight to 12 small ulcers with a gray base and inflamed periphery
   b. Numerous small vesicles precede the ulcers—often overlooked
   c. Slightly painful and sometimes difficult to swallow
   d. Sudden onset
   e. Erythematous pharynx

E. Laboratory tests/findings—throat scrapings and stool specimens to isolate coxsackievirus

F. Treatment/prognosis
1. Aspirin or acetaminophen

2. Bed rest
3. Self-limiting with few complications

Infectious Mononucleosis (Glandular Fever)

A. Etiology
1. Epstein-Barr (EB) virus
2. Transmission—intimate oral exchange of saliva; "kissing disease"
B. Age and gender affected—children and young adults; males and females equally affected
C. Clinical features
1. Systemic symptoms
a. Fever, chills, fatigue
b. Sore throat, cough
c. Headache
d. Nausea, vomiting
e. Lymphadenopathy—cervical lymph nodes
f. Enlarged spleen
2. Oral symptoms
a. Acute gingivitis and stomatitis
b. Inflamed attached gingiva
c. Ulcerations similar to those of herpes or herpangina
d. Purpura spots beneath the epithelium (thrombocytopenia—a decrease in the number of platelets)
e. Edema of the soft palate and uvula
D. Laboratory tests/findings
1. Blood count may indicate anemia, thrombocytopenia, or lymphocytosis, but lymphocytosis is very characteristic
2. Increased heterophil antibody titer—1:56 normal; 1:4096 positive for mononucleosis (Paul-Bunnell test)
3. Sharp increase in the number of white blood cells
E. Treatment/prognosis
1. Antibiotics
2. Bed rest
3. Nutritional diet
4. Course runs 2 to 4 weeks

Skin Diseases

General Characteristics

A. Characterized by various forms and sizes of ulcerative eruptions
B. Lesions may appear first or during the course of the disease
C. Reaction simulates an allergic-type reaction

Erythema Multiforme

A. Etiology
1. Unknown
2. Possibly allergy, hypersensitivity reaction, toxicity, viral or bacterial infection, drug intake
3. May be preceded by herpes simplex infection or tuberculosis
B. Age and gender affected—young adults 20 to 40 years; more common in males
C. Location
1. Extremities—hands, feet, arms, legs
2. Skin—macular, papular, or bullous eruptions; characteristic "target" or "bull's-eye" lesions
3. Mouth—lips, buccal mucosa, tongue
D. Clinical features
1. Systemic symptoms
a. Abrupt onset
b. Fatigue, malaise, fever
c. Previous occurrences
d. Has been associated with terminal cancer, nephritis, and typhoid fever
e. May be a toxic reaction to an iodide, bromide, salicylate, or antibiotic
2. Oral symptoms
a. Painful lesions
b. Macules, papules, or vesicles ulcerate and bleed easily
c. Have a raw tissue base with a grayish necrotic slough
d. Irregular shape; surrounded by a band of inflammation; encrustations
e. Edema of the lips
E. Laboratory tests/findings—biopsy for differential diagnosis
F. Histologic characteristics
1. Zone of severe liquefaction degeneration in upper layers of epithelium
2. Intraepithelial vesicle formation and thinning
3. Absence of a basement membrane
4. Dilation of capillaries and lymphatic vessels in the surface layer of connective tissue
5. Varying degree of inflammatory cell infiltration
G. Treatment/prognosis
1. Removal of the cause if known
2. Topical or systemic applications of corticosteroids
3. Antibacterial, mild mouthwashes
4. Liquid diet—Metracal, Nutriment, Instant Breakfast, Ensure
5. Antibiotics if secondary infection is present
6. Antihistamines if an allergic response
7. Lesions remain 2 to 4 weeks; can recur

Stevens-Johnson Syndrome

Severe bullous form of erythema multiforme
A. Etiology—unknown; possibly viral
B. Age and gender affected—children and young adults

under 25 years; more common in males; history of previous similar illness

C. Location—oral cavity, skin, eyes, genitalia
D. Clinical features
   1. Oral symptoms—bullae rupture, leaving thick white or yellow exudate; eating becomes impossible
   2. Skin lesions—severe, numerous; cover wide areas of the body (face, chest, abdomen)
   3. Eye involvement—severe conjunctivitis, photophobia, corneal ulceration, scarring and blindness
E. Treatment/prognosis
   1. Antibiotics and corticosteroids to control severity
   2. 1- to 4-week duration
   3. Prognosis good; some fatalities because of pneumonia

Behçet's Syndrome (Behçet's Triad, Behçet's Triple Complex)

Variant of erythema multiforme
A. Etiology—unknown; theories include
   1. Viral, hormonal, or metabolic origin
   2. Toxic mechanism
   3. Pleuropneumonia-like organisms (PPLOs)
   4. Mycoplasma (bacteria having no cell walls)
B. Age and gender affected—10 to 40 years; more common in males (6:1)
C. Location—triad location, major characteristic in the diagnostic process
   1. Oral cavity—97%
   2. Eyes
   3. Genitalia
D. Clinical features
   1. Oral lesions
      a. Painful ulcerations
      b. Large ulcers surrounded by a red border; covered with gray or yellow exudate
      c. Similar to those of recurrent ulcerative stomatitis and erythema multiforme
   2. Eye lesions
      a. Begin with photophobia and irritation
      b. Purulent conjunctivitis and uveitis
      c. Healing may be followed by scarification and consequent blindness
      d. Hypopyon (pus in the anterior chamber of the eye between the iris and cornea) in severe cases
   3. Genital lesions
      a. In females—painful ulcerations in the vulval folds, labia majora, and vaginal canal
      b. In males—painful ulcerations on the scrotum and penis
   4. Systemic symptoms
      a. Occasionally fever, pallor
      b. Complications can involve the central nervous, cardiac, and pulmonary systems

E. Laboratory tests/findings
   1. Excessive gammaglobulin in the blood
   2. Leukocytosis with eosinophilia
   3. Elevated sedimentation rate
F. Histologic characteristics
   1. Endothelial proliferation in lesions
   2. Other characteristics similar to those of recurrent ulcerative stomatitis in oral tissues
G. Treatment/prognosis
   1. Similar treatment as for erythema multiforme
   2. Lesions last 2 to 4 weeks
   3. Disease is long lasting with remission periods
   4. Complications may result in fatalities

Pemphigus Vulgaris

A. Etiology—unknown; theories include viral or streptococcal origin; severe progressive autoimmune disease
B. Age and gender affected—adults over 30 years (usually between 40 and 50 years); more common in white females
C. Location—oral cavity, anywhere on mucosa; eyes, skin
D. Clinical features
   1. Oral lesions appear first (very important point)
   2. Blisters, vesicles, or bullae collapse as soon as they are formed
      a. Vary in shape and size (from several millimeters to centimeters)
      b. Ragged peripheral borders; flat or shallow; base intensely red and raw; may extend into the lips with crusting
   3. Filmy necrotic slough of tissue can be detached from underlying tissue
   4. Neighboring soft tissue appears normal
   5. Nikolsky's sign present—epithelial tissue separates under light pressure from air syringe or tongue blade
   6. Pain may be severe with the client unable to eat
   7. Salivation is profuse; mouth odor
   8. Gingival lesions—desquamative gingivitis
E. Laboratory tests/findings
   1. Blood chemistry shows a decrease in the serum sodium level
   2. Biopsy—most conclusive
   3. Over 80% of persons with pemphigus vulgaris have circulating autoantibodies
F. Histologic characteristics
   1. Vesicle or bulla entirely intraepithelial above the basal layer, producing a distinctive "split"; acantholysis
   2. Prevesicular edema weakens the junction
   3. Intercellular bridges between epithelial cells disappear with loss of cohesiveness
   4. Clumps of epithelial cells lie free within the vesicular space

5. Tzanck cells present—swelling of nuclei
6. Increase in RNA in the cytoplasm
7. Scarcity of inflammatory cell infiltration
G. Treatment/prognosis
   1. Corticosteroids and antibiotics to control secondary infections
   2. When lesions are present, prednisolone, 100 to 175 mg/day reduced to 10 mg/day after the lesions disappear
   3. Antimicrobial or tetracycline suspension mouth rinses
   4. Prognosis poor in severe cases; persons with mild cases recover within a few days or weeks

White Lesions

General Characteristics

A. May be keratotic or hyperkeratotic
B. Vary from simple lesions to diffuse coverage; smooth to rough surfaces; elevated to flat
C. Firmly attached to mucous membranes
D. Color—white, grayish white, yellowish white
E. Painless

Stomatitis Nicotina (Nicotine Stomatitis)

A. Etiology—heavy smoking of cigarettes, cigars or pipes (but most commonly associated with pipes); "pipe smoker's palate"
B. Age and gender affected—adults 30 to 50 years; more common in males
C. Location—posterior hard and soft palates
D. Clinical features
   1. Begins with redness and inflammation of the minor salivary duct orifice; 4 to 5 mm in size
   2. Diffuse grayish white, thickened coating with a red center in each tiny nodule (indicates an inflamed, dilated, or partially occluded duct orifice)
   3. Fissures or cracks around the nodules create an overall wrinkled appearance
E. Histologic characteristics
   1. Hyperkeratosis
   2. Thickening of epithelium adjacent to the orifice
F. Treatment/prognosis
   1. Stop smoking—condition may be reversible
   2. Prognosis good if the patient permanently ceases smoking

Linea Alba

A. Etiology—pattern of occlusion may be contributory
B. Age and gender affected—any age; males and females equally affected

C. Location—buccal mucosa along the occlusal plane; usually bilateral
D. Clinical features
   1. Pink to grayish velvety swelling or clustering of tissue along the line of occlusion
   2. Localized, single line in thickness
E. Histologic characteristics—localized intracellular edema (leukoedema)
F. Treatment/prognosis—no treatment required; nonpathogenic

Leukoedema

A. Etiology—unknown; possibly a hereditary factor or defect in maturation of squamous epithelium
B. Age and gender affected—average age 45 years; males and females equally affected; blacks more affected (80% of incidence)
C. Location—buccal and labial mucosa; bilateral; extending to the inside of the lips
D. Clinical features
   1. Soft, spongy, velvety, filmy opalescence of buccal mucosa
   2. Later becomes grayish white with a coarsely wrinkled surface
E. Histologic characteristics
   1. Intracellular edema of prickle cells (spinous layer)
   2. Increased thickness of epithelium, with a superficial parakeratotic layer several cells thick
   3. Broad rete pegs that appear irregularly elongated
   4. Does not produce keratin
F. Treatment/prognosis—no treatment required; nonpathogenic

Chronic Discoid Lupus Erythematosus

A. Etiology—unknown; theories include
   1. Genetic origin
   2. Form of tuberculosis
   3. Associated with foci of infection
   4. Toxic agents
B. Age and gender affected—30 to 40 years; more common in females (3:1)
C. Location
   1. Oral mucosa—buccal
   2. Skin—face, chest, back, bridge of the nose, extremities
D. Clinical features
   1. Slow onset
   2. Oral lesions usually precede skin lesions
      a. Vary in size; may have butterfly configuration
      b. Superficial, painful ulcerations with crusting or bleeding; no actual scale as on skin lesions
      c. Margins not sharply demarcated but show a narrow zone of keratinization

3. Skin lesions—rough and circular with red or purple macules; scales form; butterfly configuration on the bridge of the nose
4. Scarred appearance shows the duration of the disease
5. Fissuring of the tongue

E. Laboratory tests/findings—blood tests are definitive; reveal
1. Lupus erythematosus cell inclusion phenomenon
2. Anemia; leukopenia; thrombocytopenia
3. Elevated sedimentation rate and serum gamma-globulin level
4. Positive Coombs test

F. Histologic characteristics
1. Hyperkeratosis or hyperparakeratosis alternating with areas of epithelial atrophy
2. Acanthosis
3. Pseudoepitheliomatous hyperplasia
4. Necrosis of the basal cell layer; thickening of the basement membrane
5. Diffuse infiltration of lymphocytes in the corium

G. Treatment/prognosis
1. Corticosteroid therapy
2. Periods of remission

Familial White Folded Dysplasia (Spongy Nevus)

A. Etiology—hereditary; autosomal dominant trait
B. Age and gender affected—progressive from childhood to adulthood; males and females equally affected
C. Location—buccal mucosa, palate, gingiva, tongue, lips (inner surface)
D. Clinical features
1. Mucosa thickened
2. Lesions diffuse and generalized
3. Grayish white; soft, spongy, velvety
4. Early years—tissues smooth and flat
5. Adolescence—tissues become increasingly folded or corrugated; appear opalescent-white when the lesion peaks

E. Histologic characteristics
1. Epithelium thickened with both hyperkeratosis and acanthosis
2. Basal cell layer intact
3. Cells of the spinous layer toward the surface exhibit intracellular edema with pyknotic nuclei
4. Lack of differentiation of epithelial cells beyond the parabasal level
5. Epithelial cells appear washed out microscopically because they do not stain well

F. Treatment/prognosis
1. No treatment required
2. Prognosis excellent; no clinical complications

Lichen Planus

A. Etiology—benign, chronic disease; exact cause unknown but emotional stress and nervousness are usually contributory
B. Age and gender affected—adults; children rarely affected; males and females equally affected
C. Location—buccal mucosa, tongue; 50% show skin lesions too
D. Clinical features
1. Size—small (several millimeters to centimeters)
2. Varied patterns/forms
   a. Reticular pattern (most common)
   (1) White, narrow, interconnecting slightly elevated lines forming a mesh, net, or lace-like pattern (Wickham's striae)
   (2) Mucous membrane between the lace pattern appears normal in color and texture
   (3) Whitish, grayish
   b. Papular pattern
   (1) Small, pinhead, raised, glistening papules; scattered or clustered
   (2) Coalescence
   (3) Radiating striae appear at the periphery
   c. Plaque pattern
   (1) Solid grayish or whitish raised patch
   (2) Varies in size and shape
   (3) Often simulates hyperkeratotis or leukoplakia
   d. Erosive or ulcerative form
   (1) Located on the buccal mucosa
   (2) Begins as an erosive, flat, or depressed lesion
   (3) Intensely red, blotching pattern
   (4) Preceded by bullous lesions or ulcerations
   (5) Malignant transformation can occur in this form
   e. Atrophic form
   (1) Smooth, red, poorly defined areas
   (2) Peripheral striae evident
3. Gingival involvement
   a. Rare; similar to desquamative gingivitis
   b. Barely detectable, disrupted, patterned, diffuse or patchy papuls papules
   c. Denuded and painfulDenuded and painful
4. Grinspan syndrome—consists of lichen planus, diabetes mellitus, and vascular hypertension
E. Histologic characteristics
1. Hyperparakeratosis or hyperorthokeratosis
2. Thickened spinous layer (acanthosis) and granular layer
3. Intracellular edema of cells in the spinous layer
4. Necrosis or degeneration of the basal cell layer with a thin band of eosinophilic coagulum in its place
5. Infiltration of lymphocytes into connective tissue
F. Treatment/prognosis

1. Bicotin T—3 or 4 times a day
2. Vitamin B complex therapy
3. Corticosteroids to decrease ulcerations and inflammation
4. Niacinamide—200 mg/day
5. Lesions are self-limiting, healing spontaneously over months or years; not considered a premalignant lesion
6. Use of dapsone

Hyperkeratosis

A. Etiology
1. Local factors (80% of incidence)—constant, low-grade irritation (e.g., from cheek biting, a denture clasp/flange, a sharp filling, or a fractured cusp)
2. Systemic factors
   a. Vitamin A deficiency
   b. Hyperestrogen medication over a prolonged period
   c. Tertiary syphilis causing keratosis of the tongue
   d. Alcoholism, malabsorptive syndromes
   e. Cirrhosis of the liver
   f. Ulcerative colitis
3. Combination of local and systemic factors
B. Age and gender affected—over 40 years; more common in males
C. Location—anywhere in the oral cavity
D. Clinical features
1. Flat, smooth, soft lesion with a diffuse boundary
2. Three layers of epithelium affected: granular, prickle, and basal
3. Fissures or ulcerations rare
E. Laboratory tests/findings—biopsy most conclusive; repeated if indicated
F. Histologic characteristics
1. Abnormal layer of keratin/parakeratosis where not normally found; thickness of keratin in areas where normally found (e.g., attached gingiva)
2. Normal underlying epithelial cells
3. Considered a premalignant lesion
4. Histologic diagnosis is definitive
G. Treatment/prognosis
1. Removal of the irritant
2. Surgical excision and biopsy
3. Slowly induced with a prolonged duration

Malignant Neoplasms of the Mouth

Mouth Cancer

A. Etiology—unknown; possibly viral; risk factors include use of all forms of tobacco; alcohol abuse
B. Age and gender affected—50 to 70 years and over; more common in males (2:1)
C. Location—98% begin in soft tissues
1. Maxilla or mandible—2%
2. Lips—25% to 30% of all oral carcinomas; 95% of lip cancers occur on lower lip; pipe smokers have a definite predilection for squamous cell carcinoma of the lower lip
3. Tongue—25% to 40% of all oral carcinomas; lateral borders at the junction of the middle and third sections; dorsum or posterior area; early metastases
4. Floor of the mouth—20%; second most common area for oral carcinoma
5. Buccal mucosa and gingiva—10%
6. Soft palate—10% to 20%
7. Hard palate—uncommon
D. Clinical features
1. Hard, firm lesion in soft tissue; feels anchored to underlying tissue
2. Stages
   a. Stage I—early; asymptomatic
   b. Stage II—intermediate; bone tenderness, pain, unexplained toothache, numbness or tingling, sudden looseness of teeth
   c. Stage III—advanced; pain and ulcerations from loss of blood; lesion moves around teeth under palpation
3. Ulcerations that do not heal
E. Radiographic appearance
1. Diffuse radiolucency with irregular borders after 40% to 60% of the bone has been destroyed; penetration into the cortex
2. Resorption of tooth roots; expansion between teeth
F. Laboratory tests/findings
1. Exfoliative cytology—not always accurate
2. Biopsy
   a. Incisional—removal of a piece of tissue
   b. Excisional—removal of the entire mass
G. Histologic characteristics
1. Proliferation of abnormal cells; nucleus denser and larger
2. Invasive to underlying tissues; metastasizes to lymph nodes, etc.
3. Types—fugating, infiltrating, papillary (growth in lateral direction)
4. Broder's classification states that the closer the malignancy to the original normal tissue from which it developed, the better the prognosis
H. Treatment/prognosis
1. Surgical excision, radiation or both; chemotherapy is not usually used since oral squamous cell carcinoma is resistant to it
2. Treatment and prognosis depend on the site and size of the tumor, the presence or absence of metastasis, the histologic grade, and the age and health of the person

Pleomorphic Adenoma (Mixed Tumor)

A. Etiology—unknown; benign salivary gland tumor
B. Age and gender affected—most common over 40; males and females equally affected
C. Location
   1. Ninety percent of all salivary gland tumors
   2. Parotid gland
   3. Hard or soft palate
D. Clinical features
   1. Parotid gland involvement
      a. Tumor arises from secreting cells of parotid gland
      b. Parotid gland is most frequent site of mixed tumors
      c. Single nodular mass with sharp borders; firm and hard to palpation
      d. Slow growing over months or years
      e. Firm painless swelling
   2. Palatal involvement
      a. Located on either side of the midline
      b. Fleshy growth similar to a fibroma
      c. Ulceration; cystic variety
      d. Intraosseous (moves bone and teeth)
E. Histologic characteristics
   1. Benign, but some are locally invasive (salivary glands)
   2. Epithelial origin
F. Treatment/prognosis
   1. Surgical excision
   2. Recurrence rate—35%
   3. Twenty-five percent can transform into a malignancy if the mixed tumor is not treated

Cystic Diseases

General Characteristics

A. True cyst is
   1. Abnormal sac or space found in hard or soft tissue
   2. Lined by epithelium and enclosed within a capsule of connective tissue
   3. Space often filled with fluid or fragments of tissues
B. Cysts are classified according to
   1. Size
   2. Location
   3. Etiology
   4. Histologic components

Radicular Cyst (Root-End Cyst, Periapical Cyst)

A. Etiology
   1. Caries
   2. Trauma
   3. Deep restoration causing pulpitis and periapical inflammation
   4. Develops from a preexisting periapical granuloma
B. Age and gender affected—any age; but more common from 30 to 60 years; more commonly observed in males
C. Location—apex of the tooth; more often maxilla
D. Clinical features
   1. Nonvital tooth
   2. Small and asymptomatic
E. Radiographic appearance—round or ovoid, well-defined radiolucent area 1 to 2 cm in size
F. Histologic characteristics—lined by stratified squamous epithelium; well-vascularized connective tissue
G. Treatment
   1. Extraction of the tooth
   2. Surgical procedure for removal of the cyst sac

Residual Cyst

A. Etiology
   1. Radicular cyst not removed after extraction of a tooth
   2. Open socket with debris acting as a stimulus
B. Age and gender affected—any age; males and females equally affected
C. Location
   1. Apices of teeth
   2. Near the alveolar ridge in edentulous mouths
D. Clinical features—small and asymptomatic
E. Radiographic appearance—well-defined radiolucent area
F. Histologic characteristics—stratified squamous epithelium lining a space or lumen
G. Treatment—removal of the cyst

Lateral Periodontal Cyst

A. Etiology—theories include
   1. Resulted from a dentigerous cyst
   2. Remnants of dental lamina
   3. Trauma
B. Age and gender affected—adults; more common in males
C. Location—between roots of mandibular canine or premolar teeth
D. Clinical features
   1. Teeth are vital
   2. Asymptomatic, no bulge
E. Radiographic appearance—small (1 cm), well-defined ovoid or elliptic radiolucent area found between teeth
F. Histologic characteristics—cystic sac composed of stratified squamous epithelial lining and a connective tissue wall
G. Treatment—surgical removal without extraction of the surrounding teeth

Developmental Cysts

A. Etiology
 1. Median mandibular cyst—develops from an area of mesenchyme elements during the growth process or type of odontogenic cyst, possibly a primordial cyst
 2. Globulomaxillary cyst—arises from odontogenic epithelium between the maxillary lateral incisor and canine
 3. Nasolabial cyst—develops from the inferior and anterior segments of the nasolacrimal duct; can occur bilaterally, thus supporting this theory of development
 4. Median alveolar cyst—represents an odontogenic cyst
 5. Nasopalatine canal cyst—presents with various types of epithelial tissue
B. Age and gender affected—adults; males and females equally affected
C. Location—names are based on location
 1. Median mandibular cyst
 2. Globulomaxillary cyst (used only as a clinical term)
 3. Nasolabial cyst
 4. Median alveolar cyst
 5. Nasopalatine canal cyst
D. Clinical features
 1. Vary in size from no evidence of a lesion to a bulge or expansion of bone
 2. All teeth vital
E. Radiographic appearance—well-defined radiolucent area
 1. Globulomaxillary cyst located between a maxillary lateral incisor and canine often is pear shaped
 2. Nasopalatine canal (incisal canal) cyst is heart shaped
F. Histologic characteristics
 1. Median mandibular cyst in the midline of the mandible has been reported as having mucous cells and ciliated epithelium
 2. Fissural cysts of the maxilla have glandular tissue or mucous glands involved
G. Treatment/prognosis
 1. Enucleation of the cystic sac and curettage of surrounding bone
 2. Prognosis excellent

Primordial Cyst

A. Etiology—neoplastic; arises from epithelium of the enamel organ or from primordial epithelium
B. Age and gender affected—under 25 years; males and females equally affected
C. Location—mandibular third molar space or posterior to an erupted mandibular third molar

D. Clinical features
 1. Tooth never present in the space occupied by the cyst
 2. Size varies from small to quite large
E. Radiographic appearance—radiolucent, well-defined oval lesion; can be multilocular
F. Histologic characteristics
 1. Four to eight cells of stratified squamous epithelium
 2. No rete pegs
 3. Parallel bundles of collagen fibers
G. Treatment/prognosis
 1. Surgical removal of bone in the area by curettage
 2. Can develop into an ameloblastoma

Dentigerous Cyst (Follicular Cyst)

A. Etiology—from reduced enamel epithelium after the crown of the tooth is completely formed (unerupted or impacted tooth); accumulation of fluid between the crown and reduced enamel epithelium; cyst *must* be associated with a tooth
B. Age and gender affected—>25 years; males and females equally affected
C. Location
 1. Mandibular third molar area—often extending to and destroying the ramus
 2. Maxillary canine region—compromising the maxillary sinus
 3. These areas also have a higher incidence of impactions
D. Clinical features
 1. Always associated with the crown of an imbedded or unerupted tooth
 2. Aggressive lesion causing expansion of bone and extreme displacement of teeth
 3. Painful
E. Radiographic appearance—smooth, unilocular radiolucency, larger than 4 mm, extending from the crown to the reduced enamel epithelium
F. Histologic characteristics—stratified squamous epithelium lining the lumen; surrounded by a thin connective tissue wall; epithelial lining is not keratinized
G. Treatment—enucleation of the cystic sac and associated tooth

Peripheral or Soft Tissue Cysts
Ranula

A. Etiology
 1. Blockage or obstruction by a salivary stone (sialolith) in the duct of a major salivary gland (sublingual or submandibular)
 2. Trauma
B. Age and gender affected—any age; males and females equally affected

C. Location—floor of the mouth, under the tongue

D. Clinical features

   1. Translucent, bluish, round, smooth-surfaced bulge 1 to 3 cm in diameter
   2. Semifirm; unilateral
   3. Increases in size between meals; decreases immediately after a meal

E. Radiographic appearance—radiopaque calculi in the duct area

F. Histologic characteristics—epithelium lining is present

G. Treatment/prognosis

   1. Surgical excision
   2. Can recur

Mucocele

A. Etiology

   1. Obstruction of a minor salivary gland duct
   2. Trauma to the salivary duct by lip biting or pinching

B. Age and gender affected—under 30 years; males and females equally affected

C. Location—most common on the lower lip; can occur on the palate, buccal mucosa, or tongue

D. Clinical features

   1. Blisterlike raised, circumscribed vesicle; pinhead to 1 cm in size
   2. Translucent and bluish
   3. Firm, movable to palpation
   4. Straw-colored fluid can be aspirated

E. Histologic characteristics

   1. Cavity rarely lined by a thin layer of epithelium; therefore, not a true cyst
   2. Wall composed of fibrous connective tissue lining and fibroblasts
   3. Numerous polymorphonuclear leukocytes present
   4. Lumen filled with many leukocytes and mononuclear phagocytes

F. Treatment/prognosis

   1. Excision of the lesion and associated gland
   2. Recurrence is possible

Soft Tissue Development Cysts

Thyroglossal Duct Cyst

A. Etiology—developmental, in the thyroglossal tract, which extends from the foramen cecum to the permanent position of the thyroid gland in the neck region; the embryonic thyroglossal tract; caused by a draining infection or trauma to lymphoid tissues

B. Age and gender affected—usually young adults, but can occur at any age; more common in females

C. Location—posterior; 75% of these lesions are below the hyoid bone

D. Clinical features

   1. Asymptomatic
   2. Firm, cystic mass; round or oval shape; few millimeters to several centimeters in size
   3. As swelling develops slowly, a fistula may form
   4. Swallowing becomes difficult (dysphagia)
   5. Inability to extend the tongue

E. Histologic characteristics

   1. Lining of stratified squamous epithelium or other types of epithelial tissue
   2. Connective tissue wall may contain lymphoid or thyroid tissue and mucous glands

F. Treatment—complete surgical excision after a thyroid scan

Lymphoepithelial Cyst, Branchial Cleft Cyst (Lateral Cervical Cyst)

A. Etiology—theories include

   1. Epithelial remnants of embryonic branchial arches
   2. Epithelium entrapped in lymph nodes in the branchial arch region
   3. Not related to the branchial arches

B. Age and gender affected—children and young adults; males and females equally affected

C. Location

   1. Lateral aspect of the second branchial arch; lateral aspect of the upper neck
   2. Usually close to the anterior border of the sternocleidomastoid muscle
   3. Area from the clavicle to the parotid gland

D. Clinical features

   1. Slow growing; asymptomatic
   2. Circumscribed, movable mass

E. Histologic characteristics

   1. Lined by stratified squamous epithelium; lymphoid tissue in the wall
   2. May contain pseudostratified columnar epithelium

F. Treatment—surgical removal

Epidermoid Cyst

A. Etiology

   1. From epithelial cells entrapped in closure lines of soft tissue during fetal development
   2. Trauma

B. Age and gender affected—young persons; males and females equally affected

C. Location

   1. Floor of the mouth above the geniohyoid muscle
   2. Mucobuccal folds
   3. Geniohyoid muscle

D. Clinical features—round, well-defined, semifirm palpable mass

E. Histologic characteristics—stratified squamous epithelium lining with a fibrous tissue wall

F. Treatment—remove surgically

Dermoid Cyst

A. Etiology—disorder of development from epithelial cells entrapped in closure lines of soft tissue during fetal life

B. Age and gender affected—young adults (depends on the stage); males and females equally affected

C. Location—anterior floor of the mouth; submaxillary or sublingual area

D. Clinical features
1. Semifirm to hard (depending on contents)
2. Two or more centimeters in diameter
3. Fistula may form for drainage

E. Histologic characteristics
1. Stratified squamous epithelial lining with a fibrous connective tissue wall
2. May contain sebaceous glands, hair follicles, sweat glands, and occasionally teeth

F. Treatment—surgical removal

Bone Cysts

Aneurysmal Bone Cyst

A. Etiology—reactive cyst, but theories include
1. Arterial venous shunt—caused by a benign fibroosseous lesion in the area, altering blood vessels; this theory is most widely believed and accepted
2. Trauma—trauma ruptures a blood vessel, with blood accumulating outside of the wall; resorbs bone

B. Age and gender affected—under 20 years; males and females equally affected

C. Location
1. Over 50% occur in the long bones or vertebral column
2. When occurrence is in the jaws, the mandible is the more common site (2:1)

D. Clinical features
1. May be asymptomatic or a slight to moderate well-defined bulge
2. Tenderness, pain on motion; may limit movement

E. Radiographic appearance—hazy, gray radiolucent area; appears cystic, with a "soap bubble" effect; multilocular pattern can be present

F. Histologic characteristics
1. No epithelial lining—a "pseudocyst"
2. Walls of fibrous connective tissue
3. Many cavernous or sinusoidal spaces filled with blood
4. Young fibroblasts line the sinusoids in the connective tissue stroma

5. Multinucleated giant cells—similar to those of a giant cell granuloma

G. Treatment/prognosis
1. Surgical exploration—on entering, if excessive bleeding is encountered, surgical enucleation and thorough curettage
2. Radical surgery
3. Low-radiation therapy—least preferred because of the possibility of a radiation sarcoma developing
4. Cryotherapy
5. Follow-up therapy and examination are required

Simple Bone Cyst (Traumatic Bone Cyst, Idiopathic Bone)

A. Etiology—theories include
1. Intramedullary hemorrhage following trauma; altered bone prevents fibroblasts and/or endothelial cells from entering the hemorrhage; clot does not form; blood never organizes, leaving a void within the bone
2. Necrotizing infection
3. Degeneration of a benign tumor
4. Bone did not develop in the area

B. Age and gender affected—around 18 years (75% in the second decade); males and females equally affected

C. Location—if found in the jaws it is more common in the mandible, but it is most common in the humerus and long bones

D. Clinical features—asymptomatic (discovered through radiographic examination)

E. Radiographic appearance—radiolucent area 1 to 7 cm in diameter; round, oval, elliptic, multilocular; projections extend between roots of teeth; lamina dura appears intact

F. Histologic characteristics
1. Thin connective tissue membrane lining the cavity; no epithelial lining (not a true cyst)
2. Center is a void

G. Treatment/prognosis
1. Surgical intervention to establish bleeding/clot
2. Lesion heals within a year

Static Bone Cyst (Lingual Mandibular Bone Concavity, Stafne's Bone Cyst)

A. Etiology—developmental; salivary gland extends laterally into the mandible

B. Age and gender affected—young persons; slightly more common in males

C. Location—angle of the mandible below the inferior alveolar canal; anterior mandible

D. Clinical features—asymptomatic; occasionally bilateral
E. Radiographic appearance—sharp, well-defined ovoid radiolucency 1 to 3 cm in diameter, anterior to angle of the mandible
F. Histologic characteristics—lymphoid, fat, submaxillary salivary gland tissues; striated muscle (not a true cyst)
G. Treatment/prognosis
   1. Surgical intervention to determine contents; once diagnosed, leave alone
   2. Prognosis excellent; no complications

Blood Dyscrasias

General Characteristics

A. Disease with numerous variations
B. Important to know normal blood levels and chemistries in order to make differential diagnosis
C. Anemias (most common type of blood dyscrasia) are categorized according to etiology
   1. Blood loss
   2. Excessive destruction of red blood cells because of a congenital or hemolytic condition
   3. Decrease in production of red blood cells
   4. Associated with congenital diseases

Sickle Cell Anemia

A. Etiology—hereditary; hemolytic
B. Age and gender affected—before 30 years; more common in females; predominantly affects blacks (1 in 600)
C. Clinical features—systemic symptoms
   1. Weakness, easily fatigued; pallor of tissues
   2. Shortness of breath; nausea, vomiting
   3. Pain in joints
D. Radiographic appearance
   1. Perpendicular trabeculations radiating outward, giving a "hair-on-end" appearance to the skull
   2. Decrease in number of trabeculae in the jaws, with large marrow spaces
   3. Lamina dura not affected
E. Laboratory tests/findings
   1. Red blood cell count reduced to $1,000,000/mm^3$ (normal—$4,000,000$ to $6,000,000/mm^3$)
   2. Decrease in the hemoglobin level (normal—males, 13.5 to 18 g/dl; females, 12 to 16 g/dl)
F. Histologic characteristics
   1. Crescent-shaped erythrocytes caused by hemoglobin S or binucleation
   2. Atypical chromatin distribution
G. Treatment/prognosis

1. Transfusions of whole blood
2. Prognosis unpredictable; many fatalities

Erythroblastosis Fetalis (Rh Anemia)

A. Etiology
   1. Congenital
   2. Antibody of the mother's Rh factor reacts against the fetal Rh factor, causing destruction of fetal blood
B. Age and gender affected—newborn (firstborn usually is not affected; chances increase with each birth); Rh factor more common in females
C. Clinical features
   1. Systemic symptoms
      a. Infants stillborn
      b. Those that live have anemia and jaundice
D. Oral symptoms
   1. Only primary teeth are affected
   2. Primary teeth have an endogenous stain that has a green, brown, or blue hue in enamel because of red blood cell hemolysis and bilirubin
   3. Enamel hypoplasia
E. Laboratory tests/findings
   1. Red blood cell count—$1,000,000/mm^3$ to normal
   2. Large number of nucleated red blood cells in circulating blood
   3. Icterus (jaundice) index may reach 100 units (normal—4 to 6 units)
   4. Positive direct Coombs test
F. Treatment/prognosis
   1. No treatment necessary for teeth because primary
   2. If undetected, infants may be stillborn

Pernicious Anemia (Primary Anemia, Addison's Anemia, Biermer's Anemia)

A. Etiology
   1. An autoimmune response
   2. Deficiency of extrinsic factor necessary for absorption of B_{12}
   3. Affects DNA synthesis
B. Age and gender affected—rarely before 30 years (increases with advancing age; in the United States, more common in males; in Scandinavia, common in females)
C. Clinical features
   1. Systemic symptoms
      a. General weakness, dizziness, pallor, anemia
      b. Numbness or tingling of extremities
      c. Gastrointestinal manifestations—nausea, vomiting, diarrhea; abdominal pain
      d. Loss of appetite and weight
      e. Shortness of breath
   2. Oral symptoms

a. Sore, painful, "beefy-red" tongue (glossitis)
   (1) Shallow ulcers
   (2) Atrophy of papillae ("bald tongue," Hunter's glossitis, Moeller's glossitis)
   (3) Distorted taste
   (4) Pallor of the oral mucosa
D. Laboratory tests/findings
   1. Red blood cell count—1,000,000/mm^3
   2. Irregularly shaped red blood cells (fewer but larger cells)
   3. Decrease in leukocytes
   4. Achlorhydria—lack of gastric hydrochloric acid secretion
E. Histologic characteristics
   1. Buccal scrapings show enlarged, irregularly shaped nuclei
   2. Variation in size of erythrocytes
F. Treatment/prognosis
   1. Vitamin B$_{12}$ (5 µg/day)
   2. Increased dietary intake of folic acid (leafy green vegetables, organ meats, wheat cereals)
   3. Five to ten percent of persons with pernicious anemia develop gastric carcinoma

Plummer-Vinson Syndrome (Iron Deficiency Anemia)

A. Etiology—iron deficiency caused by
   1. Chronic blood loss (e.g., profuse menstruation)
   2. Inadequate dietary intake
   3. Faulty iron absorption
   4. Increased iron requirements (e.g., infancy, pregnancy)
B. Age and gender affected—40 to 50 years; more common in females (5% to 30% female incidence in United States)
C. Clinical features
   1. Systemic symptoms
      a. Lemon-tinted skin; pallor
      b. Difficulty in swallowing (dysphagia)
      c. Brittle fingernails
      d. Enlarged spleen (splenomegaly) (20% to 30% of cases)
      e. Absence of free hydrochloric acid in the stomach
      f. Predisposition to the development of oral cancer
   2. Oral symptoms
      a. Cheilosis; pallor of oral tissues
      b. Smooth, red, painful tongue with atrophy of filiform and fungiform papillae
D. Histologic characteristics
   1. Altered exfoliated squamous epithelial cells of the tongue and soft tissues
   2. Deficiency of keratinized cells
   3. Abnormal cell maturation; enlarged nuclei

E. Laboratory findings
   1. Reduced hematocrit
   2. Reduced hemoglobin
   3. Low serum iron
F. Treatment
   1. Iron, vitamin B complex therapy
   2. High-protein diet

Aplastic Anemia

Primary Aplastic Anemia

A. Etiology—unknown
B. Age and gender affected—young adults; males and females equally affected
C. Clinical features—oral symptoms
   1. Spontaneous bleeding
   2. Petechiae
   3. Purpuric spots
   4. Gingival infection
   5. Pallor of oral tissues
D. Laboratory tests/findings
   1. Reduction in the number of all blood cells (pancytopenia)
   2. Reduction in the number of red blood cells (anemia)
   3. Reduction in the number of white blood cells (leukopenia)
   4. Reduction in the number of platelets (thrombocytopenia)
   5. Bone marrow changes
E. Treatment/prognosis
   1. Blood transfusions
   2. Antibiotics
   3. Rapid destruction; usually fatal

Secondary Aplastic Anemia

A. Etiology
   1. Exposure to a drug or chemical substance
   2. Exposure to radiant energy—x-rays, radium, or radioactive isotopes
B. Age and gender affected—any age; males and females equally affected
C. Clinical features—same as in primary aplastic anemia
D. Treatment/prognosis
   1. Remove cause
   2. Support therapy
   3. Prognosis good

Thalassemia (Cooley's Anemia, Erythroblastic Anemia, Mediterranean Disease)

A. Etiology—hereditary and ethnic
   1. Defect in the component controlling the rate of synthesis of adult hemoglobin
   2. Transmitted by autosomal recessive trait

3. Ethnic predilection—Mediterranean countries
B. Age and gender affected—within the first 2 years (homozygous); later in childhood, mild form (heterozygous); males and females equally affected
C. Clinical features
   1. Systemic symptoms
      a. Yellow pallor of the skin
      b. Enlarged spleen (splenomegaly); enlarged liver (hepatomegaly)
      c. Mongoloid facial features
         (1) Sunken nose bridge
         (2) Protruding zygoma
         (3) Slanting eyes
   2. Oral symptoms
      a. Malocclusion; protrusion of the maxillary anterior teeth
      b. Pallor of the mucosa
D. Radiographic appearance
   1. Peculiar trabecular pattern of the maxilla and mandible—"salt-and-pepper" effect
   2. Mild osteoporosis of the jaws
   3. Thinning of lamina dura
E. Laboratory tests/findings
   1. Elevated white blood cell count—10,000 to 25,000/mm^3
   2. Elevated serum bilirubin level
   3. Decreased hemoglobin level
F. Histologic characteristics—bone marrow shows cellular hyperplasia
G. Treatment/prognosis
   1. Splenectomy and periodic blood transfusions provide temporary remissions
   2. Prognosis poor

Polycythemia

General Characteristics

A. Abnormal increase in the number of red blood cells
B. Increased hemoglobin level
C. Three forms
   1. Relative polycythemia—temporary increase in the number of red blood cells; caused by shock, a severe burn, or excessive loss of body fluids
   2. Primary polycythemia
   3. Secondary polycythemia

Primary Polycythemia (Polycythemia Vera, Erythremia, Osler-Vasquez Disease)

A. Etiology—unknown; possibly familial; neoplastic proliferation of bone marrow stem cells
B. Age and gender affected—over 40 years; more common in males
C. Clinical features
   1. Systemic symptoms
      a. Headache, dizziness, weakness
      b. Enlarged, painful spleen
      c. Gastric complaints; peptic ulcers
      d. Tips of fingers cyanotic
      e. Nose bleeds easily (epistaxis)
   2. Oral symptoms
      a. Oral mucosa deep red to purple because of the decreased hemoglobin level
      b. Gingivae swollen and spongy; bleed easily
      c. Submucosal petechiae; ecchymosis
D. Laboratory tests/findings
   1. Red blood cell count elevated to 10,000,000 to 12,000,000/mm^3 (significant increase)
   2. Increase in
      a. Hemoglobin content
      b. Blood viscosity
      c. Platelet and white blood cell counts
      d. Hematocrit value
E. Treatment/prognosis
   1. Nonspecific treatment; phenylhydrazine to destroy or interfere with production of red blood cells
   2. Radioactive isotope phosphorus
   3. Therapy provides only temporary remissions

Secondary Polycythemia

A. Etiology—increase in number of erythrocytes
   1. Bone marrow anoxia (lack of oxygen) caused by
      a. Pulmonary dysfunction
      b. Heart disease
      c. High altitudes
      d. Carbon monoxide poisoning
   2. Stimulatory factors such as drugs or chemicals
B. Other characteristics and features similar to those of primary polycythemia

Agranulocytosis

A. Etiology
   1. Primary form—unknown
   2. Secondary form—drug ingestion or allergic reaction; toxic effect of drugs
B. Age and gender affected—any age; more common in adults; more common in females
C. Clinical features
   1. Systemic symptoms
      a. Sudden onset
      b. High fever, chills, sore throat
      c. Malaise, weakness
      d. Skin is jaundiced
   2. Oral symptoms
      a. Infection in the oral cavity
      b. Regional lymphadenitis
      c. Ulcerations of the tonsils, pharynx, palate, and gingiva

d. Hemorrhage occurs, especially from the gingiva (ulcerations of pharynx are referred to as agranulocytosis angina)

e. Excessive salivation

D. Laboratory tests/findings—severe decrease in or absence of granulocytes or polymorphonuclear cells; bone marrow has few or no granulocytes

E. Histologic characteristics

1. Necrosis of the gingiva, sulcus, free gingiva, periodontal ligament, alveolar bone

2. Rapid destruction of supporting structures of teeth

F. Treatment

1. All dental surgical procedures should be avoided

2. Removal of the causative drug or agent

3. Antibiotics

4. Transfusions

Cyclic Neutropenia

A. Etiology—inherited; autosomal dominant

B. Age and gender affected—infants and young children; males and females equally affected

C. Clinical features

1. Systemic symptoms

a. General weakness

b. Fever, sore throat, headache

c. Regional lymphadenopathy

2. Oral symptoms

a. Severe gingivitis, stomatitis, periodontitis

b. Ulcerations

c. Mild to severe loss of alveolar bone

D. Laboratory tests/findings

1. Periodic depression of granulocytes

2. Neutrophils may completely disappear in the acute stage

3. Cycles occur in intervals of 21 to 27 days

E. Treatment/prognosis

1. Nonspecific

2. Splenectomy sometimes beneficial

3. Remission periods

4. Premedication with antibiotics before dental hygiene or surgical procedures

Leukemia

General Characteristics

A. Malignant neoplastic disorder involving blood-forming cells

B. Excessive proliferation of white blood cells in the immature state

C. Etiology—unknown; theories include

1. Infections

2. Virus

3. Chronic exposure to chemicals or radiation

4. Persons with Down syndrome have a high incidence

5. Chromosome abnormalities present

Acute Leukemia

A. Age and gender affected—children and young adults; males and females equally affected

B. Clinical features

1. Systemic symptoms

a. Sudden onset

b. Weakness, fever, headache, infection

c. Swelling of lymph nodes—often the first sign

d. Hemorrhages on the skin and mucous membranes—caused by a decrease in the number of platelets

e. Enlargement of organs—spleen, liver, kidney

f. Bone and joint pain

2. Oral symptoms

a. Purpuric spots

b. Severe gingival enlargement; red, soft, spongy; spontaneous bleeding

c. Sometimes similar to Vincent's infection—ulcerations, blunted papillae, necrosis, odor

d. Pallor of tissues

e. Toothache caused by invasion and necrosis of the pulp

f. Mobility of teeth caused by a breakdown of the periodontal membrane and supporting structures

C. Laboratory tests/findings

1. Both anemia and thrombocytopenia present

2. Prolonged bleeding and coagulation times

3. White blood cell count elevated to $100,000/mm^3$

D. Treatment/prognosis

1. Transfusions

2. Antibiotics

3. Corticosteroids and antimetabolites provide periods of remission

Chronic Leukemia

A. Age and gender affected—middle age or older; males and females equally affected

B. Clinical features

1. Systemic symptoms

a. Very slow onset—disease may be present for weeks or months before symptoms lead to diagnosis

b. Pallor

c. Lymph node enlargement and enlarged spleen in the chronic lymphatic type; not in the myeloid type

d. Xerostomia (dry mouth)

e. Petechiae on the skin with nodules of leukemic cells

f. Destructive bone lesions—result in fracture

2. Oral symptoms
   a. Gingival tissues may be normal for some time, then become tender and enlarged
   b. Pallor of the gingiva and lips
   c. Purpuric spots
   d. Enlarged lymph nodes

C. Laboratory tests/findings
   1. Anemia and thrombocytopenia sometimes present
   2. White blood cell count—500,000/mm^3 (95% of the total number of blood cells)
   3. Shift to the left in maturity of the cells
   4. Differential count elevated in the cell type involved

D. Treatment/prognosis
   1. Radiation therapy to the marrow, spleen, and lymph nodes
   2. Chemotherapy
   3. Remissions occur
   4. Untreated, fatal in 2 to 3 years; if treated, fatal in 5 to 7 years

Purpura

General Characteristics

A. Purplish discoloration of the skin and mucous membranes resulting from spontaneous escape of blood into tissues

B. Caused by
   1. Defect or deficiency in blood platelets (thrombocytopenic purpura)
   2. Unexplained increase in capillary fragility (vascular or nonthrombocytopenic purpura)

Thrombocytopenic Purpura (Werlhof's Disease)

A. Etiology
   1. Primary—unknown; autoimmune mechanism in which the person is immunized against his or her own platelets; also called immune thrombocytopenic purpura
   2. Secondary—caused by a variety of conditions, including
      a. Drug toxicity
      b. Allergic reactions
      c. Infectious diseases
      d. Malignant neoplasms

B. Age and gender affected—primary in childhood; secondary at any age; males and females equally affected

C. Clinical features
   1. Systemic symptoms
      a. Spontaneous hemorrhagic lesions on the skin; vary in size (petechiae, ecchymoses, hematomas)
      b. Patient bruises easily
      c. Bleeding via the urinary tract
      d. Bleeding from the nose (epistaxis)
      e. Spleen not palpable
   2. Oral symptoms
      a. Profuse gingival hemorrhage
      b. Clustered petechiae 1 mm or less in size

D. Laboratory tests/findings
   1. Severe reduction in the platelet count—below 60,000/mm^3 (normal—150,000 to 400,000/mm^3)
   2. Bleeding time prolonged to 1 or more hours
   3. Positive capillary fragility test

E. Treatment
   1. Corticosteroids
   2. Transfusions
   3. Bed rest
   4. For secondary form—eliminate cause; splenectomy

Vascular Purpura (Nonthrombocytopenic Purpura)

A. Etiology—results from a variety of conditions that produce capillary fragility: infectious diseases, drug history, etc.

B. Clinical features—platelet count normal; other symptoms similar to those of thrombocytopenic purpura

Hemophilia

A. Etiology
   1. Hereditary; sex linked, occurring only in males
   2. Defect carried by the X chromosome
   3. Transmitted through unaffected daughters to grandsons; sons are normal and not carriers

B. Age and gender affected—present at birth, but symptoms may not appear until later; males only (except with type C)

C. Clinical features
   1. Systemic symptoms
      a. Clotting deficiency produces persistent bleeding
      b. Massive hematomas
      c. Three forms—differ in blood-clotting factor that is deficient
         (1) Type A—most common; antihemophilic globulin (AHG) factor
         (2) Type B—plasma thromboplastin component (PTC) factor
         (3) Type C—plasma thromboplastin antecedent (PTA); less severe bleeding; not sex linked
   2. Oral symptoms
      a. Gingival hemorrhage
      b. Prolonged hemorrhage following tooth eruption, exfoliation, or extraction

D. Laboratory tests/findings
   1. Prolonged coagulation and venous clotting times
   2. Normal bleeding time and blood cell count

E. Treatment
   1. Hospitalization for transfusions of whole blood
   2. Topical coagulants

Acquired Immunodeficiency Syndrome (AIDS) (See Chapter 7, Section on Immunodeficiency)

A. Etiology—human immunodeficiency virus (HIV)
   1. Syndrome includes HIV infection, cell lymphopenia, and reduced T helper cell function
B. Age—young adults 20 to 40 years; infants of infected mothers
C. Gender/ethnic characteristics
   1. Definite predilection in males
   2. Homosexuals or bisexuals
   3. Overall increased incidence among intravenous drug users
   4. Others at risk include prostitutes, prison inmates, and children of infected mothers
D. Transmission
   1. Sexual contact
   2. Blood products
   3. Mother to newborn
   4. Cofactors (e.g., other infections) may influence transmission
E. Clinical—oral
   1. At the earliest stage of the disease the oral findings are subtle
   2. Oral candidiasis occurs in more than 85% of cases
   3. History of herpes simplex; herpes zoster
   4. Acute necrotizing ulcerative gingivitis; linear gingival erythema; necrotizing ulcerative periodontitis
   5. Petechiae on attached gingiva
   6. Sudden onset of inflammation
   7. A creamy white patch covering a raw red base as seen in pemphigus
   8. Distinct odor
   9. Hairy leukoplakia
F. Clinical—general
   1. Opportunistic infections—*Candida,* cytomegalovirus, herpes simplex viruses 1 and 2, pneumocystic pneumonia
   2. Susceptible to forms of cancer—squamous cell, Kaposi's sarcoma, and non-Hodgkin lymphoma
   3. Constitutional signs including sudden, unexplained weight loss, lymphadenopathy involving cervical and submandibular nodes
   4. Health history—past and present history of long-term illness, slow healing, vital signs (fever is especially significant), and the patient profile is seen in AIDS-related complex (ARC)
   5. AIDS-related complex characteristics—HIV positive, lymphadenopathy, fatigue, diarrhea, fever, GI involvement, weight loss; oral lesions are usually manifested last
G. Laboratory—serologic testing for HIV infection
H. Histologic findings—can be extremely variable, depending on the pathologic conditions involved
I. Treatment—symptomatic
J. Prognosis—poor

Fibrous Diseases (Dysplasia)

General Characteristics

A. Rare diseases affecting bones
B. Produce swelling of bones with deformities in some forms of disease
C. Variant forms—all of unknown etiology

Monostotic Fibrous Dysplasia

A. Etiology—unknown; theories include
   1. Local infection
   2. Trauma
B. Age and gender affected—children and young adults; slightly higher incidence in females
C. Location
   1. Ribs—most common site
   2. Mandible, maxilla
   3. Can affect any bone
D. Clinical features
   1. Painless swelling; enlargement of the jaw involving the buccal plate
   2. Can cause malposition, tipping, or displacement of the dentition
   3. In the maxilla lesions are not clearly outlined, because they extend into the sinus or the floor of the orbit
E. Histologic characteristics
   1. Proliferating fibroblasts in the stroma of woven collagen fibers
   2. Irregularly shaped trabeculae; some are C-shaped
F. Treatment/prognosis
   1. Surgical removal of the deformed area
   2. Radiation therapy contraindicated because malignant transformations reported
   3. Rarely fatal

Polyostotic Fibrous Dysplasia

A. Etiology—unknown
B. Age and gender affected—childhood; more common in females (3:1)
C. Location

1. Long bones; often unilateral
2. Bones of the face and skull
3. Clavicles
4. Pelvic bones

D. Clinical features
   1. Systemic symptoms
      a. Painless to slight pain; may be unnoticed
      b. Bowing of long bones
      c. Irregular, pigmented spots on the skin; "café au lait"
      d. Females may reach premature puberty at age 2 or 3 years
      e. Dysfunction of the endocrine system—pituitary, thyroid, and parathyroid glands
   2. Oral symptoms
      a. Expansion and deformity of the jaws
      b. Disturbed eruption pattern caused by endocrine dysfunction

E. Radiographic appearance—irregular bone trabeculae; expansion of cortical bone; sometimes a multilocular cystic appearance with several radiolucencies

F. Laboratory tests/findings
   1. Serum alkaline phosphatase level sometimes elevated
   2. Moderately elevated basal metabolic rate

G. Histologic characteristics
   1. Fibrillar connective tissue
   2. Many trabeculae
   3. Irregularly shaped, coarse-woven fibers
   4. Osteocytes

H. Treatment/prognosis
   1. Surgical removal of the deformity
   2. No treatment for minor involvement
   3. Known fatal cases

Albright's Syndrome

Variant and most severe form of polyostotic fibrous dysplasia

A. Etiology—unknown
B. Age and gender affected—young persons; males and females equally affected
C. Location—same as for polyostotic fibrous dysplasia
D. Clinical features and other characteristics—same as for polyostotic fibrous dysplasia

Cherubism (Familial Fibrous Disease of the Jaws)

A. Etiology—hereditary; autosomal dominant gene
B. Age and gender affected—onset at birth or early childhood; more common in males
C. Location—only in the maxilla and mandible (more common in the mandible)

D. Clinical features
   1. Bilateral enlargement of the jaws; usually posterior area involving the ramus; firm and hard to palpation
   2. Taut facial skin; downward pull of the eyelids; "cherubic" appearance
   3. Regional lymphadenopathy
   4. Has been mistaken for an ameloblastoma or multilocular cyst
   5. Primary dentition may be prematurely shed at age 3 years
   6. Permanent dentition often defective; absence of teeth (anodontia); lack of eruption of the teeth present

E. Radiographic appearance—bilateral thinning of cortical plates; numerous unerupted, displaced teeth in cystlike spaces

F. Laboratory tests/findings—all blood levels normal

G. Histologic characteristics
   1. Fibrous tissue proliferation
   2. Numerous large multinucleated giant cells in a loose, delicate, fibrous connective tissue stroma
   3. Fibroblasts; small blood vessels
   4. Epithelial remnants from developing teeth scattered throughout

H. Treatment/prognosis
   1. Self-limiting; remission at 8 to 10 years of age
   2. No surgical intervention
   3. Prognosis good; rare malignant transformation

Periapical Cemental Dysplasia

Cementoma, Cementoblastoma, Periapical Fibrous Dysplasia, Fibrocementoma

A. Etiology—unknown; theories include
   1. Chronic trauma
   2. Infection of a tooth
   3. Past history of syphilis
   4. Endocrine or hormonal imbalance

B. Age and gender affected—mid-30s; more common in females (15:1) and blacks (8:1)

C. Location
   1. Mandible; rare in the maxilla
   2. Anterior incisor region
   3. Apex of teeth; in or near the periodontal ligament

D. Clinical features
   1. Benign, slow-growing multiple lesions
   2. Asymptomatic; teeth in the affected area vital

E. Radiographic appearance—depends on the stage of development
   1. Osteolytic—radiolucent lesion
   2. Cementoblastic—lucent with some opacities

3. Mature—cementum and/or bone densely opaque with a thin rim of lucency
F. Laboratory tests/findings—normal blood levels
G. Histologic characteristics
   1. Increase in connective tissue cells of the periodontal ligament
   2. Normal bone replaced with a fibrous mass; varying amounts of calcified material within
H. Treatment/prognosis
   1. Self-limiting; no treatment necessary
   2. Prognosis good; no complications

Paget's Disease (Osteitis Deformans, Osteitis Hyperplastica)

A. Etiology—unknown; theories include
   1. Hereditary
   2. Vascular involvement; arteriosclerosis
   3. History of syphilis; inflammatory response
   4. Endocrine imbalance
B. Age and gender affected—over 50 years; more common in males (3:1)
C. Location—bones, including the maxilla and mandible
D. Clinical features
   1. Systemic symptoms
      a. Symptoms develop slowly
      b. Enlargement of bones—spine, femur, tibia, skull (change in hat size)
      c. Affected bones are warm to the touch as a result of increased vascularity
      d. Severe headache, deafness, dizziness; bone neuralgia
   2. Oral symptoms
      a. Enlarged maxilla; spread of the dentition
      b. No change in enamel or dentin
E. Radiographic appearance
   1. Irregular radiolucent and radiopaque areas, giving a cotton-wool appearance
   2. Root resorption; hypercementosis; lamina dura may be completely absent
F. Laboratory tests/findings
   1. Serum calcium and phosphorus levels are normal
   2. Serum alkaline phosphatase level is elevated; serum acid phosphatase level is normal
G. Histologic characteristics—characterized by both bone resorption and bone deposition
   1. Areas of resorption—osteoclast activity
   2. Areas of deposition—osteoblast activity
   3. Areas of both resorption and deposition—osteoclasts and osteoblasts present; give mosaic appearance
H. Treatment/prognosis
   1. No treatment

2. Fifteen percent develop into sarcomas; prognosis poor

Metabolic Bone Diseases

General Characteristics

A. Associated with metabolic disturbances, deficiencies, or excesses
B. Disease can be caused by an internal cellular change or dietary or nutritional intake

Hyperparathyroidism

A. Etiology
   1. Primary hyperparathyroidism—parathyroid gland produces an excessive quantity of parathyroid hormone
   2. Secondary hyperparathyroidism—accompanies other systemic diseases such as renal disturbances, rickets, or extensive bone tumors
B. Age and gender affected—middle age; more common in females (3:1)
C. Clinical features
   1. Systemic symptoms
      a. Rare disease with bone pain, joint stiffness, and resorption of bone with spontaneous fractures
      b. Urinary tract stones caused by increased calcium in urine
      c. Weakness, fatigue, constipation
   2. Oral symptoms
      a. Resembles a giant cell tumor or cyst
      b. Diffuse bone loss causing malocclusion and shifting of teeth
D. Radiographic appearance
   1. Cystlike radiolucencies found posteriorly in the jaws; "ground glass" appearance
   2. Lamina dura lost or sketchy
E. Laboratory tests/findings
   1. Loss of calcium replaced by fibrous tissue
   2. Serum calcium level elevated above normal
F. Histologic characteristics
   1. Osteoclastic resorption of trabeculae of spongiosa bone
   2. Fibrosis of marrow spaces
   3. Fibroblasts replace resorbed bone
G. Treatment—surgical excision of the parathyroid gland

Osteoporosis

A. Etiology
   1. Calcium or hormone (estrogen) deficiencies over a long period of time

2. Factors producing deficiency
   a. Congenital
   b. Vitamin C deficiency; general malnutrition
   c. Senility
B. Age and gender affected—elderly; most common in postmenopausal females
C. Clinical features—systemic symptoms
   1. Lower back pain
   2. Pathologic fractures
   3. Loss of stature; deformities
D. Radiographic appearance—localized or diffuse radiolucencies
E. Laboratory tests/findings—serum calcium, phosphorus, and alkaline phosphatase levels are normal
F. Histologic characteristics—resorption of bone, which increases with age
G. Treatment—estrogen therapy; calcium supplements, protein, vitamin D, and fluoride

Osteomalacia

A. Etiology
   1. Deficiency or impaired absorption of vitamin D ($CaPO_4$) (produces osteomalacia in adults; rickets in children)
   2. Urinary loss of calcium and phosphorus
   3. Fanconi syndrome—group of diseases related to renal tubular function
B. Age affected—adults
C. Clinical features
   1. Loss of calcification of bone; soft bone
      a. Generalized weakness
      b. Bone pain and tenderness; fractures
      c. Affects gait
   2. Polyuria—urine output greatly increased
   3. Polydipsia—severe thirst
   4. No oral symptoms
D. Radiographic appearance
   1. Generalized demineralization of bone; Milkman's syndrome
   2. Lamina dura of teeth may be absent
   3. Radiopaque renal calculi in the kidney
E. Laboratory tests/findings
   1. Low serum calcium and phosphorus levels
   2. Serum alkaline phosphatase level elevated
F. Treatment
   1. Increased dosage of vitamin D; if malabsorption, water-soluble, synthetic vitamin D can be given
   2. Calcium supplements

Rickets

A. Etiology
   1. Deficiency of vitamin D, phosphorus, and calcium

2. Form of osteomalacia; failure of calcification of cartilage and bone
B. Age affected—young children
C. Clinical features
   1. Systemic symptoms
      a. Pliable bones; bowlegs, knock-knees
      b. Muscle pain
      c. Enlarged skull, spinal curvature
      d. Enlarged liver and spleen
   2. Oral symptoms
      a. Retardation of tooth eruption
      b. Malposition of teeth
      c. Retardation of growth of the mandible; class II malocclusion
D. Treatment—increased dietary intake of vitamin D, calcium, and phosphorus; supplements

Histiocytosis X (Reticulosis)
General Characteristics

A. Etiology—unknown
B. Cells accumulate in granulomatous masses
C. Includes a group of three diseases characterized by proliferation of histiocytes or reticulocytes of the reticuloendothelial system

Letterer-Siwe Disease (Acute or Subacute)

A. Age affected—first 2 years of life
B. Clinical features
   1. Skin rash on the trunk, scalp, and extremities
   2. Persistent low-grade fever; malaise, irritability
   3. Splenomegaly, hepatomegaly
   4. Anemia
   5. Oral lesions—not common
   6. Most severe form of histiocytosis
C. Prognosis—invariably fatal

Hand-Schüller-Christian Disease (Chronic Disseminated)

A. Age and gender affected—early life; more common in males
B. Clinical features
   1. Systemic symptoms—classic triad
      a. Skull and jaws affected (see radiographic appearance)
      b. Diabetes insipidus—result of pituitary dysfunction
      c. Exophthalmos—bulging eyes caused by massive infiltration of reticulocytes
   2. Oral symptoms
      a. Sore mouth without lesions
      b. Halitosis, unpleasant taste
      c. Loose, sore teeth

d. Failure to heal after extractions
C. Radiographic appearance—radiolucencies in the skull and jaws
D. Treatment/prognosis
1. Curettage
2. Radiation therapy
3. Cytotoxic drugs
4. Prognosis poor; many fatalities

Eosinophilic Granuloma (Localized)

A. Age and gender affected—older children and young adults about 20 years old; more common in males (2:1)
B. Clinical features
1. Most benign variety of histiocytosis X
2. May be asymptomatic; local pain, swelling, tenderness
3. Sore mouth, fetid breath, loosening of teeth, swollen gingiva
4. Mandible more involved than maxilla
C. Radiographic appearance—irregular radiolucencies, single or multiple; well defined, resembling a cyst
D. Treatment/prognosis
1. Curettage
2. Radiation therapy
3. Prognosis good

Abnormalities of Teeth

Loss of Tooth Structure

Attrition

A. Etiology—wearing away of tooth surfaces by active, physiologic forces
1. Mastication
2. Bruxism
3. Occlusion—heavy biting forces
4. Diet—coarse foods; tobacco chewing
B. Clinical features
1. Polished facets
2. Flat incisal edge
3. Discolored surface
4. Exposed dentin

Abrasion

A. Etiology—wearing away of tooth structure through abnormal mechanical processes
1. Improper toothbrushing technique
2. Abrasive dentifrices
3. Oral habits
B. Clinical features
1. V-shaped wedge at the cervical margin; common in the cuspid and premolar areas
2. Recession of gingiva creates sensitivity

3. Pipe smoking abrades where the pipe rests
4. Notching associated with carpenters and tailors who hold tacks, nails, and pins between their teeth

Erosion (Periomylolysis)

A. Etiology—loss resulting from chemical action
1. Acid or low-pH fluid intake
2. Acidic foods habitually used over long periods of time
3. Eating disorders (bulimia; anorexia)
B. Clinical features
1. Usually found on labial or buccal surfaces; loss of enamel on maxillary anteriors lingual surface and mesial/distal surfaces may be indicative of a person with bulimia
2. "Wear" depressions or etchings on cervical or occlusal surfaces
3. Hypersensitivity of teeth affected

Dental Caries

A. Etiology
1. Primarily *Streptococcus mutans*
2. *Lactobacillus acidophilus*—produces acid that reacts with sugars
B. Age and gender affected—highest incidence before 25 years; males and females equally affected
C. Clinical features
1. Any crown surface affected—most common
a. Occlusal pits and fissures
b. Interproximal surfaces
2. Explorer sticks in a pit, groove, or accessible surface, indicating a lesion has formed
3. Mesial and distal lesions not observable clinically until large; create a grayish shadow in the area of the marginal ridge
D. Radiographic appearance—radiolucent areas in enamel; extend into dentin and then pulp as the lesion progresses
E. Laboratory tests/findings—caries activity test (Snyder)
F. Treatment—restorative dentistry: composite, amalgam, or gold

Developmental Defects Affecting Enamel and Dentin

Amelogenesis Imperfecta (Hereditary Enamel Dysplasia, Hereditary Brown Enamel, Hereditary Brown Opalescent Teeth)

A. Etiology—malfunction of the tooth germ
B. Produces two types
1. Enamel hypoplasia—defect in formation of the matrix

a. Etiology—hereditary; environmental such as nutritional deficiency, congenital syphilis, high fever, birth injuries

b. Enamel of primary and permanent teeth appear pitted; vertical grooving; deficiency in thickness (aplasia); yellow to dark brown; open contacts; occlusal wear

c. Radiographic appearance—enamel absent or very thin layer over tips of cusps and interproximal areas

d. Histologic characteristics—thin, defective enamel; few enamel prisms; no lamellae

e. Treatment—restorations; crowns; bonding

2. Enamel hypocalcification—defect in mineralization of the formed matrix

a. Etiology—autosomal trait

b. Enamel yellow to dark brown; chalky and breaks down easily

c. Radiographic appearance—tooth shape normal; enamel and dentin have same radiodensity, which makes it difficult to differentiate

d. Histologic characteristics—broadening of interprismatic substance; distinct enamel prisms; enamel low in mineral content

e. Treatment—restorations; crowns; bonding

Dentinogenesis Imperfecta (Hereditary Opalescent Dentin)

A. Etiology
1. Hereditary
2. Disturbance of dentin formation
   a. Affects mesodermal component
   b. Enamel remains normal
B. Clinical features
1. Teeth appear "opalescent," a translucent hue
2. Gray to bluish brown color
3. Distinct constriction at the cementoenamel junction
C. Radiographic appearance
1. Partial or total obliteration of pulp chambers and root canals
2. Roots are short, blunted, and sometimes fractured
3. Cementum, periodontal membrane, and alveolar bone appear normal
D. Histologic characteristics
1. Mesoderm disturbance
2. Dentin composed of irregular tubules; uncalcified matrix
3. Tubules large in width; few in number
4. Odontoblasts degenerate easily within the matrix
5. Decrease in inorganic content
E. Treatment—cast metal crowns; caution needed with partial appliances because of root fractures

Developmental Defects Affecting Tooth Shape

Dilaceration

Sharp bend or curve in the root of a formed tooth
A. Etiology—trauma during tooth development
1. Calcified area displaced
2. Amount of tooth formed at the time of trauma will affect the angle or curve of in the root; usually affects the apical third of the root
B. Radiographic appearance—bend in the root
C. Treatment—none

Fusion

Union of two normally separated tooth germs
A. Etiology—physical force or abnormal pressure; hereditary tendency
B. Clinical features
1. If the defect occurs early in development, one large tooth
2. If the defect occurs later, fusion of roots only
3. Dentin always confluent
4. Can occur in both primary and permanent dentitions
5. Can occur between two normal teeth or one normal tooth and one supernumerary tooth
C. Radiographic appearance—can have separate or fused root canals
D. Treatment—usually none; hemisection for a crown or bridge if necessary

Gemination

Division of a single tooth germ by invagination; results in incomplete formation of two teeth
A. Etiology—possibly trauma; hereditary tendency
B. Can affect primary or permanent dentition
C. Usually have two completely or incompletely separate crowns with one root; one root canal

Concrescence

Fusion that occurs after root formation completed; roots united by cementum
A. Etiology—traumatic injury; crowding of teeth with resorption of interdental bone
B. Radiographic appearance—establishes diagnosis because teeth are joined at the root surfaces and cannot be observed clinically

Dens in Dente

Tooth within a tooth
A. Etiology—increased localized external pressure; growth retardation
B. Location—maxillary lateral incisor in the area of the lingual pit
C. Often bilateral

D. Radiographic appearance—small tooth within the pulp chamber
E. Treatment—none unless the pulp becomes inflamed or necrotic

Natal Teeth

Teeth present at birth
A. Etiology
1. Develop from part of dental lamina before the deciduous bud or from bud of accessory dental lamina
2. May represent a dental lamina cyst
B. Location—usually found in the mandibular anterior incisor area
C. Histologic characteristics—hornified epithelial structures without roots (therefore not true teeth)
D. Treatment/prognosis
1. Removal (after determining they are not prematurely erupted primary teeth)
2. Prognosis excellent; no complications

Developmental Defects Affecting the Number of Teeth

Anodontia

Missing teeth
A. Etiology—no tooth germ developed
B. Two forms
1. Total anodontia
   a. Rare condition—all teeth missing
   b. May involve both primary and permanent dentitions
   c. Usually associated with hereditary ectodermal dysplasia
2. Partial anodontia
   a. Rather common
   b. Teeth usually affected include third molars and maxillary lateral incisors
   c. Familial/hereditary tendency
   d. Odontodysplasia, "ghost-teeth"
C. Treatment
1. Space maintainers during childhood
2. Crown and bridge work
3. Prosthetic appliances
4. Dental implants

Supernumerary Teeth

More than the normal number of teeth
A. Etiology—additional tooth buds arise from dental lamina; hereditary
B. Classification
1. Mesiodent (mesiodens)—most common; cone-shaped crown; short root; located between the maxillary centrals

2. Maxillary fourth molar—distal to the third molar; occasionally find a mandibular fourth molar
3. Maxillary paramolar—usually a small molar; located buccally or lingually in the area of the maxillary molars
C. Treatment—none; observe for cystic transition; remove when interfere with normal dentition

Developmental Defects Affecting Tooth Size

Macrodontia

Abnormally large tooth; rare; possibly a result of fusion

Microdontia

Abnormally small tooth; maxillary lateral incisor and third molar most commonly affected

Abnormalities of Oral Soft Tissues

Abnormalities Affecting Mucous Membranes or Skin

Amalgam Tattoo

A. Etiology—dust or particle of an amalgam restoration embedded in the mucosa or gingiva
B. Clinical features—blue to purplish area near an amalgam restoration
C. Radiographic appearance—radiopaque if amalgam particles are present
D. Treatment—none unless inflammation results

Melanin Pigmentation

Dark pigmentation of the gingiva or mucosa
A. Etiology—hereditary; dark-complexioned persons most commonly affected
B. Treatment—none because tissue is healthy

Angular Stomatitis

A. Etiology
1. Infections; *Candida albicans*
2. Nutritional deficiency
3. Denture irritation
4. Idiopathic
B. Clinical features—inflammation and cracking at the corners of the lips; extend into facial skin
C. Histologic characteristics—inflammatory cells
D. Treatment—depends on the etiology: improve the diet; correct the vertical dimension of the denture; antifungal ointment

Fordyce's Granules

A. Etiology—developmental; aberrant sebaceous glands
B. Clinical features

1. Affects the vermilion of the lips and buccal mucosa
2. Yellow, slightly raised spots a few millimeters in size
C. Location—buccal mucosa; lips
D. Histologic characteristics—glandular tissue; not pathologic
E. Treatment—none

Abnormalities Affecting the Tongue

Geographic Tongue (Benign Migratory Glossitis)

A. Etiology—unknown; theories include
   1. Nutritional deficiency
   2. Hereditary
   3. Psychogenic origin
B. Age and gender affected—any age, but more common in children and young adults; males and females equally affected
C. Clinical features
   1. Fungiform papillae appear as red, mushroomlike projections
   2. Condition assumes variations in shape, giving a maplike appearance
   3. Discomfort
D. Histologic characteristics—characteristic inflammatory cells; keratotic cells around the borders of the lesion
E. Treatment—none

Black Hairy Tongue

A. Etiology—irritation to filiform papillae caused by
   1. Smoking
   2. Alcohol
   3. Hydrogen peroxide
   4. Antacid liquids
B. Clinical features—brownish to black appearance on the dorsal surface of the tongue
C. Histologic characteristics—elongation of filiform papillae; characteristic inflammatory cells
D. Treatment/prognosis
   1. Brushing or scraping of the tongue
   2. Prognosis good; totally reversible

SUGGESTED READINGS

Ash MM Jr: *Kerr and Ash's oral pathology,* ed 6, Baltimore, 1992, Williams & Wilkins.

Bhaskar SN: *Synopsis of oral pathology,* ed 7, St Louis, 1986, Mosby.

Eversole LR: *Clinical outline of oral pathology,* ed 3, Baltimore, Md., 1992, Williams & Wilkins.

Friedman-Kien AE: *Color atlas of AIDS,* ed 2, Philadelphia, 1996, WB Saunders.

Ibsen OAC, Phelan JA: *Oral pathology for the dental hygienist,* ed 2, Philadelphia, 1996, WB Saunders.

Lynch MA, Brightman VJ, Greenberg MS, editors: *Burket's oral medicine,* ed 9, Philadelphia, 1994, JB Lippincott.

Pindborg JJ: *Atlas of diseases of the oral mucosa,* ed 5, Philadelphia, 1992, WB Saunders.

Regezi J, Sciubba J: *Oral pathology: Clinical pathologic correlations,* ed 2, Philadelphia, 1993, WB Saunders.

Robinson HBC, Miller AS: *Colby, Kerr and Robinson's color atlas of oral pathology,* ed 5, Philadelphia, 1990, JB Lippincott.

Rose LF, Kaye D: *Internal medicine for dentistry,* ed 2, St Louis, 1990, Mosby.

Shafer WG, Hine MK, Levy BM: *A textbook of oral pathology,* ed 4, Philadelphia, 1983, WB Saunders.

Smith RM, Turner JE, Robbins ML: *Atlas of oral pathology,* St Louis, 1981, Mosby.

Sonis ST, Fazio R, Fang L: *Principles and practice of oral medicine,* ed 2, Philadelphia, 1995, WB Saunders.

Review Questions

1 The bitewing radiographs in Fig. 6-1 indicate congenital absence of the
   A. Maxillary right first premolar and maxillary left first premolars
   B. Mandibular right first premolar and mandibular left first premolar
   C. Mandibular left first premolar and mandibular right second premolar
   D. Mandibular right second premolar and mandibular left second premolar
   E. Maxillary right second premolar and maxillary left second premolar

2 A bony, hard asymptomatic swelling found on the midline of the hard palate that appears radiopaque on a radiograph is *MOST* likely a (an)
   A. Myxoma
   B. Bone cyst
   C. Odontoma
   D. Torus palatinus
   E. Ranula

Test items 3–5 refer to Fig. 6-2

3 On the panograph, Fig. 6-2, the bilateral radiolucent areas apical to the mandibular molars and identified by *A* are
   A. Stafne's bone cysts
   B. Radicular cysts
   C. Periapical abscesses
   D. Submandibular fossae
   E. Traumatic bone cysts

4 The horizontal radiopaque structure identified by *B* in Fig. 6-2 is the
   A. Anterior coronoid process
   B. Maxillary tuberosity
   C. Mandibular condyle
   D. Hamular process
   E. Zygomatic process

5 The bilateral radiolucent areas identified by *C* in Fig. 6-2 are
A. Nasal fossae
B. Orbits
C. Frontal sinuses
D. Globulomaxillary cysts
E. Maxillary sinuses

6 Mixed tumors are *MOST* often found in which of the following locations?
A. Palate
B. Mandible
C. Buccal mucosa
D. Lymph nodes
E. Fauces

7 Which of the following cysts would create difficulty when swallowing?
A. Branchial cleft
B. Thyroglossal
C. Nasopalatine
D. Mucocele
E. Residual

8 Which disease may have oral characteristics similar to those of acute necrotizing ulcerative gingivitis (ANUG)?
A. Primary herpes
B. Mononucleosis
C. Leukemia
D. Nonthrombocytopenia
E. Secondary herpes

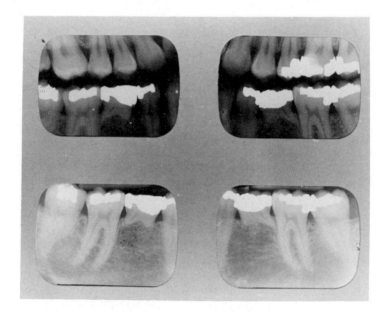

Fig. 6-1

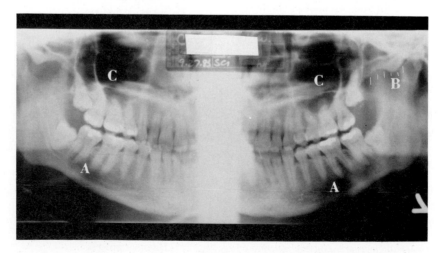

Fig. 6-2

9 A ranula is usually found in the
A. Palate
B. Inner lip
C. Buccal mucosa
D. Fauces
E. Floor of the mouth

10 Definitive dental diagnosis of oral cancer is made by a(an)
A. Complete radiographic survey
B. Panograph
C. Biopsy
D. Exfoliative cytology
E. Oral examination

11 Fig. 6-3, a periapical radiograph of the mandibular right quadrant, was taken as part of a full-mouth radiographic series. The patient was 14 years of age and asymptomatic. The periapical radiolucency indicated by the *arrow* on tooth No. 31 is *MOST* likely
A. Resorption caused by a traumatic injury
B. Periapical abscesses
C. Incomplete root formation
D. Hypercementosis
E. Stage III cementoma

12 Primordial cysts are *MOST* often found radiographically
A. In primary dentitions
B. In maxillary anterior regions
C. In the presence of supernumerary teeth
D. Posterior to erupted third molars
E. In mandibular canine and first premolar areas

13 The usual location of a true cementoma is
A. Mandibular anteriors
B. Maxillary anteriors
C. The mandibular ramus
D. Maxillary premolars
E. The midline of the hard palate

14 Which of the following is a rickettsial infection?
A. Malaria
B. Psittacosis
C. Rocky Mountain spotted fever
D. Tularemia
E. Meningitis

15 A slightly raised, noncoated, red, glossy rectangular area in the midline of the tongue has been present as long as the client can remember. It has not enlarged, changed, or caused any pain. This condition is likely
A. Geographic tongue
B. Pathologic tongue
C. Median rhomboid glossitis
D. Fissured tongue
E. Black hairy tongue

16 Which of the following provides the most conclusive diagnostic evidence in distinguishing pemphigus from pemphigoid?
A. Clinical picture
B. History of the disease
C. Biopsy and histology report
D. Race and religion
E. Age and gender of the client

17 An isolated radiopaque area in the periodontal ligament space is observed on a client's radiographs. This radiopaque structure might be a(an)
A. Epithelial rest
B. Cementum spur
C. Exostosis of alveolar bone
D. Cementicle
E. Denticle

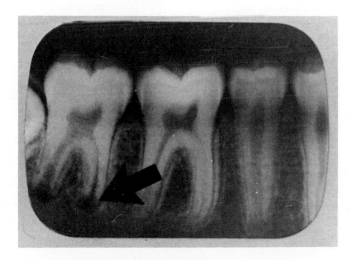

Fig. 6-3

18 A 30-year-old individual calls and complains of sudden swelling in both sides of his neck, which seems to be getting bigger. His record indicates that he has cancelled two times recently. He needs to have restorative care completed on the mandibular second molars, which have extensive decay. The client *MAY* have
   A. Actinomycosis
   B. Mumps
   C. Syphilis
   D. Ludwig's angina
   E. Pericoronitis

19 Which of the following two diseases represent different forms of infection with the same agent?
   A. Measles and German measles
   B. Chickenpox and smallpox
   C. Bacterial pneumonia and croup
   D. Shingles and chickenpox
   E. Infectious mononucleosis and cytomegalovirus (CMV)

20 While a 40-year-old woman is being seated in the dental chair, a lesion is noted on her lips. It appears as several discrete vesicles; some have ulcerated. When questioned, the woman says she always gets a sore like that before she gets a cold. The woman *MOST* likely has
   A. A chancre
   B. Perlèche
   C. An aphthous ulcer
   D. Herpes labialis
   E. Basal cell carcinoma

21 Which of the following statements *MOST* accurately describes the effect of pregnancy on the health of the mother's oral tissues?
   A. Pregnancy gingivitis is caused by hormonal changes, and nothing can be done about it
   B. Most pregnant women experience the growth of tumors in the mouth that disappear after the baby is born
   C. Hormonal changes during pregnancy result in increased gingival sensitivity to local irritants such as plaque and calculus, but pregnancy does not cause gingivitis
   D. Pregnancy results in hormonal changes, but these changes do not affect the mother's oral tissues
   E. Pregnancy results in hormonal changes that lead to decalcification of enamel

22 The hyperplasia of the gingiva shown in Fig. 6-4 was caused by a calcium channel blocker drug. The condition was *MOST* likely caused by
   A. Dilantin
   B. Vasotec
   C. Valium
   D. Prozac
   E. Procardia

23 In Fig. 6-5, the soft tissue lesion on the mandibular mucosa erupted suddenly, was filled with a clear fluid, and broke easily. The condition is *MOST* likely a
   A. Ranula
   B. Mucocele
   C. Fibroma
   D. Fistula
   E. Lipoma

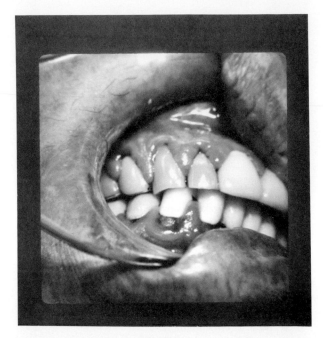

Fig. 6-4

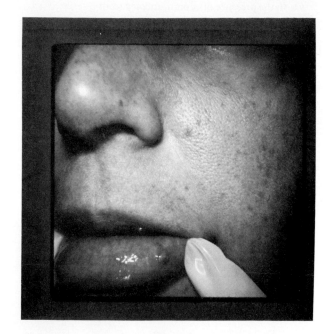

Fig. 6-5

24 Which of the following would you *NOT* be able to use the radiographic diagnostic method to detect?
   A. Dental caries
   B. Supernumerary teeth
   C. Odontoma
   D. Fibroma
   E. Cementoma

25 Which *ONE* of the diagnostic methods listed is *MOST* reliable and ensures the highest degree of accuracy?
A. Surgical
B. Differential
C. Therapeutic
D. Clinical
E. Historical

26 Which of the following does *NOT* define the term *pathogenesis*?
A. How the lesion begins
B. Behavior of the lesion
C. Clinical picture of the lesion
D. Development of the lesion
E. Evolution of the lesion

27 A pyogenic granuloma is known to *scar down* to a (an)
A. Pregnancy tumor
B. Fibrogranuloma
C. Lipoma
D. Osteoma
E. Odontoma

28 The client is a 28-year-old woman. A gingival lesion involving the interproximal papillae between teeth 7 and 8 on the labial surface is bright red, soft, and spongy; it bleeds easily, and it is caused by an irritant. The histology report shows proliferation of inflammatory cells and thin epithelium. The lesion is *MOST* likely
A. A fibroma
B. A pyogenic granuloma
C. Redundant tissue
D. A papilloma
E. Pseudopapillomatosis

29 Which one of the following cysts has the potential for developing into an ameloblastoma?
A. Lateral periodontal cyst
B. Primordial cyst
C. Stafne's bone cyst
D. Residual cyst
E. Traumatic bone cyst

30 Clinical examination reveals a possible leukoplakia. The first course of action should be to
A. Perform a biopsy
B. Perform surgical stripping
C. Give the client vitamin A therapy
D. Have the client return in 1 month to evaluate the growth
E. Perform a blood test

31 Which one of the following tests is *NOT* used for pemphigus?
A. Pels-Macht
B. Tzanck
C. Rabbit eye
D. Nikolsky's sign
E. Immunofluorescent test

32 The palatal condition of an elderly client *primarily* caused by chronic irritation from the suction chamber of a denture would be
A. A fibroma
B. A papilloma
C. Pseudopapillomatosis
D. A median palatal cyst
E. Primary aplastic anemia

33 A lesion found on the buccal mucosa of a 30-year-old white woman is pink, well defined, and soft to palpation. It has been slow growing and histologically consists of collagenous fibers, fibroblasts, and fibrocytes, but no fat cells or bone. It has a pedunculate base. The lesion is likely a
A. Fibrosarcoma
B. Fibroma
C. Fibrolipoma
D. Fibroosteoma
E. Papilloma

34 A radiolucent lesion in the posterior part of the mandible, anterior to the angle, has radiographic features of a cyst. After surgical intervention, the histology report shows submaxillary salivary gland tissue. One may conclude the lesion is likely
A. A residual cyst
B. A traumatic bone cyst
C. A Stoffer's bone cyst
D. A lingual mandibular bone concavity
E. An ameloblastoma

35 A cyst commonly found in the floor of the mouth changes size between meals. Clinically, it has a bluish hue. It may be caused by
A. A decayed tooth
B. Blockage of a major salivary duct
C. Failure of developmental fusion of the branchial arches
D. Medications that cause xerostomia
E. Chemotherapy

36 Pleuropneumonia-like organisms (PPLOs), mycoplasmas, severe systemic complications, and a triad of symptom locations (oral, eye, and genital) in a male client are specifically indicative of
A. Erythema multiforme
B. Stevens-Johnson syndrome
C. Behçet's syndrome
D. Recurrent ulcerative stomatitis (RUS)
E. Acquired immunodeficiency syndrome (AIDS)

37 For which one of the following is the etiology definitely known to be an irritant?
A. Papilloma
B. Torus
C. Granuloma
D. Lipoma
E. Polyostotic fibrous dysplasia

38 In the histology report for a granuloma the following cells are found in abundance
A. Mesenchymal cells
B. Squamous epithelial cells
C. Osteoblasts
D. Fibroblasts
E. Osteoclasts

39 There are two types of hereditary gingival fibromatosis. The one that is significant *AFTER* the eruption of permanent teeth is
A. Nodular
B. Symmetric
C. Chemical
D. Epithelial
E. Skeletal

40 An intraoral examination shows a clinical picture of punched-out papillae. The client complains of pain and a bad taste. The history indicates that the client's diet is poor and that he has been under stress. The course of action would be to
A. Do a culture and laboratory study
B. Apply a therapeutic course and debride the mouth, do a light curettage, recommend hydrogen peroxide mouth rinse, and systemic antibiotics
C. Immediately refer the client to a periodontist
D. Do a complete periodontal debridement including extensive root planing and extrinsic stain removal
E. Send client for a complete blood cell count

41 The histology reports for clinical leukoplakia could show any of the following *EXCEPT*
A. Dyskeratosis
B. Acanthosis
C. Large nuclei
D. Some necrosis
E. Osteoclasts

42 Which one of the following is *MOST* important to the pathologist when a chondroma is in question?
A. A complete personal history of the client
B. Complete removal of the tumor in question
C. Submission of a large-enough sample of tissue for histologic study because a chondroma resembles a malignant chondrosarcoma
D. Radiographs of all large bones
E. Employment of radiation and chemotherapy

43 The clinical picture of this lesion is a well-defined yellowish blisterlike eruption. It is a rare, benign neoplasm. The histology report shows a predominance of fat cells. It is likely that the lesion is a (an)
A. Papilloma
B. Osteoma
C. Lipoma
D. Fibroma
E. Myxoma

44 A tooth involved with a cyst is discovered to be nonvital on pulp testing. The cyst is probably
A. A residual cyst
B. A lateral periodontal cyst
C. A radicular cyst
D. A dentigerous cyst
E. Stafne's bone cyst

45 Which one of the following is very characteristic of pemphigus vulgaris?
A. Nikolsky's sign
B. Black females
C. Drug reaction etiology
D. White males
E. Positive rabbit eye test

46 The clinical picture reveals a palpable benign tumor in the anterior midline of the palate. The tumor arises from deeper tissue and seems to originate from the periodontal ligament. The radiograph shows the lesion infiltrating bone but no metastasis. The patient is a 35-year-old woman. A possible diagnosis is a (an)
A. Peripheral giant cell granuloma
B. Lipoma
C. Torus palatinus
D. Irritative fibroma
E. Pregnancy tumor

47 The clinical picture of this lesion shows a severe drug reaction, with the lips especially affected. There also are skin "bull's-eye" lesions, which had an abrupt onset. The diagnosis would *MOST* likely be
A. Lichen planus
B. Herpes
C. Erythema multiforme
D. Mononucleosis
E. Acquired immunodeficiency syndrome (AIDS)

48 Which one of the following cysts is the result of extracting a tooth without the cystic sac?
A. Radicular cyst
B. Residual cyst
C. Periodontal cyst
D. Primordial cyst
E. Traumatic bone cyst

49 The dental hygienist observes a clinical picture of gingival fibromatosis resulting from a chemical reaction from phenytoin (Dilantin) therapy. Which one of the following statements is correct?
A. The client should stop taking the drug
B. There is an overgrowth of connective tissue
C. There is an overgrowth of epithelium
D. A gingivectomy would "cure" the condition
E. The condition is related to hereditary fibromatosis

50 Which one of the following diagnostic methods should be applied to establish the diagnosis of stomatitis nicotina?
A. Surgical
B. Radiographic
C. Laboratory
D. Clinical and historical
E. Therapeutic

51 Clinically, this white cauliflower-like lesion is similar to a wart. The histology report shows long fingerlike projections of epithelium. The etiology is unknown. One could suspect
A. Verruca vulgaris
B. Papilloma
C. Hyperkeratotic fibroma
D. Linea alba
E. Melanoma

52 Which of the following locations based on the Palmer nomenclature system is specifically important in diagnosing a lateral periodontal cyst?
A. 4, 3 | 3, 4
B. 1 | 1
C. 4, 3 | 3, 4
D. 8 | 8
E. 8 | 8

53 A platelet count of 150,000 to 400,000/mm^3 of blood could *NOT* be indicative of
A. Thrombocytopenia
B. Anemia
C. Leukemia
D. Nonthrombocytopenic purpura
E. Mononucleosis

54 Which one of the following is *NOT* a true characteristic of acute necrotizing ulcerative gingivitis (ANUG)?
A. Punched-out papillae and craters
B. Hyperkeratinization
C. Odor
D. Pain and bleeding
E. Necrotic slough of epithelium

55 The *MOST* accepted theory in the etiology of Behçet's syndrome is
A. Viral origin
B. Metabolic origin
C. Pleuropneumonia-like organisms (PPLOs)
D. Hormonal origin
E. Sexual transmission

56 Which of the following makes Behçet's syndrome different from recurrent ulcerative stomatitis (RUS)?
A. Skin and eye lesions
B. A triad of locations of lesions (oral, eye, and genital)
C. Exudate from lesions
D. Mesenchymal proliferations
E. Osteoclastic activity

57 Herpangina is caused by
A. Chickenpox virus
B. Coxsackievirus
C. Epstein-Barr (EB) virus
D. Varicella
E. Pleuropneumonia-like organisms (PPLOs)

58 In treatment of fibrous dysplasia, which one of the following would *NOT* be advised because it can trigger a malignancy?
A. Radiation
B. Surgery
C. Chemotherapy
D. Bone marrow depressants
E. Transplants

59 Precocious puberty is *MOST* characteristic of which of the following?
A. Jaffe's syndrome
B. Monostotic fibrous dysplasia
C. Polyostotic fibrous dysplasia
D. Albright's syndrome
E. Paget's disease

60 The *MOST* conclusive diagnostic approach to a malignant lesion is
A. Complete excision
B. Radiation therapy
C. Biopsy
D. Chemotherapy
E. Stripping

61 The radiographic appearance of a malignant lesion in bone will
A. Show destruction at the earliest stages
B. Show destruction when 10% to 20% of the bone is destroyed
C. Show destruction when 40% to 60% of the bone is destroyed
D. Never be fully determined
E. Go from radiopaque to radiolucent

62 Achlorhydria, inability to absorb vitamin B$_{12}$, and lack of folic acid are characteristic of
A. Thrombocytopenia
B. Hypervitaminosis
C. Pernicious anemia
D. Hyperkeratosis
E. Herpes

63 Bone marrow anoxia occurs in
A. Secondary polycythemia
B. Pernicious anemia
C. Thalassemia
D. Aplastic anemia
E. Thrombocytopenia

64 Which one of the following is referred to as "Mediterranean anemia"?
A. Acute anemia
B. Thalassemia
C. Primary aplastic anemia
D. Thrombocytopenia
E. Acquired immunodeficiency syndrome (AIDS)

65 In leukopenia, which cell type is *PREDOMINANTLY* involved?
A. Erythrocytes
B. Granulocytes
C. Eosinophils
D. Monocytes
E. Osteocytes

66 Which of the following cysts is involved with nonvital teeth?
A. Nasoalveolar cyst
B. Lateral periodontal cyst
C. Radicular cyst
D. Cyst of the incisive papilla
E. Stafne's bone cyst

67 Which cyst could develop into an ameloblastoma?
A. Residual cyst
B. Primordial cyst
C. Median mandibular cyst
D. Lateral periodontal cyst
E. Radicular cyst

68 A tooth was extracted with a cyst left behind. The cyst would be a
A. Residual cyst
B. Primordial cyst
C. Radicular cyst
D. Dentigerous cyst
E. Lateral periodontal cyst

69 A radicular cyst is *MOST* often caused by
A. Deep restorations
B. Trauma
C. Primary occlusal traumatism
D. Dental caries
E. Food impaction

70 Epulis fissurata is caused by
A. A denture flange
B. The suction chamber of a denture
C. An allergic reaction to acrylic material
D. Denture cleaners
E. Poor oral hygiene

71 Sickle cell anemia is of hereditary origin and occurs primarily in
A. Whites
B. Native Americans
C. Mediterranean ethnic groups
D. African Americans
E. Asian Americans

72 A client with achlorhydria has
A. A low blood glucose level
B. A lack of hydrochloric acid
C. Too much hydrochloric acid
D. Xerostomia
E. Multiple skin lesions

73 A person with leukopenia has a (an)
A. Decrease in the number of white blood cells
B. Increase in the number of white blood cells
C. Decrease in the number of red blood cells
D. Decrease in the number of platelets
E. Increase in the number of platelets

Answers and Rationales

1. (D) Radiographic absence of mandibular right and left second premolars is apparent.
   (A) Maxillary right and left first premolars are present.
   (B) Mandibular right and left first premolars are present.
   (C) Although mandibular right second premolar is absent, the mandibular right first premolar is present.
   (E) Maxillary right and left second premolars are present.
2. (D) Torus palatinus is located at the midline of the hard palate and appears radiopaque.
   (A) Histologically a myxoma consists of soft tissue that appears radiolucent on radiographs.
   (B) A bone cyst appears radiolucent.
   (D) An odontoma appears as radiopaque structure of "tooth" particles.
   (E) A ranula is a soft tissue cyst caused by blockage of a major salivary duct; clinically, it is observed as a "bluish" lesion in the floor of the mouth.

3. (D) The mandible is thinner in the region of the submandibular gland and is a normal radiolucency in the panoramic image.
   (A) Stafne bone cysts are pathologic lesions and do not usually appear bilaterally; they usually have well-defined borders.
   (B) Radicular cysts are pathologic lesions with well-defined borders; they do not usually appear bilaterally.
   (C) Periapical abscesses (pathologic lesions) do not appear bilaterally.
   (E) Traumatic bone cysts are pathologic lesions and do not usually appear bilaterally; they usually have well-defined borders.
4. (E) The zygomatic process is a radiopaque structure and is imaged in the superior-posterior region of panoramic radiographs.
   (A) The anterior coronoid process is usually seen inferior to the zygomatic process.
   (B) The maxillary tuberosity is distal to most posterior molars.
   (C) The mandibular condyle is a radiopaque structure visualized posterior to the zygomatic process.
   (D) The hamular process is not usually observed in panoramic films because of superimposition of other structures.
5. (E) The maxillary sinuses are large radiolucencies located superior to the maxillary molars.
   (A) The nasal fossae are radiolucent areas near the midline.
   (B) The orbits are superior to the maxillary sinuses.
   (C) The frontal sinuses do not appear in a panoramic image.
   (D) Globulomaxillary cysts usually appear near the canine–lateral incisor area.
6. (A) The palate is the *MOST* common location for mixed tumors.
   (B) The mandible is not an appropriate location for mixed tumors.
   (C) The buccal mucosa is not the location for mixed tumors.
   (D) Lymph nodes are not common locations for mixed tumors.
   (E) Fauces are not near salivary gland tissue.
7. (B) Because of the location, from midline of the tongue to the neck area, the thyroglossal duct cyst would be most involved in the process of swallowing.
   (A) The location of the branchial cleft cyst is the lateral aspect of the upper neck region and would not affect swallowing.
   (C) The nasopalatine cyst is found in the maxillary anterior region and is developmental in nature.
   (D) Mucoceles are soft tissue cysts associated with trauma to minor salivary glands; they are usually observed on the inner surface of the lower lip mucosa.
   (E) The residual cyst is a "leftover" cyst from a radicular cyst (caused by caries) that remained after the extraction of the offending tooth.

8. (C) A person with leukemia may have oral findings similar to necrotizing ulcerative gingivitis (punched papillae, odor, ulcerations, necrosis).
   (A) Symptoms of primary herpes include fever, reddening of the oral mucosa, and numerous vesicles and ulcers on the mucous membrane.
   (B) Mononucleosis may have oral findings similar to primary herpes.
   (D) In nonthrombocytopenic purpura there is severe gingival hemorrhage due to fragile capillary walls.
   (E) Secondary herpes may have vesicles located on the hard palate, attached gingiva, or lips, but it is not similar to ANUG.

9. (E) A ranula is a soft tissue "cyst" found in the floor of the mouth and is caused by blockage or trauma to a major salivary duct.
   (A) A ranula is not found on the palate.
   (B) A mucocele may be found on the inner lip but not a ranula.
   (C) A ranula is not found on the buccal mucosa.
   (D) A ranula is not found in the area of the fauces.

10. (C) A biopsy involves removal and microscopic examination of suspicious tissues to establish a precise diagnosis.
   (A) Radiographic surveys are not diagnostic for cancer.
   (B) Panographs are not diagnostic for cancer.
   (D) Positive exfoliative cytology findings must be followed by biopsy for precise diagnosis of cancer.
   (E) Clinical examination does not involve tissue collection and evaluation.

11. (C) At age 14, incomplete root formation may be observed in dental radiographs.
   (A) There is no history of trauma in the case history.
   (B) The client was asymptomatic for periapical pathology.
   (D) Hypercementosis is radiopaque.
   (E) Stage III cementomas are radiopaque.

12. (D) Primordial cysts are found posterior to erupted third molars or in the place of a third molar that was never present.
   (A) Primordial cysts are found in the age group under 25 but not in primary dentitions.
   (B) The maxillary anterior region is not the area where primordial cysts are found.
   (C) If associated with a supernumerary tooth, the cyst is then a dentigerous cyst since a "tooth is present."
   (E) The mandibular canine and premolar region is not the common location of a primordial cyst.

13. (A) The mandibular incisor area is the most common location for a true cementoma and occurs nine times more frequently in the mandible than in the maxilla.
   (B) Cementomas are rarely found in the maxilla.
   (C) Ossifying fibroma, found in the posterior mandible, can be confused radiographically with cementoma; a cementoma is rarely found in this location.
   (D) A cementoma is rarely found in the maxilla.
   (E) A cementoma is rarely found in the maxilla; because the lesion grows up the periodontal ligament, it would not be observed in the midline of the palate.

14. (C) Rocky Mountain spotted fever is caused by *Rickettsia*.
   (A) Malaria is caused by a protozoan agent.
   (B) Psittacosis is caused by *Chlamydia psittaci*, which is not a part of *Rickettsia*.
   (D) The agent for tularemia is *Francisella tularensis*, which is not a part of *Rickettsia*.
   (E) Meningitis may be a viral or bacterial disease but is *NOT* caused by *Rickettsia*.

15. (C) Median rhomboid glossitis is thought to be developmental, or associated with *Candida albicans*.
   (A) Geographic tongue changes its "maplike" pattern frequently.
   (B) Median rhomboid glossitis is never pathologic and has never been reported to develop into a malignancy.
   (D) Fissured tongue is usually seen throughout the dorsal surface and does not have the clinical features described.
   (E) Black hairy tongue is caused by irritation to the filiform papillae; once the irritant has been removed, the tongue returns to normal.

16. (C) The histology report is *MOST* significant because in pemphigus the lesion is intraepithelial whereas in pemphigoid the lesion is subepithelial.
   (A) Clinically the lesions may be very similar.
   (B) History of the disease is noncontributory because both are autoimmune conditions.
   (D) Race and religion are noncontributory, although in pemphigus vulgaris Ashkenazic Jews are more commonly affected.
   (E) The age of those affected is usually between 40 and 55 for both lesions.

17. (D) Calcified bodies, cementicles, are sometimes found and seen radiographically in the periodontal space and appear as radiopaque structures.
   (A) An epithelial rest would not appear on a radiograph as a radiopaque structure but as radiolucent because it is a soft tissue.
   (B) A cementum spur does not float free but is attached to the cementum.
   (C) An exostosis of bone would be attached to the wall of the alveolar bone proper.
   (E) A denticle is a calcified body but is related to dentin formation and found in the pulp of the tooth, not the periodontal space.

18. (D) Ludwig's angina is a bilateral, rapidly spreading swelling, with cellulitis in the floor of the mouth and neck; it often results from infected mandibular molars.
   (A) Actinomycosis is a rare condition that usually occurs after trauma and on one side only.
   (B) The individual is somewhat old to have mumps, although it is not impossible to get mumps at his age; mumps do not produce a sudden, rapidly spreading swelling.
   (C) The gumma of syphilis does not develop suddenly.
   (E) Pericoronitis produces more pain in the mouth; it is not usually rapid swelling and creates difficulty in opening the jaw.

19. (D) Shingles and chickenpox are both caused by varicella zoster virus.
    (A) Measles and German measles are caused by two different viral agents.
    (B) Chickenpox and smallpox are caused by two different viral agents.
    (C) Bacterial pneumonia has a bacterial etiology; croup is caused by a virus.
    (E) Mononucleosis is caused by Epstein-Barr virus; CMV is caused by a different viral agent.

20. (D) The description of the lesion and client history indicates the woman has recurrent herpes labialis.
    (A) A chancre, the primary lesion in syphillis, is usually a red elevated lesion.
    (B) Perlèche occurs in the corners of the mouth with cracking, not vesicular lesions.
    (C) An apthous ulcer is usually found on the oral mucosa.
    (E) Basal cell carcinoma does not recur before colds, nor does it heal.

21. (C) Hormonal changes during pregnancy result in increased gingival sensitivity to local irritants such as bacterial plaque and calculus, but pregnancy does not cause gingivitis.
    (A) Good oral hygiene will control pregnancy gingivitis.
    (B) Oral pregnancy tumors occur infrequently.
    (D) Hormonal changes during pregnancy do alter tissue resistance.
    (E) Bacteria acids, not hormones, cause enamel decalcification.

22. (E) Procardia is a calcium channel blocker that causes gingival hyperplasia, headache, nausea, and taste changes.
    (A) Dilantin is usually prescribed for epilepsy and other neurologic disorders.
    (B) Vasotec is an ACE inhibitor indicated for hypertension.
    (C) Valium is a tranquilizer or sedative.
    (D) Prozac is a neurotransmitter that inhibits serotonin uptake; xerostomia and oral ulcerations may be observed.

23. (B) A mucocele is usually found inside the lower lip and it is caused by trauma to a minor salivary duct. It is filled with clear fluid, and the surface epithelium is thin and breaks very easily.
    (A) A ranula is a soft tissue cyst found in the floor of the mouth and is caused by trauma or blockage involving a major salivary gland or duct.
    (C) A fibroma is a soft tissue lesion that is pink in color and composed of fibrous tissue.
    (D) A fistula is a drainage point from a chronically infected area. In most cases in the oral cavity a fistula is seen on the buccal aspect of the alveolar bone and PAP is observed radiographically on the associated tooth.

24. (D) A fibroma is composed of soft tissue and does not appear radiographically.
    (A) Caries appears radiolucent.
    (B) Supernumerary teeth appear radiopaque.
    (C) An odontoma appears radiopaque.
    (E) An early cementoma appears radiolucent and then radiopaque.

25. (B) Differential diagnosis is the most complete and combines all of the other diagnostic methods.
    (A) Surgical diagnostic methods contribute only a part of the information.
    (C) Therapeutic methods contribute only minutely to the evaluative approach.
    (D) Clinical methods show the visible picture only.
    (E) Historical methods may show only the age, gender, and race, which often may be noncontributory.

26. (C) The clinical picture itself has nothing to do with the pathogenesis or growth of the lesion in question.
    (A) How the lesion begins is of vital importance; was the onset gradual or acute?
    (B) How the lesion behaves in terms of growth, expansion, etc., is of extreme importance.
    (D) The development of the lesion also describes its progression.
    (E) The evolution of the lesion is really the same as its development.

27. (B) A fibrogranuloma is often referred to as the healing stage of a pyogenic granuloma and contains fibrous cells and granulation tissue.
    (A) Pregnancy tumor is another name for a pyogenic granuloma.
    (C) A lipoma is composed primarily of fat cells.
    (D) An osteoma is composed of dense, compact bone.
    (E) An odontoma is composed of tooth structures.

28. (B) Pyogenic granuloma is another name for a pregnancy tumor, and all of the diagnostic factors presented contribute to this diagnosis.
    (A) A fibroma is composed of fibroblasts and fibrocytes, and has no gender predilection.
    (C) Redundant tissue is associated with a denture flange.
    (D) A papilloma is white in color and rare; there is no gender predilection.
    (E) Pseudopapillomatosis is associated with the suction chamber of a denture.

29. (B) Primordial cysts are neoplastic in nature, and the location in the posterior part of the mandible is also the common site for the ameloblastoma.
    (A) Lateral periodontal cysts are found in the mandibular premolar area.
    (C) Stafne's bone cysts are found in the posterior part of the mandible, are composed of salivary gland tissues, and are completely benign in nature.
    (D) A residual cyst is a "remnant" of a radicular cyst that is usually associated with caries.
    (E) Traumatic bone cysts are related to trauma. Surgical intervention stimulates healing within a year.

30. (A) Biopsy findings are the most contributory diagnostic factor for a white lesion without a cause.
    (B) Surgical stripping is performed for hyperkeratosis.
    (C) Vitamin A therapy also assists in the treatment of hyperkeratosis.
    (D) If clinical leukoplakia is suspected, 1 month is too long for the client to wait and return.
    (E) A blood test will be noncontributory.

31. (C) The rabbit eye test is used for primary herpes.
    (A) The Pels-Macht test is used to determine pemphigus.
    (B) The Tzanck test is used to determine pemphigus.
    (D) Nikolsky's sign is used to determine pemphigus.
    (E) The immunofluorescent test is used to determine pemphigus.
32. (C) Pseudopapillomatosis or papillary hyperplasia, is caused by chronic irritation of the palate from the poor suction of a denture.
    (A) A fibroma has little or nothing to do with a denture, unless irritation from a partial denture clasp irritates the buccal mucosa, where fibromas are often found.
    (B) A papilloma is rare, white, and not related to a denture or to the age of the client.
    (D) A median palatal cyst is developmental and has nothing to do with dentures.
    (E) Primary aplastic anemia has nothing to do with dentures.
33. (B) A fibroma primarily consists of fibroblasts and fibrocytes.
    (A) A fibrosarcoma has bone cells.
    (C) A fibrolipoma has fat cells.
    (D) A fibroosteoma has bone cells.
    (E) A papilloma has acanthosis of the epithelium and is most commonly observed on the palate.
34. (D) The lingual mandibular bone concavity is also called Stafne's bone cyst and is composed of salivary gland tissue.
    (A) A residual cyst is "left over" from a radicular cyst, which is found anywhere in the dentition and caused by dental caries.
    (B) A traumatic bone cyst has no salivary gland tissue. When opened, it is a void. After surgical intervention, the bone fills in within a year.
    (C) Stoffer's bone cyst is a distractor for the alternate term applied to a lingual mandibular bone concavity: *Stafne's bone cyst.*
    (E) An ameloblastoma is found in the same location but does not have salivary gland tissue. It is a very aggressive and pathologic lesion that invades surrounding tissues.
35. (B) Blockage of a major salivary duct usually causes the formation of a ranula, which has the clinical characteristics described.
    (A) A decayed tooth would not produce a blue cystic lesion in the floor of the mouth.
    (C) A ranula is not a developmental cyst; it is usually caused by trauma.
    (D) Medications do not cause cysts. Xerostomia has nothing to do with cystic formation when related to medications.
    (E) Chemotherapy may cause xerostomia, but dry mouth does not cause blue cystic lesions.

36. (C) Behçet's syndrome is specifically characterized by the triad of oral, eye, and genital symptoms.
    (A) Erythema multiforme commonly has target "bull's-eye" skin lesions.
    (B) Stevens-Johnson syndrome is a severe form of erythema multiforme.
    (D) RUS has oral lesions, but not eye or genital lesions.
    (E) AIDS has nothing to do with the triad of symptoms and characteristics described.
37. (C) A granuloma is caused by an irritant.
    (A) Papilloma—the etiology is unknown.
    (B) Torus—the etiology is heredity.
    (D) Lipoma—the etiology is unknown.
    (E) Polyostotic fibrous dysplasia—the etiology is abnormal mesenchymal cell function.
38. (D) Fibroblasts and endothelial cells are found in abundance in a granuloma.
    (A) Mesenchyme is an embryonic form of connective tissue.
    (B) Epithelial cells are very few in number in a granuloma.
    (C) Osteoblasts are found in areas of bone formation.
    (E) Osteoclasts are found in areas where bone is being resorbed.
39. (A) Nodular hereditary gingival fibromatosis is significant only after the eruption of permanent teeth.
    (B) Symmetric is also a type of gingival fibromatosis but has no relation to the dentitions.
    (C) Chemical type is related to phenytoin (Dilantin) and calcium channel blockers (Procardia).
    (D) Epithelial type is a distractor because in fibromatosis, primarily the connective tissue proliferates.
    (E) Skeletal type relates to muscles and is not hereditary; the etiology is unknown.
40. (B) Basically one would suspect acute necrotizing ulcerative gingivitis (ANUG) and treat the client with a therapeutic approach.
    (A) A culture and any laboratory study would be a waste of time since the culture would show anaerobic bacteria, confirming ANUG.
    (C) A periodontist would use the same therapeutic approach, considering the clinical and contributory signs.
    (D) Considering the client's condition, a complete periodontal debridement would be impossible and would demonstrate poor judgment in the case.
    (E) A complete blood cell count would be noncontributory in treating the client.
41. (E) Osteoclasts would not be visible because they are involved in bone formation; in clinical leukoplakia, soft tissue is involved.
    (A) Dyskeratosis can be a histologic sign of clinical leukoplakia.
    (B) Acanthosis can be a histologic sign of clinical leukoplakia.
    (C) Large nuclei can be histologic signs of clinical leukoplakia.
    (D) Some necrosis can be a histologic sign of clinical leukoplakia.

42. (C) Because the lesion is so similar to a malignancy, the histology report is of vital importance.
    (A) A personal history is noncontributory because there is no age or gender predilection in a chondroma.
    (B) Complete removal of something that one is not sure of should never be performed without a thorough diagnostic evaluation.
    (D) Radiographs of all large bones are unnecessary and expose the client to radiation; noncontributory information would result.
    (E) The tumor is resistant to radiation therapy.
43. (C) A lipoma is composed of fat cells.
    (A) A papilloma is composed of epithelial cells.
    (B) An osteoma is composed of dense, compact bone.
    (D) A fibroma is composed of fibrous cells.
    (E) A myxoma is composed of loose-textured tissues of delicate reticulin fibers.
44. (C) A radicular cyst is *MOST* often caused by dental caries, and the tooth involved would most likely be nonvital.
    (A) A residual cyst is not associated with a tooth present in the mouth. It results when a radicular cyst is left behind after extraction of the offending tooth.
    (B) Lateral periodontal cysts are always associated with vital teeth.
    (D) A dentigerous cyst is observed in the area of unerupted third molars or is associated with unerupted supernumerary teeth.
    (E) Stafne's bone cyst is not associated with a tooth. It is observed in the mandible and is composed of salivary gland tissues.
45. (A) Nikolsky's sign, in which an air syringe can "blow" the epithelium away from the connective tissue, is one of the most characteristic signs of pemphigus vulbaris.
    (B) There is no gender or racial predilection in pemphigus vulgaris.
    (C) The etiology of pemphigus vulgaris is unknown or may be viral.
    (D) There is no gender or racial predilection in pemphigus vulgaris.
    (E) The rabbit eye test is performed for herpes.
46. (A) All of the characteristics described indicate the presence of a peripheral giant cell granuloma.
    (B) A lipoma is composed of fat cells and is rare and yellowish in color.
    (C) A torus palatinus is a bony hard nonpalpable lesion, is often hereditary, and does not "infiltrate."
    (D) An irritative fibroma is really an inflammatory lesion and the "scar-down" results of a pyogenic granuloma. It is composed only of soft tissues.
    (E) A pregnancy tumor is the same as a pyogenic granuloma and is an inflammatory tumor.

47. (C) Erythema multiforme is caused by a severe drug reaction with an acute onset that seemingly is almost an allergic type of reaction. The bull's-eye description of the lesion is very characteristic.
    (A) Lichen planus is not associated with a drug reaction.
    (B) Herpes is viral in origin.
    (D) Mononucleosis is caused by the Epstein-Barr (EB) virus.
    (E) AIDS is not associated with a drug etiology.
48. (B) The residual cyst is the "leftover" of a radicular cyst when the offending tooth has been extracted with the cyst left behind. It is usually observed on the alveolar ridge.
    (A) The radicular cyst usually is caused by dental caries and is found at the apex of the tooth involved.
    (C) A periodontal cyst is found between teeth, and the associated teeth are vital (usually mandibular premolars).
    (D) A primordial cyst is neoplastic in nature and is found where a tooth was never formed.
    (E) A traumatic bone cyst is related to trauma; it is often asymptomatic but shows radiographically as a well-defined radiolucent lesion. With surgical intervention the area fills in with new bone.
49. (B) A significant overgrowth of connective tissue is present in gingival fibromatosis.
    (A) The client should never stop medication, but the physician may elect to substitute an equally effective drug.
    (C) There is a slight overgrowth of the epithelium.
    (D) A gingivectomy would temporarily enhance aesthetics; however, because the drug is causing the condition, it would return as long as the client uses the medication.
    (E) This condition is caused by the drug and has nothing to do with other types of fibromatosis.
50. (D) Stomatitis nicotina is an easily detectable pathologic condition when observed clinically, with its hyperkeratosis of the palate and marked inflammation of the salivary duct orifice. These clinical signs, coupled with the history of a client who smokes a pipe (heat in the pipe causes the hyperkeratosis), makes the diagnosis certain.
    (A) Surgical intervention would not be necessary if the irritant, the pipe, were removed and the tissues responded.
    (B) Radiographic diagnosis would be noncontributory because the soft tissues of the palate are affected.
    (C) A laboratory test would be noncontributory.
    (E) A therapeutic diagnosis would be secondary to first determining the clinical and historical pictures. Vitamin A therapy may assist in the reduction of hyperkeratosis.

51. (B) Papilloma is always defined as a cauliflower-like lesion similar to a wart. Its etiology is unknown, but warts are caused by a virus.
    (A) Verruca vulgaris is another name for a wart.
    (C) A fibroma may occasionally have some hyperkeratosis, but not as a rule. Its etiology is unknown, and it is not a white lesion.
    (D) Linea alba is a "white line" that runs along the occlusal plane of the buccal mucosa. It is not considered a lesion per se.
    (E) A melanoma is a black malignant lesion. It is one of the most aggressive lesions and is often fatal.

52. (A) The mandibular canine and premolar areas are the primary locations for a lateral periodontal cyst.
    (B) An incisal canal cyst might be observed between the maxillary central incisors.
    (C) A globulomaxillary cyst, which is developmental in nature, might be found in the area of the maxillary canine.
    (D) A dentigerous cyst, Stafne's bone cyst, or an ameloblastoma could be found in the mandibular third molar area.
    (E) The maxillary third molar area is not a prime location for any cyst.

53. (A) There is a marked decrease in the platelet count in thrombocytopenia—a count of 60,000/mm³ or less. The numbers given are normal values for platelets.
    (B) The number of red blood cells is severely decreased in anemia.
    (C) There is an increase in the number of white blood cells in leukemia.
    (D) In nonthrombocytopenic purpura, the platelet count is normal. The bleeding tendency is a result of the fragility of the capillary walls.
    (E) There is an increase in the total white blood cell count in mononucleosis. Cells called Downey cells are found in abundance. Mononucleosis can be mistaken for leukemia, but the Paul-Bunnell heterophil test will be positive in mononucleosis.

54. (B) Hyperkeratinization is never found in ANUG because there is such destruction of the epithelium.
    (A) Punched-out papillae and craters are characteristics of ANUG.
    (C) Odor is a characteristic of ANUG.
    (D) Pain and bleeding are characteristics of ANUG.
    (E) Necrosis of epithelium is a characteristic of ANUG.

55. (C) PPLOs are the most widely accepted theory concerning the etiology of Behçet's syndrome.
    (A) A viral etiology is also suspected.
    (B) Metabolic etiologic factors may also play a role.
    (D) There is a hormonal association since the disease occurs more often in males.
    (E) Sexual transmission has no relation to the etiology, although the genitalia are affected with lesions.

56. (B) The triad of locations of lesions involving oral, eye, and genital areas is specifically characteristic.
    (A) Skin and eye lesions are not common in RUS.
    (C) There can be exudate from all types of lesions in RUS or Behçet's syndrome.
    (D) Histologically, the epithelial tissues are involved; however, in Behçet's syndrome, there is also endothelial proliferation that is not observed in RUS.
    (E) There is no bone activity in either disease; all are soft tissue involvements.

57. (B) The coxsackie virus is the cause of herpangina.
    (A) The chickenpox virus causes herpes zoster.
    (C) The EB virus is associated with infectious mononucleosis.
    (D) Varicella virus is another name for the chickenpox virus, which causes herpes zoster.
    (E) PPLOs are the organisms associated with Behçet's syndrome.

58. (A) Radiation therapy has triggered malignant transformation in cases of fibrous dysplasia.
    (B) Surgery is often the mode of treatment.
    (C) Chemotherapy has not been reported.
    (D) Bone marrow depressants are not administered; however, bone recontouring via surgery is usually performed for aesthetics.
    (E) Any type of transplant or resection is seldom indicated.

59. (D) Albright's syndrome is a varient of polyostotic fibrous dysplasia, with precocious puberty in girls being the strongest diagnostic factor.
    (A) Jaffe's syndrome is a *SEVERE* form of polyostotic fibrous dysplasia.
    (B) Monostotic fibrous dysplasia is not associated with precocious puberty.
    (C) "Regular" polyostotic fibrous dysplasia is not associated with precocious puberty.
    (E) Paget's disease does not exhibit precocious puberty because the disease occurs more commonly in men over 50 years of age.

60. (C) If a determination has been made that a lesion may be malignant, the next step toward a conclusive diagnosis is to perform a biopsy. If the biopsy findings are negative but the clinician still believes that the lesion could be malignant because of its other characteristics, a second biopsy should be performed.
    (A) Complete excision of an undiagnosed lesion should not be performed.
    (B) Radiation therapy is *NOT* indicated, especially with an unconfirmed diagnosis.
    (D) Chemotherapy is *NOT* a diagnostic method.
    (E) Stripping is usually done in cases of hyperkeratosis.

61. (C) At least 40% to 60% of the bone involved must be destroyed before it can be seen radiographically.
    (A) During the earliest stages nothing is observed radiographically.
    (B) A 10% to 20% bone loss is still too little to identify a malignant lesion.
    (D) Bone destruction can be observed radiographically in the 40% to 60% bone loss stage.
    (E) There will not be a change from dense radiopacity to radiolucency. The lesion will become more and more radiolucent.

62. (C) Lack of hydrochloric acid, vitamin B_{12}, and folic acid are all related to pernicious anemia. The secretion of intrinsic factor (hydrochloric acid) does not occur, therefore preventing B_{12} from being absorbed.
    (A) Thrombocytopenia is a decrease in the number of platelets.
    (B) Hypervitaminosis indicates an excess of a particular vitamin.
    (D) Hyperkeratosis indicates thickening and the formation of a protective layer of cells over the epithelium.
    (E) Herpes is caused by a virus and has nothing to do with vitamins or gastric secretion.

63. (A) Bone marrow anoxia, caused by a particular irritant, occurs in secondary polythemia.
    (B) The etiology of pernicious anemia is related to the lack of hydrochloric acid in the stomach and B_{12} absorption.
    (C) In thalassemia, the bone marrow shows cellular hyperplasia.
    (D) There is marrow dysfunction in aplastic anemia.
    (E) There is a decrease in the number of platelets in thrombocytopenia.

64. (B) Thalassemia is often referred to as "Mediterranean anemia" because of the ethnic predilection.
    (A) Acute anemia usually results from an automobile accident.
    (C) In primary aplastic anemia the etiology is unknown.
    (D) Thrombocytopenia is a decrease in the number of platelets.
    (E) AIDS does not refer to any form of anemia.

65. (B) Granulocytes are found in abundance in leukopenia, although there is a reduction in the number of *ALL* white blood cells.
    (A) Erythrocytes form red blood cells.
    (C) Eosinophils are few in number in the normal blood, but with a decrease in the total number of white blood cells, their number also is decreased.
    (D) Large mononuclear leukocytes in the blood having a great deal of protoplasm are not involved in leukopenia.
    (E) Osteocytes are bone-forming cells and have nothing to do with the blood.

66. (C) A radicular cyst is usually caused by dental caries; the tooth involved is usually nonvital.
    (A) A nasoalveolar cyst is developmental.
    (B) A lateral periodontal cyst is found between teeth that are vital.
    (D) A cyst of the incisive papilla is developmental.
    (E) Stafne's bone cyst involves salivary gland tissues; the dentition is not affected.

67. (B) A primordial cyst is neoplastic in nature and therefore has the potential for developing into an ameloblastoma.
    (A) A residual cyst is a remnant of a radicular cyst that was not removed.
    (C) A median mandibular cyst is developmental.
    (D) A lateral periodontal cyst is not aggressive and is usually found in the mandibular canine and premolar areas.
    (E) A radicular cyst is associated with a tooth and caused by dental caries.

68. (A) A residual cyst is the cystic sac left behind after a radicular cyst was incompletely removed. Usually the offending tooth is extracted with the cyst left on the alveolar ridge.
    (B) A primordial cyst is a neoplastic cyst found *IN PLACE* of a tooth.
    (C) A radicular cyst is found at the apex of a tooth and is generally caused by dental caries.
    (D) A dentigerous cyst is a neoplastic cyst usually found around the crown of an unerupted tooth. The mandibular third molar or a supernumerary tooth is the most common location.
    (E) A lateral periodontal cyst is found between teeth, with the teeth involved all being vital.

69. (D) Dental caries is the most common etiologic factor in a radicular cyst.
    (A) A deep restoration may trigger pulpitis, which stimulates periapical pathology.
    (B) Trauma does not usually cause a radicular cyst.
    (C) Primary occlusal traumatism is a secondary etiologic factor in a radicular cyst.
    (E) Food impaction does not cause a cyst.

70. (A) A denture flange irritating the ridge area causes epulis fissurata, or redundant tissue.
    (B) Poor suction in the palatal chamber causes pseudopapillomatosis, also called papillary hyperplasia.
    (C) An allergic reaction to the acrylic would occur all over the mucosa, not in a specific area.
    (D) Denture cleaners help maintain good denture hygiene and prevent tissue response.
    (E) Poor oral or denture hygiene can contribute to any oral condition or denture response but is not the primary etiologic factor in epulis fissurata.

71. (D) One in 600 African Americans has sickle cell anemia.
    (A) Sickle cell anemia is rarely found in whites.
    (B) Sickle cell anemia has not been reported in Native Americans.
    (C) Sickle cell anemia is not a Mediterranean disease, as is thalassemia.
    (E) Sickle cell anemia has not been reported in Asians.

72. (B) Achlorhydria is a lack of production in intrinsic factor (hydrochloric acid) in the stomach.
    (A) A low blood glucose level has nothing to do with the problem.
    (C) A lack of production, not an increase in production, of hydrochloric acid occurs in achlorhydria.
    (D) Hydrochloric acid production is not related to xerostomia.
    (E) Skin lesions are not related to a lack of intrinsic factor.

73. (A) Leukopenia, an abnormality in the blood, is a marked decrease in the number of white blood cells, particularly the granulocytes.
    (B) There is no increase in the number of white blood cells.
    (C) The number of red blood cells is not changed.
    (D) The number of platelets is not changed.
    (E) The number of platelets is not changed.

Microbiology and Infection Control

Kara T. Hansen   Barbara Heckman

The practice of dental hygiene involves the risk of contracting diseases such as hepatitis, AIDS, tuberculosis, respiratory tract infections, and herpes. To recognize disease entities and understand the rationale for infection control protocols, a basic knowledge of microbiology is required.

Prevention of disease transmission in dental hygiene practice requires an understanding of the sources of contamination and infection control in the oral healthcare environments, instruments, dental materials, and radiographic equipment. Protective measures, from a *universal precautions* perspective, for all clients and oral healthcare team members are essential.

General Microbiology

Microorganisms

General Considerations

A. Present in most environments
B. Exhibit characteristics common to all biologic systems: reproduction, metabolism, growth, irritability, adaptability, mutation, and organization
C. Medically important microorganisms[1]
  1. Eukaryotes

  a. Algae—uni- or multicellular, chlorophyll-containing
  b. Protozoa—unicellular nonphotosynthetic
  c. Fungi (molds and yeast)
    (1) Nonphotosynthetic
    (2) Classified by type of spores produced, presence or absence of mycelia, mechanisms of sexual and asexual spore formation
  d. Slime molds—characterized by presence of plasmodium
  2. Prokaryotes (aerobic or anaerobic unicellular bacteria)
  a. Firmicutes
  b. Gracilicutes
  c. Tenericutes
  d. Mendosicutes
  3. Viruses; classification is still evolving but based on
  a. Type and properties of nucleic acid
  b. Morphology of nucleoproteins
  c. Presence and properties of envelopes
  4. Helminths
  a. Multicellular organisms
  b. Generally parasites of the human alimentary tract or hemolymphatic system
D. Nomenclature—the binomial system
  1. Two-word designation

a. Genus and species
b. First word capitalized and both words italicized (e.g., *Escherichia coli*)
2. Devised by Carolus Linnaeus

Methods of Observation/Measurement

A. Most commonly used units of measurement
1. Micrometer ($\mu m = 10^{-6}$ m)
2. Nanometer (nm $= 10^{-9}$ m)
3. Angstrom unit ($\mathring{A} = 10^{-10}$ m)
4. Millimeter (mm $= 10^{-3}$ m)
5. Centimeter (cm $= 10^{-2}$ m)
B. Light microscopes illuminate objects by visible light
1. Bright-field microscopy
a. Simple microscopes
b. Compound microscopes consist of at least two lens systems
(1) Objective
(a) Magnifies the specimen and is close to it
(b) Low power, high power, and oil immersion
(2) Ocular
(a) Eyepiece
(b) Magnifies the image produced by the objective lens
2. Dark-field microscopy
a. Specimens seen as bright objects against a dark background
b. Used for examination of unstained microorganisms, and hanging-drop preparations
c. Advantage—allows a view of living bacteria undisturbed in size or shape by fixing and staining techniques
3. Fluorescence microscopy
a. Used to visualize objects that fluoresce or emit light when exposed to light of a different wavelength
b. Ultraviolet light, fluorescent chemicals, and special filter systems required
c. Commonly used in the medical field to track antigen-antibody reactions
4. Phase-contrast microscopy
a. Useful in examining transparent, living cells, including their internal structure and in determining motility in a fluid medium
b. Variations in density between the microbes and surrounding medium are capitalized on to increase the contrast between the two
5. Specimen preparation
a. Viewing living organisms
(1) Methods
(a) Hanging drop
(b) Temporary wet mount

(2) Advantages
(a) Maintain shape of organisms
(b) Useful to determine size, shape, motility, and reactions to chemicals or immune sera
b. Staining
(1) Procedure
(a) Thin films of microorganisms are spread on a glass slide and allowed to dry (smear)
(b) Films are fixed, either by a chemical fixative or by passing through a flame; this coagulates the protein and kills the cell
(c) Dyes or stains are applied to the smear to allow for greater visualization; allows some differentiation of species
(d) Fixation process tends to reduce the size of cells; dye addition tends to increase the size of cells
(2) Types of dyes
(a) Acidic or negative is used to stain basic components of the cell
(b) Basic or positive is used to stain acidic components of the cell (e.g., nucleic acid polysaccharides)
(3) Simple staining procedures
(a) Use a single dye (e.g., carbolfuchsin, crystal violet, methylene blue, or safranin)
(b) Used to show shapes, sizes, arrangements of bacterial cells
(4) Differential staining procedures
(a) More than one dye preparation used
(b) Used for initial bacterial grouping
(c) Most common methods
[1] Gram stain differentiates microorganisms based on color as gram positive (purple or blue) or gram negative (red); certain characteristics of microorganisms appear correlated to their staining reactions: cell wall thickness, chemical composition, and sensitivity to penicillin; useful in diagnosis of infectious diseases
[2] Acid-fast stain is used to differentiate mycobacteria (e.g., *Mycobacterium leprae* and *Mycobacterium tuberculosis*) from other bacteria by indicating the presence or absence of special lipids in the cell wall; organisms resist decolorization

with an acidic solution of alcohol after being stained with a basic dye

    (5) Special staining procedures

      (a) Used to color and isolate specific parts of microorganisms

        [1] Negative staining for capsules

        [2] Schaeffer-Fulton spore stain (e.g., *Bacillus, Clostridium*)

        [3] Flagellar staining

C. Electron microscopy

  1. Electrons used as a source of illumination

  2. Higher magnification and better resolving power available than with a light microscope

  3. Types

    a. Transmission electron microscope—used to visualize cell and virus ultrastructure

    b. Scanning electron microscope—used to visualize three-dimensional images of cell and virus surface features

Prokaryotic (Bacterial) Cell Structure and Function

A. Bacterial morphology

  1. Cocci (singular, coccus)

    a. Spherical or ovoid shape

    b. Occur in pairs (diplococci), chains (streptococci), four-in-a-square arrangement (tetrad), eight cells in a cubic arrangement (sarcinae), and irregular clusters (staphylococci)

  2. Bacilli (singular, bacillus)

    a. Cylindric or rodlike

    b. Occur in pairs (diplobacilli); chains (streptobacilli); small, rounded rods (coccobacilli); tapered ends (fusiform bacilli)

  3. Spirilla (singular, spirillum)

    a. Spiral or curved

    b. Vary in number and fullness of turns

    c. Vibrios are portions of a spiral

B. External cell structures

  1. Appendages

    a. Provide motility

      (1) Flagella

        (a) Motility must be distinguished from brownian movement, which is caused by bacteria being hit by molecules in their surrounding medium; flagella enable bacteria to move toward favorable environments and away from adverse ones (chemotaxis)

      (2) Axial filaments

        (a) Spirochetes (e.g., *Treponema pallidum, Borrelia burgdorferi*) move by this method

    b. Provide attachments

      (1) Pili (sex pili)

        (a) Longer and fewer in number

        (b) Join bacterial cells in preparation for deoxyribonucleic acid (DNA) transfer (conjugation)

      (2) Fimbriae

        (a) Shorter and numerous

        (b) Enable a cell to adhere to surfaces (e.g., *Neisseria gonorrhoeae, Escherichia coli*)

  2. Surface coating (glycocalyx)

    a. Capsules

      (1) Condensed and well-defined masses of polysaccharides and/or polypeptides firmly attached to the cell wall

      (2) Encapsulation protects pathogenic organisms from drugs, phagocytosis, and bactericidal factors

      (3) Some bacteria need capsules to maintain virulence (e.g., *Streptococcus pneumoniae, Streptococcus mutans*)

    b. Slime layer

      (1) Unorganized, soluble mass of polysaccharides and/or polypeptides loosely attached to the cell wall

      (2) Protects microorganisms and aids in adherence

  3. Cell wall

    a. Functions

      (1) Determines and maintains the shape of the microorganism

      (2) Provides support for flagella

      (3) Prevents rupture of the cell resulting from osmotic pressure differences on either side of the cell wall

    b. Composed of the macromolecule peptidoglycan

    c. Comparison of gram-negative and gram-positive cell walls

      (1) Gram-positive cell walls consist of many layers of peptidoglycan and also contain teichoic acids

      (2) Gram-negative bacteria have a lipoprotein-lipopolysaccharide-phospholipid outer membrane surrounding a thin peptidoglycan layer

      (3) The outer membrane protects gram-negative cells from phagocytosis, penicillin, lysozyme, and other chemicals

      (4) Gram-negative cell walls are more easily broken by mechanical forces; susceptible to lysis by antibody, complement, and streptomycin

  4. Cytoplasmic (plasma) membrane

    a. Structure

      (1) Consists of phosopholipids forming a bi-

layer with proteins interspersed in a mosaic pattern (fluid mosaic)
  b. Functions
    (1) A barrier regulating movement of materials in and out of the cell
    (2) Active transport
    (3) Excretion of hydrolytic exoenzymes
    (4) Bears enzymes and carrier molecules
    (5) Bears receptors and other proteins of the chemotactic and other sensory transduction systems
  c. Lies adjacent to and beneath the cell wall and encloses the cytoplasm of the cell
5. Cell envelope
  a. Includes all external structures and appendages, including the capsule, pili, flagella, cell wall, and cytoplasmic membrane
  b. May play a role in protection from degradation, maintenance of cell shape, and cell adhesion
  c. Properties confer staining characteristics
  d. Organization and structure different in gram-positive and gram-negative bacteria
C. Internal cell structure
  1. Cytoplasm (protoplasm)
    a. Fluid compartment inside the cytoplasmic membrane
    b. Prominent site for many of the cell's biochemical and synthetic activities
    c. Contains chromatin body, ribosomes, and granules
  2. Mesosomes
    a. Irregular folds of the cytoplasmic membrane resulting from dehydration of cells in preparation for electron microscopy; considered artifacts
  3. Genetic material or genome (nucleoid)
    a. Prokaryotes lack the distinct nucleus of eukaryotes
    b. Single chromosome is composed of a single molecule of DNA, existing as a closed loop not enclosed by the nuclear membrane; located in the nucleoplasm of the cell
    c. Additional genetic material is found in plasmids, which are extrachromosomal DNA molecules; they carry information that determines drug resistance or sensitivity
  4. Ribosomes
    a. Function of synthesis of protein
    b. Composed of ribosomal protein and ribosomal ribonucleic acid (RNA)
  5. Photosynthetic apparatus
  6. Inclusions
    a. Accumulations of reserve storage materials
    b. Include polysaccharide granules, metachromatic granules, sulfur granules, lipid inclusions, carboxysomes, and gas vacuoles
D. Endospores
  1. Dormant structures formed within gram-positive bacterial cells
  2. Formed during a process called sporulation: disintegration of parent cell released endospore; then called exposure or free spore
  3. Can remain in a spore state for years; exhibit unusual resistance to heat, drying, chemical disinfection, and radiation
  4. Spores can transform back into a vegetative cell through a process called germination
  5. Ability of bacteria to produce endospores is restricted mainly to the genera *Bacillus* and *Clostridium*

Eukaryotic Cell Structure and Function (Table 7-1 and Table 7-2)

A. More complex than a prokaryotic cell; has a distinct nucleus bounded by a nuclear membrane, a nucleolus, and membrane-bound organelles
B. Animal cells
  1. Cell membrane
    a. Surrounds the cell and interconnects with the cell's internal membrane systems
    b. Functions
      (1) Regulates the passage of substances in and out of the cell through active and passive transport
      (2) Involved with phagocytosis, tumor formation, drug sensitivity, and immune response
  2. Nucleus
    a. Controls the cell's physiologic and reproductive processes
    b. Composition
      (1) Nuclear membrane
      (2) Nucleoli (involved in RNA synthesis)
      (3) Chromosomes (composed of DNA)
      (4) Nucleoprotein (chromatin)
  3. Internal structures
    a. Mitochondria are involved with adenosine triphosphate (ATP) or energy production
    b. Endoplasmic reticulum (ER)
      (1) Network of membranes involved with chemical reactions, storage, and transportation
      (2) Rough ER has ribosomes attached
    c. Golgi apparatus
    d. Lysosomes contain digestive enzymes
    e. Microtubules
C. Plant cells[2]

Table 7-1

Eukaryotic Organelles and Their Functions[3]

Organelle	Associated functions and activities
Cell membrane	1. Transport of substances into and out of cells 2. In some cells, engulfment of foreign material (phagocytosis) 3. Pinocytosis
Cell wall	1. Found only in plants, imparts shape and strength to the cell 2. Protection against certain osmotic imbalances
Chloroplast	Photosynthesis
Cilium	Motion, or movement of substances past the ciliated cell
Endoplasmic reticulum	Protein synthesis
Flagellum	Propulsion
Golgi apparatus	1. Transfer of proteins and other cellular components to a secretory cell's exterior 2. Storage and packing structure for cellular products
Microbody, or peroxisome	Enzymatic activities
Microtubule	1. Cell transport of materials 2. Development and maintenance of cell shape 3. Cell division 4. Ciliary and flagellar movement
Mitochondrion	Synthesis of the energy-rich compound adenosine triphosphate (ATP)
Nucleolus	Major site for the formation of ribosomal components
Nucleus	1. Control of cellular physiological process 2. Transfer of hereditary factors to subsequent generations
Ribosome	Protein synthesis
Vacuoles	1. Locations of water 2. Storage site for certain amino acids, carbohydrates, and proteins 3. Dumping ground for cellular wastes

From Wistreich GA, Lechtman MD: *Microbiology,* ed 5, New York, 1989, Macmillan.

1. Have some of the same organelles as animal cells, including cell membrane, nucleus, nucleolus, mitochondria, and endoplasmic reticulum
2. Cell wall is simpler in structure; major component is the polysaccharide cellulose
3. Plastids
   a. Chromoplasts impart color to flowers, fruits, and leaves
   b. Chloroplasts are necessary for photosynthesis
   c. Leukoplastids are colorless and store starch
4. Vacuoles

Microbial Growth and Cultivation

A. Definitions
   1. Culture media—nutrient preparations used to cultivate microorganisms
   2. In vitro techniques—procedures using nonliving materials in a culture vessel
   3. In vivo techniques—procedures using living cells or entire animals or plants
   4. Colony—resulting accumulation of bacteria on a medium
B. Conditions affecting growth
   1. Physical
      a. Thermal conditions
         (1) Most bacteria grow best over a range of temperature
            (a) Psychrophiles—0 to 15° C
            (b) Mesophiles—20 to 40° C
            (c) Thermophiles—45 to 60° C
         (2) Minimal, maximal, and optimal requirements are the organisms' cardinal temperatures
         (3) 30° C optimal temperature for many free-living organisms
      b. Acidity or alkalinity (pH)
         (1) Most bacteria grow best near a neutral pH, between 6 and 8
            (a) Acidophiles—pH 1 to 5.4
            (b) Neutrophiles—pH 5.4 to 8.5
            (c) Alkalinophiles—pH 9.0 to 12.0
      c. Osmotic pressure
         (1) Halophilic organisms require high salt concentration
         (2) Osmophilic organisms require high osmotic pressure
   2. Chemical
      a. Gaseous requirements
         (1) Aerobes require oxygen
         (2) Microaerophilic organisms need low concentrations of oxygen
         (3) Anaerobes do not need oxygen
         (4) Obligate (strict) anaerobes cannot tolerate any free oxygen
         (5) Facultative anaerobes can metabolize aerobically if oxygen is present or anaerobically if it is absent
         (6) Aerotolerant anaerobes metabolize substances anaerobically but are not harmed by oxygen
      b. Nutrition available
         (1) Heterotrophic organisms

Table 7-2

Major Characteristics of Eukaryotes and Prokaryotes[4]

Characteristic	Eukaryotes	Prokaryotes
Major groups	Algae, fungi, protozoa, plants, animals	Bacteria
Size (approximate)	$>5 \mu m$	$1 \times 3 \mu m$
Nuclear structures		
Nucleus	Classic membrane	No nuclear membrane
Chromosomes	Strands of DNA	Single, closed strand of DNA
Cytoplasmic structures		
Mitochondria	Present	Absent
Golgi bodies	Present	Absent
Endoplasmic reticulum	Present	Absent
Ribosomes (sedimentation coefficient)	80S	70S
Cytoplasmic membrane	Contains sterols	Does not contain sterols*
Cell wall	Absent or composed of cellulose or chitin	Complex structure containing protein, lipids, and peptidoglycans
Reproduction	Sexual and asexual	Asexual (binary fission)
Movement	Flagella, if present, are complex	Flagella, if present, are simple
Respiration	Via mitochondria	Via cytoplasmic membrane

*Except in *Mycoplasma* organisms.
From Slots J, Taubman MA: *Contemporary oral microbiology and immunology,* St Louis, 1992, Mosby.

(a) Require organic compounds for growth
(b) Most commonly cultured on a medium of glucose
(2) Autotrophic organisms
  (a) Do not require organic nutrients for growth
  (b) Use inorganic compounds such as carbon dioxide
  (c) Thrive in soils and bodies of water
(3) Hypotrophic organisms
  (a) Obligate intracellular parasites; grow only within a living host cell
  (b) Include the viruses and rickettsiae
(4) Nutrients needed include sulfur and phosphorus
(5) Nitrogen is derived from proteins and their products
(6) Certain vitamins and growth factors required
C. Types of media
  1. Synthetic media—exact chemical composition is known
  2. Rich complex media—exact chemical composition varies slightly from batch to batch (e.g., addition of blood or beef extract)
  3. Differential media
    a. Contain combinations of nutrients and pH indicators to produce visual differentiation between several microorganisms
    b. Example—blood agar is an enriched medium that allows streptococci to leave different signs on the medium; green discoloration around colonies means α-hemolytic streptococcus, clear zones mean β-hemolysis, and no effect means γ-hemolysis
  4. Selective media
    a. Allow interference with or prevention of certain microorganisms' growth while permitting others to grow
    b. Dyes and antibiotics make the media selective
  5. Selective and differential media
    a. Combine properties of the preceding two types of media
    b. Examples—mannitol, salt, agar, and MacConkey agar
  6. Enrichment media
    a. Similar to selective media but designed to increase the numbers of particular microbes to detectable levels
  7. Reducing media
    a. Contains ingredients that chemically combine with and deplete oxygen in the culture medium
    b. Used for anaerobes
D. Pure culture techniques
  1. Used to isolate and identify a bacterial species
  2. Methods
    a. Pour-plate technique
    (1) Cool the melted agar-containing medium
    (2) Inoculate the medium

(a) Use the loop or needle to transfer the organism

(b) Pass the loop through the flame and heat to redness

(c) Flame edges of tubes from which cultures are taken before and after removal of the organism

(3) Pour the inoculated medium into a sterile Petri dish

(4) Allow the medium to solidify

(5) Incubate at the desired temperature

b. Streak-plate technique

(1) Spread a loopful of material containing organisms over the surface of the solidified agar

(2) Streaking methods are shown in Figs. 7-1 and 7-2

E. Bacterial growth

1. Most bacteria reproduce by binary fission (i.e., two new cells are produced by one parent cell)

2. Growth on the culture medium

a. Typical growth curve results

b. Phases

(1) Lag phase—no increase in cell number

(2) Exponential phase (log)—cell number increases in an exponential manner; generation time is the average time for the cell to divide

(3) The maximum stationary phase—total number of viable cells is constant

(4) Phase of decline (death phase, F)—number of viable cells decreases

3. Measurement of growth

a. Made by observing an increase in mass or numbers

b. Cell mass can be measured by dry weight, chemical analysis, and turbidity

c. Cell numbers can be measured by viable counts; estimates are expressed as colony-forming units (CFU) for bacteria or plaque-forming units (PFU) for viruses

Microbial Metabolism and Cell Regulation

A. Metabolism

1. Definition—set of chemical reactions by which cells maintain life

2. Phases

a. Anabolism

(1) Synthesis of cellular constituents; energy-consuming phase

(2) Macromolecules such as nucleic acids, proteins, lipids, and polysaccharides are synthesized

b. Catabolism

(1) Breaking-down phase

(2) Complex compounds are broken down, releasing energy in the form of adenosine triphosphate (ATP) molecules

3. Energy storage and transfer

a. Conserved as chemical energy in ATP

b. May be transported by electrons (electron transport system)

c. Energy produced through oxidation-reduction reactions

(1) Aerobic oxidation (respiration)

(2) Anaerobic oxidation (fermentation)

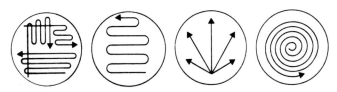

Fig. 7-1   Representative streaking patterns. (From Wistreich GA, Lechtman MD: *Microbiology,* ed 5, New York, 1989, Macmillan.)

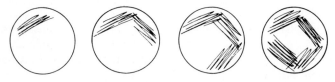

Fig. 7-2   Clock-plate method of streaking. (From Wistreich GA, Lechtman MD: *Microbiology,* ed 5, New York, 1989, Macmillan.)

4. Metabolic pathways
   a. Series of steps to complete biochemical process
   b. Glycolytic pathway
      (1) Most important way carbohydrates are metabolized
      (2) Converts glucose to pyruvic acid
      (3) Anaerobic fermentation process
      (4) Occur inside mitochondria
   c. Tricarboxylic acid (Krebs) cycle
      (1) Follows the glycolytic pathway
      (2) Responsible for complete oxidation of glucose
      (3) Important to aerobic bacteria
5. Protein synthesis
   a. DNA directs formation of proteins aided by various types of RNA
   b. Transcription—synthesis of RNA from a DNA template
   c. Translation—synthesis of protein from an RNA template
   d. Three stages of protein synthesis
      (1) Initiation
      (2) Elongation
      (3) Termination
B. Metabolic control
   1. Largely by enzymatic control
   2. Types of regulation
      a. Feedback inhibition
         (1) Allosteric enzymes—end product binds to the enzyme and distorts it so it can no longer bind to its substrate
         (2) When more end product is needed, the enzyme is released
      b. Genetic regulation—regulated by a specific unit of DNA called an operon
         (1) Enzyme repression—when the level of end product is sufficient the genetic synthesis of the enzyme is suppressed
         (2) Enzyme induction—enzymes are genetically synthesized only when substrates are present

Microbial Genetics

A. Eukaryotic genome
   1. Almost all of the eukaryotic genome is diploid
   2. Gene expression can be recessive or dominant
   3. Mitochondria and chloroplasts have a single circular DNA; function of DNA is related to that organelle
   4. Yeasts contain small circular particles of DNA called plasmids
   5. Genetic recombination is associated with sexual reproduction

B. Prokaryotic genome
   1. Most prokaryotes have a single circular chromosome
   2. Additional genes are present on plasmids (small circles of DNA)
   3. Some DNA segments move without benefit of homology (transposons)
C. Some viruses (phage) multiply in bacteria
D. Genetic recombination
   1. Conjugation
      a. Transfer of genetic material between two living bacteria that are in physical contact
      b. Plasmids are most frequently transferred
   2. Transduction—a bacterial virus (bacteriophage) transfers genetic material
   3. Transformation—the direct uptake of donor DNA by the recipient cell
E. Genetic rearrangement
   1. Transposons—small segments of DNA that can move from one region of a chromosome to another region of the same chromosome, or to a different chromosome or a plasmid
F. Mutations
   1. Result in changes in DNA strand sequence
   2. Can be caused by agents such as ultraviolet light, radiation, nitrous acid, and mustard gas

Microbial Relationships

A. Syntrophism
   1. Organisms are not intimately associated with each other but benefit from each other
   2. Examples yogurt production and organisms feeding in soil where decaying plant material is found
B. Competition
   1. Interaction between organisms resulting from a demand for nutrients and energy that exceeds immediate supply
   2. Example—molds such as *Penicillium* compete by secreting substances toxic to other organisms
C. Predation—controls the population by predators feeding on another species, the prey
D. Symbiosis—two different forms of life live in a mutually beneficial coexistence
E. Commensalism—only one organism benefits and the other neither benefits nor is harmed
F. Parasitism—one organism benefits at the expense of the other

Bacteria (Table 7-3)

A. Ternicutes
   1. Gram-positive eubacteria
B. Gracilicutes

Table 7-3

Major Categories and Groups of Bacteria that Cause Disease in Humans Used as an Identification Scheme in *Bergey's Manual of Determinative Bacteriology,* 9th ed.[1,5]

I. Gram-negative eubacteria that have cell walls	
Group 1: The spirochetes	*Treponema*
	Borrelia
	Leptospira
Group 2: Aerobic/microaerophilic, motile helical/vibroid gram-negative bacteria	*Campylobacter*
	Helicobacter
	Spirillum
Group 3: Nonmotile (or rarely motile) curved bacteria	None
Group 4: Gram-negative aerobic/microaerophilic rods and cocci	*Alcaligenes*
	Bordetella
	Brucella
	Francisella
	Legionella
	Moraxella
	Neisseria
	Pseudomonas
	Rochalimaea
	Bacteroides (some species)
Group 5: Facultatively anaerobic gram-negative rods	*Escherichia* (and related coliform bacteria)
	Klebsiella
	Proteus
	Providencia
	Salmonella
	Shigella
	Yersinia
	Vibrio
	Haemophilus
	Pasteurella
Group 6: Gram-negative, anaerobic, straight, curved, and helical rods	*Bacteroides*
	Fusobacterium
	Prevotella
Group 7: Dissimilatory sulfate- or sulfur-reducing bacteria	None
Group 8: Anaerobic gram-negative cocci	None
Group 9: The rickettsiae and chlamydiae	*Rickettsia*
	Coxiella
	Chlamydia
Group 10: Anoxygenic phototrophic bacteria	None
Group 11: Oxygenic phototrophic bacteria	None
Group 12: Aerobic chemolithotrophic bacteria and assorted organisms	None
Group 13: Budding or appendaged bacteria	None
Group 14: Sheathed bacteria	None
Group 15: Nonphotosynthetic, nonfruiting gliding bacteria	*Capnocytophaga*
Group 16: Fruiting gliding bacteria: the myxobacteria	None
II. Gram-positive bacteria that have cell walls	
Group 17: Gram-positive cocci	*Enterococcus*
	Peptostreptococcus
	Staphylococcus
	Streptococcus

From Jawetz E, Melnick JL, Adelberg EA, et al: *Jawetz, Melnick & Adelberg's medical microbiology,* ed 20, Norwalk, Conn, 1995, Appleton & Lange; and Holt JG, Krieg NR, Sneath PHA, et al: *Bergey's manual of determinative bacteriology,* ed 9, Baltimore, 1994, Williams & Wilkins.

Table 7-3		
Major Categories and Groups of Bacteria that Cause Disease in Humans Used as an Identification Scheme in *Bergey's Manual of Determinative Bacteriology*, 9th ed.[1,5]—cont'd		
Group 18: Endospore-forming gram-positive rods and cocci		*Bacillus*
		Clostridium
Group 19: Regular nonsporing gram-positive rods		*Erysepelothrix*
		Listeria
Group 20: Irregular, nonsporing gram-positive rods		*Actinomyces*
		Corynebacterium
		Mobiluncus
Group 21: The mycobacteria		*Mycobacterium*
Groups 22-29: Actinomycetes		*Nocardia*
		Streptomyces
		Rhodococcus
III. Cell wall-less eubacteria. The mycoplasmas or mollicutes		
Group 30: Mycoplasmas		*Mycoplasma*
		Ureaplasma
IV. Archaeobacteria		
Group 31: The methanogens		None
Group 32: Archaeal sulfate reducers		None
Group 33: Extremely halophilic archaeobacteria		None
Group 34: Cell wall-less archaeobacteria		None
Group 35: Extremely thermophilic and hyperthermophilic sulfur metabolizers		None

1. Gram-negative eubacteria
2. Largest group of bacteria
3. Contain many medically significant microorganisms
C. Tenericutes (Mycoplasmas)
  1. Eubacteria lacking cell walls
    a. Because they lack cell walls they are highly pleomorphic
  2. Enclosed by the plasma membrane
    a. Plasma membranes have lipids called sterols which help resist lysis
  3. Mycoplasmas are the smallest self-replicating microorganisms
D. Mendosicutes (Archaeobacteria)
  1. Conventional peptidoglycan in the cell wall is replaced with pseudomurein
  2. Often live in extreme environments
  3. Carry out atypical metabolic processes
  4. No known medically significant species

Fungi

A. Description
  1. Eukaryotic
  2. Nonphotosynthetic protist
  3. Grow well in dark, moist environments
  4. Heterotrophic sapropytes—use preexisting organic products, either living or dead

5. Few species are pathogenic to humans
B. Forms
  1. Molds (mycelial forms)
    a. Long filaments are the structural units called hyphae; multicellular hyphae result in a cobweb-like growth called mycelium
    b. Reproduce by sexual or asexual spores
  2. Yeasts
    a. Oval or spherical single cells
    b. Produce moist, shiny colonies
    c. Reproduce asexually by producing new buds or daughter cells
  3. Dimorphic fungi
    a. Some fungi exhibit characteristics of both molds and yeasts depending on growth conditions
C. Classification of medically important fungi
  1. *Zygomycotina* (the phycomyces)—include the common bread molds *Rhizopus* and *Mucor*
  2. *Ascomycotina* (sac fungi)
    a. Include *Histoplasma, Microsporum, Penicillum* (a source of antibiotics), and *Saccharomyces* (leaven bread and ferment beer and wine)
  3. *Basidiomycotina*—include *Cryptococcus neoformans*
  4. *Deuteromycotina* (the imperfect fungi)
    a. Do not produce sexual spores
D. Fungal diseases (mycoses)

Table 7-4	
Divisions of Multicellular Algae[2]	
Division Rhodophyta (~ 4000 species)	Red algae. Chlorophyll *a* phycobilins, carotenoids; store modified starch; chloroplast membranes not stacked; no flagellated cells in life history; unicellular to multicellular forms; most marine, some freshwater, a few terrestrial; e.g., *Chondrus crispus* (Irish moss), *Polysiphonia, Porphyridium*
Division Phaeophyta (~ 1500 species)	Brown algae. Chlorophylls *a* and *c* carotenoids; store laminarin: all multicellular, some very large and elaborate; almost all marine, e.g., *Fucus, Ascophyllum, Nereocystis, Laminaria*
Division Chlorophyta (~ 7000 species)	Green algae. Chlorophylls *a* and *b* carotenoids; store starch: unicellular to multicellular but not very large or elaborate; mostly freshwater, many marine, some terrestrial; e.g., *Chlorella, Chlamydomonas, Spirogyra, Ulothrix, Oedogonium, Ulva*

From Arms K, Camp PS: *Biology,* ed 4, Philadelphia, 1995, WB Saunders.

1. Generally long-lasting infections
2. Classification
   a. Systemic—can affect a number of tissues and organs
   b. Subcutaneous—beneath the skin
   c. Cutaneous—infect only the epidermis, hair, and nails
   d. Superficial—along hair shafts and in superficial epidermal cells
   e. Opportunistic—generally harmless, but can become pathogenic in a debilitated host

Slime Molds

A. Slime molds—myxomycetes or slime molds are parasitic and injure plants such as cauliflower, radish, and turnip

Protozoa

A. Description
   1. Unicellular
   2. Eukaryotic
   3. Most have a motile feeding stage called trophozoite
   4. Require organic food
   5. Many can form cysts
      a. Protective resting stage
      b. Can serve as a site for division or spreading of pathogenic protozoans (e.g., *Entamoeba histolytica,* which causes amoebic dysentery)
B. Four phyla
   1. Sarcomastigophora—contains flagellates *(Trichomonas vaginalis, Giardia lamblia)* and amoebas *(Entamoeba hystolitica)*
   2. Apicomplexa—contains the sporozoa *(Plasmodium, Toxoplasma, Cryptosporidium)*
   3. Cliophora—contains the ciliates *(Balantidium coli)*
   4. Microspora—contains microsporidial protozoa *(Nosema)*

Algae

A. Description
   1. Photosynthetic, aquatic organisms
   2. Eukaryotic cells
   3. Part of plankton population
   4. Important part of food chains
   5. Cause of environmental problems (e.g., algal blooms and algal toxins)
B. Classification—see Table 7-4

Viruses

A. Properties of a mature virus particle or virion
   1. Has a single type of nucleic acid, RNA or DNA, that contains genetic material, or a genome
   2. Nucleic acid is surrounded by a protein outer coat, the capsid; nucleic acid and capsid compose the nucleocapsid
   3. Capsids may or may not be covered by an envelope
   4. Viral nucleic acid contains the necessary information for programming an infected host cell
   5. Absence of cellular structures
   6. Lack components for energy production and protein synthesis
   7. Obligate intracellular parasites
B. Bacteriophages (bacterial viruses)
   1. Contain either RNA or DNA
   2. Virulent or lytic viruses infect and destroy host cells
   3. Temperate viruses can cause lysis or integrate their DNA into the host cell
      a. If they integrate, they are referred to as a prophage, and a stable association is established between the host and the virus
      b. Bacterial cell containing a prophage is called lysogenic; during the prophage phase cellular changes can occur
C. Plant viruses (most contain RNA)
   1. Viroids

Table 7-5

Major Groups of Viruses[6]

DNA VIRUSES

Virus family	Envelope present	Capsid symmetry	Particle size (nm)	DNA mol. wt ($\times 10^{-6}$)	DNA structure*	Medically important viruses
Parvoviridae	no	icosahedral	22	2	ss linear	B19 virus
Papovaviridae	no	icosahedral	55	3–5	ds circular, supercoiled	papilloma virus, polyomavirus (JC, BK)
Adenoviridae	no	icosahedral	75	23	ds linear	adenovirus
Hepadnaviridae	yes	icosahedral	42	1.5	ds incomplete circular	hepatitis B virus
Herpesviridae	yes	icosahedral	100†	100–150	ds linear	herpes simplex virus, varicella zoster virus, cytomegalovirus, Epstein-Barr virus
Poxviridae	yes	complex	250×400	125–185	ds linear	smallpox virus, vaccinia virus

RNA VIRUSES

Virus family	Envelope present	Capsid symmetry	Particle size (nm)	DNA mol. wt ($\times 10^{-6}$)	RNA structure*	Medically important viruses
Picornaviridae	no	icosahedral	28	2–3	ss linear, non-segmented, +ve sense	poliovirus, rhinovirus, hepatitis A virus, enteroviruses
Reoviridae	no	icosahedral	75	15	ds linear, 10 segments	reovirus, rotavirus, Colorado tick fever
Togaviridae	yes	icosahedral	40–70	4	ss linear, non-segmented, +ve sense	rubella virus, yellow fever virus
Retroviridae	yes	icosahedral	100	7‡	ss linear, 2 segments, +ve sense	HIV, HTLV
Coronaviridae	yes	helical	100	5	ss linear, non-segmented, +ve sense	coronavirus
Calciviridae	no	icosahedral	35–40	2.6	ssRNA +ve sense	Norwalk agent
Orthomyxoviridae	yes	helical	80–120	4	ss linear, 8 segments, −ve sense	influenza virus
Paramyxoviridae	yes	helical	150	6	ss linear, non-segmented, −ve sense	measles, mumps, parainfluenza, respiratory syncytial viruses

*ss, single stranded; ds, double stranded
†the herpesvirus nucleocapsid is 100 nm, but the envelope varies in size; the entire virus can be as large as 200 nm in diameter
‡retrovirus RNA contains 2 identical molecules of mol wt 3.5×10^6
Summary of major families of viruses. The scrapie type agents (responsible for kuru, Creutzfeld-Jacob disease) are not included because they are not viruses and their status remains unclear.
From Mims CA, Playfair JHL, Roitt IM, et al: *Medical microbiology*, London, 1993, Mosby Europe.

Continued

Table 7-5

Major Groups of Viruses—cont'd

RNA VIRUSES—cont'd

Virus family	Envelope present	Capsid symmetry	Particle size (nm)	DNA mol. wt ($\times 10^{-6}$)	RNA structure*	Medically important viruses
Rhabdoviridae	yes	helical	75 × 180	3–4	ss linear, non-segmented, −ve sense	rabies virus
Arenaviridae	yes	helical	80–130	5	ss circular, 2 segments with cohesive ends, −ve sense	lymphocytic choriomeningitis virus
Bunyaviridae	yes	helical	100	5	ss circular, 3 segments with cohesive ends, −ve sense	California encephalitis, sandfly fever viruses
Filoviridae	yes	complex	80 × (800–900)	4.2	ss RNA, −ve sense	Marburg, Ebola virus

    a. Small, single-stranded, circular RNA molecules
    b. Found mainly in plants
D. Human viruses (Table 7-5)
  1. Classified by structure and type of nucleic acid, and mode of replication
  2. Destructive effects to cells are termed cytopathic
  3. Prions
    a. Proteinaceous infectious particles believed to cause kuru, and Creutzfeldt-Jakob disease
    b. Organization, replication, and how they cause disease are unknown
E. Viral replication
  1. Uses biosynthetic mechanisms of the host cell
  2. Phases
    a. Attachment, penetration, and uncoating
    b. Synthesis of viral components
    c. Morphogenesis and release
F. Modes of viral transmission
  1. Direct transmission from person to person
  2. Transmission from animal to animal
  3. Transmission by an arthropod vector
G. Role of virus in cancer
  1. Oncogenous viruses can induce various types of cancer (RNA- or DNA-type viruses)
  2. Proto-oncogenes are highly conserved, "friendly" transforming genes
  3. Mechanisms of oncogene activation[1]
    a. Transduction by a virus
    b. Insertional mutagenesis
    c. Translocation
    d. Gene amplification
    e. Mutation

  4. The mechanism oncogenes play in the development of cancer is unclear

Microbial Virulence and Disease Transfer

A. Bacteria of human importance producing disease or pathologic change—see Table 7-6
B. Definitions
  1. Pathogen—agent producing disease or pathologic change
  2. Opportunist—commensal bacterium that invades the host under favorable conditions
  3. Virulence—the degree of pathogenicity; properties that determine an organism's pathogenicity include invasiveness, ability to multiply in the host, and toxin production
  4. Infection—invasion of the tissue by a pathogenic microorganism and multiplication of the organism
    a. Localized—organism remains in a particular area
    b. Generalized or systemic—microorganism invades the bloodstream and lymphatic system
    c. Acute—runs a rapid course; terminates abruptly
    d. Chronic—slow onset; infection of long duration
    e. Primary—original infection
    f. Secondary—one that follows a primary infection and is often caused by an opportunist
    g. Toxemia—presence of toxin in the blood
    h. Subclinical—no symptoms recognized

Table 7-6

Bacteria of Human Importance[7]

Organism	Diseases	Other features
GRAM-POSITIVE COCCI		
Staphylococcus aureus	Boils, septicemia, food poisoning	Common skin commensal; phage typing identifies virulent strains; enterotoxin causes food poisoning
Streptococcus pyogenes	Tonsillitis, scarlet fever, erysipelas, septicemia	Also causes glomerulonephritis and rheumatic fever, with immunopathologic basis
Streptococcus viridans group (*Streptococcus sanguis,* etc.)	Infective endocarditis	Oral commensals settle on abnormal heart valves during bacteremia
Streptococcus mutans	Dental caries	Regular inhabitant of mouth; initiates plaque on tooth surface
Streptococcus pneumoniae	Pneumonia, otitis mcningitis	Normal upper respiratory tract commensal, can spread to infected or damaged lungs
GRAM-NEGATIVE COCCI		
Neisseria gonorrhoeae	Gonorrhea	Obligate human parasite
Neisseria meningitidis	Meningitis	Obligate human parasite; increased upper respiratory carriage in epidemics
GRAM-POSITIVE BACILLI		
Corynebacterium diphtheriae	Diphtheria	Natural host humans; noninvasive disease caused by toxin
Bacillus anthracis	Anthrax	Pathogen of herbivorous animals that ingest spores; occasional human infection
Clostridium spp.	Tetanus, gas-gangrene botulism	Widely distributed in soil and intestines
GRAM-NEGATIVE BACILLI		
E. coli	Urinary tract infections, infantile gastroenteritis	Normal intestine inhabitant (humans and animals); many antigenic types
Salmonella spp.	Enteric fever; food poisoning	*Salmonella typhi*—natural host humans; invasive; other *Salmonella*—1000 species, mainly animal pathogens
Shigella spp.	Bacillary dysentery	Obligate parasites humans; local invasion only
Proteus spp.	Urinary tract and wound infection	Common in soil, feces; occasionally pathogenic
Klebsiella spp.	Urinary tract and wound infection, otitis, meningitis, pneumonia	Present in vegetation, soil, sometimes feces; pathogenic when host resistance lowered
Pseudomonas aeruginosa	Urinary tract and wound infection	Common human intestinal bacteria; resists many antibiotics
Haemophilus influenzae	Pneumonia, meningitis	Human commensal. Invades damaged lung
Bordetella pertussis	Whooping cough	Specialized human respiratory parasite

From Mims CA: *Pathogenesis of infectious disease,* ed 4, London, 1995, Academic Press, Inc.

Continued

Table 7-6

Bacteria of Human Importance—cont'd

Organism	Diseases	Other features
GRAM-NEGATIVE BACILLI—cont'd		
Yersinia pestis	Plague	Flea-borne pathogen of rodents; transfer to humans as greatest infection in history
Brucella spp.	Undulant fever	Pathogens of goats, cattle, and pigs with secondary human infection
ACID-FAST BACILLI		
Mycobacterium tuberculosis	Tuberculosis	Chronic respiratory infection in man; 10-15 million active cases in the world. Enteric infection with bovine type via milk
Mycobacterium leprae	Leprosy	Obligate parasite of humans. Attacks skin, nasal mucosa, and nerves; 15 million lepers in the world
MISCELLANEOUS		
Vibrio cholerae	Cholera	Obligate parasite of humans; noninvasive intestinal infection
Treponema pallidum	Syphilis	Obligate human parasite; sexual transmission; related nonvenereal human bacteria
Actinomyces israeli	Actinomycosis	Normal human mouth inhabitant
Leptospira spp.	Leptospirosis (Weil's disease, etc.)	Mostly pathogens of animals; human infection from urine of rats, etc.
Legionella pneumophila	Legionnaire's disease	Respiratory pathogen of humans, often acquired from contaminated air-conditioning units

i. Focal—localized in one area and spreads elsewhere
j. Bacteremia—presence of bacteria in the bloodstream
k. Latent—causative agent remains inactive for a time but then becomes active to produce symptoms of the disease
l. Sequelae—long term or permanent damage to diseased tissues or organs
m. Nosocomial—acquired as a result of a hospital stay
n. Sign—objective changes that a physician can observe and measure
o. Symptom—subjective changes in body experienced by the patient/client
5. Infectious disease—interference with the normal functioning of the host; proof by Koch's postulates
    a. Microorganisms present in every case of disease
    b. Microorganism grows in pure culture from the diseased host
    c. Same disease reproduced when pure culture is inoculated into a healthy host
    d. Microorganism recovered from the inoculated host
C. Transmission of disease
    1. Reservoir of infection—all potential sources of the disease agent
        a. Human
            (1) Active cases of infectious disease
            (2) Carriers are persons (asymptomatic) harboring infectious agents potentially pathogenic for other members of the population
            (3) Endogenous infection is one in which the causative organism is derived from the host's own microflora
        b. Animal

(1) Zoonosis—transmission of disease from animal to human
  c. Nonliving
    (1) Water, food, soil, and dust
2. Portals of exit are sources of infectious body fluids
  a. Gastrointestinal tract
  b. Genitourinary system
  c. Oral region
  d. Respiratory tract
  e. Blood and blood derivatives
  f. Skin lesions
  g. Conjunctiva
3. Routes of transmission
  a. Contact
    (1) Direct
    (2) Indirect—involves nonliving reservoir (fomite)
    (3) Droplet transmission (short distance)
  b. Vehicles
    (1) Waterborne transmission
    (2) Foodborne transmission
    (3) Airborne transmission (longer distance)
  c. Vectors
    (1) Arthropods—including ticks, lice, fleas, mosquitoes, and cockroaches

Microbial Virulence Factors

A. Capsules (*Streptococcus pneumoniae*)
  1. Resist the host's defenses by impairing phagocytosis
B. Enzyme production
  1. Include coagulases, kinases, hyaluronidases, and collagenoses
C. Toxin production
  1. Exotoxins
    a. Soluble substances secreted by gram-positive bacteria
    b. Clinically significant exotoxins are associated with botulism, tetanus, diphtheria, gas gangrene, scarlet fever, staphylococcal food poisoning, toxic shock syndrome, and traveler's diarrhea
  2. Endotoxins
    a. Heat-stable lipopolysaccharides—toxic component associated with cell wall
    b. From gram-negative bacteria
    c. Pathologic effects
      (1) Fever
      (2) Interference with hemostatic mechanisms of blood
      (3) Activation of the complement system
      (4) Leukopenia
      (5) Hypotension and shock
      (6) Organ dysfunction
      (7) Activation of complement cascade
      (8) Death

Disease Barriers

A. Normal or indigenous flora
  1. Most highly specialized bacteria; highly adapted to commensal life; cause minimal damage under normal conditions
  2. Includes beneficial microorganisms and pathogens
  3. When ecologic balance is disturbed, infection can occur (e.g., antibiotic therapy may result in *Candida albicans* infection)
B. Nonspecific resistance
  1. Mechanical and chemical barriers (Table 7-7)
    a. Intact skin
    b. Intact mucous membranes
    c. Nasal hairs
    d. Coughing and sneezing reflexes
    e. Tears and eyelashes
    f. Secretions and microorganisms of the gastrointestinal system
  2. Blood and lymphatics
    a. Leukocytes—proportionate number changes in response to infection
      (1) Granulocytes (basophils, eosinophils, neutrophils, or polymorphonuclear leukocytes)
      (2) Agranulocytes (lymphocytes and monocytes)
    b. Lymphatic system transports white blood cells and removes foreign cells and tissue debris
      (1) Consists of lymphatic vessels, lymph fluid, nodes, and lymphocytes
      (2) Reticuloendothelial system (RES)—mononuclear phagocytic cells that remove particulate matter from bloodstream and lymph—e.g., Kupffer cells in the liver
  3. Phagocytosis
    a. Digestion of the invading matter
    b. Accomplished by neutrophils and mature monocytes, or macrophages
  4. Inflammation
    a. Produced by disease agents or irritants such as chemicals, heat, or mechanical injury
    b. Cardinal signs include heat, pain, redness, swelling, and loss of function
    c. Pus formation possible
  5. Fever
    a. Bacterial endotoxins and interleukin-1 can induce fever
    b. Intensifies the effect of interferon
    c. Inhibits the growth of some microorganisms
  6. Antimicrobial substances
    a. Complement system—a defense system consist-

Table 7-7		
Host Defense Mechanisms against Microbial Invasion[8]		
Normal host defense	**Altering agent or disease**	**Possible mechanism**
Physical barriers, e.g., skin and mucous membrane	Burns, trauma, surgery, infection or inflammatory disease	Provides new portals of entry for microorganisms
		Altered physiologic defense, e.g., depressed cough reflex, deficient ciliary action in respiratory tract, defective clearing mechanism in lung, predispose to pulmonary infection
	Foreign body, prostheses	Act as nidus for infection, provide new entry portals or cause obstruction with stasis and infection
	Diagnostic procedures	Provide new portals of entry for microorganisms
	Urinary tract and intravenous catheters	Provide new portals of entry or act as nidus of infection
	Antimetabolites or radiation	Injures rapidly growing cells (e.g., in gastrointestinal tract) to produce ulceration, bleeding, and subsequent portals of entry
	Local ischemia	Alters permeability of skin or mucous membrane to produce new portals of entry, e.g., in diabetes
Normal flora	Burns, trauma	Alters normal skin flora by changing skin ecology and physiochemical properties
	Hospitalization	Host becomes colonized with new or resistant organisms
	Antibiotics	Alter normal microbial flora of skin, mucous membranes, respiratory and gastrointestinal tracts
	Heroin	Mechanism unclear; appears to alter nasal flora
Inflammatory response	Diabetes mellitus	Defects in chemotaxis and phagocytosis aggravated by marked acidosis
	Cirrhosis	Depressed chemotaxis due to serum inhibitor
	Alcohol	Defects in leukocyte mobilization, lung macrophage antibacterial activity
	Sickle cell disease	Deficiency of opsonizing antibody and probable abnormality of the alternate pathway of complement, relative asplenia
	Intrinsic leukocyte abnormalities (e.g., lazy leukocyte syndrome)	Chemotactic leukocyte defect
	Chronic granulomatous disease, myeloperoxidase deficiency	Defects in intracellular killing
	Corticosteroids, radiation and antimetabolites	Various defects in leukocyte mobilization, complement
	Hematopoietic (e.g., leukemia)	Quantitative or qualitative deficiency of polymorphonuclear cells
Immunologic system Humoral system	Multiple myeloma and chronic lymphatic leukemia	Decreased in normal immunoglobins, delayed and defective antibody response to antigenic stimuli, or production of various amounts of abnormal immunoglobulins
	Extremes of age	During first 3 to 6 mo, infant dependent on maternal antibody, possible decrease in delayed immune response in elderly
	Nephrotic syndrome, protein losing enteropathy	Excessive loss of immunoglobulins

From McGhee JR, Michalek SM, Cassell GH, editors: *Dental microbiology,* New York, 1982, Harper & Row.

Continued

Table 7-7

Table 7-7

Host Defense Mechanisms against Microbial Invasion[8]—cont'd

Normal host defense	Altering agent or disease	Possible mechanism
Immunologic system—cont'd	Ataxia telangiectasia, chronic obstructive pulmonary disease, Wiskott-Aldrich syndrome, dysproteinemia, systemic lupus erythematosus	Defective synthesis or excessive catabolism of different classes of protein and abnormalities of complement system
Cell-mediated system	Hodgkin disease Uremia Sarcoidosis Systemic lupus erythematosus Corticosteroids and antimetabolites Combined deficiency states	Depression of delayed hypersensitivity

ing of serum proteins that participate in lysis of foreign cells, inflammation, and phagocytosis

    b. Interferons (α, β, and γ)—interfere with viral replication

C. Specific defenses—Immunity (Table 7-8)

  1. Acquired

    a. Naturally

      (1) Active—person is exposed to an antigen and the body produces antibodies

      (2) Passive—antibodies of a mother are passed to her infant

    b. Artificially

      (1) Active—vaccination with killed, inactivated, or attenuated microorganisms or toxoid

      (2) Passive—injection of immune serum or γ-globulin

D. Hypersensitivity or allergy is an exaggerated response to specific substances; inciting agent is the allergen

  1. Type I (classic, immediate)

    a. Includes asthma, anaphylactic shock, hay fever, and hives

    b. Rapid release of histamines and serotonin

  2. Type II (cytotoxic)

    a. Results in cell destruction

    b. Mother-infant Rh incompatibility, blood transfusion reactions

  3. Type III (immune-complex mediated)

    a. Soluble antigens and immunoglobulins combine

    b. Serum sickness, Arthus reaction

  4. Type IV (cell mediated, delayed)

    a. Depends on T-lymphocyte reactions

    b. Includes contact dermatitis, poison ivy, graft rejection, and the tuberculin skin reaction

Immunodeficiency

See Chapter 6, section on acquired immunodeficiency syndrome.

A. Inability of the immune system to perform normally; properly functioning system recognizes and destroys that which is foreign, or nonself

B. Results in increased susceptibility to infection

C. Autoimmune disease (autoallergic)

  1. Self-antigens stimulate the production of antibodies or sensitized lymphocytes; antigen-antibody complex

  2. Mechanisms

    a. May be due to release of sequestered antigens; escape of tolerance to the "self" antigen at the T-cell level; diminished suppressor T-cell function

    b. Intolerance of "self" antigen due to cross-reactions

    c. Decreased function of suppressor T cells

  3. Includes systemic lupus erythematosus, rheumatoid arthritis, myasthenia gravis, and multiple sclerosis

D. Drug-induced immunosuppression

  1. Used as an adjunct to renal transplantation and other organ grafts; also used for the treatment of immunologically mediated disease

  2. Examples of drugs used include corticosteroids, azathioprine, and cyclosporine; common complication is infection

E. Acquired immunodeficiency syndrome (AIDS)

  1. Definition—disease that occurs because of a defect in cell-mediated immunity; cellular immunity is profoundly suppressed, allowing development of opportunistic infections and cancers; the Centers for Disease Control surveillance case definition[3]

Table 7-8

Immunology Terms[9]

Anaphylatoxin: a substance produced by complement activation (especially C3a, C5a) that results in increased vascular permeability through release of pharmacologically active mediators from mast cells

Antibody (Ab): a protein that is produced as a result of the introduction of an antigen and has the ability to combine with the antigen that stimulated its production

Antigen (Ag): a substance that can induce a detectable immune response when introduced into an animal

B cell (also B lymphocyte): strictly, a bursa-derived cell in avian species and, by analogy, a cell derived from the equivalent of the bursa in nonavian species; B cells are the precursors of plasma cells that produce antibody

Cell-mediated (cellular) immunity: immunity in which the participation of lymphocytes and macrophages is predominant; cell-mediated immunity is a term generally applied to the type IV hypersensitivity reaction (see below)

Chemotaxis: a process whereby phagocytic cells are attracted to the vicinity of invading pathogens

Complement: a system of serum proteins that is the primary mediator of antigen-antibody reactions

Cytokine: a factor such as a lymphokine or monokine produced by cells that affect other cells (e.g., lymphocytes and macrophages) and have multiple immunomodulating functions; cytokines include interleukins and interferons

Cytolysis: the lysis of bacteria or of cells such as tumor or red blood cells by insertion of the membrane attack complex derived from complement activation

Hapten: a molecule that is not immunogenic by itself but can react with specific antibody

Histocompatible: sharing transplantation antigens

Humoral immunity: pertaining to immunity in a body fluid and used to denote immunity mediated by antibody and complement

Hypersensitivity reactions: these occur in 4 types:
(1) Antibody-mediated hypersensitivity:
   Type I. Anaphylactic ("immediate"): IgE antibody is induced by allergen and binds via its Fc receptor to mast cells and basophils; after encountering the antigen again, the fixed IgE becomes cross-linked, inducing degranulation and release of mediators, especially histamine
   Type II. Cytotoxic: antigens on a cell surface combine with antibody, which leads to complement-mediated lysis (e.g., transfusion or Rh reactions) or other cytotoxic membrane damage (e.g., autoimmune hemolytic anemia)
   Type III. Immune complex: antigen-antibody immune complexes are deposited in tissues, complement is activated, and polymorphonuclear cells are attracted to the site, causing tissue damage

(2) Cell-mediated hypersensitivity:
   Type IV. Delayed: T lymphocytes, sensitized by an antigen, release lymphokines upon second contact with the same antigen; the lymphokines induce inflammation and activate macrophages

Immunity:
(1) **Natural immunity:** nonspecific resistance not acquired through contact with an antigen; it includes skin and mucous membrane barriers to infectious agents and a variety of nonspecific immunologic factors, and it may vary with age and hormonal or metabolic activity
(2) **Acquired immunity:** protection acquired by deliberate introduction of an antigen into a responsive host-active immunity is specific and is mediated by either antibody or lymphoid cells (or both)

Immune response: development of resistance (immunity) to a foreign substance (e.g., infectious agent); it can be antibody-mediated (humoral), cell-mediated (cellular), or both

Immunoglobulin: a glycoprotein composed of H and L chains that functions as antibody. All antibodies are immunoglobulins, but not all immunoglobulins have antibody function

Immunoglobulin class: a subdivision of immunoglobulin molecules based on unique antigenic determinants in the Fc region of the H chains; in humans there are 5 immunoglobulin classes: IgG, IgM, IgA, IgE, and IgD

Immunoglobulin subclass: a subdivision of the classes of immunoglobulins based on structural and antigenic differences in the H chains; for human IgG there are 4 subclasses: IgG1, IgG2, IgG3, and IgG4

Interferon: one of a heterogeneous group of low–molecular-weight proteins elaborated by infected host cells that protect noninfected cells from viral infection; interferons, which are cytokines, also have immunomodulating functions

Interleukin: a cytokine that stimulates or otherwise affects the function of lymphocytes and some other cells
   IL-1: induces T-helper cell synthesis of IL-2; activates T cells; induces chemotaxis for neutrophils
   IL-2: stimulates antibody synthesis, T cytotoxic cells, and natural killer cells
   IL-3: stimulates hematopoiesis
   IL-4: induces isotype switching
   IL-5: promotes the growth and differentiation of B cells
   IL-6: antiviral activity; stimulates B cell differentiation; activates T cells
   IL-7: promotes pre-B cell growth
   IL-8: stimulates chemotaxis of neutrophils
   IL-9: promotes T cell growth
   IL-10: induces IL-2 and IL-4 proliferation

Modified from Stites DP, Stobo JD, Wells JV, editors: *Basic & Clinical Immunology*, ed 8, East Norwalk, Conn, 1994, Appleton & Lange.

Table 7-8

Immunology Terms[9]—cont'd

Lymphocyte: a mononuclear cell 7-12 μm in diameter containing a nucleus with densely packed chromatin and a small rim of cytoplasm; lymphocytes include the T cells and B cells, which have primary roles in immunity

Lymphokine: a cytokine that is a soluble product of a lymphocyte; lymphokines are responsible for multiple effects in a cellular immune reaction

Macrophage: a phagocytic mononuclear cell derived from bone marrow monocytes and found in tissues and at the site of inflammation; macrophages serve accessory roles in cellular immunity

Major histocompatibility complex (MHC): a cluster of genes located in close proximity that determines histocompatibility antigens of members of a species

Membrane attack complex: the end product of activation of the complement cascade, which contains C5, C6, C7, and C8 (and C9); the membrane attack complex makes holes in the membranes of gram-negative bacteria, killing them and, in red blood or other cells, resulting in lysis

Monocyte: a circulating phagocytic blood cell that develops into tissue macrophages

Opsonin: a substance capable of enhancing phagocytosis; antibodies and complement are the 2 main opsonins

Opsonization: the coating of an antigen or particle (e.g., infectious agent) by substances such as antibodies, complement components, fibronectin, and so forth, that facilitate uptake of the foreign particle into a phagocytic cell

Polymorphonuclear cell (PMN): also known as a neutrophil or granulocyte, a PMN is derived from a hematopoietic cell of bone marrow and is characterized by a multilobed nucleus; PMNs migrate from the circulation to a site of inflammation by chemotaxis and are phagocytic for bacteria and other particles

T cell (also T lymphocyte): a thymus-derived cell that participates in a variety of cell-mediated immune reactions

T_H (Helper) or CD4 cell–activates cytotoxic and other helper T cells and also helps B cells respond to antigens

T_C (Cytotoxic) or CD8 cell–destroys target cells

T_D (Delay hypersensitivity) cell–causes inflammation associated with allergic reactions and tissue transplant rejection

T_S (Suppressor) or CD8 cell–regulates the immune response

---

includes all HIV-infected persons with CD4+ T-lymphocyte counts of <200 cells/μL or a CD4+ percentage of <14. This definition includes the following clinical conditions and is to be used by all states for AIDS case reporting effective January 1993[3]

a. Candidiasis of bronchi, trachea, or lungs
b. Candidiasis, esophageal
c. Cervical cancer, invasive
d. Coccidioidomycosis, disseminated or extrapulmonary
e. Cryptococcosis, extrapulmonary
f. Cryptosporidiosis, chronic intestinal (>1 month duration)
g. Cytomegalovirus disease (other than liver, spleen, or nodes)
h. Cytomegalovirus retinitis (with loss of vision)
i. Encephalopathy, HIV related
j. Herpes simplex: chronic ulcer(s) (>1 month duration); or bronchitis, pneumonitis, or esophagitis
k. Histoplasmosis, disseminated or extrapulmonary
l. Isosporiasis, chronic intestinal (>1 month duration)
m. Kaposi sarcoma
n. Lymphoma, Burkitt (or equivalent term)

o. Lymphoma, immunoblastic (or equivalent term)
p. Lymphoma, primary, of brain
q. *Mycobacterium avium* complex or *M. kansasii*, disseminated or extrapulmonary
r. *Mycobacterium tuberculosis*, any site (pulmonary or extrapulmonary)
s. *Mycobacterium*, other species or unidentified species, disseminated or extrapulmonary
t. *Pneumocystis carinii* pneumonia
u. Pneumonia, recurrent
v. Progressive multifocal leukoencephalopathy
w. *Salmonella* septicemia, recurrent
x. Toxoplasmosis of brain
y. Wasting syndrome due to HIV

2. Irreversible acquired defect
3. Etiology
   a. Lentivirus subfamily of human retroviruses[10]
   b. Infects lymphocytes, macrophages, promyelocytes, and epidermal Langerhans cells[10]
4. High fatality rate
5. Virus isolated from blood, semen, vaginal secretions, saliva, tears, breast milk, cerebrospinal fluid, amniotic fluid, and urine[10]
6. Transmission
   a. Susceptible exposure to infected blood (e.g., intravenous drug use)

b. Sexual contact

c. Mother to newborn (perinatal)

d. Cofactors (e.g., genital herpes) may influence transmission

7. Centers for Disease Control classification system for HIV-infected adolescents and adults categorizes persons based on CD4+ T-lymphocyte counts and clinical conditions associated with HIV infection[11]

   a. CD4+ T-lymphocyte categories

      (1) Three CD4+ T-lymphocyte categories

         (a) Category 1: ≥500 cells/µL

         (b) Category 2: 200-499 cells/µL

         (c) Category 3: <200 cells/µL

      (2) These categories correspond to CD4+ T-lymphocyte counts per microliter of blood and guide clinical and therapeutic actions in the management of HIV-infected adolescents and adults. The revised HIV classification system also allows for the use of the percentage of CD4+ T cells

      (3) Classification of HIV-infected persons should be based on existing guidelines for the medical management of HIV-infected persons. Thus, the lowest accurate but not necessarily the most recent CD4+ T-lymphocyte count should be used for classification purposes

   b. Clinical categories of HIV infection

      (1) Category A—consists of one or more of the conditions listed below in an adolescent or adult (≥13 years) with documented HIV infection. Conditions listed in categories B and C must not have occurred

         (a) Asymptomatic HIV infection

         (b) Persistent generalized lymphadenopathy

         (c) Acute (primary) HIV infection with accompanying illness or history of acute HIV infection

      (2) Category B—consists of symptomatic conditions in an HIV-infected adolescent or adult that are not included among conditions listed in clinical category C and that meet at least one of the following criteria: the conditions are attributed to HIV infection or are indicative of a defect in cell-mediated immunity, or the conditions are considered by physicians to have a clinical course or to require management that is complicated by HIV infection. **Examples** of conditions in clinical category B include, **but are not limited to**

         (a) Bacillary angiomatosis

         (b) Candidiasis, oropharyngeal (thrush)

         (c) Candidiasis, vulvovaginal; persistent, frequent, or poorly responsive to therapy

         (d) Cervical dysplasia (moderate or severe)/cervical carcinoma in situ

         (e) Constitutional symptoms such as fever (38.5° C) or diarrhea lasting >1 month

         (f) Hairy leukoplakia, oral

         (g) Herpes zoster (shingles), involving at least two distinct episodes or more than one dermatome

         (h) Idiopathic thrombocytopenic purpura

         (i) Listeriosis

         (j) Pelvic inflammatory disease, particularly if complicated by tubo-ovarian abscess

         (k) Peripheral neuropathy

         (l) For classification purposes, category B conditions take precedence over those in category A. For example, someone previously treated for oral or persistent vaginal candidiasis (and in whom a category C disease has not developed) but who is now asymptomatic should be classified in clinical category B

      (3) Category C—includes the clinical conditions listed in the AIDS surveillance case definition. For classification purposes, once a category C condition has occurred, the person will remain in category C

8. Secondary neoplasms

   a. Kaposi sarcoma—skin lesions; may be oral; multiple small reddish blue, purple, or hyperpigmented brown papules, plaques, or nodules (Fig. 7-3)

   b. B-cell lymphomas

9. Opportunistic infections

   a. Cytomegalovirus (CMV)—frequently involves the eye, causing retinal lesions

   b. Tuberculosis

   c. *Pneumocystis carinii*

   d. Oral and esophageal infection from *Candida albicans*

   e. Herpes simplex viruses I and II

10. Incidence/prevalence

   a. About 14 million people have been infected with the AIDS virus worldwide; the number could rise as high as 40 million by the year 2000

   b. About 223,000 people living with AIDS in the United States

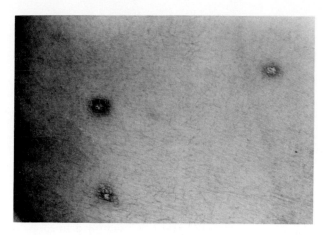

Fig. 7-3 Kaposi sarcoma. (Courtesy Dr. Charles Barr, Beth Israel Medical Center, New York.)

c. As of 1997, leading cause of death among men (25-44 years) and the fifth among women (15-44 years) in the United States

d. Mortality is approximately 50%

e. Risk factors

(1) Unsafe sexual practices

(2) Exposure to blood or blood products

(3) Intravenous drug use

(4) Infant of infected individual

f. Transmission to healthcare personnel providing care to infected individuals is rare[6]

11. Treatment

a. No known cure or vaccine

b. Vaccine will need to be targeted both to free virus in bloodstream and to virus present in infected host cells

c. The one class of drugs the FDA has approved for HIV therapy are the synthetic nucleotide analogues

(1) azidothymidine (AZT)

(2) dedeoxyinosine (ddI)

(3) dedeoxycytidine (ddC)

(4) dedeoxythymidine (D4T)

d. Some success being observed with protease inhibitors

12. Oral manifestations

a. Hairy leukoplakia

b. Herpetic lesions

c. Oral and esophageal candidiasis

d. Kaposi sarcoma

e. Linear gingival erythema and necrotizing ulcerative periodontitis

f. Human papillomavirus

g. Lymphoma

h. Recurrent aphthous ulcers

Infections of the Skin, Nails, and Hair

A. Bacterial infections

1. Tetanus

a. Etiology—*Clostridium tetani*

b. Pathogenesis/transmission—by spores that germinated in the wound and produce tetanus-causing toxin

c. Clinical findings/symptoms

(1) Trismus (stiff jaw); eventually locked jaw

(2) Spasms of facial muscles

(3) Dysphagia

(4) Difficulty in breathing

2. Leprosy

a. Etiology—*Mycobacterium leprae*

b. Pathogenesis/transmission—transmitted by prolonged direct contact or inhalation of organisms

c. Clinical findings/symptoms

(1) Skin lesions

(2) Oral lesions are tumorlike masses of tissue involving the oral lining, tongue, lips, or palate

3. *Pseudomonas aeruginosa* infections

a. Pathogenesis

(1) Low pathogenicity for humans, except in debilitated persons (e.g., burn victims or those taking antibiotics or immunosuppressive drugs)

(2) Ubiquitous in nature

b. Clinical findings/symptoms

(1) *Pseudomonas* dermatitis

(a) Self limiting rash associated with swimming pools, hot tubs, and saunas

(2) Otitis externa

(a) Infection of the external ear canal

4. Staphylococcal infections

a. Etiology—*Staphylococcus aureus*

b. Pathogenesis—determined by extracellular factors and invasion properties of the strain

c. Clinical findings/symptoms

(1) Most *S. aureus* strains are resistant to penicillin

(2) Causes furuncles (boils), carbuncles, and impetigo

5. Streptococcal infections

a. Etiology—*Streptococcus pyogenes* (group A β-hemolytic)

b. Pathogenesis

(1) Determined by portal of entry

(2) Diffuse and rapidly spreading infection

c. Clinical findings/symptoms

(1) Scarlet fever

(a) Acute inflammation of the upper respiratory tract

(b) Generalized rash caused by erythrogenic exotoxin

(c) Oral mucosa is red; "strawberry tongue"

(d) Sequelae from group A streptococcal infection include rheumatic fever and hemorrhagic glomerulonephritis

(2) Erysipelas

6. Acne

a. Etiology-*Propionibacterium acnes*

b. Pathogenesis—*P. acnes* metabolizes sebum trapped in hair follicles and sets up an inflammatory response

B. Fungal infections

1. Etiology—dermatophytes most important

2. Pathogenesis—grow only within dead keratinized tissue

3. Clinical findings/symptoms

a. Inflammatory response, especially at the border of lesions; patching; scaling

b. Antigens can cause an allergic response

4. Candidiasis

a. Etiology—*Candida albicans*

b. Pathogenesis

(1) Dissemination and sepsis in compromised patients (opportunistic infection)

(2) Normal inhabitant of the skin and mucosal surfaces

(3) Predisposing factors include diabetes mellitus, pregnancy, obesity, vitamin deficiency, use of broad-spectrum antibiotics, and immunologic defects

c. Clinical findings/symptoms

(1) Angular cheilitis or perleche

(a) Infection in corners of the mouth

(b) Can also be caused by *Staphylococcus aureus*

5. Other dermatophytes include tineas ("ringworms") and *Sporothrix schenckii*

C. Viral infections

1. Herpes simplex

a. Etiology—herpes simplex virus

b. Pathogenesis

(1) Transmission through oral and ocular secretions

(2) Virus is present in saliva even in apparent good health

(3) Indirect contact (e.g., fomites)

(4) Infects epithelial cells

(5) Establishes a latent infection from retroviruses

c. Clinical findings/symptoms

(1) Types

(a) Type I—generally above the waist; commonly found in and around the mouth

(b) Type II—herpes genitalis

(2) Frequently asymptomatic

(3) Most commonly acute gingivostomatitis; usually in children—fever, malaise, irritability, local lymphadenopathy, and anorexia; red, edematous gingiva and adjacent mucosa; lesions are vesicles with yellowish contents that rupture and ulcerate; bright margin of erythema; sharply defined; pain may be severe; duration of about 7 days; self-limiting

(4) Herpetic whitlow infection of fingers; can be caused by herpes simplex type I or II; abrupt onset; local irritation; tenderness, edema, erythema, and vesicles; difficult to differentiate from bacterial pyoderma caused by staphylococci

(5) Recurrent secondary infections by type I

(a) Virus now latent but permanently established in nerve ganglia (carrier)

(b) Infections may be induced by stress, sun, or colds

(6) Herpes labialis is the most common clinical manifestation of recurrent infection

(a) Cold sores, fever blisters

(b) Vesicles on an erythematous base

(c) Prodromal burning and hyperesthesia

(d) Swollen lymph nodes

(7) Intraoral lesions

(a) Usually found on the mucosa or hard palate overlying bone

(b) Small, discrete lesions; vesicles of clear fluid; ulcerate with a red base

(8) Keratoconjunctivitis (ocular herpes)

(a) Conjunctiva and cornea

(b) Repeated attacks may result in blindness

2. Chickenpox

a. Etiology—varicella zoster virus

b. Pathogenesis

(1) Route of infection via the mucosa of the upper respiratory tract

(2) Highly infectious

(3) Virus probably circulates in the blood and localizes on the skin

(4) Incubation period 2 weeks

c. Clinical findings/symptoms

(1) Earliest symptoms are malaise and fe-

ver, followed by a rash and formation of vesicles

(2) Oral lesions may occur throughout the mouth and appear like small canker sores or aphthae; vesicles rupture quickly

3. Shingles
   a. Etiology—varicella zoster virus
   b. Pathogenesis
      (1) Reactivation of latent virus in dorsal root ganglion
      (2) Closely follows area of innervation
      (3) Chickenpox and shingles represent different forms of infection by the same agent
      (4) Virus resides in ganglia; usually affects sensory nerves (thoracic area is the most often involved; ophthalmic division of the trigeminal nerve is the next most involved)
   c. Clinical findings/symptoms
      (1) Mostly found in adults
      (2) Malaise, fever, followed by severe pain in area
      (3) Rash and vesicles along the nerve trunk

4. Warts
   a. Etiology—papillomaviruses
   b. Pathogenesis—tropic for epithelial cells of skin and mucous membranes
   c. Clinical findings/symptoms
      (1) Skin warts, plantar warts, flat warts, genital condylomas, laryngeal papillomas
      (2) Oral warts are papular or nodular lesions covered with papilliferous projections; also may look like common warts

5. Measles
   a. Etiology—rubeola virus
   b. Pathogenesis
      (1) Access by the respiratory tract
      (2) Spreads to regional lymphoid tissue
      (3) Primary viremia disseminates the virus
      (4) Secondary viremia seeds the epithelial surfaces of the body
   c. Clinical findings/symptoms
      (1) Koplik's spots
         (a) Small bluish white spots with a red surrounding zone; cannot be wiped off
         (b) Occur on the buccal mucosa opposite the molars
      (2) Followed by a diffuse skin rash and fever
      (3) Bacterial secondary infections occur, such as middle ear infections or pneumonia

6. German measles
   a. Etiology—rubella virus
   b. Pathogenesis
      (1) Occurs through the upper respiratory tract
      (2) Incubation period 2 to 3 weeks
   c. Clinical findings/symptoms
      (1) Malaise, low-grade fever, rash, and lymphadenopathy
      (2) Rash starts on face; extends to trunk and extremities

7. Lyme disease
   a. Etiology—*Borrelia burgdorferi* (spirochetes)
   b. Pathogenesis
      (1) Transmitted by ticks
      (2) Antigen-antibody complexes may be responsible for arthritic or neurologic difficulties
   c. Clinical findings/symptoms
      (1) Skin lesion, headache, fever, myalgia, lymphadenopathy, cardiac disease
      (2) Recurring neurologic symptoms and/or arthritis

Infections of the Respiratory Tract

A. Bacterial infections
   1. Diphtheria
      a. Etiology—*Corynebacterium diphtheriae*
      b. Pathogenesis
         (1) Droplets or by contact to susceptible individuals
         (2) Bacilli grow on mucous membranes or in skin abrasions
         (3) Damage caused by the systemic distribution of toxin
      c. Clinical findings/symptoms
         (1) Enlarged lymphadenopathy of the neck, possibly edema
         (2) Pseudomembrane forms on tonsils
   2. Streptococcal pharyngitis ("strep" throat)
      a. Etiology—*Streptococcus pyogenes*
      b. Pathogenesis: transmitted by the respiratory route and contaminated food, water, and milk
      c. Clinical findings/symptoms: severe inflammation of the throat and tonsils; fever

B. Viral infections—common cold (Table 7-9)

Lower Respiratory System Infections

A. Bacterial infections
   1. Bacterial pneumonia
      a. Inflammation of the lungs
      b. Caused by several species
      c. Legionnaire's disease
         (1) Etiology—*Legionella pneumophila*
         (2) Pathogenesis
            (a) Inhalation of bacteria from aerosols
            (b) Bacteria multiply in lungs and produce pneumonia

Table 7-9

Viral Infections of the Respiratory Tract[1]

Syndromes	Main symptoms	Most common viral causes		
		Infants	Children	Adults
Common cold	Nasal obstruction, nasal discharge	Rhino Adeno	Rhino Adeno	Rhino Corona
Pharyngitis	Sore throat	Adeno Herpes simplex	Adeno Coxsackie	Adeno Coxsackie
Laryngitis/croup	Hoarseness, "barking" cough	Parainfluenza Influenza	Parainfluenza Influenza	Parainfluenza Influenza
Tracheobronchitis	Cough	Parainfluenza Influenza	Parainfluenza Influenza	Influenza Adeno
Bronchiolitis	Cough, dyspnea	Respiratory syncytial Parainfluenza	Rare	Rare
Pneumonia	Cough, chest pain	Respiratory syncytial Influenza	Influenza Parainfluenza	Influenza Adeno

From Jawetz E et al: *Jawetz, Melnick & Adelberg's medical microbiology*, ed 20, East Norwalk, Conn, 1995, Appleton & Lange.

(3) Clinical findings/symptoms
   (a) Influenza-like illness with pneumonia
   (b) Complications include renal failure, gastrointestinal hemorrhage, and respiratory failure
d. Pneumococcal pneumonia
   (1) Etiology—most common agent is *Streptococcus pneumoniae*
   (2) Pathogenesis
     (a) Spread by droplets from nasal or pharyngeal secretion
     (b) Person may contract the disease or become an asymptomatic carrier
     (c) Predisposing factors include age, impaired resistance, and bacteremia
   (3) Clinical findings/symptoms: symptoms include sudden onset of high fever, chills, chest pain, dry cough, and rust-colored sputum
2. Tuberculosis
a. Etiology—*Mycobacterium tuberculosis*
b. Pathogenesis
   (1) Transmitted by inhalation of droplets, ingestion, or direct inoculation; disseminated by coughing, sneezing, or contaminated dust
   (2) Predisposing factors include advanced age, chronic alcoholism, poor nutrition, diabetes mellitus, and prolonged stress
   (3) Incubation period is generally 28 to 47 days; can be as long as 6 months

c. Clinical findings/symptoms
   (1) Symptoms vary but include fever, general discomfort, weight loss, tubercle formation (nodule in lung tissue), night sweats, persistent cough
   (2) Oral lesions may appear as an ulcerated lesion on the tongue or mucosa (rare)
   (3) Diagnosis by a skin test and a radiograph
3. Whooping cough (pertussis)
a. Etiology—*Bordetella pertussis*
b. Pathogenesis—transmitted by inhalation of droplets; produce toxins
c. Clinical findings/symptoms—spasmodic coughing and gasping noise with inhalation
4. Psittacosis
a. Etiology—*Chlamydia psittaci*
b. Pathogenesis—humans infected by inhaling dust contaminated with excreta of infected birds
c. Clinical findings/symptoms—symptoms in humans include fever and pneumonitis; spread from the lungs to the spleen, brain, or other organs; mild, coldlike illness; may be asymptomatic
5. Mycoplasmal pneumonia
a. Etiology—*Mycoplasma pneumonia*
b. Pathogenesis—transmitted in airborne droplets. Binds respiratory epithelium and inhibits ciliary action.
c. Clinical findings/symptoms—mild symptoms of low fever, cough, and headache which persist for 3 weeks or longer

B. Fungal infections
1. Histoplasmosis
   a. Etiology—*Histoplasma capsulatum*
   b. Pathogenesis—transmitted by inhalation of spores, especially in excreta of wild birds, poultry, and bats
   c. Clinical findings/symptoms
      (1) Skin lesions are common
      (2) Meningitis
2. Pneumocystis pneumonia
   a. Etiology—*Pneumocytis carinii*
   b. Pathogenesis—inhalation of spores; more common disease among immunodepressed persons, especially those with AIDS
C. Viral infections
1. Influenza virus infection
   a. Etiology—Orthomyxoviruses
   b. Pathogenesis
      (1) Genome can undergo sudden genetic reassortment
      (2) Spread by airborne droplets or contact with contaminated objects
      (3) Virus attaches to the respiratory epithelium
   c. Clinical findings/symptoms
      (1) Chills, headache, dry cough, fever, malaise, muscular ache, and inflammation of the soft palate
      (2) Secondary infection by *S. aureus., H. influenzae, S. pyogenes,* and *S. pneumoniae;* may result in bronchitis and pneumonia
      (3) Reye syndrome may be a complication[1]
2. Hantavirus pulmonary syndrome
   a. Etiology—Hantavirus
   b. Pathogenesis—inhalation of excretions from deer mice
   c. Clinical findings/symptoms—severe cold followed by an internal hemorrhage of blood plasma in the lungs

Infections of the Gastrointestinal Tract

A. Bacterial infections
1. Cholera
   a. Etiology— *Vibrio cholerae*
   b. Pathogenesis
      (1) Transmitted by unsanitary living conditions and the ingestion of the organisms
      (2) Organisms attach to microvilli of epithelial cells; produce toxin
   c. Clinical findings/symptoms: nausea, vomiting, profuse diarrhea, and abdominal cramps
2. Salmonellosis
   a. Etiology—several species of *Salmonella*
   b. Pathogenesis—organisms enter via the oral route usually by contaminated food or drink
   c. Clinical findings/symptoms—organisms cause enteric fevers, bacteremia, followed by focal lesions or endocarditis
3. Shigellosis (bacillary dysentery)
   a. Etiology—*Shigella dysenteriae, Shigella flexneri, S. boydii,* and *S. sonnei*
   b. Pathogenesis
      (1) Transmitted through contaminated food or water
      (2) Invades mucosal epithelium
   c. Clinical findings/symptoms—abdominal pain, fever, and watery diarrhea
4. Traveler's diarrhea
   a. Etiology—*Escherichia coli*
   b. Pathogenesis—member of the normal intestinal flora
5. Typhoid fever
   a. Etiology—*Salmonella typhi*
   b. Pathogenesis—transmitted through contaminated food or water
   c. Clinical findings/symptoms
      (1) Fever, severe headache, abdominal pain, and abdominal rash
      (2) Complications include carrier state, relapses, inflammation of the gallbladder, and intestinal bleeding
6. Helicobacter peptic disease syndrome
   a. Etiology—*Helicobacter pylori*
   b. Pathogenesis—*H. pylori* produce ammonia, which neutralizes stomach acid, allowing the bacteria to colonize the stomach mucosa
   c. Clinical findings/symptoms—peptic ulcers
7. Food poisoning
   a. Botulism
      (1) Etiology—*Clostridium botulinum*
      (2) Pathogenesis
         (a) Regularly contaminates human, plant, and animal food products
         (b) Produces a deadly toxin that acts on nerves
         (c) Transmitted through improperly preserved foods and uncooked fish and meats; foods do not appear contaminated
      (3) Clinical findings/symptoms
         (a) Difficulty in speaking, blurred vision, inability to swallow, heart failure, and respiratory paralysis
         (b) Infant botulism may be one of the causes of sudden infant death syndrome

Table 7-10

Characteristics of the Various Types of Viral Hepatitis[12]

Characteristic	Hepatitis A	Hepatitis B	Hepatitis C	Hepatitis D	Hepatitis E	Hepatitis G*
Transmission	Fecal–oral (ingestion of contaminated food, ice, and water)	Parenteral (injection of contaminated blood or other body fluids)	Parenteral	Percutaneous, permucosal, or parenteral (host must be coinfected with hepatitis B or as a superinfection in persons with chronic HBV infection)	Fecal–oral (contaminated drinking water most common)	Bloodborne and co-infection with HCV
Agent	Hepatitis A virus (HAV); single-stranded RNA; no envelope	Hepatitis B virus (HBV); double-stranded DNA; envelope	Hepatitis C virus (HCV); single-stranded RNA; envelope	Hepatitis D virus (HDV); defective single-stranded RNA; envelope from HBV	Hepatitis E virus (HEV); single-stranded RNA; no envelope	Hepatitis G virus, although causal association remains to be confirmed
Incubation period	15 to 50 days	45 to 160 days	2 to 26 weeks	Uncertain	15 to 60 days	Acute disease spectrum unknown
Manifestations or symptoms	Children under 6 years may not have signs of illness; severe cases: fever, headache, malaise, jaundice, fatigue, loss of appetite, nausea, dark urine	Clinical manifestations are age-dependent; anorexia, nausea, malaise, vomiting, jaundice, dark urine, clay-colored stools, abdominal pain, and more likely to progress to severe liver damage	Similar to HBV	Severe liver damage; high mortality rate	Similar to HAV, but pregnant women may have high mortality rate; less common symptoms include arthralgia, diarrhea, pruritis, urticaria	
Chronic liver disease	No	Yes	Yes	Yes	No	No
Vaccines	Vaccine is a sterile suspension of inactivated virus	Genetically engineered	None	HBV vaccine is protective because coinfection required	None	None

From Tortora GJ, Funke BR, Case DL: *Microbiology: An introduction*, ed 5, Menlo Park, NJ, 1995, Benjamin/Cummings.
*Information on Hepatitis G from Centers for Disease Control and Prevention, 1997.

b. Staphylococcal food poisoning
  (1) Etiology—toxin produced by staphylococci (usually *S. aureus*) in unrefrigerated foods such as dairy products, custard, cream-filled products, fish, or processed meats
  (2) Pathogenesis
    (a) Caused by ingestion of preformed enterotoxin
    (b) Incubation period is from 1 to 8 hours
    (c) Symptoms include violent nausea, vomiting, diarrhea; no fever
    (d) Rapid convalescence; self-limiting
c. Perfringens poisoning
  (1) Etiology—*Clostridium perfringens*
  (2) Pathogenesis
    (a) Precise mechanism is unknown
    (b) Organism produces an enterotoxin
    (c) Incubation period is 8 to 16 hours
  (3) Clinical findings/symptoms
    (a) Symptoms are similar to those of staphylococcal food poisoning

    (b) Usually self-limiting
B. Viral infections
  1. Hepatitis A (Table 7-10)
    a. Etiology—hepatitis A virus (HAV)
    b. Pathogenesis
      (1) Oral-fecal route in unsanitary conditions; contaminated food and water; close intimate contact
      (2) Rarely through the blood
      (3) Incubation period is from 15 to 50 days
      (4) Usually occurs in children and young adults
    c. Clinical findings/symptoms
      (1) Preicteric (before jaundice appears)—similar to influenza; fever, headache, nausea, vomiting, fatigue, and abdominal pain, loss of appetite, dark urine
      (2) Icteric—jaundice (rare in children); other symptoms continue
      (3) Anicteric—without jaundice; two to three times more prevalent than icteric state; symptoms resemble those of influenza

(4) Recovery and immunity
  (a) Antibody to hepatitis A virus (anti-HAV) is usually in the blood 2 weeks after onset
  (b) Most individuals recover completely in 4 to 6 weeks
  (c) Immunity develops following recovery
  (d) No carrier state develops
  (e) Usually self-limiting
d. Active immunization
  (1) Hepatitis A vaccine (Havrix) at least 2 weeks before expected exposure; booster dose recommended 6 to 12 months later for adults
  (2) Vaccine may be administered concomitantly with immune globulin in persons exposed to hepatitis A
2. Hepatitis B infection (Table 7-10)
  a. Etiology
    (1) Hepatitis B virus
    (2) Terminology
      (a) Hepatitis B virus (HBV)
      (b) Hepatitis B surface antigen (HBsAg) (Australian antigen)—serologic indicator found in the blood during an acute, chronic, or carrier state of hepatitis B
      (c) Hepatitis B core antigen (HBcAg)
      (d) Hepatitis B "e" antigen (HBeAg)—considered an indicator of infectivity; may indicate development of chronic liver disease
      (e) Antibody to HBsAg (anti-HBs or HBsAb)—present after clinical or subclinical infection; represents immunity
      (f) Antibody to HBcAg (anti-HBc or HBcAb)—found during the active phase of acute hepatitis; "with anti-HBs" means immunity
      (g) Antibody to HBeAg (anti-HBe or HBeAb)—indicates a low infectivity rate but not necessarily complete elimination of infectivity
    (3) Pathogenesis
      (a) Infected blood or serum through parenteral inoculation (e.g., blood transfusions, contaminated dental or medical instruments, needles and syringes used by drug abusers, and accidental self-inoculation by health care professionals)
      (b) Other body fluids, including saliva, semen, tears, urine, sweat, and nasopharyngeal secretions
      (c) Oral or sexual contact or other close personal contact
      (d) Coughing or sneezing and aerosols
      (e) Salivary transmission by way of hands, instruments, and other equipment is important in the practice of dental hygiene
    (4) Incubation
      (a) Between 45 and 160 days
      (b) Presence of HBsAg indicates ability to be infective
    (5) Symptoms
      (a) Similar to hepatitis A
      (b) Slower in onset; longer duration
      (c) Asymptomatic to severe and debilitating
      (d) Person may have subclinical disease and remain undiagnosed
      (e) May result in chronic liver disease; strong evidence for link between chronic hepatitis B infection and hepatocellular carcinoma (liver cancer)
    (6) Recovery
      (a) Development of anti-HBs indicates immunity
      (b) Approximately 3% of those infected develop a chronic carrier state; HBsAg still present after 6 months; carriers are usually asymptomatic and often undetected
    (7) Risk factors
      (a) Exposure to virus at birth (e.g., newborn infants born to mothers with HBV)
      (b) Exchange of blood or blood products (e.g., hemodialysis, blood transfusions, or intravenous drug use)
      (c) Exposure to blood or blood products (e.g., health care workers)
      (d) Close intimate contact
      (e) Unsafe sexual practices
      (f) Institutionalization (e.g., Down syndrome and prisoners)
      (g) Immunosuppressive therapy
    (8) Immunization
      (a) Two types of HBsAg vaccines
        (1) Obtained from HBsAg-positive carriers (Heptavax)
        (2) Obtained from recombinant DNA in yeast cells (Recombivax)
      (b) Passive immunization results from hepatitis B immune globulin (HBIg); used for postexposure prophylaxis; preferably within 24 to 48 hours; partially effective
3. Hepatitis D (formerly delta hepatitis) (Table 7-10)
  a. Pathogenesis

(1) Similar to HBV

(2) Infection dependent on HBV replication

b. Clinical findings—may produce acute exacerbations of chronic HBV and fulminant hepatitis

4. Hepatitis type C (Table 7-10)

a. Pathogenesis—hepatitis C virus

(1) Originally named non-A, non-B hepatitis virus

(2) Risk factors include blood transfusion, intravenous drug use, and heterosexual transmission

b. Clinical findings/symptoms

(1) Mild symptoms; most asymptomatic

(2) Development of chronic hepatitis in 50%; may develop into cirrhosis and hepatocellular carcinoma

5. Hepatitis type E (Table 7-10)

a. Pathogenesis—hepatitis E virus

(1) Originally named non-A, non-B hepatitis virus

(2) Enteric transmission

(3) Epidemic outbreaks occurring in developing countries

6. Hepatitis G (Table 7-10)

7. Cytomegalovirus infections

a. Etiology—cytomegalovirus

b. Pathogenesis[1]

(1) Cytomegalic inclusion disease is caused by intrauterine or perinatal infection

(2) Virus may persist in organs in a latent state or as a chronic infection

(3) Cytomegalovirus mononucleosis occurs spontaneously or through blood transfusions

(4) Route of infection is unknown in older infants, children, and adults

c. Clinical findings/symptoms

(1) In infants may result in death

(2) In infants, prematurity, jaundice, pneumonitis, CNS damage, and mental or motor retardation can occur

(3) Acquired infection in children results in hepatitis, pneumonitis, and anemia

(4) Cytomegalovirus mononucleosis produces a mononucleosis-like disease

Infections of the Circulatory System
Diseases of the Heart

A. Rheumatic fever

1. Etiology

a. β-Hemolytic group A *Streptococcus* infection

2. Pathogenesis

a. Rheumatic fever—hypersensitivity state developing after streptococcal infection; associated with β-hemolytic group A *Streptococcus*

b. Heart valves become inflamed; subsequent abnormal growths of connective tissue; scarring of valves occurs, resulting in rheumatic heart disease

3. Clinical findings/symptoms

a. Fever, malaise, polyarthritis, inflammation of heart

b. Defective heart valves are a result of carditis

c. Heart valve damage

(1) Stenosis—narrowing of the valve opening

(2) Valvular insufficiency—failure of the valve to close completely

4. Antibiotic premedication is necessary before dental treatment

B. Bacterial endocarditis

1. Etiology—most often associated with the normal flora of respiratory or intestinal tract

2. Pathogenesis

a. Inflammatory condition of the heart; microbial colonization of the endothelial membrane that covers the inner surface of the heart and valves

b. Predisposing factors

(1) Heart valves scarred by rheumatic fever

(2) Arteriosclerosis

(3) Individuals who have had cardiac surgery (valve replacement)

(4) Narcotic abusers

(5) Individuals with low resistance to infection

c. Dental and dental hygiene procedures may allow bacteria to enter the bloodstream (bacteremia) and lodge in the heart valves

3. Clinical findings/symptoms

a. Fever, anemia, weakness, and heart murmur

b. Inflammation of the heart

c. May result in death

4. Antibiotic prophylaxis is recommended for all dental clients with predisposing factors (see Chapter 8, section on antiinfectives and Appendix B)

Other Microbial Diseases of the Circulatory System

A. Bacterial infections

1. Tularemia

a. Etiology—*Francisella tularensis*

b. Pathogenesis

(1) Transmitted by biting arthropods, contact with infected tissue, aerosols, and ingestion of contaminated food or water

c. Clinical findings/symptoms

(1) Enlargement of lymph nodes

(2) Fever, malaise, headache, regional pain

2. Rickettsial infections

a. Etiology—obligate intracellular parasites
b. Pathogenesis
  (1) Transmitted by arthropods such as fleas, lice, mites, and ticks
  (2) Rocky Mountain spotted fever (tick vector)
  (3) Typhus (flea-borne, common in rats)
  (4) Rickettsialpox (mouse-mite vector)— usually involves fever, rash, and vasculitis
B. Protozoan infections—malaria
  1. Spread by mosquitoes
  2. Symptoms include shaking, chills, fever, headache, and nausea
C. Infectious mononucleosis
  1. Etiology—Epstein-Barr virus (EBV)
  2. Pathogenesis
    a. Transmitted by kissing or sharing drinking glasses
    b. Involves the lymph nodes and spleen; increase in lymphocytes
  3. Clinical findings/symptoms
    a. Acute leukemia-like infection
    b. Primarily found in young adults
    c. Symptoms include mild jaundice, fever, enlarged and tender lymph nodes, sore throat, bleeding gingiva, and general weakness

Infections of the Reproductive and Urinary System

Urinary Tract Infections

A. Etiology—primarily caused by *E. coli*
B. Pathogenesis
  1. Predisposing conditions
    a. Diabetes mellitus
    b. Neurologic diseases (e.g., polio and spinal cord injury)
    c. Lesions (e.g., kidney stones) interfering with urine flow
    d. Eclampsia of pregnancy
C. Clinical findings/symptoms
  1. Blood in urine
  2. Accumulation of fluid in tissue
  3. Pain

Reproductive System Infections

A. Venereal diseases
  1. Gonorrhea
    a. Etiology—*Neisseria gonorrhoeae,* a gram-negative aerobic bacteria
    b. Pathogenesis
      (1) Risk of infection is 20% to 30% from a single exposure for men; higher percentage in women
      (2) Grow primarily in the genitourinary tract;

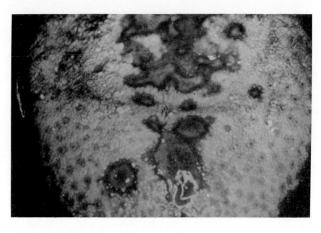

Fig. 7-4 Gonococcal glossitis. (Courtesy Beverly Entwistle Inman, formerly with Department of Applied Dentistry, University of Colorado School of Dentistry, Denver, Colo.)

possess pili that allow attachment to mucosal cells and resist phagocytosis; can infect the eye, rectum, and throat
      (3) Type of host epithelium influences invasiveness
        (a) Columnar and transitional epithelium highly susceptible
        (b) Stratified squamous epithelium highly resistant
    c. Clinical findings/symptoms
      (1) Sometimes found in the pharynx; localized yellow or gray-white raised patches or generalized lesions with a gray membrane; membrane sloughs, leaving a bright area; seen on the gingiva, tongue, and soft palate; may have itching or burning
      (2) Gonococcal glossitis (Fig. 7-4)
      (3) Newborn's eyes may be infected on passing through the birth canal (ophthalmia neonatorum); use of silver nitrate or antibiotic after birth reduces incidence
      (4) Men experience painful, frequent urination and mucous- and pus-containing discharge
      (5) Women often do not have symptoms; may have urethral or vaginal discharge, backache, or abdominal pain
      (6) Oral infection results in pharyngitis, glossitis, or stomatitis including some areas of ulceration (see Fig. 14-13, p. 592)
      (7) Complications include sterility, disseminated infection, and meningitis
  2. Syphilis (Fig. 7-5)
    a. Etiology
      (1) *Treponema pallidum*
      (2) Spirochete, anaerobic

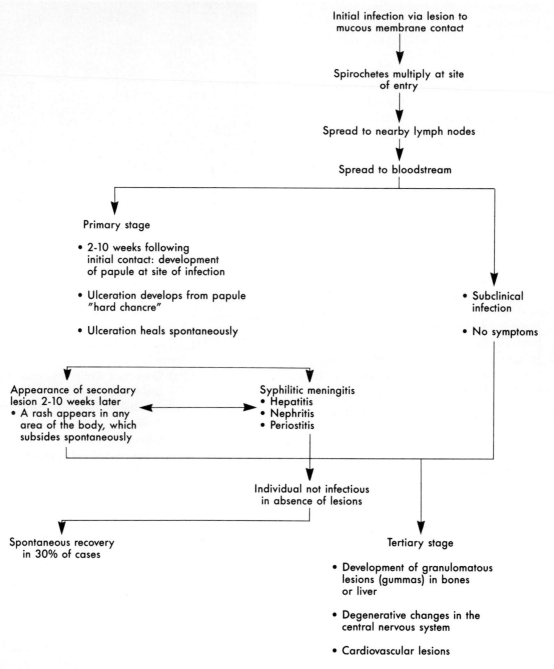

Fig. 7-5   Stages of infection for syphilis.

b. Pathogenesis
(1) Usually transmitted by sexual contact with skin or mucous membrane lesions
(2) Infection limited to the human host
(3) Congenital syphilis occurs when organism crosses the placenta
(4) *T. pallidum* can pass through abraded skin and can probably pass through intact mucous membranes

(5) Organisms gain access to the circulatory system; affect all organs; rapidly spread to the lymphatic system and bloodstream
c. Clinical findings/symptoms (Fig. 7-6)
(1) Primary stage
(a) Chancre—single granulomatous lesion; often asymptomatic; common on the lips; may involve the tongue and oral mucosa; highly contagious; occurs 2 to 3

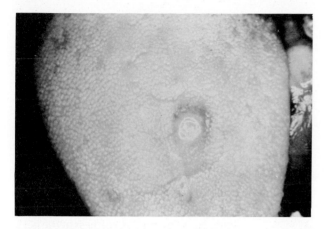

Fig. 7-6   Chancre lesion of primary syphilis. (Courtesy Beverly Entwistle Inman, formerly with Department of Applied Dentistry, University of Colorado, Denver, Colo.)

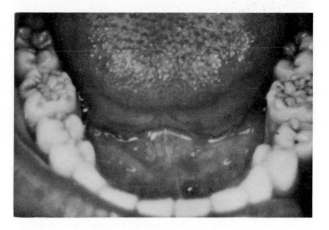

Fig. 7-8   "Mulberry molars" of congenital syphilis. (Courtesy Beverly Entwistle Inman, formerly with Department of Applied Dentistry, University of Colorado, Denver, Colo.)

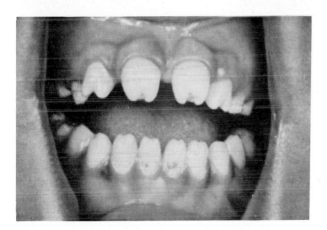

Fig. 7-7   Hutchinson's incisors of congenital syphilis. (Courtesy of Beverly Entwistle Inman, formerly with Department of Applied Dentistry, University of Colorado, Denver, Colo.)

weeks after exposure and lasts 3 to 5 weeks; red, small, elevated nodule; heals spontaneously; no scarring

(2) Secondary stage
    (a) Appears 6 to 8 weeks after exposure; patient can be asymptomatic for 2 to 6 months and then have secondary lesions appear
    (b) Flulike symptoms
    (c) Skin rashes—maculopapular rash on the face, hands, and feet
    (d) Mucous patches on the lips, soft palate, and tongue—painless shallow ulcers; grayish white areas may be removed, leaving red areas of erosion; highly contagious
    (e) Swollen lymph nodes

(3) Tertiary stage
    (a) Gumma—inflammatory granulomatous lesion with a central zone of necrosis; may be on the tongue, palate (perforation), or facial bones; soft, swollen areas or tumors; not contagious and usually asymptomatic
    (b) Often takes 5 to 20 years to develop
    (c) Involvement of the central nervous system and spinal cord leads to paresis, loss of fine muscle coordination, or personality changes
    (d) Involvement of the cardiovascular system—major cause of death

(4) Congenital syphilis
    (a) Hutchinson's incisors—notched, bell-shaped (Fig. 7-7)
    (b) "Mulberry molars"—first molars are irregular with poorly developed cusps (Fig. 7-8)
    (c) Skin, mucous membrane lesions
    (d) High mortality

3. Genital herpes
  a. Etiology
    (1) Herpesvirus
    (2) Type II—herpes genitalis (genital herpes)
  b. Pathogenesis
    (1) Transmitted by sexual contact
  c. Clinical findings/symptoms
    (1) Lesions appear 2 to 7 days after exposure
    (2) Lesions appear in or on the genitalia and skin
    (3) Lesions may ulcerate early and be painful or crust over
    (4) Fever, lymphadenopathy, malaise, anorexia

(5) Initial lesions subside and heal in 2 to 3 weeks

(6) Recurrent lesions follow a milder course

(7) Highly infectious

(8) Primary and recurrent infections

(a) Most (90%) primary infections are sub-clinical

(b) Recurrent infections in women often serve as a source of neonatal herpes

4. Toxic shock syndrome (TSS)

a. Etiology—*S. aureus*

b. Pathogenesis

(1) Short incubation period of 1 to 8 hours

(2) Toxin is produced by organism

c. Clinical findings/symptoms

(1) Rash, violent nausea, vomiting, and diarrhea but no fever

(2) Rapid convalescence

(3) Often occurs within 5 days of the onset of menses

(4) Can recur

Infections of the Central Nervous System

A. Bacterial infections

1. Meningitis

a. Etiology

(1) Aseptic meningitis—caused by a variety of agents including viruses, spirochetes, bacteria, mycoplasmas, or chlamydias

(2) Meningococcal meningitis—caused by *Neisseria meningitidis*

b. Pathogenesis—meningococcal meningitis is transmitted by droplet inhalation

c. Clinical findings/symptoms

(1) Aseptic meningitis produces an acute onset, fever, headache, and stiff neck

(2) Meningococcal meningitis produces headache, vomiting, stiff neck, and a coma within a few hours

B. Viral infections

1. Poliomyelitis

a. Etiology—poliomyelitis virus

b. Pathogenesis—transmitted via the mouth and intestines

c. Clinical findings/symptoms

(1) Flaccid paralysis; destruction of motor neurons in the spinal cord

(2) Acute inflammation of the meninges

(3) May range from mild illness to paralysis

2. Rabies

a. Etiology—rabies virus

b. Pathogenesis

(1) Transmitted to humans from the bite of a rabid animal

(2) Incubation period is from 4 to 6 weeks or longer

c. Clinical findings/symptoms—include visual difficulties, painful throat spasms, convulsions, and respiratory paralysis

3. Viral encephalitis

a. Etiology—commonly caused by arboviruses

b. Pathogenesis—replicate in and spread by arthropods, usually mosquitoes or ticks

c. Clinical findings/symptoms

(1) Cause extensive nervous tissue damage and encephalitis

(2) Symptoms include fever, chills, nausea, fatigue, drowsiness, pain, stiffness of the neck, general disorientation, blindness, deafness, and paralysis

C. Protozoan infection—Toxoplasmosis

1. Etiology

a. *Toxoplasma gondii*

b. Sources include infected cat feces, contaminated raw meat and soil, and rodents (cats may eat infected mice)

2. Pathogenesis

a. Inhaling or ingesting cysts when handling cat litter or sandboxes frequented by the infected cat

b. Eating raw meat

c. Through the placenta (especially important for pregnant women not to eat raw or undercooked meat and not to handle litter boxes)

3. Clinical findings/symptoms

a. Resembles infectious mononucleosis in adults

b. Congenital infection can lead to stillbirth, psychomotor dysfunction, blindness, and other congenital defects

D. Fungal infection—cryptococcoses

1. Etiology—*Cryptococcus neoformans*

2. Pathogenesis

a. Organism favors pigeon droppings

b. Transmitted by inhalation of dehydrated yeasts

3. Clinical findings/symptoms

a. Meningitis most common; often associated with immunocompromised patients

b. Disseminated disease can affect the skin, lungs, or other organs

Infections of the Eye

A. Bacterial infections

1. Conjunctivitis

a. Etiology—*Haemophilus aegyptius*

b. Clinical findings

(1) Purulent conjunctivitis

(2) Epidemic in warmer climates

B. Viral diseases

1. Trachoma/inclusion conjunctivitis

a. Etiology—*Chlamydia trachomatis*
b. Pathogenesis—transmitted by person-to-person contact; associated with poor sanitation and personal hygiene
c. Clinical findings/symptoms
  (1) Inflammation of conjunctiva; scarring of eyelids and/or cornea; can lead to secondary infection; can lead to partial or complete blindness
  (2) "Swimming pool conjunctivitis," which results in conjunctiva inflammation, is usually self-limiting
2. Adenovirus infection
a. Etiology—adenoviruses
b. Pathogenesis
  (1) Hand-to-eye contact is most important
  (2) "Swimming pool conjunctivitis" most likely caused by waterborne route
c. Clinical findings/symptoms
  (1) Inflammation of conjunctiva, excessive lacrimation, periorbital edema
3. Coxsackievirus A24 is one of the causes of acute hemorrhagic conjunctivitis
4. Herpetic keratitis
a. Etiology—primarily due to HSV-I; occasionally due to HSV-II
b. Pathogenesis—cytolytic
c. Clinical findings/symptoms
  (1) Severe keratoconjunctivitis; corneal ulcers or vesicles on the eyelids
  (2) May recur
  (3) May cause blindness
5. Conjunctivitis caused by Newcastle disease virus
a. Etiology—an avian paramyxovirus
b. Clinical findings/symptoms
  (1) Inflammation of conjunctiva
  (2) Recovery in 10 to 14 days

Helminths (Worms) as Human Parasites

A. Nematodes (roundworms)
1. Hookworm infection
a. Adult worm lives in the human small intestine
b. Transmitted through contaminated soil, skin, or contaminated water
c. Symptoms include iron deficiency anemia, abdominal pain, and protein deficiency; mild infections are asymptomatic
2. Pinworm (seatworm, *Enterobious vermicularis* infection)
a. Adult worm lives in the intestine
b. More common in children
c. Tickling or intense itching in the perianal area
d. Transmission
  (1) Ingestion of larvae

  (2) Handling of fomites (infected bedding and clothes)
  (3) Contaminated hands
  (4) Inhalation of eggs
3. Trichinosis
a. Adult worm lives in the intestine
b. Transmitted by eating improperly cooked or inadequately processed pork
c. Symptoms include diarrhea, muscular pain, and nervous disorders; many light infections are asymptomatic
B. Platyhelminthes (flatworms)
1. Tapeworms (cestodes)
a. Adult worm lives in the small intestine
b. Transmitted by contaminated or inadequately cooked beef, pork, lamb, or fish
c. Symptoms include nausea and abdominal discomfort; many cases are asymptomatic or have poorly defined symptoms
2. Flukes (trematodes)
a. Adults can live in the liver, lungs, bladder, or large intestine, causing various diseases
b. Transmitted by inadequately cooked or contaminated fish, vegetation, or crayfish; also by swimming or working in contaminated water

Microbiology of the Oral Cavity

Normal Oral Flora

A. Composition (Table 7-11)
1. Flora of mucous membranes (Tables 7-12 and 7-13)—different types of surfaces affect the number and variety of organisms present[13]
2. Tongue—papillae allow for a large surface area for colonization
3. Saliva—organisms derived mainly from the dorsum of the tongue and plaque
4. Tooth surfaces (plaque)
a. Interproximal surfaces
  (1) Inaccessible to routine oral hygiene
  (2) Plaque bacteria can proliferate undisturbed
  (3) Common site for caries
b. Occlusal pits and fissures
  (1) Morphologic condition allows for proliferation
  (2) Common site for caries
c. Gingival sulcus is an area of stagnation and bacterial proliferation—environmental influences include an increase in crevicular fluid, desquamation of epithelial cells, and bacterial acid products
d. Remaining coronal surfaces

Table 7-11

Genera Found in the Oral Cavity

Streptococcus	Neisseria
Micrococcus	Veillonella
Peptostreptococcus	Haemophilus
Peptococcus	Bacteroides
Actinomyces	Fusobacterium
Lactobacillus	Capnocytophage
Bacterionema	Actinobacillus
Rothia	Eikenella
Arachnia	Campylobacter
Propionibacterium	Vibrio (Camphylobacteria
Leptotrichia	rectus)
Bifidobacterium	Selenomonas
Eubacterium	Leptotrichia
Prevotella	Treponema
Enterobacteriaceae	Porphyromonas
(rare)	Clostridium (rare)
	Corynebacterium (rare)
	Bacillus (rare)

    (1) Can be covered with plaque if oral hygiene is absent
    (2) Plaque formation limited by the cleansing action of saliva, soft tissue movement, and the action of food particles
    (3) Oral bacteria colonize in a predictable succession

B. Factors influencing microbial composition
  1. Nutrient requirements include fermentable carbohydrates and amino acids
  2. Nutrient sources
    a. Exogenous sources include the host's diet, especially dietary sugar needed for acid and polysaccharide production
    b. Endogenous sources
      (1) Saliva
      (2) Gingival exudate
      (3) Epithelial cells and leukocytes
      (4) Flora continues to exist even when humans and animals are fed by a stomach tube
      (5) Certain bacteria use metabolic by-products from other bacteria
  3. pH requirements
    a. Dietary sugars provide a selective force favoring predominance of certain organisms that tolerate an acidic medium
    b. Strains of S. mutans, related streptococci, and lactobacilli are both acidogenic (produce acid) and aciduric (tolerate low pH values)
  4. Oxygen concentration—plaque is a predominantly anaerobic mass, even on exposed surfaces

  5. Microbial interactions
    a. Oral bacteria colonize in a predictable succession
    b. Interspecies antagonisms—acid-producing and hydrogen peroxide–producing bacteria inhibit staphylococci and corynebacteria; acid producers include S. mutans and lactobacilli; hydrogen peroxide producers include S. mitis, S. sanguis, and viridans streptococci
    c. Microbial aggregation
      (1) Certain species undergo reactions between cell surfaces
      (2) Such reactions may contribute to the formation and accumulation of plaque
  6. Saliva
    a. Flow rate bears some relationship to caries susceptibility
    b. Rate of secretion is correlated to the buffering capacity
    c. Components aid in bacterial attachment to teeth
    d. Immunologic and nonimmunologic components may adversely affect attachment to teeth or inhibit bacterial growth
      (1) High molecular weight glycoproteins inhibit adherence
      (2) Antibacterial components include lysozyme, lactoperoxidase, lactoferrin, and salivary thiocyanate
      (3) Secretory IgA inhibits microbial attachment
    e. Flow of saliva removes bacteria from oral surfaces

Development of Oral Microflora

A. Oral cavity usually sterile at birth
B. Number of organisms increases 8 hours after birth
C. At 12 months most children have
  1. Streptococci
    a. S. salivarius predominate
    b. S. mutans and S. sanguis are not established until teeth erupt
    c. S. mutans disappears when full-mouth extractions occur; reappears with dentures
  2. Staphylococci
  3. Veillonella organisms
  4. Neisseria organisms
  5. Actinomyces organisms
  6. Lactobacilli
  7. Nocardia organisms
  8. Fusobacterium organisms
D. Preschool-age child
  1. Resembles flora of adult
  2. Prevotella melaninogenicus and spirochetes not common

Table 7-12

Intraoral Site Distribution of Various Indigenous and Supplemental Members of the Oral Flora[13]

Species	Saliva	Tongue	Plaque Supragingival	Plaque Subgingival
S. salivarius	+++	+++		
S. sanguis	++	++	+++	+
S. mitior	++	++	++	++
S. milleri	±	±	+ to +++	0
S. mutans	± to +	±	+ to +++	0
Lactobacillus sp.	± to +	+	+	±
Actinomyces sp.	+	+	++	± to ++
Fusobacterium sp.	0	0	±	± to ++
Capnocytophaga	0	0	±	± to +
Treponema sp.	0	0	±	± to +++
B. melaninogenicus	0	0	±	± to +
Porphyromonae gingivalis	0	0	0	0 to +
A. actinomycetemcomitans	0	0	±	0 to +
Veillonella	+	+	++	++

0 = not usually detected; ± = rarely present; + = usually present in low proportions; ++ = usually present in moderate proportions; +++ = usually present in high proportions.
From Newman MG, Nisengard R: *Oral microbiology and immunology,* ed 2, Philadelphia, 1994, WB Saunders.
Adapted from following sources: Gibbons RJ, van Houte J: *J Periodontol* 44:347, 1973; Loesche WJ: *J Periodontol* 6:245, 1968; Mejare B, Edwardsson S: *Arch Oral Biol* 20:757, 1975; Slots, et al: *Infect Immun* 29:1013, 1980; Loesche WI, Syed SA: Unpublished data.

Table 7-13

Percentage Distribution of Bacteria in Different Sites in the Oral Cavity[13]

Bacterium	Location Tongue	Location Gingival crevice	Location Saliva	Location Cheek	Location Supragingival plaque
S. mutans	0.3	—	0.2	0.5	3.9
S. sanguis*	9.0	—	47.0	29.0	75.0
S. salivarius*	55.0	0.5	47.4	10.7	0.7
B. melaninogenicus†	0.4	4.5	0.4	0.3	0.3
Treponema sp‡	—	1.5	—	—	>0.1
Lactobacillus sp.	—	—	0.01	—	>0.01

From Newman MG, Nisengard R: *Oral microbiology and immunology,* ed 2, Philadelphia, 1994, WB Saunders.
(Data taken from Socransky and Manganiello: *J Peridontol* 42:486, 1971, with permission.)
*% of facultative streptococci.
†% of total cultivable flora.
‡% of microscopic counts.

Bacterial Plaque

See Chapter 11, section on bacterial plaque.
A. Definition
  1. Deposit formed by the colonization of teeth by members of the normal oral flora
  2. Complex of bacteria in the matrix mainly of bacterial polysaccharides

B. Stages of formation
  1. Cell-free pellicle
    a. High molecular weight salivary glycoproteins
    b. Quickly colonized by bacteria
  2. Bacterial colonization
    a. Streptococci show early dominance
    b. *S. sanguis* is usually one of the first colonizers,

Table 7-14

Factors Influencing the Composition and Maturation of Bacterial Plaque[13]

I. *Factors of bacterial origin*
   A. Extracellular products: Glucans (skeleton of plaque)
                               Fructans (energy resources)
   B. Bacterial interactions: Coaggregation reactions
   C. Plaque ecology:
      Dietary changes: Sucrose intake—aciduric bacteria
      Oxygen environment—anaerobic bacteria
      Nutritional interactions—bacterial succession
      Bacteriocin production
II. *Host-derived factors*
   A. Mechanical oral cleansing mechanisms
   B. Saliva:
      pH, lactoperoxidase, lactoferrin, lysozyme
      Salivary glycoproteins: adhesion mechanisms
   C. Host-immune responses:
      Oral secretions—IgA
      Crevicular fluid: leukocytes, IgG, IgM, complement, etc.

From Newman MG, Nisengard R: *Oral microbiology and immunology,* ed 2, Philadelphia, 1994, WB Saunders.

Table 7-15

Predominant Subgingival Bacteria Associated with Gingival Health[13]

Streptococcus mitis
Streptococcus sanguis
Staphylococcus epidermidis
Rothia dentocariosus
Actinomyces viscosus
Actinomyces naeslundii
Small spirochetes

From Newman MG, Nisengard R: *Oral microbiology and immunology,* ed 2, Philadelphia, 1994, WB Saunders.

---

but lactobacilli, nocardiae, veillonellae, or neisseriae may be found in the beginning
   c. Filamentous bacteria (*Veillonella* and *Actinomyces* species) appear in 7 to 14 days
   d. Complexity increases
   e. Respiration becomes increasingly anaerobic (increase in *Bacteroides, Actinomyces, Capnocytophaga, Treponema, Prevotella melaninogenicus,* and *Fusobacterium* organisms)
C. Factors affecting adherence and retention
   1. Salivary glycoprotein
      a. Affinity for hydroxyapatite
      b. Causes bacteria to aggregate
   2. Specific bacterial attachment mechanisms
      a. Electrostatic forces
      b. Bacterial surface components (adhesions) bind specific sites of the pellicle
      c. Hydrophobic interactions
   3. Bacterial competition
      a. Relative numbers of a species may affect colonization patterns
      b. *S. sanguis* has a stronger affinity for enamel than *S. mutans;* fewer numbers of *S. mutans* are in saliva and available to compete for tooth sites
   4. Bacterial interactions—some evidence that *S. mutans* and *S. sanguis* are antagonistic
   5. Natural local cleansing activity and retentive areas

6. Diet
D. Plaque polysaccharides
   1. Extracellular dextrans—structural component of plaque
      a. Synthesized from sucrose
      b. Properties
         (1) Insoluble
         (2) May mediate attachment of bacteria to dental tissues
         (3) May entrap bacterial enzymes or metabolic products
         (4) Ability of *S. mutans* to produce glucans appears essential for cariogenicity
   2. Levans (fructans)—produced by *S. mutans, S. sanguis, S. salivarius, Lactobacillus casei,* and *Lactobacillus acidophilus*
      a. Soluble
      b. Reserve nutrients
E. Microbial composition of plaque (Table 7-14)
   1. Bacterial composition of supragingival (supramarginal) plaque
      a. Thin layer; 1 to 20 cells thick
      b. Mostly gram-positive facultative anaerobic organisms
      c. Most predominant organisms are *S. sanguis, A. viscosus,* and *A. naeslundii*
      d. Other species found include *Actinomyces israelii, S. mutans, Veillonella, Fusobacterium* organisms, and *Treponema capnocytophaga*
   2. Bacterial composition of normal gingival crevicular plaque (Table 7-15)
      a. Predominantly gram-positive filamentous bacteria; some gram-positive and gram-negative cocci and rods
      b. Quantity of species relatively constant; proportions of species vary among people and even within the same mouth

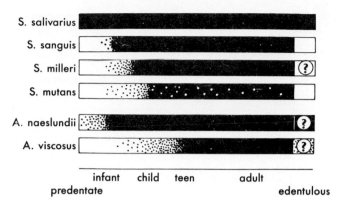

S. salivarius

S. sanguis

S. milleri

S. mutans

A. naeslundii

A. viscosus

| infant | child | teen | adult |

predentate · edentulous

Fig. 7-9 Comparative oral isolation frequencies for *A. viscosus, A. naeslundii,* and oral streptococci during the human life span. (From Ellen RP: Oral colonization by gram-positive bacteria significant to periodontal disease. In Genco RJ, Mergenhagen SE, editors: *Host-parasite interactions in periodontal diseases,* Washington, DC, 1982, ASM Publications.)

3. Bacterial composition associated with age (Fig. 7-9)
4. Calculus
    a. Inorganic salts, 70% to 90%
    b. Microbes similar to those of the gingival crevicular area
    c. Main role in periodontal disease is to serve as a collection site for more bacteria

Dental Caries

A. Prerequisites for caries development
    1. Cariogenic bacteria
    2. Supply of substrate for acid production
    3. Susceptible host
B. Cariogenic bacteria
    1. Essential properties
        a. Acidogenic and aciduric; acid must be produced and low pH maintained for a long period
        b. Ability to attach to tooth surfaces
        c. Formation of protective matrix
    2. Streptococci
        a. *S. mutans*
            (1) Most strongly cariogenic bacteria in animals
            (2) Hard surfaces are a prerequisite for presence; organisms disappear if teeth are extracted; reappear with dentures
            (3) Homofermentive lactic acid former
            (4) Produces insoluble glucans
            (5) High-sucrose diet is generally associated with an increased *S. mutans* population
            (6) Usually found in early stages of plaque formation
            (7) Association of *S. mutans* is based on epidemiologic findings
        b. *S. sanguis*
            (1) Produces glucans
            (2) Some strains are cariogenic in animals
            (3) Colonizes teeth
            (4) Present in plaque and sometimes tongue
        c. *S. mitior*
            (1) Synthesizes intracellular polysaccharides
            (2) Cariogenic in animals
            (3) Found on nonkeratinized mucosa: cheek, lip, ventral surfaces of the tongue
        d. *S. milleri*
            (1) Cariogenic in animals
            (2) Generally found near the gingival crevice
        e. *S. salivarius*
            (1) Usually has a strong affinity for oral soft tissues
            (2) Minor degree of cariogenic significance in humans
            (3) Found in plaque, throat, nasopharynx, oral mucosa, and dorsum of tongue
    3. Lactobacilli
        a. Present in small numbers in plaque
        b. Increase in number in the mouth when the sugar content in the diet is high
            (1) Sites in the mouth where sugar is retained
            (2) Carious lesions act as retention sites
        c. Strongly acidogenic and aciduric
        d. Cariogenic in animals; found mainly in fissures
        e. Evidence for causative role in human caries does not appear to be strong
    4. *Actinomyces*
        a. *A. viscosus* and *A. naeslundii* cause root-surface caries in animals
        b. Plaque former
        c. Ferment glucose to produce mostly lactic acid
        d. *A. naeslundii* is present in tongue, saliva, and young children
        e. *A. viscosus* is present in supragingival plaque
C. Acid production in plaque
    1. Decalcification of teeth occurs by acids produced through bacterial fermentation
    2. Cariogenic plaque, when exposed to sugar, shows a decrease in pH that is low enough to decalcify enamel within minutes; pH returns to resting levels after approximately 40 minutes; even though sugar is washed away by saliva, pH can remain at a low level for 20 minutes
    3. Important features of the acid production process
        a. Amount of plaque
        b. The predominant microflora
        c. Rate of salivary flow
        d. Substrate characteristics
        e. Location of plaque

Table 7-16

Bacterial Types in Health, Gingivitis, and Periodontitis[13]

	Health		Gingivitis		Periodontitis	
	Freq*	Prop*	Freq	Prop	Freq	Prop
Small spirochetes	25%	2%	82%	13%	100%	32%
Medium spirochetes	0	0	41	3	100	8
Large spirochetes	0	0	24	1	38	2
Small motile rods	13	1	12	1	75	7
Large motile rods	6	1	47	2	50	3
Curved motile rods	19	1	71	5	94	16
Filaments	31	4	53	4	63	2
Fusiforms	44	7	94	17	81	9
Small nonmotile rods	69	18	100	38	94	13
Cocci	94	66	92	15	50	4
Other nonmotile rods	5	2	3	2	4	7

*Freq = frequency (percent) of detection in sites by dark-field microscopy; Prop = proportion (mean percent) of dark-field groups per site.
From Newman MG, Nisengard R: *Oral microbiology and immunology,* ed 2, Philadelphia, 1994, WB Saunders.
Adapted from Savitt ED, Socransky SS: *J Periodontol Res* 19:111, 1984.

4. More lactic acid present than any other acid
D. Bacterial substrates and diet
  1. Sucrose
    a. Main substrate for cariogenic bacteria
    b. Important in the formation of smooth-surface caries
    c. Metabolized to form acids and glucans
    d. Essential for caries production in animals
    e. Epidemiologic evidence established its role in human caries
    f. Increase in frequency of sucrose; consumption is associated with an increase in caries
    g. High cariogenic effect when retained on teeth for a long period
  2. Starches
    a. Low cariogenicity
    b. Probably influences plaque microflora
E. Host factors
  1. Tooth surface
    a. Caries formation influenced by tooth morphology and arch form
    b. Enamel surfaces are probably more caries-resistant than the subsurface
  2. Saliva
    a. Functions affecting the carious process
      (1) Clearance of food
      (2) Buffer activity
      (3) Bacterial aggregation
      (4) Antibacterial function (e.g., IgA, lysozyme, salivary peroxidase)
    b. Rate of flow and buffering abilities
      (1) As flow rate increases, pH rises

      (2) High salivary flow rates and buffering are associated with low caries activity

Inflammatory Periodontal Diseases

See Chapter 11, section on diseases of the periodontium.
A. Types
  1. Gingivitis (Table 7-16)
    a. Inflammation of gingiva in response to the bacteria in plaque
    b. Early gingivitis
      (1) Plaque is thicker and more complex than in health; 100 to 300 cells thick
      (2) *Actinomyces* organisms predominate
      (3) Mostly gram-positive organisms
    c. Chronic gingivitis
      (1) Gram-negative anaerobic organisms increase; rods form 75% of the subgingival flora
      (2) Presence of *Actinomyces, Fusobacterium,* and *Bacteroides* organisms
      (3) Spirochetes elevated at affected sites
  2. Adult periodontitis
    a. Extension of inflammatory changes into deeper periodontal structures with resulting bone loss
    b. May be multiple diseases that share similar characteristics
    c. Pockets provide a favorable environment for bacteria
    d. Different bacterial populations associated with destructive periodontitis have been described (Table 7-17)

Table 7-17

Principal Bacteria Associated with Periodontal Disease

Adult periodontitis	*Porphyromonas gingivalis, Prevotella intermedia, B. forsythus, Campylobacter rectus*
Refractory periodontitis	*Bacteroides forsythus, P. gingivalis, Campylobacter rectus, P. intermedia*
Localized juvenile periodontitis (LJP)	*Actinobacillus actinomycetemcomitans, Capnocytophaga*
Periodontitis in juvenile diabetes	*Capnocytophaga, A. actinomycetemcomitans*
Pregnancy gingivitis	*P. intermedia*
ANUG	*P. intermedia*, intermediate-sized-spirochetes

From Newman MG, Nisengard R: *Oral microbiology and immunology,* ed 2, Philadelphia, 1994, WB Saunders.

e. Progression is usually episodic
f. Suspected organisms include
  (1) *Prevotella intermedia*
  (2) *Porphyromonas gingivalis*
  (3) *Eubacterium* sp.
  (4) *Fusobacterium nucleatum*
  (5) Spirochetes
  (6) *Bacteroides forsythus*
  (7) *Campylobacter rectus*
3. Juvenile periodontitis
  a. Onset at puberty (12 to 14 years)
  b. Associated with functional defects in neutrophils or monocytes; familial distribution
  c. Lesions localized to permanent first molars and/or incisors
  d. Sparse amounts of plaque
  e. Prominent microflora
    (1) *Capnocytophaga ochraceus*
    (2) *Actinobacillus actinomycetemcomitans*
    (3) *Prevotella intermedius* and *Eikenella corrodens* may be involved
4. Acute necrotizing ulcerative gingivitis (ANUG)
  a. Anaerobic infection of gingival margins causing ulceration and, if allowed to progress, destruction of gingivae and underlying bone; acute sudden onset
  b. Interproximal areas affected first
  c. Appears to be opportunistic infection based on predisposing factors
  d. Predominant microflora
    (1) *Prevotella intermedia*
    (2) Intermediate-sized spirochetes

(3) *Fusobacterium* sp.
  (4) *Selenomonas* sp.
5. Linear gingival erythema (formerly HIV-gingivitis)
  a. Appearance
    (1) Extensive and/or spontaneous bleeding
    (2) Fiery red color of the alveolar and attached gingival tissues; petechiae may be present
    (3) A red outline following the free gingival margin
    (4) May be similar to ANUG but does not respond as readily to local therapy
  b. Pain
  c. Evidence indicates that gingivitis may progress to periodontitis if left untreated
  d. Occurs in persons infected with HIV
6. Necrotizing ulcerative periodontitis (formerly HIV-periodontitis)
  a. Appearance
    (1) Rapid destruction of periodontal attachment and bone; may lead to exposure of alveolar bone and sequestration
    (2) Lack of pocketing due to destructive nature of the disease
    (3) Localized or generalized
  b. Jaw pain or deep aching pain; fever
  c. May be episodic
  d. Occurs in persons infected with HIV
B. Bacterial plaque and periodontal disease
  1. Factors determining the severity of periodontal disease
    a. Level of oral hygiene
    b. Nature of bacterial flora of plaque
    c. Host resistance and immunity
  2. Evidence supports a microbial etiology of periodontal disease
    a. Gram-negative microorganisms are the principal bacteria associated with disease
    b. Plaque associated with gingivitis and periodontitis has different bacterial populations
    c. Current approaches (Table 7-18)
  3. Pathogenic mechanisms of plaque bacteria
    a. Attachment mechanisms—attachment to the tooth surface may depend on early colonizers of tooth surface and pellicle (e.g., *Streptococcus* and *Actinomyces* organisms, which are gram-positive)
    b. Products of bacteria
      (1) Bacteria themselves may invade tissue
      (2) Products may result in tissue destruction
        (a) Endotoxins
        (b) Enzymes (collagenase, lysozyme, and hyaluronidase)
  4. Immunologic aspects of periodontal disease

Table 7-18

Identification of the Bacterial Etiology in Periodontal Diseases

1. Large numbers of the bacteria are *associated* with the disease state and absence or reduced numbers associated with health
2. *Elimination* or suppression of the organism reverses or reduces the disease
3. Elevated *host responses* are associated with the disease
4. *Animal pathogenicity* similar to periodontal disease occurs upon implantation of the organism(s) into germ-free animals
5. The bacteria possess potentially *pathogenic mediators* that could contribute to the disease process

From Newman MG, Nisengard R: *Oral microbiology and immunology,* ed 2, Philadelphia, 1994, WB Saunders.

a. Bacteria of plaque are antigenic in varying degrees; present a challenge to the immune system
b. Immune responses are just as likely to be protective as they are injurious to tissue
c. Mechanisms of tissue destruction may involve anaphylactic, cytotoxic, immune complex, and cell-mediated or delayed hypersensitivity reactions
d. Participation of the humoral immune system
    (1) Lymphocytes and plasma cells are the predominant cells in the gingiva in the vicinity of plaque
    (2) Antibody production is stimulated
    (3) Complement system is activated
        (a) Mediates inflammatory response and immunologic reactions
        (b) Complement is activated by plaque bacteria, either by endotoxin (lipopolysaccharide) or by bacterial antigen–antibody complexes
        (c) Involved with chemotaxis (directed migration of inflammatory cells)
e. Participation of the cell-mediated immune system
    (1) Cell-mediated immunity leads to release of lymphokines (e.g., osteoclast activating factor)
    (2) Conflicting reports when correlating the cell-mediated reactivity with the severity of periodontal disease
    (3) Clinically not possible to distinguish between cell-mediated immunity (resistance) and delayed hypersensitivity (damaging) re-

Table 7-19

Prevotella and *Porphyromonas* in Necrotic Root Canals

	Incidence
Positive culture	60-80%
Black pigmenting species	4-67%
P. endodontalis	1-16%
P. gingivalis	5-11%
P. intermedia	5-28%
P. melaninogenicus	4-50%

From Newman MG, Nisengard R: *Oral microbiology and immunology,* ed 2, Philadelphia, 1994, WB Saunders.

Table 7-20

Prevotella and *Porphyromonas* in Periapical Abscesses

	Incidence
Positive culture	89-100%
Black pigmenting species	14-100%
P. denticola	38%
P. endodontalis	2-69%
P. gingivalis	5-10%
P. intermedia	8-20%
P. melaninogenicus	30-50%

From Newman MG, Nisengard R: *Oral microbiology and immunology,* ed 2, Philadelphia, 1994, WB Saunders.

actions in humans; both reactions depend on the same cellular participants

Periapical Infections and Oral-Facial Tissue Infections

A. Infections
   1. Abscesses (periodontal and periapical)
   2. Postsurgical and extraction wound infections
   3. Endodontically involved infections
   4. Sinus tract infections
   5. Cellulitis
   6. Traumatic injuries
   7. Osteomyelitis
   8. Postextraction alveolar osteitis (dry socket)
   9. Pericoronitis
   10. Periodontally involved infections
B. Bacteria cultivated from such infections (Tables 7-19 and 7-20)
   1. Predominantly gram-negative bacilli

2. Obligate anaerobic bacteria predominate in acute endodontic infections

C. Ludwig's angina
   1. Mixed infection
      a. Aerobic or facultative organisms in conjunction with anaerobic flora
      b. Often caused by the normal oral flora gaining access through the infected tooth
   2. Symptoms
      a. Rapidly spreading, diffuse bilateral cellulitis of the floor of the mouth and neck
      b. Swelling may block air passages
      c. Fever and malaise
   3. Predisposing factors
      a. Infected mandibular molars
      b. Thin lingual cortical plate of the mandible

Opportunistic Infections of the Oral Cavity

A. Definition—organisms that take advantage of a compromised situation in the host and subsequently invade and cause infection

B. Actinomycosis
   1. Etiology
      a. *A. israelii* most common
      b. *A. naeslundii*, *A. viscosus*, *Arachnia propionica* found in some lesions
   2. Pathogenesis
      a. Gram-positive bacteria; member of the normal oral flora
      b. Infection may follow injury with introduction of contaminated debris into the tissues
   3. Clinical findings/symptoms
      a. Facial swelling, most commonly in soft tissues below the angle of the jaw
      b. Small, chronic, superficial mass
      c. Abscess with sinus and chronic discharge develops

C. Oral candidiasis
   1. Four clinically distinct forms
      a. Pseudomembranous candidiasis
         (1) A removable soft, creamy, white plaque; red and/or bleeding base
         (2) Predominantly found on the buccal and labial mucosa, tongue, hard and soft palate
      b. Erythematous candidiasis
         (1) A smooth, flat, red lesion on the dorsum of the tongue; associated with loss of papillae
         (2) Can also be found on the hard palate
      c. Angular cheilitis—cracking or redness around the corners of the mouth
      d. Hyperplastic candidiasis
         (1) A raised, white nonremovable plaque

      (2) Appears on the buccal mucosa, hard palate, or dorsum of the tongue

D. Staphylococci
   1. Etiology—*S. aureus* and *S. epidermidis*
   2. Pathogenesis—normal flora of the skin, oral cavity, and anterior nares
   3. Clinical findings/symptoms
      a. Localized infections
         (1) Cellulitis
         (2) Carbuncles
      b. Systemic infections
         (1) Endocarditis
         (2) Pneumonia
      c. Mandibular osteomyelitis
      d. Acute suppurative parotitis

E. Other oral diseases
   1. Mumps
      a. Etiology—mumps virus
      b. Clinical findings/symptoms
         (1) Painful, swollen parotid or submaxillary glands
         (2) Fever and malaise
         (3) Papilla of Stensen's duct is red and swollen
         (4) Prevention through vaccine
   2. Herpangina (vesicular pharyngitis)
      a. Etiology—Coxsackievirus A
      b. Pathogenesis
         (1) Transmitted by ingestion of contaminated materials
         (2) Primarily occurs in children
      c. Clinical findings/symptoms—fever and vomiting; vesicles and later ulcers on the mucous membrane of the throat, palate, or tongue
      d. Recovery in 7 to 10 days; complications rare
   3. Recurrent apthous ulcers
      a. Etiology unknown; evidence suggests immunologic role
      b. Clinical findings/symbols
         (1) Canker sore, small ulcer
         (2) Covered by pseudomembrane
         (3) Surrounding erythematous halo
         (4) Occur on nonkeratinized mucosa
   4. Hand, foot, and mouth disease
      a. Etiology—Coxsackievirus A
      b. Pathogenesis
         (1) Highly infectious
         (2) Typically affects many children, particularly in schools
      c. Clinical findings/symptoms
         (1) Vesicular stomatitis and rash
         (2) Affects the buccal mucosa, tongue, gingiva, lips, hands, and feet
         (3) Pain

Prevention of Disease Transmission in Oral Healthcare

Primary Considerations

A. Universal precautions
   1. All clients' blood and body fluids are considered potentially infectious with HIV, HBV, and other bloodborne pathogens
   2. During oral healthcare procedures
      a. Contamination of saliva with blood is predictable
      b. Trauma to oral healthcare personnels' hands is common
   3. To prevent exposures to oral healthcare personnel, universal precautions are used for all clients regardless of their bloodborne infectious status
   4. Universal precautions also protect the client's oral mucous membranes from exposures to blood that may occur from breaks in skin of oral health workers' hands
B. Pathogens transmissible through the oral cavity (Table 7-21)
C. Health history
   1. Obtain, review, and update at subsequent visits
   2. Specific questions related to present health status, physician care, hospitalizations, history of childhood and adult diseases, pertinent family or experiential history, medications, allergies, current and recurrent illness, unintentional weight loss, the review of major organ systems, lymphadenopathy, oral soft tissue lesions, other infections, and history of hepatitis
   3. Health history, physical examinations, or laboratory tests cannot be expected to identify all infectious clients; clients may suppress some information purposely or unknowingly, so each client must be considered potentially infectious; therefore, the blood of all clients should be treated as if it were infective (universal precautions)
   4. Health history is essential for identifying conditions that will require
      a. Consultations
      b. Premedication
      c. Diagnostic evaluation; it is not a reliable identifier of clients likely to put oral healthcare personnel at risk—80% of persons infected with hepatitis B virus (HBV), 75% of hepatitis C (HCV) cases, and many with HIV are asymptomatic[14]
   5. Laboratory tests—limitations
      a. HIV antibody status—a period of 2 months to 6 months between time person infected and time when tests can detect antibodies (window period of seronegativity)
      b. Person may test HIV negative but still be infectious (false-negative results)[14]
      c. Newer HIV diagnostic methods now allow for earlier detection before serologic[14] evidence[15] (Polymarase chain reaction technique [PCR])
   6. Role of health history in selection of a treatment setting
      a. Hospital dental environment is best for client who is incapacitated; selection of treatment setting or specific infection control protocol is not based on past history of disease or diagnosis of AIDS; care and setting are based on client needs and level of debilitation[20]
      b. For individuals infected with HIV, two categories of needs
         (1) Special care—oral soft tissue complications, periodontitis, candidiasis, hairy leukoplakia, apthous ulcers, Kaposi sarcoma
         (2) General dental care—including routine dental hygiene, periodontal, restorative, orthodontic, and prosthodontic care
      c. Determination of *Mycobacterium tuberculosis* (TB) includes tuberculin skin test (Mantoux), chest x-ray, bacteriologic workup, and other diagnostic tests over and above the health history and physical exam; most individuals will become noninfectious after 2 to 3 weeks on antituberculin medications (confirm with sputum culture)[15]

General Considerations

A. Sources of contamination in the oral healthcare environment
   1. Dust-borne organisms
   2. Aerosols created by
      a. Breathing, speaking, coughing, and sneezing
      b. Prophylaxis angles, cups, and brushes
      c. Handpieces, airbrasive (air-polishing) devices
      d. Ultrasonic and sonic scalers
      e. Air-water syringes—capillary action and spatter contaminate the ends and insides of tips[33]
   3. Dental unit water lines (DUWL)[16]
      a. Normally occurring aquatic bacteria (e.g., *P. aeruginosa*)
      b. Water allowed to stand in lines will have some bacteria that may attach to and accumulate on the inside of the water lines, forming an adherent biofilm
      c. Water drops contaminated with oral flora (*Staphylococcus* and *Streptococcus*) may be retracted back into the DUWL[14]
      d. High concentrations of bacteria have been found in the dental unit water lines of handpieces, air-water syringes, and ultrasonic scal-

Table 7-21

Infectious Hazards for Both Oral Healthcare Provider and Client in the Treatment Area[14]

Infectious organism	Habitat	Transmission	Potential pathology	Vaccine[a]
		BACTERIA		
Bordetella pertussis (B)[c]	Nasopharynx	Nasopharyngeal secretions[c]	Whooping cough	Yes
Cardiobacterium hominis (A)	Nasopharynx	Nasopharyngeal secretions[c]	Endocarditis	No
Corynebacterium diphtheriae	Nasopharynx	Nasopharyngeal secretions[c]	Diphtheria	Yes
Enterobacteriaceae (A)				
Escherichia coli *Proteus vulgaris* *Klebsiella* *pneumoniae*	Mouth, gastrointestinal (GI) tract	Blood, lesion exudate[d]	Pneumonia, bacteremia, abscesses, wound infections	No
Haemophilus *influenzae* (C)	Mouth, nasopharynx	Blood, nasopharyngeal secretions[c]	Pneumonia, meningitis, otitis	Yes
parainfluenzae (A)			Conjunctivitis, endocarditis	No
paraphrophilus (A)			Endocarditis	No
Mycobacterium *tuberculosis* (D)	Pharynx	Pharyngeal secretions[c]	Tuberculosis	No
Mycoplasma *pneumoniae* (A)	Pharynx	Pharyngeal secretions[c]	Primary atypical pneumonia	No
Neisseria *meningitidis* (C)	Mouth, nasopharynx	Blood, nasopharyngeal secretions[c]	Cerebrospinal meningitis	Yes
gonorrhoeae (D)	Mouth, nasopharynx	Blood, lesion exudate, nasopharyngeal secretions[d]	Oral lesions, conjunctivitis	No
Pseudomonas *aeruginosa* (A)	Ubiquitous, sink and drain contaminant	Lesion exudate[c]	Pneumonia, wound infections	No
Staphylococcus *aureus* (A)	Mouth, skin, nasopharynx	Lesion exudate[c]	Suppurative lesions, bacteremia	No
epidermidis (A)			Endocarditis	No
Streptococcus *pyogenes* (A)	Nasopharynx	Blood, nasopharyngeal secretions[d]	Rheumatic and scarlet fever, otitis media, cervical adenitis, mastoiditis, peritonsillar abscesses, meningitis, pneumonia, acute glomerulonephritis	No
pneumoniae (A)			Pneumonia, endocarditis	Yes
viridans group (A)			Endocarditis	No

Adapted from American Dental Association Research Institute, Department of Toxicology: *J Am Dent Assoc* 117:374, 1988.
References: Jawetz E, Melnick JL, Adelberg EA: *Review of medical microbiology,* ed 17, Norwalk, Conn, 1987, Appleton & Lange.
[a]Inactivation: always use heat sterilization when possible. All of the above organisms can be killed by autoclaving at 121° C, 15 min, 15 psi. Dry heat sterilization: 170° C, 60 min. Heat-sensitive instruments and surfaces may be disinfected using phenolic or glutaraldehyde-based solutions.
[b]Centers for Disease Control reported new U.S. cases for 1987. Key: A = nonreportable; B = less than 1000; C = 1000-9999; D = greater than 9999.
[c]Infected droplet contact: inhalation, ingestion, direct inoculation.
[d]Direct inoculation to tissue surface.
[e]Control—The Infectious Disease Newsletter: Hepatitis A: a vaccine at last, Vol 7, No 6, June 1992.
[f]Inoculation into circulatory system.
[g]Kelen GD, Green GB, et al: Hepatitis B and Hepatitis C in emergency department patients, *N Engl J Med,* 326:1399-1404, 1992.
[h]Control—The Infectious Disease Newsletter: NA-NBH—the fourth hepatitis, Vol 3, No 5, 1988.
[i]American Liver Institute.
[j]Cottone JA, Terezhalmy GT, Molinairi JA: *Practical Infection Control in Dentistry,* ed 2, Media, Penn, 1996, Williams & Wilkins.

Continued

Table 7-21

Infectious Hazards for Both Oral Healthcare Provider and Client in the Treatment Area[14]—cont'd

Infectious organism	Habitat	Transmission	Potential pathology	Vaccine[a]
Treponema pallidum (D)	Blood, oral mucosa	Exudate from oral lesions[d]	Syphilis	No
Actinomycosis sp. *Bacterioides* sp. *Eubacterium* sp. *Fusobacterium* sp. (A)	Gingival crevice (normal oral flora)	Crevicular exudate[d]	Abscesses	No
Peptococcus sp. *Peptostreptococcus* sp. *Propionibacterium* sp.				
VIRUSES				
Coxsackie virus (A)	Oropharyngeal mucosa	Ingestion	Hand-foot-mouth disease, vesicular pharyngitis	No
Cytomegalovirus (A)	Salivary gland	Saliva, blood[d]	Cellular enlargement and degeneration in immunocompromised individuals	No
Epstein-Barr (A)	Parotid gland	Saliva, blood[d]	Infectious mononucleosis	No
Hepatitis				
A (D)	Liver, GI tract	Blood (rare), ingestion	Liver inflammation, jaundice	Yes[e]
B (D)	Liver	Blood, saliva, tears, semen[f]	Eventual hepatocellular carcinoma in chronic antigen carriers	Yes
C[g] (formerly parenterally transmitted[j], non-A, non-B)(C)	Liver?	Blood[d], sexual activity?	Many develop chronic carrier state; many will have chronic active hepatitis and cirrhosis	No
D[i] (formerly delta)(A)	Liver	Blood[d]	Coinfection with hepatitis B virus (HBV) required	Yes (HBV vac)
E (formerly enterically transmitted non-A, non-B)[j]	Liver	Ingestion	Liver inflammation caused by a virus that resembles hepatitis A	?
Herpes simplex 1 and 2 (A)	Nasopharynx	Lesion exudate, saliva[d]	Oral lesions, hepatic whitlow, conjunctivitis	No
Human immunodeficiency virus (HIV)(D)	T4 lymphocyte	Blood[f]	Acquired immunodeficiency syndrome (AIDS)	No
Measles				
Rubeola (C) Rubella (B)	Nasopharynx	Nasopharyngeal secretions, blood, saliva, vesicle exudate[c]	Generalized vesicular rash	Yes Yes
Mumps virus (D)	Parotid gland	Saliva, ingestion	Parotitis, meningitis	Yes
Poliovirus (B)	Oropharyngeal mucosa, GI tract	Ingestion	CNS paralysis	Yes

Table 7-21

Infectious Hazards for Both Oral Healthcare Provider and Client in the Treatment Area[14]—cont'd

Infectious organism	Habitat	Transmission	Potential pathology	Vaccine[a]
Respiratory viruses (A)				
Influenza A and B			Flu, common cold	Yes
Parainfluenza	Nasopharynx	Nasopharyngeal secretions[c]		No
Rhinovirus				No
Adenovirus				Yes
Coronavirus				No
Varicella (A)	Skin	Vesicle exudate[d]	Chicken pox	No
FUNGI				
Candida albicans (A)	Mouth, skin	Nasopharyngeal secretions[c]	(Opportunistic) candidiasis, cutaneous infections	No
PROTOZOA				
Pneumocystis carinii (A)	Mouth	Nasopharyngeal secretions[c]	(Opportunistic) interstitial pneumonia in immunocompromised individuals	No

ers; they are a source of contamination for the client directly and the dental team via aerosols

    e. *Pseudomonas* (opportunistic pathogen) has been found and can survive in water and biofilms for extended periods[17]

    f. Presence of microorganisms in DUWL has not been seen as a major threat to clients/dental team; studies on actual occurrence of disease have not been performed; immunocompromised individuals are at greatest risk[17]

  4. Suction devices

    a. Residues of infected material form

    b. Lead to permanent bacterial growth on the insides of tubes

  5. Dental air lines—research required to investigate the presence of organisms such as *Legionella* and the tubercle bacilli (TB) in air lines[18]

B. Transmission

  1. Chain of infection—a cyclic process that depends on six elements for an infection to take place

    a. Infectious agent or pathogens

    b. Source of growth (reservoir: oral cavity, hands)

    c. Portal of exit (skin, mucous membrane, oral cavity, GI tract, respiratory tract, genitourinary system, blood, blood derivatives)

    d. Means of transmission

    e. Portal of entry to the host (same routes as exit)

  2. Occupational exposure to infectious blood or serum and saliva—transmission via direct contact

    a. Parenteral exposure (i.e., exposure occurring as a result of piercing the skin barrier, e.g., needlestick or cut with a sharp instrument)

    b. Percutaneous inoculation (exposure via either needle or sharp object or through nonintact skin [dermatitis, scratches, burns])

    c. Contact with mucous membrane[19] (intraoral, nasal, ocular)

  3. Organisms from the oral cavity enter the air of the operatory (aerosolization, airborne transfer)

  4. Modes of transmission

    a. Client to oral healthcare provider (direct contact resulting in cross-infection)

    b. Oral healthcare provider to patient (direct contact resulting in cross-infection)

    c. Client to client (indirect contact)—no documented indirect contact transmission of infection by contaminated instruments, equipment, or records, yet the potential exists so precautions must be taken

C. Autogenous infection

  1. A local or systemic posttreatment infection caused by introducing the microflora of clients into injured tissues

  2. May develop if the host's defense mechanisms are reduced

3. Examples of possible infections
   a. Bacteremia
   b. Abscess
   c. Infections developing after oral surgery or treatment of fractures
4. Prevention
   a. Antibiotic premedication where indicated
   b. Lower the oral microbial count by rinsing with an antimicrobial rinse, e.g., chlorhexidine and phenol mouthwashes. Peridex by Procter & Gamble or Listerine by Warner Lambert results in a 98% reduction; even rinsing with plain water results in a 75% reduction
   c. Preparation of the injection site
      (1) Dry tissue with sterile gauze to reduce the number of microorganisms at the injection site
      (2) Apply a topical antiseptic, e.g., iodophore solutions with 1% iodine

D. Definitions
1. Sterilization—destroys or removes all forms of life, including bacterial spores and viruses
2. Disinfection
   a. Kills pathogenic organisms but not necessarily spores; disinfectants are applied to inanimate objects; antiseptics to living tissues
   b. Levels of disinfection
      (1) *High level* can kill some but not necessarily all bacterial spores and is tuberculocidal; EPA-registered disinfectant/sterilizant agents are high-level disinfectants
      (2) *Intermediate level* kills *Mycobacterium tuberculosis* var. *bovis,* hepatitis B (HBV), and human immunodeficiency (HIV) viruses but not spores
      (3) *Low level* kills most bacteria, some fungi, some viruses; does not kill spores or *Mycobacterium tuberculosis* var. *bovis*
3. Sanitization—reducing microbials to levels judged safe by public health requirements; generally a cleaning process of inanimate objects
4. -cide—suffix indicates agents that kill; germicides kill most vegetative bacteria, especially pathogens, but not all spore forms; terms *viricide, fungicide,* and *sporicide* kill viruses, fungi, and spores, respectively
5. -static—indicates agents that prevent growth but do not necessarily kill organisms
6. Sepsis—pathogenic microorganisms are present
7. Asepsis—living pathogenic microorganisms are absent
8. Infection control protocol—procedures to avoid infection or microbial contamination
9. Aerosols—air-suspended liquid or solid particles that measure less than 50 μm in diameter, remain airborne for extended periods, and are subject to inhalation unless protective measures are implemented
10. Spatter—droplets measure more than 50 μm in diameter and can be observed on protective eyewear and operating lights; quickly settle and can contaminate operatory surfaces and operator's clothing

Precautions for Oral Healthcare Personnel

A. Immunizations
1. Personnel risks warrant vaccinations to develop protective immunity for diseases they have not had or have not been immunized against
   a. Hepatitis B, measles, mumps, rubella, tetanus, polio
   b. Consider influenza vaccine as well to prevent possible transmission to older or medically compromised persons
2. Vaccines alone are insufficient protection
   a. Hepatitis B (HBV) vaccine does not produce absolute immunity in those who receive it
   b. Where effective vaccine is feasible, cross-infection potential for client-to-client, indirect transmission, contaminated equipment, etc, still present risks
   c. Many blood-borne pathogens with no vaccine (e.g., HIV, HCV, CMV, EBV)
3. ADA Council on Scientific Affairs recommends that all dental personnel involved in client care (including laboratory technicians) receive hepatitis B vaccine; OSHA requires employers to make hepatitis B vaccine available to all employees who have occupational exposure
   a. Critical occupational hazard study shows that 24% of oral surgeons, 17% of prosthodontists, 16% of general dentists, and 13% of auxiliaries had HVB markers indicating previous exposure
   b. Two types (both safe and effective)
      (1) Plasma-derived HB vaccine (1982) (Heptavax-B: Merck, Sharp, and Dohme [discontinued in 1989.])
      (2) Recombinant DNA HB vaccine (1986) (Recombivax-HB: Merck, Sharp, and Dohme; Engerix-B: SmithKline Biologicals [1988])
   c. Process
      (1) Prevaccine testing for the antibody to hepatitis B surface antigen—value of pretesting questioned because of issues of effectiveness, false positives, and cost-effectiveness;

pregnancy not contraindication for HB vaccine

(2) Vaccine administered unless assured antibody present (most common regime is a series of three inoculations in the deltoid muscle given at 0, 1, and 6-months)

(3) Postvaccination testing should follow the last in the series of three injections to ensure a positive response to the vaccine; the specific postvaccination time interval recommendation for evaluation for appropriate antibody (Anti-HBs) levels ranges from 1 month, 6 weeks, 3 months, to 6 months[17]

(4) Booster—the CDC states that hepatitis B vaccine protection lasts at least 7 years; a specific time interval recommendation will require more information being available; if vaccinated over 5 years ago without postscreening, recommendation is for a single injection before antibody titer evaluation; no postvaccination cases of anyone developing clinical hepatitis B[17]

B. Handwashing

1. Rationale

   a. Reduce microorganisms in folds and grooves of skin by lifting and rinsing from surface

   b. Prevents transfer of microorganisms from one person to another; or if break in skin, prevents autogenous infection

   c. Resident microorganisms (*Staphylococcus epidermidis,* micrococci, and diptheroids) are those that survive and multiply on the skin and can be repeatedly cultured; may inhabit surface epithelium of deeper areas

   d. Transient microorganisms are recent contaminants that can survive or remain on skin for a limited period of time; temporary residents that may be washed away or, in event of skin break (dermal defects), cause autogenous infection; also can contaminate sterile instruments, dental equipment, or environmental surfaces

   e. Use of gloves does not serve as a substitute for routine handwashing

   f. Wash hands before gloving to minimize number of organisms that multiply rapidly when enclosed in warm and moist environment (moisture accumulates between gloves and skin, causing bacteria and yeast to grow; can cause skin irritation)

   g. Wash hands after carefully removing gloves; defects exist in about 1.5% to 9% of unused gloves; in addition, tears and punctures may occur during treatment and permit microorganisms to be transferred to hands or from hands to client

   h. Rings, even smooth bands, should be removed to prevent possible perforation of gloves or creation of area to harbor resident or transient microorganisms

   i. If gloves are torn, cut, or punctured during course of care, remove, discard as soon as possible, wash hands thoroughly, and reglove before completing procedure

   j. Use of an effective liquid antiseptic soap has an antimicrobial effect that is maximized with repeated washings and leaves a residual inhibiting benefit against common skin contaminants

2. Methods of handwashing (antimicrobial soap with substantivity)

   a. Short handwash

   (1) Begin day with *two* consecutive 15-second handwashes with soap and water; repeated lathering serves to loosen debris and microorganisms and rinsing washes them away

   (2) Between clients, wash hands for a full 15 seconds and also before and after lunch, lavatory, or any time hands become contaminated

   b. Surgical hand scrub

   (1) Use before surgical procedure

   (2) Five-minute scrub of hands, arms up to elbows (repeated scrub and rinse cycles)

   (3) Use antimicrobial soap and soft sterile brush

   (4) Dry with sterile towel

   (5) Specific protocol for surgical scrub usually posted over sinks

3. Recommendations

   a. Use a gentle (non-irritating) and effective antimicrobial liquid antiseptic soap

   b. Do not use a brush on hands more than once a day because it can cause dermatitis; the skin is a natural defense to be preserved

   c. Sterilize brushes after each use

   d. If the sink does not have foot- or knee-operated controls, use paper towels or elbow to turn off after handwashing

   e. If using cloth towels for drying, use a new one for each client

   f. Maintain cleanliness by touching only sterile instruments or disinfected surfaces

   g. Keep nails short and clean and cuticles well-groomed to prevent breaks

   h. Personnel who have exudative lesions or weeping dermatitis should refrain from all direct or indirect contact with blood and saliva

i. Hand lotions can be helpful to prevent hands from chapping
4. Soaps (hand antiseptic agents)
   a. Liquid soaps or detergents effective in removing many transient (possible pathogens) and most resident microorganisms found in top layer of skin
   b. Liquid antiseptic soap may kill resident microorganisms in deeper layers of skin
      (1) Recommended antimicrobial soaps
         (a) Chlorhexidene gluconate (CHG), 2% or 4%, with isopropyl, 4% (e.g., BactoShield 4, Hibiclens)
            [1] Use throughout day; 90% reduction in hand microbes
            [2] Has substantivity, a residual inhibiting effect
         (b) Para-chlorometaxylenol (PCMX), 3% (e.g., Banique 3, Derm-Aseptic, Ultradex)
         (c) Povidone iodine (PI), 7.5% to 10.00% (e.g., Betadine); broad spectrum
         (d) Triclosan (TI)
      (2) Comparison of infection rates with plain versus antimicrobial soaps hindered by lack of well-controlled studies[19]
C. Gloves[19]
1. Use of gloves provides a high level of protection for both oral health care provider and client
   a. Prevents direct skin contact with blood, saliva, mucous membranes, and contaminated items
   b. Bare hands provide numerous small cuts and abrasions that provide portals of entry for the skin's natural transient microbes and pathogenic organisms
   c. Risks
      (1) Ungloved hands are probably the route by which oral healthcare personnel have acquired HBV from clients
      (2) Documentation of transmissions of HBV from provider to client; largest outbreak involved an ungloved dentist who infected 55 of his clients
      (3) Ungloved hygienist with herpetic lesions on hands (herpetic whitlow) transmitted herpes simplex virus to 20 clients
      (4) HIV antibody present in one dentist who, with no other risk factor except occupation but had a history of sustaining needle-stick injuries and trauma to hands, did not routinely wear gloves when providing dental care

(5) Cytolomegalovirus (CMV) DNA family, high concentration in saliva, linked to birth defects
(6) Additional risk: contact with chemicals that may irritate skin
   d. Watches should not be worn unless completely covered by gloves; bracelets should be removed during working hours
2. Protocol for glove use
   a. Gloves must be worn *whenever* anticipating contact with blood, saliva, mucous membranes, or blood-contaminated objects or surfaces
   b. Wash hands before and after glove use (see section on handwashing)
   c. Gloves should cover the cuff of a long-sleeved gown
   d. Gloves must be changed between clients and during long appointments
   e. Defects in gloves dramatically increase with use beyond 60 minutes, particularly when washed with antiseptics; washing/disinfecting glove may cause "wicking," i.e., enhanced penetration of liquids through undetected holes in gloves
   f. Repeated use of a single pair of gloves by disinfecting them is not acceptable
   g. Double gloving (wearing two pairs of gloves to enhance safety)—if chosen, it should be used universally and *not selectively,* i.e., based on a client's health history; double thickness of latex reduces dexterity and increases cost; CDC, ADA, and OSHA do not recommend double gloving in their guidelines
   h. Torn or punctured gloves should be removed as soon as client safety permits, hands washed and gloves replaced with new gloves[17]
3. Types of gloves
   a. Descriptions
      (1) Single-use nonsterile gloves, often called "examination gloves," fit both hands and are sized small, medium and large, provide an adequate level of protection for most procedures
      (2) Single-use sterile gloves or sized "sterile surgical gloves" are recommended for surgical procedures involving contact with normally sterile areas of the body
      (3) Multiple-use utility gloves, "heavy-duty puncture-resistant gloves," are made of polynitrile or heavy latex and are recommended for handling of contaminated instruments for sterilization or exposure to chemicals

(4) Single-use plastic overgloves (nontreatment) or "food-handler" type gloves are worn over treatment gloves to prevent cross-contamination of items such as charts, drawers, telephones, etc.

(5) Heat-resistant gloves are to be worn when handling hot items, e.g., unloading sterilizers[17]

b. Materials[19]

(1) Latex gloves (sterile and nonsterile), vulcanized, "straight dip" type, minimal manufacturing defects

(2) Vinyl gloves (sterile and nonsterile) useful for personnel with latex allergies; generally not as elastic as latex, may tear more easily

(3) Nonvinyl alternative for oral healthcare personnel with latex sensitivity—hypoallergenic gloves; offer greater elasticity and better fit[19]

(4) Overgloves—plastic

(5) Heavy-duty utility gloves, rubber, neoprene, polynitrile (heat sterilizable) gloves

4. Latex hypersensitivity

a. Providers must be aware of latex hypersensitivities (immediate and delayed), associated risks, document in medical/dental records and provide latex-free gloves and armamentarium[14]

b. Allergy to latex gloves[14]

(1) Symptoms include eye itching and watering, coughing, wheezing, decreased blood pressure, dizziness; symptoms develop within minutes of latex exposure

(2) Potential exists for anaphylaxis and death

(3) Type IV reaction most common; appears 48 to 72 hours after exposure in the form of dry, cracked, and pruritic skin[14]

D. Protective barriers for mouth, nose, and eyes

1. Objective—to prevent exposure of easily infected mucous membranes to droplets of blood and saliva as well as bacteria-laden particles of debris, polishing agent, calculus, and water

a. Spatter containing blood and saliva is associated with all instrumentation, with the greatest amount generated by air-turbine handpiece, air-water syringe, ultrasonic scaler, airpolishing delivery system

b. Spatter represents greater risk of exposure than aerosols (artificially generated collection of invisible solid or liquid particles suspended in air and capable of airborne infection), e.g., *Mycobacterium,* tubercle bacillus (MTB)

2. Masks must be worn to protect mucous membranes of nose and mouth

a. An effective mask will

(1) Prevent inhalation and direct contact with potentially infectious aerosols and spatter[28]

(2) Filter particles during procedures (95% of droplets 3.0 to 3.2 μm)

(3) Have minimal marginal leakage

b. Types of masks:

(1) Glass fiber mat and synthetic fiber mat most effective filters[14]

(2) Dome mask with elastic band

(a) Distance from face decreases rate of moistness

(b) Moist mask compromises effectiveness of barrier

(3) Surgical tie-on mask or ear loop mask

(a) Better filtration of smaller particle size

(b) Closer adaptation to face

(c) Becomes moist quickly; wet fabric serves as vehicle for microbial transfer through mask

(4) Disposable particulate respirator (PRM)

(a) Alternative to standard surgical mask to provide increased protection when treating person who has infectious TB

(b) Designed for tight face seal, proper fit is imperative to protect against inhalation of droplet nuclei[14]

(c) Greater filtration efficiency—99% efficiency for particles 1 μm in diameter

c. Maximize effectiveness and minimize cross-contamination[20]

(1) New mask for each patient or change if mask gets wet during procedure

(2) Put on mask before handwash

(3) Adjust mask so it fits snugly against face; poor fit may allow aerosols and spatter to enter edges of mask

(4) Avoid touching mask during appointment

(5) Keep mask on after completing a procedure in presence of aerosols to prevent direct exposure to airborne organisms *Mycobacterium* tubercle bacillus (MTB)

(6) Protect from exposure to chemicals (splashes, droplets, e.g., disinfectants)

(7) Remove mask overhead; handle it only by elastic or cloth tie strings; avoid dangling mask around neck (contaminated mask may contaminate neck)

3. Protective eyewear must be worn during client care, laboratory, disinfection, and sterilization procedures

a. Objective is to protect eyes and mucous membranes from physical projectiles, chemical damage, and microbial injury

b. Risks associated with exposure of eyes to debris, blood, and body fluids
   (1) Conjunctivitis
   (2) Ocular herpes (herpes simplex), second to injury as leading cause of blindness
   (3) Hepatitis B (eye as portal of entry)[14]
   (4) *Staphylococcus aureus*
   (5) Penetrating eye injury
   (6) Chemicals used in dentistry incompatible with ocular tissue (e.g., chlorides with low pH and chemicals associated with sterilization/disinfection)[21]

c. Type of eyewear
   (1) Traditional prescription glasses offer limited coverage (open top and sides) resulting in poor side splash/side impact protection
   (2) Safety glasses or goggles
      (a) Cover entire eye orbit (top and side shields)
      (b) Frame extensions for expanded facial coverage all around the eye
      (c) Possible to wear over prescription glasses
      (d) More shatter resistant than regular eyewear
   (3) Face shields
      (a) Ensure maximum coverage
      (b) Alternative to protective glasses or goggles, not substitute for mask
      (c) Adjunct to glasses and mask for high aerosol-generating procedures

d. Maximize effectiveness and minimize cross-contamination
   (1) Wear as part of clinic attire; selective use could lead to forgetting or misplacing protective glasses
   (2) Shatter-resistant quality with minimal visual distortion
   (3) Able to withstand immersion disinfection
   (4) Wash with soap and water and disinfect between clients
   (5) Have multiple pairs available to accommodate disinfection
   (6) Recognize nontreatment risks such as laboratory procedures, mixing and pouring of chemicals, and use of disinfectants
   (7) Face shield limitation as substitute does not provide "fit" of mask; increases inhalation of aerosols and spatter may come up behind shield

      (8) Protective eyewear also should be routinely provided for clients to wear during procedures that create aerosols/spatter and propel objects
      (9) Eyewear designed to protect against damage from ultraviolet irradiation

E. Protective clothing
   1. Rationale—provides additional protection for skin and attire from exposure to blood and saliva
   2. Risks
      a. Potential exposure of clothing and skin to aerosols, spatter sprays, and droplets of oral fluids and associated pathogens; greatest risk if skin is nonintact
      b. Large numbers of certain pathogenic microorganisms have been found on soiled linen, but actual risk of disease transmission is negligible
      c. Clothing exposed to HIV may be safely used after a normal laundry cycle
   3. Types of protective clothing
      a. Reusable or disposable
      b. Surgical/"isolation" type gown is ideal
         (1) Covers street clothing
         (2) Fits closely around neck, high coverage
         (3) Covers arms
         (4) Fitted cuffs
      c. Laboratory coats or uniforms with long sleeves and high collars
   4. To maximize effectiveness and minimize cross-contamination
      a. Wear protective attire made with synthetic material; contaminants are not easily absorbed into synthetic material (more fluid resistant)
      b. Wear protective attire with sleeves, reinforced material with fitted cuffs at wrist, and high collar; long sleeves with fitted cuffs permit gloves to extend over cuffs for complete coverage
      c. Seams, buttons, and buckles should be kept to a minimum
      d. Avoid wearing protective attire outside practice setting to prevent problem with contaminants at home and in other non–client care areas
      e. Consider having work shoes worn only in the oral health care area
      f. Change protective clothing daily or if visibly soiled
      g. Avoid touching clothing throughout the day
      h. Consider additional coverage during invasive procedures that are likely to result in the splashing of blood and saliva
         (1) Plastic aprons

(2) Fluid-proof fabric
(3) Head covers
(4) Shoe covers
  i. Laundry/disposal
    (1) Handle as little as possible
      (a) Sort in separate non–client care area
      (b) Bag in leakproof sealed laundry/disposal bags for disposal or transport to or from client care area
    (2) Laundering
      (a) Launder separately
      (b) High temperature (60° to 70° C or more)
      (c) Wash cycle with normal bleach concentration
      (d) Machine-dry (100° C or more)[19]

Oral Healthcare Environment and Promotion of Infection Control

A. Design and equipment selection
  1. Minimize the surfaces requiring contact with contaminated hands of oral healthcare team
    a. Smooth construction—eliminate knobs, hooks, and crevices
    b. Client chairs and operator stools
      (1) Minimize buttons and seams
      (2) Controls—easily disinfected control panel and operator stool height adjustment lever
    c. Tubings—avoid fabric-covered, coiled, or mechanically retracted tubing
    d. Sink faucets—knee, electronic, or forearm controlled
    e. Soap dispensers—knee, foot, or forearm controlled
    f. Paper towel dispenser designed to avoid touching hardware
    g. Plastic-lined waste containers recessed under cabinet with opening on countertop
  2. Surfaces must be compatible with disinfectants and/or detergents
    a. Vinyl upholstery for chairs and stools
    b. Plastic laminate cabinets, countertops versus wood
    c. Vinyl flooring and walls that are smooth
    d. Carpeting not recommended in treatment or laboratory areas
  3. Dental unit water lines (DUWL) should have water check valves to prevent aspiration of microorganisms into the water lines (capillary retraction of fluid); contamination in dental unit water lines may be reduced by: self-contained dedicated supply system (reservoir for sterile water inserted into water line for handpiece and air/water syringe); insertion of small bacterial filtration unit in water line; flushing lines in unit with disinfectant followed by a rinse. Research and development needed for more reliable and low maintenance solution to DUWL contamination.[17]
  4. Reduce airborne microbes by air circulation exchange system or single-room filtration units; ventilation systems should be designed to control noxious sterilization and laboratory vapors and to prevent recirculation of contaminated air (microbes transported via ventilation system); filters in heating, ventilation and air conditioning systems should prevent transfer of microbes; dental facilities should have filters with a minimal particle removal efficiency rate greater than the normal work setting (60%) and less than hospital grade range of 99.9% efficiency[14]
B. Housekeeping
  1. Walls, floors, furnishings, and sinks are not associated with disease transmission to clients or oral healthcare workers
  2. Environmental surfaces not associated with client treatment should be cleaned routinely with detergent and water
  3. Keeping treatment area free of unnecessary or seldom used equipment and items facilitates post-care cleaning and disinfection

Preparation of Treatment Area for Client Care

A. Surface disinfection procedures[22-23]: disinfect items that do not normally penetrate or contact mucous membranes (noncritical items) but are exposed to spatter, spray, and splashing of blood and saliva or touched by contaminated hands
  1. Strategy
    a. Identify and list surfaces that will be contaminated by blood or saliva during treatment; post the list in the treatment area to increase effectiveness and efficiency
    b. Devise methods to avoid contact with objects that must be handled
      (1) Use disposable covers (e.g., aluminum foil, impervious backed paper, plastic wrap, and commercially available polyethylene sheets and tubing) for light handles, chairback with control buttons, headrest, chair arms, hoses, etc.
      (2) Have sterile pliers or forceps, overgloves (food handler type) or additional exam gloves, gauze, and paper towels readily accessible for use as a barrier between con-

taminated gloved hands and uncontaminated supply, drawer, or record area

2. Typical list of surfaces to disinfect
   a. Countertops, cabinet surfaces, mobile cabinets, tray table, and x-ray unit and controls
   b. Air-water syringe, high- and low-volume evacuator (because these items are used intraorally and touched frequently, they should be removable for cleaning and sterilization; consider future purchase of equipment with these features)
   c. All hose ends, controls, and tubing attached to handpieces
   d. Supports for handpiece, air-water syringe, and suction devices
   e. Chair, including switches and levers
   f. Control switches (power, water, air, light, and ultrasonic scalers)
   g. Lamp handle
   h. Cuspidor and controls
   i. Sink handles, soap dispenser (if manually operated)
   j. Instrument tray (if cannot be sterilized)
   k. Blood pressure equipment: stethoscope earpieces
   l. Large or bulk dispensers of floss, topical fluoride, or other items should not be touched with contaminated gloves; items must be disinfected if they have been touched or in zone of aerosols, spatter

3. Effectiveness of surface disinfection procedure influenced by several factors
   a. Number and type of organisms present
   b. Amount of organic matter or other debris present on item being disinfected
   c. Selection of an intermediate-level disinfectant that is registered by the Environmental Protection Agency as a tuberculocidal hospital disinfectant, with appropriate viricidal activity[14]
   d. Concentration and length of exposure to disinfecting agent; follow manufacturer's directions for dilution
   e. Initial precleaning of surface to maximize removal of "bioburden" (blood, saliva, and microorganisms) before disinfection

4. Surface disinfection technique (spray/wipe/spray)
   a. *Preparation*—wear heavy-duty polynitrile gloves (heat sterilizable)
   b. *Preclean* (first spray)
      (1) Apply (pump spray bottle best) cleaner or cleaner/disinfectant (aqueous-based disinfectants that contain a detergent are preferred because they are used for both cleaning and disinfection); disinfectants containing more than 50% alcohol are not suitable for precleaning, and alcohol-based products are inefficient for removing protein-containing debris; therefore, another product should be selected to preclean surface
      (2) Brush particularly soiled or rough surfaces
   c. *Wipe*—Use paper towels to remove cleaner; paper towels are preferred over 4 × 4 gauze because they are large, fast, and inexpensive; mechanical action (wiping) important for effectiveness
      (1) Use *dry* paper towel or gauze to wipe wet surface; gauze stored in chemicals reduces the effectiveness of agent over the course of a day
   d. *Apply disinfectant* or reapply cleaner/disinfectant (EPA-registered tuberculocidal hospital disinfectant)
   e. Leave surface undisturbed for specified moist contact time

5. Chemical disinfectants for surface disinfection
   a. Criteria for an ideal disinfectant for oral healthcare (no single product meets all criteria)[14]
      (1) Sporicidal, tuberculocidal, and viricidal in the times stated for each (broad spectrum)
      (2) Effective in 3 minutes or less for surfaces
      (3) Nontoxic/hypoallergenic
      (4) Odorless
      (5) Reasonable cost
      (6) Residual effect on treated surfaces
      (7) Retains most of its stability and activity in the presence of organic matter and in heavy use for the periods described
      (8) Good penetrating and cleaning ability
      (9) Surface compatibility, not damaging to painted, plastic, or metal surfaces
      (10) Must be effective in killing vegetative forms of pathogenic organisms, influenza and enteroviruses, and the *tubercle bacillus* usually in 10 minutes
   b. Critical to select EPA-registered hospital disinfectant
      (1) EPA number on label
      (2) Label claim—"kills *M. tuberculosis*," "is tuberculocidal," "kills tubercle bacillus" (very resistant because of outer cellular wax and lipid layers)
      (3) If capable of killing *Mycobacterium* var. *bovis*, will destroy less resistant organisms as well
      (4) Labeled viricidal and fungicidal
      (5) ADA seal of acceptance—approved by the Council on Scientific Affairs for use in den-

tistry; the American Dental Association no longer has a formal acceptance program for disinfectants; products that have previously or may currently carry the seal of acceptance have withstood the scrutiny of evaluation required to display the seal[24]

(6) Neither ADA nor CDC recommends alcohol or quaternary ammonium compounds as surface disinfectants for use in dentistry

c. Preparation of disinfectant

(1) Precisely follow label directions

(a) Use
(b) Mixing dilution
(c) Method of duration of application
(d) Temperature requirements
(e) Shelf life
(f) Activated use life
(g) If applicable, reuse life

(2) Exercise care with use; read label

(a) Prevent irritation to eyes, skin (protective eyewear and nitrile gloves)
(b) Avoid breathing vapors (adequate ventilation)

d. Recommended chemicals for environmental surface disinfection (Table 7-22)

B. Care and maintenance of dental unit water lines

1. Bacteria may grow or accumulate within the water lines (adherent biofilm colonies) on internal tubing walls of the air-water syringe, handpiece, hose, and the ultrasonic scaler

a. Water is often contaminated with gram-negative bacteria
b. Water contaminated with *Legionella pneumophila* (a gram-negative bacterium that causes a type of pneumonia) and *Pseudomonas* (opportunistic pathogen) can be infectious in persons with altered resistance

2. Check the anti-retraction valves in the handpiece and other water lines with antiretraction valves (valves can stick open with age)[14]

a. Until 1981, most units were fitted with retraction valves to prevent water dripping
b. Water retraction valves can draw saliva and aerosols back up the waterline when the handpiece is stopped
c. All retraction valves should have been replaced with anti-retraction valves

3. Flush water lines at the beginning of each day for 3 to 5 minutes to reduce bacterial counts; this includes handpiece, air-water syringe, and ultrasonic scalers

4. Between clients, flush waterlines for 20 to 30 seconds and several minutes if system has been idle[17]

5. Sterile water should be used for surgery and irrigating pockets (separate sterile water supply or use of heat-sterilized bulb syringes with sterile water)[14]

C. Other preparations for patient care procedures

1. Preplanning materials (unit dose), instruments, and medications increases efficiency, prevents risk of contamination of other supplies

2. Prearranged tray setups/cassettes

a. Ultrasonic, sterilizable, instrument cassette
b. Eliminate need to go to storage areas and cabinets
c. Individual sterilized bur blocks

3. Use of disposables whenever possible saves time and solves problem of decontaminating hard-to-clean items

4. Surface barriers (single-use covers)

a. Placed for quick and easy surface protection
b. More expensive alternative to surface disinfection
c. Minimize drawbacks associated with chemicals that stain, corrode, and are toxic
d. May be selected for rough and odd-shaped surfaces only

During Client Care

A. Droplet, spatter, and aerosol reduction

1. Client preparation, toothbrushing, and rinsing with antibacterial mouthrinse will reduce microbial count in aerosols
2. Use air and water separately instead of a combined spray
3. Use a rubber cup instead of brushes for polishing; use a toothbrush for occlusal surfaces
4. Use ventilation system with filters to prevent recirculation of contaminated air[14]
5. Use high-volume suction
6. Use proper client position

B. Reduce risk of infection and minimize cross-contamination

1. Contaminated and noncontaminated zones—designate uncontaminated areas to limit field of contamination, then always use overgloves when going into noncontaminated zone
2. Avoid touching unprotected switches, handles, and other equipment once gloves have been contaminated; *anything touched with contaminated hands* during the appointment must be carefully cleaned and disinfected at the end of procedure[19]
3. Avoid entering drawers, cabinets, and other storage areas *once gloves have been contaminated*
4. Protect dental records, charts, radiographs from handling and contamination during client treatment

a. Ask for assistance

Table 7-22

Chemical Agents for Environmental Surface Cleaning and Disinfection

Chemical classification	Product examples (1)	Scope	Advantages	Limitations*
Iodophors	Biocide, Bi-Arrest, Surf-A-Cide, Asepti-IDC Iodofive	Broad spectrum of antimicrobials	Residual film of iodine—effective antimicrobials; minimizes stains and allergic reactions	Starch-based wipes deactivate; repeated use or long exposure stains white or pastel vinyls and corrodes metals
Chlorines Sodium hypochlorite	Household bleach, 5.25%, 1 : 10 solution approved by American Dental Association Dispatch (0.55%)	Broad spectrum; bactericidal; viricidal, tuberculocidal	Household bleach: inexpensive; effective for precleansing also; good surface disinfectant, even though not an EPA-registered disinfectant; dispatch EPA registered	Dilution is unstable (mix daily); inactivated by organic matter, precleaning essential corrodes some metals (chrome, cobalt alloy, aluminum, highly oxidizable metals); irritation to skin and eyes; strong odor
Chlorine dioxide	Exspor	Viricidal	Rapid action (2-min disinfection); for sterilization also (min. 6 hr)	Corrosiveness and irritation to skin and mucosa; limit use to well-ventilated areas; fresh solutions needed; corrodes most metals
Phenolic combinations Complex phenol (combination synthetic phenolics)	• Water-based pump spray: Omni II, Prophene Vital Defense-D, Pro-Spray • Alcohol-based pump spray: CoeSpray-The Pump • Alcohol-based aerosol: Lysol IC disinfectant	Broad antimicrobial spectrum: tuberculocidal; most are capable of hydrophilic virucide (check label)	Synergistic; economical; for cleansing also; compatible with most metals, plastics (Note: alcohol-based products are poor to fair in cleaning ability)	Not sporicidal; prolonged exposure degrades certain plastics, glass; film accumulation; irritating to skin and mucous membranes, epithelial tissues

*All are considered toxic substances, so minimize risk of exposure to potential hazardous effects by wearing nitrile gloves, mask, and protective eyewear when using or mixing chemicals.

b. Use overgloving technique—a second pair of disposable gloves such as examining gloves or food handling gloves to prevent contamination of charts, telephones, and cabinets
c. Use barriers such as folded paper squares and plastic sleeves; last resort, remove gloves, wash, rewash, put on new pair of gloves
5. Do not wash gloves; this may cause gloves to tear or increase their permeability; instead change or overglove[17]
6. Recording assessments
   a. Request assistance
   b. Recording only, not passing contaminated equipment
   c. Overgloves
   d. Future trend—voice-activated computers

7. Avoid touching mask after hands are prepared; remove and reposition by elastic ties
8. Position clients so that they do not come in contact with your gown or apron
9. Only equipment and supplies necessary for immediate treatment should be inside the treatment areas to avoid unnecessary contamination
10. Individual prepackaged sterilized bags of cotton rolls, gauze, swabs, and pellets; ensure that disposable supplies are sterile
11. Waste disposal during treatment
    a. Immediately discard saliva- or blood-soaked contaminated waste in small biohazard waste bag
    b. Do not allow contaminated waste to accumulate on instrument tray
    c. Wipe instruments before returning to the tray (minimize bioburden)
C. Precautions and care in handling syringes with needles or reusable sharp instruments
    1. Needlestick injuries are a major cause of infection of healthcare personnel
    2. Special precautions for handling of syringe with needle and sharp instruments
       a. Keep sharp end angled away from dental healthcare provider
       b. Never permit point of needle to be moved in direction of body
       c. Do not allow uncovered needles to remain on instrument tray
       d. Never recap needle with a two-handed technique
          (1) Use "scoop" technique in which cap is scooped up from the tray with one hand only
          (2) Use commercially available sheath holder
          (3) Hold cap with cotton pliers for resheathing
       e. Needles should not be bent, broken, or otherwise manipulated by hand
D. Exposure incident protocol
    1. All contaminated needlesticks, puncture wounds, and cuts occurring during the course of treating clients or while decontaminating instruments should be treated as potentially infectious; contamination of open wounds or mucous membranes by blood and/or saliva should be given the same consideration
    2. Immediately administer first aid treatment
       a. Squeezing (bleeding) the wound
       b. Cleansing by running under tap water and using antimicrobial soap
       c. Disinfecting with iodophor or bleach
    3. Source individual—if source client can be identi-

fied, consult and request consent and cooperation for blood testing on same day as exposure (antibodies for HIV and hepatitis B surface antigen); results of source individual's tests are only to be confidentially directed to the exposed employee, not the employer
4. Inform employer of incident as soon as possible after incident; employer responsible for providing confidential medical evaluation and follow-up at a reasonable time and place and performed or supervised by a physician or other licensed healthcare professional (e.g., nurse, practitioner) (HCP)
5. The exposed healthcare worker should have laboratory testing, counseling, and blood assessments for HIV and HBV status on day of exposure incident, with employee's consent; if the exposed employee declines testing, the blood sample is to be preserved 50 days should the employee later consent to testing
6. Postexposure evaluation and vaccination for the employee is provided according to recommendations from the U.S. Public Health Service; the employee is informed of his or her own and source individual's test results by HCP; the HCP also tells employee of any conditions that require further evaluation and treatment[14]
7. The employer should receive a written report verifying that the *employee* was counseled, tested, informed of results and any further evaluation or treatment needed; also administration of Hep B vaccine; no findings or diagnoses are included in report to the employer because they are confidential between HCP and employee[14]

Prevention of Disease Transmission During Radiographic Procedures

See Chapter 5, section on infection control
A. Although radiographic procedures are generally noninvasive, the potential for disease transmission does exist
    1. Surface cleaning and disinfection
       a. Spray-wipe-spray should be performed only when operator is protected from potential pathogens as well as associated chemicals by wearing heavy-duty nitrile gloves, mask, protective clothing, and eyewear
       b. Include all surfaces touched and not otherwise protected with impervious barriers
       c. Machine control panel and any other equipment with electrical connections should not be sprayed directly with cleaner/disinfectant
    2. Use of barriers for radiographic equipment will prevent contamination and promote efficiency
       a. Placement of polyethylene bag over cone (posi-

tion indicating device, PID) tube head and swivel arms to turn tube head
  b. Exposure control switch and panel for various kVp and millamperage settings should be protected with plastic covering (set kVp before barrier placement; static charge may affect accuracy of reading[25])
  c. Cover headrest and adjustment levers, armrest, and chair controls
  d. Surface disinfection is more time-consuming alternative approach
3. Film and film holders
  a. Options for handling of exposed contaminated film before processing:
    (1) Clean and disinfect film (plastic-covered film only)
    (2) Place film in specifically designed plastic pouches before placing film in mouth and carefully remove barrier to avoid contaminating film covering
    (3) Unwrap contaminated film wrap *without* contaminating film
  b. Types of film holders and recirculation indications
    (1) A number of reusable film holders may be heat sterilized (e.g., RINN X-C-P instruments, Precision [Masel Inc.], and panoramic bite-block and holders); check manufacturer's recommendations
    (2) Disposable film holders (tabs for bite-wing films and Styrofoam bite blocks for periapical films); discard after use
    (3) If heat or ethylene oxide sterilization is not possible, rinse, decontaminate, and immerse heat-sensitive materials in an EPA-registered liquid chemical sterilant
B. Universal precautions for imaging of film
  1. Prepare *all* necessary materials to eliminate need to leave area during treatment which increases risk of cross-contamination
  2. Drape client with leaded apron and thyroid shield, and place client bib to act as barrier covering surfaces of the protective equipment; if shields become contaminated with blood or saliva, use surface cleaner/disinfectant
  3. Personnel's consistent use of gloves, gown, mask, and protective eyewear all decrease chance of disease transmission as well as chemically related injury
  4. Following radiograph exposure, wipe film with tissue to remove excess saliva (minimize bioburden)
  5. Drop film in disposable cup used to contain exposed contaminated film without contaminating the outside of the cup

6. After all films have been exposed, put on overgloves or remove gloves and wash hands before transporting film from the operatory
7. Proceed to processing area without contaminating surfaces en route to darkroom or automatic processor with daylight loader
C. Universal precautions for processing film
  1. Darkroom
    a. Prepare counter area adjacent to processor with surface barrier; designate contaminated/noncontaminated zones.
    b. Carefully pour out the contaminated exposed film on the surface area designated as contaminated
    c. Remove overgloves, or if not gloved, put on a new pair of gloves before handling the contaminated film packaging
    d. Open each film packet with care to touch only the packaging and not the film itself
    e. Hold the partially opened packet over the noncontaminated barrier area so that the noncontaminated film will fall out onto the noncontaminated surface
    f. Once all the films have been removed from the packets
      (1) Remove gloves, wash hands before picking up the noncontaminated films for placement into the processor, or
      (2) Don new gloves (preferably examination gloves without powder) and use caution to handle the films only by the edges when placing the films into the processor; requires very careful handling to prevent artifacts from gloves on uncovered films
    g. Discard contaminated waste, gloves; wash hands and exit darkroom
    h. Note: developer and fixer, even when contaminated, do not sustain bacterial or fungal growth[14]
  2. Daylight loading box with automatic processor
    a. Prepare processor by placing a barrier (plastic wrap) lining in the daylight loading box
    b. Place two cups inside the box, one holding the exposed film packets and the other cup to be used as a waste receptacle
    c. Prevent contamination of the fabric-covered hand portals (light-tight baffles) by entering portals while wearing a new pair of examination gloves
    d. Open film packets, handle films by the edges, and put them into the processor
    e. After all films have been fed into processor, remove gloves (pull them inside out), and place in the waste cup

f. Remove hands from light baffles, lift lid, and dispose of cups and waste

g. Wash hands

Infection Control for the Dental Laboratory

All aspects of oral healthcare delivery require prevention of disease transmission; dental impressions, prostheses, and appliances and related materials are contaminated with saliva and possibly blood and present special problems for infection control in and between the treatment area and dental laboratory; protection of dental laboratory personnel from bloodborne pathogens is also mandated by OSHA regulations

A. Protective attire and barrier techniques in the dental laboratory

1. When performing laboratory procedures, protective attire and gloves should be worn; use caution with lathes when wearing gloves to avoid hazard of injury

2. Wear masks and protective eyewear when performing procedures that produce aerosols; spatter and projectiles; or involve hazardous chemicals (e.g., disinfectants)[14,17]

B. Preparation of materials and transport to laboratory

1. Dental impressions, prostheses, and casts from the mouth can serve as potential sources of infectious microorganisms such as hepatitis B and herpetic whitlow

2. Clean and disinfect impressions, prostheses, and casts contaminated with blood and saliva before transporting them to the laboratory

   a. Rinse with running tap water before and after disinfection, partially to remove blood and saliva; attempt to remove any residual disinfectant

   b. Selection of a disinfectant should be based on the following considerations

      (1) Type of material

      (2) EPA registered as a hospital disinfectant with tuberculocidal activity and that kills both hydrophilic and lipophilic viruses

      (3) Disinfectants available/use in office (multipurpose)

      (4) Compatibility recommended by manufacturer/ADA

      (5) Available research data

      (6) Cost

      (7) Time required

3. Minimize contamination of common areas in laboratory

   a. Paper countertop covers

   b. Plastic covers over "high touch" areas

   c. Polishing lathe supplies

      (1) Fresh pumice

      (2) Clean disposable tray

      (3) Sterile or disposable ragwheel

   d. Use of shielding device and high-volume suction with polishing lathe, model trimmer, or grinding bench to minimize aerosolization

C. Disinfection of impressions

1. Thoroughly rinse *all* impressions under gently running water to remove blood, saliva, and organic matter before disinfection

2. Consult the impression material manufacturer for disinfection recommendations and to assess compatibility with the specific chemical disinfectant

3. The ADA recommends the immersion of impressions into a disinfectant as the disinfection method of choice in order to maximize effectiveness.[26] Immerse for the time recommended for TB disinfection; recommended disinfectants for specific types of impression materials[27,28]

   a. *Alginate:* Iodophors, chlorine compounds

   b. *Silicon rubber and polysulfide rubber base:* iodophors, chlorine compounds, glutaraldehydes, complex phenolics

   c. *Polyether:* Chlorine compounds, others may be used with caution

   d. *ZOE impression paste:* iodophors, glutaraldehydes

   e. *Reversible hydrocolloid:* iodophors, chlorine compounds

   f. *Compound:* iodophors, chlorine compound

D. Disinfection of complete dentures, fixed and removable prostheses[29]

1. Indications for disinfecting prostheses

   a. Before delivery to client

   b. Before return to laboratory after insertion in mouth

   c. When making adjustments in office

2. No ideal disinfectant currently exists for this purpose

   a. Selection depends on material[30]

      (1) Glutaraldehydes not recommended because potential for irritation and harm to intraoral tissues

      (2) Iodophors and chlorine compounds could damage metal; use minimal exposure time (10 min) to avoid damage to metal

   b. Removable (acrylic/porcelain)—iodophors and chlorine compounds recommended[29]

   c. Removable (metal/acrylic)

      (1) Recommendation for disinfectant needs further study

      (2) Study suggests that iodophors and chlorine dioxide may damage chrome-cobalt alloy within 3 minutes and that 1:10 sodium hypochlorite solution has a less corrosive effect[30]

(3) Use iodophor or phenol compound for disinfection of nonnoble alloys (nonprecious metals)

3. Use *minimum* essential exposure time with selected disinfectant along with thorough rinsing under running tap water to remove any residual disinfectant[30]; after disinfecting dental appliance, place it in mouthrinse to ensure pleasant taste and comfort for the client; orthodontic appliances should be handled in a similar manner

4. If removable prostheses need to be brushed, scrubbed, scaled, or polished to remove softened calculus or stain, equipment including brushes will need to be sterilized following procedure

E. Professional cleaning of removable prostheses
1. Commercial denture cleaning solutions recommended for stain and bacterial plaque removal are not a substitute for disinfection; some of these products have incorporated some antimicrobial activity, but it is limited and will not provide hospital-level elimination of microorganisms[14]
2. To eliminate need for disinfection of prostheses to be cleaned and to prevent contamination of ultrasonic bath or other "high touch" equipment associated with the cleaning procedure
   a. Use self-sealing disposable bag
   b. Use single unit dose of stain, bacterial plaque, and calculus removal solution for one time only
3. Place sealed bag in disinfected beaker in ultrasonic cleaning unit for specified time
4. Remove bag and beaker from ultrasonic unit, and use care in handling to avoid cross-contamination
5. Pour off solution; with gloved hand remove appliance and rinse thoroughly; brush if deposits remain
6. After calculus and stain removal, place appliance in mouthrinse in a bag to ensure pleasant taste
7. Rinse and return to client for reinsertion

F. Return prosthesis to treatment area from dental laboratory
1. Always disinfect appliance before sending it to another location (e.g., going from lab to treatment area)
2. Use new packing material each time prosthesis is sent between lab and dental office to prevent cross-contamination of shipping materials[19]
3. Communicate infection control protocol for laboratory procedures to lab and dental office personnel
4. Due to the porous nature of acrylic, dentures and other acrylic appliances that have been worn by clients should be handled as if contaminated even after disinfection; adequate disinfection is difficult with acrylic appliances[14]

Postclient Care of the Oral Healthcare Environment

A. Decontamination of treatment room
1. Wear protective eyewear, a mask, and puncture-resistant nitrile gloves
2. If local anesthetic was administered, the recapped needle should be removed from the syringe, and the syringe end of the needle should be recapped with the one-handed scoop technique and immediately placed in the sharps container located in each operatory; the glass cartridge is also considered an infectious potential sharp and object is to be disposed of in the sharps container as well
3. The small biohazard bag used during the appointment to contain blood-soaked gauze should be immediately sealed for transport to the workplace biohazardous waste container
4. Remove all disposable surface barriers; use care to avoid contacting the clean uncovered surface during removal
5. Flush all water lines for 20 seconds between clients
6. Instrument cassette should be closed or procedure trays covered to control airborne microorganisms[14] and immediately transported to the instrument recirculation area
7. If instrument sterilization processing is delayed instruments should be placed in a holding solution to keep blood, saliva, protein (bioburden) from drying on the instruments in order to promote ease in decontamination procedures[14]
8. Disposable single-use items such as disposable air-water syringe tips and saliva ejectors should be discarded
9. Clean and disinfect the interior surfaces of the suction tubing by flushing the high- and low-volume suction with a commercial cleansing and disinfecting solution

B. Infectious waste[31,32]
1. U.S. Environmental Protection Agency (EPA) *regulates* the management and disposal of infectious waste for three categories
   a. Sharps
   b. Tissue and extracted teeth
   c. Blood and blood-soaked items
2. Other state and local regulations may differ from the EPA in categories and amount of waste to qualify for small generator exemption[31]
3. ADA Council on Government Affairs and Federal Dental Services created four categories of waste to consider
   a. Regulated waste (biohazardous)—three categories:

(1) Sharps (used and unused needles, disposable syringes, broken instruments, suture needles, scalpel blades, burs, and local anesthetic cartridges

(2) Soft tissues, teeth, and other body tissues

(3) Blood and blood-soaked items (gauze, cotton rolls); liquid or semiliquid blood or saliva (other potentially infectious material–OPIM)[14]

(4) Items that are caked with dried blood or OPIM (saliva)[14]

b. Biomedical waste—a broad spectrum of medical solid waste that is generated through healthcare and research and includes all disposable items *other* than sharps, tissues, and blood/saliva soaked items (fourth category)

(1) Gloves, masks

(2) Saliva ejectors

(3) Client bibs and cups

(4) Surface barriers

(5) Disinfection wipes and paper towels

(6) Rubber cups, rubber dams

c. Biomedical or solid waste may be disposed of as common trash unless restricted by state and local ordinances[32]

4. State and local governments have developed waste disposal and handling rules; check with local department of health to determine regulations and definitions of what is considered biohazardous wastes

5. Waste management

a. Do not allow saliva or blood-coated material to accumulate on the bracket tray

b. Tape a small biohazard bag to the back of the dental unit; seal and dispose as biohazardous waste

c. Line trash cans with plastic or paper bags

d. Place disposable needles, scalpels, and other sharp items intact into puncture-resistant containers for disposal; sharps container must be in each treatment area

e. When the trash can is full, seal in sturdy, impervious bags and send for incineration

6. Waste disposal

a. Containment of biohazardous waste must be separated from other wastes and must be distinguished with warning signs

b. Disposal options—incineration, burial in sites approved for hazardous wastes, sterilization; if liquid, discharge into sewer system. Check state and local ordinance and EPA regulations

C. Instrument care[33]

1. Organization of sterilization area

a. Instrument recirculation area should be centrally located to all treatment rooms for efficiency

b. Design to allow for linear progression of instrument processing

c. Design to allow for separation of contaminated/noncontaminated zone

d. Recirculation center should be divided into six clearly designated areas:

(1) Containment—receiving area for contaminated instruments (presoaking and waste disposal)

(2) Decontamination—rinsing, ultrasonic cleaning, rinsing, drying

(3) Packaging—preparation of instruments (wrapped or bagged) before renewal

(4) Renewal—sterilization (usually more than one method because no one method suitable for all instruments)

(5) Maintenance—storage of instruments until ready to use

(6) Dispensing—tray preparation and distribution

e. Adhere to protocol for path instruments are to follow, which includes specific directions for procedures at each function area

f. Recessed countertop trash chutes for quick disposal of contaminated material

2. Instrument containment and decontamination

a. Handle contaminated instruments with heavy-duty nitrile gloves

b. Recessed ultrasonic unit facilitates access, cleaning, draining, and noise reduction

c. Use an area separate from the treatment area to clean instruments; spatter occurs and increases the potential of environmental pathogens

d. Instrument preparation

(1) Precleaning is the most important step in instrument sterilization; organic debris acts as a barrier to the sterilant and sterilization process

(2) Both surface disinfection and sterilization are multiple-step procedures

(a) Step 1—efficient initial and terminal precleaning

(b) Step 2—effective sterilization

(c) These two steps ensure sterilizing equipment and/or chemicals function as designed

(3) Dry instruments before sterilization—water interferes with dry heat and ethylene oxide sterilization

e. If time lapses before cleaning (decontamina-

tion), rinse in cold water and use disinfectant as holding solution
(1) Prevents adherence of organic debris
(2) Prevents rust and discoloration

f. Ultrasonic instrument cleaning
(1) Safest and most efficacious method of pre-cleaning; eliminates handscrubbing
(2) Action of ultrasonic cleaning
(a) Ultrasonic vibrations initiate cavitation; minute bubbles are produced; bubbles expand and collapse, creating vacuum areas that are responsible for cleaning by dislodging, dispersing, or dissolving the organic material on instruments
(b) Cleans by physical agitation and chemical dissolution
(3) Advantages
(a) Cleans more thoroughly
(b) Less chance of injury
(c) Less time consuming
(d) Less spatter of aerosols
(e) Penetrates grooves in instruments
(4) Procedure
(a) Follow the manufacturer's instructions
(b) Cassettes are ideal for encasement of a functional set of instruments through entire recirculation process
(c) Rinse
(d) Do not overload; keep the unit covered to prevent aerosols from contaminating sterilization area
(e) Time from 1 to 10 minutes, depending on the unit, solution, and material being cleaned, longer for cassettes—15 minutes
(f) Rinse instruments and carefully dry by air, dryer, convection oven, or heat lamp as alternatives to hand drying
(g) Promptly package and sterilize
(h) Change the solution daily
(i) Wipe the unit with 1% sodium hypochlorite

g. Manual scrubbing alternative—only used when ultrasonic would damage equipment (e.g., some handpieces or ultrasonic) cleaning unit malfunctions
(1) Wear puncture-resistant heavy-duty nitrile gloves
(2) Scrub with a long-handled, heat-sterilizable stiff brush; concentrate on grooved areas
(3) Scrub instruments submerged in water to minimize spatter and aerosols
(4) Use detergent, not soap
(5) Rinse and dry
(6) Sterilize brushes; brushes used for hand cleansing should be sterilized separately
(7) Disadvantages
(a) Increased risk for injury
(b) Less effective than ultrasonic cleaning
(c) Spatter
(d) Time consuming

3. Handpieces[34]
a. Sterilization of handpieces between clients has been recommended by the CDC and ADA for years,[35] handpiece sterilization will be mandated in near future[36]
(1) Flush water lines of high-speed handpieces
(2) Scrub thoroughly with detergent and water to remove adherent material
(3) Heat-sterilize
b. Some handpieces currently in use cannot be heat-sterilized without being damaged and should not be used
(1) If handpiece cannot be heat-sterilized, it is a compromise to infection control to disinfect because there is no way to decontaminate the interior of the handpiece[19]
(2) Some disinfectants cause damage; check label directions carefully (e.g., fiber-optic handpieces not compatible with iodophors)
(3) Investigate to determine whether handpieces that are not heat tolerant can be modified with replacement of parts with heat-stable components (retrofitting)
c. When purchasing new equipment, an important consideration should be whether or not the item can be sterilized (heat-sterilizable handpiece purchase should be a top priority)

4. Prophylaxis angles, contraangles, and air-water syringes[34]
a. Sterilizing these pieces of equipment is recommended according to the manufacturer's instructions
b. Most manufacturers now make equipment that can be sterilized
c. For effective routine sterilization, several items are needed for each treatment area
d. For angles
(1) Disassemble before sterilization
(2) Clean with grease solvent
(3) Sterilize
(4) Lubricate
(5) Reassemble
e. For air-water syringes[34]

(1) Flush water lines

(2) Remove entire syringe if it is readily disconnected and heat sterilizable, preferred option

(3) Alternative approach if air-water syringe permanently attached

    (a) Remove air-water tip and heat-sterilize

    (b) Spray and scrub syringe with an EPA-registered hospital cleaner/disinfectant

    (c) Wipe

    (d) Spray and let air-dry for the time specified by the manufacturer for tuberculocidal effect

5. Instrument packaging and storing[33]

  a. Packaging of items

    (1) Unpackaged instruments are immediately exposed to the environment and associated contaminants post sterilization; packaging prevents contamination post sterilization during storage and distribution

    (2) Packaging materials vary according to the type of sterilization method (Table 7-23); the packaging material selected must not melt, prevent sterilizing agent from penetrating to reach instruments, or release unwanted chemicals into the sterilization chamber[17]

    (3) Cleaned instruments are placed in heat-stable poly/paper pouches (see through plastic biofilm material on one side and heavy sterilization paper on the other); plastic tubing, cassettes, or trays to be wrapped with sterilization wrap, sealed with appropriate tape, and dated

    (4) Heat-stable, slotted instrument cassettes are ideal because the cassette may be placed in ultrasonic cleaner for instrument cleaning, handled with minimal risk of puncture (instruments not exposed), and stored in sealed wrap after sterilization and cassette may serve as sterile instrument tray

    (5) Pins, staples, or paper clips should not be used because they make holes in the wrap that permit entry of microorganisms

    (6) Instruments should be packaged loosely to allow maximum contact with steam or chemical vapors; too many instruments in package can lead to incomplete sterilization

  b. Storage of instruments

    (1) After sterilization, allow time for instruments to dry, if wet, and cool down before they are stored in the sealed packages until they are used

    (2) To ensure continued protection from recontamination, sealed packages should be kept on shelves protected by glass doors for dry, low-dust storage

    (3) Many commercial wraps and sealed plastic pouches can maintain sterility for months if unopened (maximum storage, 30 days); sterile packages that are dropped on floor, punctured, torn, or become wet must be considered contaminated

    (4) Taking instruments out of package and placing them in disinfected cabinet drawers for later use is not recommended; instruments are no longer sterile if unwrapped because they come into contact with microorganisms in the atmosphere or storage area

D. Guidelines on what to sterilize, disinfect, or clean—items associated with the oral care environment may be classified as critical, semicritical, or noncritical items[17,37]

  1. *Critical items* are those that penetrate oral soft tissue or bone and must be sterilized (e.g., probe); heat or heat pressure sterilization methods are preferred because they are

    a. Effective

    b. Relatively easy to use

    c. Comparatively inexpensive

    d. Readily monitored for effectiveness

  2. *Semicritical items* are instruments that come in contact with mucous membranes and must be heat sterilized between uses (e.g., handle component of ultrasonic handpiece) if heat sensitive, select an alternative method for sterilization

  3. *Noncritical items* are items or equipment that do not normally penetrate or contact mucous membrane but are exposed to spatter, spray, or splashing of blood or touched by contaminated hands (e.g., x-ray tube head); require intermediate-level disinfection

E. Sterilization methods.[14,33,39] No single method of sterilization will be suitable for all items used in the oral healthcare environment (Table 7-23)

  1. Steam autoclave (moist heat under pressure)

    a. Action

      (1) Moist heat denatures and coagulates microbial protein; pressure serves only to elevate temperature[28]

      (2) Steam must be able to penetrate

        (a) Air must be adequately removed to allow steam penetration and heat transfer

        (b) Steam travels vertically

        (c) Pack loosely; arrange load to allow free passage of steam

Table 7-23

Sterilization of Dental Instruments, Materials and Some Commonly Used Items[a]

Instrument, material or item	Steam autoclave	Dry heat oven	Chemical vapor	Ethylene oxide[b]	Other methods & comments
Angle Attachments[a]	c	c	c	d	
Burs					
Carbon steel	e	f	f	f	Discard
Steel	c	f	f	f	Discard
Tungsten-carbide	c	f	c	f	Discard
Condensers	f	f	f	f	
Dapen Dishes	f	c	c	f	
Endodontic Instruments (Broaches, Files, Reamers)	f	f	f	f	
Stainless steel handles	c	f	f	f	
Stainless w/ plastic handles	f	f	e	f	
Fluoride Gel Trays					
Heat-resistant plastic	f	d	e	f	
Non–heat-resistant plastic	d	d	e	f	Discard (f)
Glass Slabs	f	f	f	f	
Hand Instruments					
Carbon steel (steam autoclave with chemical protection [2% sodium nitrite])	e	f	f	f	
Stainless steel	f	f	f	f	
High-speed Handpieces[a]	(f)a	e	(c)a	d	
Contra-angles	f	e	f	d	
Prophylaxis Angles[a] (disposable preferred)	c	c	c	d	Discard (f)
Impression Trays					
Aluminum metal	f	c	f	f	
Chrome-plated	f	f	f	f	
Custom acrylic resin	d	d	d	f	Discard (f)
Plastic	d	d	d	f	Discard preferred (f)
Instruments in Packs	f	c Small packs	f	f Small packs	
Instrument Tray Setups					
Restorative or surgical	c Size limit	c	c Size limit	f Size limit	
Mirrors	e	f	f	f	
Needles					
Disposable	d	d	d	d	Discard (f) Do not reuse
Nitrous Oxide					
Nose piece	(f)a	d	(f)a	d	
Hoses	(f)a	d	(f)a	d	

From: ADA Council on Scientific Affairs and ADA Council on Dental Practice: Infection control recommendations for the dental office and dental laboratory. *J Am Dent Assoc* 127:5:676-677, 1996.
[a]Because manufacturers use a variety of alloys and materials in these products, confirmation with the equipment manufacturers is recommended, especially for handpieces and their attachments
[b]Ethylene oxide should only be used to sterilize instruments that can be thoroughly cleaned and dried
[c]Effective and acceptable method
[d]Ineffective method
[e]Effective method, but risk of damage to materials
[f]Effective and preferred method

Table 7-23

Sterilization of Dental Instruments, Materials and Some Commonly Used Items—cont'd

Instrument, material or item	Steam autoclave	Dry heat oven	Chemical vapor	Ethylene oxide[b]	Other methods & comments
Orthodontic Pliers					
High-quality stainless	f	f	f	f	
Low-quality stainless	e	f	f	f	
With plastic parts	d	d	d	f	
Pluggers and Condensers	f	f	f	f	
Polishing Wheels & Disks					
Garnet and cuttle	d	e	e	d	
Rag	f	e	c	d	
Rubber	c	e	e	d	
Prostheses, Removable	e	e	e	d	
Rubber Dam Equipment					
Carbon steel clamps	e	f	f	f	
Metal frames	f	f	f	f	
Plastic frames	e	e	e	f	
Punches	e	f	f	f	
Stainless Steel Clamps	f	f	f	f	
Rubber Items					
Prophylaxis cups	e	e	e	d	Discard (f)
Saliva Evacuators, Ejectors (Plastic)	e	e	e	e	Discard (f) (single use/ disposable)
Stones					
Diamond	c	f	f	f	
Polishing	f	c	f	f	
Sharpening	f	f	f	e	
Surgical Instruments					
Stainless steel	f	f	f	f	
Ultrasonic Scaling Tips	c	d	d	f	
Water air Syringe Tips	f	f	f	d	Discard (f)
X-ray Equipment					
Plastic film holders	(f)a	d	(c)a	f	
Collimating devices	e	d	d	f	

      (d) Place jars on sides
    b. Operation
      (1) Autoclave at 121° C (250° F) at 15 pounds pressure for 15 to 20 minutes (wrapped)
      (2) Flash sterilization with autoclave[17,33]
        (a) Flash sterilization—process uses higher-than-standard temperature and shorter time
        (b) Autoclave at 134° C (273° F), 3.5 to 12 minutes; rubber, plastic, or items with lumens (porous) require longer time
        (c) Use perforated tray
        (d) Restrict use for emergency situations or unplanned urgent need

        (e) Since instrument is unwrapped, deliver for immediate use only
      (3) timing begins when the temperature gauge reaches the recommended temperature
      (4) Heavy loads may require twice the time
    c. Advantages
      (1) Time-efficient
      (2) Allows loads to be packaged, eases maintenance
      (3) Penetrates fabric and paper wrappings
      (4) Nontoxic
      (5) Can be readily monitored for effectiveness
    d. Disadvantages/precautions
      (1) Nonstainless steel items may rust and cor-

rode; corrosion inhibitors (e.g., sodium nitrite) may reduce this problem
        (2) May damage plastics and rubber
        (3) May dull sharp items
2. Dry heat
    a. Action
        (1) Oxidation of cell parts
        (2) Heat conducted from the exterior surface to the interior of the object; time required for heat penetration varies among materials
    b. Operation
        (1) Dry heat sterilizers
            (a) Static-air type dry heat sterilizer; similar to oven used for cooking; dental use requires FDA approved medical sterilizer that has higher standards for insulation and temperature criteria[14]
            (b) Rapid heat transfer dry heat sterilizer (forced-air convection unit) circulates heated air throughout chamber at high velocity which permits more rapid transfer of heat
        (2) Dry heat (static-air)—sterilize at 160° C (320° F) for 60 to 120 min; rapid heat: 191° C (375° F), 12 minutes for wrapped and 6 minutes for unwrapped instruments[33]
        (3) Properly time sterilization interval
            (a) Chamber and instruments must be preheated to sterilization temperature
            (b) Keep airspaces between packages
            (c) If cycle interrupted (sterilizer opened) must start timing over again[14]
        (4) Verification of temperature
            (a) Oven thermometer only indicates the oven temperature, not the instruments' temperature
            (b) Load temperature should be checked with a thermocouple and pyrometer
    c. Advantages
        (1) Nontoxic
        (2) Does not dull cutting edges
        (3) Does not rust and corrode (items must be dry before sterilization)
        (4) Easy to use with very little maintenance required
        (5) Can be readily monitored for effectiveness
    d. Disadvantages
        (1) Usually requires longer cycle for sterilization (except for rapid heat transfer)
        (2) Damages heat labile items (e.g., some rubber/plastics)
        (3) May discolor or char fabric

        (4) Poor penetration requires careful loading
        (5) Cannot sterilize liquids
        (6) Generally not suited for handpieces
        (7) Unwrapped items quickly contaminated post sterilization
3. Unsaturated chemical vapor
    a. Action
        (1) Alcohols, formaldehyde, ketone, acetone and water heated under pressure to produce gas that permeates and destroys the microbes and viruses
    b. Operation
        (1) Sterilize at 134° C (273° F) with 20 to 40 pounds pressure for 20 minutes;[33] follow manufacturer's directions
        (2) Start timing after the correct temperature is reached
        (3) Heavy wrapping and large loads greatly increase time
        (4) Need the manufacturer's chemical solution
        (5) Heavy, tightly wrapped packages do not allow vapor penetration (e.g., muslin packs will not sterilize); must select packaging pouches, bags, wraps indicated as appropriate for unsaturated chemical vapor
        (6) Adequate ventilation required
    c. Advantages
        (1) Relatively short cycle time
        (2) Does not corrode or rust metal items
        (3) Very reliable
        (4) Does not dull cutting edges
        (5) Items dry quickly
    d. Disadvantages
        (1) Uses hazardous chemicals (ethanol and formaldehyde); good ventilation required
        (2) Vapor must penetrate through all materials (fabric packs incompatible)
        (3) Damages some materials sensitive to chemicals, temperature, and pressure
        (4) Requires special solution increasing cost
4. Ethylene oxide (ETO)
    a. Action
        (1) Ethylene oxide vapor sterilization creates a gas toxic for all viruses and bacteria at relatively low temperature
        (2) Has unusual powers of penetration of organic material[33]
    b. Operation
        (1) Sterilize at room temperature 25° C (75° F) for 10 to 16 hours
        (2) Preferably overnight processing
        (3) Well-ventilated area required

(4) Because of potential for explosion during sterilization cycle, in certain units, a special container with spark shield is required

(5) Aeration of materials after sterilization

(a) Metal instruments can be used immediately

(b) Aerate absorbent materials (plastics and rubber) for 24 to 48 hours for complete dissipation of ethylene oxide (residual gas can cause burning of epithelial tissues)

c. Advantages

(1) Many types of materials can be sterilized with minimal or no damage (including rubber and handpieces)

(2) High capacity for penetration

d. Disadvantages

(1) Requires long processing times

(2) High cost of equipment and operation

(3) Use of ethylene oxide gas, toxic/hazardous chemical

(4) Gas absorption requires aeration of plastic, rubber, and cloth items for 24 to 48 hours

5. Prolonged immersion in liquid chemical sterilants[38]

a. Immersion in a chemical sterilant is used only when items cannot be sterilized by heat, ethylene oxide (biologically verifiable) is preferred for many heat-sensitive items over liquid sterilant

b. Overall requirements if selecting chemical sterilant

(1) Must be registered by Environmental Protection Agency (EPA) as a sterilant (reuse for 28 to 30 days)

(2) Contact time determines difference between whether solution will sterilize or just disinfect

(3) Must follow manufacturer's directions

c. Chemical products available for immersion sterilization

(1) Glutaraldehyde—action effective against bacteria, viruses; sporicidal in 10 hours

(2) Chloride dioxide—rapid action as a disinfectant in 3 minutes and as a sterilant in 6 hours (e.g., Exspore)

d. Process

(1) Wear protective eyewear and heavy-duty nitrile gloves when preparing and using sterilants

(2) Prepare solution according to manufacturer's explicit instructions

(3) Avoid diluting solution with water from precleaning process

(4) Instruments must be precleaned and remain undisturbed and immersed for the prescribed length of time

(5) Remove instruments with sterile forceps, rinse with sterile water, dry and at once cover with sterile towel

e. Advantages[14]:

(1) Can be used to sterilize items sensitive to heat

(2) Active in presence of organic matter

(3) Prolonged activated life

f. Disadvantages[14]

(1) Reuse life varies with bioburden

(2) Toxicity from fumes and severe tissue irritation

(3) Allergenic

(4) Cannot package items[42]

(5) Items must be rinsed with sterile water

(6) Not time saving when compared with steam autoclaving or unsaturated chemical vapor

(7) Solutions may be diluted or inactivated by water, other soaps, and chemicals

(8) Effectiveness cannot be biologically monitored

(a) Cannot determine whether sterilization has been achieved

(b) Systems are available for assessing concentrations of these agents[17]

(9) No liquid chemical can be considered a substitute for sterilization by steam, dry heat, chemical vapor, or ethylene oxide[14]

F. Verification of sterilization

1. Routine use of biologic indicators for verification of the adequacy of sterilization cycles is recommended by the American Dental Association (ADA) and Centers for Disease Control (CDC); destruction of the heat-resistant bacterial spores during sterilization procedures is used to infer that *all* microorganisms exposed to the same conditions have been destroyed[14]

2. Needed because failure of sterilization can occur as a result of

a. Overloading

b. Improper packaging

c. Improper timing

d. Improper unit operation

e. Unit malfunction

f. Improper maintenance

3. Methods[39]

a. Biologic indicators (spore tests)

(1) Bacterial endospores are either sealed in vials or ampules or impregnated in paper strips

(2) Most reliable test of sterilization, testing for actual killing of bacterial spores

(3) Test the sterilization equipment weekly and when:
(a) Equipment repaired
(b) New packaging material implemented
(c) New sterilizer initially used
(d) Staff training (during and after)
(e) Change in loading arrangement
(f) Implant device is sterilized and hold until test results known[39]

(4) Biologic monitoring system must be compatible with the method of sterilization[19]

(5) Steam and chemical vapor—use spores of *Bacillus stearothermophilus*
(a) Steam autoclave—spores packaged in filter paper *strips* encased in an envelope, in *vials* that contain a small disk with spores plus a small ampule of culture media, or in a sealed ampule with spores suspended in a culture medium
(b) Unsaturated chemical vapor—requires strip biomonitoring

(6) Dry heat and ethylene oxide—use spores of *Bacillus subtilis*
(a) Ethylene oxide—packaged in strips or vials

(7) Biologic indicators should be placed inside packs, bags, or cassettes to test penetration of the sterilization agent

(8) Incubate an unexposed (unsterilized) ampule, vial, or strip in media at the same time to provide a control; growth of spores from control monitor and no growth from the sterilized monitor indicate that the sterilizer is functioning properly

b. Internal chemical indicators, also called "slow change" indicator

(1) Dyes that change color when heat, steam, or gas has reached inside of the load for prolonged time and probable sterilization

(2) Sensitive to certain combinations of exposure; cannot be relied on for proof of sterility

(3) Provide a warning of gross sterilizer malfunction

(4) Place inside each multiple instrument pack to confirm heat penetration to all instruments during each cycle[14]

(5) Use with each load or pack, place inside instrument package

c. Chemical process indicators

(1) Dyes that change color upon short exposure to sterilizing conditions, generally printed on packaging materials or in tape form

(2) Not proof of sterilization

(3) Distinguishes those instruments that have been in the sterilizer from those that have not

(4) Use on each pack in each load

4. Documentation of monitoring procedures
a. Records results of process and biologic monitoring procedures
b. Documents compliance with federal regulations
c. Provides a safeguard against a potential liability suit by documenting quality assurance practices

Occupational Safety and Health Administration (OSHA) and Occupational Exposure to Bloodborne Pathogens

A. Goal is protection of healthcare employees against exposure to blood-borne infectious diseases; requires employers at healthcare facilities to provide a safe working environment

B. OSHA standards

1. In 1987 OSHA developed interim regulations that resulted in the Final Bloodborne Pathogen Standards published in December 1991.

2. The standards are based on CDC and ADA guidelines for prevention of HIV/HBV and other bloodborne diseases

C. Bloodborne pathogen standards and the responsibilities of the employer

1. Determine employee's occupational exposure risk status by identifying tasks and procedures where contact with blood may occur

2. Develop an infection control plan that incorporates universal precautions along with specific controls and procedures to address all regulations within the standard

3. Provide training program that incorporates content to prevent occupational exposure to bloodborne pathogens appropriate to the employee's language, and educational and literacy levels

4. Make available appropriate personal protective equipment (gloves, masks, eye protection, and gowns) and take responsibility to arrange disposal, cleaning, repair, and replacement of such equipment

5. Ensure cleanliness of work site with emphasis on surface cleaning and disinfection, laundry handling

protocol, and infectious waste disposal according to federal, state, and local regulations

6. Offer and assume costs for hepatitis B vaccination and if the employee refuses vaccination, a signed statement to that effect must be placed in the employee's file

7. Provide exposure incident medical and laboratory procedures without cost to employees

8. Maintenance of records to include training sessions (participants, trainers, summary of content), employee's HBV immunization status, and reports on postexposure evaluation (confidential)

9. Post signs, biohazardous waste labels, and/or red containers that indicate infectious materials or waste

D. Inspections conducted by OSHA[40,41]
   1. Types
      a. Employee complaint inspections
      b. Programmed inspections of randomly selected work sites employing 11 or more people
   2. Process
      a. OSHA representative would request infection control records from employer and documentation of needlestick and/or illness records
      b. If office has no formal infection control program with documentation and/or did not keep injury and illness records, emphasis of inspection would be on interviewing employees and evaluation of work site
      c. OSHA inspection of oral healthcare environment would focus on client care areas and employee hazard communication program
   3. Violation consequences
      a. Employer issued citation
      b. Citation letter will include
         (1) Abatement date
         (2) Penalties incurred
         (3) Deadline by which recommended changes must be made and fines paid

REFERENCES

1. Jawetz E, Melnick JL, Adelberg EA, et al: *Jawetz, Melnick & Adelberg's medical microbiology,* ed 20, Norwalk, Conn, 1995, Appleton & Lange.
2. Arms K, Camp PS: *Biology,* ed 4, Philadelphia, 1995, WB Saunders.
3. Wistreich GA, Lechlman MD: *Microbiology,* ed 5, New York, 1989, Macmillan.
4. Slots J, Taubman MA: *Contemporary oral microbiology and immunology,* St Louis, 1992, Mosby.
5. Holt JG, Krieg NR, Sneath PHA, et al: *Bergey's manual of determinative bacteriology,* ed 9, Baltimore, 1994, Williams & Wilkins.
6. Mims CA, Playfair JHL, Roitt IM, et al: *Medical microbiology,* London, 1993, Mosby Europe.
7. Mims CA: *Pathogenesis of infectious disease,* ed 4, London, 1995, Academic Press.
8. McGhee JR, Michalek SM, Cassell GH, eds: *Dental microbiology,,* New York, 1982, Harper & Row.
9. Stites DP, Stobo JD, Wells JV, editors: *Basic and clinical immunology,* ed 8, East Norwalk, Conn, 1994, Appleton & Lange.
10. Levy JA: The human immunodeficiency virus and its pathogenesis. In Medical management of AIDS, *Infect Dis Clin North Am* 2:285, 1988.
11. Centers for Disease Control: 1993 revised classification system for HIV infection and expanded surveillance case definition for AIDS among adolescents and adults, *MMWR Morb Mortal Wkly Rep* 41:17, 1992.
12. Tortora GJ, Funke BR, Case CL: *Microbiology: An introduction,* ed 5, Menlo Park, NJ, 1995, Benjamin/Cummings.
13. Newman MG, Nisengard R: *Oral microbiology and immunology,* ed 2, Philadelphia, 1994, WB Saunders.
14. Cottone JA, Terezhalmy GT, Molinari JA: *Practical infection control in dentistry,* ed 2, Baltimore, 1996, Williams & Wilkins.
15. Bednarsh H, Eklund KJ: TB prevention calls for a national standard, *ACCESS,* 8:8-11, 1994.
16. Shearer BG: Biofilm and the dental office. *J Am Dent Assoc* 127: 181-189, 1996.
17. Miller CH, Palenik CJ: *Infection control and the management of hazardous materials for the dental team,* St Louis, 1994, Mosby.
18. King LJ: AIDS awareness, *ACCESS* 7:4, 6, 1993.
19. Miller CH: Routine gloving common practice, *RDH* 1991.
20. Runnells RR: *Handbook of dental infection control,* New York, 1988, Johnson & Johnson.
21. MacDonald G: Chemical hazards: Regulations, identification, and resources, *Calif Dent Assoc* 17:32, 1989.
22. Molinari JA, Gleason MJ, Cottone JA, et al: Cleaning and disinfectant properties of dental surface disinfectants, *J Am Dent Assoc* 117.179, 1988.
23. Molinari JA, Gleason MJ, Cottone JA, et al: Comparison of dental surface disinfectants, *Gen Dent* 35:171, 1987.
24. Office Sterilization and Asepsis Procedures (OSAP) Research Foundation: April 1993, OSAP Research Foundation.
25. Jeffries D, Morris JW, White VP: KVP meter errors induced by plastic wrap, *J Dent Hyg* 2:91-93, 1991.
26. Council on Dental Therapeutics, Council on Prosthetic Services and Dental Laboratory Relations: Guidelines for infection control in the dental office and the commercial dental laboratory, *J Am Dent Assoc* 110:969, 1985.
27. Merchant VA: Update on disinfection of impressions, prostheses and casts, *Calif Dent Assoc* 10:31-35, 1992.
28. Merchant VA: Disinfection of dental impressions, *Dent Teamwork* 3:13, 1989.
29. Merchant VA, Molinari JA: Infection control in prosthodontics: A choice no longer, *Gen Dent* 37: 1, 1989.
30. Merchant VA: Prosthodontics and infection control—it's a whole new ballgame, *Calif Dent Assoc* 17:49, 1989.

31. Fan PL, McGill SL: How much waste do dentists generate? *Calif Dent Assoc* 17:39, 1989.

32. Shaefer ME: Hazardous waste management, *Dent Clin North Am* 35:383-390, 1991.

33. Office Sterilization and Asepsis Procedures (OSAP) Research Foundation: *Instrument processing position paper,* January 1997, OSAP Research Foundation.

34. Office Sterilization and Asepsis Procedures (OSAP) Research Foundation: *Dental unit waterlines position paper,* January 1997, OSAP Research Foundation.

35. Centers for Disease Control: HIV transmission in dental settings, *MMWR Morb Mortal Wkly Rep* 41:344-346, May 15, 1992.

36. Control: The Infectious Disease Newsletter: Current status of handpiece sterilization, 6:1, 1991.

37. Office Sterilization and Asepsis Procedures (OSAP) Research Foundation: *Chemical agents for surface cleaning and disinfection,* 1995, OSAP Research Foundation.

38. Office Sterilization and Asepsis Procedure (OSAP) Research Foundation: *Glutaraldehydes for instrument sterilization,* 1995, OSAP Research Foundation.

39. Miller CH: Sterilization and disinfection: What every dentist needs to know, *J Am Dent Assoc* 123:46-54, 1992.

40. Fay MF: OSHA infection control rule, inspections make compliance by dentists mandatory, *New Silverman's News* 1:10, 1989.

41. Miyasaki CM, et al: Demystifying OSHA inspection guidelines, *Calif Dent Assoc* 17:28, 1989.

Review Questions

1 Microscopy that does *NOT* illuminate objects by visible light includes
   A. Fluorescence
   B. Phase-contrast
   C. Dark-field
   D. Bright-field
   E. Compound

2 Which early microbiologist was *MOST* responsible for proving microorganisms can cause disease?
   A. Louis Pasteur
   B. Robert Koch
   C. Joseph Lister
   D. Robert Hooke
   E. Carolus Linnaeus

3 Microscopy used to produce three-dimensional images of a virus surface is
   A. Transmission electron
   B. Scanning electron
   C. Phase-contrast
   D. Fluorescence
   E. Dark-field

4 Stains used for initial bacterial grouping include
   A. Negative and gram stains
   B. Flagellar and negative stains
   C. Acid-fast and flagellar stains
   D. Acid-fast and gram stains
   E. Gram and flagellar stains

5 Structures used for bacterial locomotion are
   A. Fimbriae and flagella
   B. Cilia and fimbriae
   C. Axial filaments and flagella
   D. Pili and axial filaments
   E. Flagella and pili

6 A glycocalyx that is loosely attached to the cell is the
   A. Cell wall
   B. Cytoplasmic membrane
   C. Outer membrane
   D. Capsule
   E. Slime layer

7 Gram-positive and gram-negative cell walls both contain
   A. Lipopolysaccharides
   B. Peptidoglycan
   C. Techoic acid
   D. Outer membranes
   E. Endotoxin

8 What division of bacteria has a gram-negative cell wall?
   A. Firmicutes
   B. Gracilicutes
   C. Tenericutes
   D. Archaeobacteria
   E. Mendosicutes

9 Chemical conditions affecting microbial growth include
   A. Oxygen concentration and vitamin sources
   B. Temperature and osmotic pressure
   C. pH and nutrient sources
   D. Osmotic pressure and oxygen concentration
   E. Vitamin sources and pH

10 Which of the following are *MOST* likely to be pathogenic for humans?
   A. Mesophiles
   B. Thermophiles
   C. Acidophiles
   D. Psychrophiles
   E. Alkalinophiles

11 Which microorganisms require low concentrations of oxygen for growth?
   A. Aerotolerant anaerobes
   B. Facultative anaerobes
   C. Microaerophilic
   D. Aerobes
   E. Strict anaerobes

12 *Streptococcus pyogenes* cultured on blood agar would have a _____ zone around colonies
   A. Red
   B. Green
   C. Black
   D. Yellow
   E. Clear

13 Psychrophiles would be expected to grow *BEST*
A. At low pH
B. At high pH
C. In hot springs
D. In the refrigerator
E. At room temperature

14 Penicillin is *MOST* effective during which phase of bacterial growth?
A. Lag
B. Log
C. Stationary
D. Decline
E. Death

15 Metabolic control by feedback inhibition is activated by a build-up of
A. End-product
B. Substrate
C. Enzyme
D. Reactant
E. Operon

16 Biosynthesis within microorganisms is also called
A. Anabolism
B. Catabolism
C. Metabolism
D. Glycolysis
E. Respiration

17 Plasmids are most commonly transferred by
A. Transposons
B. Transduction
C. Transformation
D. Conjugation
E. Mutation

18 The relationship between a pathogen and a human is termed
A. Commensalism
B. Parasitism
C. Predation
D. Symbiosis
E. Syntrophism

19 The relationship between vitamin K producing intestinal flora and a human is termed
A. Syntrophism
B. Parasitism
C. Commensalism
D. Symbiosis
E. Competition

20 Fungi that do *NOT* produce sexual spores are
A. Zygomycotina
B. Basidiomycotina
C. Sac fungi
D. Dimorphic fungi
E. Imperfect fungi

21 The active feeding stage of a protozoa is a
A. Cyst
B. Sporozoa
C. Trophozoite
D. Pseudopodia
E. Ciliophora

22 Small, single-stranded, circular RNA molecules that primarily infect plants are
A. Virions
B. Viroids
C. Operons
D. Prions
E. Phages

23 What are the general steps in a viral multiplication cycle?
A. Penetration, attachment, uncoating, synthesis, release
B. Penetration, attachment, synthesis, release, uncoating
C. Attachment, penetration, uncoating, synthesis, release
D. Attachment, uncoating, penetration, synthesis, release
E. Uncoating, release, synthesis, attachment, penetration

24 After use, the preferred method of cleaning instruments is by
A. Placing instruments in an ultrasonic cleaning unit
B. Scrubbing instruments with a stiff brush
C. Soaking instruments in a blood solvent
D. Holding instruments under a hard spray of water
E. Placing instruments directly in an autoclave

25 Before sterilizing the prophylaxis angle, it must be
A. Soaked in a grease solvent
B. Disassembled and soaked in a disinfectant
C. Soaked in a disinfectant
D. Disassembled and decontaminated
E. Disassembled and soaked in a grease solvent

26 If instruments are sterilized without being wrapped, they must be
A. Placed in a drawer that has been disinfected
B. Placed on a disinfected tray for use within 18 hours
C. Wrapped in sterile towels within 2 hours
D. Directly transported to the treatment area for immediate use
E. Put into a plastic bag and stapled for closure

27 Most plastics can be renewed by which biologically verifiable method of sterilization?
A. Steam autoclaving
B. Soaking in glutaraldehyde
C. Dry heat
D. Chemical vapor
E. Ethylene oxide

28 In the autoclave, wrapped instrument packs should be arranged loosely and placed as upright as possible so that
A. Steam can penetrate
B. Instruments will not be bent or broken
C. Moisture will not collect and cause rust
D. A vacuum can be created
E. The temperature reaches the correct range

29 The dental hygienist is using a standard dry-heat oven to sterilize instruments. The oven is preheated, and the instruments have reached the same temperature as the oven. Approximately how long will it take until sterilization is achieved?
A. 3 hours
B. 2 hours
C. 30 minutes
D. 20 minutes
E. 60 minutes

30 What is one disadvantage of chemical vapor pressure sterilization?
  A. Materials must be aerated
  B. Rusting can occur
  C. Adequate ventilation is necessary
  D. Instruments are wet at the end of the cycle
  E. The process is too long

31 The oral healthcare team uses a steam autoclave for sterilization. If you are responsible for purchasing spore strips to test sterility, which of the following would you order?
  A. *Clostridium botulinum*
  B. *Bacillus stearothermophilus*
  C. *Clostridium tetani*
  D. *Bacillus anthracis*
  E. *Bacillus subtilis*

32 What is one reason for selecting a chemical sterilant for instruments?
  A. It is faster than heat sterilization
  B. Verification of sterilization is possible
  C. For limited sterilization of a few heat-sensitive items if ethylene oxide is not available
  D. It is inexpensive
  E. The good penetrating ability when instruments are soaked

33 In designing a sterilization area, what is the *MOST* crucial requirement?
  A. Availability of glutaraldehyde
  B. Allowance for adequate counter space
  C. Availability of instrument storage areas
  D. Separation of contaminated and noncontaminated areas
  E. Purchase of a dry-heat oven

34 Radiographs have been taken on a client. After dismissing the client, the *FIRST STEP* should be to
  A. Process the radiographs
  B. Remove surface barriers and disinfect the unit
  C. Label the radiographic mount
  D. Reassemble the film holders
  E. Wipe the film holders with disinfectant

35 Dental employers must provide at-risk employees with protection from
  A. Hepatitis A, hepatitis B, and hepatitis C
  B. Hepatitis B
  C. Tuberculosis and hepatitis A
  D. Hepatitis B and hepatitis C
  E. Hepatitis B and tuberculosis

36 The personnel in the office where you have just accepted employment do not wear uniforms but instead wear regular street clothing. Your action should be to
  A. Soak and wash clothes worn at the office in bleach
  B. Refuse to conform and wear uniforms
  C. Launder clothes worn at the office with your other street clothing
  D. Discuss OSHA regulations regarding protective clothing with your employer
  E. Try to convince other office personnel to purchase uniforms

37 When considering factors to prevent disease transmission, which of the following is *MOST* acceptable?
  A. Wristwatches
  B. Bracelets that do not dangle
  C. Small earrings
  D. Wedding bands
  E. Other rings

38 How often should face masks be changed?
  A. After each client
  B. Three to four times a day
  C. At noon
  D. When damp
  E. At midmorning and midafternoon

39 The dental hygienist is about to perform nonsurgical periodontal therapy on a client who has no medical complications as indicated by the health history and interview. For this appointment the dental hygienist should wear
  A. Protective eyewear
  B. Protective eyewear and a face mask
  C. Protective eyewear and gloves
  D. Protective eyewear and gloves for the initial examination
  E. Protective eyewear, gloves, and a face mask

40 You wear gloves routinely for all clients and are trying not to be wasteful with office supplies. What is the *BEST* alternative to changing gloves for each client?
  A. Wash and rinse gloved hands one time between clients
  B. Perform a short scrub on the gloved hands between clients
  C. Perform a surgical scrub before gloving
  D. Lather and rinse gloved hands two to three times between clients
  E. No acceptable alternative

41 Which of the following behaviors associated with hand washing is recommended?
  A. Use cloth towels for drying
  B. Use a brush on hands two times a day
  C. Perform a short scrub at the beginning of each day
  D. Disinfect the scrub brush
  E. Perform a surgical scrub at the beginning of each day

42 Which of the following is a *PRIORITY* in the selection of a hand cleanser?
  A. Gentleness
  B. Viricidal ability
  C. Bacteriostatic ability
  D. Bactericidal ability
  E. Cost

43 Which of the following forms of hand cleansers is *LEAST* likely to contribute to disease transmission?
  A. Liquid or powdered
  B. Bar or liquid
  C. Liquid only
  D. Powdered or bar
  E. Powdered only

44 After a known carrier of hepatitis B has been treated, dental instruments should be
   A. Soaked in sodium hypochlorite
   B. Processed the same as other instruments
   C. Handled with two pairs of household rubber gloves
   D. Scrubbed with iodine surgical scrub
   E. Sterilized twice as long

45 Wearing protective eyewear during professional oral health-care helps prevent
   A. Conjunctivitis and hepatitis A
   B. Hepatitis B and ophthalmia neonatorum
   C. Herpes and injury
   D. Ophthalmia neonatorum and herpes
   E. Injury and hepatitis A

46 The mature virus particle is called a
   A. Bacteriophage
   B. Capsid
   C. Genome
   D. Prophage
   E. Virion

47 Which of the following is likely to be found on the tongue and in saliva?
   A. *S. salivarius*
   B. *S. milleri*
   C. *S. sanguis*
   D. *S. mitior*
   E. *S. mutans*

48 The virulence of many gram-negative bacteria is enhanced by their
   A. Endotoxin production
   B. Invasiveness
   C. Lysogenic action
   D. Interferon production
   E. Capsule formation

49 Human diseases caused by protozoans include
   A. Malaria and toxoplasmosis
   B. Ameobic dysentery and ringworm
   C. Toxoplasmosis and botulism
   D. Malaria and diptheria
   E. Amoebic dysentery and thrush

50 The transfer of genetic material by a bacteriophage is termed
   A. Lysogenic conversion
   B. Sexduction
   C. Conjugation
   D. Transduction
   E. Transformation

51 A major distinction between the prokaryotic cell and the eukaryotic cell is that the eukaryotic cell has a
   A. Cell wall
   B. Distinct nucleus
   C. Chromosome
   D. Flagellum
   E. Cell membrane

52 The greatest possibility of contracting herpetic whitlow would be by touching an infected patient's
   A. Vesicular lesions and blood
   B. Clothing and saliva
   C. Blood and saliva
   D. Blood and clothing
   E. Saliva and vesicular lesions

SITUATION: Your client is a 40-year-old man who has worked in a blood bank for 15 years and frequently works without gloves. He is scheduled for a 6-month continued care appointment. As you are seating the client, he mentions he is just recovering from influenza. You now notice his eyes are somewhat yellowish. Questions 53 and 54 refer to this situation.

53 What disease might this client have?
   A. Hepatitis A
   B. Influenza
   C. Infectious hepatitis
   D. Hepatitis B
   E. Infectious mononucleosis

54 The *BEST* choice of treatment for this client at this appointment would be to
   A. Wear gloves and a face mask and perform an intraoral and extraoral examination
   B. Refer to a physician and reschedule in 6 months
   C. Refer to a hospital equipped to treat the client dentally with maximal precautions
   D. Wear gloves and face mask and render nonsurgical periodontal therapy
   E. Refer to a physician and reschedule according to the physician's recommendation

55 One of the most important human disease barriers for the protection of the dental hygienist is the
   A. Phagocytic mechanism
   B. Normal oral flora
   C. Coughing reflex
   D. Inflammatory response
   E. Intact skin

56 Some gram-positive bacteria can form a spore state. Spores are fragile and can be destroyed easily.
   A. Both statements are *TRUE*.
   B. Both statements are *FALSE*.
   C. The first statement is *TRUE*; the second statement is *FALSE*.
   D. The first statement is *FALSE*; the second statement is *TRUE*.

57 Infectious mononucleosis is caused by which of the following microorganisms?
   A. Rubella virus
   B. Epstein-Barr virus
   C. Herpes zoster virus
   D. Varicella zoster virus
   E. Variola virus

58 A herpetic lesion of the finger is called
   A. Herpetic whitlow
   B. Herpes labialis
   C. Herpes keratoconjunctivitis
   D. Angular cheilitis
   E. Conjunctivitis

59 The human immunodeficiency virus (HIV) can be transmitted by saliva. The presence of HIV antibodies indicates immunity for acquired immunodeficiency syndrome (AIDS).
  A. Both statements are *TRUE*.
  B. Both statements are *FALSE*.
  C. The first statement is *TRUE*; the second statement is *FALSE*.
  D. The first statement is *FALSE*; the second statement is *TRUE*.
60 A virus cannot replicate outside a living organisms. A virus has a single strand of nucleic acid.
  A. Both statements are *TRUE*.
  B. Both statements are *FALSE*.
  C. The first statement is *TRUE*; the second statement is *FALSE*.
  D. The first statement is *FALSE*; the second statement is *TRUE*.

Answers and Rationales

1. (A) Microscopy that uses ultraviolet light
   (B) Microscopy that uses visible light
   (C) Microscopy that uses visible light
   (D) Microscopy that uses visible light
   (E) A type of microscopy consisting of at least a two-lens system. Used with both ultraviolet and visible light
2. (B) Developed Koch's postulates that are used to relate a specific microorganism to a specific disease
   (A) Developed aseptic techniques
   (C) First to use disinfectants in surgical procedures
   (D) First to observe cells
   (E) Designed the two-name nomenclature system of genus and species
3. (B) SEM is used to visualize three-dimensional images of cell and virus surface features
   (A) TEM is used to visualize cell and virus ultrastructure
   (C) Viruses cannot be seen with phase-contrast microscopy
   (D) Viruses cannot be seen with fluorescence microscopy
   (E) Viruses cannot be seen with dark-field microscopy
4. (D) Acid-fast and gram stains are used for initial bacterial grouping (e.g., gram positive versus gram-negative)
   (A) Negative stains are used to visualize capsules and are a special staining procedure
   (B) Flagellar stains are used to visualize flagella and are a special staining procedure
   (C) Flagellar stains are a special staining procedure
   (E) Flagellar stains are a special staining procedure
5. (C) Flagella are used by bacteria for locomotion and axial filaments are used by some spirochetes for locomotion
   (A) Fimbriae provide bacterial attachment
   (B) Cilia provide locomotion for eukaryotic cells
   (D) Pili provide bacterial attachment
   (E) Pili provide bacterial attachment.

6. (E) The slime layer is a glycocalyx loosely attached to the cell wall
   (A) The cell wall is not a glycocalyx
   (B) The cytoplasmic membrane is not a glycocalyx
   (C) The outer membrane is not a glycocalyx
   (D) The capsule is a glycocalyx firmly attached to the cell wall
7. (B) Gram-positive cell walls have many layers of peptidoglycan and gram-negative cell walls have a thin peptidoglycan layer
   (A) Lipopolysaccharides (LPS) are found in the outer membrane of gram-negative cells
   (C) Techoic acid is found in gram-positive cell walls
   (D) Outer membranes are found in gram-negative cells
   (E) Endotoxin is another name for LPS found in gram-negative cells
8. (B) Gracilicutes are eubacteria with a gram-negative cell wall
   (A) Firmicutes are eubacteria with a gram-positive cell wall
   (C) Tenericutes are bacteria lacking a cell wall
   (D) Archaeobacteria are bacteria with an atypical cell wall
   (E) Mendosicutes are bacteria with an atypical cell wall
9. (A) Oxygen concentration and vitamin source are two chemical conditions that affect microbial growth
   (B) Temperature and osmotic pressure are physical conditions that affect microbial growth
   (C) Nutrient source is a chemical condition; however, pH is a physical condition
   (D) Osmotic pressure is a physical condition
   (E) pH is a physical condition
10. (A) Mesophiles grow best from 20° to 40° C. The human body temperature is 37° C
   (B) Thermophiles grow best from 45° to 60° C, above the average human body temperature
   (C) Acidophiles grow best from pH 1 to 5.4, below the average human body pH
   (D) Psychrophiles grow best from 0° to 15° C, below the average human body temperature
   (E) Alkalinophiles grow best from pH 9.0 to 12.0, above the average human body pH
11. (C) Microaerophilic organisms require low concentrations of oxygen for growth
   (A) Aerotolerant anaerobes metabolize substances anaerobically, but are not harmed by oxygen
   (B) Facultative anaerobes can metabolize aerobically if oxygen is present or anaerobically if it is absent
   (D) Aerobes require oxygen
   (E) Strict anaerobes cannot tolerate any free oxygen
12. (E) *S. Pyogenes* is a beta-hemolytic group A streptococcius; beta-hemolysis leaves a clear zone around *S. pyogenes* colonies on blood agar
   (A) A red zone is not typical of any type of hemolysis on blood agar
   (B) A green zone is typical of alpha-hemolysis on blood agar
   (C) A black zone is not typical of any type of hemolysis on blood agar
   (D) A yellow zone is not typical of any type of hemolysis on blood agar

13. (D) Psychrophiles grow best from 0° to 15° C.
    (A) Psychrophiles describe temperature requirements, not pH requirements
    (B) Psychrophiles describe temperature requirements, not pH requirements
    (C) Psychrophiles grow best at lower temperatures, not higher temperatures
    (E) Psychrophiles grow best at lower temperatures, not at room temperature

14. (B) Penicillin inhibits cell wall synthesis; it requires actively growing cells; cells are increasing in number exponentially during the log phase
    (A) Cells are not actively growing during the lag phase
    (C) Cell growth is not as great during the stationary phase
    (D) The number of viable cells is decreasing in the decline phase
    (E) The decline phase is also called the death phase

15. (A) In feedback inhibition the build-up of end product promotes the binding of end-product to the enzyme; the resultant distortion of the enzyme prevents it from binding to its substrate
    (B) A buildup of substrate will not activate feedback inhibition
    (C) A buildup of enzyme will not activate feedback inhibition
    (D) A reactant is the same as a substrate
    (E) An operon is a specific unit of DNA involved in metabolic control by enzyme repression or induction

16. (A) Anabolism is the synthesis of cellular constituents
    (B) Catabolism is the breaking down of cellular constituents
    (C) Metabolism is the set of chemical reactions by which cells maintain life; this includes both anabolism and catabolism
    (D) Glycolysis is the energy-yielding breakdown of glucose
    (E) Respiration is the oxidative breakdown and release of energy from nutrient molecules by reaction with oxygen

17. (D) Conjugation is the transfer of genetic material between two living bacteria in physical contact; plasmids are transferred most often by this method
    (A) Transposons are small segments of DNA that can move within a chromosome, to a different chromosome or to a plasmid
    (B) Transduction is the transfer of genetic material by bacteriophages
    (C) Transformation is the direct uptake of donor DNA by the recipient cell
    (E) Mutations are changes in the DNA caused by UV light, radiation, nitrous acid, and other mutagenic agents

18. (D) Parasitism occurs if one organism benefits at the expense of the other
    (A) Commensalism occurs if one organism benefits and the other neither benefits nor is harmed
    (C) Predation occurs as a means to control the population; predators feed on another species, their prey
    (D) Symbiosis occurs if two different forms of life live in a mutually beneficial coexistence
    (E) Syntrophism occurs if organisms that are not intimately associated with each other benefit from each other

19. (D) Symbiosis occurs if two different forms of life live in a mutually beneficial coexistence; the intestines of a human host support the growth of the bacteria and the bacteria provide the host with vitamin K
    (A) Syntrophism occurs if organisms that are not associated intimately with each other benefit from each other
    (B) Parasitism occurs if one organism benefits at the expense of the other
    (C) Commensalism occurs if only one organism benefits and the other neither benefits nor is harmed
    (E) Competition occurs if there is an interaction between organisms resulting from demand for nutrients and energy that exceeds immediate supply

20. (E) Imperfect fungi (Deuteromycotina) do not produce sexual spores
    (A) Zygomycotina produce asexual and sexual spores
    (B) Basidiomycotine produce asexual and sexual spores
    (C) Sac fungi (Ascomycotina) produce asexual and sexual spores
    (D) Dimorphic fungi describes fungi that exhibit characteristics of both mold and yeasts depending on growth conditions

21. (C) A trophozoite is the motile feeding stage of protozoa
    (A) A cyst is the protective resting stage of protozoa
    (B) Sporozoa is a protozoan found in the Apicomplexa phylum
    (D) Pseudopodia are a means by which protozoa are motile
    (E) Ciliophora is one of the four phyla of protozoa

22. (B) Viroids are small, single-stranded, circular RNA molecules found to infect primarily plants
    (A) Virions are a mature virus particle; they can be RNA or DNA, and can infect plants, animals, or bacteria
    (C) Operons are specific units of DNA that regulate enzyme repression and induction
    (D) Prions are proteinaceous infectious particles believed to cause kuru and Creutzfeldt-Jakob disease
    (E) Phages are bacterial viruses

23. (C) Attachment, penetration, uncoating, synthesis, release
    (A) These steps are not in proper order
    (B) These steps are not in proper order
    (D) These steps are not in proper order
    (E) These steps are not in proper order

24. (A) An ultrasonic cleaner more thoroughly cleans instruments in less time, with less chance of injury, with less spatter, and penetrates grooves more thoroughly.
    (B) Scrubbing instruments with a sterile brush is *not* preferred. Disadvantages of this technique include the length of time necessary to clean instruments, a greater chance of injury, and increased spatter.
    (C) Instruments should be soaked in a holding solution that acts as a blood solvent if there is a time lapse before using an ultrasonic cleaner.
    (D) Too much spatter is produced when holding instruments under a hard spray of water.
    (E) Organic debris acts as a barrier, so instruments should be cleaned first before placing them in an autoclave.

25. (E) If the prophylaxis angle is not disassembled according to manufacturer recommendations before sterilizing, steam may not penetrate all areas. If grease is not removed first, the sterilant cannot penetrate, and the grease becomes caked on.
  (A) The prophylaxis angle should be decontaminated by ultrasonic cleaning with an all-purpose detergent, but it must also be disassembled for proper sterilizing.
  (B) It is not necessary to soak a prophylaxis angle in a disinfectant, but it is necessary to disassemble it per manufacturer recommendations and remove accumulated grease.
  (C) Merely soaking a prophylaxis angle in a disinfectant will not allow proper sterilization.
  (D) A prophylaxis angle should be disassembled and ultrasonically cleaned before sterilizing. Scrubbing the exterior of the prophylaxis angle is not sufficient to remove grease.

26. (D) Maintaining postrenewal sterility is extremely difficult with unwrapped instruments. Once instruments are exposed, they become recontaminated and have a zero shelf life. Unwrapped sterilized instruments must be used immediately.
  (A) Unwrapped sterilized instruments have a zero shelf life.
  (B) Unwrapped sterilized instruments have a zero shelf life.
  (C) Unwrapped sterilized instruments have a zero shelf life.
  (E) The sterility of unwrapped instruments is compromised immediately after sterilization. Staples do not totally seal as well.

27. (E) Ethylene oxide is the only verifiable method of sterilization applicable to almost any material including plastics.
  (A) Most plastics cannot withstand steam autoclaving.
  (B) Plastics will withstand immersion in chemical sterilants, yet this is not a preferred method of sterilization because there is no biologic monitoring test for any liquid chemical sterilants.
  (C) Most plastics cannot withstand dry-heat sterilizing.
  (D) Most plastics cannot withstand a chemical vapor.

28. (E) Moist heat travels vertically and coagulates protein. It must be able to reach all items for sterilization to take place. Therefore items must be arranged within the autoclave to accomplish this.
  (B) Properly wrapped and arranged instrument packs may prevent bent and broken instruments, but this is secondary to accomplishing proper sterilization.
  (C) Moisture can collect even if the instrument packs are in an upright position.
  (D) A vacuum is not created in an autoclave.
  (E) If the autoclave is operating properly, the correct temperature range should occur whether instrument packs are vertical or horizontal.

29. (E) It may take up to 60 minutes for the instruments to reach the sterilization temperature, and another 60 minutes is required for sterilization to occur. Once the load temperature has been reached, the sterilization time must be sufficient and sustained without opening the oven; otherwise, cycle must be restarted.
  (A) Even without preheating the oven, a total of 3 hours would probably be a waste of time.
  (B) After the instruments have actually reached the sterilization temperature, it takes 60 minutes for sterilization to take place. (Preheating may take 15-60 minutes.)
  (C) Even after the instruments have reached the sterilization temperature, 60 minutes is required for sterilization to be achieved.
  (D) Even after the instruments have reached the sterilization temperature, 60 minutes is required for sterilization to be achieved.

30. (C) Chemical vapors should not be inhaled; therefore adequate ventilation is required when chemical vapor pressure sterilization is used.
  (A) Materials must be aerated when ethylene oxide is used but not when chemical vapors are used.
  (B) Rusting instruments can occur when a steam autoclave is used, but this is not true for chemical vapor pressure sterilization.
  (D) When a steam autoclave is used, instruments are sometimes wet at the end of the cycle, but this is not true for chemical vapor pressure sterilization.
  (E) Because it requires only 20 minutes for chemical vapor pressure sterilization, the time required is not a disadvantage of this method.

31. (B) The spores of *B. stearothermophilus* are extremely resistant to moist heat, so they are used for testing a steam autoclave sterilizer.
  (A) The spores of *C. botulinum* are *not* recommended for use in testing sterilization devices.
  (C) The spores of *C. tetani* are *not* recommended for use a testing sterilizing devices.
  (D) The spores of *B. anthracis* are *not* recommended for use in testing sterilizing devices.
  (E) The spores of *B. subtilis* are recommended for use in testing dry-heat and ethylene oxide sterilizers.

32. (C) Although use of a chemical sterilant (nonverifiable) is not a preferred method of sterilization, limited use with a few heat-sensitive items is acceptable if ethylene oxide (verifiable) sterilization isn't available.
  (A) Use of a chemical sterilant is *not* faster than heat sterilization. Instruments require at least 10 hours to be sterilized. Steam autoclaves can sterilize in 20 minutes, and sterile packages are produced. Additional time is required after soaking instruments in a sterilant to rinse, dry, and place in storage areas with the challenge being to maintain sterility.
  (B) Verification of sterilization is *not* possible with sterilants.
  (D) Chemical sterilants *are* expensive.

33. (D) The most important consideration in designing the sterilization area is preventing contamination or routes of cross-infection by separating contaminated and non-contaminated areas.
    (A) The availability of glutaraldehyde is a factor depending on the dental instruments and equipment used for heat-sensitive instrument sterilization.
    (B) Although adequate counter space is important, it is not the first priority in designing a sterilization area.
    (C) Instrument storage areas may or may not be located in the sterilization area because their location depends on individual office instrument flow patterns.
    (E) Although a dry-heat oven may be needed, it depends on the individual office—what equipment must be sterilized.

34. (B) Any part of the radiograph unit that has been touched by saliva-coated hands has the potential for disease transmission, and barriers should be removed and surfaces disinfected before the next client is seated.
    (A) Before developing the radiographs, the radiographic unit must be disinfected before the next client is seated.
    (C) Labeling the radiographic mount can be done later. The unit should be cleaned and disinfected so that other clients can use the x-ray room.
    (D) The film holders must be disassembled and sterilized before they are reused.
    (E) The film holders must be sterilized, not merely wiped with disinfectant.

35. (B) The federal standard for occupational exposure to bloodborne pathogens requires employers to provide the vaccination for hepatitis B.
    (A) Oral healthcare personnel are not at great risk of contracting hepatitis A. There is no vaccine specifically for hepatitis C.
    (C) It is not recommended to vaccinate oral healthcare personnel for hepatitis A.
    (D) There is no vaccine specifically formulated for hepatitis C.
    (E) It is recommended that oral healthcare personnel be routinely tested for tuberculosis; however, the only vaccination employers are required to provide is for hepatitis B.

36. (D) OSHA federal rule requires employer to provide protective clothing and laundry service for employees with occupational exposure to bloodborne pathogens.
    (A) Protective clothing and laundry service are provided by the employer.
    (B) The employer is required to provide protective clothing and laundry service.
    (C) Laundry service is a responsibility of the employer.
    (D) OSHA federal rule requires employers to provide and launder protective clothing.

37. (C) It is recommended not to wear any jewelry on the hands or wrists, but small earrings are not in an operating zone in dental procedures.
    (A) Wristwatches are worn on the wrist and are therefore not acceptable.
    (B) Bracelets are worn on the wrist and are not acceptable.
    (D) Wedding bands are worn on the fingers and are not acceptable.
    (E) Rings are worn on the fingers and are not acceptable.

38. (D) Face masks should be changed after every client or whenever they become damp because they are not effective when damp.
    (A) There is no set time schedule to change face masks, only when they become damp.
    (B) There is no set time schedule to change face masks, only when they become damp.
    (C) There is no set time schedule to change face masks, only when they become damp.
    (E) There is no set time schedule to change face masks, only when they become damp.

39. (E) Wearing gloves, protective eyewear, and a face mask is recommended for all client treatments. It is impossible to detect from a health history all clients who have tuberculosis, hepatitis, or AIDS or who are in the incubation stage or carrier state of a disease.
    (A) Wearing gloves and a face mask is also recommended.
    (B) Wearing gloves is also recommended.
    (C) Wearing a face mask is also recommended.
    (D) Wearing a face mask, protective eyewear, and gloves is recommended for the initial examination and also for the rest of the treatment.

40. (E) Universal precautions for bloodborne pathogens require changing gloves between *all* clients. Gloves are a critically important barrier protecting client and operator.
    (A) Washing and rinsing compromises the quality of gloves' effectiveness as a barrier.
    (B) One does not want to use a brush to scrub if gloves are on, and it is impractical to remove gloves to scrub. The need is to remove germs from the gloves.
    (C) It is recommended to perform a short scrub at the beginning of the day. A surgical scrub is not necessary. Handwashing is very important before gloving and after removing gloves.
    (D) Washing gloves compromises the effectiveness of the barrier because they become permeable.

41. (C) The recommended procedure is to perform a short scrub at the beginning of the day. It is too time consuming and harsh on the hands to scrub between clients.
    (A) Cloth towels can be used for drying instead of paper towels *if* a new towel is used for each client.
    (B) Using a brush on the hands more than once a day is too irritating to the skin.
    (D) Scrub brushes need to be sterilized, not disinfected.
    (E) Only before surgery is a surgical scrub required.

42. (A) Gentleness in a hand cleanser must be a high priority because the intact skin is a natural defense.
    (B) A hand cleanser will never sterilize the hands, so it is important to choose one that is nonirritating and nonallergenic. Friction in cleaning is the most important factor in reducing microbes.
    (C) A hand cleanser will never sterilize the hands, so it is important to choose one that is nonirritating and nonallergenic. Friction in cleaning is the most important factor in reducing microbes.
    (D) A hand cleanser will never sterilize the hands, so it is important to choose one that is nonirritating and nonallergenic. Friction in cleaning is the most important factor in reducing microbes.
    (E) Although cost is important, preserving the intact skin is the first priority.

43. (C) A liquid hand cleanser is the fastest and least likely to become contaminated.
    (A) Powdered hand cleansers take longer to form a liquid, soapy state.
    (B) Bar hand cleansers accumulate microorganisms and are not recommended.
    (D) Powdered hand cleansers take longer to form a liquid, soapy state, and bar hand cleansers accumulate microbes.
    (E) Powdered hand cleansers take longer to form a liquid, soapy state.

44. (B) Dental instruments used on a known carrier of hepatitis B should be processed for sterilization by using the same universal approach for all instruments because most HBV carriers are unknown.
    (A) Sodium hypochlorite is corrosive to metals.
    (C) One pair of heavy household rubber gloves is adequate for protection.
    (D) Instruments used on a known carrier of hepatitis B should be handled according to universal precautions and protocol for instrument recirculation.
    (E) It is not recommended that instruments used on known carriers of hepatitis B be sterilized twice as long as normal for added protection.

45. (C) Wearing protective eyewear during dental treatment helps prevent herpes and injury. Herpes is present in saliva even without clinical infection. Ocular herpes is a leading cause of blindness.
    (A) Conjunctivitis could be caused by spatter, but the eyes are not a likely route for contracting hepatitis A.
    (B) The eyes are not a likely route for hepatitis B transmission; ophthalmia neonatorum is acquired congenitally.
    (D) Ophthalmia neonatorum is acquired congenitally.
    (E) The eyes are not a likely route for hepatitis A transmission.

46. (E) A virion is a mature virus particle.
    (A) A bacteriphage is a bacterial virus.
    (B) A capsid is a protein outer coat of virus.
    (C) A genome is genetic viral material.
    (D) Prophage is the integration of a temperate bacteriophage into the host cell.

47. (A) *S. salivarius* is most likely to be found on the tongue and in saliva.
    (B) *S. milleri* is generally found near the gingival crevice.
    (C) *S. sanguis* is found mostly in bacterial plaque and on the tongue.
    (D) *S. mitior* is found mostly on nonkeratinized mucosa.
    (E) *S. mutans* is found mostly on hard surfaces.

48. (A) The virulence of gram-negative bacteria is enhanced by their endotoxin production. Endotoxin has a direct pathologic effect on human tissues.
    (B) Many gram-negative bacteria that produce endotoxins do not directly invade tissue.
    (C) Lysogenic action applies to viruses and their destructive effects.
    (D) Interferon production is a protective mechanism and induces a state of resistance to viruses.
    (E) Capsule formation maintains virulence of some bacteria but not gram-negative bacteria as a group.

49. (A) Malaria and toxoplasmosis are both caused by protozoans.
    (B) Ringworm is caused by a fungus.
    (C) Toxoplasmosis and botulism are both caused by bacteria.
    (D) Diptheria is caused by bacteria.
    (E) Thrush is caused by a fungus.

50. (D) Transduction is the transfer of genetic material by a bacteriophage.
    (A) Lysogenic conversion occurs as a result of viral infections.
    (B) Sexduction involves transfer by an F particle.
    (C) Conjugation requires two living bacteria in physical contact.
    (E) Transformation is caused by soluble extracts of DNA.

51. (B) A distinct nucleus is not present in the prokaryotic cell and is the major distinguishing factor between the two cell types.
    (A) Both cell types have a cell wall.
    (C) The prokaryotic cells have one chromosome, whereas the eukaryotic cells have more than one chromosome.
    (D) Both types of cells can have flagella.
    (E) Both types of cells have cell membranes.

52. (E) Saliva and vesicular lesions are the known routes of transmission for herpetic whitlow and are where the highest counts of virus are available.
    (A) Blood is not a route of transmission for herpetic whitlow.
    (B) Whitlow is not likely to be transmitted by touching clothing because the virus survives only seconds to minutes on surfaces.
    (C) Blood is not a route of transmission for herpetic whitlow.
    (D) Blood and contact with clothing are not routes of transmission for herpetic whitlow.

53. (D) Persons working with blood are in a high-risk group; hepatitis B often is transmitted through the blood. The longer a person works around blood products, the greater the chance of contracting hepatitis B. A yellowish tint to the eyes is suggestive of hepatitis symptoms; other symptoms can be similar to influenza.
    (A) Hepatitis A is not usually transmitted through blood products but is usually transmitted in unsanitary conditions.
    (B) Influenza is a possible choice, but the yellow color of the eyes is suggestive of hepatitis.
    (C) Infectious hepatitis is hepatitis A, but the occupation noted suggests hepatitis B.
    (E) Infectious mononucleosis is a possible choice, but the yellow color of the eyes suggests hepatitis B.

54. (E) Hepatitis B can be transmitted by all body fluids with the risk of contracting the disease or passing it on to other patients. Universal precautions are essential. The client needs to be evaluated by physician for laboratory tests and diagnosis. The client's health may be compromised.
    (A) The disease is transmitted through all body secretions; gloves are not foolproof, and hepatitis B virus survives months on surfaces. It is also very resistant to chemical disinfectants
    (B) Rescheduling should not be done until the status of blood tests is known.
    (C) It cannot be assumed that the patient has hepatitis B.
    (D) Gloves and a face mask are not foolproof against contracting the disease.

55. (E) Without considering artificial protective measures, intact skin of the hands is the first line of defense.
    (A) Phagocytic mechanisms are human disease barriers but not the first line of defense for a dental hygienist's most vulnerable area, the hands.
    (B) The normal oral flora is a human disease barrier but not the first line of defense against disease.
    (C) The coughing reflex is a human disease barrier but not the body's first line of defense against disease.
    (D) The inflammatory response is a human disease barrier but not the first line of defense against disease.

56. (C) Some gram-positive bacteria can form endospores that are also resistant to heat, drying, chemical disinfection, and radiation.
    (A) Spores are not fragile and cannot be destroyed easily because they are resistant to heat, drying, chemical disinfection, and radiation.
    (B) Some gram-positive bacteria have the ability to form endospores.
    (D) Some gram-positive bacteria have the ability to form endospores. Spores cannot be destroyed easily and are resistant to harsh conditions.

57. (B) Epstein-Barr virus is the etiologic agent that causes infectious mononucleosis.
    (A) Rubella virus is the etiologic agent that causes German measles.
    (C) Herpes zoster virus is the etiologic agent that causes "cold sores" (herpes labialis), herpes keratoconjunctivitis, herpetic whitlow, and genital herpes.
    (D) Varicella-zoster virus is the etiologic agent that causes chicken pox and shingles.
    (E) Variola virus is the etiologic agent that causes smallpox.

58. (A) A herpetic lesion on the finger is called herpetic whitlow.
    (B) A herpetic lesion on the lip is called herpes labialis.
    (C) A herpetic lesion of the eye is called herpes keratocon junctivitis.
    (D) A yeast infection (Candida) of the corners of the lip is called angular cheilitis.
    (E) A bacterial or viral infection of the eye is called conjunctivitis.

59. (B) HIV cannot be transmitted by saliva, and the presence of HIV antibodies does not indicate immunity for AIDS.
    (A) HIV cannot be transmitted by saliva, and the presence of HIV antibodies does not indicate immunity for AIDS.
    (C) HIV cannot be transmitted by saliva.
    (D) The presence of HIV antibodies does not indicate immunity for AIDS.

60. (A) A virus can replicate only inside a living organism and contains a single strand of RNA or DNA.
    (B) It is not possible for a virus to replicate outside a living organism, and a virus contains a single strand of nucleic acid.
    (C) Viruses contain only a single strand of RNA or DNA.
    (D) A virus can replicate only inside a living organism.

Pharmacology

Barbara Requa-Clark

As the healthcare provider who often assesses the health history, the dental hygienist needs to have an understanding of the drugs a client may be taking and the conditions for which these drugs are used. The health history is the basis on which decisions regarding client care rest; therefore, before dental treatment is planned, the client's medical conditions and the medications used to manage them should be recorded in the client's permanent record. The use of contraindications or cautions to professional care from these agents should be determined using an appropriate reference.

Knowing the client's medical conditions is important because some people may need prophylactic antibiotics before dental and dental hygiene care. Also, by being aware of the condition a person has, one may prevent foreseeable emergencies. If an emergency does occur, the oral health team can act appropriately if they are prepared.

This chapter reviews the effects of a wide variety of drugs, including their pharmacologic effects, adverse drug reactions, and their usual indications and contraindications. When special oral implications or considerations are applicable, they too are listed.

General Considerations

Definitions

A. Pharmacology—knowledge of various properties of drugs
B. Drugs

1. Drug—substance used in prevention, diagnosis, alleviation, treatment, or cure of disease
2. Nomenclature (names)—one drug can have several names
   a. Chemical—name based on the drug's chemical formula, e.g., N-acetyl paraamino phenol
   b. Trade (proprietary) name—each drug company producing a drug makes up its own trade name (e.g., Tylenol, Peridex)
   c. Brand name—technically name of the drug company itself, but often used interchangeably with trade name (e.g., either Astra [company that makes Xylocaine] or Xylocaine can be considered the brand name)
   d. Generic name—one name chosen by the U.S. Adopted Name Council that is used by all manufacturers of a particular drug (e.g., acetaminophen)

References

A. Books
1. *Physicians' Desk Reference* (PDR)[1]—drugs organized by drug manufacturer; updated yearly; most common reference in oral healthcare environment; inclusion in book paid for by manufacturer (little used products not listed), similar to package insert (information not updated regularly), biased
2. *Facts and Comparisons*[2]—drugs organized by pharmacologic classes; very complete listing, updated monthly; contains both prescription and

		Table 8-1		
		Drug Enforcement Administration Schedules Used in Dentistry (II through IV)		

Schedule	Abuse potential	Examples	Handling
II	Great	Morphine, meperidine, oxycodone mixtures (Percodan, Percocet)	Prescription must be signed by the prescriber, can't be telephoned to pharmacist; no refills
III	Some	Codeine mixtures (Tylenol and codeine), hydrocodone mixtures (Vicodin), "weaker" stimulants and sedatives	Prescriptions may be telephoned to pharmacy; may be refilled 5 times within 6 months
IV	A little	Dextropropoxyphene (Darvon) diazepam (Valium)	Same as schedule III

over-the-counter drugs; prepared by independent editors

3. *Applied Pharmacology for the Dental Hygienist*[3] and *Pharmacology for Dental Hygiene Practice*[4]—basic pharmacology textbooks for the dental hygienist; more detailed than this review

4. *Gage and Pickett: Mosby's 1997 Dental Drug Reference*[5]—dentally related comments on a limited number of drugs. Includes dental drug interactions, oral side effects, and dental considerations (e.g., for xerostomia may produce candidiasis, increases caries potential)

5. Wynn R.L., Miller T.E., Crossley H.L.: *Drug Information Handbook for Dentistry 1996-7*, Hudson, Ohio, 1996, Lexi-Comp.[6]

B. CD Rom titles are becoming more available. It is important to preview CD-Roms because user friendliness varies considerably; many can be purchased with quarterly updates included

C. Internet sites—millions and growing; use a search engine to explore sites related to your profession

Agencies/Legislation

A. Food and Drug Administration (FDA)—determines drugs to be marketed in the United States; requires proof of both safety and efficacy

B. Drug Enforcement Administration (DEA)—branch of the Department of Justice; determines degree of control for substances with abuse potential; Schedules I through V (Table 8-1)

Drug Action

A. *Log dose-effect curve*—as the dose of a drug increases (x-axis), the percent of maximum response rises (y-axis) until increasing the dose further produces no increase in the percent of response (it plateaus) (Fig. 8-1)

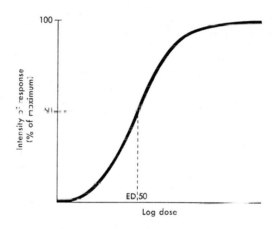

Fig. 8-1   Log dose-effect curve.

B. Definitions

1. Structure-activity relationships (SAR)—drugs with similar structures often exert similar actions

2. Effective dose $(ED)_{50}$—dose that produces 50% of the maximum response; or the dose of a drug that produces a specific response in 50% of the subjects

3. Lethal dose $(LD)_{50}$—dose that is lethal (kills) 50% of the subjects; laboratory animals are used

4. Therapeutic index (TI)—the LD_{50}/ED_{50}, a measure of the safety of a drug

5. Onset—time required for a drug's effect to begin; very short if given intravenously, longer if administered orally

6. Duration—length of time a drug's effect lasts; related to a drug's half-life

7. Half-life $(t_{1/2})$—time required for the serum concentration at any point in time to decrease by 50%; five half-lives are required for a drug to be eliminated from the body.

8. Potency—amount (e.g., in milligrams) needed to get an effect; the more potent an agent, the less it takes to produce an effect (Fig. 8-2)

9. Efficacy—effect elicited by drug, independent of dose (Fig. 8-2)

10. Tolerance—same dose produces less effect or larger dose required for same effect

C. Routes of administration

1. Oral (PO)—by mouth; easiest to use; good client acceptance, latent period

2. Rectal—suppository, enema; either local or systemic effect

3. Intravenous (IV)—into vein; shortest onset of action; most dangerous

4. Intramuscular (IM)—into the muscle; sometimes painful

5. Subcutaneous (SC, SQ)—beneath skin (e.g., insulin)

6. Intradermal—into dermis (e.g., skin test for tuberculosis—makes a bleb [bump])

7. Intrathecal—into the spinal fluid (e.g., for meningitis)

8. Intraperitoneal—into peritoneal cavity (abdomen)

9. Inhalation—into lungs; particles, volatile liquids, or gas; all inhaled (e.g., nitrous oxide-oxygen analgesia)

10. Topical—applied to the skin or mucous membranes; ointments or creams (e.g., hydrocortisone)

11. Sublingual—under the tongue, tablet dissolves or solution sprayed (for systemic effect)

12. Parenteral—other than an oral route; usually refers to an injection

D. Dosage forms

1. Capsule—gelatin shell

2. Tablet—compressed, or molded dosage form

3. Ointment or cream—semisolid for topical application

4. Suppository—penile, rectal or vaginal; systemic or local

5. Solution—one-phase system of more than one constituent

6. Suspension—insoluble particles in liquid (e.g., milk of magnesia)

7. Emulsion—two immiscible (not mixable) liquids (e.g., oil and water)

8. Elixir—sweetened and hydroalcoholic (water and alcohol mixture)

9. Tincture—usually alcoholic

E. Dosage

1. Varies depending on the client's

a. Age—geriatric person may require smaller doses because they may metabolize and excrete drugs more slowly

b. Weight

c. Condition (disease)

d. Route of administration

2. Child's dose

a. Less than the adult dose

b. Based on

(1) Manufacturer's recommendations—best method

(2) Surface area—good

(3) Weight—OK

(4) Age—very poor

Adverse Reactions

A. Manifestations

1. Exaggerated effect on the target organ—more of the effect than desired, (e.g., an antianxiety agent producing too much sleepiness), predictable, dose-related

2. Effect on a nontarget organ—effect on an organ other than that intended to be altered (e.g., insomnia [inability to sleep] from a bronchodilator)

3. Teratogenic effect—adverse effect on fetus in a pregnant woman (e.g., alcohol intake during pregnancy produces fetal alcohol syndrome)

4. Allergic reaction—varies from mild rash to anaphylaxis; involves an antigen-antibody reaction (e.g., rash from penicillin); can include urticaria, soft tissue swelling, difficulty in breathing; not predictable, not dose-related

5. Idiosyncrasy—unexpected reaction to a drug; not predictable

6. Interference with natural defense mechanisms—body is less able to fight infection (e.g., steroids)

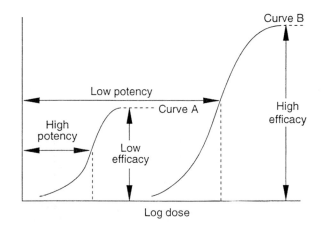

Fig. 8-2 Potency and efficacy of a drug. Curve A has high potency and low efficacy; curve B has low potency and high efficacy

B. Safety

$$\text{Therapeutic index} = \left[\frac{LD_{50}}{ED_{50}}\right]$$

The measure of a drug's safety—the larger the number of this ratio, the safer the drug

Pharmacokinetics (ADME)

Pharmacokinetics is how the body handles drugs
A. **Absorption** depends on
   1. Degree of ionization—the more ionized (charged), the less absorbed; the less ionized (charged) the more absorbed; with weak acids or bases this is a function of pH [H^+]
   2. Lipid solubility—the more lipid-soluble, the more absorbed; the less lipid-soluble, the less absorbed orally
B. **Distribution** of the drug (Fig. 8-3)
   1. Drug to the site of action
   2. Only the free drug can cross membranes (*arrows between boxes*)
   3. In each compartment an equilibrium between the bound and unbound (free) drug occurs
   4. Redistribution—moves from one tissue (exerts effect) to another tissue (inactive); one method of terminating a drug's effect
C. **Metabolism** (biotransformation)—takes place in the liver (mainly by hepatic microsomal enzymes; metabolites are more polar and less protein-bound, more easily excreted; drugs can affect metabolism of themselves or other drugs (either increase [i.e., barbiturates] or decrease [i.e., cimetidine, erythromycin] metabolism), source of drug interactions

D. **Excretion**—usually via the kidneys (urine); can also be via the feces (enterohepatic circulation), sweat, tears, or lungs (e.g., N_2O)

Receptors

An area in the body where a drug binds
A. Agonist—has affinity for receptor and binds to it producing an effect (e.g., opioid [narcotic] analgesic agent)
B. Antagonist—has affinity for receptor and binds to it, but produces **no** effect; competitively blocks the effect of an agonist (e.g., naloxone, an opioid [narcotic] antagonist [blocks the effect of the agonist an opioid])

Autonomic Nervous System Agents

The autonomic nervous system agents fall into four groups—including both stimulation (+) and inhibition (−) of the parasympathetic (P) and the sympathetic (S) nervous systems [P+, P−, S+, S−]

P+ Cholinergic (Parasympathomimetic) Agents

"Mimic" the action of the parasympathetic autonomic nervous system (PANS); PANS stimulation
A. Receptors—Fig. 8-4 illustrates a typical cholinergic nerve labelled PANS
   1. *"Muscarinic"*—receptor stimulated by the compound found in the poisonous mushroom *Amanita muscaria* (Fig. 8-4, *A*)
      a. Areas affected (*A*)
         (1) Smooth muscle
         (2) Cardiac muscle
         (3) Gland cells
      b. Neurotransmitter—acetylcholine (ACh)

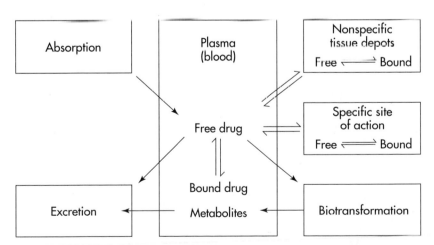

Fig. 8-3   Absorption and fate of drug. (From Holroyd SV: *Clinical pharmacology in dental practice,* ed 4, St. Louis, 1989, Mosby.)

c. Location—synapse between postganglionic fiber and the neuroeffector organ in the PANS
d. Stimulated by muscarine
e. Blocked by atropine

2. *"Nicotinic"*—receptor stimulated by nicotine; found in cigarettes (Fig. 8-4, *B* and *C*)
   a. Areas affected
      (1) Postganglionic neurons *(B)*
      (2) Skeletal muscle end-plates *(C)*
   b. Neurotransmitter—acetylcholine (ACh)
   c. Location—autonomic ganglia *(B)* and neuromuscular junction *(C)*
   d. Stimulated by nicotine
   e. Blocked by hexamethonium (autonomic, *B*) and *d*-tubocurarine (neuromuscular junction, *C*)

B. Acetylcholine—synthesis and inactivation

$$\underset{\substack{A \\ \text{Acetyl} \\ \text{(CoA)}}}{} + \underset{\substack{Ch \\ \text{Choline}}}{} \underset{\substack{\text{acetylcholinesterase} \\ \text{(AChE)}}}{\overset{\substack{\text{Choline} \\ \text{acetyltransferase}}}{\rightleftharpoons}} \underset{\substack{ACh \\ \text{Acetylcholine}}}{}$$

C. Classification/mechanism of action
   1. Direct acting—drug acts at the receptor just like acetylcholine
      a. Choline derivatives

b. **Pilocarpine** (Salagen)

2. *Indirect* acting—drug increases the amount of acetylcholine indirectly; blocks acetylcholine inactivation by inhibiting acetylcholinesterase (AChE, enzyme that normally destroys acetylcholine)
   a. *Reversible cholinesterase inhibitors*—drugs that block action of AChE, but whose action is terminated (ACh then destroyed)
      (1) Edrophonium (Tensilon)
      (2) Physostigmine (Eserine)
      (3) Neostigmine (Prostigmin)
   b. *"Irreversible" cholinesterase inhibitors*—drugs attach to and inactivate AChE; e.g., organophosphates used as insecticides (malathion, parathion)

D. Pharmacologic effects—similar to PANS stimulation
   1. Smooth muscle stimulation
      a. Increase in gastrointestinal (GI) motility—diarrhea may result; used to treat postoperative ileus (GI/GU—gastrointestinal/genitourinary)
      b. Bronchoconstriction—stimulates bronchial smooth muscle
   2. Glands—**increased secretion of saliva;** used to treat xerostomia
   3. Eye—decreased intraocular pressure; used to treat glaucoma

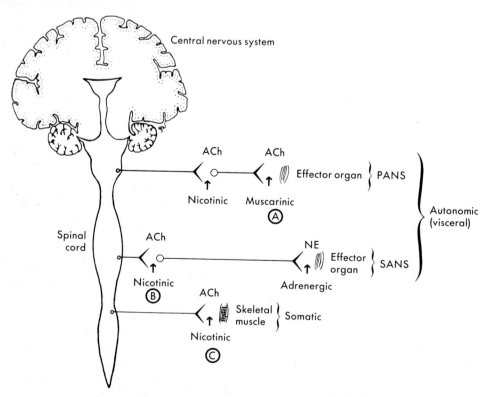

Fig. 8-4   Typical neurons with neurotransmitters. (*ACh,* acetylcholine; *NE,* norepinephrine) and typical PANS, SANS, and somatic nerves and muscarinic *(A)* and nicotinic *(B)* and *(C)* receptors.

E. Toxic reactions—extension of the pharmacologic effects; "too much" effect
   1. SLUD—salivation, lacrimation (tearing), urination, and defecation (bowel movement)
   2. Treatment of overdose
      a. Pralidoxime (2-PAM, Protopam)—regenerates acetylcholinesterase
      b. Atropine—antimuscarinic; blocks the muscarinic effects of acetylcholine excess (not the nicotinic effects)
F. Dental use—treatment of xerostomia
   1. Pilocarpine tablets may increase saliva flow

P— Anticholinergic (Parasympatholytic, Cholinergic Blocking) Agents

Block muscarinic actions of the PANS
A. Basic principles
   1. Used to dry up saliva
   2. Many drugs can have an anticholinergic or *atropine-like* or *atropinic* effect
   3. Block the muscarinic receptors
B. Pharmacologic effects
   1. Heart—tachycardia (increased heart rate [HR]; useful during general anesthesia when the HR may fall too low)
   2. Eye
      a. Mydriasis (dilation of the pupils; results in photophobia)
      b. Cycloplegia (paralysis for distant vision—cannot read up close)
      c. Avoid repeated doses in **narrow**-angle glaucoma (only autonomic drug group relatively contraindicated in certain glaucoma)
   3. Decreased secretions—**saliva flow reduced;** useful in dentistry (Table 8-2 lists several drug groups producing xerostomia)
   4. Central nervous system (CNS)—sedation or excitation
C. Adverse reactions and toxicity; contraindications to use
   1. Dry mouth/skin/eyes; caution in persons wearing contact lenses; agent reduces milk flow in nursing mothers
   2. Eye—blurred vision; avoid in narrow-angle glaucoma; careful use in persons with wide-angle glaucoma using eye drops usually no problem
   3. Urinary retention—avoid in persons with prostatic hypertrophy (enlarged prostate)
   4. Dizziness/fatigue—delirium, hallucinations, coma, and convulsions (toxicity)
   5. Tachycardia—watch with persons who have cardiovascular disease
   6. Reduced GI motility—avoid in persons with gastric retention or intestinal obstruction

D. Clinical uses
   1. Gastrointestinal—has "antispasmodic" activity (reduces GI overactivity) and secretions (e.g., stomach acid)
   2. Ophthalmology—dilates the eyes and paralyzes the muscles of accommodation (person can see far away only); used for eye exam
   3. Dental
      a. Before general anesthesia to dry up saliva and prevent vagal slowing of the heart
      b. To prepare the mouth for impressions or equilibrations; to decrease secretions; agent produces a "drier field"
E. Examples

Atropine	} Natural, tertiary
Propantheline (Pro-Banthine)	
Methantheline (Banthine)	} Synthetic, quaternary
Glycopyrrolate (Robinul)	

S+ Adrenergic (Sympathomimetic) Agents

"Mimic" the action of the sympathetic autonomic nervous system (SANS); act like norepinephrine (NE) in the SANS; SANS stimulation; epinephrine produces same effect (Fig. 8-2)
A. Basic principles
   1. SANS is activated by fear; **"fight or flight"** response
   2. Catecholamine—chemical structure of some adrenergic agents
   3. Receptors (SANS)
      a. α_1-receptors—constriction of the skin and mucosal blood vessels (vasoconstriction)
      α_2-receptors—decrease sympathic outflow by decreasing vasoconstriction, leading to vascular relaxation
      b. β-receptors
         (1) β_2—relaxes smooth muscles
            (a) Dilation of the skeletal muscle blood vessels (vasodilation)
            (b) Bronchodilation (we have 2 lungs = β_2)
         (2) β_1—stimulates the heart (we have 1 heart = β_1), increases the HR, contractility, and conduction velocity
B. Pharmacologic effects/adverse reactions
   1. Central nervous system—increased alertness; anxiety, anorexia (loss of appetite) (e.g., the amphetamines)
   2. Stimulation of the heart—S+ produces
      a. Positive chronotropic effect (increased HR)
      b. Positive inotropic effect (increased strength of contraction of the heart)
      c. Arrhythmias with higher doses
      d. α-Receptor stimulation—decreased HR because of the indirect (reflex vagal) effect

Table 8-2
Xerostomia-producing Drug Groups with Examples

Drug group	Examples
Anticholinergics* [P−]	Atropine, Donnatal, Artane
Antihypertensives*	Clonidine, guanethidine, methyldopa
Antipsychotics, phenothiazines*	Thorazine, Mellaril, Stelazine
Antidepressants,* tricyclic	Elavil, Tofranil
Antihistamines	Benadryl, Chlor-Trimeton
Adrenergic agents [S+]	Amphetamine, Preludin
Diuretics	Hydrochlorothiazide, Dyazide
Benzodiazepines	Valium, Librium

*More likely to produce xerostomia; effect still dose-related.

3. Vascular effects (effects on the arterial tree)
   a. α-Receptors—vasoconstriction of skin and mucosal blood vessels
   b. β-Receptors—vasodilation of skeletal muscle blood vessels
   c. Total peripheral resistance (TPR)
      (1) α-Receptors—increased TPR
      (2) αβ-Receptors and β-receptors—decreased TPR
4. Mydriasis (pupil dilation) and reduced intraocular pressure; useful in treating glaucoma
5. Bronchodilation (β₂-agonist); useful in treating asthmatic patients
6. Alterations in the blood glucose level; watch persons with diabetes mellitus
7. Production of thick, viscid saliva
C. Drug interactions—reasonable quantities, administered carefully to persons taking the drugs listed below should not cause problems; adrenergic agents plus
   1. Tricyclic antidepressants (e.g., Elavil, Tofranil)—increase blood pressure; produce dysrhythmias
   2. β-Blockers (e.g., Inderal)—produce hypertension and bradycardia (slowed HR)
   3. Antidiabetic agents (e.g., insulin, Orinase, Diabinese)—increase blood glucose level
   4. Monoamine oxidase inhibitors (MAOI)—no problem with epinephrine; indirect-acting amines (e.g., pseudoephedrine) *must* be avoided.
   5. General anesthetics (halogenated hydrocarbons, e.g., halothane [Fluothane]) sensitize the myocardium to catecholamines; epinephrine is a catecholamine; increase the chance of arrhythmias
D. Therapeutic uses

1. Medical—treatment of
   a. Anaphylaxis
   b. Cardiac arrest
   c. Nasal congestion—decongestant
   d. Asthma (β₂-agonist)
   e. Attention deficit disorder
   f. Glaucoma
2. Dental
   a. Local anesthetic additive (vasoconstrictor)
   b. Hemostatic to reduce bleeding; provide adequate tissue retraction (cord)
E. Examples

Adrenergic agent	Receptor stimulated	Comments
Epinephrine (Adrenalin)	αβ	Endogenous catecholamine; local anesthetic additive
Isoproterenol (Isuprel)	β	Endogenous catecholamine
Phenylephrine (Neo-Synephrine)	α	Nasal decongestant
Levonordefrin (Neo-Cobefrin)	α > β	Local anesthetic additive
Amphetamine	αβ	Diet pill (abused)
Pseudoephedrine (Sudafed)	αβ	Orally active nasal decongestant
Phenylpropanolamine (PPA)	αβ	All above apply; OTC diet ingredient

F. Adrenergics as vasoconstrictors in local anesthetic solutions
   1. Examples
      Epinephrine (Adrenalin)
      Levonordefrin (Neo-Cobefrin)
   2. Advantages
      a. Prolong duration of anesthesia
      b. Reduce systemic toxicity
      c. Provide hemostasis
      d. Reduce absorption (vasoconstriction)
      e. Increase concentration at nerve membrane
   3. Disadvantages
      a. Systemic toxicity with excess
      b. Persons with cardiovascular disease
         (1) Can use reasonable amounts as local anesthetic additives in stable cardiovascular patients
         (2) Avoid epinephrine-impregnated retraction cord
         (3) Maximum safe dose (MSD) for normal and cardiovascular patients
            (a) Epinephrine—normal person, 0.2 mg; cardiovascular client, 0.04 mg
            (b) Levonordefrin (Neo-Cobefrin)—normal person, 1 mg; cardiovascular client, 0.2 mg (some say 1 mg)
      c. Hyperthyroid clients—vasoconstrictors may

produce thyroid storm in **untreated** or drug-treated hyperthyroid persons or those receiving drug therapy

    4. Minimize toxicity

      a. Inject slowly

      b. Aspirate before injecting

      c. Calm client

      d. Use smallest effective dose

S— β-Adrenergic Blockers (β-Blockers)

See cardiovascular drugs for more discussion

A. Mechanism of action—drug blocks SANS action (β-receptors); some β-blockers are more selective for the β_1-receptor than others ($\beta_1 > \beta_2$) (specific)

B. Used to treat hypertension, angina, arrhythmias, congestive heart failure, anxiety, and glaucoma; used to prevent migraine and myocardial infarction (MI, heart attack)

C. Examples (note "olol" ending with generic names)
    Propranolol (Inderal)
    Metoprolol (Lopressor)
    Atenolol (Tenormin)

Neuromuscular Blocking Agents

A. Pharmacologic effects—paralysis of voluntary skeletal muscles; can include muscles of respiration; **not** autonomic nervous system (ANS) agent

B. Therapeutic use—paralyzing skeletal muscles at start of general anesthesia to facilitate intubation (passing an orotracheal or nasotracheal tube)

C. Examples
    Tubocurarine ("curare")—poison arrow
    Succinylcholine (Anectine)

Local Anesthetic Agents

A. Properties of the ideal local anesthetic (LA)

    1. Potent

    2. Reversible

    3. No local anesthesia

    4. No local, systemic, or allergic reactions

    5. Rapid onset

    6. Satisfactory duration

    7. Adequate tissue penetration

    8. Low cost

    9. Stable in solution (long shelf-life)

    10. Sterilized by autoclave

    11. Metabolism and excretion easy

B. Chemistry

    1. Three components common to LA

      a. Aromatic lipophilic group—contains a benzene ring

      b. Intermediate chain—either **ester** or **amide**

      c. Hydrophilic amino group—secondary or tertiary amine

    2. Intermediate chain

      a. Esters

        (1) Cocaine

        (2) Ethyl aminobenzoate (Benzocaine)

        (3) Tetracaine (Pontocaine)

        (4) Procaine (Novocain)

        (5) Propoxycaine (in Ravocaine)

      b. Amides

        (1) Lidocaine (Xylocaine)

        (2) Mepivacaine (Carbocaine)

        (3) Prilocaine (Citanest)

        (4) Bupivacaine (Marcaine)

        (5) Etidocaine (Duranest)

C. Mechanism

    1. Nerve fiber susceptibility—nerves generally affected in this order: autonomic, cold/warmth, pain, touch pressure, vibration, proprioception, and motor; regain function in reverse order

    2. Specific receptor theory—bind to receptors on the sodium channel; permeability to sodium ions is decreased and nerve conduction is interrupted

    3. Base and salt forms of local anesthetics (Fig. 8-5)—both forms needed; base penetrates the lipid membranes, salt traverses the cellular fluid

    4. Inflammation—reduces LA effect

      a. Acid environment (pH 5.5) of inflammation increases ionized form and reduces effect

      b. Edema—dilutes LA because of an increase in fluids present

      c. Increased tissue vascularity—increased blood supply carries away LA; duration of action is shortened

D. Pharmacokinetics

    1. Absorption

      a. Effect on the vasculature

        (1) LAs produce vasodilation (except cocaine); vasoconstrictors are added to counteract dilation

      b. Absorption and distribution of local anesthetic determined by pH of environment

$$\text{Inflammation} \rightarrow \downarrow pH \rightarrow \uparrow [H^+] \rightarrow \uparrow \text{ charged form } \circledS \rightarrow \downarrow \text{unionized}$$
$$\text{(more acid)} \quad \text{(more hydrogen ions)}$$
$$\text{form } \circledB \rightarrow \updownarrow \text{ charged distribution}$$

      c. Solubility

        (1) Lipid soluble—nonionized form penetrates membranes

        (2) Water soluble—ionized form crosses cell and exerts its effect at the nerve

      d. Rate of absorption

(1) Faster absorption—greater chance of systemic toxicity and shorter duration of action

(2) Route of administration alters the rate of absorption; topical anesthetic can be absorbed quickly

2. Distribution—level of local anesthetic in the blood is determined by movement of LA around body; side effects occur if LA reaches a high enough level in other organs (e.g., CNS, heart); blood level determined by:

a. Rate of injection

b. Speed of absorbtion depends on proximity to blood vessels

c. Speed of distribution to other tissues

d. Speed of metabolism and/or excretion

3. Metabolism (biotransformation)

a. Esters—hydrolyzed by plasma pseudocholinesterases

(1) Procaine—metabolized to para-aminobenzoic acid (PABA) (allergenic)

(2) Congenital cholinesterase deficiency—ester LAs are absolutely contraindicated

b. Amides—metabolized in the liver

(1) Liver dysfunction—give amide LAs cautiously, may be metabolized more slowly, toxic levels build up if repeated doses are administered

(2) Prilocaine—metabolized to orthotoluidine, which can produce methemoglobinemia more methemoglobin in blood, less oxygen

carrying capacity (not usually a problem in healthy clients)

4. Excretion capacity

a. Esters are almost completely metabolized before being excreted

b. Amides are mostly metabolized before being excreted

c. Significant renal disease can cause all local anesthetic metabolites to accumulate

E. Adverse reactions

1. Factors influencing toxicity

a. Drug

b. Concentration

c. Route

d. Vascularity (inflamed?)

e. Vasoconstrictor

f. Weight of client

g. Rate of metabolism and excretion (repeated doses)

2. Symptoms of LA toxicity—central nervous system (CNS) and cardiovascular system (CVS) are affected most; severity of effects is related directly to blood levels

a. Central nervous system—stimulation followed by depression

(1) CNS stimulation (excitatory)—restlessness, shivering, tremors, convulsions

(2) CNS depression—sedation, drowsiness, respiratory and cardiovascular depression, coma; CNS depression can occur without previous excitation

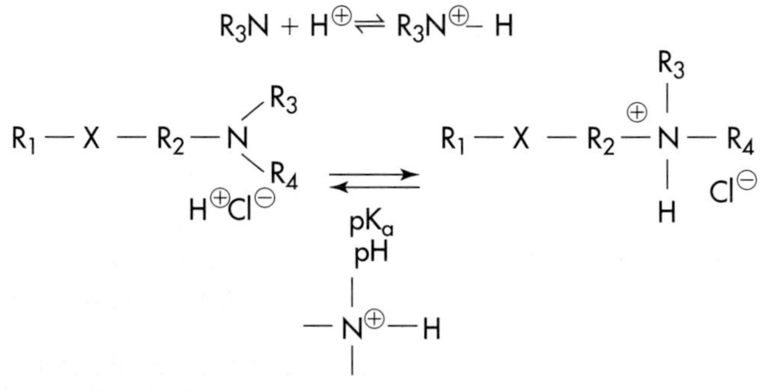

$$R_3N + H^{\oplus} \rightleftharpoons R_3N^{\oplus}\!- H$$

Free base
Uncharged, unionized
Fat soluble (lipophilic)
Penetrates nerve tissue

Salt
Charged, cation (ionized)
Water soluble (hydrophilic)
Form present in dental cartridge (pH 4.5-6.0)
Infection, doesn't penetrate

Fig. 8-5   Base and salt forms of local anesthetics. pH determines amount on each side (in equilibrium).

b. Cardiovascular system
  (1) Antidysrhythmic action—lidocaine used IV to treat dysrhythmias
  (2) Vasodilation produces hypotension (releases vascular smooth muscle, lowers resistance)
3. Toxicity—the higher the number, the more likely it is that an LA agent is toxic; "absolute" considers only the drug, whereas "relative" considers the concentration available (%)

Drug	Toxicity Absolute	Relative
Procaine (Novocain)	1	1
Lidocaine (Xylocaine, Octocaine)	2	2
Mepivacaine (Carbocaine, Isocaine)	1.5	1.5
Prilocaine (Citanest)	1+	2+
Tetracaine (Pontocaine—topical)	10	5
Propoxycaine (in Ravocaine)	10	2
Bupivacaine (Marcaine)	4	3+
Etidocaine (Duranest)	4	3+

4. Malignant hyperthermia
5. Allergic reactions
  a. Range of reactions—mild rash to anaphylaxis
  b. Esters—much more allergenic than amides; presence of true allergic reactions to the amides in question
  c. Skin testing—poor; false-positive and false-negative results; need emergency equipment and trained personnel on hand
  d. Other ingredients may produce allergic reactions (preservatives, sulfiting agents)
  e. Client allergic to ester, give amide and vice versa (if allergic to both may use diphenhydramine [Benadryl], an antihistamine)
F. Drug interactions
  1. Esters plus sulfonamides—esters may interfere with the sulfonamides' antiinfective action locally
  2. Cimetidine (Tagamet)—prolongs liver metabolism of lidocaine; lidocaine blood levels may increase with repeated doses; not important to dentistry
G. Composition of local anesthetic solutions
  1. Other ingredients
    a. Vasoconstrictor—epinephrine (Adrenalin), levonordefrin (Neo-Cobefrin)
    b. Preservatives (antiseptics)—methylparabens and propylparabens no longer present in dental cartridges
    c. Antioxidant—sodium bisulfite or sodium metabisulfite; present if contains vasoconstrictor; may precipitate asthma attacks in susceptible persons; "salad-bar" reaction
    d. Alkalinizing agent—sodium hydroxide; adjusts pH, keeps LA in salt form so soluble in water
    e. Sodium chloride—makes isotonic
  2. For LAs in dental cartridges, see Table 8-3
H. Topical LAs
  1. Cocaine—high abuse potential; *never* indicated for dental use
  2. Benzocaine—used topically because it cannot be used systemically; some sensitization occurs (ester), especially before gloves, e.g., rash
  3. Lidocaine—topically effective

Table 8-3
Local Anesthetic Agents in Dental Cartridges*

Local anesthetic	Concentration (%)	Vasoconstrictor	
ESTER			
Propoxycaine (Ravocaine) mixed with procaine (Novocain)	0.4	Levonordefrin (Neo-Cobefrin)	1:20,000
	2	Norepinephrine (Levophed)	1:30,000
AMIDES			
Lidocaine (Xylocaine, Octocaine)	2	Epinephrine	1:100,000
	2	Epinephrine	1:50,000
Mepivacaine (Carbocaine, Isocaine, Polorcaine)	2	Levonordefrin (Neo-Cobefrin)	1:20,000
	3	None	
Prilocaine (Citanest, Citanest Forte)	4	Epinephrine	1:200,000
	4	None	
Bupivacaine (Marcaine, Sensorcaine)	0.5	Epinephrine	1:200,000

*1 cartridge = 1.8 ml

4. Tetracaine—avoid use because of toxicity and slow onset

I. Dosage calculation—if LA 2% and $\% = \frac{g}{100}$, then

$$LA\ 2\% = \frac{2\ g}{100\ ml} = \frac{2000\ mg}{100\ ml} = \frac{20\ mg}{1\ ml}$$

If cartridge is 1.8 ml, then 1 cartridge of 2% LA would contain

$$\frac{20\ mg}{1\ ml} \times \frac{1.8\ ml}{1\ cartridge} = 36\ mg/cartridge$$

J. Other local anesthetic—diphenhydramine (Benadryl) 1%
   1. Antihistamines—weak local anesthetic action
   2. Used as a last resort (e.g., if the client is allergic to all other LA agents)

General Anesthetics

General Considerations

A. Dental use—uncooperative clients with multiple dental procedures; client hospitalized
B. Stages and planes of anesthesia
   Stage I—Analgesia, three planes; nitrous oxide alone
   Stage II—Excitement, delirium; avoid if possible
   Stage III—Surgical anesthesia, four planes
   Stage IV—Respiratory paralysis (medullary paralysis); death without treatment
C. Routes of administration
   1. Intravenous anesthetics; fixed anesthetics (cannot be removed by respiration)
      a. Barbiturates (e.g., thiopental [Pentothal])
      b. Dissociative—ketamine (Ketalar, Ketaject)
      c. Neuroleptanalgesic—fentanyl (Sublimaze) plus droperidol (Inapsine, Innovar)
   2. Inhalation gases
      a. Nitrous oxide–oxygen
      b. Cyclopropane
   3. Inhalation volatile liquids
      a. Diethyl ether (ether)
      b. Halogenated hydrocarbons (e.g., halothane [Fluothane])

Specific Agents

A. Nitrous oxide–oxygen analgesia (N_2O–O_2)
   1. Incomplete anesthetic; used alone cannot reach stage III
   2. Usual concentration—30% to 50% to prevent O_2 deprivation
   3. Advantages
      a. Rapid onset and recovery
      b. Least toxic; safe when used appropriately
      c. May be used in children
      d. Nonflammable
      e. Nonirritating to the GI tract
      f. Good analgesia, anxiolytic effect
   4. Disadvantages
      a. "Misuse" potential with both clients and oral healthcare professionals
      b. Reduces fertility (more difficult to get pregnant)
      c. Improper use (without concomitant local anesthetic block injection) gives N_2O a "bad name"; analgesia from N_2O–O_2 is insufficient to omit the use of a local anesthetic agent
      d. Nausea—most common complaint; rapid changes in N_2O concentration in inspired air, change levels slowly
      e. *Diffusion hypoxia* (low O_2 in lungs due to diffusion of O_2 into blood supply) rarely occurs; give 100% oxygen at end of procedure to prevent it
   5. Contraindications
      a. Respiratory problems
         (1) Upper respiratory tract infection (URI)—nasal passages are congested, difficult to administer N_2O–O_2 analgesia
         (2) Chronic obstructive pulmonary disease (COPD), such as emphysema or bronchitis
            (a) administering oxygen (O_2) at the usual concentration with nitrous oxide could produce apnea (cessation of respiration)
            (b) client's respiration is driven by carbon dioxide (CO_2) levels
      b. Pregnancy—first trimester is the most critical; greatest number of spontaneous abortions (especially in oral healthcare personnel); teratogenic? (probably not)
      c. Lack of communication
         (1) Psychologic—patients with psychologic problems may respond inappropriately
         (2) Language—patient cannot comprehend your language; speaks a foreign language
      d. Contagious disease—tuberculosis, hepatitis (if can't sterilize entire tubes)
B. Diethyl ether—unpopular because
   1. Explosive
   2. Slow induction and recovery
   3. Gastrointestinal—nausea and vomiting common
C. Halogenated hydrocarbons
   1. Examples:
      Halothane (Fluothane)
      Enflurane (Ethrane)
      Isoflurane (Forane)
   2. No mucous membrane irritation; not explosive; poor muscle relaxation; no analgesia; little nausea or vomiting

3. Sensitize the myocardium to catecholamines (epinephrine)—dysrhythmias
4. Hepatotoxic; greater with more exposures

D. Ultrashort-acting barbiturates
1. Examples
   Thiopental (Pentothal); also known as truth serum
   Methohexital (Brevital)
   Thiamylal (Surital)
2. Rapid onset; short duration secondary to *redistribution* (to brain, muscles, then fat)
3. Used to induce general anesthesia; advances to stage III rapidly
4. Adverse reaction—laryngospasm
5. Contraindicated in porphyria

E. Ketamine (Ketalar, Ketaject) produces *dissociative* anesthesia
1. *Not* a complete anesthetic
2. Can produce a trance
3. Emergence reactions—bad dreams, "bad trip"; more likely in adults; related to phencyclohexylpiperidine (PCP, angel dust)
4. Can produce hyperactive reflexes, such as cough, gag, or tongue movement

F. Innovar produces *neuroleptanalgesia*
1. Fentanyl (opioid) plus droperidol (major tranquilizer)
2. Produces "lead pipe" chest as an adverse reaction, CPR difficult if needed

Central Nervous System Depressants

General Considerations

A. Several pharmacologic groups possess antianxiety properties: sedative-hypnotic agents, minor tranquilizers, nitrous oxide, opioid (narcotic) analgesic agents and antihistamines

B. Definitions
1. Sedative—provides relaxation during daytime
2. Hypnotic—induces sleep at bedtime
3. Tranquilizers—major versus minor
   a. Minor tranquilizers (e.g., benzodiazepines) produce the following effects
      (1) Anxiety relief
      (2) Sedation and disinhibition
      (3) Anesthesia and death
      (4) Anticonvulsant effect
      (5) Voluntary muscle relaxation
      (6) Physical dependence and addiction
   b. Major tranquilizers (e.g., phenothiazines) produce the following effects
      (1) Control of psychotic behavior
      (2) Easy arousal
      (3) Convulsions
      (4) Extrapyramidal effects (parkinsonian)
      (5) Anticholinergic effect
      (6) *No* addiction

Sedative-Hypnotics (Barbiturates and Nonbarbiturates)

A. Pharmacologic effects
1. Sedation and anxiety relief, sleep, anesthesia—a continuum with increasing doses
2. Anticonvulsant—long-acting agents are usually the most useful
3. Muscle relaxation—this action is inseparable from CNS (sedation) effects
4. *No* analgesic action—in the presence of pain agitation may result if an analgesic is not also given

B. Adverse reactions
1. CNS depression—drowsiness, impaired performance and judgment; caution required when driving a car (see box for drugs producing sedation)
2. Abuse—euphoria, habituation, withdrawal, tolerance
3. Acute overdose—suicide attempt produces respiratory arrest (depression of respiratory center)
4. Barbiturates—contraindicated in porphyria; stimulate liver microsomal enzymes (drugs metabolized by the liver disappear more quickly)

C. Therapeutic uses
1. Medical—treatment of epilepsy, sedation, or antianxiety
2. Dental
   a. Preoperative anxiety reduction—oral or intramuscular injections
   b. Induction of general anesthesia—intravenous barbiturates

D. Examples
1. Barbiturates

SELECTED PHARMACOLOGIC GROUPS PRODUCING SEDATION

- Alcohol, ethyl
- Antihistamines
- Antipsychotics (phenothiazines)
- Barbiturates
- Benzodiazepines
- Centrally acting muscle relaxants
- Nonbarbiturate sedative-hypnotics
- Nonsteroidal antiinflammatory drugs (NSAIDs)
- Opioid (narcotic) analgesic agents
- "Tranquilizers"
- Tricyclic antidepressants

	Anticonvulsant Agents of Choice for Seizures		
Seizure type	**First choice agent**	**Alternatives**
Absence (petit mal)	Ethosuximide (Zarontin) Valproate (Depakote)	Clonazepam (Clonopin)
Tonic-clonic (grand mal)	Carbamazepine (Tegretol) Phenytoin (Dilantin)	Phenobarbital (Luminal) Primidone (Mysoline)
Status epilepticus	Diazepam (Valium)	Phenytoin (Dilantin) Phenobarbital (Luminal)

Table 8-4

a. Ultrashort acting—for induction of general anesthesia
   Thiopental (Pentothal)
   Methohexital (Brevital)
b. Short acting—for insomnia; most abused
   Pentobarbital (Nembutal)
   Secobarbital (Seconal)
c. Intermediate acting—for insomnia/daytime sedation; abused
   Amobarbital (Amytal)
   Butabarbital (Butisol)
d. Long acting—for daytime sedation and as an anticonvulsant; little abuse
   Phenobarbital (Luminal)
   Mephobarbital (Mebaral)
   Primidone (Mysoline)
2. Other sedative-hypnotic agents
   a. Chloral hydrate (Noctec)
      (1) Produces GI irritation
      (2) Used with children
   b. Meprobamate (Equanil, Miltown)—tranquilizer
   c. Zolpidem (Ambien)—newer non-benzodiazepine sedative hypnotic

Benzodiazepines

A. Mechanism of action—more specific anxiolytic (antianxiety) action than the barbiturates; potentiate GABA-ergic (γ-aminobutyric acid—an inhibitory neurotransmitter) neurotransmission producing more sedation (antianxiety)
B. Wide therapeutic index when ingested alone; much safer than the barbiturates
C. Adverse reactions
   1. Sedation—warn patients about driving a car
   2. Addiction potential—some, less than barbiturates
   3. Teratogenicity—increased incidence of birth defects if taken during the first trimester; FDA category D or X
   4. Thrombophlebitis—intravenously (local irritation with diazepam due to use of propylene glycol as

diluent); midazolam (Versed) soluble in H_2O, so no propylene glycol
   5. Overdose treated with flumazenil (Mazicon), a benzodiazepine antagonist
D. Specific agents
   1. Examples

Drug	Usual dose (mg)
Alprazolam (Xanax)	0.25-0.5
Chlordiazepoxide (Librium)	5-20
Diazepam (Valium)	2-10
Flurazepam (Dalmane)	15-30
Lorazepam (Ativan)	2-4
Midazolam (Versed)	IV
Oxazepam (Serax)	15-30
Temazepam (Restoril)	15-30
Triazolam (Halcion)	0.25-0.5

   2. Differences
      a. Equivalent dose—usual dose varies with agent
      b. Duration varies—few hours to a few days; shorter-acting agents are listed first under examples
      c. Metabolism (1) Most metabolized by oxidation to active metabolites, (2) Few (oxazepam, lorazepam, and temazepam) inactivated by glucuronidation
   3. Drug interactions—cimetidine and age reduce metabolism of oxidized benzodiazepines; clients who smoke have less sedation (smoking induces liver enzymes)

Anticonvulsants

A. General properties of anticonvulsants
   1. Pharmacologic effects—reduction of frequency or elimination of seizures (Table 8-4)
   2. Gastrointestinal—common side effect
   3. Teratogenicity—variable teratogenic potential (pregnant women with epilepsy need to be treated)
   4. Sedation—tolerance to sedative effect occurs without tolerance to anticonvulsant effect
   5. Blood dyscrasias—can be serious, laboratory monitoring important

Table 8-5

Analgesic Summary

Pharmacologic effect and adverse reactions	Aspirin	NSAIDs	Acetaminophen	Opioids (narcotics)
Analgesic	+	++	+	+++++
Antipyretic	+	+/O	+	O
Antiinflammatory	+	++	O	O
CNS effects (drowsiness)	++[a]	++	O[b]	++
GI effects	++[c]	+[c]	O	+[d]
Bleeding	++	+[g]	O	O
Hepatotoxic	+[e]	+	+[f]	O
Nephrotoxic	+[g]	+[g]	+[g]	O
Addicting effects	O	O	O	+++++

[a] Poisoning—salicylism.
[b] Very high doses.
[c] Stomach upset, ulcers, pain.
[d] Nausea, constipation.
[e] Hepatitis in persons with systemic lupus erythematosus or rheumatoid arthritis.
[f] With acute overdose.
[g] Aspirin or NSAIDs and acetaminophen.

B. Phenytoin (Dilantin)
   1. **Gingival enlargement (hyperplasia)**—meticulous oral hygiene reduces enlargement frequency
   2. Vitamin deficiencies—D and folate
   3. Fetal hydantoin syndrome—teratogenicity
C. Valproic acid (Depakene, Depakote)
   1. Hepatic failure—monitor liver function tests
   2. **Thrombocytopenia**—bleeding
      a. Watch with aspirin or Coumadin use
D. Carbamazepine (Tegretol)
   1. Induces metabolism of itself and other drugs
   2. CNS—drowsiness, dizziness
   3. Gastrointestinal—nausea and vomiting
   4. Hemopoietic—monitor platelets, reticulocytes, serum iron
   5. Hepatic—monitor liver function tests
   6. Indications—various seizures and **trigeminal neuralgia**
   7. Drug interactions—carbamazepine increases metabolism of warfarin, theophylline, doxycycline; metabolism is inhibited by erythromycin, verapamil, diltiazem; increases the effect of lithium
E. Benzodiazepines
   1. Diazepam (Valium)—used for status epilepticus and emergency treatment of seizures
   2. Clonazepam (Clonopin)—orally for absence seizures and psychiatric conditions

Antihistamines

A. Antihistamines are histamine$_1$ (H$_1$)-receptor antagonists
B. Pharmacologic effects—reduce allergic symptoms; block most actions of histamine (increased capillary permeability and edema, flares, and itching)
C. Adverse reactions
   1. Sedation—CNS depression, drowsiness; active ingredient in over-the-counter (OTC) sleep aids; children can exhibit excitation; newer nonsedating antihistamines listed below (±)
   2. Xerostomia—weak anticholinergic effect
   3. Extrapyramidal—see antipsychotics for promethazine; lip smacking, tremors, stiffness, restlessness
D. Examples—incidence of adverse effects varies

Drug	Degree of sedation
Diphenhydramine (Benadryl)	+++
Promethazine (Phenergan)*	+++
Chlorpheniramine maleate (Chlor-Trimeton)	+
Triprolidine (in Actifed)	+
Loratadine (Claritin)	±
Fenoxaferadine (Allegra)	±

*Exhibits some phenothiazine-like action

Analgesics (Table 8-5)

General Considerations

A. Pain
   1. Perception—uniform through nerve (signal from site of pain to CNS)
   2. Reaction—varies greatly from person to person (interpretation within the CNS of the signal)
B. Variables—client's age, gender, race, ethnic group, fatigue, fear
C. Placebo effect occurs (inert ingredient produces phar-

macologic effect)—clinical trials must include a placebo; expressing confidence in medication often makes it more effective

Salicylates (Aspirin)

A. Mechanism of action—primarily peripheral; prostaglandin synthesis inhibitor (inhibits the enzyme cyclooxygenase or prostaglandin synthetase)
B. Pharmacologic effects—"the three A's"
  1. Analgesic—reduces pain
  2. Antipyretic—therapeutic dose reduces an elevated body temperature
  3. Antiinflammatory—higher dose reduces inflammation
C. Adverse reactions
  1. Gastrointestinal—minimize by ingesting with food, glass of water, or antacids
  2. Bleeding altered
    a. Platelet adhesiveness—reduced platelet adhesiveness for the life of the platelets (4 to 7 days); normal clotting appears 72 hours after aspirin ingestion requires only a single small dose; useful in small doses to prevent clotting
    b. Hypoprothrombinemia—reduced prothrombin levels; requires several consecutive doses
  3. Salicylate toxicity ("salicylism") tinnitus, hyperthermia (increased body temperature), electrolyte and glucose problems, and an altered sensorium
  4. Allergies—**true** allergy is uncommon, if person is allergic, some cross-reactivity exists with other agents (e.g., nonsteroidal antiinflammatory drugs [NSAIDs]); can produce acute asthmatic attack; asthmatic persons with nasal polyps more susceptible
  5. Reye syndrome—children with chickenpox or influenza should *not* be given aspirin; avoid aspirin in children and adolescents up to 18 years of age
D. Drug interactions—aspirin plus
  1. Warfarin (Coumadin) (used as an anticoagulant)—bleeding or hemorrhage
  2. Probenecid (Benemid) (used to treat gout)—acute attack of gout
  3. Tolbutamide (Orinase) (used to control diabetes)—altered blood glucose level
  4. Methotrexate (MTX) (used to treat cancer or control arthritis)—MTX toxicity of bone marrow

Nonsteroidal Antiinflammatory Agents/Drugs (NSAIAs/NSAIDs)

A. Mechanism—like aspirin, drug inhibits prostaglandin synthesis (cyclooxygenase)
B. Pharmacologic effects—"the three A's" (similar to aspirin)
  1. Analgesic
  2. Antipyretic
  3. Antiinflammatory
C. Adverse reactions
  1. Gastrointestinal—greater than aspirin; abdominal discomfort to ulcers
    a. Treated or managed with prostaglandin—misoprostil (Cytotec)
  2. Central nervous system—dizziness, sedation; caution required when driving a car
  3. Blood coagulation—reduction in platelet aggregation and possible prolongation of bleeding time; alteration (reversible; unlike aspirin whose effect is not reversible)
  4. Teratogenic effects—contraindicated in pregnant or nursing woman
D. Therapeutic uses
  1. Pain control—analgesic; stronger than aspirin, equal to or stronger than some opioids (dose dependent); antiinflammatory effect makes NSAIDs especially useful in dentistry
  2. For arthritis—antiinflammatory action
  3. For dysmenorrhea (painful menstruation)—effective because mechanism of action specific for problem excess prostaglandins due to excessive uterine contractions
E. Examples
  Ibuprofen (Motrin-IB, Rufen, Nuprin, Advil*)
  Naproxen (Naprosyn)
  *Naproxen sodium (Anaprox; Aleve)
  Ketoprofen (Orudis [KT])
  Indomethacin (Indocin)

Acetaminophen (*N*-Acetyl-*p*-aminophenol [NAPAP]; Tylenol)

A. Pharmacologic effects ("The Two A's")
  1. Analgesic
  2. Antipyretic
  3. *NOT* antiinflammatory
B. Adverse reactions
  1. Analgesic nephropathy—adversely affects the kidneys; more likely to occur if chronic use in combination with aspirin
  2. Hepatotoxicity—with acute or chronic overdose; delayed reaction; treated with *N*-acetylcysteine; can require liver transplant or be fatal

Opioid (Narcotic) Analgesic Agents

A. Pharmacologic effects—proportional to the "strength" of the opioid
  1. Analgesia

---

*Available OTC.

2. Sedation (anxiety relief)
B. Adverse reactions—proportional to the "strength" of the opioid
   1. Sedation/euphoria—may lead to abuse
   2. Respiratory depression—dose related; cause of death in overdose; reversed with naloxone
   3. Gastrointestinal—nausea, vomiting, constipation; Diphenoxylate can be useful therapeutically
   4. Abuse—can occur with *all* opioid analgesics; tolerance develops to all the pharmacologic effects except miosis (pupillary constriction) and constipation; withdrawal produced if drug abruptly stopped
C. Therapeutic uses
   1. Pain relief—central mechanism; agent affects person's perception of pain; some can relieve severe pain
   2. Sedation and anxiety relief—not main use; used preoperatively
   3. Cough suppression—have antitussive action (suppress cough); small dose needed, e.g., codeine-containing cough syrups
   4. Diarrhea—symptomatic relief only; reduce GI motility by increasing tone and spasm; diphenoxylate (in Lomotil)
D. Examples of agonists (combine with opioid receptor and produce an effect)

Drug	Usual dose (mg)	"Strength"
Morphine	10	Stronger
Hydromorphone (Dilaudid)	2-4	
Meperidine (Demerol)	50-100	
Oxycodone (in Percodan)	5	
Hydrocodone (in Vicodin)	5	
Codeine (in Tylenol #3, Empirin #3)	30-60	Weaker

E. Other opioids
   1. Agonist-antagonists
      a. e.g., Pentazocine (Talwin-NX)
      b. Principle
         (1) Maintain analgesic properties
         (2) Have lower abuse potential
      c. Can precipitate withdrawal in opiate addicts
   2. Antagonists
      a. e.g., Naloxone (Narcan)
      b. Combines with opioid receptor; produces no effect
      c. Therapeutic uses
         (1) Treat opioid overdose
         (2) Counteract respiratory depression
         (3) Include in any dental emergency kit

Drugs Used for Gout

A. Disease—metabolic problem with increased serum uric acid, episodes of acute attacks of pain in joints (big toe, knee) due to deposition of monosodium urate resulting in severe inflammation
B. Prevention
   1. Probenecid (Benemid)—uricosuric (promotes uric acid excretion); aspirin interferes with this effect of probenecid
   2. Allopurinol (Zyloprim)—xanthine oxidase inhibitor (inhibits uric acid synthesis); also used in cancer patients before chemotherapy or radiation to prevent gouty attack that can occur when many cells are killed and release their amino acids (end product is uric acid)
C. Treatment
   1. Colchicine—binds to microtubular protein tubulin (prevents leukocyte migration and phagocytosis); inhibits formation of leukotriene B_4; GI toxicity—nausea, vomiting, diarrhea is endpoint of treatment
   2. Nonsteroidal antiinflammatory drugs—antiinflammatory action, ameliorates symptoms, e.g., indomethacin

Antiinfectives (Antibiotics)

General Considerations

A. Prevention of infection (see Chapter 7)
   1. Sterilization measures (e.g., autoclaving) prevent infection
   2. Many infections—handle with local measures (i.e., incision and drainage) antibiotics often not needed; host (client) resistance must be considered
   3. Antibiotic administration carries risk
   4. Prophylaxis is rarely indicated except for prevention of infective endocarditis, even this case in question as to effectiveness
B. Definitions
   1. Antimicrobial—against microbes
   2. Antiinfective—against organisms causing infections
   3. Antibacterial—against bacteria
      a. Bactericidal—kills bacteria
      b. Bacteriostatic—retards or incapacitates bacteria (reversible); if bacteria removed from the environment, they can multiply
   4. Antiviral—against viruses
   5. Antifungal—against fungi
   6. Antibiotic—effective in low concentrations; produced by microorganisms; suppresses or kills growth of other organisms

7. Spectrum—range of an antibiotic's antiinfective properties; narrow (few organisms) to wide or broad (many organisms); may include gram-positive and gram-negative

8. Resistance—organism unaffected by an antiinfective agent; may be either natural (always has been resistant) or acquired (the resistance developed); prolonged exposure to antibiotics can select out resistant strains (survival of the "fittest")

9. Suprainfection (superinfection)—a new infection with other than the original organism occurs after taking antimicrobial agent; new infection is usually more difficult to treat; are common when spectrum is widest; example: *Candida* infection in person taking tetracycline

10. Synergism—more than additive $(1 + 1 > 2)$

11. Antagonism—less than additive $(1 + 1 < 2)$

C. General side effects
1. Gastrointestinal side effects—variable, depends on antibiotic
2. Suprainfection
3. Drug interactions
   a. Oral contraceptives—antibiotics may reduce effectiveness; warn client
   b. Warfarin (Coumadin)—antibiotics alter GI flora (makes vitamin K) potentiates warfarin's effect
   c. Bacteriostatic and bactericidal antibiotics mixed—the "static" stops the bacteria from growing so the "cidal" cannot work properly (on cell wall) to kill bacteria; e.g., erythromycin and penicillin

D. Treatment versus prophylaxis
1. Treatment—antiinfective is used to treat an infection that is present
2. Prophylaxis (to prevent)—used to prevent some potential future infection; only proved beneficial in a few instances (even those are questionable); remember that a condom used to prevent pregnancy is also called a prophylactic.

E. Tables 1, 2, and 4 of Appendix B (on pages 794, 797, and 799) summarize the conditions, the dental procedures, and the antibiotics and their dosing regimens, respectively

Penicillins

A. Mechanism—inhibits cell wall synthesis; bactericidal
B. Spectrum—three penicillin subgroups
1. Penicillin G/penicillin V
2. Penicillinase-resistant penicillins
3. Extended-spectrum penicillins
   a. Ampicillin-like
   b. Carbenicillin-like
C. Stability
1. Acid labile—degrade in stomach acid; therefore used parenterally (e.g., penicillin G, methacillin, carbenicillin)
2. Acid stable—may be used orally (e.g., penicillin VK, amoxicillin)
D. Pharmacokinetics (body handling)
1. Peak—blood levels peak in 30 minutes to 1 hour by oral or intramuscular route; peak immediately when used intravenously
2. Half-life $(T_{1/2})$—between 30 minutes and 1 hour
3. Excretion very rapid, actively secreted; duration prolonged by concomitant probenecid (Benemid) administration
E. Adverse effects
1. Relatively nontoxic except for allergy
2. Allergic reactions—from mild rash to anaphylaxis
3. Nephrotoxicity (kidney damage) occurs occasionally; more likely with broader-spectrum penicillins

Penicillin G/Penicillin V

A. Examples
   Penicillin G potassium
   Penicillin G procaine (Wycillin, Crysticillin)
   Penicillin G benzathine (Bicillin)
   Penicillin VK (V-Cillin K, Pen-Vee K)
B. Spectrum—versus many gram-positive aerobic organisms, such as *Streptococcus* and *Staphylococcus,* and certain Gram-negative aerobic cocci, such as *Neisseria gonorrhoeae;* same anaerobes; *NOT* resistant to penicillinase
C. Penicillin G—parenteral; (1) dosed in units (e.g., 5 million unit) (2) intramuscular salts (procaine and benzathine) provide longer duration of action than sodium and potassium salts
D. Penicillin V—more acid stable than penicillin G so can be used orally; potassium (K) salt better absorbed; therefore, penicillin VK is the most used antibiotic in dentistry; 400,000 units = 250 mg

Penicillinase (β-lactamase)–Resistant Penicillins

A. Examples
   Methicillin (Staphcillin)
   Nafcillin (Unipen, Nafcil)
   Oxacillin (Prostaphlin, Bactocill)
   Cloxacillin (Tegopen, Cloxapen)
   Dicloxacillin (Dynapen, Pathocil)
B. Therapeutic use—limited; used against penicillinase-producing staphylococci

Extended-Spectrum ("Broader" or "Wider" Spectrum) Penicillins

A. Ampicillin-like
   1. Examples
   Ampicillin (Omnipen, Totacillin, Polycillin)
   Amoxicillin (Amoxil, Larotid, Polymox)
   2. Spectrum—work against many gram-positive organisms and also some gram-negative bacteria, such as *Haemophilus influenzae,* some *Escherichia coli,* and *Proteus mirabilis*
   3. *Not* penicillinase resistant
   4. Augmentin—amoxicillin + clauvulanic acid (CA); CA binds with penicillinase so amoxicillin is *NOT* inactivated, can be used with penicillinase-producing organisms
B. Carbenicillin-like
   1. Examples
   Ticarcillin (Ticar)
   Carbenicillin (Geopen, Pyopen)
   2. Spectrum—gram-negative coverage, such as against *Pseudomonas aeruginosa, Proteus,* and organisms resistant to ampicillin-like drugs
   3. Used parenterally (in hospitalized patients) for systemic action

Macrolides

A. Mechanism—interferes with protein synthesis (binds to the 50S ribosomal subunit); bacteriostatic
B. Spectrum
   1. Erythromycin
      a. Work primarily against gram-positive microorganisms (e.g., penicillin V); poor against anaerobes
      b. Also used against certain strains of *Rickettsia, Chlamydia,* and *Actinomyces,* as well as the drug of choice for *Mycoplasma pneumoniae* and *Legionella pneumophila*
   2. Azithromycin (Zithromax)
      a. Recently recommended by the American Heart Association for use in prevention of bacterial endocarditis prior to certain dental procedures in people who are allergic to penicillin (see Appendix B)
      b. Adverse effects—stomatitis, candidiasis, angioedema (allergy), heart palpitations, chest pain, nausea, vomiting, diarrhea, abdominal pain, hepatotoxicity, heartburn, flatulence
      c. Alternative drug of choice for mild infection due to susceptible organisms in persons allergic to penicillin
   3. Clarithromycin (Biaxin)
      a. Recently recommended by the American Heart

Association for use in the prevention of bacterial endocarditis prior to certain dental procedures in persons who are allergic to penicillin (see Appendix B)
      b. Adverse effects—abnormal taste, candidiasis, stomatitis, nausea, abdominal pain, diarrhea, hepatotoxicity, heartburn, anorexia, vomiting, vaginitis, moniliasis, urticaria, rash, pruritus
      c. Alternative drug of choice for mild infection due to susceptible organisms in persons allergic to penicillin
C. Pharmacokinetics (body handling) of erythromycin
   1. Erythromycin—acid lability (instability), so enteric coated (does not dissolve in the stomach; dissolves in the intestine) or formulated as esters to protect against stomach acid (e.g., ethylsuccinate, EES)
   2. Effect peaks in 2 to 4 hours
D. Adverse effects
   1. GI upset is *very* common; take with food to decrease
   2. Cholestatic jaundice is primarily associated with the estolate ester
E. Examples
   1. Erythromycin
   Erythromycin base (E-mycin)
   Erythromycin stearate (Erythrocin)
   Erythromycin ethylsuccinate (EES, Pediamycin)
   Erythromycin estolate (Ilosone)
   2. Others
F. Therapeutic use (1) Treatment of dental infections in penicillin-allergic persons (2) Specific suspected infections (see spectrum), also for (3) Other macrolides

Cephalosporins

A. Mechanism—similar to penicillins; inhibits cell wall synthesis; bactericidal
B. Chemistry similar to penicillins
C. Spectrum—work against many gram-positive and gram-negative organisms; the *third*-generation cephalosporins and the newest 4th generation cephalosporins have the *widest* spectrum of action
D. Adverse reactions
   1. GI upset common (33%)
   2. Other—similar to those of the broader-spectrum penicillins (e.g., nephrotoxicity, suprainfection)
   3. Allergy—some cross-hypersensitivity (10%) with penicillin allergy (possess a similar structure)
E. Examples
   Cephalexin (Keflex)
   Cephradine (Velosef, Anspor)
   Cefuroxime (Ceftin)
F. Suggested oral antibiotic regimen for the client with joint prosthesis (soon not recommended)

Clindamycin (Cleocin)

A. Mechanism—inhibits protein synthesis (binds to the 50S ribosomal subunit); generally bacteriostatic
B. Spectrum—gram-positive organisms and many anaerobes, such as *Bacteriodes* species
C. Adverse reactions
1. Gastrointestinal—diarrhea; pseudomembranous colitis (PMC) or antibiotic associated colitis (AAC); incidence up to 10%; discontinue drug if bloody stools with mucus occur
2. Food and Drug Administration says "reserved for serious anaerobic infections"
D. Dental use—certain anaerobic infections thought to be due to *Bacteroides* species; jaw infections, periodontal infections; infective endocarditis prophylaxis (Table 8-7)

Tetracyclines

A. Mechanism—inhibits protein synthesis (binds to the 30S ribosome); bacteriostatic
B. Spectrum—truly broad spectrum; work against many gram-positive and many gram-negative organisms
C. Pharmacokinetics
1. Tetracyclines—divalent and trivalent cations (e.g., Ca^{++} [in dairy products], Mg^{++} and Al^{+++} [in antacids], Fe^{++}); inhibit absorption of tetracycline (by chelation)
2. Doxycycline (Vibramycin) and minocycline (Minocin) less affected by food or dairy products than tetracycline itself, avoid taking antacids or Ca^{++} supplementation concomitantly
D. Resistance—cross-transference can occur; organisms can become resistant without being exposed to drug
E. Adverse effects
1. GI upset—is relatively common
2. Suprainfection—very common because wide spectrum of action; drug alters normal flora (e.g., vaginal candidiasis)
3. Photosensitivity—exaggerated sunburn with exposure to sunlight (watch tanning booths)
4. Teeth—both hypoplasia and discoloration can occur if given during enamel development; primary teeth affected from the last half of the pregnancy to age 4 to 6 months; permanent teeth are affected from age 2 months to 7 to 12 years
F. Examples
Tetracycline (Achromycin-V)
Doxycycline (Vibramycin)
Minocycline (Minocin)
G. Therapeutic uses
1. Medical—treatment of acne, respiratory tract infections in patients with COPD (emphysema or bronchitis), certain sexually transmitted diseases (STD)
2. Dental—manage periodontal diseases; drug placed in periodontal pocket, e.g., tetracycline fibers (Actisite)

Quinolone

A. Mechanism—inhibition of the bacteria's gyrase so that daughter segment of DNA cannot acquire the proper configuration to divide
B. Spectrum—works against gram-negative bacteria including *Enterobacter* species, *Escherichia coli, Morganella morganii*
C. Adverse reactions—abdominal pain, nausea, vomiting, diarrhea, rash, urticaria, angioedema
D. Example—nalidixic acid

Aminoglycosides

A. Mechanism—drug inhibits protein synthesis (binds to the 30S ribosomal subunit); bactericidal (only group that combines inhibition of protein synthesis with cidal action)
B. Spectrum—work against some gram-positive and many gram-negative organisms
C. Pharmacokinetics—not effective systemically if given orally; must be given parenterally (IM or IV)
D. Adverse reactions—toxicity usually results from excessive blood levels
1. Ototoxicity—adverse effect on cranial nerve VIII; both vestibular (balance) and auditory (hearing functions)
2. Nephrotoxicity—adverse effect on kidney
E. Examples
Neomycin (Mycifradin)
Kanamycin (Kantrex)
Gentamicin (Garamycin)
Tobramycin (Tobrex)

Sulfonamides ("Sulfa" Drugs)

A. Mechanism—competitive antagonist of PABA; prevents use of PABA to make folic acid needed in organism
B. Adverse reactions
1. Allergic reactions—rash
2. Photosensitivity (sun)
C. Examples
Sulfisoxazole (Gantrisin)
Trimethoprim-sulfamethoxazole (Bactrim, Septra)
D. Therapeutic uses
1. Urinary tract infections
2. Otitis media (children's ear infections)
3. Respiratory infections
4. Dental use unclear but probably not useful

Metronidazole (Flagyl)

A. Mechanism—breaks DNA structure, which inhibits protein synthesis; bactericidal
B. Spectrum
   1. Trichomonocidal (works against *Trichomonas vaginalis*)
   2. Bactericidal (works against anaerobes, such as *Bacteroides* species)
C. Adverse reactions
   1. GI—anorexia, nausea, vomiting, headache, dizziness
   2. CNS—Disulfiram (Antabuse)-like reaction—alcohol ingestion produces nausea and vomiting (avoid alcoholic beverages)
   3. Carcinogenic in animals; mutagenic in organisms—significance to cancer unknown
D. Dental use—periodontal clients with anaerobes; good against organisms, inexpensive

Antituberculosis Agents

A. Tuberculosis (TB)—a chronic disease
   1. Resistant organisms easily develop
   2. Treatment difficult, drug combinations frequently required; MDR (multiple drug resistant) organisms common
   3. Duration of therapy 6 to 9 months
B. Drugs
   1. Isoniazid (INH)—used alone as prophylaxis; used in combination with 2 and 5 other agents, hepatitis is side-effect
   2. Rifampin (Rifadin, Rimactane)
   3. Pyrizinamide
   4. Ethambutol (Myambutol)
C. Dental implications—universal precautions, persons treated for 6 weeks to 2 months, not contagious (if compliant), direct observation needed

Antifungal Agents

A. Disease—candidiasis, *Candida albicans* present, thrush in infants
B. Nystatin (Mycostatin, Nilstat)
   1. Dosage forms—oral suspension, pastille, (rubbery lozenge)
C. Clotrimazole (Mycelex)—lozenges available
D. Ketoconazole (Nizoral)
   1. Tablets—once/day
   2. Acid environment required for adequate absorption—watch H_2-blockers
   3. Adverse reactions
      a. Nausea and vomiting
      b. Hepatocellular dysfunction
      c. Teratogenic potential
      d. Drug interactions
E. Fluconazole (Diflucan)
   1. Tablets, oral suspension and IV
   2. Therapeutic use—systemic
   3. Adverse reactions—headache, abdominal pain, nausea, diarrhea, hepatic toxicity
F. Itraconazole (Sporanox)
   1. Capsules
   2. Therapeutic use—indicated for treatment of certain fungal infections in immunocompromised and nonimmunocompromised persons
   3. Adverse reactions—nausea, vomiting, diarrhea, abdominal pain, anorexia, edema, rash, fatigue, fever, malaise
   4. Warning—coadministration with terfenadine can cause serious cardiovascular events including death

Antiviral Agents

A. Acyclovir (Zovirax)
   1. Topical (ointment), oral (capsules or tablets), and IV
   2. Therapeutic use
      a. Initial genital herpes in nonimmunocompromised persons
      b. Recurrent genital herpes in immunocompromised persons
      c. po is prophylactic with continuous use
   3. Indications—HIV + and AIDS
      a. Zidovudine (AZT, Retrovir)
      b. Didanosine (ddI, Videx)
      c. Zalcitabine (ddC, Hivid)
B. Ganciclovir (Cytovene, Cytovene IV, DHPG)
   1. Inhibits replication of most herpes viruses
   2. Therapeutic use
      a. To prevent and treat cytomegalovirus disease in persons with AIDS
   3. Adverse effects—fever, coma, chills, confusion, abnormal thoughts, dizziness, bizarre dreams, headaches, psychosis, tremors, paresthesia, dysrhythmia, hypertension, hypotension, hemorrhage, anorexia, blood dyscrasia

Cardiovascular Agents

See Chapters 7 and 14 for contraindications and cautions involving dental treatment in persons with cardiovascular disease

Digitalis Glycosides

A. Pharmacologic effects—heart beats stronger (positive chronotropic effect), usually more slowly (bradycardia), so efficiency increased
B. Adverse reactions
   1. GI disturbances (nausea, vomiting)

2. CV (arrhythmias)
3. CNS (yellow-green vision, halos around lights)
C. Therapeutic uses—congestive heart failure, certain arrhythmias
D. Dental considerations—hypokalemia [K↓] due to diuretics; digitalis toxicity may exacerbate the dysrhythmias, epinephrine exacerbates dysrhythmias
E. Example
Digoxin (Lanoxin)

Antidysrhythmics

A. Pharmacologic effects—suppress dysrhythmias
B. Dental considerations—cardiac problems; watch local anesthetics with epinephrine
C. Examples
Quinidine
Procainamide
Propranolol (Inderal)
Lidocaine (Xylocaine)*

Antianginal Agents

A. Pharmacologic effects—reduce "work" of the heart because nonspecific vasodilator (by reducing amount of blood returning to heart)
B. Adverse reactions—hypotension, and severe headache common; patient should sit to take nitroglycerin (NTG)
C. Therapeutic use—angina pectoris
D. Dental considerations
1. Storage—unstable products; store properly; heat, light, and moisture degrade more; opened container should be discarded after 2 months
2. Acute anginal attack
a. Sublingual (SL)† nitroglycerin (tablets or spray)
3. Routes of nitroglycerin
a. Sublingual—tablets or spray
b. Transdermal—patches applied to chest or arm
c. Ointment—in ointment applied to skin
E. Examples
Nitroglycerin (NTG) (Nitrostat), SL† tablet
Isosorbide dinitrate (Isordil) or mononitrates
Nitroglycerin lingual spray (Nitrolingual SL spray)

Antihypertensives (Table 8-6; see also Table 4 in Appendix B, on page 799)

A. Pharmacologic effects—reduce elevated blood pressure
B. Adverse reactions—CNS depression (fatigue), dry mouth (xerostomia), orthostatic hypotension (patient suddenly arises from a supine position—blood pressure falls resulting in dizziness or syncope), constipation/diarrhea, sexual dysfunction
C. Therapeutic use—treatment of hypertension
D. Dental considerations
1. Take blood pressure to ensure that it is normal
2. Observe for dry mouth—counsel patient on use of sugarless products and artificial saliva
3. Help client arise from dental chair slowly

Diuretics

A. Pharmacologic effects—removes excess water and sodium via kidneys; direct vasodilating action on blood vessels, lowers total peripheral resistance, lowers blood pressure
B. Adverse reactions—hypokalemia (low potassium); patient may be taking potassium replacement; hyperglycemia, hyperuricemia
C. Therapeutic uses—hypertension, edema
D. Dental considerations
1. Hypokalemia (K↓) potentiates epinephrine-induced arrhythmias
2. Client may urinate more frequently after taking medicine (usually in the morning)
E. Examples
1. Thiazide diuretics: Hydrochlorothizide (HCTZ, HydroDIURIL)
2. Loop diuretics: Furosemide (Lasix)
3. Combinations of thiazide diuretics with potassium-sparing diuretics: Dyazide, Maxzide, reduces side effect of hypokalemia (K↓)

Anticoagulants

A. Mechanism—drug interferes with vitamin K–dependent clotting factors (II, VII, IX, X)
B. Pharmacologic effects—reduces ability of blood to clot; latent time required before full effect is seen (several days); time required for effect to subside after discontinuing treatment
C. Adverse reactions—bleeding, hemorrhage
D. Therapeutic uses—after myocardial infarction, thrombophlebitis, atrial fibrillation, emboli, valve replacement (any condition where too much blood clotting occurs)
E. Dental considerations
1. Excessive bleeding may result; obtain good health history (every appointment)
2. Monitoring international normalized ratio (INR); older test is prothrombin time (PT)
a. Clients with INRs ≤ 3 can safely receive periodontal debridement
F. Example
Warfarin (Coumadin)
G. Drug interactions—warfarin plus

---

*Local anesthetic used parenterally as an antidysrhythmic agent.
†Sublingual—tablets or spray.

Table 8-6

Selected Antihypertensives: Examples, Mechanisms, and Adverse Reactions

Drug group	Examples	Mechanism	Adverse reactions
Diuretics-thiazides	Hydrochlorothiazide (HCTZ)	Inhibits Na reabsorption, direct vasodilator, moderate potency	Hypokalemia Hyperuricemia Hyperglycemia NSAIDs* ↓ effect
Loop diuretic	Furosemide (Lasix)	Loop of Henle, high potency	Similar to thiazides
Thiazides combined with K^{++} sparing	Maxzide Dyazide	K-sparing, low potency	Hyperkalemia
β-Blockers	Propranolol (Inderal) Atenolol (Tenormin) Metoprolol (Lopressor)	Blocks sympathetic effect on heart (↓ CO*); ↓ PVR*, inhibits stimulation of renin	NSAIDs↓ effect
Angiotensin converting enzyme (ACE) inhibitor	Captopril (Capoten) Lisinopril (Zestril) Prinivil Enalapril Quinapril	Inhibits ACE*, angiotensin II (vasoconstriction; aldosterone secretion) production inhibited	Neutropenia Bone marrow depression Cough Dysgeusia (altered taste) NSAIDs* ↓ effect
Calcium channel blocking agents	Verapamil (Isoptin, Calan) Diltiazem (Cardizem) Nifedipine (Procardia) Nimodepine Isradapine	Blocks calcium channel: relax vascular smooth muscle, decrease myocardial contractility (force)	Gingival enlargement Hyperkalemia Renal failure Dysgeusia
Adrenergic blockers			
Centrally acting antiadrenergic agents	Clonidine (Catapres) Methyldopa (Aldomet) Terazocin	Stimulates arteriolar and CNS (medulla) α-receptors	Transdermal patch Xerostoma Sedation D/C* gradually
Cardura tenex α Selective blockers	Prazosin (Minipress)	Blocks α_1-receptor in arterioles/venules	Also used for benign prostatic hypertrophy
Postganglionic sympathetic blockers	Guanethidine (Ismelin)	Inhibits release of NE*, replaces NE (false neurotransmitter)	Postural hypotension Diarrhea Impaired ejaculation
	Reserpine	Blocks uptake and storage of amines	Mental depression Sedation
Vasodilators	Hydralazine (Apresoline)	Relaxes smooth muscles of arterioles	Combined with sympathetic blockers, β-blockers, and diuretics
	Minoxidil (Loniten)		Hirsutism

*NSAIDs, nonsteroidal antiinflammatory drugs; CO, cardiac output; PVR, peripheral vascular resistance; ACE, angiotensin converting enzyme; D/C, discontinue; NE, norepinephrine; **bold type,** one of the "Big 5" to be used initially for treatment of hypertension.

1. Aspirin—potentiates bleeding problems; do not use concomitantly; alternative is acetaminophen
2. Vitamin K—helps blood to clot; used to treat overdose or reduce latent period for improving the clotting status; antibiotics may reduce vitamin K by altering intestinal flora (potentiate anticoagulant's effect)

Psychotherapeutic Agents

Antipsychotics (Major Tranquilizers)

A. Pharmacologic effects
   1. Antipsychotic—manages psychotic patient; patient may perceive comments as threats (paranoia)

2. Sedation/drowsiness—additive CNS depression with other CNS depressants
3. Antiemetic—depression chemoreceptor trigger zone (CTZ), reduces nausea and/or vomiting

B. Adverse reactions
1. Orthostatic hypotension—dizziness or fainting on arising
2. Extrapyramidal (areas in the brain affecting bodily movements) effects
   a. Dyskinesia—uncontrollable movements of the tongue or face
   b. Tardive dyskinesia—dyskinesia that is irreversible; chronic use required
   c. Parkinsonian—tremors and rigidity, like the disease Parkinsonism
   d. Akathisia—motor restlessness (e.g., swinging legs)
   e. Difficulty in opening the mouth (jaw); jaw muscles are contracted; dislocation possible
3. Anticholinergic—dry mouth may produce a high caries rate

C. Drug interaction—antipsychotic agent plus
1. CNS depressants—additive CNS depression
2. Anticholinergic—additive anticholinergic toxicity

D. Therapeutic uses
1. Psychosis (e.g., schizophrenia)
2. Nausea or vomiting (antiemetic)
3. Opioid potentiation—combined with opioid to potentiate analgesia and sedation; reduce dose of the opioid if antipsychotic added

E. Examples

Drug	Group
Chlorpromazine (Thorazine) Trifluoperazine (Stelazine) Thioridazine (Mellaril)	Phenothiazines
Haloperidol (Haldol)	Not a phenothiazine; but acts in a similar fashion

Antidepressants

A. Pharmacologic effects/adverse reactions—similar to the phenothiazines also
1. Pharmacologic effects—reduces endogenous (no known cause) depression; onset slow (4 to 6 weeks)
2. Adverse reaction
   a. Cardiotoxic in overdose—dysrhythmias; usual cause of death when used in a suicide attempt
   b. Xerostomia
   c. Sedation
   d. GI—nausea-SSRI

B. Drug interactions—antidepressant plus
1. Epinephrine—results in hypertension (increased vasopressor response); small doses contained in LA solutions can be used safely in normotensive (normal blood pressure) persons

2. Anticholinergic—results in additive anticholinergic action (excessive xerostomia)

C. Therapeutic uses
1. Endogenous depression
2. Migraine headache prophylaxis
3. Nocturnal enuresis (bed-wetting) in children
4. Chronic pain adjuvant

D. Drugs
1. Tricyclic antidepressants (TCA)
   a. Amitriptyline (Elavil)
   b. Imipramine (Tofranil)
2. Other antidepressants
   a. Trazodone (Desyrel)—less anticholinergic effects
   b. Fluoxetine (Prozac)—less sedative effects over years of use
3. SSRI

Other Psychotherapeutic Agents

A. Lithium—for bipolar affective disorder (manic depressant); blood level difficult to maintain; sodium balanced affects; NSAIDs increase serum lithium levels
B. Monoamine oxidase inhibitors (MAOI)
1. Infrequently used for depression
2. Potential for **numerous severe** drug and food interactions (e.g., wine, sausage, cheese; indirect-acting adrenergic agents, meperidine)

Endocrine Agents

Adrenocorticosteroids (Steroids)

A. Classification
1. Glucocorticoids—regulate glucose metabolism and have an antiinflammatory effect
2. Mineralocorticoids—regulate sodium (minerals) and water

B. Pharmacologic effect—antiinflammatory
C. Adverse reactions
1. Cushing's syndrome—long-term, high-dose steroids produce symptoms including
   a. Metabolic effects—moon face, buffalo hump, truncal obesity
   b. Peptic ulcers—exacerbation and/or stimulation of stomach acid secretion
   c. Skin—bruising, striae, delayed healing
   d. Mental changes—euphoria when medication started or increased; depression when dose is being tapered (reduced)
   e. Infection—mask symptoms; watch closely, treat aggressively; suppresses immunity
   f. Osteoporosis (reduced bone density)—bones break more easily
   g. Hypertension (elevated blood pressure)—water

and sodium retention (mineralocorticoid action)

    h. Hyperglycemia (elevated blood glucose)—exacerbates diabetes

2. Adrenal crisis—abrupt withdrawal or stress (e.g., a dental appointment) can precipitate crisis; prevent by premedicating with additional steroids; potentially serious situation

D. Contraindications/cautions

  1. Ulcers—ulcerogenic

  2. Cardiovascular disease—congestive heart failure, edema (mineralocorticoid effect)

  3. Acute psychoses

  4. Infection—bacterial, fungal, or viral

  5. Diabetes—hyperglycemia

E. Therapeutic uses

  1. Medical—treatment of many inflammatory conditions (e.g., arthritis, asthma, dermatitis)

  2. Dental

    a. Aphthous lesions—palliative treatment; topical or intralesional (into the lesion) therapy

    b. Oral lesions secondary to collagen vascular diseases—topical, intralesional, or systemic therapy

    c. Temporomandibular joint disease (TMD)—intraarticular injection (into the joint) if arthritic

F. Examples

Steroid	Comments	Equivalent dose (mg)
Hydrocortisone	Some mineralocorticoid action	20
Prednisone	Most commonly used orally	5
Triamcinolone (Kenalog)	Used topically and into joints	2-20
Dexamethasone (Decadron)	Very potent, so lower dose used	.75

Agents for Diabetes Mellitus

See Chapter 14, section on diabetes mellitus

A. Disease

  1. Symptoms

    a. Polyuria—increased urination

    b. Polydipsia—increased thirst

    c. Polyphagia—increased hunger

    d. Weight loss

    e. Xerostomia—dry mouth

  2. Classification

    a. Insulin-dependent diabetes mellitus (IDDM), or type I diabetes—because circulating insulin is absent; requires insulin therapy

    b. Non–insulin-dependent diabetes mellitus (NIDDM), or type II diabetes—decreased tissue sensitivity to insulin and impaired β cell response to glucose; controlled by diet, oral hypoglycemia agents and/or insulin

  3. Complications—associated with vascular system (microangiopathy and atherosclerosis) and peripheral nervous system

    a. Cardiovascular problems—circulation problems, heart problems, myocardial infarction, stroke

    b. Retinopathy—vision problems, cataracts, blindness

    c. Neuropathy—reduced sensations in the extremities

    d. Renal failure—nephropathy (kidney problems)

    e. Immunity—reduced ability to fight infections

    f. Healing—slower, delayed

    g. Oral manifestations—reduced immunity (ability to fight infections due to WBC dysfunction), reduced vascular supply (small vessel disease), or other unknown alterations in function predispose the patient to periodontal disease; loss of alveolar bone

B. Adverse reactions

  1. Hypoglycemia—too much drug or too little food (in balance)

    a. Symptoms—nervousness, sweating, tremulousness, talking, mental confusion, nausea, convulsions, coma

    b. Treatment—glucose orally if patient conscious and able to swallow; glucose IV if unconscious (or glucagon SQ or IM)

  2. Hyperglycemia—less common cause of problems with the diabetic person; treated in emergency room with insulin and fluids

C. Examples

  1. Insulin

Insulin	Activity (hr) Peak	Activity (hr) Duration
Rapid: Regular (crystalline)	½-3	5-7
Intermediate: Isophane (NPH) or Lente	8-12	18-24

    a. Combine regular plus NPH—one or two times/day

    b. Human insulin—from gene splicing (*E. coli* makes it) or alters pork insulin

  2. Oral hypoglycemic agents (sulfonylureas)

Agent	$t_{1/2}$ (hr)	Duration
First generation		
Tolbutamide (Orinase)	4-5	6-12
Chlorpropamide (Diabinese)	36	60
Second generation		
Glyburide (Diabeta, Micronase)	10	24
Glipizide (Glucotrol)	3	10-24
Glucophage (Metformin HCL)	2-2.5	17.6

  3. Other new agents

Thyroid Agents

A. Hypothyroidism
  1. Thyroid replacements used; becomes euthyroid (normal thyroid)
  2. Examples
     Levothyroxine (Synthroid, Levothroid)
     Liotrix (Euthroid, Thyrolar)
  3. No special handling if dose adequate
B. Hyperthyroidism
  1. Partial thyroidectomy (cut out) or radioactive iodine (I^{131}) ablates part of thyroid function—patient requires supplemental thyroid, no unusual considerations if on treatment
  2. Patients awaiting surgery or poor surgical candidates—maintained on a regimen of thyroid suppressants
     a. Drugs suppress thyroid function—Propylthiouracil (PTU)
     b. β-Blockers given to reduce elevated HR, e.g., propranolol
     c. Dental implications—avoid epinephrine because can trigger thyroid storm

Respiratory System Agents

Agents for Asthma

A. Disease—dyspnea, cough, and wheezing secondary to bronchospasm (hyperirritable bronchioles), inflammation of bronchioles with secretions; two types
B. Drugs
  1. Adrenergic agents (sympathomimetics)—see ANS
     a. PO, IH (inhalation)
     b. Inhalers
        Metaproterenol (Alupent, Metaprel)
        Albuterol (Proventil, Ventolin)
     c. Bronchodilators
     d. Epinephrine IV for an acute attack
  2. Methylxanthines
     a. Examples
        Theophylline (Theo-Dur, Slo-bid)
        Aminophylline (theophylline ethylenediamine)
        Caffeine (in coffee)—relative of theophylline
     b. Pharmacologic effects
        (1) Bronchodilation (smooth muscle relaxation) helps asthma
        (2) CNS stimulation—alertness, insomnia
        (3) Diuresis—increased urination
  3. Cromolyn sodium (Intal, Nasalcrom)—used for asthma prophylaxis by inhalation and for allergic rhinitis
  4. Ipratropium (Atrovent)—anticholinergic bronchodilator inhaler; used more with emphysema
  5. Adrenocorticosteroids—see section on adrenocorticosteroids
C. Dental considerations
  1. Disease considerations
     a. Degree of control—avoid elective treatment if poorly controlled
     b. Client's anxiety may precipitate acute attack, antianxiety agent may be useful (e.g., benzodiazepine)
  2. Analgesic choice—no easy answer
     a. Aspirin-containing compounds—may precipitate attack
     b. NSAIDs—if aspirin causes bronchospasm, NSAIDs are contraindicated
     c. Opioids—produce bronchoconstriction (histamine release) and respiratory depression; can use with care in lower doses or strengths
     d. Acetaminophen—best choice; may use mixed with weak opioid (e.g., Tylenol #3)

Gastrointestinal Agents

Agents Affecting GI Motility

A. Laxatives—increase GI motility; symptomatically treat constipation (e.g., milk of magnesia)
B. Antidiarrheals—reduce GI motility; symptomatically treat diarrhea (e.g., Lomotil, Imodium, any opioid)

Agents for GERD—Histamine (H_2)-Blocker

A. Mechanism—agent blocks secretion of stomach acid reflux of stomach [HB] contents, then doesn't hurt
B. Examples (all OTC now)
   Cimetidine (Tagamet)
   Ranitidine (Zantac HB 75)
C. Dental considerations
  1. Interferes with absorption of drugs that need acid for absorption (e.g., ketoconazole [Nizoral])
  2. Avoid ulcerogenic medications unless needed (e.g., aspirin, NSAIDs, and glucocorticoids)
  3. Cimetidine
     a. Reduces hepatic blood flow
     b. Inhibits metabolism of certain drugs (diazepam, warfarin)

Emetics and Antiemetics

A. Emetics—induce vomiting; used to treat most poisonings (e.g., syrup of ipecac—available without a prescription); abused by bulemics
B. Antiemetics
  1. Reduce nausea or vomiting

2. Examples
Prochlorperazine (Compazine)
Trimethobenzamide (Tigan)
Benzquinamide (Emete-Con)

Antineoplastic Agents

A. Mechanism—drug interferes with metabolism or the reproductive cycle of malignant cells; also affects host cells
B. Drugs
1. Alkylating agents
a. Nitrogen mustards
Cyclophosphamide (Cytoxan)
Chlorambucil (Leukeran)
Melphalan (Alkeran)
b. Nitrosoureas
Carmustine (BiCNU)
c. Bisulfan (Myleran)
2. Antimetabolites
a. Folic acid analog
Methotrexate (MTX)
b. Purine antagonists
Mercaptopurine (6-MP)
Thioguanine (6-TG)
c. Pyrimidine antagonists
Fluorouracil (5-FC)
Cytarabine (Cytosar-U, ara-C)
3. Other antineoplastics
a. Plant alkaloids
Vinblastine (Velban)
Vincristine (Oncovin)
b. Antibiotics
Daunorubicin (Cerubidine)
Doxorubicin (Adriamycin)
Dactinomycin (actinomycin D, Cosmegen)
Mitomycin (Mitocin-C)
c. Hormones
Androgens
Estrogens
Tamoxifen (Nolvadex)—antiestrogen
Progestin
Adrenocorticosteroids
d. Miscellaneous
Asparaginase (Elspar)
Hydroxyurea (Hydrea)
Cisplatin (Platinol)
Bleomycin (Blenoxane)
C. Adverse reactions
1. Lack of specificity against tumor cells; normal cells are destroyed; cells with quickest turnover affected first
2. Bone marrow suppression
a. Leukopenia (lowered white blood cell count; infection more likely)
b. Thrombocytopenia (lowered platelets, bleeding increased)
c. Anemia
3. Gastrointestinal—stomatitis, mucosal sloughing
4. Infection—reduced immunity (ability to fight infection)
5. Skin/hair—rash, alopecia (baldness)
6. Oral effects
a. Symptoms—pain, ulcers, dryness, impaired taste, gingival hemorrhage, sensitivity of teeth and gingiva
b. Treatment—avoid mouthwashes with alcohol; substitute saline or sodium bicarbonate; avoid alcohol
c. Candidiasis—use antifungal agents, e.g., Nystatin
d. Xerostomia—use artificial salivas (Xero-lube, Salivart), use sips of H_2O or H_2O spray, chew sugarless gum, use fluoride agent to reduce caries incidence
D. Dental considerations
1. Improve oral hygiene before chemotherapy, if possible
2. Avoid elective procedures during chemotherapy; timing is important, best time is day beginning chemotherapy (highest blood counts)
3. Check coagulation status before emergency surgery
4. Prophylactic antibiotic premedication is controversial

Substance Abuse

See Chapter 14, section on chemical dependency.

Definitions

A. Tolerance—large dose required to produce same effect; same dose produces less effect; occurs with repeated administration
B. Physical dependence—symptoms of withdrawal occur if drug is abruptly discontinued
C. Psychologic dependence—craving occurs if drug stopped; no physical withdrawal syndrome; psychologic dependence just as likely to result in relapse (e.g., cocaine)
D. Abuse—self-administration of a drug in a socially unacceptable manner that results in an adverse outcome
E. Addiction—pattern of abuse that continues despite medical or social complications
F. Withdrawal—a physical reaction attributable to physical dependence

G. Abstinence—drug-free state

H. Enabling—pattern of coping methods used by associates of addict that allows continued drug use, e.g., making excuses for absences

Drugs of Abuse

A. Depressants
   1. Alcohol—impaired judgment, slurred speech, ataxia, seizures, coma, death; withdrawal produces autonomic hyperactivity, hallucinations, or seizures; cirrhosis with chronic use
   2. Opioids (heroin, codeine, morphine)—euphoria, abscesses, constipation, respiratory depression; withdrawal produces "cold turkey"; methadone maintenance used to suppress "high" from injecting heroin; naltrexone (acts like orally active naloxone) blocks "high"
   3. Barbiturates—secobarbital, pentobarbital
   4. Volatile solvents—glue sniffing; paint, solvent inhaling, called "huffing"
   5. Benzodiazepines—diazepam
   6. Anesthetics—nitrous oxide; oxygen analgesia; PCP
B. Stimulants
   1. Amphetamines—"ice" (methamphetamine) highly addicting
   2. Cocaine—"coke," "crack," most psychologically addicting drug; euphoria, hyperactive, paranoia, acute MI
   3. Nicotine—in cigarettes, spit tobacco, and cigars
   4. Caffeine—in soft drinks, coffee, tea
C. Psychedelics
   1. Lysergic acid diethylamide (LSD)—"bad trip," treat with reassurance; flashbacks occur (without drug)
   2. Psilocybin—derived from some mushrooms
   3. Phencyclidine (PCP)—disorientation, seizures; treatment—"talking down"
   4. Marijuana (cannabis) active ingredient is THC-tetrahydrocannabinol—silliness, relaxation, euphoria, paranoia, confusion, chronic amotivational syndrome; entrance drug (used first before trying other addictive drugs)
D. Dental implications
   1. Cocaine—cardiac stimulant effect, addictive effect on heart with local anesthetics
   2. Nitrous oxide—euphoria, dental personnel abuse (unsupervised use), abuse produces neuropathy (sometimes irreversible); without adequate oxygen hypoxia produced
   3. Addicts—"shoppers" attempt to obtain prescriptions for controlled substances (see Introduction section) from dental office, feign or harbor real dental pain, refuse definitive treatment; be suspicious

Drug Use During Pregnancy

A. General
   1. Avoid any unnecessary drugs
   2. Check with obstetrician
   3. First trimester worse
      a. Organogenesis active
      b. Second trimester best for elective dental treatment
      c. Third trimester—avoid because of proximity to delivery, and client comfort
B. Dental drugs probably safe
   1. Amoxicillan
   2. Penicillin
   3. Erythromycin
   4. Lidocaine
   5. Epinephrine (limit dose)
C. Dental drugs to avoid
   1. Aspirin
   2. Nonsteroidal antiinflammatory drugs (NSAIDs)
   3. Metronidazole
   4. Nitrous oxide—mainly dental personnel, limit dose while pregnant, improve room air, turnover, evacuate system

REFERENCES

1. Physician's desk reference, ed 48, Oradell, NJ, 1997, Medical Economics.
2. Olin BR, Hebel SK, Dombek CE, editors: *Facts and Comparisons*, St Louis, 1996, Facts and Comparisons.
3. Requa-Clark BS: Applied pharmacology for the dental hygienist, ed 4, St Louis, Mosby (in press).
4. Haveles, EB: *Pharmacology for dental hygiene practice*, 1996, Albany, Delmar.
5. Gage TW, Pickett FA: *Dental drug reference*, 1996, St Louis, Mosby.
6. Wynn RL, Miller TF, Crossley HL: *Drug information handbook for dentistry* Hudson, Ohio, 1996-7, Lexi-Comp.
7. Holroyd SV: *Clinical pharmacology in dental practice*, ed 4, St Louis, 1989, Mosby.
8. Dajani AS, Bisno AL, et al: Prevention of bacterial endocarditis, *JAMA* 264(22):2919-2922, 1990.
9. American Hospital Formulary Service: Drug Information, Bethesda, Md, 1996, American Society of Hospital Pharmacists, Inc.

Review Questions

1 Drugs with teratogenic effects can produce
   A. Tumors
   B. Hypoglycemia
   C. Hepatotoxicity
   D. An abnormal fetus
   E. Excessive hirsutism

2 Chronic temporomandibular joint disease (TMD) is *NOT* managed well with
A. Opioids
B. Antidepressants
C. Muscle relaxants
D. Relaxation techniques
E. Nonsteroidal antiinflammatory drugs

3 Persons taking which two agents may reduce their ability to fight infection and prolong the duration of healing? (choose two responses)
A. Glyburide
B. Diazepam
C. Cimetidine
D. Prednisone
E. Theophylline

4 Which is *LEAST* likely to produce gingival enlargement (formerly hyperplasia)?
A. Nifedipine
B. Phenytoin
C. Verapamil
D. Cyclosporin
E. Hydrochlorothiazide

5 Persons who have chronic constipation should be given _____ with caution.
A. Codeine
B. Ibuprofen
C. Amoxicillin
D. Tetracycline
E. Acetaminophen

6 The *MOST* important side effect related to valproic acid (Depakote) for the dental practitioner is
A. Constipation
B. Thrombocytopenia
C. Grand mal seizures
D. Trigeminal neuralgia
E. Gingival enlargement

7 As used in the oral healthcare environment, nitrous oxide-oxygen analgesia should keep a patient in Stage
A. I
B. II
C. III
D. IV

8 In which type of diabetes mellitus is insulin always required?
A. Type I
B. Type II
C. Type III

9 Which is *NOT* used to treat glaucoma?
A. Cholinergic agent (P+)
B. Anticholinergic agent (P−)
C. Adrenergic agonists (S+)
D. Adrenergic blockers (S−)

10 Which pharmaceutical agent may reduce the effectiveness of oral contraceptives?
A. Antibiotics
B. Epinephrine
C. Acetaminophen
D. Opioids (narcotics)
E. Nonsteroidal antiinflammatory drugs

11 Periodontal disease is more common in persons (choose two responses)
A. Who smoke
B. With hypertension
C. With hyperthyroidism
D. With diabetes mellitus
E. Who are postmenopausal

12 If patients with asthma who are taking theophylline are given _____ , theophylline toxicity may result.
A. Penicillin
B. Amoxicillin
C. Tetracycline
D. Clindamycin
E. Erythromycin

13 Which could *MOST SAFELY* be given to a person who is allergic to codeine?
A. Vicodin
B. Percocet
C. Tylenol #3
D. Empirin #3
E. Darvocet-N 100

14 What is the *MOST* common side effect associated with the oral antidiabetic agents (sulfonylureas) such as glyburide?
A. Sedation
B. Hepatoxicity
C. Hypoglycemia
D. Blood dyscrasias
E. Gastrointestinal upset

15 What should *NOT* be given to a person with a history of aspirin hypersensitivity (allergy)?
A. Codeine
B. Ibuprofen
C. Oxycodone
D. Hydrocodone
E. Acetaminophen

16 Corticosteroids are used to treat oral manifestations of
A. Cushing syndrome
B. Herpes simplex or herpes zoster
C. ANUG (acute necrotizing ulcerative gingivitis)
D. Dry socket secondary to dental extractions
E. Connective tissue diseases such as lichen planus

17 Which medication has the "strongest" analgesic effect?
A. Codeine 30 mg
B. Aspirin 650 mg
C. Codeine 60 mg
D. Ibuprofen 600 mg
E. Acetaminophen 650 mg

18 Lithium is indicated for the treatment of
A. Psychoses
B. Gouty arthritis
C. Parkinsonism
D. Endogenous depression
E. Bipolar affective disorder

19 What is the drug of choice to treat an opioid overdose?
A. 2-PAM (protopam)
B. Naloxone (Narcan)
C. Epinephrine (Adrenalin)
D. Diphenhydramine (Benadryl)
E. N-acetylcysteine (Mucomyst)

20 What effect can aspirin produce in the body?
  A. Dependence
  B. Hypothermia
  C. Hyperuricemia
  D. Gastrointestinal side effects
  E. Increased platelet adhesiveness

21 Which of the following phrases is true about warfarin (Coumadin)
  A. Has a quick onset of action
  B. Can cause a client to bleed
  C. Is monitored using PT or INR
  D. Is monitored using clotting time
  E. Has a drug interaction with acetaminophen

22 What should patients who are given metronidazole be warned about?
  A. Drowsiness if driving
  B. Avoid taking with milk
  C. May cause sun sensitivity
  D. Using alcoholic beverages
  E. Taking on an empty stomach

23 Nitrous oxide–oxygen (N_2O–O_2) analgesia is contraindicated in clients who
  A. Have epilepsy
  B. Are on steroids
  C. Have severe COPD
  D. Have diabetes mellitus
  E. Are on birth control pills

24 What is nitroglycerin's (NTG) *MOST* common side effect?
  A. Arrhythmias
  B. Gastric upset
  C. Hypertension
  D. Angina pectoris
  E. Severe headache

25 What immunization does the dental hygienist need in order to practice safely in the oral healthcare environment?
  A. Tetanus
  B. Influenza
  C. Hepatitis A
  D. Hepatitis B

26 Certain drugs such as carbamazepine, phenobarbital, and rifampin reduce the effectiveness of both themselves and other drugs by
  A. Enhancing their excretion
  B. Inhibiting their absorption
  C. Binding irreversibly to them
  D. Stimulating hepatic microsomal enzymes

27 With few exceptions, generic drugs produced today are of _____ quality than the equivalent brand name drug.
  A. Lower
  B. Equal
  C. Higher

28 If a client has a vague history of an allergy to a drug, he/she should be given a tiny amount of the drug to see if it is a true allergy.
  A. True
  B. False

29 If a person taking a phenothiazine such as chlorpromazine (Thorazine) for 25 years exhibits constant movement of her tongue, lips, and mouth, she may have
  A. Xerostomia
  B. Restlessness
  C. Acute psychoses
  D. Tardive dyskinesia
  E. Bipolar affective disorder

30 Before dental hygiene care, what should be given to a client with a history of infective (bacterial) endocarditis who is allergic to penicillin and has severe gastric upset with erythromycin?
  A. Amoxicillin
  B. Augmentin
  C. Tetracycline
  D. Clindamycin
  E. Metronidazole

31 A person who has no pulse, no blood pressure, cyanosis, and dilated pupils should be treated with
  A. Naloxone (Narcan)
  B. Phenytoin (Dilantin)
  C. Epinephrine (Adrenalin)
  D. Aromatic spirits of ammonia
  E. Cardiac pulmonary resuscitation (CPR)

32 Which is used to treat an *acute* asthmatic attack in the oral care environment?
  A. Albuterol
  B. Diazepam
  C. Prednisone
  D. Nitroglycerin
  E. Theophylline

33 Epinephrine is indicated for the emergency treatment of
  A. Epilepsy
  B. Hypoglycemia
  C. Angina pectoris
  D. Myocardial infarction
  E. Anaphylactic reaction

34 Which drug group can be abused?
  A. Antihistamines
  B. Phenothiazines
  C. Anticholinergics
  D. Antidepressants
  E. Benzodiazepines

35 Because of the lack of specificity, most antineoplastic drugs (cancer chemotherapy agents) commonly produce
  A. Oral ulcers
  B. Hepatotoxicity
  C. Bone marrow suppression
  D. Oral ulcers and bone marrow suppression

36 A person taking isoniazid (INH), rifampin, and pyrazinamide is being treated for
  A. Epilepsy
  B. Anaphylaxis
  C. Tuberculosis
  D. Peptic ulcers
  E. Adrenal crisis

37 Opioids can be used to manage or treat
A. Diarrhea
B. Diarrhea and pain
C. Pain and cough
D. Diarrhea, pain, and cough

38 Which drug has antiinflammatory, antipyretic, analgesic, and antiplatelet action?
A. Aspirin
B. Codeine
C. Hydrocodone
D. Propoxyphene
E. Acetaminophen

39 Which would be *BEST* to treat xerostomia?
A. Atropine
B. Ibuprofen
C. Pilocarpine
D. Probenecid
E. Propranolol

40 The maximum cardiac dose of epinephrine is ___ mg.
A. 0.02
B. 0.04
C. 0.2
D. 0.4

41 What is the effect of giving epinephrine to a person pretreated with a β blocker?
A. Hypotension and tachycardia
B. Hypotension and bradycardia
C. Hypertension and tachycardia
D. Hypertension and bradycardia

42 Nonsteroidal antiinflammatory drugs like ibuprofen, indomethacin, and naproxen can reduce the pharmacologic effect of
A. Lithium
B. Probenecid
C. ACE inhibitors
D. Oral contraceptives
E. Calcium channel blockers

43 Which adverse reaction is associated with antihypertensive agents?
A. Anxiety
B. Drooling
C. Impotence
D. Hepatotoxicity
E. Stomach upset

44 What should be given to a person with a history of rheumatic heart disease who is to have an oral prophylaxis?
A. Amoxicillin
B. Clindamycin
C. Doxycycline
D. Erythromycin
E. Metronidazole

45 Anticholinergics are relatively contraindicated in persons with
A. Diarrhea
B. Prostatic hypertrophy
C. Sulfite hypersensitivity
D. Congestive heart failure
E. Congenital cholinesterase deficiency

46 What is used to decrease salivary flow to prevent choking during general anesthesia?
A. α-blockers
B. β-blockers
C. Sympathomimetics
D. Parasympatholytics
E. Parasympathomimetics

47 In which emergency situation does the client remain conscious?
A. Syncope
B. Hypoglycemia
C. Cardiac arrest
D. Angina pectoris
E. Tonic-clonic convulsions

48 A sign of epinephrine toxicity is
A. Miosis
B. Nausea
C. Sedation
D. Sweating
E. Tachycardia

49 What is the *MOST* common symptom associated with untreated hypertension?
A. Fatigue
B. Nothing
C. Nausea
D. Headache
E. Palpitations

50 Carbamazepine (Tegretol) is the drug of choice for the treatment of
A. Peptic ulcers
B. Absence seizures
C. Trigeminal neuralgia
D. Cushing syndrome
E. Temporomandibular joint dysfunction

Answers and Rationales

1. (D) Drugs with teratogenic effects can produce an abnormal fetus; terato- is monster and -genic is produce or make.
   (A) This is not the correct definition of teratogenic; tumors are abnormal growths that may or may not be cancer.
   (B) This is not the correct definition of teratogenic; hypoglycemia means low blood sugar.
   (C) This is not the correct definition of teratogenic; hepatotoxicity means liver toxicity.
   (E) This is not the correct definition of teratogenic; hirsutism means hairiness.

2. (A) Chronic temperomandibular joint disease (TMD) is *NOT* managed well with opioids because long-term management of non-terminal pain with opioids is *NOT* indicated and chronic pain does not usually respond well to opioids.
   (B, C, D, E) These are the agents used to manage TMD; warm, moist heat is also useful.

3. (A and D) Persons taking either glyburide (oral sulfonylurea, for diabetes) or prednisone (steroid) may reduce their ability to fight infection and prolong the duration of healing.
   (B) Diazepam, a benzodiazepine for sedation, does not affect infections or healing.
   (C) Cimetidine, an H_2-blocker for GERD, does not affect infections or healing.
   (E) Theophylline, a xanthine bronchodilator for asthma, does not affect infections or healing.

4. (E) Gingival enlargement has *NOT* been associated with hydrochlorothiazide
   (A, B, C, D) Nifedipine and verapamil (calcium channel blockers), phenytoin (anticonvulsant), and cyclosporin (prevents rejection of kidney transplants) have been associated with gingival enlargement.

5. (A) Persons who have chronic constipation should be given opioids (e.g., codeine) with caution because opioids can cause constipation by paralyzing the intestines so that the fecal matter becomes excessively dry and defecation is difficult.
   (B) Ibuprofen usually has little effect on the bowels, but can occasionally produce diarrhea.
   (C and D) Antibiotics can often produce diarrhea because they alter the normal flora (bacteria).
   (E) Acetaminophen has no effect on the intestines.

6. (B) The most important side effect related to valproic acid (Depakote) is thrombocytopenia, which may cause bleeding.
   (A) Constipation is *NOT* an important side effect related to valproic acid (Depakote).
   (C) Grand mal seizures are associated with agents that lower the convulsion threshold such as the antipsychotics.
   (D) Trigeminal neuralgia is usually produced by a disease process, not a drug; drugs are used to treat trigeminal neuralgia.
   (E) Gingival enlargement is produced by agents such as nifedipine, verapamil, phenytoin, and cyclosporine.

7. (A) As used in the oral healthcare environment, nitrous oxide should keep a patient in Stage I; consciousness is maintained and reflexes are active.
   (B) In Stage II the patient has sympathetic release resulting in an increase in heart rate and flailing with loss of consciousness; in general anesthesia, Stage II is quickly bypassed to progress into Stage III.
   (C) Stage III is surgical anesthesia; this is where most surgical procedures are performed.
   (D) Stage IV is when respiration stops; this is never a stage into which it is desirable for the patient to go; respiration can be mechanically maintained during this stage, but quickly moving to Stage III is important.

8. (A) In Type I diabetes mellitus (juvenile onset) insulin is always required because the individual does not produce any insulin.
   (B) In Type II diabetes mellitus (adult onset), the individual usually produces some or even excessive insulin, but the timing is poor; this type is treated with sulfonylureas (oral hypoglycemic agents).
   (C) In Type III diabetes mellitus the diabetes is caused by another abnormality (anatomic) or drug; treatment usually focuses on correcting the primary source of the problem.

9. (B) Anticholinergic agents (P–) are *NOT* used to treat glaucoma, they are contraindicated in NARROW angle glaucoma (OK in WIDE angle glaucoma, which is the most common type of glaucoma).
   (A) Cholinergic agents (P+), such as pilocarpine, are used to treat glaucoma (constrict pupil so that aqueous humor can drain, more room in the trabecula).
   (C) Adrenergic agonists (S+), like propine, are used to treat glaucoma (dilate blood vessels to allow drainage of aqueous humor).
   (D) Adrenergic blockers (S–), like timolol, are used to treat glaucoma (reduce formation of aqueous humor).

10. (A) Some antibiotics can reduce the effectiveness of the oral contraceptives so clients on birth control pills should be warned when antibiotics are prescribed.
    (B, C, D, E) These do not reduce the effectiveness of oral contraceptives.

11. (A, D) Persons who smoke and those with diabetes are more likely to have periodontal disease. The degree of periodontal disease with a specific diabetic person is related to the degree of control of the patient's blood sugar as well as the duration of the disease.
    (B, C) Hypertension and hyperthyroidism do not result in an increase in periodontal disease.
    (E) Women who are postmenopausal have less estrogen and progesterone (progestin) unless ERT (estrogen replacement therapy) is instituted. Although it is known that high doses of estrogen can affect the gingiva, whether postmenopausal women on ERT have more periodontal problems is controversial.

12. (E) Erythromycin and some of the other macrolides inhibit the liver (hepatic) metabolism of many drugs such as theophylline.
    (A, B, C, D) None of these antibiotics affects the metabolism of other drugs.

13. (E) Darvocet-N 100 contains propoxyphene which is in a chemical class unrelated to codeine.
    (A) Vicodin contains acetaminophen and hydrocodone, which is chemically related to codeine.
    (B) Percocet contains acetaminophen and oxycodone, which is chemically related to codeine.
    (C) Tylenol #3 contains acetaminophen and codeine.
    (D) Empirin #3 contains acetaminophen and codeine.

14. (C) Hypoglycemia is a common side effect of the sulfonyl-ureas; occurs because the person's medication, exercise, and food intake are unbalanced.
  (A) Sedation is not a side effect of oral sulfonylureas.
  (B) Hepatotoxia can occur with oral sulfonylureas, but is not as common as hypoglycemia.
  (D) Blood dyscrasias can occur with the oral sulfonylureas, but are not as common as hypoglycemia.
  (E) Gastrointestinal upset can occur with the oral sulfonyl-ureas but is not as common as hypoglycemia.

15. (B) Nonsteroidal antiinflammatory drugs such as ibupro-fen are contraindicated in persons allergic to aspirin because there is cross hypersensitivity between the NSAIDs and aspirin.
  (A, C, D) These are opioids and are not related chemically to aspirin; therefore, they can be given to aspirin allergic clients.
  (E) Acetaminophen (Tylenol) can be given to aspirin-allergic clients.

16. (E) Corticosteroids are used to treat oral manifestations of connective tissue diseases such as lichen planus.
  (A) Cushing syndrome is produced by excess corticoste-roids; giving more steroids would make the condition worse.
  (B, C, D) These are infective processes and corticosteroids are contraindicated in infections because they inhibit the cellular immunity and the body's ability to fight infection.

17. (D) Ibuprofen 600 mg produces the "strongest" analgesic effect.
  (A, B, C, E) The order of analgesic effect from least to most is A, C, B, E; adding nonopioids to opioids can increase the analgesic effect of each individual agent.

18. (E) Lithium is the drug of choice for the treatment of bipolar affective disorder (manic depressive).
  (A) Psychoses are treated with antipsychotics.
  (B) Gouty arthritis is treated with colchinine and nonste-roidal antiinflammatory drugs such as ibuprofen and indomethacin.
  (C) Parkinsonism is treated with Sinemet (levodopa and carbidopa) among others.
  (D) Depression is treated with antidepressants.

19. (B) Naloxone (Narcan), an opioid antagonist, is the drug of choice for the treatment of opioid overdoses. Given IV, it reverses the respiratory depression that occurs.
  (A) 2-PAM is used with atropine to treat poisoning from an irreversible cholinesterase inhibitor (cholinergic).
  (C) Epinephrine is used to treat anaphylactic reactions.
  (D) Diphenhydramine, an antihistamine, is used to treat mild allergic reactions such as rash.
  (E) N-acetylcysteine, by providing SH groups to the liver, is used to treat an overdose of acetaminophen which can produce hepatotoxicity.

20. (D) Aspirin can produce gastrointestinal side effects that are reduced by taking with food or antacids.
  (A) Aspirin does not produce dependence or habituation, nor does tolerance develop.
  (B) Aspirin produces hyperthermia in overdose.
  (C) Aspirin alone in higher doses is a uricosuric (enhances secretion of uric acid); actually low doses of aspirin can inhibit uric acid secretion.
  (E) Aspirin decreases platelet adhesiveness by binding with the platelets irreversibly; enough new platelets are formed so that normal bleeding is restored in 72 hours after using aspirin.

21. (B) The most serious adverse reaction to Warfarin (Cou-madin) is hemorrhage.
  (A) Warfarin has a slow onset of action because the clotting factors present must be exhausted and the long half-life (60 hr) requires several days for a steady state condition (plateau of blood level).
  (C) Warfarin (Coumadin) is monitored using the Interna-tional Normalized ratio (INR). The older measurement was with the prothrombin time (PT). The INR is a PT corrected for the activity of the specific tissue throm-boplastin used in the laboratory.
  (D) Warfarin (Coumadin) is monitored using the Interna-tional Normalized Radio (INR).
  (E) Many drugs interact with Warfarin (Coumadin) to increase or decrease its effects, but acetaminophen is not one of them.

22. (D) Patients who are given metronidazole should be warned about using alcoholic beverages because of the potential for the disulfiram (Antabuse)—like reaction producing nausea and vomiting.
  (A) Metronidazole does not produce drowsiness.
  (B, E) Metronidazole should be taken with food to reduce gastrointestinal upset.
  (C) Metronidazole does not produce photosensitivity (sun sensitivity) but the tetracyclines do.

23. (C) Nitrous oxide–oxygen analgesia (N_2O–O_2) is contrain-dicated in clients who have severe COPD (chronic obstructive pulmonary disease) because the high concentration of oxygen may produce apnea (quit breathing).
  (A) Nitrous oxide–oxygen analgesia (N_2O–O_2) is NOT con-traindicated in clients who have epilepsy.
  (B) Nitrous oxide–oxygen analgesia (N_2O–O_2) is NOT con-traindicated in clients who are on steroids.
  (D) Nitrous oxide–oxygen analgesia (N_2O–O_2) is NOT con-traindicated in clients who have diabetes mellitus.
  (E) Nitrous oxide–oxygen analgesia (N_2O–O_2) is NOT con-traindicated in clients who are on birth control pills.

24. (E) NTG can produce severe headaches because it is a nonspecific vasodilator (dilates vessels in brain).
  (A) NTG doesn't have this effect.
  (B) This is not a major side effect.
  (C) NTG doesn't have this effect, in fact it can produce hypotension (lowered blood pressure)
  (D) NTG is used to treat angina pectoris.

25. (D) The dental hygienist should have a series of Hepatitis B immunizations to practice because hepatitis B is a bloodborne infection.
    (A) Tetanus immunizations are required for school children.
    (B) An influenza immunization is useful, especially in chronic illness, because persons with the flu may infect the dental office staff.
    (C) Hepatitis A immunization is useful before traveling to certain foreign countries where food handling is problematic.

26. (D) Carbamazepine, phenobarbital, and rifampin stimulate hepatic microsomal enzymes thereby reducing the blood level and effectiveness of both themselves and other drugs.
    (A) Carbamazepine, phenobarbital, and rifampin do not affect the excretion of other drugs.
    (B) Carbamazepine, phenobarbital, and rifampin do not inhibit the absorption of other drugs.
    (C) Carbamazepine, phenobarbital, and rifampin do not bind irreversibly to other drugs.

27. (B) Generic drugs of today are of equal quality to their equivalent brand name drug for almost all drugs; for a limited list of drugs question exists as to equivalency; no dental drugs are on this list (few anticonvulsants and heart medications).
    (A) Before the FDA began testing drugs for bioavailability (getting into the body), some generics did not equal their brand name equivalents.
    (C) Some generic products made were more bioequivalent than the brand name products; the amount of drug in these dosage forms had to be reduced to equal the brand name product.

28. (B) If a true allergy exists, then even a small amount could produce a serious reaction because allergic reactions are *NOT* dose related. Allergy testing should *NEVER* be done without the support of staff trained in advanced life support with adequate equipment.
    (A) Giving a client even a tiny amount of a drug can cause anaphalaxis and death, if the person is allergic to the drug.

29. (D) Taken chronically, phenothiazines can result in tardive dyskinesia which exhibits itself as uncontrollable constant mouth and tongue movements.
    (A) Phenothiazines can produce xerostomia, but the symptoms are inconsistent with this reaction.
    (B) Phenothiazines can produce restlessness, but the symptoms are inconsistent with this reaction.
    (C) Phenothiazines are used to treat acute psychoses.
    (E) Lithium is used to treat bipolar affective disorder (manic depression).

30. (D) Clindamycin is used prophylactically before any dental procedure that can produce bleeding (such as scaling and root planning) for persons who have a history of infective endocarditis.
    (A, B) Persons with penicillin allergies should not be given amoxicillin because of the almost complete cross-hypersensitivity. Augmentin contains amoxicillin plus clavulanate.
    (C, E) Neither tetracycline nor metronidazole is useful for antibiotic prophylaxis for infective endocarditis.

31. (E) Cardiac pulmonary resuscitation (CPR) is indicated to treat cardiac arrest (symptoms include no pulse, no blood pressure, cyanosis and dilated pupils).
    (A) Naloxone is used to treat an opioid overdose.
    (B) Phenytoin is used to treat epilepsy.
    (C) Epinephrine is used to treat anaphylaxis.
    (E) Aromatic spirits of ammonia is used to treat simple syncope.

32. (A) Albuterol, by inhalation, is used to treat an acute asthmatic attack in the dental office.
    (B) Diazepam (Valium) is used to treat seizures that do not subside.
    (C) Prednisone, a steroid, is used to treat severe asthma or connective tissue diseases (autoimmune diseases).
    (D) Nitroglycerin is used as an explosive and to treat angina pectoris.
    (E) Theophylline is used to manage asthma.

33. (E) Epinephrine is indicated for the emergency treatment of anaphylactic reaction.
    (A) The emergency treatment for epilepsy is a benzodiazepine such as diazepam.
    (B) The emergency treatment for hypoglycemia is oral glucose or IV dextrose.
    (C) The emergency treatment for angina pectoris is SL nitroglycerin.
    (D) The emergency treatment for a myocardial infarction (MI, heart attack) is CPR.

34. (E) Benzodiazepines such as diazepam (Valium) can be abused. Other abusable prescription drug groups include sedative-hypnotics (including barbiturates), amphetamines and methylphenidate, and opioids (codeine).
    (A, B, C, D) These are not abusable drug groups; most pyschotropic drug groups (other than the benzodiazepines) are not abusable (e.g., B & D.)

35. (D) Antineoplastic drugs (cancer chemotherapy agents) commonly produce both oral ulcers and bone marrow suppression (lowered platelets and white blood cells) because they suppress the fastest growing cells (bone marrow and oral mucosa).
    (A) Oral ulcers is only a partial answer.
    (B) Hepatoxicity can occur with a few antineoplastic agents, but not for all of them, and it is much less common than the other side effects.
    (C) Bone marrow suppression is only a partial answer.

36. (C) Isoniazid (INH), rifampin, and pyrazinamide are used in combination to treat tuberculosis. Sometimes even more drugs are added with resistant cases.

    (A) Epilepsy is treated with valproic acid (Depakote), phenytoin (Dilantin), or carbamazepine (Tegretol).

    (B) Anaphylaxis is treated with epinephrine IV.

    (D) Peptic ulcers are treated with specific antibiotic combinations (amoxicillin, doxycycline, and others) plus an acid reducer (either H_2-blockers or omeprazozle), sometimes Pepto-Bismol is used too (several weeks of therapy).

37. (D) Opioids can be used to manage or treat diarrhea, pain, and cough (opioids have antitussive effects).

    (A, B, C) These choices don't include all uses.

38. (A) Aspirin, like ibuprofen and naproxen has antiinflammatory, antipyretic, analgesic, and antiplatelet action.

    (B) Codeine does not have antiinflammatory, antipyretic, or antiplatelet action.

    (C, D) Neither hydrocodone nor propoxyphene have antiinflammatory, antipyretic, or antiplatelet action.

    (E) Acetaminophen does not have antiinflammatory or antiplatelet action.

39. (C) Pilocarpine, a cholinergic or parasympathomimetic, is best to treat xerostomia because it stimulates saliva flow.

    (A) Atropine, an anticholinergic or parasympatholytic, produces xerostomia (inhibits saliva flow).

    (B) Ibuprofen, a NSAID, has little effect on saliva flow (xerostomia occasionally reported).

    (D) Probenecid, a uricosuric, has little effect on saliva flow (xerostomia occasionally reported).

    (E) Propranolol, a β blocker, has little effect on saliva flow (xerostomia occasionally reported).

40. (B) The maximum cardiac dose of epinephrine is 0.04 mg (⅕ dose is the normal). This is the amount contained in 2 cartridges of 1 : 100,000 epinephrine. The maximum dose of epinephrine for the normal person is 0.2 mg.

    (A, C, D) These are not the correct dose.

41. (D) If epinephrine is given to a person pretreated with a β-blocker, hypertension and bradycardia result. The β-blocker blocks the β effect of epinephrine leaving the unopposed α effect. The α effect produces vasoconstriction producing hypertension (an increase in blood pressure), this leads to reflex bradycardia (via the vagus).

    (A) The opposite of hypotension and tachycardia occur.

    (B) Hypotension does not occur, but bradycardia does occur.

    (C) Hypertension does occur, but tachycardia does not occur.

42. (C) Nonsteroidal antiinflammatory drugs can reduce the pharmacologic effect of ACE inhibitors.

    (A) Nonsteroidal antiinflammatory drugs can increase the pharmacologic effect of lithium.

    (B) Nonsteroidal antiinflammatory drugs do not alter the effect of probenecid (but probenecid can increase the blood level of the NSAID).

    (D) Nonsteroidal antiinflammatory drugs do not alter the effect of oral contraceptives.

    (E) Nonsteroidal antiinflammatory drugs do not alter the effect of calcium channel blockers.

43. (C) Antihypertensive agents can produce adverse reactions such as impotence (sexual problems), intestinal problems (diarrhea or constipation), and orthostatic hypotension (dizziness upon arising abruptly from a lying or sitting position).

    (A) Antihypertensive agents do not usually produce anxiety, in fact they can sometimes produce sedation.

    (B) Antihypertensive agents do not usually produce drooling, in fact they can sometimes produce xerostomia.

    (D) Antihypertensive agents do not usually produce hepatotoxicity.

    (E) Antihypertensive agents do not usually produce stomach upset, but can occasionally.

44. (A) A client with a history of rheumatic heart disease without any allergies who is to have an oral prophylaxis should be given amoxicillin. The adult dose is 3 g 1 hour before the procedure and 1.5 g 6 hours after the initial dose.

    (B) A client with a history of rheumatic heart disease can be given clindamycin before the oral prophylaxis if allergic to penicillin.

    (C) Doxycycline is never indicated to prevent infective endocarditis (too many resistant strains).

    (D) Erythromycin, although not nearly as effective as the other two recommended agents (amoxicillin and clindamycin) is still recommended to prevent infective endocarditis.

    (E) Metronidazole is never indicated to prevent infective endocarditis (does not cover the correct spectrum).

45. (B) Anticholinergics are relatively contraindicated in clients with prostatic hypertrophy (enlarged prostate) because they can produce difficulty in urinating and urinary retention.

    (A) Diarrhea due to hypermotility can be treated with anticholinergics because they block the increase in motility produced by the PANS.

    (C) Persons with sulfite hypersensitivity should avoid using local anesthetic agents with vasoconstrictors because they contain sulfiting agents to increase the stability in solution of the vasoconstrictors; the sulfites act as antioxidants.

    (D) Persons with congestive heart failure (CHF) can tolerate small doses of anticholinergics, but higher doses could result in tachycardia which would not be good for the individual with CHF.

    (E) Persons with congenital cholinesterase deficiency should avoid the ester local anesthetic agents because they are metabolized by this enzyme.

46. (D) Parasympatholytics or anticholinergics are used to decrease saliva flow to prevent choking during general anesthesia.

    (A, B) Both α- and β-blockers are sympatholytics or adrenergic blockers.

    (C) Sympathomimetics or adrenergic agents do not affect saliva flow but its consistency.

    (E) Parasympathomimetics or cholinergic agents increase saliva flow.

47. (D) During an acute anginal attack, the person remains conscious.

    (A) A person loses consciousness during a simple syncopal attack (fainting).

    (B) A person loses consciousness during a hypoglycemic episode (blood glucose is decreased).

    (C) During a cardiac arrest, a person loses consciousness.

    (E) During a tonic-clonic seizure (convulsions), a person loses consciousness.

48. (E) A sign of epinephrine toxicity is tachycardia (fast heart rate), palpitations, anxiety, and mydriasis (dilated pupils).

    (A) Epinephrine toxicity produces miosis (constricted pupils).

    (B) Epinephrine toxicity does not produce nausea.

    (C) Epinephrine toxicity can produce excitement, not sedation.

    (D) Epinephrine toxicity does not produce much sweating.

49. (B) Because untreated hypertension produces no symptoms, it is called the "silent killer."

    (A, C, D, E) Hypertension does not have these symptoms.

50. (C) Carbamazepine (Tegretol) is the drug of choice for the treatment of trigeminal neuralgia, also known as tic douloureux. It is effective for epilepsy because it is an anticonvulsant.

    (A) The drugs of choice for the treatment of peptic ulcers include specific antibiotic combinations plus an acid reducer; sometimes Pepto-Bismol is used too.

    (B) The drug of choice for the treatment of absence seizures is ethosuximide.

    (D) Cushing syndrome is due to excessive corticosteroids; withdrawal of the steroids reverses the syndrome, patient often cannot stop using the steroids because of their primary condition so Cushing syndrome is managed by treating the adverse reactions that occur (e.g., oral hypoglycemics or insulin for hyperglycemia, antiinfective agents for increased infections).

    (E) TMD is treated with muscle relaxants, antidepressants, steroids, and antiinflammatory agents.

Biochemistry, Nutrition, and Nutritional Counseling

Dianne M. Frazier   Sally Mauriello

Humans are multicellular organisms who require an intake of specific chemicals or nutrients from food to grow and maintain homeostasis and optimal health. An understanding of cellular biochemistry and nutrition is essential for all health professionals actively involved in preventing and treating disease in humans. The science of nutrition includes the intake of food and all the processes involved in the digestion, absorption, transportation, metabolism, and excretion of nutrients in food. Nutrition is also an applied science that involves counseling people to adapt food patterns to nutritional needs within the framework of a particular cultural, economic, and psychosocial environment. Nutritional counseling can be done effectively in the practice setting to motivate individuals in modifying food habits so that optimal oral and general health can be achieved.

This chapter covers the six major nutrient groups and their metabolic activities in mammalian cells, dietary modifications for diseases, nutritional diseases and disorders, and oral manifestations of nutritional deficiencies and toxicities. Also described are the effects of nutrients on oral tissues and the dietary assessment tools and techniques available for counseling individuals with various types of oral diseases. Because nutritional problems in the U.S. population are a result of overeating and undereating,

the chapter includes a review of energy balance and weight control.

Cellular biochemistry is fundamental in studying nutrition; therefore, the reader is referred first to Chapter 2, section on general histology, and Chapter 3, section on cellular structures and organelles, for a review of the structural and functional similarities in cells.

Six Major Classes of Essential Nutrients

Carbohydrates (CHO)

A. Definition—polyhydroxy aldehydes or ketones that serve as the body's primary source of quick energy; they are composed of basic units, monosaccharides, that contain carbon, hydrogen, and oxygen
B. Basic chemical structure
   1. Ratio of carbon, hydrogen, and oxygen is 1:2:1
   2. Reactive portion of the molecule may be in a ketose or aldose form

Ketose	Aldose
H_2COH	$HC = O$
$\|$	$\|$
$C = O$	$HCOH$
$\|$	$\|$
R	R

Table 9-1

Digestive Action at Various Points along the Gastrointestinal Tract

	Carbohydrates	Proteins	Fats
Mouth	Salivary amylase: starch → maltose	No action	No action
Stomach	Salivary amylase*: starch → maltose	Pepsin: proteins → smaller peptides HCl: activates pepsin and denatures proteins	Gastric lipase†: short- and medium-chain triglycerides → fatty acids + monoglycerides
Small intestine Pancreatic enzymes	Pancreatic amylase: starch → maltose	Trypsin, chymotrypsin, carboxypeptidase: proteins, polypeptides → dipeptides, amino acids	Pancreatic lipase: triglycerides → fatty acids + monoglycerides
Bile salts	No action	No action	Bile salts: emulsification of fats
Brush border enzymes	Disaccharidases: disaccharides → monosaccharides	Aminopeptidases, dipeptidases: dipeptides → amino acids	Lecithinase: lecithin → monoglyceride + fatty acid + PO_4 + choline
Large intestine	Some fermentation of undigested nutrients but with negligible absorption of the fermentation products		

*A small amount of action within the bolus of swallowed food.
†A minor role in total fat digestion.

3. Position of the hydroxyl (—OH) groups determines properties such as sweetness and absorbability
C. Classification
  1. Simple carbohydrates
    a. Monosaccharides
      (1) Trioses (C_3) and tetroses (C_4)—usually formed during intermediary metabolism and are not important dietary components
      (2) Pentoses (C_5)—important in nucleic acids and coenzymes, do not occur free (uncombined), and are not important dietary components (e.g., ribose)
      (3) Hexoses (C_6)—most important group physiologically
        (a) Glucose—blood sugar; primary energy source
        (b) Galactose—seldom found free but found in lactose
        (c) Fructose—fruit sugar; sweetest sugar; found in honey and fruits
    b. Disaccharides—composed of two monosaccharide units
      (1) Sucrose—glucose plus fructose (cane and beet sugar)
      (2) Lactose—glucose plus galactose (milk sugar)
      (3) Maltose—glucose plus glucose (intermediate of starch hydrolysis [digestion])
    c. Oligosaccharides—composed of two to six monosaccharide units
  2. Complex carbohydrates
    a. Homopolysaccharides—made up of more than six identical monosaccharide units
      (1) Starch—plant storage form of glucose; source of half of dietary carbohydrates
        (a) Amylose—straight chain
        (b) Amylopectin—branched chain
      (2) Glycogen—animal storage form of glucose; found in the liver and muscle of living animals; insignificant source of dietary carbohydrates
      (3) Cellulose—chief constituent of the framework of plants; glucose units are in β-linkages, not capable of being hydrolyzed by human digestive enzymes; provides bulk and fiber to the diet
      (4) Insulin—starch-like polymer made up of fructose units; used in kidney function tests

b. Heteropolysaccharides—carbohydrates associated with noncarbohydrates or carbohydrate derivatives
  (1) Pectin, lignin—important contributors to fiber in the diet
  (2) Glycoproteins—carbohydrate and protein in a specific, functional arrangement (e.g., blood group substances and many hormones)
  (3) Glycolipids—carbohydrate and lipid, as in gangliosides
  (4) Mucopolysaccharides—protein and carbohydrate in a loose binding
    (a) Hyaluronic acid—vitreous humor and joint lubricant
    (b) Heparin—anticoagulant
    (c) Chondroitin sulfate—cartilage, skin, bone, and teeth
    (d) Keratin sulfate—nails and teeth
D. Digestion, absorption, and transport
  1. Digestion (Table 9-1)
    a. Mouth
      (1) Teeth and tongue—mechanical breakdown and mixing of food
      (2) Saliva—hydration and lubrication of food
      (3) Salivary amylase (ptyalin)—initial enzymatic hydrolysis of starch
    b. Stomach—no digestive enzymes for carbohydrates; initial enzymatic hydrolysis of starch by salivary amylase may continue
    c. Small intestines
      (1) Pancreatic juices—pancreatic amylases
      (2) Intestinal villi (brush border) enzymes—disaccharidases
        (a) Sucrase—converts sucrose to glucose and fructose
        (b) Lactase—converts lactose to glucose and galactose
        (c) Maltase—converts maltose to glucose
    d. Large intestine—bacterial "fermentation" of some undigested carbohydrates
      (1) No significant contribution to absorbable carbohydrates
      (2) May be the cause of gas production and bloating during primary or secondary disaccharidase deficiency (e.g., "lactose intolerance")
  2. Absorption (Fig. 9-1)
    a. Factors affecting absorption
      (1) Intestinal motility
      (2) Type of food mixture
      (3) Integrity of intestinal mucosa
      (4) Endocrine activity
    b. Mechanism
      (1) Passive diffusion along the osmotic gradient (when the intestinal concentration of carbohydrates is greater than the blood level)
      (2) Facilitated diffusion allows only certain molecules to pass as recognized by a carrier
      (3) Active transport with the aid of a carrier at the brush border, which requires energy and allows molecules to pass against a concentration gradient
    c. Route
      (1) Carbohydrates are water soluble and are absorbed directly into the capillaries of the intestinal mucosa
      (2) Carried via the portal circulation to the liver
E. Metabolism—glucose is the main immediate source of energy for the body; a glucose level of 80 to 120 mg/100 ml blood is maintained by most healthy persons (Fig. 9-2)
  1. Sources of blood glucose
    a. Dietary carbohydrates—sugars, starches
    b. Stored liver glycogen breakdown—glycogenolysis
    c. Synthesis from intermediary metabolites such as pyruvic acid—gluconeogenesis
    d. Synthesis from noncarbohydrate sources—gluconeogenesis
      (1) Deaminated (glucogenic) amino acids
      (2) Glycerol portion of lipids
  2. Reactions of blood glucose—"burned" for energy
    a. Glycolysis—end product is pyruvate or lactic acid in the absence of oxygen (anaerobic conditions) or acetylcoenzyme A (acetyl-CoA) in the presence of oxygen (aerobic conditions)
    b. Tricarboxylic acid cycle (TCA) or Krebs cycle—burning of acetyl-CoA with the release of carbon dioxide (CO_2)
    c. Oxidative phosphorylation and electron transport production of adenosine triphosphate (ATP) (a high-energy molecule) and water (H_2O)
  3. Storage for reserve use
    a. Glycogenesis—glycogen is the short-term storage form of glucose in liver and muscle (6 to 18 hours)
    b. Lipogenesis—excess carbohydrate in the diet is converted to fat to be stored in adipose tissue as a long-term energy storage form
  4. Conversion to other molecules
    a. To other carbohydrates needed for structural or functional molecules

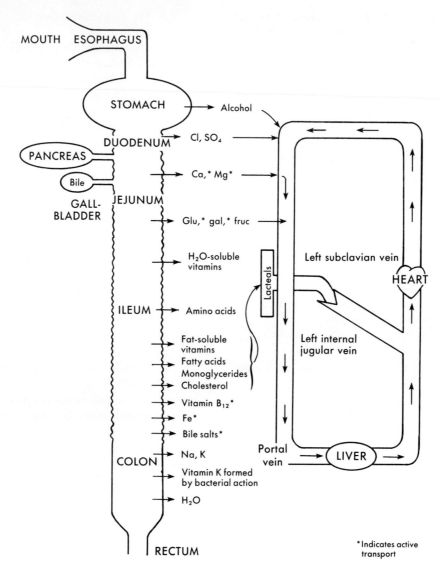

Fig. 9-1 Absorption of major nutrients, vitamins, and minerals.

b. To ketoacids to be used in the synthesis of amino acids for protein synthesis

F. Metabolic regulators
1. Anabolic hormones (lower the blood glucose level)—insulin
   a. Increases entry of glucose into cells
   b. Increases glycogenesis
   c. Increases lipogenesis
2. Catabolic hormones (raise the blood glucose level)
   a. Glucagon—stimulates glycogenolysis
   b. Steroid hormones—stimulate gluconeogenesis
   c. Epinephrine—stimulates glycogenolysis
   d. Growth hormone and adrenocorticotropic hormone (ACTH)—act as insulin antagonists

e. Thyroxine—increases insulin breakdown, glucose intestinal absorption, and epinephrine release
3. Coenzymes—B-complex vitamins are important precursors of the coenzymes involved in the catabolism of carbohydrates

G. Fiber in the diet
1. Definition—substances, usually non-starch polysaccharides, found in plants that are not broken down by human digestive enzymes; some may be digested by G.I. tract bacteria
   a. Crude fiber—plant residue that remains unhydrolized after laboratory treatment with strong acid or strong alkali

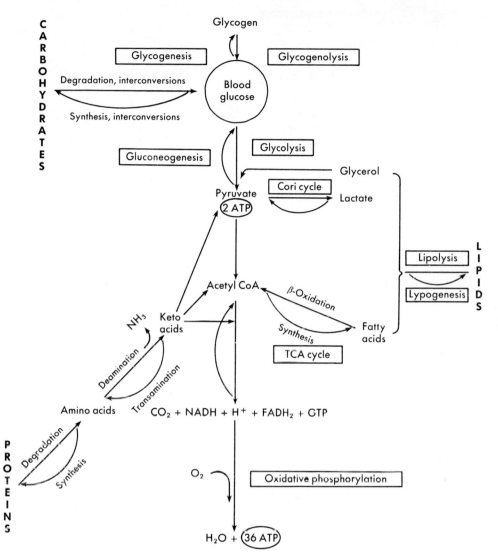

Fig. 9-2 Overview of metabolism.

b. Dietary fiber—plant residue that remains unhydrolized after human digestion
2. Epidemiologic studies indicate that individuals whose diets include a significant amount of fiber have a low incidence of chronic "Western" diseases
3. Specific fibers are believed to play roles in decreasing the incidence of obesity, irregularity, hemorrhoids, appendicitis, diverticulosis, colon cancer, hyperlipidemia, and fluctuations in blood glucose (Table 9-2)
4. Excess dietary fiber
   a. Bulky diets for persons with a limited intake may cause a nutrient deficiency
   b. Use of large doses of purified fiber may inhibit absorption of Ca, K, Zn, Fe

c. Phytic acid, often found in high fiber foods such as cereal grains, can bind and prevent absorption of minerals
5. Recommended fiber intake—for adults, 20 to 35 g/day
H. Biologic role and functions of carbohydrates
   1. Provide precursors of structural and functional molecules (e.g., gangliosides)
   2. Energy source (4 kcal/g)
   3. Spare protein
   4. Provide bulk and palatability to the diet
I. Oral biology
   1. Preeruptive effect on teeth
      a. Energy source for growth and development
      b. Protein-sparing nutrient

Table 9-2

Role of Dietary Fiber

Fiber type	Effect	Food source
Oat bran, pectin	Lowers blood cholesterol	Apples, raw whole oats
Wheat bran	Stool softener	Whole wheat
Pectin, guar gums	Slows gastric emptying	Apples
	Slows carbohydrate absorption	Legumes
Cellulose	Decreases transit time	Raw fruits and vegetables

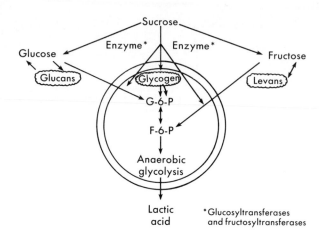

Fig. 9-3 Streptococcal cell. (From Lee M, Stanmeyer W, Wight A: *Nutrition and dental health, part II. Diet and dental bacteriology,* Carrboro, NC, 1982, Health Sciences Consortium.)

2. Posteruptive effect on teeth (Fig. 9-3)
   a. Energy source for oral cariogenic bacteria (e.g., *Streptococcus mutans*)
   b. Acidogenic bacteria metabolize monosaccharides and disaccharides, particularly sucrose, for the production of energy through glycolysis that results in the formation of lactic acid and other acids
   c. *S. mutans* synthesizes polysaccharides (glucans, levans, and glycogen) from sucrose
      (1) Polysaccharides are used for energy when sucrose is unavailable
      (2) Glucans form insoluble complexes with *S. mutans* and have a strong affinity for enamel, thus enhancing bacterial plaque formation
      (3) The organic acids are liberated into the interface between the bacterial plaque and surface enamel
      (4) At pH 5.5, decalcification and demineralization begins
   d. Firm texture of some complex carbohydrates, such as found in raw fruits and vegetables, can help to remove food debris retained between teeth; chewing action can also stimulate salivary flow
3. Dietary sweeteners (Table 9-3)
   a. Nutritive sweeteners are used by the body as an energy source; they provide calories
      (1) Sugar alcohols (xylitol, sorbitol, and mannitol) are noncariogenic nutritive sweeteners that are slowly fermented through anaerobic metabolism by oral bacteria; excessive intake of these polyols can cause diarrhea because of the osmotic transfer of water into the bowel

   (2) Aspartame is a noncariogenic nutritive sweetener consisting of two amino acids: aspartic acid and phenylalanine; because it is at least 100 times sweeter than sucrose, the amount needed as a sugar substitute provides negligible calories; it has a large margin of safety for human consumption; because it is unstable and loses its sweetening power in low-pH and high-temperature environments, it is not used in frying and baking
   b. Nonnutritive sweeteners are calorie-free and have no nutritive value; saccharin and acesulfame-K are nonnutritive sweeteners approved by the Food and Drug Administration (FDA); they are noncariogenic
   c. Food labels often list sugar content in its various forms (e.g., invert sugars, dextrose corn sweeteners) to give appearance of lower sugar content
4. Cariogenicity factors of diet habits (in order of importance)
   a. Frequency of intake of simple sugars—the more frequent the exposure to sugar, the more cariogenic the diet; six candy bars eaten at six different times during the day are more harmful in terms of acid and bacterial plaque formation than if the six candy bars were consumed at one time
   b. Form of simple sugars (liquid or retentive)—liquid sweets clear the oral cavity faster than solid or retentive sweets and therefore are less cariogenic
   c. Time of ingestion of simple sugars—combining

Table 9-3

Dietary Sweeteners

Type	Nutritive (N)/ Nonnutritive (NN)	Sweetener	Relative sweetness*	Relative acid production (cariogenicity)*
Sugars	N	Sucrose	1.0	1.0
		Glucose (dextrose)	0.7	†
		Fructose	1.1 to 1.7	0.8 to 1.0
		Lactose	0.2	0.4 to 0.6
		Maltose	0.4	†
		Galactose	0.6	†
Sugar alcohols	N	Sorbitol	0.7	0.1 to 0.3
		Mannitol	0.7	0
		Xylitol	0.9	0
Natural	N	Honey (fructose and glucose)	0.7 to 0.9	1.0
		Molasses (sucrose and invert sugar)	1.0	1.0
		Brown sugar (sugar and molasses)	1.0	1.0
Others	N	Glucose syrups	0.3 to 0.6	1.0
		High-fructose corn syrups	1.0 to 1.5	1.0
		Corn sweeteners	1.0	1.0
Dipeptides	N	Aspartame	120 to 280	0
Artificial	NN	Sodium saccharin	200 to 700	0
	NN	Acesulfame-K	200	0

From Lee M, Stanmeyer W, Wight A: Nutrition and dental health, part II, *Diet and dental bacteriology,* Carrboro, NC, 1982, Health Sciences Consortium.
*Relative to sucrose = 1.0.
†Information not available.

sweets with liquids and other noncariogenic foods during a meal is less cariogenic than a concentrated exposure to sweets between meals as a snack

  d. Total intake of simple sugars—annual consumption of sugar for each American is over 100 pounds; 60% of the sugar intake is from processed foods (e.g., cereal), which are often called "hidden sugars"

  e. Starch-rich foods that are retained on the teeth for prolonged periods of time are ultimately degraded to organic acids and can contribute to dental caries production

  f. Combining cariogenic foods with noncariogenic foods—recent studies indicate that certain cariogenic foods (e.g., canned pears in syrup) are less cariogenic when combined with a particular noncariogenic food (e.g., cheese)

 5. Carbohydrate importance in periodontal health

  a. Energy source for the growth and repair of periodontal tissues

  b. Protein-sparing nutrient

  c. Firm texture of complex carbohydrates can promote circulation in gingival tissue

  d. Dietary monosaccharides and disaccharides enhance supragingival bacterial growth and plaque

formation; these bacteria set the stage for the growth and development of subgingival bacteria and plaque, which are responsible for the destructive effects of periodontitis

J. Requirements

 1. Minimum adult intakes (60 to 100 g) prevent use of body protein as an energy source; children and infants need additional carbohydrates to provide energy and spare protein for growth and development

 2. Recommendations

  a. Calories from simple carbohydrates (monosaccharides and disaccharides)—10% or less of the total caloric intake

  b. Calories from complex carbohydrates (including fiber)—48% or more of the total caloric intake

K. Dietary modifications for disease

 1. Obesity—cut total calories and percentage of simple carbohydrates (concentrated sweets) to increase the nutrient density of a lower-calorie diet

 2. Genetic defects

  a. Lactose intolerance (inability to hydrolyze lactose)—eat fewer milk products, use fermented products, or add a commercial lactase enzyme to milk

(1) Primary—congenital absence of the lactase enzyme (a brush border enzyme)

(2) Secondary—temporary or permanent loss of lactase activity resulting from intestinal injury or disease

b. Galactosemia (congenital inability to metabolize galactose)—remove lactose and milk products from the diet

c. Fructose intolerance (congenital inability to metabolize fructose)—remove fructose as well as sucrose from the diet; individuals with fructose intolerance have significantly fewer dental caries

3. Dental caries and periodontal disease—protective diet

a. Eat a diet that is low in retentive carbohydrates

b. Do not eat cariogenic snacks

c. Eat a diet that is adequate in all nutrients

d. Include foods of firm or hard texture

4. Diabetes (inability to regulate glucose because of insufficiency or relative ineffectiveness of insulin)—dietary treatment (see Chapter 15, section on diabetes mellitus)

a. Eat a high–complex carbohydrate, low–simple sugar diet

b. Limit fat intake to 30% of kcal

c. Provide consistent carbohydrate intake and meal spacing throughout the day

d. Coordinate food intake and exercise with medication

e. Control weight—80% of patients with type II diabetes are overweight

5. Reactive hypoglycemia—rare; symptoms of dizziness, hunger, and heart palpitations are lessened with a low-carbohydrate diet

6. Dumping syndrome—after gastric surgery; postprandial symptoms of nausea, dizziness, cramping, and diarrhea are lessened by a low-monosaccharide, low-disaccharide diet

7. Alcoholism—overconsumption of alcohol may cause malnutrition (see Chapter 15, section on alcoholism)

a. Depresses the appetite

b. Empty-calorie food

c. Causes vitamin B depletion because the liver needs niacin and thiamine to metabolize alcohol

d. Causes folate and iron deficiency

e. Depresses the antidiuretic hormone, causing loss of magnesium, potassium, and zinc in the urine

8. Alcohol consumption during pregnancy—appears to have a direct teratogenic effect on the developing fetus (fetal alcohol syndrome) (see Chapter 15, section on fetal alcohol syndrome)

9. Carbohydrate regulation in some hyperlipoproteinemias—total carbohydrate and alcohol intake is controlled; concentrated sweets are restricted

Proteins

A. Definition—complex biologic compounds of high molecular weight containing nitrogen, hydrogen, oxygen, carbon, and small amounts of sulfur; each protein (PRO) has a specific size and is made up of amino acid building blocks linked through peptide bonds in a specific arrangement

B. Classifications

1. Chemical

a. Simple proteins—contain amino acids only

b. Compound proteins (conjugated)—contain simple proteins and a nonprotein group

(1) Nucleoproteins

(2) Metalloproteins

(3) Phosphoproteins

(4) Lipoproteins

c. Derived—fragments produced during digestion or hydrolysis (e.g., peptides, peptones, and proteoses)

2. Biologic

a. Complete proteins contain sufficient amounts of the essential amino acids for normal metabolic reactions; found in foods of animal origin

(1) Essential amino acids cannot be synthesized by humans and must be provided in the diet in sufficient amounts to meet needs

(a) Adult—histidine, isoleucine, leucine, lysine, methionine, phenylalanine, threonine, tryptophan, and valine

(b) Infant—all of the above plus histidine and probably taurine

(c) Premature infant—all of the above plus cysteine

(2) Nonessential amino acids can be synthesized by the body and need not be provided by the diet but are necessary for normal metabolic reactions

b. Incomplete proteins have insufficient quantities of one or more essential amino acids to support protein synthesis in humans; plant proteins are often incomplete (e.g., corn protein is low in lysine; legume protein is low in methionine)

c. Complementary proteins are proteins that, when ingested singly, are incomplete but, when combined, provide sufficient essential amino acids

(1) In a vegan (or strict vegetarian) diet, the complementary of plant proteins can be

accomplished by combining appropriate incomplete proteins in the same meal; vegans are at risk for developing deficiencies in vitamin B_{12}, iron, and essential amino acids; major foods for these nutrients are from animal sources

    (2) In an ovolacto vegetarian diet, milk and egg proteins can provide the essential amino acids that are inadequate in incomplete plant proteins

  d. Protein quality is a measure of a protein's ability to support protein synthesis; it is measured by comparing the test protein with a reference protein, usually egg protein

    (1) Amino acid or protein chemical score (CS)—compares the essential amino acid content in a dietary protein to that of a reference protein

    (2) Protein efficiency ratio (PER)—measures a protein's ability to support growth

    (3) Biologic value (BV)—expression of the percentage of nitrogen retained for maintenance and growth compared with the amount absorbed

    (4) Net protein utilization (NPU)—expression of the percentage of nitrogen retained compared with the amount ingested; differs from BV because it takes into account the protein's digestibility

    (5) Protein-digestibility–corrected amino acid score (PDCAAS)—compares the amino acid balance of a food protein with the amino acid requirements of preschool-aged children and then corrects for digestibility; used by the FDA for labeling

C. Structure

  1. Primary—linear sequence of the component amino acids

  2. Secondary—steric relationship of amino acids that are close to one another in the linear sequence (e.g., the α-helix and the collagen helix)

  3. Tertiary—steric relationship between amino acids far apart in the linear sequence that causes folding and the ultimate functional structure of the protein (e.g., globular, fibrous, and pleated sheet)

  4. Quaternary—steric interaction between subunits of proteins with more than one polypeptide chain (e.g., hemoglobin; this is also a functional form)

D. Digestion, absorption, and transport (see Table 9-1 and Fig. 9-1)

  1. Mouth—mechanical breakdown and moistening

  2. Stomach

    a. Hydrochloric acid from the parietal cells denatures or unfolds proteins and activates pepsinogen to give pepsin

    b. Pepsin begins the hydrolysis of the peptide bonds of proteins to form peptides and proteoses

  3. Small intestine

    a. Pancreas secretes bicarbonate into the duodenum to neutralize the acidic products from the stomach and proteolytic enzymes in an inactive form; enzymes activated by trypsin through a hormonal feedback mechanism are chymotrypsin, aminopeptidase, and carboxypeptidase; each hydrolyzes peptide bonds formed by different classes of amino acids

    b. Enzymes of the brush border are dipeptidases that hydrolyze dipeptides to amino acids

  4. Absorption—at the brush border of the microvilli of the small intestine, absorption occurs by both simple diffusion along a concentration gradient and by active transport at specific amino acid sites involving carrier enzymes, a sodium-ATP pump, and vitamin B_6

  5. Transport—absorbed amino acids are collected by the portal blood system and transported to the liver

E. Metabolism (see Fig. 9-2)

  1. Amino acid pool—collection of amino acids in a dynamic equilibrium in the liver, blood, and other cells that provides the raw material for the body's protein and amino acid needs

    a. Input into the pool comes from proteins in the diet, breakdown of body proteins, and synthesis of nonessential amino acids

    b. Output from the pool is for synthesis of body structures, specialized substances (e.g., melanin from tyrosine), and energy as needed

  2. Anabolism

    a. De novo synthesis—requires deoxyribonucleic acid (DNA), messenger ribonucleic acid (mRNA), and ribosomal ribonucleic acid (rRNA)

    (1) In the nucleus the DNA carries the genetic information in groups of three bases that provide the code for the individual amino acids that make up a specific protein

    (2) mRNA transports a copy of the code from the DNA into the cytoplasm

    (3) mRNA attaches to a ribosome and acts as a template for the alignment of amino acids that are attached to transfer RNA (tRNA)

    (4) If the proper amino acids are in the correct proportions and the synthetic enzymes and energy are available, the polypeptide chain is synthesized

b. Transamination
   (1) Nonessential amino acids can be synthesized from the corresponding α-keto acids, an α-amino acid (as the NH_3^+ donor), a specific transaminase enzyme, and the coenzyme pyridoxal phosphate (vitamin B_6)
   (2) Intermediate complex formed in this reaction is called a Schiff base
3. Catabolism—amino acids in excess of those needed for the synthesis of proteins and other biomolecules cannot be stored or excreted; they may, however, be deaminated and the α-keto acid used as a metabolic fuel for immediate energy needs or for long-term energy storage as fat
   a. Amino group
      (1) Deamination—loss of the α-amino group, usually in the liver, through transfer to α-ketoglutarate to form glutamate; glutamate is then oxidatively deaminated to yield ammonia (NH_3)
      (2) Urea cycle—series of steps whereby the ammonia produced during deamination is converted to urea for excretion
   b. α-Keto acid
      (1) Ketogenic amino acids are those whose carbon skeleton, after deamination, yields acetyl-CoA or acetoacetyl-CoA, which then yields ketone bodies; high concentrations of ketone bodies lead to some of the undesirable side effects of high-protein, low-carbohydrate diets
      (2) Glucogenic amino acids are those that yield pyruvate, α-ketoglutarate, and other intermediates of the citric acid cycle that can, if needed, be converted to glucose
4. Nitrogen balance—comparison of the amount of nitrogen ingested with the amount excreted (e.g., urinary nitrogen plus about 1 g/day for nail, hair, skin, and perspiration losses) to determine whether there is net protein catabolism, anabolism, or equilibrium
   a. Positive balance—intake is greater than output; indicates net protein synthesis and is the normal situation for anyone building protein-containing tissue, such as during childhood, pregnancy, and recovery from undernutrition, surgery, or illness
   b. Negative balance—intake is less than output; indicates net protein breakdown, when the body must break down its own protein to meet energy or metabolic needs; can result from insufficient protein (or essential amino acids) or energy intake or from fever, infection, anxiety, or prolonged stress

F. Metabolic regulation
   1. Hormones
      a. Anabolic—growth hormone, insulin, normal thyroid hormone, and sex hormones
      b. Catabolic—adrenocortical hormones and large amounts of thyroid hormone
   2. Vitamins—pyridoxine and riboflavin are necessary for protein synthesis; when they are deficient in the diet, synthesis may be limited
G. Functions
   1. Structural
      a. Collagen and elastin
      b. Bone and tooth matrix
      c. Myosin fibrils
      d. Keratin
   2. Dynamic
      a. Transport of nutrients
         (1) Lipids and fat-soluble vitamins
         (2) Iron—transferrin
         (3) Oxygen—hemoglobin and myoglobin
         (4) Protein-bound molecules
         (5) Membrane transport
      b. Regulation and control
         (1) Immunoglobulins
         (2) Buffers
         (3) Hormones
         (4) Enzymes
         (5) Blood coagulation—fibrin
         (6) Muscle contraction—actin and myosin
   3. Energy source (4 kcal/g)
   4. Oral biology
      a. Preeruptive effects on teeth—essential for all cells and therefore necessary for normal tooth bud and pulp formation and synthesis of protein matrix for enamel and dentin
      b. Posteruptive effects on teeth
         (1) Essential for maintaining the integrity of pulpal tissue throughout life
         (2) Chemical nature of protein foods can neutralize acids produced by oral bacteria
      c. Periodontal health and disease
         (1) Essential for all cells in growth, development, and maintenance of the periodontium
         (2) Essential for the normal function of cellular defenses against subgingival bacteria and toxins
         (3) Necessary in the healing and repair of injured tissues from periodontitis or periodontal surgery
H. Requirements
   1. Determination and estimates of protein requirements
      a. Nitrogen-balance studies are used to determine

the lowest protein intake that will support homeostasis or equilibrium

b. Average requirement for reference proteins of 0.8 g/kg/day for young adult males; other groups by extrapolation or interpolation

c. Estimates for growth needs in infants are based on the amount of protein provided by that quantity of human milk that ensures a satisfactory growth rate

2. 1989 Recommended Dietary Allowances (RDAs)—developed by the National Research Council; based on 1985 WHO recommendations, which utilize nitrogen balance data; these allowances assume ingestion of a good-quality protein in a mixed diet; adjustments are made for growth, pregnancy, and lactation (Table 9-4)

3. Food sources—protein needs of an average adult can be met by choosing two or more servings per day from any of the following groups: meats, poultry, fish, eggs, milk and dairy products, dried beans and peas, and nuts

I. Dietary modifications for disease

1. Genetic disorders

a. Phenylketonuria (PKU)—inherited enzyme defect in which individuals cannot metabolize the phenylalanine found in nearly all proteins; prescribed diet provides only enough phenylalanine to meet growth and maintenance needs; dietary protein is restricted, but amino acids are provided by a synthetic, formula from which the phenylalanine has been removed

b. Maple syrup urine disease, homocystinuria, tyrosinemia, methylmalonic aciduria, propionic acidemia, and isovaleric acidemia—other genetic disorders in which amino acid metabolism is altered, and patients are treated with low-protein diets and synthetic amino acid formulas

c. Gout—characterized by excessive uric acid production leading to the formation of urate crystals deposited in the joints; treatment often includes restriction of protein to limit purine (and uric acid) production

2. Protein needs are increased during fever, after severe injury and surgery, intestinal malabsorption, increased protein loss from the kidneys, or diminished protein synthesis by the liver

3. Dietary protein must be restricted when the kidneys can no longer remove nitrogenous wastes from the body or in severe liver disease when the nitrogenous by-products of protein catabolism can no longer be synthesized

4. Protein-energy (calorie) malnutrition (PEM or PCM)

a. Kwashiorkor (classic)—failure of the young child to grow because of an insufficient protein intake (usually because of weaning from the mother's milk); often edema masks muscle wasting

b. Marasmus (classic)—failure of the infant or young child to grow because of partial starvation; total caloric intake, as well as protein intake, is insufficient

c. Adult PCM or PEM—seen even in industrialized countries among alcoholics and long-term hospitalized patients with AIDS, tuberculosis and anorexia nervosa, for example

Lipids (Fats)

A. Definition—biochemical compounds composed of carbon, hydrogen, oxygen, and small amounts of phosphorus; they are insoluble in water and soluble in fatty substances and organic solvents

B. Classification

1. Simple lipids

a. True fats—contain fatty acids attached to glycerol (a trihydroxy alcohol) through an ester linkage; these may be monoglycerides, diglycerides, or triglycerides, depending on the number of glycerol-hydroxyl groups esterified; chemical and biochemical characteristics of the glycerides depend on the number, order, and kind of fatty acids attached

(1) Saturated fatty acids—contain no double bonds and are found in lipids from animal sources; are solids at room temperature (high melting point)

(2) Unsaturated fatty acids—contain one or more double bonds and come from plant sources; are usually liquids at room temperature (low melting point)

(3) Hydrogenation—addition of hydrogen to some or all of the double bonds; this is done in making margarine or butter substitutes from vegetable oils; in partial hydrogenation, some *trans* bonds are formed that may present a health risk

(4) Rancidity—addition of oxygen to some of the double bonds of fatty acids that contributes to spoilage; occurs spontaneously in foods and can be lessened by the addition of antioxidants, such as butylated hydroxytoluene (BHT)

(5) Iodine number—chemical indication of the degree of unsaturation of a fatty acid; the more molecules of iodine bound by the fatty acid, the more unsaturated and the higher the iodine number

b. Waxes—esters of a fatty acid and an alcohol

Table 9-4

Food and Nutrition Board, National Academy of Sciences—National Research Council Recommended Dietary Allowances,[a] Revised 1989
Designed for the maintenance of good nutrition of practically all healthy people in the United States

Category	Age (years) or condition	WEIGHT[b] (kg)	WEIGHT[b] (lb)	HEIGHT[b] (cm)	HEIGHT[b] (in)	Protein (g)	FAT-SOLUBLE VITAMINS Vitamin A (μg RE)[c]	Vitamin D (μg)[d]	Vitamin E (mg α-TE)[e]	Vitamin K (μg)
Infants	0.0–0.5	6	13	60	24	13	375	7.5	3	5
	0.5–1.0	9	20	71	28	14	375	10	4	10
Children	1–3	13	29	90	35	16	400	10	6	15
	4–6	20	44	112	44	24	500	10	7	20
	7–10	28	62	132	52	28	700	10	7	30
Males	11–14	45	99	157	62	45	1000	10	10	45
	15–18	66	145	176	69	59	1000	10	10	65
	19–24	72	160	177	70	58	1000	10	10	70
	25–50	79	174	176	70	63	1000	5	10	80
	51+	77	170	173	68	63	1000	5	10	80
Females	11–14	46	101	157	62	46	800	10	8	45
	15–18	55	120	163	64	44	800	10	8	55
	19–24	58	128	164	65	46	800	10	8	60
	25–50	63	138	163	64	50	800	5	8	65
	51+	65	143	160	63	50	800	5	8	65
Pregnant						60	800	10	10	65
Lactating	1st 6 months					65	1300	10	12	65
	2nd 6 months					62	1200	10	11	65

[a]The allowances, expressed as average daily intakes over time, are intended to provide for individual variations among most normal persons as they live in the United States under usual environmental stresses. Diets should be based on a variety of common foods in order to provide other nutrients for which human requirements have been less well defined. See text for detailed discussion of allowances and of nutrients not tabulated.
[b]Weights and heights of Reference Adults are actual medians for the U.S. population of the designated age, as reported by NHANES II. The median weights and heights of those under 19 years of age were taken from Hamill P.V.V., T.A. Dvizd, C.L. Johnson, R.B. Reed, A.F. Roche, and W.M. Moore. 1979. Physical growth: National Center for Health Statistics Percentiles. Am. J. Clin. Nutr. 32:607-629. The use of these figures does not imply that the height-to-weight ratios are ideal.
[c]Retinol equivalents. 1 retinol equivalent = 1 μg retinol or 6 μg β-carotene. See text for calculation of vitamin A activity of diets as retinol equivalents.
[d]As cholecalciferol. 10 μg cholecalciferol = 400 IU of vitamin D.
[e]α-Tocopherol equivalents. 1 mg d-α tocopherol = 1 α-TE. See text for variation in allowances and calculation of vitamin E activity of the diet as α-tocopherol equivalents.
[f]1 NE (niacin equivalent) is equal to 1 mg of niacin or 60 mg of dietary tryptophan.

other than glycerol; body is unable to use waxes because digestive enzymes do not hydrolyze their ester linkage
2. Compound lipids contain compounds added to the glycerol and fatty acids
   a. Phospholipids

   Glycerol + 2 Fatty acids + Phosphate group + R group

   (1) Water-soluble emulsifiers (e.g., lecithin, with choline as the R group)
   (2) Membrane constituents (e.g., sphingomyelin)
   (3) Active intermediates in metabolism of lipid compound (e.g., CoA)
   b. Glycolipids—contain a carbohydrate component and are found in the brain and nervous tissue (e.g., cerebrosides)

   c. Lipoproteins—are water soluble and are responsible for carrying lipids throughout the body
   (1) Chylomicrons—about 2% protein; carry exogenous (absorbed from the diet) triglycerides around the body
   (2) Very low density lipoproteins (VLDLs)—9% protein; carry endogenous triglycerides around the body
   (3) Low-density lipoproteins (LDLs)—21% protein; carry mostly cholesterol from the liver to peripheral sites
   (4) High-density lipoproteins (HDLs)—50% protein; carry cholesterol back to the liver; can be elevated by exercise
3. Derived lipids are compounds whose synthesis begins like that of fatty acid synthesis with acetyl groups added on one at a time

Table 9-4

Food and Nutrition Board, National Academy of Sciences—National Research Council Recommended Dietary Allowances,[a] Revised 1989
Designed for the maintenance of good nutrition of practically all healthy people in the United States—cont'd

WATER-SOLUBLE VITAMINS							MINERALS						
Vita-min C (mg)	Thia-min (mg)	Ribo-flavin (mg)	Niacin (mg NE)[f]	Vita-min B_6 (mg)	Fo-late (µg)	Vita-min B_{12} (µg)	Cal-cium (mg)	Phos-phorus (mg)	Mag-nesium (mg)	Iron (mg)	Zinc (mg)	Iodine (µg)	Sele-nium (µg)
30	0.3	0.4	5	0.3	25	0.3	400	300	40	6	5	40	10
35	0.4	0.5	6	0.6	35	0.5	600	500	60	10	5	50	15
40	0.7	0.8	9	1.0	50	0.7	800	800	80	10	10	70	20
45	0.9	1.1	12	1.1	75	1.0	800	800	120	10	10	90	20
45	1.0	1.2	13	1.4	100	1.4	800	800	170	10	10	120	30
50	1.3	1.5	17	1.7	150	2.0	1200	1200	270	12	15	150	40
60	1.5	1.8	20	2.0	200	2.0	1200	1200	400	12	15	150	50
60	1.5	1.7	19	2.0	200	2.0	1200	1200	350	10	15	150	70
60	1.5	1.7	19	2.0	200	2.0	800	800	350	10	15	150	70
60	1.2	1.4	15	2.0	200	2.0	800	800	350	10	15	150	70
50	1.1	1.3	15	1.4	150	2.0	1200	1200	280	15	12	150	45
60	1.1	1.3	15	1.5	180	2.0	1200	1200	300	15	12	150	50
60	1.1	1.3	15	1.6	180	2.0	1200	1200	280	15	12	150	55
60	1.1	1.3	15	1.6	180	2.0	800	800	280	15	12	150	55
60	1.0	1.2	13	1.6	180	2.0	800	800	280	10	12	150	55
70	1.5	1.6	17	2.2	400	2.2	1200	1200	320	30	15	175	65
95	1.6	1.8	20	2.1	280	2.6	1200	1200	355	15	19	200	75
90	1.6	1.7	20	2.1	260	2.6	1200	1200	340	15	16	200	75

a. Sterols—all have a polycyclic nucleus as shown below

Cholesterol is a precursor for the synthesis of many steroid compounds and a constituent of cell membranes

(1) Sources

  (a) Exogenous—average dietary intake is 400 to 600 mg from foods of animal origin

  (b) Endogenous—average synthesis in the body is 1 to 2 g/day

(2) Regulation of cholesterol—dietary cholesterol, percentage of fat, ratio of poly- to mono- to unsaturated fat, and amount of certain fibers in the diet

b. Steroids—similar to sterols but with side-chain modification (e.g., bile acids, sex hormones, adrenocortical hormones, and vitamin D)

4. Artificial fats—substances developed for use in foods that have the flavor, appearance, and feel of dietary fats but do not have the physiologic effects

  a. Olestra—a 0-kcal artificial fat made from an indigestible combination of sucrose and fatty acids; may help serum cholesterol levels by directly interfering with cholesterol absorption; may increase the requirement for vitamin E; approved for use in snack foods

  b. Simplesse—has about 15% of the kcal as the fat it replaces; made by microparticulation of protein; the small protein particles have the feel of fat; not suitable for cooking, but used in fat-free dairy products and salad dressings

  c. Oatrim and maltodextrim—carbohydrate-based fat replacements; mimic texture and feel of fat by forming gels; are digestible and contribute some calories

C. Digestion, absorption, and transportation (see Table 9-1 and Fig. 9-1)

1. Digestion
   a. Mouth—no enzymatic action; mechanical and moistening action only
   b. Stomach—gastric lipase hydrolyzes some short- and medium-chain fatty acids from triglycerides
   c. Small intestine
      (1) Gallbladder—bile salts emulsify fats before digestion
      (2) Pancreas—pancreatic lipase (steapsin) hydrolyzes fatty acids from triglycerides to form diglycerides and monoglycerides
      (3) Intestinal mucosa—lecithinase converts lecithin to fatty acids, monoglyceride, phosphate, and choline
2. Absorption and transport
   a. Short-chain fatty acids can be absorbed into the portal system
   b. Medium- and long-chain fatty acids are water insoluble, require bile as a carrier (emulsifier), and are absorbed in stages
      (1) Bile separated out at the intestinal wall and recirculated
      (2) Complete breakdown of triglycerides within the mucosal cells by mucosal lipase
      (3) Resynthesis of new triglycerides that combine with protein carriers to form chylomicrons
      (4) Passage into the lymph system (lacteals) and the blood via the thoracic duct
      (5) At its destination, lipoprotein lipase hydrolyzes the triglycerides, clearing chylomicrons from the blood
      (6) Lipoprotein carriers (VLDLs, LDLs, and HDLs) carry endogenous lipids and cholesterol
D. Metabolism (occurs in liver and adipose tissue; see Fig. 9-2)
   1. Anabolism
      a. Lipogenesis—synthesis of triglycerides for long-term storage of energy; starting material is acetyl-CoA, which can come from glucogenic amino acids, carbohydrates, or breakdown of dietary lipids; lipogenesis takes place in nearly all cells but is most active in adipose cells
      b. Synthesis of steroids occurs in all cells
      c. Synthesis of lipoproteins occurs mainly in the liver
   2. Catabolism
      a. β-Oxidation—fatty acids are broken down in a stepwise manner to yield one molecule of acetyl-CoA for every two carbon atoms; acetyl-CoA can be catabolized further via the TCA and oxidative phosphorylation

   b. Ketone production—when the body's supply of carbohydrates is low, the TCA is depressed and acetyl-CoA from β-oxidation accumulates; alternate route for acetyl-CoA is ketone production; acetoacetone, acetone, and β-hydroxyl butyrate are the ketone bodies; excess ketone production can cause ketosis, ketonuria, and ketoacidosis (a sometimes fatal condition)
E. Metabolic regulators
   1. Vitamins as coenzyme precursors
      a. Anabolism—biotin, riboflavin (in flavin adenine dinucleotide [FAD]), niacin (in nicotinamide-adenine dinucleotide [NAD]), and pantothenic acid (in CoA) (see Fig. 9-2)
      b. Catabolism—riboflavin, niacin, and pantothenic acid
   2. Hormones
      a. Anabolism—insulin
      b. Catabolism—ACTH, thyroid-stimulating hormone (TSH), epinephrine, and glucagon
   3. Enzymes necessary for the metabolism of lipids are synthesized or inhibited in response to the relative amounts of substrates and products available
F. Biologic role and functions
   1. Structural components of cell membrane
   2. Energy source
      a. Provides 9 kcal/g (compared with 4 kcal/g for protein or carbohydrates)
      b. Long-term storage form of energy
   3. Carrier of fat-soluble vitamins
   4. Protective padding for body organs
   5. Insulation for the maintenance of body temperature
   6. Oral biology
      a. Cariostatic properties
         (1) Oils in fats provide a coating on the tooth's surface and prevent retention of food particles
         (2) Oils provide a fatty protective layer over plaque and prevent fermentable sugars from entering bacterial plaque or acids from leaving bacterial plaque
      b. No fat-periodontal relationship
G. Requirements
   1. Essential fatty acids (EFAs)—cannot be synthesized in sufficient amounts to meet needs; must be supplied in the diet; for humans the only EFAs are linoleic (ω-6) and linolenic (ω-3); requirement is about 3% of total kilocalories
      a. Function—necessary for the synthesis of membranes and prostaglandins (local hormone)
      b. Deficiency symptoms—seen in infants on low-polyunsaturated fatty acid (PUFA) diets and

adults receiving total parenteral nutrition feedings without lipids; characterized by slow growth, reproductive failure, and skin lesions
2. Recommendations (U.S. dietary goals)
   a. Total fats less than or equal to 30% of total kilocalories
   b. Cholesterol less than or equal to 300 mg/day
   c. Saturated fats less than or equal to 10% of total kilocalories, with an approximately equal amount of polyunsaturated and monounsaturated fats
3. The Committee on Diet and Health and Healthy People 2000 make similar recommendations for healthy people over the age of 2
4. 1990 Canadian RNI recommends that ω-3 and ω-6 fatty acid should be consumed in a ratio of 1:4

H. Dietary modifications for disease
1. Cardiovascular disease (CVD)—blood vessel lumens become narrower and sometimes completely blocked because of the plaques caused by accumulation of fatty substances, cellular debris, and calcium; blood pressure and the work required of the heart are increased, formation of clots is increased, and the result may be a heart attack (myocardial infarction) or stroke
   a. Hyperlipoproteinemias—elevation of serum VLDL, LDL, and chylomycron levels is a diagnostic tool that indicates a patient is at risk for CVD; there is a genetic predisposition for certain hyperlipoproteinemias; elevated HDL levels may exert a protective effect against CVD; routine exercise elevates HDL levels in most people
   b. Dietary factors that may increase serum lipids—high intakes of cholesterol, saturated fats, total fats, sucrose, fructose, and ethanol (alcohol)
   c. Dietary factors that may decrease serum lipids—monounsaturated and polyunsaturated fatty acids, omega fatty acids (fish oils), and pectin; ethanol in moderate amounts may have a protective effect by increasing HDL levels; unidentified substances in garlic, yeast, onions, and some wines may also have a protective effect
2. Obesity—because fats are a concentrated source of calories (9 kcal/g), most reducing diets recommend a decrease in fat intake; fat should not be too severely restricted because it adds to the palatability and satiety of the diet
3. Gallbladder disease and chronic pancreatitis—often cause pain after lipid ingestion; diet may have to be restricted in fats until the conditions are corrected
4. Cystic fibrosis and malabsorption disorders—often treated by using synthetic medium-chain triglyceride formulas that are more easily absorbed
5. Dumping syndrome and gastric ulcers—often treated by increasing fat in the diet to delay gastric emptying
6. Epilepsy—children with some types of epilepsy may be effectively treated with a ketogenic diet that is high in fats, low in carbohydrates, and causes a ketotic condition

Vitamins
A. Definition—organic substances that are essential to life and are needed in very small amounts; serve regulatory functions and often act as coenzymes or precursors of coenzymes; vitamins are present in food, but some can be produced in precursor form or activated in the body
B. Classification
1. Water-soluble vitamins
   a. Vitamin C
   b. B-complex vitamins
2. Fat-soluble vitamins
   a. Vitamin A
   b. Vitamin D
   c. Vitamin E
   d. Vitamin K
C. Chemistry and general properties
1. Water-soluble vitamins
   a. Soluble in water
   b. Sensitive to heat, light, and oxygen
   c. Contain the elements carbon, hydrogen, oxygen, and nitrogen and in some cases other elements such as cobalt or sulfur
   d. Absorbed into the blood by both active and passive transport from the upper portion of the digestive tract (see Fig. 9-1); vitamin B_{12} requires intrinsic factor for absorption
   e. Transported free and unbound to cells in the blood
   f. Minimal storage of dietary excesses except for
      (1) Vitamin C—stores may last 30 to 90 days
      (2) Vitamin B_{12}—stores may last many years in absence of pernicious anemia
      (3) Folic acid—stores may last 4 to 5 months
   g. Excreted in urine
   h. Should be supplied in the diet nearly every day
   i. Deficiency symptoms often develop rapidly
   j. Relatively nontoxic with excessive dietary intakes, although the increased use of over-the-counter megavitamin preparations has caused the appearance of toxic symptoms
2. Fat-soluble vitamins
   a. Soluble in fat and fat solvents (some water-soluble derivatives are available)

Table 9-5

Estimated Safe and Adequate Daily Dietary Intakes of Selected Vitamins and Minerals*

		VITAMINS	
Category	Age (years)	Biotin (μg)	Pantothenic acid (mg)
Infants	0–0.5	10	2
	0.5–1	15	3
Children and	1–3	20	3
adolescents	4–6	25	3–4
	7–10	30	4–5
	11+	30–100	4–7
Adults		30–100	4–7

		TRACE ELEMENTS†				
Category	Age (years)	Copper (mg)	Manganese (mg)	Fluoride (mg)	Chromium (μg)	Molybdenum (μg)
Infants	0–0.5	0.4–0.6	0.3–0.6	0.1–0.5	10–40	15–30
	0.5–1	0.6–0.7	0.6–1.0	0.2–1.0	20–60	20–40
Children and	1–3	0.7–1.0	1.0–1.5	0.5–1.5	20–80	25–50
adolescents	4–6	1.0–1.5	1.5–2.0	1.0–2.5	30–120	30–75
	7–10	1.0–2.0	2.0–3.0	1.5–2.5	50–200	50–150
	11+	1.5–2.5	2.0–5.0	1.5–2.5	50–200	75–250
Adults		1.5–3.0	2.0–5.0	1.5–4.0	50–200	75–250

*Because there is less information on which to base allowances, these figures are not given in the main table of RDA and are provided here in the form of ranges of recommended intakes.
†Because the toxic levels for many trace elements may be only several times usual intakes, the upper levels for the trace elements given in this table should not be habitually exceeded.

b. More stable in light, heat, and oxygen than water-soluble vitamins
c. Contain only elements of carbon, hydrogen, and oxygen
d. Must be emulsified and carried across the membranes of the intestinal cells in the presence of fat and bile (see Fig. 9-1); any conditions that decrease the digestion, absorption, or transport of lipids will lower the usable amount of fat-soluble vitamins
e. Absorbed into the lymphatic system and transported by attachment to protein carriers
f. Intake in excess of the daily need is stored in the body
g. Not readily excreted
h. Not absolutely necessary in the diet every day
i. Deficiency symptoms slow to develop
j. Toxic with chronic excessive intake
D. General functions
1. Water-soluble vitamins
a. Coenzymes for energy metabolism
b. Synthesis of red blood cells and DNA
2. Fat-soluble vitamins

a. Vision
b. Maintenance of the body's mucosal linings and epithelial cells
c. Integrity of mineralized tissues of bone and teeth by regulating calcium and phosphorus levels in the body
d. Cellular antioxidant
e. Normal blood clotting
E. Requirements (Tables 9-4 and 9-5)—note that the RDAs are based on vitamin and mineral intakes from foods and not supplements
F. Dietary sources, specific body functions, and symptoms of deficiencies and toxicities (Table 9-6)
G. Oral biology
1. Functions
a. Tooth formation (Table 9-7)
b. Periodontium (Table 9-8)
2. Oral manifestations of deficiencies and toxicities (Table 9-9)

Minerals

A. Definition—inorganic elements that are essential to life; serve both structural and regulatory functions

Table 9-6

Dietary Sources and Functions of Vitamins

Vitamin	Dietary sources	Major body functions	Deficiency	Excess
Water Soluble				
Vitamin B_1 (thiamin)	Meat (especially pork and organ meats), grains, dry beans and peas, fish, poultry	Coenzyme (thiamine pyrophosphate) in reactions involving the removal of carbon dioxide in carbohydrate metabolism	Beriberi (peripheral nerve changes, edema, heart failure)	Nervous system hypersensitivity reaction
Vitamin B_2 (riboflavin)	Widely distributed in both animal and vegetable foods	Constituent of two flavin nucleotide coenzymes involved in energy metabolism (FAD and FMN)	Cracks at corner of mouth (cheilosis), inflammation of lips, glossitis, photophobia	None reported
Niacin (can be formed from tryptophan)	Liver, meat, fish, grains, legumes, poultry, peanut butter	Constituent of two coenzymes involved in oxidation-reduction reactions (NAD and NADP)	Pellagra (skin and gastrointestinal lesions, nervous, mental disorders, glossitis)	Flushing, burning, and tingling around neck, face, and hands
Vitamin B_6 (pyridoxine)	Meats (liver), vegetables, whole-grain cereals, egg yolks	Coenzyme (pyridoxal phosphate) involved in amino acid metabolism	Irritability, convulsions, muscular twitching, kidney stones, microcytic hypochromic anemia, glossitis, cheilosis	Severe impairment of the sensory nerves
Pantothenic acid	Widely distributed in all foods; organ meats and whole-grain cereals	Constituent of coenzyme A, which plays a central role in energy metabolism	Fatigue, sleep disturbances, impaired coordination, nausea (rare in humans), GI distress	None reported
Folacin	Liver, kidney, yeast, mushrooms, green vegetables	Coenzyme (reduced form) involved in transfer of single-carbon units in nucleic acid and amino acid metabolism	Macrocytic anemia; gastrointestinal disturbances, diarrhea, glossitis	None reported
Vitamin B_{12} (cobalamin)	Muscle and organ meats, eggs, dairy products (not present in plant foods)	Coenzyme involved in synthesis of single-carbon units in nucleic acid metabolism	Pernicious anemia, neurologic disorders, glossitis	None reported
Biotin	Liver, kidney, milk, egg yolk, yeast	Coenzymes required for synthesis and oxidation of fats, carbohydrates, and deamination	Fatigue, depression, nausea, dermatitis, muscular pains, loss of hair	Not reported

From Lee M, Stanmeyer W, Wight A: *Nutrition and dental health, part I, Assessment of human nutrition requirements,* Carrboro, NC, 1982, Health Sciences Consortium.

Continued

Table 9-6

Dietary Sources and Functions of Vitamins—cont'd

Vitamin	Dietary sources	Major body functions	Deficiency	Excess
Vitamin C (ascorbic acid)	Citrus fruits, tomatoes, green peppers, broccoli, spinach, strawberries, melon	Maintains intercellular matrix of cartilage, bone and dentin; important in collagen synthesis, utilization of iron, calcium, and folic acid	Scurvy (degeneration of skin, teeth, blood vessels, epithelial hemorrhages), delayed wound healing, anemia	Induced scurvy, nausea, abdominal cramps, diarrhea; possible kidney stones
Fat Soluble				
Vitamin A (retinol)	Provitamin A (beta-carotene) widely distributed in green and yellow vegetables and fruits; retinol present in milk, butter, cheese, fortified margarine, egg yolk	Constituent of rhodopsin (visual pigment); maintenance of epithelial tissues; role in mucopolysaccharide synthesis, bone growth, and remodeling	Xerophthalmia (keratinization of ocular tissue), night blindness, folliculosis, respiratory infections	Headache, vomiting, peeling of skin, anorexia, swelling of long bones, resorption of bones
Vitamin D	Fish-liver oil, eggs, dairy products, fortified milk, and margarine	Promotes growth and mineralization of bones and teeth, increases absorption of calcium at intestines	Rickets (bone deformities) in children; osteomalacia in adults	Vomiting, diarrhea, weight loss, kidney damage, hypercalcemia
Vitamin E (tocopherol)	Vegetable oils and seeds, green leafy vegetables, margarines, shortenings	Functions as an antioxidant, in cellular respiration, synthesis of body compounds	Possibly anemia	Relatively nontoxic; possible GI disturbances
Vitamin D (phylloquinone)	Green and yellow vegetables; small amount in cereals, fruits, and meats	Important in blood clotting (involved in formation of active prothrombin)	Conditioned deficiencies associated with severe bleeding, internal hemorrhages	Relatively nontoxic; synthetic forms at high doses may cause jaundice

B. Classification (Table 9-10)
　1. Macrominerals—present in relatively high amounts in body tissues
　2. Microminerals or trace elements—present at less than 0.005% of body weight
C. Chemistry and general functions
　1. Exist as inorganic ions
　2. Chemical identity not altered in the body or food
　3. Indestructible
　4. Soluble in water and tend to form acidic or basic solutions
　5. Vary in amounts absorbed and in pathways of excretion (see Fig. 9-1)
　6. Some readily absorbed into the blood and transported freely
　7. Some require carriers for absorption and transportation
　8. Excessive intakes can be toxic
D. General functions
　1. Maintenance of acid-base balance
　2. Coenzymes or catalysts for biologic reactions
　3. Components of essential body compounds
　4. Maintenance of water balance
　5. Transmission of nerve impulses
　6. Regulation of muscle contraction
　7. Growth of oral and other body tissues
E. Requirements (see Tables 9-4 and 9-5)
F. Dietary sources, specific body functions, and symptoms of deficiencies and toxicities (see Table 9-10)
G. Oral biology

Text continued on p. 379

Table 9-7

Nutrients and Their Preeruptive Effects on Oral Health

Nutrient	Role in tooth formation	Deficiencies*
Vitamin A	1. Normal growth of dentin and enamel	1. Hypoplastic enamel formation 2. Atrophy of odontoblasts with abnormal dentin tubular arrangement
Vitamin C	1. Integrity of blood vessels 2. Hydroxylation of proline and lysine in collagen synthesis	1. Atrophy of odontoblasts 2. Dentin laid down irregularly and at a greatly reduced rate 3. Fragility of vessels in pulpal tissue
Protein	1. Major organic substance in enamel and dentin 2. Collagen formation	1. Small size teeth 2. Late eruption of third molars 3. Altered canine patterns 4. Increased susceptibility to carious lesions 5. Poorly calcified dentinal matrix
Calcium-phosphorus ratio	1. Normal tooth mineralization	1. Decreased molar size 2. Decreased mineralization of enamel and dentin
Vitamin D	1. Control of calcification of dentin and enamel by regulating calcium absorption at intestines	1. Non-functioning ameloblasts with poor enamel mineralization 2. Disturbances in calcification of dentin and cementum 3. Delays in tooth eruption 4. Small size molars
Fluoride	1. Forms strong dentin and enamel apatite crystals through a systemic action	1. Increases solubility of enamel and dentin

From Lee M, Stanmeyer, Wight A: *Nutrition and dental health, part III, Diet and teeth,* Carrboro, NC, 1982, Health Sciences Consortium.
*Many of these deficiencies have been demonstrated in animal research only.

Table 9-8

Nutrients and Their Effects on Oral Soft and Hard Tissues

Nutrient	Function
Proteins (amino acids)	1. Synthesis of epithelial and connective tissues 2. Synthesis of collagen, essential for integrity of connective tissue fibers in soft tissues and the protein matrix in mineralized tissues 3. Synthesis of antibodies and leukocytes, essential for tissues to defend against bacterial irritants 4. Synthesis of new epithelial and connective tissue in the healing process
Vitamin A	1. Synthesis and function of epithelial cells 2. Maintenance of the integrity of sulcus, an important part of the epithelial barrier 3. Normal growth and function of salivary glands 4. Essential for activity of epiphyseal cartilage cells and normal endochondral bone growth 5. Release of proteolytic enzymes (lysosomes) in bone remodeling
Vitamin C	1. Synthesis of connective tissue; essential for hydroxylation of lysine and proline in collagen synthesis 2. Essential for integrity of capillaries and oral mucosa 3. Needed for normal bone matrix formation 4. Needed for normal phagocytic function and antibody synthesis in host defense system
B-complex	1. Function as coenzymes for essential metabolic reactions in epithelial and connective tissues 2. Essential for integrity of gingiva, tongue, buccal mucosa, hard and soft palate 3. Needed for normal phagocytic function and antibody synthesis in host defense system

From Lee M, Stanmeyer W, Wight A: *Nutrition and dental health, part IV, Diet and periodontics,* Carrboro, NC, 1982, Health Sciences Consortium.

Continued

Table 9-8

Nutrients and Their Effects on Oral Soft and Hard Tissues—cont'd

Nutrient	Function
Iron	1. Synthesis of hemoglobin; essential for the transport of oxygen to cells for metabolic activity 2. Essential for normal antibody formation and healing 3. Essential part of many enzymes
Zinc	1. Stabilizes cell membranes 2. Functions in taste acuity 3. Needed in collagen formation 4. Essential in cell-mediated immunity
Calcium	1. Functions in mineralization of protein matrix in oral hard tissues 2. Essential for normal blood clotting, cell membrane function, muscle contraction, and nerve impulse transmission
Vitamin D	1. Essential for absorption and utilization of calcium and phosphorus
Retentive sugars	1. Enhances growth of acidogenic bacteria 2. Results in increased formation of bacterial irritants, such as acids, enzymes, and endotoxins 3. Acts as a substrate for supragingival acidogenic bacteria

Table 9-9

Oral Manifestations of Nutritional Deficiencies and Toxicities

Tissue	Nutrient	Deficiency symptoms	Toxicity symptoms
Oral mucosa	Vitamin A	Keratinizing of epithelium (squamous metaplasia) with hyperkeratotic white patches; generalized gingivitis	Thinning of epithelium resulting in inflamed, hemorrhagic membranes, reddened gingiva
	Vitamin C	Deep red to purple inflamed gingiva with edema, hyperplasia, spontaneous hemorrhaging, ulceration, and necrosis	None
	Thiamin (B_1)	Hypersensitivity and burning sensations	None
	Riboflavin (B_2)	Occasional bluish to purple mucosa	None
	Niacin	Thin and parakeratotic epithelium, inflammation of mucosa (stomatitis); reddened and inflamed marginal and attached gingiva; nonspecific burning sensation	None
	Pyridoxine (B_6)	Stomatitis	None
	Vitamin B_{12}	Stomatitis; pale or yellow-tinged mucosa	None
	Folic acid	Inflamed gingiva; erosion and ulcerations on mucosa; pale mucosa with anemia	None
	Iron	Painful, sore mouth; stomatitis; thinned buccal mucosa with ulcerations and pale to ashen gray color	None
	Zinc	Thickening of epithelium	Stomatitis
Tongue and lips	Vitamin A	None	Cracking and bleeding of lips
	Thiamin (B_1)	Painful or burning tongue; loss of taste acuity	None
	Riboflavin (B_2)	Inflammation, fissures, and ulcers at cornea of the lips (angular cheilitis); dry, scaly lips; red to purple color tongue; atrophy and inflammation of tongue papillae; enlarged fungiform papillae giving the tongue surface a pebbly appearance	None

From Lee M, Stanmeyer W, Wight A: *Nutrition and dental health, part IV, Diet and periodontics,* Carrboro, NC, 1982, Health Sciences Consortium.

Table 9-9

Oral Manifestations of Nutritional Deficiencies and Toxicities—cont'd

Tissue	Nutrient	Deficiency symptoms	Toxicity symptoms
Tongue and lips	Niacin	Atrophy of tongue papillae resulting in a fiery, red, smooth, shiny surface; edematous or enlarged tongue; ulcerations of tongue on central surface; angular cheilitis; loss of appetite	None
	Pyridoxine (B$_6$)	Inflamed and atrophic tongue with a red, smooth appearance; angular cheilitis	None
	Vitamin B$_{12}$	Atrophy and inflammation of tongue; bright red, painful, edematous tongue with glossy appearance; altered taste sensations and decreased appetite	None
	Folic acid	Smooth, bright red tongue; patchy surface of tongue as papillae atrophy; ulcerations along edges of tongue; angular cheilitis	None
	Iron	Angular cheilitis; burning, painful tongue with atrophy of papillae; reddening at tip and around margins of tongue; ulcerations of tongue; pallor to ashen gray color of lips and tongue	None
	Zinc	Impaired taste; thickening and parakeratotic tongue with underlying muscle atrophy	None
	Protein	Red, smooth, edematous tongue; angular cheilitis; fissures on lower lip; depigmentation along buccal border of lips	None
Skin, eyes, salivary glands	Vitamin A	Drying of conjunctiva and cornea of eyes; decreased salivary flow	Dry, scaly skin lesion; a high carotene intake results in a yellow color skin
	Riboflavin (B$_2$)	Greasy, scaly dermatitis of nasolabial folds; keratinizing of corneal surface of eyes, resulting in opacities and ulcerations	None
	Niacin	Scaly and inflamed skin; skin thickening with dark pigmentation of sunlight-exposed skin	None
	Pyridoxine (B$_6$)	Seborrheic lesions of face	None
Bone	Vitamin D and calcium	Failure to mineralize bone matrix resulting in soft, fragile bones with pathologic fractures and skeletal deformities; thinning of cortical bone, resorption of cancellous bone, and enlargement of medullary cavity resulting in overall bone loss; osteomalacia manifested in loss of lamina dura around roots of tooth and increased width of cortical bone	Calcium deposits in bone
	Vitamin C	Defect in collagen formation of osteoid matrix resulting in resorption of alveolar bone	None
Teeth	Fluoride	Less resistant tooth structure to oral irritants	Fluorosis
	Refined carbohydrate	None	Dental caries Bacterial plaque formation
	Vitamin A	Abnormal formation of ameloblasts and odontoblasts during early stages of tooth formation; results in hypoplastic enamel and dentin	None
	Vitamin D, calcium	Abnormal calcification of enamel and dentin	None

Table 9-10

Dietary Sources and Functions of Minerals

Mineral	Dietary sources	Major body functions	Deficiency	Excess
Macrominerals				
Calcium	Milk, cheese, dark-green vegetables, dried legumes, bread	Bone and tooth formation, blood clotting, nerve transmission, muscle contraction	Stunted growth, rickets, osteoporosis, convulsions	Not reported in humans
Phosphorus	Milk, cheese, meat, poultry, grains, eggs	Bone and tooth formation, acid-base balance, release of energy (ADP, ATP)	Weakness, demineralization of bone, loss of calcium	Erosion of jaw (phossy jaw)
Sulfur	Sulfur amino acids (methionine and cystine) in dietary proteins	Constituent of active tissue compounds, cartilage, and tendon	Related to intake and deficiency of sulfur amino acids	Excess sulfur amino acid intake leads to poor growth
Potassium	Meats, milk, many fruits, fish, eggs	Acid-base balance, body water balance, nerve function, muscle relaxant	Muscular weakness, paralysis, heart abnormalities	Muscular weakness, death
Chlorine	Table salt, cured and pickled foods, broth	Formation of gastric juice, acid-base balance	Muscle cramps, mental apathy, reduced appetite	Vomiting
Sodium	Table salt, cured and pickled foods, broth, canned foods	Acid-base balance, body water balance, nerve function	Muscle cramps, mental apathy, reduced appetite	Possibly high blood pressure
Magnesium	Whole grains, green leafy vegetables, cocoa, nuts, soybeans	Activates enzymes involved in protein synthesis	Growth failure, muscle tremors and convulsions	Diarrhea
Microminerals				
Iron	Eggs, lean meats, liver, legumes, whole grains, green leafy vegetables, dried fruit	Constituent of hemoglobin and enzymes involved in energy metabolism	Iron-deficiency anemia (weakness, reduced resistance to infection)	Siderosis, cirrhosis of liver
Fluorine	Drinking water, tea, seafood	May be important in maintenance of bone structure, forms strong apatite crystals during tooth formation	More susceptible to tooth decay	Mottling of teeth, increased bone density, neurologic disturbances
Zinc	High protein foods, whole grains	Constituent of enzymes involved in digestion and metabolism	Growth failure, small sex glands	Loss of iron and copper, anemia
Copper	Meats, drinking water, shellfish, nuts, whole grains	Constituent of enzymes associated with iron metabolism and nerve function	Anemia, bone changes (rare in humans)	Rare metabolic condition (Wilson's disease)
Selenium	Seafood, meat, grains	Functions in close association with vitamin E as an antioxidant	Anemia (rare)	GI disorders, lung irritation, increased tooth decay

From Lee M, Stanmeyer W, Wight A: *Nutrition and dental health, part I, Assessment of human nutrition requirements*, Carrboro, NC, 1982, Health Sciences Consortium.

	Table 9-10			
	Dietary Sources and Functions of Minerals—cont'd			
Mineral	**Dietary sources**	**Major body functions**	**Deficiency**	**Excess**
Manganese	Whole grains, legumes, nuts, tea, green leafy vegetables	Normal skeletal development; involved in fat synthesis, urea formation, energy release	In animals: poor growth, disturbances of nervous system, reproductive abnormalities	Poisoning in manganese mines: generalized disease of nervous system, abnormal iron metabolism
Macrominerals				
Iodine	Marine fish and shellfish, dairy products, table salt, eggs	Constituent of thyroid hormones, regulates energy metabolism	Goiter (enlarged thyroid), cretinism, myxedema	Very high intakes depress thyroid activity
Molybdenum	Legumes, cereals, organ meats	Constituent of enzymes involved in uric acid formation and oxidation of aldehydes	Not reported in humans	Inhibition of enzymes, bone abnormalities
Chromium	Vegetables, grains and cereals, fruit	Involved in glucose and energy metabolism, protein synthesis	Impaired ability to metabolize glucose	Occupational exposures: skin and kidney damage
Cobalt	Organ and muscle meats, milk, poultry, shellfish	Constituent of vitamin B_{12}	Not reported in humans	Enlarged thyroid gland, hyperplasia of bone marrow, polycythemia

1. Function
   a. Tooth formation (Table 9-11; see also Table 9-7)
   b. Periodontium (see Table 9-8)
2. Oral manifestations of deficiencies and toxicities (see Table 9-9)

Water

A. Definition—essential nutrient abundantly found in foods and beverages; makes up 50% to 60% of the total body weight; survival without water is limited to 2 or 3 days
B. Total body water
   1. Body water as a percentage of body weight decreases with age, ranging from 69% in newborn infants to 49% in women
   2. Distribution
      a. Intracellular compartment
         (1) Enclosed within the cell membrane
         (2) Accounts for two thirds of the total
         (3) Increases with increased body cell mass
      b. Extracellular compartment
         (1) Intravascular
            (a) Approximately 3 L
            (b) Includes water in blood vessels
         (2) Intercellular (interstitial)
            (a) Approximately 12 L

         (b) Fluids that leave blood vessels
         (c) Fluids present in spaces between and surrounding each cell
C. Biologic role and functions
   1. Medium in which most of the body's reactions take place
   2. Means for transporting vital materials to cells and waste products away from cells
   3. Regulates a constant body temperature
   4. Maintains a constant composition of elements in body fluids (e.g., calcium, sodium, and fluoride)
   5. Part of the chemical structure of compounds that forms cells (e.g., proteins)
   6. Active in many chemical reactions (e.g., digestion of a disaccharide)
   7. Serves as a solvent (e.g., amino acids dissolve in water, and this permits their transport to body cells)
   8. Lubricates and protects sensitive tissue around joints and mucosal linings
D. Water balance
   1. Intake—controlled by thirst sensations; total daily intake ranges from 1500 to 3000 ml
      a. Sources
         (1) Ingested beverages and foods—1200 to 2000 ml

Table 9-11

Nutrients and Their Posteruptive Effect on Oral Health

Nutrient	Effect on dental caries	Mode of action
Carbohydrates	Cariogenic (sucrose)	1. Substrate for glycolytic organisms to form complex organic acids 2. Substrate for bacterial synthesis of intra- and extracellular polysaccharides (glucan, levan, glycogen) 3. Predisposes implantation of caries-inducing streptococci 4. Predisposes formation and attachment of bacterial plaque on tooth's surface
Fluoride	Cariostatic	1. Favors formation of fluorapatite crystal structure during remineralization of enamel 2. Antimicrobial action 3. Increases rate of maturation of enamel surface 4. Reduces enamel solubility
Phosphate	Cariostatic	1. Iso-ionic exchange of phosphate in oral environment 2. Acts as a buffer 3. Complexes calcium
Other mineral elements	Cariostatic	1. Reduces enamel solubility 2. Enhances maturation process
Fats	Cariostatic	1. Produces a protective oily film on enamel 2. Antimicrobial action
All nutrients and firm textured foods	Salivary glands	1. Normal development 2. Increases flow rate by mastication 3. Influences composition of saliva

From Lee M, Stanmeyer W, Wight A: *Nutrition and dental health, part III, Diet and teeth,* Carrboro, NC, 1982, Health Sciences Consortium.

(2) Metabolic water from the oxidation of foods—200 to 300 ml
2. Elimination—total water output is 1500 to 3000 ml daily
   a. Sensible or measurable losses through the kidneys as urine and through the bowel as feces; constant daily losses amount to 650 to 1800 ml
   b. Insensible or unmeasurable losses through the lungs with expired air and skin as perspiration; daily losses vary considerably with an average of 850 to 1200 ml
E. Regulation
   1. Potassium (K) and sodium (Na) concentrations are responsible for maintaining the water balance; when extracellular sodium equals intracellular potassium, water will not move into or out of the cell
   2. Mechanisms of regulation
      a. Thirst response—when the sodium increases, it stimulates the hypothalamus and induces drinking behavior
      b. Excretion regulation
         (1) Increased sodium stimulates the hypothalamus to signal the pituitary to release the antidiuretic hormone (ADH), and water is reabsorbed in the kidney tubules
         (2) Decreased sodium causes the release of al-

dosterone, which causes a reabsorption of sodium at the kidney tubules
F. Requirements
   1. Adults—1000 ml/1000 calories
   2. Infants—1500 ml/1000 calories
G. Etiology of deficiency and toxicity conditions
   1. Dehydration
      a. Malfunction of kidneys
      b. Blood loss
      c. Vomiting
      d. Diarrhea
      e. No water supply
   2. Water intoxication
      a. Edema
      b. Hypertension
      c. Sodium retention

Specialized Cells of Oral Tissues—Effects of Nutrients

A. Epithelial cells
   1. Important in tooth formation during the embryonic period
   2. Make up the outer layers of tissue in the oral mucosa
      a. Rapid cell renewal, especially in the sulcus area
      b. Cell renewal more frequent as age increases

3. Important in the normal development of salivary glands
4. Vitamin A and protein are essential for the normal proliferation of epithelial cells

B. Fibroblasts
1. Synthesize collagen fibrils in connective tissues of the gingiva, periodontal ligament, and pulp
2. Throughout life, fibroblasts maintain a rate of collagen synthesis equal to that of collagen breakdown; nutrient deficiencies can interfere with this equilibrium and cause a net loss of collagen tissue
3. Vitamin C, zinc, copper, and protein are important in collagen formation

C. Cementoblasts and cementocytes
1. Synthesize the protein matrix for cementum; vitamin C, zinc, copper, and protein are essential
2. Calcify the protein matrix; protein, calcium, phosphorus, and vitamin D are essential
3. Cementum is avascular and part acellular
4. Cellular cementum consists of cementocytes that depend on diffusion from the periodontal ligament for their nutrient supply

D. Ameloblasts
1. Synthesize the protein matrix for enamel; vitamins A and C, zinc, copper, and protein are essential
2. Calcify the protein matrix; protein, calcium, phosphorus, and vitamin D are essential; fluoride improves the quality of the apatite crystals formed
3. Once enamel is formed, no metabolic cells are present

E. Odontoblasts
1. Synthesize the protein matrix for dentin; vitamins A and C, zinc, copper, and protein are essential
2. Calcify the protein matrix; protein, calcium, phosphorus, and vitamin D are essential; fluoride improves the quality of the apatite crystals formed
3. Once dentin is formed, no metabolic cells are present, except in reaction to trauma; with trauma, new odontoblasts can form (possibly from pulpal tissue) and secondary dentin can be laid down

F. Osteocytes—osteoblasts and osteoclasts
1. Function in the synthesis of the alveolus
2. Function in the lifelong process of bone apposition (osteoblasts) and resorption (osteoclasts) in the alveolus
3. Nutrients important in the formation and maintenance of the alveolus are protein, vitamins A, C, and D, zinc, copper, calcium, and phosphorus

Energy Balances and Weight Control

A. Definition—energy balance is a dynamic state in which the energy or calories from food are equal to the energy needs of the body; changes or disturbances in energy balance result in a relative gain or loss in body weight

B. Measurement of energy
1. By calorimetry—food sample is burned in oxygen in an enclosed vessel surrounded by water; 1 kilocalorie is the amount of heat produced sufficient to raise the temperature of 1 kg of water 1° C; (the term *calorie* as commonly used has the same definition)
2. In the body—carbon, hydrogen, and oxygen (from protein, carbohydrates, or fats) are converted to carbon dioxide, water, and energy; energy (kcal) produced is "stored" in ATP until needed; when needed, each ATP molecule loses a high-energy phosphate bond and becomes adenosine diphosphate (ADP) with a release of approximately 7.3 kcal/mole

C. Energy-producing systems
1. Blood glucose—immediate and preferred source of energy for cellular metabolism; glycogen stores provide glucose through glycogenolysis during the short periods of fasting between meals and in response to hormonal signals during sudden movement or intense exercise
   a. Protein—can be used as an energy source when the blood glucose level falls; glucogenic amino acids are converted into glucose after deamination by gluconeogenesis; in starvation, body proteins are used for energy, and this may cause irreversible damage if the essential protein components of the body are catabolized
   b. Fat—mobilized from adipose tissue; triglycerides are broken down into glycerol and fatty acids in the liver; fatty acids are catabolized by β-oxidation to acetyl-CoA
   c. Ethanol (alcohol)—can be oxidized to acetaldehyde, which is then converted into acetyl-CoA
2. Acetyl-CoA—enters the TCA from all sources
3. ATP—made during the process of oxidative phosphorylation in the mitochondria; because of their difference in molecular structure, proteins, carbohydrates, and fats do not all yield the same number of ATP molecules per molecule of starting material; the following can be used as a general guide when estimating the potential energy of foods; protein, 4 kcal/g; carbohydrate, 4 kcal/g; fat, 9 kcal/g; and ethanol, 7 kcal/g

D. Energy-using systems—ATP produced during catabolism is used by the body for biosynthetic activities, muscle contraction, ion transport, nerve conduction, and maintenance of body temperature
1. Energy for basal metabolism—basal metabolic rate (BMR) is a measure of the energy required to

Table 9-12

Median Heights and Weights and Recommended Energy Intake

Category	Age (years) or condition	WEIGHT (kg)	WEIGHT (lb)	HEIGHT (cm)	HEIGHT (in)	REE* (kcal/day)	Multiples of REE	AVERAGE ENERGY ALLOWANCE (kcal)† Per kg	AVERAGE ENERGY ALLOWANCE (kcal)† Per day‡
Infants	0.0–0.5	6	13	60	24	320		108	650
	0.5–1.0	9	20	71	28	500		98	850
Children	1–3	13	29	90	35	740		102	1300
	4–6	20	44	112	44	950		90	1800
	7–10	28	62	132	52	1130		70	2000
Males	11–14	45	99	157	62	1440	1.70	55	2500
	15–18	66	145	176	69	1760	1.67	45	3000
	19–24	72	160	177	70	1780	1.67	40	2900
	25–50	79	174	176	70	1800	1.60	37	2900
	51+	77	170	173	68	1530	1.50	30	2300
Females	11–14	46	101	157	62	1310	1.67	47	2200
	15–18	55	120	163	64	1370	1.60	40	2200
	19–24	58	128	164	65	1350	1.60	38	2200
	25–50	63	138	163	64	1380	1.55	36	2200
	51+	65	143	160	63	1280	1.50	30	1900
Pregnant	1st trimester								+0
	2nd trimester								+300
	3rd trimester								+300
Lactating	1st 6 months								+500
	2nd 6 months								+500

*Calculation based on FAO equations, then rounded.
†In the range of light to moderate activity, the coefficient of variation is ±20%.
‡Figure is rounded.

maintain a living state while at rest and without food; includes respiration, circulation, maintenance of body temperature, muscle tone, glandular activities, and cellular metabolism
  a. Conditions for BMR measurement—postabsorptive state, muscles totally relaxed, awake, environmental temperature between 20° C and 25° C (68° F and 77° F), free of emotional stress, and not during ovulation
  b. Factors influencing the BMR—age, gender, body size, nutritional state, muscular training, pathologic conditions, climate, and altitude
 2. Energy for activity—activity component of the energy requirement is for voluntary physical activity and varies from 20% of the BMR for sedentary activity to 50% or more of the BMR for heavy activity; factors influencing energy needs for the activity component include the size of the individual and the intensity and duration of the activity
 3. Energy for metabolizing food, or the specific dynamic energy (SDE), is the energy required to "gear up" to digest, absorb, and metabolize food; also called "nonshivering thermogenesis" because there is a slight elevation in body temperature after eating; not a clearly defined phenomenon; believed to include the energy needed to increase muscular contractions of the digestive tract, increase synthesis of digestive enzymes, and transport molecules; amounts to about 10% of the BMR and activity energy components
E. Requirements
 1. Determination—by an intake of food energy that allows maintenance of ideal weight; data have been gathered from animal studies, balance studies, and intake surveys
  a. Recommendations represent average needs of people in each age group and within a given activity category (Table 9-12)
  b. Recommendations are influenced by body size, gender, climate, age, and activity level
 2. Empty-calorie foods—provide energy but few other nutrients (e.g., concentrated sweets, alcohol, and fats)

F. Weight-reduction programs
1. Calculation of caloric intake needs
   a. Determine the ideal body weight (IBW) from published tables (see Table 9-12) or by using the following rule of thumb
      (1) Males IBW = 106 + (6 × inches over 5 feet tall)
      (2) Females IBW = 100 + (5 × inches over 5 feet tall)
   b. Determine the caloric requirement (kilocalories/pound)

	ACTIVITY LEVEL		
	Sedentary	Moderate	Very active
Overweight	10	11	12
Normal	13	14	15
Underweight	16	17	18

   c. Alternate method—decrease in usual caloric intake by 500 kcal/day usually allows a 1 pound/week weight loss; this loss may plateau as the body adjusts to a new BMR
2. Types of diet modifications
   a. Balanced, low calorie—if calories are about 1000 kcal/day and the intake is balanced and varied, this is the safest and healthiest reducing diet (e.g., Weight Watchers Diet)
   b. Low carbohydrate—may risk developing ketosis (e.g., Stillman's Diet)
   c. Low fat—may deprive the individual of essential fatty acids and fat-soluble vitamins; causes rapid emptying of the stomach (low satiety) and may make food seem flavorless; most individuals can decrease their usual fat intake without any harmful effects
   d. High fiber—increases fiber and bulk in the diet and allows a more rapid transit time for food in the gastrointestinal tract; fiber also binds other nutrients so they are not completely absorbed; moderate increases in the fiber content of the diet (e.g., in well-designed vegetarian diets) appear to be helpful in treating diabetes, diverticulosis, and hypercholesterolemia, as well as decreasing the total calorie intake in reducing diets; very high fiber diets cause gastrointestinal discomfort and may induce mineral deficiencies (e.g., Beverly Hills Diet)
   e. Single food (monotonous)—no one food by itself can provide a balance of nutrients; one must eat a variety of foods from the basic four food groups; diets that promote a single food with unrealistic claims are not recommended (e.g., the grapefruit diet)
   f. Liquid formulas (protein)—are very low calorie diets, and although they have been successfully used in treating very obese patients in a carefully monitored hospital setting, they are not recommended for the individual (e.g., Cambridge Diet)
3. Activity in weight management—even moderate activity such as walking will increase caloric expenditure and should be considered in every weight-loss program; moderate exercise also improves muscle tone, stimulates circulation, increases BMR, and often creates a sense of well-being
4. Behavior modification—often eating habits and attitudes must be changed to prevent weight regain; many successful diet programs combine decreased food intake and increased activity with an analysis and modification of eating behaviors; group programs, such as Weight Watchers, help provide behavioral changes
5. Dietary aids—represent a multimillion dollar business, and although they may help cause an initial rapid weight loss, they are no more effective than mere calorie cutting in long-term weight maintenance; moreover, most diet drugs have the potential for serious side effects if used habitually over a long period or by persons with certain medical conditions; types most often used are appetite suppressants, stimulants, laxatives, diuretics, and bulk-producing agents
6. Long-term success in weight reduction by any plan is poor, with an estimated average success rate of only 5%
7. Recent studies indicate that genetic factors may play a greater factor in obesity and the inability to maintain a satisfactory weight loss than had previously been assumed
G. Underweight conditions
1. Treatment
   a. Correct any underlying physiologic causes of weight loss
   b. Increase caloric intake with foods that are concentrated sources of energy and with several small meals per day
   c. Limit weight-gain goals to 1 to 2 pounds/week
2. Anorexia nervosa—state of protein energy malnutrition (PEM) brought on by voluntary starvation (and often with the use of diet aids, intense exercise, and self-induced vomiting); seen most often in middle- and upper-income adolescent females who are typically described as perfectionists, overachievers, and models of good behavior; they begin dieting

because they have a distorted perception of body shape and weight; death may occur due to multiple organ system failure; treatment usually includes specially tailored counseling and hospitalization before voluntary weight gain is possible

3. Bulimia—condition of alternate food gorging and purging by vomiting and/or use of laxatives to maintain weight; most often found in adolescent females who appear to be of normal weight; is more prevalent than anorexia nervosa; treatment involves counseling; self-induced vomiting can cause swelling of the salivary glands and esophagus and acid-destruction of tooth enamel

Nutritional Counseling

Malnutrition

A. Overconsumption of nutrients
1. Fat—can result in excess calories and weight; associated with coronary heart disease (CHD), obesity and certain types of cancer
2. Sugar—can result in excess calories and weight; associated with obesity, dental caries, and plaque-induced gingivitis
3. Salt or sodium—can result in excess body fluid retention; associated with high blood pressure; increased sodium may also decrease calcium
4. Calories—can result in excess weight and obesity; associated with CHD, hypertension, and diabetes mellitus type II
5. Vitamin and mineral supplementation—megadoses (500% to 1000% of RDAs) can result in toxicity of one or many nutrients and inhibition of others
B. Nutrient deficiencies—health of a person is at risk because of the unavailability of nutrients for cellular activities; end result of deficiencies is the same, but the multiple causes can be classified as primary or secondary
1. Primary deficiency is a result of an inadequate food intake and can result from the following conditions
   a. Fad diets—low calorie or imbalanced diet plans
   b. Economics—inadequate resources to provide a healthy diet
   c. Illness—loss of appetite
   d. Improper food preparation—destruction of nutrients because of delayed storage and overcooking of foods
   e. Accessibility to food—nutritious foods unavailable because of patient transportation problems or market supplies
   f. Ignorance—lack of nutritional knowledge

g. Flavor preferences—palatability of sweets and fats can lead to a diet high in empty-calorie foods
h. Time constraints—inadequate time for food preparation can lead to the use of highly processed convenience foods, which have a lower nutrient density than the basic foods
i. Poor oral health—inability to masticate food because of edentulism or oral disease; altered taste perceptions result from oral disease
2. Secondary deficiency is a result of an inability to digest, absorb, and use foods consumed; person may eat a balanced diet, but other factors interfere with the use of nutrients in foods; examples of these conditioning factors include
   a. Disease—any gastrointestinal or metabolic disease can interfere with the digestion and use of foods and nutrients (e.g., ulcers, lactase deficiency, partial obstruction of the gastrointestinal tract, and inborn errors of metabolism)
   b. Drug-nutrient interactions—certain drugs can interfere with and reduce the absorption, transportation, and metabolism of nutrients
   c. Nutrient-nutrient interactions—excess or deficiency of certain nutrients can affect absorption of other nutrients (e.g., vitamin C and iron)
   d. Allergies—sensitivity to certain foods or chemicals in foods can lead to malabsorption syndromes (e.g., gluten sensitivity such as in celiac disease)
3. Manifestations of primary and secondary deficiencies
   a. Gradual decreases in the tissue level of nutrients
      (1) Earliest sign of malnutrition
      (2) Determined by blood and urine analysis for each nutrient
   b. Biochemical disturbances
      (1) Duration of deficiency is long enough to deplete body stores and interfere with cellular metabolism
      (2) Determined by blood and urine analysis for alterations in cellular levels of enzymes and metabolites
   c. Anatomic lesions
      (1) Signs of chronic and severe malnutrition, leading to destruction of body tissues
      (2) Determined by clinical examination of body tissues

Complete Nutritional Assessment

A. Health history
1. Factors that influence food intake
   a. Socioeconomic conditions—food-purchasing power

Table 9-13

Some Laboratory Blood and Urine Tests Used in the Evaluation of Nutritional Status*

Body fluid	General level of nutrient or metabolite tested	Nutrient imbalance suggested†
Whole blood	Low ascorbate	↓ Ascorbate
	Low hemoglobin	
	Low erythrocytes (hematocrit)	↓ Iron
Erythrocytes	Low folate	↓ Folate
Blood serum	High cholesterol	
	High triglycerides	↑ Lipids
	High lipoproteins	↑ Kcal
	High albumin	↓ Protein
	Low total protein	
	Low vitamin B_{12}	↓ Vitamin B_{12}
	Low thymidylate synthase	
	Low vitamin A	
	Low carotene	↓ Vitamin A
	Low 25-OH cholecalciferol	
	Low alkaline phosphatase	↓ Vitamin D
	Low calcium and phosphorus	
Blood plasma	Low amino acids	↓ Protein
Urine	Low urea/creatinine	↓ Protein
	Low thiamin	
	Low erythrocyte transketolase	↓ Thiamin
	Low riboflavin	
	Low erythrocyte glutathione reductase	↓ Riboflavin
	Low methylmalonic acid	↓ Vitamin B_{12}
	Low iodine	↓ Iodine
	High FIGLU	↓ Folate
	High xanthurenic acid	↓ Vitamin B_6

From Reed P: *Nutrition: An applied science*, Edinburgh, 1980, Churchill Livingstone.
*The type of imbalance suggested by the general level of the nutrient or metabolite is included.
† A downward arrow (↓) indicates an undersupply of the nutrient; an upward arrow (↑) indicates an oversupply.

b. Home environment—culture, family values, and eating practices

c. Client motivation and education—interest and awareness of the principles for eating a nutritious diet

2. Factors that influence food use

   a. Oral health—ability to masticate, saliva production, and presence of oral disease

   b. Medical health—ability to digest, absorb, and metabolize nutrients in food; therapeutic diets for disease control

B. Assessment of dietary intakes

1. Collection of objective data on what a patient eats

   a. Assessment tools—screening questionnaire for food intake frequency, 24-hour recall method, and food record or diary

   b. Specific amounts or quantities of foods eaten must be recorded to use assessment tools

2. Analysis and evaluation of food intake

   a. Methods of analysis—Daily Food Guide of the Food Guide Pyramid, computer analysis for specific nutrients

   b. Methods of evaluation—comparing results of diet analysis with standards of adequacy

3. Diet modifications

   a. Adding foods to the diet to correct for nutrient deficiencies

   b. Eliminating or reducing excessive nutrient intakes for disease control and prevention (e.g., sugar, fat, or sodium)

C. Biochemical evaluation (Table 9-13)

1. Blood and urine analysis

   a. Most objective and precise assessment data

   b. Determines marginal nutritional deficiencies before overt clinical signs appear by measuring either the concentration of a nutrient or the functional activity of the nutrient

2. Delayed cutaneous hypersensitivity skin tests

Table 9-14

Some Classical Symptoms of Poor Nutritional Status and the Nutrient Imbalances They Indicate

Area examined	Symptom	Nutrient imbalance suggested*
Skin	Follicular hyperkeratosis	↓ Vitamin A
	Petechiae	↓ Vitamin C
	Dark dermatitis in areas exposed to sunlight	↓ Niacin
	Flaky dermatitis	↓ Protein-energy (kwashiorkor)
	Pallor	↓ Iron, folate, vitamin B$_{12}$, copper
Eyes	Xerosis	↓ Vitamin A
	Keratomalacia	
	Bitot's spot	
	Inflamed conjunctiva	↓ Vitamin A, riboflavin
Mouth and tongue	Cheilosis	↓ Riboflavin
	Glossitis (magenta tongue)	
	Glossitis (red, raw tongue)	↓ Niacin, folacin, iron
	Gingivitis (bleeding, spongy gums)	↓ Vitamin C
	Carious teeth	↓ Fluoride
		↑ Sugar
Hair	Depigmentation	↓ Protein-energy
	Thin, sparse, poor texture	↓ Protein-energy
Nails	Koilonychia (spoon nails)	↓ Iron
Subcutaneous fat	Little fat	↓ Protein-energy (marasmus, starvation)
	Excessive fat	↑ Energy nutrients
	Edema	↓ Protein-energy (kwashiorkor), thiamin
Musculature	Wasted muscles	↓ Protein-energy (marasmus, starvation)
	Paralysis at extremities	↓ Thiamin, B$_{12}$
Skeletal structure	Bowed legs, knock-knees	↓ Vitamin D
	Rosary beading of ribs	↓ Vitamin C

From Reed P: *Nutrition: An applied science,* Edinburgh, 1980, Churchill Livingstone.
*↓ Indicates an undersupply of the nutrient; ↑ indicates an oversupply.

a. Assessment of the host defense mechanisms by evaluating the patient's reaction to common skin test antigens as a nonspecific indicator of malnutrition
b. Most useful for evaluating the critically ill patient's ability to withstand the stresses of surgery
3. Multielemental hair analysis
a. Chemical analysis of hair for mineral status
b. Questionable usefulness as a reliable and accurate assessment
(1) Lack of information correlating hair mineral concentrations with body levels of minerals
(2) Lack of information on normal ranges for mineral concentration in hair
(3) Lack of control for hair changes because of environmental factors (e.g., shampoos and air pollution)
D. Clinical examination of body tissues—indicator of

general health and nutritional status (Table 9-14; see also Table 9-9)
1. Oral tissues
a. Dental caries—excessive sugar or acid exposure
b. Gingivitis and periodontal disease—excessive sugar intake and nutritional deficiencies
c. Glossitis—nutritional deficiencies affecting tongue papillae and color
d. Stomatitis—nutritional deficiencies affecting oral soft tissues
e. Cheilosis—nutritional deficiencies affecting the lips and corners of the mouth
f. Acute necrotizing ulcerative gingivitis—excessive sugar and caffeine intakes combined with nutritional deficiencies result in stress and lowered tissue resistance to bacterial plaque and bacterial insults
2. Anthropometric analysis—determines the body structure, form, and composition (e.g., content of

lean body mass and fat tissue); the following tools are useful, but each has its limitations
  a. Height and weight standards based on body frame size
  b. Skinfold thickness measurements
    (1) Obtained by using skinfold calipers to measure subcutaneous fat in millimeters in selected areas (e.g., triceps and subscapular regions)
    (2) Measurements are compared with standards to estimate total body fat composition
  c. Arm muscle circumference
    (1) Sensitive indicator of the muscle mass that reflects protein stores
    (2) Determined by measuring the arm circumference at the midpoint of the upper arm and triceps skinfold measurements
  d. Bioelectrical impedance and ultrasound methods
    (1) Potential predictors of total body fat
    (2) Currently being tested for reliability and validity
  3. Other body tissues (Table 9-14)

Methods for Assessment of Dietary Intake

A. Dietary intake standards
  1. RDAs (see Table 9-4)
    a. "The levels of intake of essential nutrients considered, in the judgment of the Committee on Dietary Allowances of The Food and Nutrition Board on the basis of available scientific knowledge, to be adequate to meet the known nutritional needs of practically all healthy persons"[1]
    b. Appropriate use
      (1) Planning and evaluating food supplies for groups
      (2) Standards for evaluating food-consumption records
      (3) Guidelines for new food products
      (4) Basis for regulatory standards of nutritional quality
      (5) Standards for nutritional labeling: the percent of daily value (% DV) used in labelling is based on the RDA values
  2. Dietary goals for the United States—recommendations made by the U.S. Senate Select Committee on Nutrition and Human Needs in 1977 to modify the intake of those foods associated with the leading causes of mortality and morbidity in the United States
    a. Consume only enough calories to balance energy expenditures
    b. Increase the consumption of complex carbohydrates to 48% of the total energy intake
    c. Reduce the intake of refined and processed sugars to 10% of the total energy intake
    d. Reduce fat consumption to 30% or less of the total energy intake
    e. Reduce saturated-fat consumption to 10%, and balance it with equal amounts of polyunsaturated and monounsaturated fats
    f. Reduce cholesterol to 300 mg/day
    g. Limit sodium intake by reducing the intake of salt (NaCl) to about 5 g each day
  3. Dietary Guidelines for Americans (USDA, USDHEW, 1995)
    a. Eat a variety of foods
    b. Balance the food you eat with physical activity; maintain or improve your weight
    c. Choose a diet with plenty of grain products, vegetables, and fruits
    d. Choose a diet low in fat, saturated fat, and cholesterol
    e. Choose a diet moderate in sugars
    f. Choose a diet moderate in salt and sodium
    g. If you drink alcoholic beverages, do so in moderation
  4. Food and Nutrition Board's recommendations for healthy adult Americans
    a. "Adjust dietary energy intake and energy expenditure so as to maintain appropriate weight for height; if overweight, achieve appropriate weight reduction by decreasing total food and fat intake and by increasing physical activity"[1]
    b. If the requirement for energy is low (e.g., reducing diet), reduce the consumption of foods such as alcohol, sugars, fats, and oils that provide calories but few other essential nutrients
    c. Use salt in moderation; adequate salt intakes are considered to range between 3 and 8 g of sodium chloride daily
    d. Select a nutritionally adequate diet from the foods available by each day consuming appropriate servings of dairy products, meats or legumes, vegetables and fruits, and cereals and breads (Table 9-15)
    e. Select as wide a variety of foods in each of the major food groups as is practicable to ensure a high probability of consuming adequate quantities of all essential nutrients
  5. Food Guide Pyramid (USDA and DHHS) (Fig. 9-4)
    a. Graphically organizes foods into five groups and conveys three essential elements of a healthy diet

Table 9-15

Daily Guide to Food Choices

Food group	DAILY RECOMMENDED SERVINGS			Foods and portion sizes for one serving	Nutrient contribution
	1600 kcal	2200 kcal	2800 kcal		
Dairy	2-3	2-3	2-3	Milk (skim, whole, low fat, buttermilk)—1 cup	Calcium
					Riboflavin
				Cheese—1½ oz	Protein
				Cheese food—2 oz	Phosphorus
				Cottage cheese—1 cup	*When fortified:*
				Ice cream—1½ cup	Vitamin D
				Yogurt—1 cup	Vitamin A
				Pudding or custard—1 cup	
Meat (oz)	5		7	Meat, fish, poultry—lean	Protein
				Hot dogs, luncheon meats	Niacin, thiamin
					Iron, zinc
Alternatives (equiv to 1 oz meat)				Eggs (1), peanut butter (2 Tbsp)	Magnesium
				Legumes cooked (½ cup)	Phosphorus
				Tofu (4 oz), nuts (2 Tbsp)	Vitamin B_6, B_{12}
Fruits	2	3	4	Fresh fruit—1 med size or ½ cup	Vitamin A, C
				Cooked fruit—½ cup	Potassium
				Juice—¼ cup	Fiber
				Dried fruit—¼ cup	Iron (dried fruits)
Vegetables	3	4	5	Cooked or raw—½ cup	Vitamin A, C
				Leafy raw—1 cup	Folate
				Juice—¾ cup	Potassium
					Magnesium
					Fiber
					Iron (legumes, some dark green)
Breads, cereal and grains	6	9	11	Bread—1 slice	Complex carbohydrates
				Cooked cereal, rice, pasta—½ cup	Riboflavin
					Thiamin
				Dry cereal—1 oz	Niacin
				Bagel, small bun, English muffin—½	Iron
					Protein
				Small roll, biscuit, muffin—1	Magnesium
				Cracker—2 large, 4 small	
Total fat	53 gm	73 gm	93 gm		Essential fatty acids
					Energy
Added sugar	6 tsp	12 tsp	18 tsp		Energy

    (1) The relative amounts of foods to choose from each group
    (2) The variety within each group
    (3) Moderation in eating fats, oils, and sweets
  b. Recommendations
    (1) 6-11 servings of breads, cereals, rice and pasta
    (2) 3-5 servings of vegetables
    (3) 2-4 servings of fruit
    (4) 2-3 servings of dairy products
    (5) 2-3 servings of meat, eggs, beans, and nuts

    (6) sparing use of fats, oils, and sweets
B. Methods for collecting data on food intakes
  1. Nutritional screening questionnaire (see box on p. 390)
    a. Description—patient indicates frequency of sugar and food-group intake over a day or week
    b. Advantages
      (1) Can be filled out by the patient while waiting in the oral healthcare setting
      (2) Requires 15 to 20 minutes to complete
      (3) Allows analysis of food-group consumption

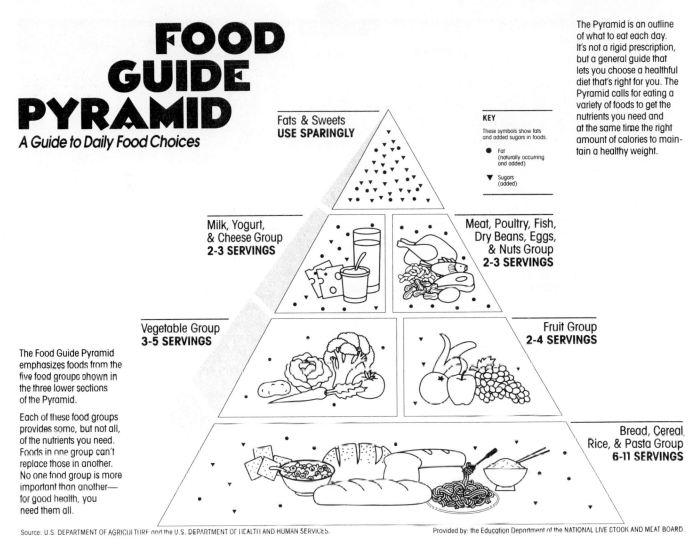

Fig. 9-4   The Food Group Pyramid.

(4) Allows sugar-intake evaluation
  c. Limitations
    (1) No nutrient analysis
    (2) Relies on the patient's memory
2. Twenty-four-hour dietary recall
  a. Description—interviewer collects data from the patient on all food consumed over a 24-hour period
  b. Advantages
    (1) Requires 20 minutes for the interview
    (2) Allows nutrient analysis
    (3) Allows analysis of food-group consumption
    (4) Allow sugar-intake evaluation
  c. Limitations
    (1) Requires a trained interviewer
    (2) Relies on the patient's memory

(3) Represents only 1 day of food consumption
    (4) Requires a nutrient data file on foods to analyze nutrients
3. Three- to seven-day food record or diary
  a. Description—patient keeps a record of food and eating times for 3 to 7 days
  b. Advantages
    (1) No interviewer required except to give directions on how to fill out the record
    (2) Allows for both nutrient and food-group analysis
    (3) Allows for sugar-intake evaluation
    (4) An average intake of several days may be more representative of the patient's food intake than 1 day

NUTRITIONAL SCREENING QUESTIONNAIRE

Name _____ Date _____

Chart No. _____

1. How many meals do you have a day? _____
   About what times are these eaten? _____
2. Would you consider your appetite to be:
   Good _____
   Fair _____
   Poor _____
3. How often do you eat between meals?
   Never _____
   Occasionally _____
   Often _____
   What foods do you usually eat between meals? _____
   _____

4. How often do you drink soft drinks, fruit drinks, or any other sweetened beverages?
   Never _____
   Occasionally _____
   Often _____ (times/day)
   When do you drink these beverages?
   With meals _____
   Between meals _____
   At both/either time(s) _____
5. How often do you drink coffee and/or tea?
   Never _____
   Occasionally _____
   Often _____ (cups/day)
   How do you drink your coffee/tea? With:
   Milk/cream _____
   Cremora _____
   Sweetener _____
      (Specify the kind)
6. How often do you use gum and/or mints?
   Never _____
   Occasionally _____
   Often _____
   What brand do you use?
   _____

7. How often do you use cough drops, throat lozenges, and/or antacid tablets? (Please circle which ones)
   Never _____
   Occasionally _____
   Often _____
8. How often do you take vitamin or mineral supplements?
   Never _____
   Occasionally _____
   Daily _____
   What is your supplement? _____
      (Specify the type of vitamins or minerals?
9. Are you presently on any special or restricted diet? Yes _____ No _____
   If so, what kind? _____

Modified from DePaola D, Cheney H: *Preventive dentistry,* Littleton, Mass, 1979, PSG/Wright Publishing.

NUTRITIONAL SCREENING QUESTIONNAIRE—cont'd

	Never	Times/day	Times/week
10. a. How often do you eat/drink milk, cheese, yogurt, or other dairy foods?			
b. How often do you eat whole-grain or enriched breads, cereals, or pasta?			
c. How often do you eat cooked or raw vegetables?			
d. How often do you eat/drink citrus fruit or juice (orange, grapefruit, tomato)?			
e. How often do you eat one of the following: carrots, pumpkin, sweet potatoes, greens, broccoli, spinach (or other dark yellow or green vegetable or fruit)?			
f. How often do you eat meat, fish, poultry, or eggs?			
g. How often do you eat peanut butter, nuts, dried peas or beans, or soybean products?			
h. How often do you eat your meals in restaurants or fast-food places?			

   c. Limitations
     (1) Represents the food consumption of only the days included in the record
     (2) Relies on the cooperation and ability of the patient to keep the record
     (3) Requires a nutrient data file for nutrient analysis
C. Methods for evaluating food intake
  1. Daily Food Guide
    a. Nutrient contributions (Table 9-16)
     (1) Role in general health
     (2) Role in oral health
    b. Advantages for use in counseling
     (1) Patient participation
     (2) Simple
     (3) Inexpensive
     (4) Fairly accurate
     (5) Patient can use at home after a session for self and for family
    c. Limitations
     (1) No provisions made for combination foods (e.g., pizza or casseroles); need to break down into ingredients that correspond to the five food groups
     (2) No nutrient analysis
  2. Computer diet analysis
    a. Definition—foods are individually entered into a computer, and the specific amounts of each nutrient for each food consumed are calculated

    b. Nutrient data file (software)—contains food with their nutrients
    c. RDAs—used as a standard for comparison with the patient's daily nutrient intake (see Table 9-4)
    d. Advantages
     (1) Accurate
     (2) Specific
     (3) Cost-efficient when hardware available
       (a) Microcomputers in oral healthcare settings
       (b) Services available outside the oral healthcare setting for a fee
    e. Limitations
     (1) Limited patient participation and home use
     (2) Hardware and software availability
     (3) Expensive
  3. Sugar analysis and evaluation
    a. Dental caries and periodontal disease are multifactorial diseases that result from the interaction of the resistance of oral tissues (host factor) to the destructive effects of bacterial plaque and acids (agent factor) produced from metabolism of dietary sugars (diet or environment factor); dental disease occurs when all three factors exist simultaneously and is often called the "triad" of dental disease; nutritional assessment of sugar exposure is an essential part of nutritional counseling in preventive dentistry programs and can

Table 9-16

Nutrient Contribution and Functions of the Food Groups

Food group	Nutrient contribution	Function in the body	Function in oral health
Milk	Proteins	4 kcal per gram, constituent of every cell; builds and repairs tissues and forms antibodies to resist infection	Collagen formation; formation of the matrix of dentin and enamel, maintains the integrity of periodontal tissues
	Calcium and phosphorus	Calcification of the body's hard tissues, involved in blood clotting, muscle and nerve activity	Normal tooth and bone mineralization
	B_{12} (B-complex)	Coenzyme involved in synthesis of single-carbon units in nucleic acid metabolism	Integrity of nerve tissue and normal red blood cell formation in oral tissues
	Riboflavin (B-complex)	Constituent of two flavin nucleotide coenzymes (FAD, FMN) in energy metabolism	Energy metabolism of oral tissues
	Vitamin D	Necessary for the absorption of calcium from the intestines; regulation of calcium and phosphorus homeostasis	Needed for calcium absorption which is important for tooth and bone mineralization
Meat	Proteins	(See milk group)	(See milk group)
	Pyridoxine (B-complex)	Coenzyme in carbohydrate and amino acid metabolism, cofactor in formation of porphyrin in hemoglobin synthesis	Normal carbohydrate and protein metabolism and hemoglobin synthesis in oral tissues
	Niacin (B-complex)	Constituents of two coenzymes involved in oxidation-reduction reactions (NAD, NADP)	Integrity of oral tissues
	Folacin (B-complex)	Coenzyme involved in transfer of single-carbon units in nucleic acid and amino acid metabolism	Normal synthesis of protein compounds in oral tissues (e.g., enzymes, hemoglobin)
	Thiamin (B-complex)	Coenzyme (thiamine pyrophosphate) in reactions involving the removal of carbon dioxide	Normal energy metabolism during development and maintenance of oral tissues
	B_{12} (B-complex)	(See milk group)	(See milk group)
	Iron	Combines with protein to form hemoglobin, constituent of enzymes involved in energy metabolism	Normal hemoglobin formation and oxygen transportation to oral tissues
	Vitamin A	Integrity of epithelial tissues; synthesis of mucopolysaccharides and rhodopsin (visual purple)	Normal growth of enamel and dentin; normal growth of periodontal tissues and maintenance of epithelium
Fruits and vegetables	Vitamin A	(See meat group)	(See meat group)
	Vitamin C	Hydroxylation of lysine and proline in collagen formation; wound healing and resisting infection	Collagen formation; integrity of blood vessels in gingival and pulpal tissues; normal formation of dentin
	Folacin (B-complex)	(See meat group)	(See meat group)
	Pyridoxine (B-complex)	(See meat group)	(See meat group)
	Fiber (indigestible carbohydrate)	Adds bulk to diet	Stimulates salivary flow; integrity of periodontal tissues
Bread and cereal	Thiamin	(See meat group)	(See meat group)
	Riboflavin	(See milk group)	(See milk group)
	Niacin	(See meat group)	(See meat group)
	Iron	(See meat group)	(See meat group)
	Fiber	(See fruit and vegetable group)	(See fruit and vegetable group)

From Lee M, Stanmeyer W, Wight A: *Nutrition and dental health, part V, Nutrition counseling,* Carrboro, NC, 1982, Health Sciences Consortium.

be conducted by using precise or simplified methods

(1) Precise analysis—computer analysis of the diet for carbohydrate content: total carbohydrate in grams, monosaccharides and disaccharides in grams (e.g., grams of sucrose), and fiber in grams; percentage of the total daily calorie intake from simple and complex carbohydrates can be calculated and compared with the recommendations: 48% complex, 10% simple

(2) Simplified analysis—dietary sugars (sweets and foods processed with sugars; see Table 9-3) are circled on the food record or recall; cariogenicity of the diet is assessed based on the frequency and form of sugar exposure; frequent exposure to retentive solid sugars, especially between meals, is harmful; acid production potential of the diet can be calculated by using the following formula

Total daily solid sugar exposures × 40 minutes + Total daily liquid sugar exposures × 20 minutes =
Total minutes of acid exposure to oral tissues from dietary sugars; should not exceed 100 min

Formula is based on research that shows glucose rinses result in a drop of oral pH below the critical level (5.5 pH—where acids decalcify enamel) and that it takes 20 minutes for saliva to neutralize acids and raise the pH to a safe level; solid sugars adhere to teeth and have approximately double the acid production potential

b. Caries-activity tests—often involve counting the number of acidogenic bacteria or measuring the acids produced by these bacteria; provide information about the current oral environment and help to detect dental caries activity; are valuable adjuncts in patients' plaque control programs and can be used to monitor a patient's progress in oral home care and diet modifications; names of some tests include the Snyder, Sim, and Grainger tests

Nutritional Counseling Techniques

A. Direct approach—counseling technique that focuses on the dietary problem
   1. Role of the patient—patient provides information on the diet; is passive and listens to the counselor
   2. Role of the counselor—counselor controls the session; analyzes and evaluates the patient's diet and makes recommendations for improvement
   3. Advantages—easier for the counselor and often requires less time than a more patient-oriented approach
   4. Limitations—fosters patient dependence; little chance of success if the patient is not committed to dietary changes

B. Nondirect or behavior modification approach—counseling technique that focuses on the patient
   1. Role of the patient—patient actively participates in the diet analysis, evaluation, and modification program
   2. Role of the counselor—counselor provides information on the etiology of dental disease, the role of the diet, and the use of dietary assessment tools
   3. Method
      a. Assumption—dietary habits are learned behaviors and can be "unlearned" and replaced with new behaviors
      b. Collection of baseline data
      c. Patient takes ownership of the dietary problems and is committed to change
      d. Patient determines the behavior changes and goals; develops own reward system to use when goals are met
      e. Changes are gradually made in small steps; appropriate changes are rewarded and failures ignored
      f. Close monitoring of progress until new behaviors become self-reinforcing
   4. Advantages—fosters patient independence; success is more likely because the patient is in control of the change process
   5. Limitations—more time and effort needed to arrive at appropriate solutions to dietary problems and rewards for behavior modification

C. Factors that influence the patient's food intake—any combination of the following influences affects food choices and needs to be addressed in a modification program
   1. Environmental influences—economics, lifestyle, geography, seasons, markets
   2. Social influences—family, culture, religion, social pressures, marketing strategies
   3. Psychologic influences—self-image, emotions, stresses, values, priorities

D. Determinants for dental patient selection
   1. High-risk patients—patients with conditions that would benefit most from nutritional counseling
      a. Pregnancy—nutrient needs are high; hormonal changes may lead to exaggerated responses to plaque and bacterial toxins; maternal diet affects the formation of fetal oral tissues
      b. Adolescence—nutrient needs are high; vulner-

able to nutritional problems from fad diets for weight loss and muscle building; frequent snacking on empty-calorie foods; problems of anorexia and bulimia can lead to enamel erosion (permolysis), irritation to oral mucosa, and infected or swollen salivary glands with possible xerostomia

c. Rampant caries—high bacterial plaque and calculus and/or a positive caries-activity test may indicate a frequent sugar-exposure problem

d. Periodontal disease or necrotic ulcerated gingivitis—frequent exposure to sugar and nutritional deficiencies can contribute to the development and progression of these conditions

e. Oral surgery—nutritional counseling before and after surgery is important for optimal surgical recovery; postsurgical nutrient needs are high because of blood loss, tissue repair, and host defense activities; modifications in food texture (e.g., soft foods) are made according to the ability to masticate

f. Edentulism—inability to masticate can result in nutrient deficiencies because of the limited nutrient content in soft and liquid foods

g. Oral cancer—nutrient needs are high because of host defense activities and tissue repair from cancer and its treatment; cancer or treatment may result in inadequate food intake because of decreased appetite, altered taste perceptions, irritated oral tissues, and xerostomia

2. Office resources—availability of trained personnel, time, and facilities to conduct nutrition counseling services

3. Patient factors—level of patient motivation to use and benefit from nutritional counseling and patient financial and intellectual capabilities for using nutritional counseling services

Dietary Modifications for Specific Dental Conditions

A. Dental caries (see Tables 9-7 and 9-11)
1. Role of nutrients in tooth formation
   a. Preeruptive effects—nutrients are used systemically for enamel, dentin, and pulp formation; tooth bud formation begins at 6 weeks in utero, and calcification is completed at 13 years
   b. Posteruptive effects—fluoride aids in the remineralization of small enamel lesions; there is evidence that specific minerals or combinations of minerals and fats have local cariostatic properties
2. Local effect of dietary carbohydrates on bacteria growth and plaque formation (see pp. 357-367)

3. Role of diet and nutrients in salivary gland function
   a. Nutrients are used systemically for the normal development and secretory function of salivary glands
   b. Foods of firm texture (e.g., raw vegetables) enhance mastication, stimulate the salivary flow rate, and modify the concentration of constituents in saliva, possibly improving antibacterial properties and the buffering capacity to neutralize decalcifying acids
B. Periodontal disease (see Table 9-8)
1. Role of nutrients in the formation of periodontal tissues
   a. Nutrients are used systemically for the normal development of the gingiva, periodontal ligament, cementum, and alveolus
   b. Periodontal tissues are metabolically active throughout the patient's life, and nutrients are constantly needed for maintenance (e.g., the cell population of the sulcular epithelium completely renews itself within 3 to 6 days)
2. Local effect of dietary carbohydrates on bacteria growth and plaque formation
3. Role of nutrients in the host defense system
   a. During the initial stages of periodontitis the nutritional status of the patient is important in cellular immunocompetence for combating bacterial insults to the periodontium
   b. After periodontal surgery, cellular immunocompetence is important for optimal healing and preventing infection
C. Oral surgery
1. Presurgical nutritional counseling
   a. Adequate nutrient intake is needed to build up nutrient reserves in tissues to cope with postsurgical nutrient demands and complications
   b. Counseling is helpful for advising the patient to plan and purchase appropriate food products before surgery for the convalescent period
2. Postsurgical nutritional counseling
   a. Nutrient requirements are high because of blood loss, increased catabolism, tissue repair, and host defense activities
   b. Dietary intakes will be influenced by surgical complications of anorexia, dysphagia, and oral discomfort; a liquid diet should be used initially for the first few days, followed by a soft diet until the patient can eat normally; during convalescence, high-protein liquid products fortified with vitamins and minerals (e.g., Ensure, Sustacal, and Instant Breakfast) are helpful but contain cariogenic sweeteners; safe levels of vitamin

and mineral supplements (100% to 200% of RDAs) can be used also

D. Prosthodontics
  1. Nutritional counseling in the preparation of the mouth for a prosthesis
     a. Nutrients—systemically important for the health of oral soft tissues and the alveolar ridge
        (1) Surgery—if surgery is necessary, nutrient requirements will be higher for postsurgical healing
        (2) Tissue state—if any inflamed or soft tissue injuries and bone resorption conditions exist, nutrient requirements will be higher for repair and host defense activities
     b. Dietary sugars—condition of the remaining dentition is important for maintaining the use of a new prosthesis; cariogenic sugars need to be restricted to control bacterial growth, acid production, and bacterial plaque formation
     c. Texture of foods—partial or fully edentulous patients will often need to eat chopped, soft foods; if nutrient intake is compromised, fortified liquid products or nutrient supplements are helpful
  2. Nutritional counseling after prosthesis insertion
     a. Food texture—liquid foods for the first 24 hours, followed by soft foods and chopped or cut-up foods; this minimizes biting and chewing and allows time for the muscles and tongue to adjust to the new prosthesis
     b. Counter-dislodgement forces—for every bite of food, food should be evenly divided in the right and left sides of the mouth before chewing to equalize occlusal forces
     c. Nutrients—adequate intake for the integrity of the oral mucosa and alveolar ridge
     d. Dietary sugars—restrict to prevent bacterial growth, acid production, and bacterial plaque formation on the remaining dentition and prosthesis
     e. Food flavors—initially, flavors of foods will be altered because of the new prosthesis, but this side effect will eventually disappear with denture use

E. Orthodontics
  1. Role of nutrients—systemically important for the integrity of periodontal tissues; requirements are higher as stresses of tooth movement result in more bone apposition and the synthesis of a new periodontal ligament; nutrients are needed for the healing and repair of gingival injuries and irritations from orthodontic bands
  2. Role of sugars—to prevent enamel erosion and decay; dietary sugars (especially retentive sweets) must be restricted during the wearing of appliances
  3. Role of food textures—when appliances or bands are tightened, chewing hard-textured foods may be painful, and liquid and soft foods should be eaten temporarily; retentive and sticky foods should be avoided because they become trapped in appliances and are difficult to remove

F. Oral cancer
  1. Nutritional support for healing and cellular immunocompetence
     a. Compromised nutritional status—weight loss and nutrient deficiencies increase the risk of not withstanding the physiologic stresses of cancer and anticancer therapies
     b. Surgical treatment—primary method in treating cancer; nutrient requirements are higher as a result of the increased catabolic activities, tissue repair, and host defense activities
     c. Chemotherapy and radiation treatment—nutrient needs are higher because of the destruction of healthy cells and tissues that occurs during these types of treatments
  2. Diet modifications useful in treating complications from cancer and/or cancer treatments
     a. Patient unable to ingest or digest food
        (1) Home enteral feedings can furnish nutrients (e.g., nasogastric tube feedings)
        (2) Home parenteral feedings can furnish nutrients (e.g., intravenous feedings)
     b. Eating problems arising from complications or side effects of anticancer therapies
        (1) Nausea and vomiting—suck on ice chips; eat frequently; eat dry, bland foods; eat and drink slowly; avoid highly spiced and fatty foods; new antinausea medications are quite effective
        (2) Loss of appetite—use foods and recipes that are appealing; make up nutrient requirements at times when the appetite is good; use foods with a high nutrient density
        (3) Food aversions and alterations in taste and smell—eliminate offending foods; use highly spiced and distinctive textures to improve taste perceptions; cook and serve food with plastic rather than metal utensils
        (4) Dry mouth or xerostomia—chew sugar-free gum, suck on ice chips, or use synthetic saliva; drink liquids with meals; use cold-temperature foods rather than hot-temperature foods; concentrate on highly nutritious liquids

(5) Radiation caries—restrict cariogenic foods

(6) Glossitis and stomatitis—eat a variety of soft, easy-to-chew foods; use stewed foods rather than broiled and fried foods; avoid highly spiced or acidic foods; use moderate-temperature foods; use straws if swallowing is difficult

G. Special-needs individual (see Chapter 14)

1. Dental problems—unmet oral healthcare needs for this population significantly exceed that of the general population

a. Oral caries rate may be higher than that of the general population because of poor oral hygiene and cariogenic food habits

b. Increased periodontal disease as compared with the general population because of the following

(1) Poor oral hygiene; limited self-care behaviors

(2) Diets consisting of soft-textured foods

(3) Frequent exposures to sweets

(4) Metabolic disturbances affecting disease resistance and the reparative process

(5) Nutritional deficiencies associated with diet or metabolic disturbance

(6) Malocclusion and developmental defects

c. Barriers to health care

2. Nutritional problems—slow growth, excessive weight loss or gain, and nutrient deficiencies can occur in the following situations

a. Inability to consume an adequate diet

(1) Absence or weak sucking response (e.g., cleft lip and palate)

(2) Poor arm and head control (e.g., cerebral palsy)

(3) Inadequate jaw, lip, and tongue control (e.g., tongue thrust and tonic bite)

(4) Attention deficit (e.g., mental retardation and hyperactivity)

b. Impaired nutrient use

(1) Malabsorption conditions (e.g., cystic fibrosis)

(2) Inborn errors of metabolism (e.g., phenylketonuria)

(3) Drug-nutrient interactions (e.g., anticonvulsant medications can interfere with calcium and phosphorus use)

(4) Poor muscle control (e.g., constipation)

c. Excessive intake of foods, calories, and sweets

(1) Food, especially sweets, used as reinforcer for good behavior

(2) Overfeeding because of parental guilt

(3) Overemphasis on feeding because it is the major time for parent-child interaction

(4) Excessive calorie intake resulting from inactivity and the pleasurable aspects of eating

H. The immunocompromised individual

1. Causes of malnutrition in HIV-infected persons

a. Reduced food intake

(1) Drug treatments cause vomiting, nausea, and food aversions

(2) Fatigue, depression, and fear cause anorexia

(3) Oral infections alter taste, cause pain, and reduce saliva flow

(4) Esophageal infections and respiratory complications hamper swallowing

b. Increased nutrient loss

(1) Cancers of the GI tract cause malabsorption

(2) Drugs cause diarrhea and malabsorption

(3) PEM leads to malabsorption

c. Altered metabolism

(1) Cancer, infections, and fevers increase BMR

(2) Drug therapy alters nutrient utilization

2. Nutrient support

a. Correct any subclinical nutrient deficiencies and/or weight loss at the time of positive HIV test

b. Provide at least 100% of the RDA of all vitamins and minerals

c. Avoid food-borne illness

d. Design the nutrition plan based on the individual complications, with emphasis on controlling weight loss using nutrient-dense foods given throughout the day

REFERENCE

1. Food Nutrition Board, Committee on Dietary Allowances: Recommended dietary allowances, ed 10, Washington, DC, 1989, National Academy of Sciences.

SUGGESTED READINGS

Alpers D, Clouse R, Stenson W: *Manual of nutritional therapeutics,* ed 2, Boston, 1988, Little, Brown & Co.

Alverez JO: Nutrition, tooth development, and dental caries, *Am J Clin Nutr* 61:410-416, 1995.

Christakis G: *Nutritional assessment in health programs,* Washington, DC, 1973, American Public Health Association.

Curricular guidelines on biochemistry and nutrition for dental hygienists, *J Dent Educ* 53:256, 1989.

Nizel A: *Nutrition in clinical dentistry,* ed 3, Philadelphia, 1989, WB Saunders.

Pollack R, Kravitz E: *Nutrition in oral health and disease,* Philadelphia, 1985, Lea & Febiger.

Whitney E, Hamilton E, Rolfes S: *Understanding nutrition,* ed 7, St Paul, 1995, West Publishing.

Wilkins E: *Clinical practice of the dental hygienist,* ed 7, Philadelphia, 1994, Lea & Febiger.

Yamamoto J, Fannon ME, McKenzie M: Dental hygiene care: Caries prevention and control. In Darby ML, Walsh MM, eds, *Dental hygiene theory and practice.* Philadelphia, 1995, WB Saunders.

Review Questions

1 Carbohydrates may be chemically defined as
 A. Polyhydroxyl aldehydes
 B. Polyhydroxyl ketones
 C. Compounds with carbon, hydrogen, and oxygen in a ratio of 1:2: 1
 D. None of the above
 E. All of the above

2 Which of the following is an example of a monosaccharide?
 A. Sucrose
 B. Galactose
 C. Lactose
 D. Maltose

3 Which of the following complex carbohydrates *CANNOT* be digested by humans?
 A. Starch
 B. Glycogen
 C. Amylose
 D. Cellulose

4 Which of the following is (are) an important site(s) for carbohydrate digestion?
 A. Mouth
 B. Stomach
 C. Small intestine
 D. A and B
 E. B and C

5 Which of the following are potential sources of glucose via the gluconeogenic pathway?
 A. Glycogen
 B. Fatty acids
 C. Pyruvic acid
 D. Ketogenic amino acids

6 In the absence of oxygen, glucose is catabolized to
 A. Lactic acid
 B. Acetyl CoA
 C. Carbon dioxide
 D. A and B
 E. B and C

7 In a healthy individual, if the amount of glucose in the blood exceeds the body's immediate energy needs
 A. Glucose will be stored as glycogen in liver and muscle
 B. Glucose will be converted to fat and stored in adipose tissue
 C. Excess glucose will be excreted in the urine
 D. A and B
 E. B and C

8 Which of the following hormones lowers blood glucose?
 A. Tyroxine
 B. Growth hormones
 C. Epinephrine
 D. Insulin
 E. Glucagon

9 Of the dietary fibers, which plays a role in lowering blood cholesterol?
 A. Oat bran
 B. Wheat bran
 C. Guar gums
 D. Cellulose

10 Which of the following is an *INACCURATE* statement about fiber in the diet?
 A. Bulky diets, high in fiber, for persons with a limited intake may cause a nutrient deficiency
 B. Large doses of purified fiber may inhibit absorption of Fe
 C. Phytic acid, found in some high fiber foods, can inhibit the absorption of Fe
 D. The recommended fiber intake for adults is 70 to 90 g/day

11 Which of the following are important posteruptive effects of the carbohydrates on teeth?
 A. Carbohydrates are an energy source for *S. mutans*
 B. The end product of glycolysis for acidogenic bacteria is lactic acid
 C. *S. mutans* synthesizes polysaccharides from sucrose which have a strong affinity for enamel
 D. A, B, and C
 E. B and C

12 An example of a nonnutritive sweetener is
 A. Xylitol
 B. Sorbitol
 C. Aspartame
 D. Acesulfame-K
 E. Mannitol

13 Which *ONE* of the following characteristics of sugar intake is the *MOST* important factor in determining cariogenicity?
 A. Form of simple sugar—liquid or retentive
 B. Frequency of intake of simple sugar
 C. Timing of intake of simple sugar—alone or with a meal
 D. Total intake of simple sugars

14 The recommended amount of complex carbohydrates in the diet is
 A. <10%
 B. 15%
 C. 30%
 D. >48%

15 If a person is lactose intolerant
 A. He or she was born without the lactase enzyme
 B. He or she may be able to drink milk if he or she adds a commercial lactase enzyme to it
 C. He or she may be able to eat fermented dairy products
 D. A and B
 E. B and C

16 Which of the following is *NOT* a dietary recommendation for a diabetic person?
A. Eat a low complex-carbohydrate diet
B. Limit fat intake to 30% of kcal
C. Regulate carbohydrate and meal spacing during the day
D. Coordinate food intake, exercise, and medication
E. Limit simple sugars

17 Vegans are at risk for developing deficiencies in which of the following nutrients?
A. Carbohydrates
B. Vitamin B_{12}
C. Protein
D. Vitamin A
E. Vitamin C

18 Which of the following measures of protein quality take into account both its digestibility and its ability to support growth?
A. CS
B. PER
C. BV
D. PDCAAS

19 Nitrogen balance is
A. Positive when output is greater than intake
B. Negative during childhood
C. Positive when recovering from surgery
D. Negative during pregnancy
E. Positive when there is a net loss of protein

20 Which of the following is an important component of protein digestion in the stomach?
A. Hydrochloric acid
B. Bicarbonate
C. Trypsin
D. Chymotrypsin
E. Dipeptidase

21 The important nucleic acids that carry the genetic message for protein synthesis to the cytoplasm are
A. DNA
B. cDNA
C. mRNA
D. rRNA
E. tRNA

22 The protein requirement for the average adult male who weighs 70 kg is
A. 210 g
B. 140 g
C. 70 g
D. 56 g
E. 35 g

23 Saturated fatty acids
A. May contain one or more double bonds
B. Are liquids at room temperature
C. Usually come from plant sources
D. May contain some *trans* bonds if hydrogenated from unsaturated fatty acids
E. Have a low melting point

24 Of the following lipoproteins, which can be evaluated by exercise?
A. VLDL
B. HDL
C. LDL
D. Chylomicrons

25 Which of the following statements is true about cholesterol?
A. Intake in the average diet is 200 mg/day
B. Synthesis by the body is 200 mg/day
C. Levels in the blood are increased by increased percentage of total fat in the diet
D. Levels in the blood are decreased by the amount of saturated fat in the diet

26 Which of the following organs is (are) important for the digestion of fat?
A. Pancreas
B. Stomach
C. Gall bladder
D. Intestinal mucosa
E. All of the above

27 The body can synthesize triglycerides from
A. Dietary fat
B. Dietary protein
C. Dietary carbohydrate
D. A and C only
E. A, B, and C

28 If an individual ate 180 g of ice cream that was 33% fat (by weight), how many kilocalories came from fat?
A. 60 kcal
B. 180 kcal
C. 270 kcal
D. 540 kcal
E. Not enough information given to calculate fat kcal.

29 Which of the following statements is true about essential fatty acids?
A. Are linoleic and linolenic in humans
B. Should compose approximately 20% of total kcal
C. Are necessary for the synthesis of prostaglandins
D. A and B
E. A and C

30 Which of the following disorders *DO NOT* interfere with digestion and absorption of dietary fats?
A. Gallbladder disease
B. Pancreatitis
C. Cystic fibrosis
D. Gastric ulcers

31 Characteristics of fat-soluble vitamins include all of the following *EXCEPT*
A. Contain the elements carbon, hydrogen, and oxygen
B. Must be emulsified before they can be absorbed from the diet
C. Deficiency symptoms are slow to develop
D. Unstable to light, heat, and oxygen
E. Toxic with chronic excessive intake

32 Which one of the following is a general function of water soluble vitamins?
A. Function as coenzymes for energy metabolism
B. Are important for vision
C. Are important for regulating Ca and P levels in the body in bones and teeth
D. Are important for normal blood clotting
E. Function to maintain epithelial cells and mucosal linings

33 A phossy jaw may be related to an excess in the intake of which of the following minerals?
A. Phosphorus
B. Potassium
C. Magnesium
D. Chloride

34 Which of the following statements is true about water?
A. Is a nonessential nutrient because it provides 0 calories
B. Makes up 97% of the total body weight
C. Is contained in intracellular, intravascular, and intercellular spaces
D. Is regulated by calcium concentrations
E. Is required in an amount equal to 3 ml/kcal

35 In the body, energy is produced when which of the following is (are) oxidized?
A. Carbon
B. Hydrogen
C. Nitrogen
D. All of the above
E. A and B only

36 Which of the following statements is true about the basal metabolic rate?
A. Should be measured while a person sleeps
B. Is influenced by climate and altitude
C. Includes the energy necessary for normal muscle activity
D. Includes the specific dynamic energy (SDE)
E. Should be measured at an environmental temperature of 98.6° F

37 Which of the following is recommended for a healthy weight-loss diet?
A. Less than 60 mg/day carbohydrate
B. More than 60 g/day fiber
C. Less than 600 kcal/day
D. Less than 6 g/day fat
E. None of the above

38 Increasing activity level in an attempt to help weight loss has all of the following benefits *EXCEPT*
A. Activity increases energy expenditure
B. Activity decreases BMR
C. Activity stimulates circulation
D. Activity improves muscle tone

39 Which of the following statements is false about anorexia nervosa?
A. A state of protein-energy malnutrition
B. More prevalent in females than males
C. Treated with psychiatric and/or psychological counseling
D. More prevalent than bulimia
E. Often seen in individuals described as perfectionists

40 Which of the following can be described as a cause of a primary nutrient deficiency?
A. Lactose deficiency
B. Drug-nutrient interaction
C. Partial obstruction of the gastrointestinal tract
D. Overcooking vegetables
E. Nutrient-nutrient interaction

41 The Food Guide Pyramid has all the following features *EXCEPT*
A. It organizes foods into 4 groups
B. It shows relative amounts of foods to choose from each group
C. It stresses variety within each group
D. It stresses moderation in the use of fats and sweets
E. It recommends 6 to 11 servings of bread, cereals, rice and pasta

42 Gathering information about a client's food intake by using a nutritional screening questionnaire has all of the following advantages *EXCEPT*
A. It relies on the client's memory
B. It can be done while client is waiting in the oral healthcare setting
C. It requires 15 to 20 minutes to complete
D. It allows for evaluation of sugar consumption
E. It allows for evaluation of food group consumption

43 Acid production potential of a diet can be assessed
A. If the number of dietary sugar exposures per day is known
B. If the form (liquid or solid) of the dietary sugar exposures per day is known
C. If one assumes that solid sugars have approximately double the acid production potential of liquids
D. A and B
E. A, B, and C

44 In the "triad" of dental disease, the host factor includes
A. The presence of oral bacteria
B. The acid produced by the oral bacteria
C. The presence of dietary sugars
D. The frequency of eating dietary sugars
E. The congenital formation of the teeth

45 Causes of malnutrition in HIV-infected patients include
A. Reduced food intake
B. Increased nutrient loss
C. Altered metabolism
D. A and B
E. A, B, and C

46 A complete and accurate nutritional assessment includes all of the following *EXCEPT*
A. Health history
B. Bacteriologic assessment
C. Biochemical assessment
D. Clinical assessment
E. Food intake assessment

47 Which of the following statements is true about body water?
A. Composes 95% of the body's weight
B. Can be found in the extracellular spaces only
C. Is the product in many of the body's chemical reactions
D. Is lost by adults, from the kidneys, at a rate of approximately 100 to 150 ml/day

48 Which of the following is the healthiest type of weight-loss diet?
A. Very low carbohydrate, 1000-kcal diet
B. Very low fat, 1000-kcal diet
C. Very high fiber, 1000-kcal diet
D. Balanced nutrition, 1000-kcal diet
E. Single food, 1000-kcal diet

49 Which of the following is *NOT* a concern for feeding a cancer patient?
A. Altered taste perception
B. Decreased energy requirement
C. Irritated oral tissues
D. Nausea and vomiting treatment
E. Decreased appetite

50 Cancer patients who have had radiation treatments to the abdomen may have the added complication of not being able to digest foods. Patients who can no longer digest their food can be fed by nasogastric tube.
A. Both statements are *TRUE*
B. Both statements are *FALSE*
C. The first statement is true; the second is *FALSE*
D. The first statement is false; the second is *TRUE*

Answers and Rationales

1. (E) Carbohydrates are polyhydroxyl with a carbon, hydrogen, oxygen ratio of $1:2:1$. They may be in either the aldehyde or ketone form.
2. (B) Galactose is a monosaccharide. It is usually found combined with glucose in the disaccharide lactose, found in milk.
3. (D) Because the glucose units in cellulose are in a B linkage, they cannot be broken down by human digestive enzymes.
4. (D) Starches are partially digested in the mouth by salivary amylase. There is essentially no starch digestion in the stomach. Digestion is completed in the small intestine by the pancreatic amylase and the disaccharidases of the brush border.
5. (C) Pyruvic acid can be converted to glucose via the gluconeogenic pathway. Pyruvic acid can come from glucogenic amino acids or carbohydrates.
   (A) Although glycogen can break down into glucose, it does so via the glycogenolysis pathway.
   (B) Fatty acids can be broken down into acetyl CoA, but acetyl CoA cannot be converted to pyruvate. Pyruvate can be converted to acetyl CoA and then to fatty acids, however.
   (D) Ketogenic amino acids are converted to acetyl CoA, not to pyruvate.
6. (A) In the absence of oxygen, glucose cannot be completely oxidized. The end product of anaerobic catabolism of glucose is lactic acid.
   (B, C) Acetyl CoA and CO_2 can be formed from glucose only in the presence of sufficient oxygen.

7. (D) In a healthy (nondiabetic) individual, excess glucose can be stored as glycogen for short term storage or converted to fat.
   (A, B) See D
   (C) Glucose is not excreted in the urine unless an individual is diabetic or has renal disease.
8. (D) Insulin is released from the B cells of the pancreas in response to elevated levels of blood glucose. It facilitates the entrance of glucose into the cells from the blood.
   (A) Thyroxine increases insulin breakdown, absorption of glucose from the intestine, and epinephrine release.
   (B) Growth hormone acts as an insulin antagonist.
   (C) Epinephrine stimulates glycogenolysis, which increases blood glucose.
   (E) Glycogen stimulates glycogenolysis, which increases blood glucose.
9. (A) Oat bran plays a role in lowering blood cholesterol.
   (B) Wheat bran, found in whole wheat, acts as a stool softener to prevent constipation.
   (C) Guar gums slow gastric emptying and carbohydrate absorption. They may be helpful in maintaining a constant blood glucose level in diabetes.
   (D) Cellulose, which comes mainly from raw fruits and vegetables, decreases the transit time of foods in the intestine, thus helping to prevent constipation.
10. (D) The recommended fiber intake for adults is 20 to 30 grams/day.
    (A) When an individual is on a limited diet, a very high intake of fiber may inhibit the absorption of some minerals already in limited supply.
    (B) Large doses of fiber have been shown to inhibit absorption of Ca, Zn, and Fe.
    (C) Phytic acid is found in some high-fiber cereals. It has been shown to inhibit Fe absorption.
11. (C) Statements A, B, and C are true.
    (A) Carbohydrates are the main energy source for *S. mutans*, thus allowing them to multiply in the oral cavity.
    (B) Because of the anaerobic environment within the plaque on the teeth, the glycolytic end products are lactic and other acids.
    (C) The polysaccharides formed by *S. mutans* have a strong affinity for teeth and enhance plaque formation.
12. (D) Acesulfame-K is calorie-free and has no nutritive value. It is also noncariogenic.
    (A) Xylitol, sorbitol, and mannitol are all sugar alcohols that are noncariogenic but can be used as a carbohydrate source by the body.
    (B) See A
    (C) Aspartame is an artificial sweetener made from the two amino acids phenylalanine and aspartic acid.
13. (B) The most important factor in determining the cariogenicity of a simple sugar is the frequency of intake.
    (A) The timing, retentiveness, and total intake of the simple sugars are all important factors in determining cariogenicity.

14. (D) The recommended amount of complex carbohydrate in the diet is >48%.
    (A) It is recommended that the amount of simple sugar be >10%.
    (B) It is recommended that the amount of protein be about 15%.
    (C) It is recommended that the amount of fat be about 30%.
15. (D) If a person is lactose intolerant, he or she may be able to drink milk if a commercial lactase enzyme is added or consume fermented dairy products such as yogurt.
    (A, C) Very few people are born without the lactase enzyme. Most lactose intolerant individuals lose the lactase activity in early childhood.
16. (A) Complex carbohydrates are believed to be more slowly digested and absorbed. This should prevent the blood glucose levels from having wide fluctuations.
    (B) Fat intake should be limited to no more than 30% of kcal to help prevent the cardiovascular problems that are a complication of diabetes.
    (C) By regulating carbohydrates, meals, exercise, and medication throughout the day, there is less opportunity for wide fluctuations of blood glucose levels.
17. (B) Vegans consume no products of animal origin so they are at risk for vitamin B_{12} deficiency; vitamin B_{12} cannot be synthesized by plants.
    (A) Carbohydrates in the diet come mostly from plant sources.
    (C) Very good sources of proteins can be found in plants as well as animals.
    (D) Vitamin A can be found in deep-colored fruits and vegetables.
    (E) Vitamin C in the diet comes mainly from plant sources.
18. (D) The protein-digestibility corrected amino acid score (PDCAAS) compares the amino acid balance of a food protein with the amino acid requirements of preschool-age children and then corrects for digestibility.
    (A) The chemical score (CS) compares the essential amino acid content of a dietary protein with that of a reference protein.
    (B) The protein deficiency ratio (PER) measures a protein's ability to support growth.
    (C) The biological value (BV) is an expression of the percentage of nitrogen retained compared with the amount absorbed.
19. (C) Nitrogen balance is positive when recovering from surgery because the body is using protein to synthesize new tissue.
    (A) Nitrogen balance is negative when output is greater than intake.
    (B) Nitrogen balance is positive during childhood when growth is occurring.
    (D) Nitrogen balance is positive during pregnancy because of the growth of the fetus.
    (E) Nitrogen balance is negative when there is a net loss of protein.

20. (A) Hydrochloric acid in the stomach denatures proteins so that they can be hydrolyzed more easily by digestive enzymes. HCl also activates pepsin, a proteolytic enzyme in the stomach.
    (B) Bicarbonate is produced in the pancreas and released into the small intestine to neutralize the food that empties from the stomach.
    (C) Trypsin and chymotrypsin are produced in the pancreas and act in the small intestines to digest proteins.
    (D) Dipeptidase is produced by the brush border cells to carry out the final step of protein (dipeptide) hydrolysis before absorption.
21. (C) mRNA or messenger RNA carries the genetic information from the nucleus to the cytoplasm.
    (A) DNA is the genetic material in the nucleus.
    (B) cDNA is a copy of a portion of the DNA.
    (C) rRNA is ribosomal RNA.
    (D) tRNA is transfer RNA that attaches to the individual amino acids, which then become incorporated into the growing protein chain.
22. (A) The protein requirement for the average adult male who weighs 70 kg to 56 g or 0.8 g/kg. However, most Americans eat at least 2 to 3 times the requirement.
23. (D) Saturated fatty acids may contain some *trans* bonds if formed by hydrogenation from unsaturated fatty acids.
    (A) Saturated fatty acids do not contain double bonds.
    (B) Saturated fatty acids are usually solids at room temperature.
    (C) Saturated fatty acids usually come from animal sources.
    (E) Saturated fatty acids melt at a higher temperature than do unsaturated fatty acids.
24. (B) HDL (or good) cholesterol can be raised by increasing the amount of physical exercise.
    (A, C, D) Exercise has no effect on VLDL, LDL, or chylomicrons.
25. (C) Cholesterol levels in the blood are increased by increasing the total fat in the diet; increasing the saturated fat, increasing dietary cholesterol, and increasing total kilocalories.
    (A) The recommended cholesterol intake is 300 mg/day; the average intake in the U.S. is 300 to 450 mg/day.
    (B) The body synthesizes 2000 to 3000 mg of cholesterol per day.
    (D) See C.
26. (E) The complete digestion of fats requires processes that take place in the stomach, pancreas, gall bladder, and intestinal mucosa.
    (A) The pancreas produces pancreatic lipase, important for hydrolyzing medium and long chain fatty acids.
    (B) The stomach produces gastric lipase, important for hydrolyzing short and medium chain fatty acids.
    (C) The gallbladder stores bile, which is important for emulsifying dietary fats.
    (D) The final stage in the digestion of fats takes place in the intestinal mucosa where the monoglycerides and fatty acids are absorbed.

27. (E) The body can synthesize triglycerides from fat, protein, or carbohydrate. When any of these are eaten in excess the body converts to fat for long term storage.
    (A, B, C, D) See E.
28. (D) If 33% of the 180 g are fat and each fat gram has 9 kcal, the total grams from fat are 540.
29. (D) The essential fatty acids, linoleic and linolenic, should compose approximately 2% to 3% of the total kcal. One of the most important roles of the essential fatty acids is as precursors of the prostaglandins.
30. (D) Gastric ulcers do not interfere with the digestion of fats.
    (A) Gallbladder disease may interfere with the release of bile and therefore the emulsification of the fats, which is necessary before digestion can take place.
    (B) Pancreatitis can interfere with the synthesis and release of pancreatic digestive enzymes.
    (C) Cystic fibrosis causes blockage in many ducts in the body, often blocking the pancreatic duct. This prevents the release of pancreatic digestive enzymes.
31. (D) Most fat soluble vitamins, unlike water soluble vitamins, are stable to light, heat, and exposure to oxygen.
    (A, B, C, E) Are true statements about fat soluble vitamins.
32. (A) The B vitamins are very important as coenzymes for the reactions of energy metabolism.
    (B) Vitamin A is important for vision.
    (C) Vitamin D is important in regulating Ca and P.
    (D) Vitamin K is important for clot formation.
    (E) It is a characteristic of vitamin A, not the water soluble vitamins, to be important in maintaining epithelial cells and mucosal linings.
33. (A) Erosion of the jaw (phossy jaw) can be caused by an excessive intake of phosphorus.
    (B) Excessive potassium can cause muscle weakness and death.
    (C) Excessive magnesium can cause diarrhea.
    (D) Excessive chloride can cause vomiting.
34. (C) Water is contained in intracellular, intravascular, and intercellular spaces.
    (A) Water is an essential nutrient even though it provides 0 kcal.
    (B) Water makes up between 50% and 70% of the human body.
    (D) Water is regulated by potassium and sodium concentrations.
    (E) Water is required in an amount equal to 1 ml/kcal.
35. (E) Energy is produced in the human body when hydrogen is oxidized to water and carbon is oxidized to carbon dioxide.
    (A, B, D) See E.
    (C) The human body cannot oxidize nitrogen as some plants can.
36. (B) The basal metabolic rate (BMR) is influenced by climate and altitude. The BMR is increased at higher altitudes.
    (A) The BMR should be measured while an individual is awake, but at rest.
    (C) The BMR does not include the energy necessary for normal muscle activity.
    (D) The BMR does not include SDE.
    (E) The BMR should be measured at room temperature.

37. (E) None of the choices would be recommended in a healthy weight-loss diet.
    (A) Carbohydrate intake should be at least 60 to 100 g.
    (A) A fiber intake of greater than 60 would be excessive; it could bind essential nutrients and cause gastrointestinal distress.
    (C) A 600 kcal diet would not provide enough of the essential nutrients; 1000 kcal is a more appropriate goal.
    (D) Fat intake should be about 30% of total kcal.
38. (B) Increased physical activity increases energy expenditure, stimulates circulation, improves muscle tone, and *increases* BMR.
    (A, C, D) See B.
39. (D) Anorexia is seen less often than bulimia.
    (A, B, C, E) are true.
40. (C) Overcooking vegetables may destroy some of the water-soluble vitamins. Therefore an insufficient intake of these nutrients is the cause of the deficiency.
    (A) An individual with lactase deficiency may ingest sufficient nutrients but lose them because of the diarrhea associated with lactase deficiency.
    (B) Phosphates and drugs such as antacids inhibit the nutrient from being absorbed.
    (C) Partial obstruction may prevent adequate absorption of ingested nutrients.
    (E) Nutrients may compete for the same transport molecules so that an excess of one may cause a deficiency of another (e.g., Fe and Zn).
41. (A) The Food Pyramid organizes food into five groups: dairy, grains, meats/meat alternatives, fruits, and vegetables.
    (B, C, D, E) are true.
42. (A) The main disadvantage of using the screening questionnaire to gather information about the client's food intake is that it relies on the client's memory.
    (B, C, D, E) are advantages.
43. (E) The acid production potential of the diet is based on the total number of minutes of exposure. This is calculated by multiplying the number of liquid exposures by 20 and adding that to the number of solid exposures times 40.
    (A) Not only do you need to know the number of exposures, you also need to know the type of exposure.
    (B) You need to know the number of each form of exposure.
    (C) The assumption is correct; however, to calculate acid production potential, you need both type and number of exposures.
    (D) See E.
44. (D) The congenital formation or structure of the teeth is a host factor in the triad of dental disease.
    (A) The oral bacteria are agent factors.
    (B) The acid produced is an agent factor.
    (C) The dietary sugars are an environmental factor.
    (D) The frequency of sugar intake is an environmental factor.
45. (E) Causes of malnutrition in HIV-infected persons include reduced food intake, increased nutrient loss, and altered metabolism.
    (A, B, C, D) See E.

46. (B) A bacteriologic assessment is not part of a complete nutritional assessment.

(A) A health history gives information about altered nutritional needs due to illness.

(C) Biochemical assessment can detect levels of certain nutrients before their excess or deficiency causes clinical signs.

(D) Clinical signs are important indicators of deficiencies or excesses.

(E) Food intake records, over several days and in conjunction with the other means of assessment, can complete the nutritional assessment.

47. (C) Water is the end product of many oxidative reactions. This water, sometimes referred to as "metabolic water," contributes approximately 200 to 300 ml to total body water.

(A) The percentage of the body's weight that is water ranges from 69% in newborns to 49% in adult women.

(B) Approximately two thirds of the body's water is found within the cells; the remaining third (or approximately 15 L) is in the extracellular space and vascular system.

(D) Water loss from kidneys averages about 1000 ml/day in adults.

48. (D) A balanced nutrient, 1000-kcal diet is the best choice in a healthy weight reduction plan.

(A) A very low carbohydrate diet puts the dieter at risk of developing ketosis and using essential body proteins for energy.

(B) A very low fat diet may cause the person to become deficient in the essential fatty acids and fat soluble vitamins. A very low fat diet lacks satiety and taste appeal and is difficult to maintain.

(C) A very high fiber diet can cause GI distress with bloating and diarrhea. The fiber also may inhibit the absorption of essential minerals.

(E) Single-food or monotonous diets cannot provide all the nutrients required for optimal health. This type of diet does not help the person learn healthy food choices for maintaining weight loss.

49. (B) Cancer patients nearly always have increased energy needs to support the synthetic processes needed to rebuild tissue after destruction by the cancer cells themselves or by the treatment regimen.

(A) Both the cancer and its treatments (chemotherapy and radiation) can affect taste perceptions. Patients may refuse certain foods.

(C) Cancer treatments often irritate oral tissues, so acidic and rough-textured foods should be avoided.

(D) Nausea and vomiting are common after treatments. Sometimes bland foods are better tolerated.

(D) Decreased appetite is often a problem with cancer patients. They often do better if offered several small meals and snacks throughout the day and evening rather than a few large meals.

50. (C) The first statement is true. Radiation treatments in the abdominal area may destroy some of the healthy cells that line the gastrointestinal tract; this will make the digestion of ordinary foods and absorption of nutrients impossible. The second statement is false because passing food directly into the stomach will not make it any more digestible or absorbable if the lining of the small intestine has been damaged. These patients need intravenous feeding that bypasses the gastrointestinal tract.

Dental Materials

Stephen C. Bayne   Edward J. Swift, Jr.   Jeffrey Y. Thompson

To render quality dental hygiene care, it is important to understand the dental materials used and the restorative materials encountered in a client. A variety of metallic, ceramic, polymeric, and composite materials are used for both preventive and restorative procedures. The introduction is a review of the general considerations, structure, and properties that are helpful in understanding specific dental materials. General considerations include applications, terminology, and classifications for each dental materials topic. The structure of materials is reviewed in terms of the starting components, the reactions involved for use, and the manipulation procedures. The properties of materials are divided into important physical, chemical, mechanical, and biological properties. Properties critically depend on the structure produced by manipulation and the effects of preventive procedures. Both direct and indirect applications of restorative and preventive dental materials are reviewed with the same organizational approach.

Direct applications (preventive/restorative) of these materials include dental amalgams, dental composites, pit-and-fissure sealants, bonding agents, varnishes, liners, cement bases, temporary filling materials, permanent cement filling materials, fluoride gels, and polishing agents. Indirect applications (preventive/restorative) include impression materials, models, casts, dies, waxes, investment materials, casting alloys, dental solders, chromium alloys for partial dentures, porcelain fused to metal (PFM) alloys,

dental and PFM porcelains, cement luting agents, acrylic denture bases, denture teeth, denture liners, denture cleansers, veneers, mouth protectors, milled restorations (CAD/CAM; copy milled), and implants.

Introduction

General Considerations

A. Applications for dental materials
  1. Direct preventive and restorative procedures for teeth
  2. Indirect preventive and restorative procedures for teeth
B. Definitions and terminology
  1. Materials science terminology
  2. Dental materials terminology for classification
C. Classification of materials for applications
  1. Classification by key parts of composition-influencing properties
  2. Classification by extent of cavity preparation

Structure

A. Composition
  1. Generally two components in special ratio
     a. Powder and liquid (P/L)
     b. Powder and powder (P/P)
     c. Water and powder (W/P)

d. Paste and paste (p/p)

e. Paste (and light)

2. Generally the liquid part is the major reactant

B. Reaction during use

1. Physical reaction—solidification by drying or cooling with no chemical reaction

2. Chemical reaction—solidification by creation of new primary bonds within composition

C. Manipulation

1. Proportioning variables

a. Ratio of parts

b. Temperature

c. Relative humidity

2. Mixing variables

a. Method of combining components (e.g., stirring and stropping)

b. Rate of mixing (e.g., fast and slow)

3. Stages of manipulation

a. Definitions of times

(1) Mixing time—the elapsed time from the onset to the completion of mixing

(2) Working time—the elapsed time from the onset of mixing until the onset of the initial setting time

(3) Initial setting time—time at which sufficient reaction has occurred to cause the materials to be resistant to further manipulation

(4) Final setting time—time at which the material practically is set as defined by its resistance to indentation

b. Definitions of intervals

(1) Mixing interval—length of time of the mixing stage

(2) Working interval—length of time of the working stage

(3) Setting interval—length of time of the setting stage

c. All water-based materials lose their gloss at the time of setting

Properties

A. Physical properties—events that do not involve changes in composition or primary bonds

1. Descriptive properties

a. Weight—gravitational force that attracts a body

b. Mass—resistance of a body to being accelerated

c. Volume—a defined region in three-dimensional space

d. Density—a body's weight per unit of volume

2. Thermal properties

a. Linear coefficient of thermal expansion (LCTE, α)

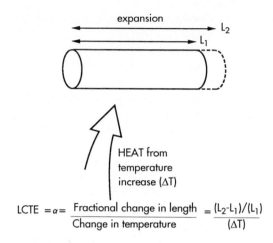

$$LCTE = \alpha = \frac{\text{Fractional change in length}}{\text{Change in temperature}} = \frac{(L_2-L_1)/(L_1)}{(\Delta T)}$$

Fig. 10-1   Linear coefficient of thermal expansion.

(1) Rate of expansion or contraction of one dimension of a material with temperature (Fig. 10-1)

(2) $LCTE = [(L_2 - L_1)/(L_1)]/T_2 - T_1$

L_1 = original length

L_2 = new length

T_1 = original temperature

T_2 = new temperature

(3) Values reported as in/in°F (inch per inch per °F), cm/cm/°C, 10^{-6}/°C, or ppm/°C

(4) When thermal expansion of restorative material does not match tooth structure, percolation of fluids occurs at the margins during cyclic heating and cooling

(5) LCTE values—tooth, 9 to 11 ppm/°C; amalgam, 25 ppm/°C; composite, 35 to 45 ppm/°C; inlay wax, 300 ppm/°C

b. Thermal conductivity

(1) Insulators transmit heat poorly (examples are dental enamel, dental cements, acrylic polymers, dental porcelain, and ceramic restorations)

(2) Conductors transmit heat easily (examples are dental amalgam and cast gold alloys)

(3) Teeth with metal restorations may be sensitive to hot and cold foods because of their good thermal conduction

(4) Individuals wearing dentures may not sense normal temperature differences attributable to thermal insulation of the acrylic denture base

(5) To be an effective insulator, the material must be at least 0.5 mm thick

3. Electrical properties

a. Electrical conductivity

(1) Conductors transmit electrons easily (examples are metals)

(2) Semiconductors transmit electrons sometimes (examples are ceramics)

(3) Insulators transmit electrons poorly (examples are ceramics and polymers)

4. Surface properties

   a. Contact angle—internal angle of liquid droplet with solid surface

     (1) Good wetting (angle = 0 degrees)

     (2) Spreading (angle <90 degrees)

     (3) Poor wetting (angle ≥90 degrees)

   b. Reflection—degree of surface backscattering

5. Color properties

   a. Perception—physiologic response to physical stimulus by the eye, which can distinguish 3 parameters

     (1) Dominant wavelength—blue, green, yellow, orange, and red

     (2) Luminance—lightness of color from black to white

     (3) Excitation purity—saturation of light

   b. Measurement

     (1) Munsell Color System (e.g., 5R 6/4)

       (a) Hue—color family (R, YR, Y, GY, G, BG, B, PB, P, RP)

       (b) Value—lightness from black to white (0/ to 10/)

       (c) Chroma—saturation from gray upward (/0 to /18)

     (2) Instrumentation techniques—record the spectral reflectance versus wavelength curves (405 to 700 nm)

     (3) L*a*b* color system

   c. Definitions

     (1) Metamerism—colors with different spectral energy distributions that look the same under certain lighting conditions but that look different with different light sources

     (2) Fluorescence—emission of light by a material when a beam of light is shined on it

     (3) Opacity—degree of light absorption by a material

     (4) Translucency—degree of internal light reflection

     (5) Transparency—degree of light transmission through a material

B. Chemical properties

1. Primary chemical bonding types

   a. Types

     (1) Metallic (e.g., metals)

     (2) Ionic (e.g., ceramics)

     (3) Covalent (e.g., ceramics and polymers)

   b. Events related to changes in primary chemical bonding

     (1) Contraction attributable to chemical reaction

       (a) Rate of contraction of size of material during chemical reaction or phase change at constant temperature

       (b) Linear change (%) = $[(L_1 - L_0)/(L_0)] \times 100\%$

         L_0 = original length

         L_1 = final length (after 24 hours)

       (c) Values reported as percentage changes

     (2) Corrosion of surfaces

2. Secondary chemical bonds

   a. Types

     (1) Hydrogen bonding

     (2) Van der Waals forces

   b. Events related to changes in secondary chemical bonding

     (1) Adsorption—uptake "onto" the surface of the solid

     (2) Absorption—uptake "into" the solid

       (a) Example—water absorbed by denture

       (b) Example—moisture absorbed by alginate (imbibition)

     (3) Desorption—fluid lost from solid

       (a) Example—water lost from alginate (syneresis)

     (4) Solubility—material loss by dissolution of surface

     (5) Disintegration—material loss by disruption of solid, usually by absorbed water

3. Corrosion:

   a. Chemical corrosion—chemical reaction at surface

     (1) Products may be soluble

     (2) Products may be insoluble and form layer (tarnish)

   b. Electrochemical corrosion—chemical reaction that requires anode (e.g., dental amalgam), cathode (e.g., gold crown), an electrolyte (e.g., saliva), and an electrical circuit (e.g., contact) for electron flow (Fig. 10-2)

     (1) Galvanic corrosion—dissimilar metals in contact (e.g., example above)

     (2) Local galvanic corrosion (structure-selective corrosion)—dissimilar phases in the same metal in contact

     (3) Crevice corrosion—corrosion in crack under plaque, between a restoration and tooth structure, or in scratch on surface of restoration where the metals may be the same but locally the electrolytes are different

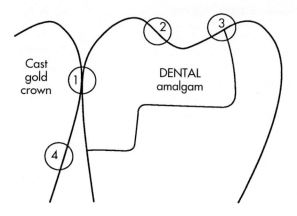

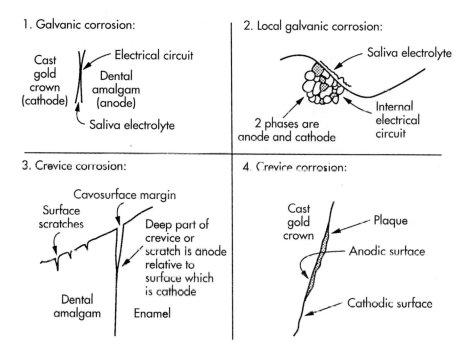

1. Galvanic corrosion:

Cast gold crown (cathode)

Electrical circuit

Dental amalgam (anode)

Saliva electrolyte

2. Local galvanic corrosion:

Saliva electrolyte

2 phases are anode and cathode

Internal electrical circuit

3. Crevice corrosion:

Cavosurface margin

Surface scratches

Deep part of crevice or scratch is anode relative to surface which is cathode

Dental amalgam

Enamel

4. Crevice corrosion:

Cast gold crown

Plaque

Anodic surface

Cathodic surface

Fig. 10-2 Electrochemical corrosion.

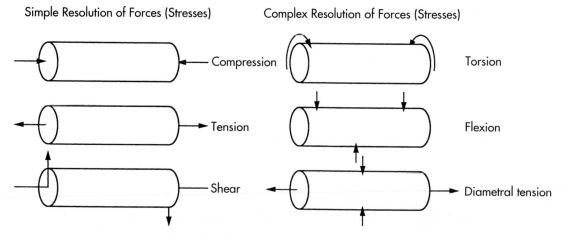

Simple Resolution of Forces (Stresses)

Compression

Tension

Shear

Complex Resolution of Forces (Stresses)

Torsion

Flexion

Diametral tension

Fig. 10-3 Resolution of forces.

c. Corrosion potential
  (1) Immune—does not corrode (i.e., cathodic)
  (2) Active—corrodes readily (i.e., anodic)
  (3) Passive—corrosion produces protective film (e.g., chromium oxide film on stainless steel)
C. Mechanical properties
  1. Resolution of forces (Fig. 10-3)
    a. Uniaxial (one-dimensional) forces—compression, tension, and shear
    b. Complex forces—torsion, flexion, and diametral
  2. Normalization of forces and deformations
    a. Stress
      (1) Applied force (or material's resistance to force) per unit area
      (2) Stress = force/area (in lb/in^2, kg/cm^2, or MN/m^2)
    b. Strain (Fig. 10-4)
      (1) Change in length per unit of length because of force
      (2) Strain = $(L - L_0)/(L_0)$; dimensionless units
  3. Stress-strain diagrams
    a. Plot of stress (vertical) versus strain (horizontal)
      (1) Allows convenient comparison of materials
      (2) Different curves for compression, tension, and shear
      (3) Curves depend on rate of testing and temperature
    b. Analysis of curves (Fig. 10-4)
      (1) Elastic behavior
        (a) Initial response to stress is elastic strain

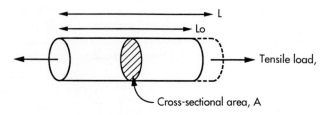

Stress = Load/Area = P/A

Strain = Fractional Change in Length = ((L-Lo)/(Lo))

Modulus = Stress/Strain = Stiffness = E

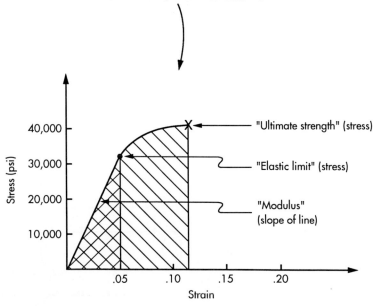

Fig. 10-4 Stress-strain curve.

(elastic = when stress is removed, the strain returns to zero and material becomes original length)

(b) Elastic modulus—slope of first part of curve and represents stiffness of material or the resistance to deformation under force

(c) Elastic limit (proportional limit)—stress above which the material no longer behaves totally elastically

(d) Yield strength—stress that is an estimate of the elastic limit at 0.002 permanent strain

(e) Hardness—value on a relative scale that estimates the elastic limit in terms of a material's resistance to indentation (Knoop hardness scale, Diamond pyramid, Brinnell, Rockwell hardness scale, Shore A hardness scale, Mohs hardnes scale [Table 10-1]); hardness values are used to determine the ability of abrasives to alter the substrates they contact.

(f) Resilience—area under the stress-strain curve up to the elastic limit (and it estimates the total elastic energy that can be absorbed before the onset of plastic deformation)

(2) Elastic and plastic behavior

(a) Beyond the stress level of the elastic limit, there is a combination of both elastic and plastic strain

(b) Ultimate strength—highest stress reached before fracture; the ultimate compressive strength is greater than the ultimate shear strength and the ultimate tensile strength

(c) Elongation (percent elongation)—percent change in length up to the point of fracture = strain × 100%

(d) Brittle materials—<5% elongation at fracture

(e) Ductile materials—>5% elongation at fracture

(f) Toughness—area under the stress-strain curve up to the point of fracture (it estimates the total energy absorbed up to fracture)

(3) Time-dependent behavior

(a) Strain rate sensitivity = the faster a stress is applied, the more likely a material is to store the energy elastically and not plastically

(b) Creep (i.e., strain relaxation with time in response to a constant stress—such as dental wax deforming due to built in stresses created during cooling)

(c) Stress relaxation (with time in response to a constant strain)

(d) Fatigue = failure due to cyclic loading at low stress levels that would not produce demonstrable strain after a single cycle

4. Principles of cutting, polishing, and surface cleaning

a. Terminology

(1) Cutting = gross removal of excess material from the surfaces of restorations or teeth

(2) Finishing = fine removal of surface material in an effort to produce finer and finer surface scratches

(3) Polishing = smoothing of surfaces by removal of fine scratches

(4) Debriding = removal of unwanted material attached to surfaces

b. Surface mechanics for materials (Table 10-2)

(1) Cutting—requires highest possible hardness materials to produce the cuts

(2) Finishing—requires highest possible hardness materials to produce finishing, except at margins of restorations where tooth structure may be inadvertently affected

(3) Polishing—requires only materials with Mohs hardness that is only 1 to 2 units above that of substrate

(4) Debriding—requires materials with Mohs hardness that is less than or equal to that of substrate to prevent scratching

Table 10-1

Mohs Scale for Hardness (Standards for Checking the Hardness of Abrasives and Substrates)

Number	Hardness
10	Diamond
9	Corundum
8	Topaz
7	Quartz
6	Orthoclase
5	Apatite
4	Fluorite
3	Calcite
2	Gypsum
1	Talc

Table 10-2

Hardness Values for Dental Substrates (Mohs Scale)

Hardness value	Number
CAD/CAM ceramic	6-7
Porcelain	6-7
Composite	5-7
Glass	5-6
Dental enamel	5-6
Dental amalgam	4-5
Dentin	3-4
Hard gold alloys	3-4
Pure gold	2-3
Acrylic	2-3

    c. Factors affecting cutting, polishing, and surface cleaning
      (1) Applied pressure
      (2) Particle size of abrasive
      (3) Hardness of abrasive
      (4) Hardness of substrate
    d. Precautions
      (1) During cutting, heat will build up and change the mechanical behavior of the substrate from brittle to ductile and encourage smearing
      (2) Instruments may transfer debris onto the cut surface from their own surfaces during cutting, polishing, or cleaning operations (this is important for cleaning implant surfaces)
D. Biologic properties
  1. Definitions of biohazards
    a. Toxicity—cell or tissue death attributable to material concentration
    b. Sensitivity—systemic reaction to substance
      (1) Allergy—reaction to relatively small amounts of material
      (2) Hypersensitivity—reaction to minute amounts of material
  2. Definitions of local tissue interactions with biomaterials
    a. Fibrous tissue capsule formation (tissue encapsulation)
    b. Integration at the interface
      (1) Bone ingrowth (osseointegration)
      (2) Bone ongrowth (osseointegration)
    c. Biodegradation (desorption or resorption)
  3. Classification of biologic materials/tissue interfaces

    a. Intraoral and supragingival—in enamel or dentin
    b. Intraoral, pulpal, or periapical
    c. Transcutaneous
    d. Subcutaneous
    e. Intraosseous
  4. Clinical analysis of biocompatibility
    a. Risk versus benefits
    b. Safety and efficacy
  5. Agencies overseeing materials, devices, and therapeutics
    a. Regulatory agencies
      (1) Food and Drug Administration (FDA)
    b. Standards development for manufacturing practices; for physical, chemical, mechanical, and biological properties; and for clinical testing
      (1) American Dental Association (ADA)—Council on Scientific Affairs
      (2) American National Standards Institute (ANSI)
      (3) International Standards Organization (ISO)
      (4) Federation Dentaire Internationale (FDI)

Direct Preventive/Restorative Materials

Dental Amalgam

A. General considerations
  1. Applications
    a. Load-bearing restorations for posterior teeth (class I, II)
    b. Pin-retained restorations
    c. Buildups (foundations) or cores for cast restorations
    d. Retrograde canal filling material
    e. Some class V restorations
  2. Terminology
    a. Amalgam alloy—powder particles of Ag-Sn-(Cu)-(Zn) or Ag-Sn-Cu-(Zn). NOTE: minor elements indicated in parentheses
    b. Amalgam—reaction product of anything with mercury
    c. Dental amalgam—reaction product of amalgam alloy (Ag-Sn or Ag-Sn-Cu) with mercury
  3. Classification of dental amalgam
    a. By powder particle shape
      (1) Irregular (comminuted, filing, or lathe-cut)
      (2) Spherical (spherodized)
      (3) Blends (e.g., irregular-irregular, irregular-spherical, or spherical-spherical)
    b. By total amount of copper

Before Reaction   After Reaction

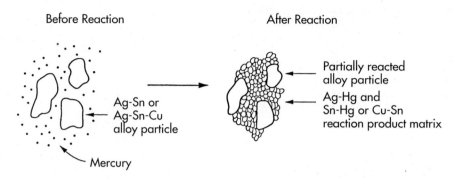

Fig. 10-5   Schematic view of amalgam reaction.

(1) Low-copper alloys (conventional, traditional); <5% copper (Ag-Sn-Cu)
(2) High-copper alloys (corrosion resistant); 12% to 28% copper (Ag-Sn-Cu)
  c. By presence of zinc
  d. By other modifications
4. Examples
  a. Low-copper, irregular-particle alloy—Ag (70%)-Sn (26%)-Cu (4%)
  b. High-copper, blended-particles alloy—irregular particles, Ag (70%)-Sn (26%)-Cu (4%); spherical particles, Ag (72%)-Cu (28%)
  c. High-copper, spherical-particles alloy Ag (60%)-Sn (27%)-Cu (13%)
B. Structure
  1. Components
    a. Mercury mixed with amalgam alloy
    b. Mercury reacts with periphery of alloy particle to produce crystalline silver-mercury, tin-mercury, and/or copper-tin phases
  2. Reaction (Fig. 10-5)
    a. Setting reactions
      (1) Low-copper dental amalgam

      Hg + Ag-Sn →
      Ag-Sn + Ag-Hg + Sn-Hg

      (2) High-copper dental amalgam

      Hg +Ag-Sn-Cu →
      Ag-Sn-Cu + Ag-Hg + Cu-Sn
      Hg + Ag-Sn + Ag-Cu→
      Ag-Sn + Ag-Cu +Ag-Hg + Cu-Sn

    b. Phases in set amalgams
      (1) Residual alloy (Ag-Sn, Ag-Sn-Cu, or Ag-Cu)—strongest; most corrosion resistant
      (2) Ag-Hg ($= \gamma_1$) = major matrix phase in low- or high-copper dental amalgams
      (3) Sn-Hg ($= \gamma_2$) = second matrix phase in low-copper dental amalgams

(4) Cu-Sn (η or ϵ) = second matrix phase in high-copper dental amalgams
3. Manipulation
  a. Selection—based on clinical requirements for strength
  b. Packaging
    (1) Powder or pressed tablets; mercury
    (2) Precapsulated powder and mercury
  c. Mixing
    (1) Mercury/alloy specific to each product but generally less than 1:1 so that amalgam contains 43% to 50% mercury
    (2) Mechanical amalgamators—variable time, speed (frequency and amplitude), and amalgamator motion for different equipment, which affects the mixing process
    (3) Each amalgamator has specific settings for each different amalgam alloy (low-copper amalgams require 10 to 20 seconds; high-copper amalgams require 5 to 10 seconds)
    (4) Amalgamator capsules are reusable or disposable
    (5) Pestle may be included in capsule for mixing efficiency
    (6) Overmixed mass difficult to remove from capsule
    (7) Undermixed mass is crumbly
  d. Condensation
    (1) Adaptation of amalgam to cavity walls
    (2) Removal of excess mercury-rich matrix produces a stronger and more corrosion-resistant amalgam because it minimizes the formation of the matrix phase of amalgam, which are the least desirable parts of the set material
    (3) Amalgams with spherical alloys are more fluid and require larger-tipped condensers

(4) Condense in small increments, overpack restoration, avoid delays, and avoid saliva contamination

e. Finishing
(1) Carve anatomy within a few minutes after condensing
(2) Burnish surface and/or final finish at least 24 hours later

C. Properties
1. Physical
   a. Coefficient of thermal expansion = 25 ppm/°C (thus amalgams allow percolation during temperature changes)
   b. Thermal conductivity—high (therefore, amalgam may need insulating liner or base in very deep cavity preparations)

2. Chemical
   a. Dimensional change on setting, less than ±20µm (excessive expansion can produce postoperative pain)
   b. Cavity varnish or bonding agent electrically insulates a dental amalgam restoration, but it does not prevent corrosion
   c. Chemical corrosion produces black or green tarnish on the surface that is aesthetically displeasing but not detrimental
   d. Electrochemical corrosion produces penetrating corrosion of low-copper amalgams but only produces superficial corrosion of high-copper amalgams, so they last longer

3. Mechanical
   a. Compressive strength = 45,000 to 70,000 psi, comparable with enamel but is not important to prevent marginal fracture
   b. Because of low tensile strength, enamel support is needed at margins
   c. Spherical high-copper alloys develop high tensile strength faster and can be polished sooner
   d. Excessive creep is associated with Ag-Hg phase of low-copper amalgams and contributes to early marginal fracture
   e. Marginal fracture correlated with creep and electrochemical corrosion in low-copper amalgams (Fig. 10-6)
   f. Bulk fracture (isthmus fracture) occurs across thinnest portions of amalgam restorations because of high stresses during traumatic occlusion and/or the accumulated effects of fatigue
   g. Dental amalgam is relatively resistant to abrasion (i.e., wear)

4. Biologic
   a. Mercury hygiene
      (1) Do not contact mercury with skin

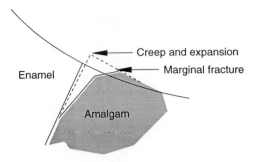

Fig. 10-6 Schematic view of marginal ditching in an amalgam restoration, produced by creep and expansion elevating the margins of the amalgam, and functional stresses producing marginal fracture.

(2) Clean up spills to minimize mercury vaporization
(3) Store mercury or precapsulated products in tight containers
(4) Only triturate amalgam components in tightly sealed capsules
(5) Use amalgamators with covers
(6) Store spent amalgam under water or fixer in a tightly sealed jar
(7) Use high vacuum suction during amalgam alloy placement, setting, or removal when mercury may be vaporized
(8) Polishing amalgams generally causes localized melting of Ag-Hg phase with release of mercury vapor, so water cooling and evacuation must be used
(9) Beware of aerosols created by vacuuming materials spilled on floor or carpet
(10) Replace floor coverings every 5 years to eliminate accumulation of spilled material

b. Mercury bioactivity
(1) Depends on whether it is metallic, inorganic, or organic mercury
(2) Metallic mercury is the least toxic form and is absorbed primarily through the lungs rather than the GI tract or skin
(3) Mercury in the body may come from air, water, food, dental (a low amount), or medical sources
(4) Half-life for mercury elimination from body is 55 days on average
(5) OSHA level for mercury *toxicity* is <50 µm/m³ on average per 40-hour work week
(6) Mercury *hypersensitivity* is estimated as less than 1 per 100,000,000 persons

c. Amalgam alternatives
(1) Indium-containing amalgams can have

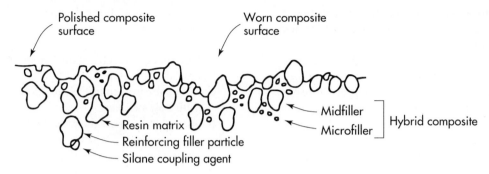

Fig. 10-7 Schematic view of hybrid dental composite.

lower mercury vapor pressures than conventional dental amalgam
   - (2) Gallium alloys except that they have poor corrosion resistance and may become toxic
   - (3) Esthetic filling materials (composites, ceramic restorations, compomers)
   - (4) Cast-gold or PFM restorations

Dental Composites

A. General considerations
   1. Applications
      a. Anterior restorations for aesthetics (class III, IV, V, cervical erosion/abrasion lesions)
      b. Low-stress posterior restorations (small class I, II)
      c. Veneers
      d. Cores for cast restorations
      e. Cements for porcelain restorations
      f. Cements for resin-bonded bridges
      g. Repair systems for composites or porcelains
   2. Terminology (Fig. 10-7)
      a. Composite—physical mixture of materials to average the properties of the materials involved
      b. Dental composite—restoration resulting from the mixture of ceramic reinforcing filler particles in a monomer matrix that is converted to polymer on setting
      c. Polymerization—reaction of small molecules (monomers) into very large molecules (polymers)
      d. Cross-linking—tying together of polymer molecules by chemical reaction between the molecules to produce a continuous three-dimensional network
   3. Classification
      a. Amount of filler—25% to 65% volume, 45% to 85% weight
         - (1) High—restorative composite
         - (2) Low—flowable composite
      b. Filler particle size (diameter in microns)
         - (1) Macrofill—10 to 100 μm (traditional composites)
         - (2) Midifill—1 to 10 μm (small particle composites)
         - (3) Minifill—0.1 to 1 μm
         - (4) Microfill—0.01 to 0.1 μm (fine particle composites)
         - (5) Hybrid—blend (usually midifill or minifill with microfill)
      c. Polymerization method
         - (1) Auto-cured (self-cured; SC)
         - (2) Visible light-cured (VLC)
         - (3) Dual-cured (VLC and SC)
         - (4) Staged cure (2-stage cure)
      d. Matrix chemistry
         - (1) BIS-GMA (= bis-GMA) type
         - (2) Urethane dimethacrylate (UDM or UDMA) type
         - (3) TEGDMA—diluent monomer to reduce viscosity

B. Structure
   1. Components
      a. Filler particles—colloidal silica, crystalline silica (quartz), or silicate glasses (non-crystalline) of various particle sizes (containing Ba, Li, Al, Zn, Yr, ...)
      b. Matrix—BIS-GMA (or UDMA) with lower molecular weight diluents (e.g., TEGDMA) that co-react during polymerization
      c. Coupling agent—silane that chemically bonds the surfaces of the filler particles to the polymer matrix
   2. Reaction
      a. Free radical polymerization
         - (1) Monomers + initiator + accelerators → polymer molecules
      b. Initiators—start polymerization by decomposing and reacting with monomer

c. Accelerators—speed up initiator decomposition
  (1) Amines used for accelerating self-curing systems
  (2) Light used for accelerating light-curing systems
d. Retarders or inhibitors—prevent premature polymerization

3. Manipulation
  a. Selection
    (1) Microfilled composites or hybrids for anterior class III, IV, V
    (2) Hybrids or midifills or special microfills for class I, II, III, IV, V
  b. Conditioning of enamel and/or dentin
    (1) Do not apply fluorides before etching
    (2) Acid-etch (see bonding agents)
    (3) Rinse for 20 seconds with water
    (4) Air-dry enamel for 20 seconds but do not desiccate or dehydrate
    (5) Apply bonding agent and polymerize
  c. Mixing (if required)—mix two pastes for 20 to 30 seconds
    (1) Self-cured composite—working time is 60 to 120 seconds after mixing
    (2) Light-cured composite—working time is nearly unlimited (used for most anterior and some posterior composite restorations)
    (3) Dual-cured composite—working time is 5 to 8 minutes
    (4) Two-stage cured composite—working time is >5 minutes
  d. Placement—use plastic instrument or syringe
  e. Light curing
    (1) Cure incrementally in <2 mm thick layers
    (2) Use matrix strip where possible to produce smooth surface and contour composite
    (3) Postcure to improve hardness (i.e., light-cure a second time after polishing)
  f. Finishing and polishing
    (1) Remove oxygen-inhibited layer
    (2) Use stones, carbide burs, or diamonds for gross reduction
    (3) Use multi-fluted carbide burs or special diamonds for fine reduction
    (4) Use aluminum oxide strips or disks for finishing or rubber points, cups, and disks
    (5) Use fine aluminum oxide finishing pastes
    (6) Microfills develop smoothest finish because of small size of filler particles

C. Properties—improve with filler content
  1. Physical
    a. Radiopacity depends on ions in silicate glass
    b. Coefficient of thermal expansion is 35 to 45 ppm/°C and decreases with increasing filler content
    c. Thermal and electrical insulators
  2. Chemical
    a. Water absorption is 0.5% to 2.5% and increases with polymer level
    b. Acidulated topical fluorides (e.g., APF) tend to dissolve glass particles, and thus composites should be protected with petroleum jelly (Vaseline) during those procedures or a different topical fluoride such as neutral sodium fluoride should be chosen for use
    c. Color changes occur in resin matrix with time because of oxidation, which produces colored by-products
  3. Mechanical
    a. Compressive strength is 45,000 to 60,000 lb/in^2, which is adequate
    b. Wear resistance—improves with higher filler content, higher percentage of conversion in curing, and use of microfiller, but it is not adequate for some posterior applications
    c. Surfaces rough from wear retain plaque and stain more readily
  4. Biologic
    a. Components may be cytotoxic, but cured composite is biocompatible as restorative filling material

Pit-and-Fissure Dental Sealants

A. General considerations
See Chapter 12, section on dental sealants
  1. Applications
    a. Occlusal surfaces of newly erupted posterior teeth
    b. Lingual surfaces of anterior teeth with fissures
    c. Occlusal surfaces of teeth in older persons with reduced saliva flow (because low saliva increases the susceptibility to dental caries)
  2. Classification
    a. Polymerization method
      (1) Self-curing (amine accelerated)
      (2) Light-curing (light accelerated)
    b. Filler content
      (1) Unfilled—many systems are unfilled because filler tends to interfere with wear away from self-cleaning occlusal areas (sealants are designed to wear away, except where there is no self-cleaning action; a common misconception is that sealants should be wear resistant)
      (2) Lightly filled (10 to 30 wt %)

B. Structure
  1. Components
    a. Monomer—BIS-GMA with TEGDM diluent to facilitate flow into pits and fissures before cure
    b. Initiator—benzoyl peroxide (in self-cured) and diketone (in light-cured)
    c. Accelerator—amine (in light-cured)
    d. Opaque filler—1% titanium dioxide or other colorant to make the material detectable on tooth surfaces
    e. Reinforcing filler—generally not added because wear resistance is not required within pits and fissures
    f. Fluoride—may be added for slow release
  2. Reaction—free radical reaction (see Composites)
  3. Manipulation
    a. Preparation
      (1) Clean pits and fissures of organic debris
      (2) Do not apply fluoride before etching because it will tend to make enamel more acid resistant
      (3) Etch occlusal surfaces, pits, and fissures with 37% phosphoric acid
      (4) Wash occlusal surfaces for 20 seconds
      (5) Dry etched area for 20 seconds with clean air spray
      (6) Apply sealant and polymerize
    b. Mixing or dispensing
      (1) Self-cured—mix equal amounts of liquids in Dappen dish for 5 seconds with brush applicator
      (2) Light-cured—dispense from syringe tips
    c. Placement—pits, fissures, and occlusal surfaces
      (1) Allow 60 seconds for self-cured materials to set
      (2) Light-cure following manufacturer's directions
    d. Finishing
      (1) Remove unpolymerized and excess material
      (2) Examine hardness and marginal adaptation of sealant
      (3) Make occlusal adjustments where necessary in sealant; some sealant materials are self-adjusting

C. Properties
  1. Physical
    a. Wetting—low-viscosity sealants wet acid-etched tooth structure the best
  2. Mechanical
    a. Wear resistance should not be too great because sealant should be able to wear off of self-cleaning areas of tooth
    b. Be careful to protect sealants during polishing

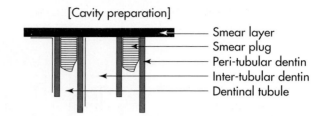

Fig. 10-8 Schematic view of the surface of cut dentin, with a smear layer and smear plugs occluding the dentinal tubules.

    procedures with air abrading units to prevent sealant loss
  3. Biologic—no apparent biologic problems
  4. Clinical efficacy
    a. Effectiveness is 100% if retained in pits and fissures
    b. Requires routine clinical evaluation for resealing of areas of sealant loss attributable to poor retention
    c. Sealants resist most effects of topical fluorides

Bonding Agents

A. General considerations
  1. Applications—composites, resin-modified glass ionomers, ceramic bonded to enamel restorations, veneers, orthodontic brackets, and desensitizing dentin by covering exposed tubules, resin-bonded bridges, composite and ceramic repair systems, amalgams and amalgam repair, and pin amalgams
  2. Definitions
    a. Smear layer—thin layer of compacted debris on enamel and/or dentin from the cavity preparation process (Fig. 10-8) that is weakly held to the surface (5 to 6 MPa) and that limits bonding agent strength if not removed
    b. Etching (or conditioning)—smear layer removal and production of microspaces for micromechanical bonding by dissolving minor amounts of surface hydroxyapatite crystals
    c. Priming—micromechanical (and possibly chemical) bonding to the microspaces created by conditioning step
      (1) Conditioning/priming agent—agent that accomplishes both actions
    d. Bonding—formation of resin layer that connects the primed surface to the overlying restoration (e.g., composite)
      (1) Enamel bonding system—for bonding to enamel (although dentin bonding may be a second step)
      (2) Dentin bonding system—for bonding to

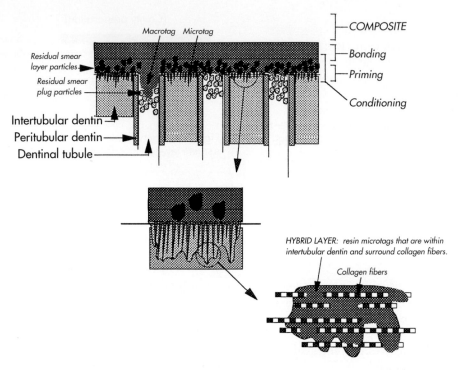

Fig. 10-9 Schematic view of adhesion in new-generation dentin bonding system.

dentin (although enamel bonding may have been a first step)

  (a) First-generation dentin bonding system—for bonding to smear layer
  (b) Current generation dentin bonding system—for removing smear layer and etching intertubular dentin to allow primer and/or bonding agent to diffuse into spaces between collagen fibers and form hybrid zone (see Fig. 10-9)
  (3) Enamel and dentin bonding system—for bonding to enamel and dentin surfaces with the same procedures
  (4) Amalgam bonding system—for bonding to enamel, dentin, and amalgam during an amalgam placement procedure or for amalgam repair
  (5) Universal bonding system—for bonding to enamel, dentin, amalgam, porcelain, or any other substrate intraorally that may be necessary for a restorative procedure using the same set of procedures and materials
3. Classification
  a. Major substrate
    (1) Enamel bonding system
    (2) Dentin bonding system
    (3) Amalgam bonding system
    (4) Universal bonding system
  b. Number of components
    (1) Three-component (conditioner, primer, bonding agent)
    (2) Two-component
      (a) Conditioning agent and combined primer/bonding agent (called a one-component system if the conditioning agent is not supplied directly in the kit)
      (b) Conditioning/priming agent and bonding agent
B. Structure
  1. Components of bonding systems
    a. Conditioning agent—mineral or organic acid
      (1) Enamel only—37% phosphoric acid
      (2) Dentin only or enamel and dentin—37% phosphoric acid, EDTA, polyacrylic acid, citric acid, maleic acid, or nitric acid
    b. Priming agent
      (1) Alcohol and/or acetone solvent and light-cured monomer
      (2) Water and light-cured monomer
    c. Bonding agent
      (1) BIS-GMA–type monomer system
      (2) UDMA-type monomer system

2. Reaction
   a. Bonding occurs primarily by intimate micromechanical retention with the relief created by the conditioning step
   b. Chemical bonding is possible but is not recognized as contributing significantly to the overall bond strength
3. Manipulation (follow manufacturer's directions)
   a. Conditioning
      (1) Apply 37% phosphoric acid solution or equivalent
      (2) Rinse and dry without desiccation (keep dentin moist with "glistening" appearance)
      (3) In case of overdrying, moisten dentin with water for 30 to 60 seconds
   b. Priming
      (1) Apply priming agent and gently dry to remove excess solvent
      (2) Apply multiple layers until dentin fully impregnated to surface
   c. Bonding
      (1) Apply single coat of bonding agent when bonding composites
      (2) Apply multiple coats of bonding agent and/or mix with thickening agent in preparation for bonding with amalgam restorations

C. Properties
   1. Physical—thermal expansion and contraction may create fatigue stresses that debond the interface and permit microleakage
   2. Chemical—water absorption into the bonding agent may chemically alter the bonding
   3. Mechanical—mechanical stresses may produce fatigue that debonds the interface and permits microleakage
      a. Enamel bonding—adhesion occurs by macrotags (between enamel prisms) and microtags (into enamel prisms) to produce micromechanical retention
      b. Dentin bonding—adhesion occurs by removal of smear layer and formation of microtags into intertubular dentin (Fig. 10-9) to produce a hybrid zone (interpenetration zone or diffusion zone) that microscopically intertwines collagen bundles and bonding agent polymer
   4. Biologic
      a. Conditioning agents may be locally irritating if they come into contact with soft tissue
      b. Priming agents (uncured), particularly those based on HEMA, may be skin sensitizers after several contacts with dental personnel

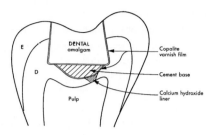

Fig. 10-10 Schematic view of varnish, liner, and base applications for use with dental amalgam that is not bonded to the cavity preparation walls.

      (1) Protect skin on hands and face from inadvertent contact with unset materials and/or their vapors
      (2) HEMA and other priming monomers may penetrate through rubber gloves in relatively short times (60 to 90 seconds)

Solution Liners (Varnishes)

A. General considerations (limited use; being replaced by bonding agents)
   1. Applications (Fig. 10-10)
      a. Enamel and dentin lining for amalgam restorations
      b. Enamel and dentin lining for cast restorations that are used with nonadhesive cements
      c. Coating over materials that are moisture sensitive during setting
B. Structure
   1. Components of copal resin varnish
      a. 90% solvent mixture (e.g., chloroform, acetone, and alcohol)
      b. 10% dissolved copal resin
   2. Reaction
      a. Varnish sets physically by drying
      b. Solvent loss occurs in 5 to 15 seconds (a film forms the same way as drying fingernail polish)
   3. Manipulation
      a. Apply thin coat over dentin, enamel, and margins of the cavity preparation
      b. Dry lightly with air for 5 seconds
      c. Apply a second thin coat
      d. Final thickness is 1 to 5 μm
C. Properties
   1. Physical
      a. Electrically insulating barrier that prevents shocks
      b. Too thin to be thermally insulating
      c. Decreases degree of percolation attributable to thermal expansion

2. Chemical
   a. Forms temporary barrier that prevents microleakage into dentinal tubules until secondary dentin formation occurs
   b. Decreases initial tendency for electrochemical corrosion
3. Mechanical
   a. Very weak and brittle film that has limited lifetime
   b. Film adheres to smear layer
4. Biologic
   a. Solvent is potentially toxic but has never been shown to cause problems to dentin
   b. Solvent should not be inhaled by client or operator

Suspension Liners

A. General considerations (limited use; being replaced by bonding agents)
   1. Applications
      a. Dentin lining under amalgam restorations
      b. Stimulation of reparative dentin formation
B. Structure
   1. Components
      a. Calcium hydroxide powder
      b. Water
      c. Modifiers
   2. Reaction
      a. Physical reaction of drying
   3. Manipulation
      a. Used as W/P or pastes
      b. Paint thin film on dentin
      c. Use forced air for 15 to 30 seconds to dry
      d. Film is thicker (15 μm) than varnishes
      e. Do not use on enamel or cavosurface margins
C. Properties
   1. Physical
      a. Electrically insulating barrier
      b. Too thin to be thermally insulating
   2. Chemical
      a. High basicity for calcium hydroxide (pH is 11)
      b. Dissolves readily in water and should not be used at exposed cavosurface margins or gaps may form
   3. Mechanical—weak film
   4. Biologic—calcium hydroxide dissolves, diffuses, and stimulates odontoblasts to occlude dentin tubules below cavity preparation

Cement Liners

A. General considerations (limited use)
   1. Applications (if remaining dentin thickness is <0.5 mm)

   a. Used for thermal insulation where cavity preparation is close to the pulp
   b. Used for delivering medicaments to the pulp
      (1) Calcium hydroxide stimulates reparative dentin or
      (2) Eugenol relieves pain by desensitizing nerves
   c. Used to deliver F ion to enamel and dentin
B. Structure (for zinc oxide—eugenol types, see section on dental cements)
   1. Components
      a. Paste of calcium hydroxide reactant powder, ethyl toluene sulfonamide dispersant, zinc oxide filler, and zinc stearate radiopacifier
      b. Paste of glycol salicylate reactant liquid, titanium dioxide filler powder, and calcium tungstenate radiopacifier
   2. Reaction
      a. Chemical reaction of calcium ions with salicylate to form methylsalicylate salts
      b. Moisture absorbed to allow calcium hydroxide to dissociate into ions to react with salicylate
      c. Mixture sets from outside surface to inside as water diffuses
   3. Manipulation
      a. Dentin should not be dehydrated or material will not set
      b. Mix drop of each paste together for 5 seconds
      c. Apply material to dentin and allow 1 to 2 minutes to set
C. Properties
   1. Physical—good thermal and electrical insulator
   2. Chemical—poor resistance to water solubility and may dissolve
   3. Mechanical—low compressive strength (100 to 500 psi)
   4. Biologic—releases calcium hydroxide constituents, which diffuse toward the pulp and stimulate reparative dentin formation

Cement Bases

A. General considerations (limited use)
   1. Applications
      a. Thermal insulation below a restoration
      b. Mechanical protection where there is inadequate dentin to support amalgam condensation pressures
   2. Classification (many types have been used)
      a. Zinc phosphate cement bases
      b. Polycarboxylate cement bases
      c. Glass ionomer cement bases (self-curing and light-curing)

B. Structure (see section on luting cements)
1. Components
a. Reactive powder (chemically basic)
b. Reactive liquid (chemically acidic)
2. Reaction
a. Acid-base reaction that forms salts or cross-linked matrix
b. Reaction may be exothermic
3. Manipulation—consistency for basing includes more powders, which improves all of the cement properties
C. Properties
1. Physical—excellent thermal and electrical insulation
2. Chemical—much more resistant to dissolution than cement liners
a. Polycarboxylate and glass ionomer cements are mechanically and chemically adhesive to tooth structure
b. Solubility of all cement bases is lower than cement liners if they are mixed at higher powder-to-liquid ratios
3. Mechanical—much higher compressive strengths (12,000 to 30,000 psi)
a. Light-cured hybrid glass ionomer cements are the strongest
b. Zinc oxide—eugenol cements are the weakest
4. Biologic (see section on luting cements for details)
a. Zinc oxide—eugenol cements are obtundent to the pulp
b. Polycarboxylate and glass ionomer cements (that are properly manipulated) are kind to the pulp

Other Cement Applications

A. Root canal sealers
1. Applications
a. Cementation of silver cone or gutta-percha point
b. Paste filling material
2. Classification
a. Zinc oxide—eugenol cement types
b. Noneugenol cement types
c. Therapeutic cement types
3. Important properties
a. Physical—radiopacity
b. Chemical—insolubility
c. Mechanical—flow; tensile strength
d. Biologic—inertness
B. Gingival tissue packs
1. Application—provide temporary displacement of gingival tissues

2. Composition—slow setting zinc oxide–eugenol cement mixed with cotton twills for texture and strength
C. Surgical dressings
1. Application—gingival covering after periodontal surgery
2. Composition—modified zinc oxide–eugenol cement (containing tannic acid, rosin, and various oils)
D. Orthodontic cements
1. Application—cementation of orthodontic bands
2. Composition—zinc phosphate cement (see luting cements or bonding agents)
3. Manipulation
a. Zinc phosphate types are routinely mixed (see luting cements) with cold or frozen mixing slab to extend the working time
b. Enamel bonding agent types use acid etching for improved bonding
c. Band, bracket, or cement removal requires special care

Temporary Filling Materials

A. General considerations
1. Applications
a. While waiting for lab fabrication of cast restoration
b. While observing reaction of pulp tissues
2. Objectives
a. Provide pulpal protection
b. Provide medication to reduce pulpal inflammation
c. Maintain the tooth position
d. Be esthetic
3. Classification
a. Temporary filling cements
b. Temporary filling resins
B. Structure
1. Components
a. Temporary filling cements
(1) Zinc oxide–eugenol cement with cotton fibers added
(2) Polymer powder–reinforced zinc oxide–eugenol cement
b. Temporary filling resins
(1) MMA/PMMA filling materials
(2) Bis-acryl filling materials
2. Reaction (see section on cements and composites)
3. Manipulation (see section on cements and composites)
C. Properties
1. Physical
a. Excellent thermal and electrical insulation

b. Percolation resistance is good for cements but poor for resins
2. Chemical—generally good resistance to dissolution
3. Mechanical
   a. Good short-term resistance to fracture
   b. Poor resistance to abrasion
4. Biologic—cements are biocompatible, but resins with low–molecular-weight monomers may cause pulpal inflammation if cured in situ without caution

Permanent Cement Filling Materials

A. General considerations
   1. Applications for glass ionomer cements
      a. Class V restorations—resin-modified glass ionomers for geriatric dentistry
      b. Class I and II restorations—resin-modified glass ionomers, metal-modified glass ionomers in pediatric dentistry
      c. Class III restorations—resin-modified glass ionomers
   2. Classification by composition
      a. Conventional glass ionomer—limited use
      b. Metal-modified glass ionomer—limited use
      c. Resin-modified glass ionomer—popular use
      d. Compomer (hybrid of composite and glass ionomer)—popular use (see Fig. 10-11)
B. Structure—glass ionomer cements

1. Components
   a. Powder—aluminosilicate glass
   b. Liquid—water solution of copolymers (or acrylic acid with maleic, tartaric, or itaconic acids) and water-soluble monomers (e.g., HEMA)
2. Reaction (may involve several reactions and stages of setting)
   a. Glass ionomer reaction (acid-base reaction of polyacid and ions released from aluminosilicate glass particles)
      (1) Calcium, aluminum, fluoride, and other ions released by outside of powder particle dissolving in acidic liquid
      (2) Calcium ions initially cross-link acid functional copolymer molecules
      (3) Calcium cross-links are replaced in 24 to 48 hours by aluminum ion cross-links, with increased hardening of system
      (4) If there are no other reactants in the cement (e.g., resin modification), then protection from saliva is required during the first 24 hours
   b. Polymerization reaction (polymerization of double bonds from water-soluble monomers and/or pendant groups on copolymer to form cross-linked matrix)
      (1) Polymerization reaction can be initiated

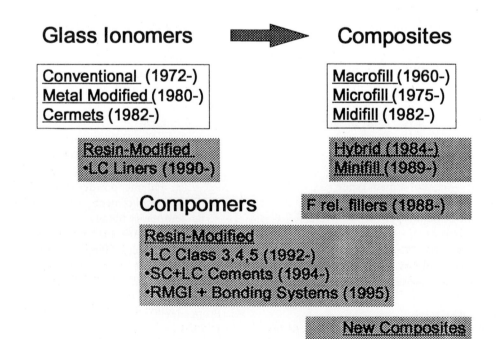

Fig. 10-11 Evolution of glass laminate compositions toward composites over 25 years.

with chemical (self-curing) or light-curing steps

   (2) Cross-linked polymer matrix ultimately interpenetrates glass ionomer matrix

  3. Manipulation

   a. Mixing—powder and liquid components may be manually mixed or may be precapsulated for mechanical mixing

   b. Placement—mixture is normally syringed into place

   c. Finishing—can be immediate if system is resin-modified (but otherwise must be delayed 24 to 72 hours until aluminum ion replacement reaction is complete)

   d. Sealing—sealer is applied to smooth the surface (and to protect against moisture affecting the glass ionomer reaction)

C. Properties

  1. Physical

   a. Good thermal and electrical insulation

   b. Better radiopacity than most composites

   c. Linear coefficient of thermal expansion and contraction is closer to tooth structure than for composites (but is less well matched for resin-modified systems)

   d. Aesthetics of resin-modified systems are competitive with composites

  2. Chemical

   a. Reactive acid side groups of copolymer molecules may produce chemical bonding to tooth structure

   b. Fluoride ions are released

    (1) Rapid release at first due to excess fluoride ions in matrix

    (2) Slow release after 7 to 30 days because of slow diffusion of fluoride ions out of aluminosilicate particles (see Figure 10-11)

   c. Solubility resistance of resin-modified systems is close to that of composites

  3. Mechanical properties

   a. Compressive strength of resin-modified systems is much better than that of traditional glass ionomers but not quite as strong as composites

   b. Glass ionomers are more brittle than composites

  4. Biologic properties

   a. Ingredients are biologically kind to the pulp

   b. Fluoride ion release may discourage secondary caries (see Fig. 10-12)

Fluoride Gels

A. General considerations (see Chapter 12, section on professionally administered topical fluoride treatments)

  1. Applications—used to prevent smooth surface caries

  2. Classification

   a. Acidulated phosphate fluoride gels (acid pH)

   b. Neutral gels (sodium fluoride at neutral pH)

B. Structure for APF

  1. Composition

   a. Fluoride ion concentration ranges from 1.22% to 1.32%

   b. Ingredients—2% sodium fluoride, 0.34% hydrogen fluoride, 0.98% orthophosphoric acid, thickening agent, flavoring agent, coloring agent, and aqueous gel

   c. pH ranges from 3 to 4 (and may dissolve glass in restorations so those surfaces must be protected)

  2. Reactions

   a. Acid demineralization of outer layer of enamel

   b. Fluoride accelerates remineralization of demineralized enamel

   c. Fluoride ions incorporated to produce fluoride-substituted hydroxyapatite

  3. Manipulation

   a. Gels are applied in a soft, spongy tray after prophylaxis

   b. Teeth should be free from saliva

   c. Maxillary and mandibular trays are loaded, placed in position, and squeezed to mold the trays tightly around the teeth

   d. Tray is held in position for 4 minutes (shorter applications are not effective)

   e. Patient is told not to eat or drink for 30 minutes

C. Properties

  1. Chemical—enamel solubility is decreased by fluoride ion incorporation

  2. Biologic—enamel is more resistant to carious dissolution

Tooth Polishing and Cleansing Agents

A. General considerations

  1. Cleansing—removal of exogenous stains, pellicle, materia alba, and other oral debris without causing undue abrasion to tooth structure

  2. Polishing—smoothing surfaces of amalgam, composite, glass ionomers, porcelain, and other restorative materials

  3. Factors influencing cleaning and polishing

   a. Hardness of abrasive particles versus substrate (see Tables 10-1 and 10-2)

   b. Particle size of abrasive particles

   c. Pressure applied during procedure

   d. Temperature of abrasive materials

B. Structure

  1. Composition—contain abrasives, such as kaolinite, silicon dioxide, calcined magnesium silicate, diato-

maceous silicon dioxide, pumice, sodium-potassium aluminum silicate, or zirconium silicate; some pastes also may contain sodium fluoride or stannous fluoride, but they have never been shown to produce positive effects
2. Reactions—abrasion for cleansing and polishing
3. Manipulation (see section on abrasion)

C. Properties

1. Mechanical
   a. Products with pumice and quartz produce more efficient cleansing but also generate greater abrasion of enamel and dentin
   b. Coarse pumice is the most abrasive
   c. The abrasion rate of dentin is 5 to 6 times faster than the abrasion rate of enamel, regardless of the product

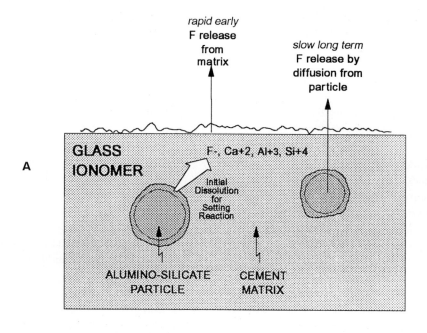

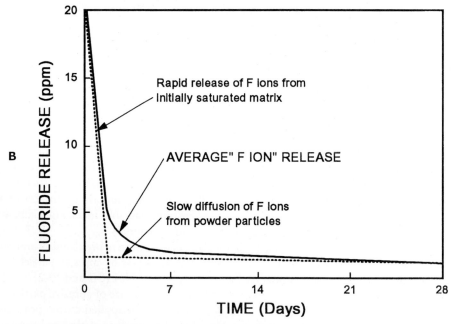

Fig. 10-12   A, Schematic view of fluoride ion diffusion from glass ionomer cement. **B,** Schematic summary of fluoride concentration released by glass ionomer cement over time. From Bayne SC: In Sturdevant CM. Dental materials. Art and science of operative dentistry, ed 3, St. Louis, 1995, Mosby.)

d. Polymeric restorative materials, such as denture bases, denture teeth, composites, PMMA veneers, and composite veneers, can be easily scratched during polishing
e. Do not polish cast porcelain restorations (e.g., Dicor) that are externally characterized or the color will be lost
2. Biologic—no known problems

Indirect Preventive/Restorative Materials

Impression Materials

A. General considerations
1. Applications
   a. Dentulous impressions for casts for prosthodontics
   b. Dentulous impressions for pedodontic appliances
   c. Dentulous impressions for study models for orthodontics
   d. Edentulous impressions for casts for denture construction
2. Terminology
   a. Rigid—inflexible and will not remove from undercut area
   b. Flexible—capable of removal from undercut area
   c. Hydrocolloid—gel produced by interconnection of small particles (colloid, <1 μm) dispersed in water
   d. Rubber or elastomer—based on polymeric material that is flexible
3. Classification
   a. Rigid impression materials
      (1) Plaster
      (2) Compound
      (3) Zinc oxide–eugenol
   b. Flexible hydrocolloid impression materials
      (1) Agar-agar (reversible hydrocolloid)
      (2) Alginate (irreversible hydrocolloid)
   c. Flexible, elastomeric, or rubber impression materials
      (1) Polysulfide rubber (mercaptan rubber)
      (2) Silicone rubber (condensation silicone)
      (3) Polyether rubber
      (4) Polyvinyl siloxane (addition silicone)
B. Structure
1. Components (Table 10-3)
   a. Fillers added to most to control shrinkage
   b. Matrix
2. Reaction (Table 10-3)

Table 10-3

Impression Materials

Materials	Type	Reaction	Composition	Manipulation	Initial setting time
Plaster	Rigid	Chemical	Calcium sulfate hemihydrate, water	Mix P/L in bowl	3-5 min
Compound	Rigid	Physical	Resins, wax, stearic acid, and fillers	Soften by heating	Variable (sets on cooling)
Zinc oxide–eugenol	Rigid	Chemical	Zinc oxide powder, oils, eugenol, and resin	Mix pastes on pad	3-5 min
Agar-agar	Flexible	Physical	12-15% agar, borax, potassium sulfate, and 85% water	Mix P/L in bowl	Variable (sets on cooling)
Alginate	Flexible	Chemical	Sodium alginate, calcium sulfate, retarders, and 85% water	Mix P/L in bowl	4-5 min
Polysulfide	Flexible	Chemical	Low MW mercaptan polymer, fillers, lead dioxide, copper hydroxide, or peroxides	Mix pastes on pad	5-7 min
Silicone	Flexible	Chemical	Hydroxyl functioanl dimethyl siloxane, fillers, tin octoate, and orthoethyl silicate	Mix pastes on pad	4-5 min
Polyether	Flexible	Chemical	Aromatic sulfonic acid ester and polyether with ethylene imine groups	Mixing gun or mixing machine	2-4 min
Polyvinyl siloxane	Flexible	Chemical	Vinyl silicone, filler, chloroplatinic acid, low MW silicone, and filler	Mixing gun or mixing machine	4-5 min

Table 10-4

Gypsum Products

Characteristics	Plaster	Stone	Diestone
Chemical name	Beta-calcium sulfate hemihydrate	Alpha-calcium sulfate hemihydrate	Alpha-calcium sulfate hemihydrate
Formula	$CaSO_4 \cdot \frac{1}{2}H_2O$	$CaSO_4 \cdot \frac{1}{2}H_2O$	$CaSO_4 \cdot \frac{1}{2}H_2O$
Uses	Plaster models, impression plaster	Cast stone, investments	Improved stone, diestone
Water (W)			
Reaction water	18 ml	18 ml	18 ml
Extra water	32 ml	12 ml	6 ml
Total water	50 ml	30 ml	24 ml
Powder (P)	100 g	100 g	100 g
W/P ratio	0.50	0.30	0.24

a. Physical reaction—cooling causes reversible hardening
b. Chemical reaction—irreversible reaction during setting
3. Manipulation
  a. Mixing
    (1) P/L types mixed in bowl (plaster and alginate)
    (2) Thermoplastic materials not mixed (compound and agar-agar)
    (3) Hand-mix: paste/paste types hand mixed on pad (zinc oxide–eugenol, polysulfide rubber, silicone rubber, polyether rubber, and polyvinylsiloxane)
    (4) Auto-mix: paste/paste mixed through a nozzle on an auto-mixing gun (polyvinyl siloxane)
    (5) Machine mix: components mixed and extruded using small machine (e.g., Pentamix)
  b. Placement
    (1) Mixed material carried in tray to mouth (full arch tray, quadrant tray, or triple tray)
    (2) Materials set in mouth more quickly because of higher temperature
  c. Removal—rapid removal of impression encourages deformation to take place elastically rather than permanently (elastic deformation requires about 20 minutes)
  d. Cleaning and disinfection of impressions (see Chapter 7, section on infection control for the dental laboratory)
  e. Problems: polyvinyl siloxane may be surface inhibited by dentin bonding agent from preparation wall and may be dissolved by subsequent infection control solutions

Model, Cast, and Die Materials

A. General considerations
  1. Applications
    a. Gold casting, porcelain, and porcelain-fused-to-metal veneer fabrication procedures
    b. Orthodontic and pedodontic appliance construction
    c. Study models for occlusal records
  2. Terminology
    a. Models—replicas of hard and soft tissues for study of dental symmetry
    b. Casts—working replicas of hard and soft tissues for use in the fabrication of appliances or restorations
    c. Dies—working replicas of one tooth (or a few teeth) used for the fabrication of a restoration
    d. Duplicates—second casts prepared from original casts
  3. Classification by materials
    a. Models (model plaster or orthodontic stone; gypsum product)
    b. Stone casts (regular stone; gypsum product)
    c. Stone dies (diestone; gypsum product)—may be electroplated
    d. Epoxy dies (epoxy polymer)—abrasion-resistant dies
B. Structure of gypsum products
  1. Components (Table 10-4)
    a. Powder (calcium sulfate hemihydrate = $CaSO_4 \cdot \frac{1}{2}H_2O$)
    b. Water (for reaction with powder and dispersing powder)
  2. Reaction
    a. Calcium sulfate hemihydrate (one-half water) crystals dissolve and react with water

b. Calcium sulfate dihydrate (two waters) form and precipitate new crystals
c. Unreacted (excess) water is left between crystals in solid
3. Manipulation
  a. Selection—based on strength for models, casts, or dies
  b. Mixing
    (1) Proportion the water and powder (Table 10-4)
    (2) Sift powder into water in rubber mixing bowl
    (3) Use stiff blade spatula to mix mass on side of bowl
    (4) Complete mixing in 60 seconds
  c. Placement
    (1) Use vibration to remove air bubbles acquired through mixing
    (2) Use vibration during placement to help mixture wet and flow into the impression
C. Properties
1. Physical
  a. Excellent thermal and electrical insulator
  b. Very dense
  c. Excellent dimensional stability
  d. Good reproduction of fine detail of hard and soft tissues
2. Chemical
  a. Heating will reverse the reaction (decompose the material into calcium sulfate hemihydrate, the original dry component)
  b. Models, casts, and dies should be wet during grinding or cutting operations to prevent heating
3. Mechanical
  a. Better powder packing and lower water contents at mixing lead to higher compressive strengths (plaster < stone < diestone)
  b. Poor resistance to abrasion
4. Biologic
  a. Materials are safe for contact with external epithelial tissues
  b. Masks should be worn during grinding or polishing operations that are likely to produce gypsum dust

Waxes

A. General considerations
1. Applications
  a. Making impressions
  b. Registering of tooth or soft tissue positions
  c. Creating restorative patterns for lab fabrication
  d. Aiding in laboratory procedures
2. Terminology

  a. Inlay wax—used to create a pattern for inlay, onlay, or crown for subsequent investing and casting in a metal alloy
  b. Casting wax—used to create a pattern for metallic framework for a removable partial denture
  c. Baseplate wax—used to establish the vertical dimension, plane of occlusion, and initial arch form of a complete denture
  d. Corrective impression wax—used to form a registry pattern of soft tissues on an impression
  e. Bite registration wax—used to form a registry pattern for the occlusion of opposing models or casts
  f. Boxing wax—used to form a box around an impression before pouring a model or cast
  g. Utility wax—soft pliable adhesive wax for modifying appliances, such as alginate impression trays
  h. Sticky wax—sticky when melted and used to temporarily adhere pieces of metal or resin in laboratory procedures
3. Classification
  a. Pattern waxes—inlay, casting, and base registration waxes
  b. Impression waxes—corrective and biteplate waxes
  c. Processing waxes—boxing, utility, and sticky waxes
B. Structure
1. Components
  a. Base waxes—hydrocarbon (paraffin) or ester waxes
  b. Modifier waxes—carnauba, ceresin, beeswax, rosin, gum dammar, or microcrystalline waxes
  c. Additives—colorants
2. Reaction—waxes are thermoplastic
C. Properties
1. Physical
  a. High coefficients of thermal expansion and contraction
  b. Insulators (cool unevenly); should be waxed in increments to allow heat dissipation
2. Chemical
  a. Degrade prematurely if overheated
  b. Designed to degrade into CO_2 and H_2O during burnout
3. Mechanical—stiffness, hardness, and strength depend on modifier waxes used

Investment Materials

A. General considerations
1. Applications

3. Classification by materials
   a. Laminate veneers—PMMA outer surface
   b. Direct composite resin veneer
   c. Indirect composite resin veneer (laboratory processed)
   d. Porcelain veneer
   e. CAD/CAM or copy-milled ceramic veneer
B. Structure
   1. Components—PMMA, composite, porcelain, or other ceramic
   2. Manipulation
      a. Bonding—enamel etching and bonding agents
      b. Finishing and polishing must be done with care to avoid scratching the surfaces
   3. Maintenance
      a. Do not polish or scale with abrasive materials
      b. Protect during topical APF fluoride treatments or use neutral sodium fluoride
C. Properties
   1. Physical—good aesthetics, but some color may be provided by composite resin used for bonding the veneer
   2. Chemical
      a. PMMA and composite veneers have good acid resistance
      b. Porcelain and CAD/CAM veneers should be protected from APF or other acids
   3. Mechanical
      a. PMMA and composite veneers are subject to scratching
      b. Porcelain and CAD/CAM veneers have good abrasion resistance
   4. Biologic—no known problems

CAD/CAM and Copy-Milled Restorations

A. General considerations
   1. Applications—inlays, onlays, veneers, crowns, bridges, implants, and implant prostheses
   2. Stages of fabrication for CAD/CAM
      a. CSD—computerized surface digitization
      b. CAD—computer-aided (assisted) design
      c. CAM—computer-aided (assisted) machining
   3. Stages of fabrication for copy-milling
      a. Fabrication of wax or composite dies
      b. Dies and ceramic blocks mounted in tandem for copy-milling operation
   4. Classification
      a. Chairside or in-office systems
         (1) Cerec II (Siemens system)—inlays, onlays, veneers, and crowns
      b. Laboratory systems
         (1) DentiCAD (Rekow system)—inlays, onlays, veneers, crowns

      (2) Cicero (Elephant system)—porcelain-fused-to-metal crowns
      (3) Celay (Vident)—copy-milling of inlays, onlays, veneers, crowns, and bridges
B. Structure
   1. Materials
      a. Feldspathic porcelains (Vita)
      b. Machinable glass ceramics (Dicor MGC)
      c. Machinable high strength ceramics (Inceram)
      d. Metal alloys (limited use)
   2. Cementing
      a. Etching enamel and/or dentin for micromechanical retention
      b. Bonding agent for retention to etched surface
      c. Composite as a luting cement for reacting chemically with bonding agent and with silanated surfaces of restoration
      d. Silane for bonding to etched ceramic (or metal) restorations and to provide chemical reaction
      e. Hydrofluoric acid etching to create spaces for micromechanical retention on surface of restoration
C. Properties
   1. Physical properties
      a. Thermal expansion coefficient well matched to tooth structure
      b. Good resistance to plaque adsorption or retention
      c. Superior esthetics (for shade matching)
   2. Chemical properties—not resistant to hydrofluoric acid and should be protected from APF
   3. Mechanical properties
      a. Excellent wear resistance (but may abrade opponent teeth)
      b. Some wear of luting cements but self-limiting
      c. Excellent toothbrush abrasion
      d. Limited fatigue resistance due to brittleness and initiation and propagation of cracks
   4. Biologic properties—excellent properties

Dental Implants

See Chapter 11, section on dental implants.
A. General considerations
   1. Applications
      a. Single-tooth implants
      b. Abutments for bridges (freestanding, attached to natural teeth)
      c. Abutments for overdentures
   2. Terminology
      a. Subperiosteal—below the periosteum but above the bone (second most frequently used types)
      b. Intramucosal—within the mucosa

    c. Endosseous—into the bone (80% of all current types)

    d. Endodontic—through the root canal space and into the periapical bone

    e. Transosteal—through the bone

    f. Bone substitutes—replacing bone

  3. Classification by geometric form

    a. Blades

    b. Root forms

    c. Screws

    d. Cylinders

    e. Staples

    f. Circumferential

    g. Others

  4. Classification by materials type

    a. Metallic—titanium, stainless steel, and chromium/cobalt

    b. Polymeric—PMMA

    c. Ceramic—hydroxyapatite, carbon, and sapphire

  5. Classification by attachment design

    a. Bioactive surface retention by osseointegration

    b. Nonactive porous surfaces for micromechanical retention by osseointegration

    c. Nonactive, nonporous surface for ankylosis by osseointegration

    d. Gross mechanical retention designs (e.g., threads, screws, channels, or transverse holes)

    e. Fibrointegration by formation of fibrous tissue capsule

    f. Combinations of the above

B. Structure

  1. Components

    a. Root (for osseointegration)

    b. Neck (for epithelial attachment and percutaneous sealing)

    c. Intramobile elements (for shock absorption)

    d. Prosthesis (for dental form and function)

  2. Manipulation

    a. Selection—based on remaining bone architecture and dimensions

    b. Sterilization—radiofrequency glow discharge leaves biomaterial surface uncontaminated and sterile; autoclaving or chemical sterilization is contraindicated for some designs

C. Properties

  1. Physical—should have low thermal and electrical conductivity

  2. Chemical

    a. Should be resistant to electrochemical corrosion

    b. Do not expose surfaces to acids (e.g., APF fluorides)

    c. Keep in mind the effects of adjunctive therapies (e.g., Peridex)

  3. Mechanical

    a. Should be abrasion resistant and have a high modulus

    b. Do not abrade during scaling operations (e.g., with metal scalers or air-power abrasion systems like the Prophy jet)

  4. Biologic—depend on osseointegration and epithelial attachment

SUGGESTED READINGS

Anusavice KJ, Phillips RW: *Science of dental materials,* ed 10, Philadelphia, 1996, WB Saunders.

Bayne SC, Taylor DF, Zardiackas LD: *Biomaterials science,* Chapel Hill, NC, 1992, Brightstar.

Barton RE, Matteson SR, Richardson RE: *The dental assistant,* ed 6, Philadelphia, 1988, Lea & Febiger.

Craig RG: *Dental materials: A problem-oriented approach,* St Louis, 1978, Mosby.

Craig RG, editor: *Restorative dental materials,* ed 10, St Louis, 1997, Mosby.

Craig RG, O'Brien WJ, Powers JM: *Dental materials Properties and manipulation,* ed 3, St Louis, 1983, Mosby.

Dentists' desk reference: Materials, instruments, and equipment, ed 2, Chicago, 1983, American Dental Association.

Ferracane JL: *Materials in dentistry,* Philadelphia, 1995, JB Lippincott.

Leinfelder KF, Barton RE, Taylor DF: *Dental assisting manual, VI, Dental materials and technical application,* ed 3, Chapel Hill, NC, 1980, The University of North Carolina Press.

Leinfelder KF, Lemons JE: *Clinical restorative materials and techniques,* Philadelphia, 1988, Lea & Febiger.

O'Brien WJ: *An outline of dental materials and their selection,* ed 6, Philadelphia, 1989, WB Saunders.

Phillips RW, Moore BK: Elements of dental materials, ed 5, Philadelphia, 1994, WB Saunders.

Review Questions

1 Which *ONE* of the following is *NOT* a packaging method for dental materials?

  A. Three components mixed in an auto-mixing syringe

  B. Two components mixed in a machine mixer

  C. One component that sets when water is added

  D. One component that sets when VLC is added

  E. A powder and liquid that are mixed by spatulation

2 What is the setting time?

  A. Time elapsed from the onset of mixing until the beginning of setting

  B. Time elapsed from the end of mixing until the end of the working interval

  C. Length of the working interval

  D. Length of the setting interval

  E. Time elapsed from the onset of mixing until the end of the setting process

3 Which *ONE* of the following requires VLC (visible light curing) for setting?
A. Dental amalgam
B. Polyvinyl siloxane
C. Calcium sulfate hemihydrate
D. Traditional glass ionomer
E. Posterior composite

4 Which *ONE* of the following procedures does *NOT* involve a loss of gloss during setting?
A. Pit-and-fissure sealant
B. Plaster
C. Glass ionomer cement
D. Dental amalgam
E. Alginate

5 What is the linear coefficient of thermal expansion for tooth structure?
A. 5 ppm/°C
B. 10 ppm/°C
C. 15 ppm/°C
D. 20 ppm/°C
E. 60 ppm/°C

6 Which *ONE* of the following is a poor thermal insulator?
A. Dentin
B. Enamel
C. Gold alloy restorations
D. Glass ionomer cement
E. Ceramic inlays

7 Which *ONE* of the following is most important for good pulpal insulation?
A. Liners that are good thermal insulators
B. Dentin sealing
C. 1 to 2 mm thickness of insulation below a restoration
D. Low optical conductivity
E. High density

8 Which *ONE* of the following terms is not related to color?
A. Fluoresence
B. Luminance
C. Dominance
D. Translucency
E. Resilience

9 Which *ONE* of the following is not associated with electrochemical corrosion events?
A. Stress
B. Crevices
C. Plaque
D. Passivation
E. Metamerism

10 Engineering stress is computed as:
A. Applied load divided by the original cross-sectional area of the object
B. Applied load divided by the volume of the object
C. Modulus multiplied by the plastic deformation
D. Difference between the total strain and the plastic strain
E. Percent elongation

11 Engineering strain is computed as:
A. Change between the initial and final strain divided by the time
B. Area under the stress-strain curve
C. Modulus multiplied by the plastic deformation
D. Applied load divided by the original cross-sectional area of the object
E. Deformation divided by the original length of the object

12 What is another name for a material's modulus?
A. Stiffness
B. Resilience
C. Toughness
D. Fatigue resistance
E. Strain rate sensitivity

13 Loading of a restoration beyond the material's elastic limit produces:
A. Only plastic deformation
B. Only elastic deformation
C. Fatigue fracture
D. Elastic and plastic deformation
E. Stress relaxation

14 The point at which loading begins to produce both plastic and elastic strain at the same time is called any of the following terms except:
A. Elastic limit
B. Yield point
C. Proportional limit
D. Hardness
E. Breaking point

15 Which *ONE* of the following statements is not true about the Moh's hardness scale?
A. Scale involves units of 1 to 10
B. Diamond is the hardest reference value
C. Talc is the softest reference value
D. Enamel is 7-8 on the scale
E. Dentin is 3-4 on the scale

16 Which *ONE* of the following biologic reactions is concentration-dependent?
A. Hypersensitivity
B. Fibrous capsule formation
C. Toxicity
D. Inflammation
E. None of the above

17 Which *ONE* of the following phases in dental amalgam restorations is most prone to electrochemical corrosion?
A. Ag-Sn
B. Ag-Sn-Cu
C. Sn-Hg
D. Cu-Sn
E. Ag-Hg

18 Which *ONE* of the following phases in dental amalgam restorations has the best mechanical properties and highest corrosion resistance?
A. Ag-Sn
B. Cu-Sn
C. Sn-Hg
D. Ag-Hg
E. All of the above

19 Which *ONE* of the following mixing methods permits the escape of dental amalgam mercury vapor?
A. Mixing in a mortar and pestle
B. Proportioning mercury and alloy into a friction-fit-capsule
C. Triturating pre-capsulated alloy and mercury
D. A cover over the mixing arms on a triturator
E. All of the above

20 Low copper dental amalgam alloys involve what ranges of copper in their composition?
A. 0.1% to 0.5%
B. 0.5% to 1%
C. 1% to 5%
D. 6% to 12%
E. 12% to 15%

21 Which *ONE* of the following is not true about high copper dental amalgam restorations?
A. Better corrosion resistance than low copper dental amalgams
B. Contain both Sn and Ag in the composition as well
C. Produce excessive creep
D. Restorations are more brittle than low copper versions
E. Contain 12% to 30% copper in the original alloy composition mixed with Hg

22 What is the melting temperature of the Ag-Hg matrix phase in a set dental amalgam restoration?
A. 127°C
B. 227°C
C. 327°C
D. 427°C
E. 527°C

23 Which *ONE* of the following is the criterion for a failed high copper dental amalgam restoration?
A. Accumulation of black or green tarnish on the exposed surfaces
B. Marginal ditching along occlusal margins
C. Creep of the restoration out of the cavity preparation in proximal areas
D. Wear facets along the occlusal contact areas
E. None of the above

24 Surface wear on posterior dental composite restorations should be managed by:
A. Replacing the composite with a dental amalgam
B. Repairing the worn areas with resin-modified glass ionomer
C. Replacing the restoration with a new high-strength ceramic
D. Adjustment of the occlusion of the opponent tooth
E. Resurfacing of the old composite with new composite

25 Which *ONE* of the following procedures is standard for conditioning tooth structure before bonding procedures for composite restorations?
A. Phosphoric acid conditioning of enamel only
B. Phosphoric acid conditioning of dentin only
C. Phosphoric acid conditioning of enamel and dentin
D. EDTA conditioning of enamel and dentin
E. Polyacrylic acid conditioning of enamel and dentin

26 The smear layer is all of the following except:
A. 2 to 5 micron layer of debris from enamel and dentin cavity preparation
B. Primarily hydroxyapatite in composition
C. Loosely adherent to tooth structure with about 4 to 6 MPa of bond strength
D. Capable of partially sealing dentinal tubules
E. Soluble in HEMA in priming agents for dentin bonding procedures

27 Strong bonding to dentin requires:
A. Extensive conditioning
B. Very dry dentin
C. Pre-application of chlorhexidine
D. Scrubbing during conditioning
E. Hybrid layer formation

28 Which *ONE* of the following items is *NOT* related to the others?
A. Resin-interpenetration zone
B. Hybrid layer
C. Resin interdiffusion zone
D. Collagen impregnation zone
E. Silanation zone

29 Water-miscible acrylic monomers are most likely found in:
A. Liquid conditioners
B. Gel conditioners
C. Pit-and-fissure sealants
D. Dentin primers
E. Dentin adhesives

30 Which *ONE* of the following is *NOT* required for good dentin bonding?
A. Conditioning
B. Dentin with a glistening appearance after conditioning
C. Dentin with a glistening appearance after priming
D. Use of adhesive
E. Air thinning to eliminate excess primer or adhesive

31 Recent version of dentin bonding systems for composites are simpler because:
A. Conditioning is not required for bonding
B. No mixing of components is required
C. Bonding agents have already been added directly to the dental composite
D. Only one layer is applied rather than two to five coats
E. There are two steps rather than three in the procedure

32 Which *ONE* of the following restorations does not require protection with vaseline during APF application procedures?
A. High-strength ceramics
B. Hybrid dental composites
C. Resin-modified glass ionomers
D. PFM
E. Cast gold

33 Which *ONE* of the following is the *LEAST* effective method of sealing a cavity preparation?
1. Copalite
2. Dentin bonding system
3. Amalgam bonding system
4. Glass ionomer liner
5. Bonded composite cement

34 Which *ONE* of the following constituents may produce palliative action if it can diffuse to the dental pulp?
A. Calcium hydroxide
B. Eugenol
C. HEMA
D. BIS-GMA
E. 4-META

35 Which *ONE* of the following cavity preparation liners provides no practical thermal insulation for the pulp?
A. Glass ionomer liner
B. Zinc phosphate cement base
C. Polycarboxylate cement base
D. Calcium hydroxide liner
E. Dentin bonding systems

36 The largest component of zinc phosphate, polycarboxylate, and ZOE dental cements is:
A. Water
B. Silica
C. Mineral acid
D. Eugenol
E. Zinc oxide

37 Glass ionomer cement may chemically adhere to tooth structure as a result of what event?
A. Aluminum ions released from the particles of cement powder
B. Chelation of calcium by ionized polyacrylate groups
C. Electrostatic attraction to aluminosilicate powder
D. Hydration of the set materials
E. Fluoride ion release

38 In dental cements, increasing the powder-to-liquid ratio of components produces:
A. Lower strength
B. Higher modulus
C. Increased water absorption
D. Improved toughness
E. Increased solubility

39 Compomers are:
A. Very slightly modified glass ionomers
B. Composites that set by a new chemical reaction
C. Composites that contain excessive free monomer after visible light-curing
D. Extensively modified glass ionomers approaching composites
E. Biologically compatible glass ionomers

40 The principal advantage of resin-modified glass ionomers over traditional ones is:
A. Immediate finishing is possible
B. Mixing is much easier
C. All post-operative sensitivity is eliminated
D. Better adhesion to tooth structure
E. No shrinkage occurs on setting

41 The major use of glass ionomer restorations is for which application?
A. Class III restorations in older adults
B. Thin, saucer-shaped Class V restorations
C. Class II restorations in children
D. Class IV restorations in permanent teeth
E. Root caries lesions

42 In addition to the hardness of an abrasive material, what is also a key factor in the cutting effectiveness of the abrasive?
A. Particle size of the abrasive
B. Fluoride in the abrasive paste
C. Cooling water during the procedure
D. Vibration of the paste
E. Thickness of the abrasive paste against the surface

43 All of the following are flexible impression materials *EXCEPT:*
A. Alginate
B. Polyether
C. Polyvinyl siloxane
D. Polysulfide
E. ZOE

44 Which *ONE* of the following impression materials does not set via a chemical reaction?
A. Agar-agar hydrocolloid
B. ZOE
C. Polysulfide
D. Polyether
E. Polyvinyl siloxane

45 Which *ONE* of the following impression materials may be machine mixed?
A. Alginate
B. ZOE
C. Polyether
D. Silicone
E. Polysulfide

46 What is the removable piece from a working cast that contains the prepared tooth information called?
A. Die
B. Master cast
C. Negative
D. Duplicate
E. Model

47 What is the chemical composition of gypsum products that have fully reacted with water?
A. Calcium sulfate hemihydrate
B. Calcium sulfate monohydrate
C. Calcium sulfate dihydrate
D. Calcium sulfate trihydrate
E. Calcium sulfate tetrahydrate

48 Gypsum powder that is to be reacted to form working casts is composed primarily of:
A. Aluminosilicate glass
B. Calcium sulfate hemihydrate
C. Calcium carbonate
D. Sodium fluoride
E. Calcium phosphate

49 How much water of reaction is required for the setting of 100 grams of calcium sulfate hemihydrate powder?
A. 10 ml
B. 18 ml
C. 24 ml
D. 32 ml
E. 50 ml

50 What is the major difference between plaster and stone powders?
   A. Degree of water hydration
   B. Color
   C. Different chemical reactions on setting
   D. Different powder particle packing
   E. Different setting times

51 What is the reason that different types of gypsum-based powders require different amounts of water for mixing?
   A. Powder particles pack differently
   B. Different reactions are involved
   C. Some powder particles are porous and imbibe water
   D. Water controls the viscosity and flow-ability of the mixture
   E. Some materials are naturally more hygroscopic in air

52 What is the reason that wax application to dies to create patterns for onlays and crowns should be accomplished slowly and in thin layers allowing each increment to cool?
   A. Low elastic modulus of wax
   B. Poor adhesion of wax to the dies
   C. Distortion from thermal contraction
   D. Susceptibility to water absorption
   E. Porosity

53 What is the major component in most dental waxes?
   A. Carnauba wax
   B. Colorant
   C. Paraffin
   D. Rosin
   E. Beeswax

54 Dental inlay waxes are primarily formulated with what goal in mind?
   A. High modulus
   B. Minimizing the thermal expansion coefficient
   C. Complete pyrolysis on heating to CO_2 and H_2O
   D. Color matched to application or use
   E. Cost

55 What is the classification scheme for dental investment materials?
   A. Composition of the matrix phase
   B. Amount of water involved in mixing the materials
   C. Extent of expansion on heating
   D. Compatibility with casting alloy types
   E. Ranges of strength

56 What is the investment material used primarily with high gold casting alloys for all metal crowns?
   A. Gypsum bonded investment
   B. Silicate bonded investment
   C. Phosphate bonded investment
   D. Magnesia investment
   E. Ceramming investment

57 What is the karatage of an alloy that is 50% Au by weight?
   A. 10 karat
   B. 12 karat
   C. 20 karat
   D. 24 karat
   E. 50 karat

58 In high-gold casting alloys, which element is primarily responsible for good corrosion resistance?
   A. Au
   B. Cu
   C. Ag
   D. Zn
   E. Pd

59 In high-gold casting alloys, which element is primarily responsible for counteracting the effect of copper on the color?
   A. Au
   B. Pt
   C. Ag
   D. Zn
   E. Pd

60 What is the effect of chromium oxide for stainless steel alloys?
   A. Aid in production of alloy
   B. Produces the shiny color for the alloy
   C. Increases the modulus
   D. Passivating film that prevents corrosion
   E. Material for polishing stainless steel orthodontic brackets

61 Which ONE of the following materials does not involve passivation?
   A. Stainless steel
   B. Cr-Ni
   C. Cr-Co
   D. Titanium
   E. Lithium aluminosilicate glass

62 The difference between soldering and brazing is:
   A. Temperature
   B. Type of solder
   C. Method of fluxing
   D. Acid pretreatment
   E. Corrosion resistance

63 Which ONE of the following terms is related to dental solders?
   A. 650 fine
   B. Low gold alloys
   C. Passivation
   D. Welding
   E. Vitrification

64 Gold alloys for porcelain-fused-to-metal applications versus all gold crown applications require:
   A. Better electrochemical corrosion resistance
   B. Lower thermal conductivity
   C. Whiter color
   D. High melting temperatures
   E. None of the above

65 Nickel sensitivity could occur with all of the following compositions except:
   A. Stainless steel orthodontic wires and brackets
   B. Stainless steel crowns on primary teeth
   C. Ni-Cr PFM restorations
   D. Co-Cr partial dentures
   E. All of the above

66 What is the general incidence of nickel sensitivity for men?
   A. 1%
   B. 4%
   C. 8%
   D. 11%
   E. 20%

67 What are the main components in typical dental porcelains?
   A. Silica, calcium carbonate, and alumina
   B. Silica, alumina, and potassium oxide
   C. Alumina, zinc oxide, and fluoride
   D. Alumina, potassium oxide, and calcium oxide
   E. Calcium oxide, magnesium oxide, and chromium oxide

68 Which *ONE* of the following is *NOT* an advantage for dental ceramics?
   A. Excellent color and translucency
   B. Low coefficient of thermal expansion
   C. Low plastic deformation
   D. Low thermal and electrical conductivity
   E. High hardness

69 Which *ONE* of the following is true about traditional dental cements?
   A. Requires mixing in a triturator only
   B. Reactions are endothermic
   C. Based on mixture of acidic liquids with basic powder components
   D. Materials are extremely hydrophobic
   E. Set materials are generally stronger than dental composites

70 Which *ONE* of the following cements does *NOT* contain zinc oxide as part of the chemical composition?
   A. ZOE
   B. EBA-modified ZOE
   C. Zinc phosphate
   D. Polycarboxylate
   E. All of the above

71 Which *ONE* of the following dental cement compositions requires staged additions of powder to the liquid during mixing on a chilled glass slab to control the reaction?
   A. Polycarboxylate cement
   B. Composite resin cement
   C. Resin-modified glass ionomer cement
   D. Zinc phosphate cement
   E. Zinc oxide eugenol cement

72 Denture bases are fabricated from acrylic resin based primarily on what monomer?
   A. Ethyl methacrylate
   B. Methyl methacrylate
   C. BIS-GMA
   D. UDM
   E. HEMA

73 Acrylic resin teeth are preferred for denture construction because of their:
   A. Light weight
   B. Bondability to the denture base
   C. Wear resistance
   D. Ease of cleaning
   E. Excellent esthetics

74 What is the *MAJOR* reason that tissue conditioners used with denture bases quickly become harder over several days?
   A. Desorption of plasticizer into the patient's saliva
   B. Mineralization of the material by calcium phosphate from the saliva
   C. Continuing chemical reactions in the tissue conditioner
   D. Chemical effects of cleaning solutions on the tissue conditioner
   E. Fungal growth along the surface of the tissue conditioner

75 CAD/CAM operations collect detailed tooth surface information using:
   A. Micro-tomography
   B. Automated contact digital profilometry
   C. Laser profilometry
   D. Intraoral digital cameras
   E. Silverized impressions

76 Which *ONE* of the following applications is most challenging for CAD/CAM and copy-milling procedures?
   A. Inlays
   B. Onlays
   C. Crowns
   D. Bridges
   E. Veneers

77 Which *ONE* of the following materials is most suitable for CAD/CAM restorations?
   A. Dental composite
   B. Dental porcelain
   C. Dicor
   D. Dicor MGC
   E. Gold alloys

78 What is copy-milling?
   A. Production of secondary dies for indirect procedures
   B. Production of replacements for failed CAD/CAM restorations
   C. Generation of milled restorations by copying a master model
   D. Generation of standard sized inlays and onlays
   E. Method of mass production of denture teeth

79 Where is wear most likely with a CAD/CAM MOD inlay restoration?
   A. Interproximal contact areas
   B. Occlusal surfaces
   C. Marginal ridges
   D. Cemented margins
   E. Cavosurface inlay margins

80 Which *ONE* of the following is the main reason for milled ceramic restoration failure?
   A. Poor fatigue fracture resistance
   B. Color change over time
   C. Failure of composite resin bonding system
   D. Inadequate hardness
   E. Poor wear resistance

81 What type of dental materials will *MOST* likely disappear by the turn of the century?
   A. Glass ionomers
   B. Dental composites
   C. CAD/CAM or copy-milled restorations
   D. Gold alloy crowns
   E. All-ceramic crowns and bridges

Answers and Rationales

1. (A) Three components are never required to be mixed for dental materials.
   (B) Two polyether impression materials components (base and catalyst) are mixed with a machine mixer.
   (C) Plaster, stone, gypsum bonded investment, and alginate impression materials are examples of systems in which one component is mixed with water.
   (D) Dental composite, pit-and-fissure sealant, and dentin bonding systems are examples of a single component being set by visible light-curing.
   (E) Zinc phosphate, ZOE, and polycarboxylate dental cements are examples of systems in which powders and liquids are mixed by spatulation.

2. (A) The setting time is the clock time from the onset of the mixing process until the time that setting begins.
   (B) This is only the working interval and does not include the mixing interval.
   (C) The length of the working interval must be added to the mixing interval to know the clock time for the start of setting.
   (D) The setting interval begins at the setting time.
   (E) The setting time only involves the mixing and working intervals and not the setting interval.

3. (E) Posterior composite is generally cured by visible light curing (although it may also be supplied in chemical curing versions as well).
   (A) Dental amalgam sets by a chemical reaction that starts during the trituration process.
   (B) Polyvinyl siloxane sets by a chemical reaction that starts during manual or machine mixing of the base and catalyst components.
   (C) Calcium sulfate hemihydrate reacts chemically when mixed with water.
   (D) Traditional glass ionomer undergoes a series of complicated chemical reactions when the powder and liquid components are mixed together.

4. (A) Pit and-fissure sealant retains a thin layer of air-inhibited (uncured) sealant that makes the material continue to look glossy after curing.
   (B) Plaster loses its gloss after setting.
   (C) Glass ionomer cement loses its gloss after setting.
   (D) Dental amalgam loses its gloss after setting until it is burnished or polished.
   (E) Alginate loses its gloss after setting.

5. (B) The LCTE for tooth structure is 9 to 11 ppm/°C.
   (A) Aluminosilicates have low values for LCTE, such as 5 ppm/°C.
   (C) Values of 15 ppm/°C are typical of PFM systems.
   (D) 20 ppm/°C are not typical for any dental materials.
   (E) 60 ppm/°C is close to linear acrylic resin systems like PMMA.

6. (C) Gold alloy restorations, being metallic, are poor thermal insulators.
   (A) Dentin, with its high water content and hydroxyapatite, is a reasonably good insulator.
   (B) Enamel, with its very high hydroxyapatite content, is a good thermal insulator.
   (D) Glass ionomer cement, with its high ceramic filler content and ceramic matrix, is a good thermal insulator.
   (E) Ceramic inlays are good thermal insulators.

7. (C) 1 to 2 mm of thickness (dentin and other liners or bases) of insulation below a restoration provides sufficient thickness to discourage heat transport during short periods of temperature difference.
   (A) Liners are typically very thin and on their own do not provide much thermal insulation.
   (B) Sealing dentin, such as with dentin bonding agents, practically provides no increase in thermal insulation.
   (D) Optical conductivity is not related to thermal insulation.
   (E) Density is not related to thermal insulation.

8. (E) Resilience is the total elastic energy absorption during mechanical loading up to the elastic limit.
   (A) Fluoresence is the emission of light when light is shined on the object.
   (B) Luminance is the lightness of color from black to white.
   (C) Dominance is the major wavelength associated with a color of light.
   (D) Translucency is the degree of internal light reflection.

9. (E) Metamerism is the appearance of being the same color when two objects in fact have different spectral energy distributions.
   (A) Stress on a restoration can produce regions with locally different stress concentrations and therefore regions acting as anodes or cathodes for corrosion.
   (B) At a crevice associated with a metallic restoration, the portion within the tip of the crevice acts as a local anode and the rest of the material acts as a cathode.
   (C) The region below plaque on a metallic restoration acts as a local anode while the uncovered portion of a restoration acts as a cathode.
   (D) Passivation is corrosion that produces a thin protective film that then prevents further corrosion.

10. (A) Stress is computed as the applied load divided by the original cross-sectional area of the object being loaded.
    (B) The applied load divided by the volume of the object is a nonsense answer.
    (C) The modulus multiplied by the plastic deformation is a nonsense answer.
    (D) The difference between the total strain and plastic strain is the elastic strain.
    (E) The percent elongation is the strain multiplied by 100%.

11. (E) Engineering strain is the deformation divided by the original length of the object, or the fractional change in length of the object.
    (A, B, C) These are nonsense answers.
    (D) The stress is the applied load divided by the original cross-sectional area of the object.

12. (A) The modulus is the slope of the stress-strain curve, or the stress it takes to produce a certain amount of strain, or the stiffness.
    (B) Resilience is the area under the stress-strain curve up to the elastic limit.
    (C) Toughness is the area under the stress-strain curve up to the breaking point.
    (D) Fatigue resistance is the ability to resist many cycles of stress under all loading conditions.
    (E) Strain rate sensitivity is the relative difference between ultimate strengths for different rates of loading during testing.

13. (D) Up to the elastic limit only elastic deformation is involved, but beyond that, there is a combination of elastic and plastic deformation, with the plastic portion increasing and the elastic portion decreasing, up to the breaking point.
    (A) There is no time that only plastic deformation is involved during loading of a solid object.
    (B) There is only elastic deformation at all points up to the elastic limit.
    (C) Fatigue fracture is failure caused by multiple cycling to loads below the breaking point and typically well below the elastic limit.
    (E) Stress relaxation occurs when a material is under constant strain and could occur at any strain value up to failure.

14. (E) The breaking point is the stress at the time of failure, beyond the elastic limit.
    (A, B, C, D) The elastic limit, yield point, proportional limit, and hardness are ways of describing the limit of totally elastic behavior.

15. (D) Dental enamel is 5 to 6 on the Moh's hardness scale.
    (A) The scale does involve units from 1 (talc) to 10 (diamond).
    (B) Diamond is the hardness reference value (=10).
    (C) Talc is the softness reference value (=1).
    (E) Dentin is 3-4 on the scale.

16. (C) Toxicity is generally a concentration-dependent event, although there may be critical threshold level that must be exceeded first.
    (A) Hypersensitivity is considered an immune system response that is concentration-independent for all practical purposes.
    (B) Fibrous tissue capsule formation is independent of the concentration or magnitude of the initiating event.
    (D) Inflammation occurs because the substance in question exceeds a critical threshold level for cells to manage the problem.
    (E) This is incorrect because the answer is toxicity.

17. (C) Sn-Hg is the corrosion-prone phase in low copper dental amalgams and is the most prone to corrosion of all amalgam phases.
    (A) Ag-Sn is the alloy that reacts with Hg, and residual Ag-Sn is relatively corrosion-resistant.
    (B) Ag-Sn-Cu is the alloy that reacts with Hg, and residual Ag-Sn-Cu is relatively corrosion resistant.
    (D) Cu-Sn is a phase in high copper dental amalgams that is more corrosion resistant than Sn-Hg but is capable of some corrosion.
    (E) Ag-Hg is the principal matrix phase in both low and high copper dental amalgams, and is more corrosion-resistant than Sn-Hg or Cu-Sn but less than that of the original alloy particles used for the reaction.

18. (A) An Ag-Sn alloy that is mixed with Hg remains after the setting reaction and has the best mechanical properties and corrosion resistance.
    (B) Cu-Sn is much less corrosion-resistant than Ag-Sn.
    (C) Sn-Hg is much less corrosion-resistant than Ag-Sn and mechanically much weaker.
    (D) Ag-Hg is less corrosion-resistant and weaker than Ag-Sn.
    (E) This is wrong because Ag-Sn has good properties.

19. (E) None of the above is correct.
    (A) Exposure of unreacted Hg during the mortar and pestle mixing procedure allows mercury to be vaporized.
    (B) Friction-fit and screw-fit capsules still leak during the trituration process.
    (C) Pre-capsulated alloy and mercury minimize but do not prevent mercury losses during trituration.
    (D) Covers over the mixing arms on a trituration device eliminate the aerosol of material leaking from the mixing capsule but do not prevent air contamination by the material dropping below the mixing cover.

20. (C) Low copper dental amalgams involve ≤5% copper.
    (A) 0.1% to 0.5% copper is too little to affect amalgam properties.
    (B) 0.5% to 1% is too little to affect amalgam properties.
    (D) 6% to 12% copper is beyond the low copper range but insufficient to produce the major corrosion resistance of high copper compositions.
    (E) 12% to 15% copper is in the broad range of 12% to 30% copper for high copper dental amalgams.

21. (C) High copper dental amalgams are much more corrosion resistant and do not undergo nearly as much creep as low copper amalgams.
    (A) High copper dental amalgams do have better corrosion resistance because of the elimination of the Sn-Hg phase during the reaction by the presence of Cu.
    (B) All amalgams have both Sn and Ag in their composition.
    (D) High copper dental amalgams are more brittle than low copper ones.
    (E) High copper dental amalgams are defined as containing between 12% and 30% copper in the original alloy that is mixed with Hg.

22. (A) 127°C is the temperature at which the Ag-Hg phase of the matrix begins to melt.
    (B) 227°C is well above the temperature at which the Ag-Hg phase melts.
    (C) 327°C is well above the temperature at which the Ag-Hg phase melts.
    (D) 427°C is well above the temperature at which the Ag-Hg phase melts.
    (E) 527°C is well above the temperature at which the Ag-Hg phase melts.

23. (E) None of the above is predictive of clinical failure. In fact, most failure of high copper dental amalgams occurs at interproximal margins as a result of secondary caries or from fatigue failure.
    (A) Accumulation of green or black tarnish is not important to the success of a dental amalgam, although it may be esthetically displeasing.
    (B) Marginal ditching along occlusal margins occurs because of creep and corrosion, but is never considered predictive of failure for high copper dental amalgam, even though it was predictive for low copper amalgams.
    (C) Dental amalgam slowly continues to react and expand over long periods of time, therefore extruding itself above original margins in areas where there is little natural wear occurring. These overhangs should simply be polished back to contour.
    (D) Wear facets along the occlusal surface are indicative only of functional contact areas.

24. (E) Composite restorations can be easily resurfaced with new composite using dentin bonding systems to bond the interface.
    (A) Composites can be easily repaired and do not require replacement for wear.
    (B) Composites should be repaired with composite because it is stronger and more wear resistant than resin-modified glass ionomer.
    (C) Composites can be easily repaired and do not require replacement for wear.
    (D) Most wear is related to food bolus abrasion and not opponent tooth wear.

25. (C) Enamel and dentin are both routinely conditioned (etched) at the same time.
    (A) Enamel and dentin are both routinely conditioned (etched) at the same time.
    (B) Enamel and dentin are both routinely conditioned (etched) at the same time.
    (D) EDTA is no longer used for conditioning enamel.
    (E) Polyacrylic acid is only rarely used to condition enamel and does not work nearly as effectively on dentin as phosphoric acid.

26. (E) Hydroxyapatite crystals in the smear layer can be dissolved in strong acids but are very resistant to dissolution in routine organic species such as HEMA.
    (A) The smear layer is produced from cavity preparation debris and forms a 2 to 5 micron thick layer on enamel and dentin.
    (B) During cavity preparation the heat from bur cutting decomposes the collagen and vaporizes most of the water from the debris, leaving mostly hydroxyapatite.
    (C) The smear layer is loosely adherent and can be removed with about 4 to 6 MPa of shear stress.
    (D) The layer also involves debris that is pushed into dentinal tubules to form smear plugs, and in combination, the dentin surface becomes partially sealed.

27. (E) Hybrid layer is key to the formation of strong bonding, approximately 20 to 22 MPa.
    (A) Conditioning is only required to dissolve the smear layer and decalcify a small portion of the dentin for potential impregnation and hybrid layer formation. This occurs with very short conditioning times.
    (B) Dentin that is dried after conditioning is very resistant to impregnation and results in poor bonding.
    (C) Pre-application of chlorhexidine will sterilize the field but should be completely rinsed away so as not to interfere with conditioning, priming, and bonding events.
    (D) Scrubbing for conditioning used to be routine during enamel etching but is no longer recommended for conditioning.

28. (E) Silanation zone is not related to the rest of the terms. It involves silane bonding to ceramic materials containing silica.
    (A) Resin-interpenetration zone is another name for hybrid layer.
    (B) Hybrid layer can be called an interpenetration or inter-diffusion or impregnation zone.
    (C) Resin interdiffusion zone is another name for hybrid layer.
    (D) Collagen impregnation zone is another description of a hybrid layer.

29. (D) Dentin primers include water-miscible monomers that will easily diffuse into decalcified wet dentin and surround remaining collagen fibers before polymerizing.
    (A) Liquid conditioners contain acidic materials in water, generally strong mineral acids, such as phosphoric acid.
    (B) Gel conditioners contain acidic materials in water with gelling agents.
    (C) Pit-and-fissure sealants are unfilled monomer mixtures, usually containing BIS-GMA–like monomers that are not water miscible.
    (E) Dentin adhesives could contain small amounts of water-miscible monomer, but they are primarily hydrophobic monomers such as BIS-GMA to bridge the gap between the primer and composite resin.

30. (E) Air thinning had been recommended by some manufacturers to spread primer or adhesive, but generally produces layers that are too thin and prohibit good bonding.
    (A) Conditioning is key to the elimination of the smear layer and decalcification of the surface region of intertubular dentin.
    (B) Dentin that is properly conditioned should not be dehydrated. The clinical sign of proper moisture content is the glistening appearance.
    (C) Dentin that is primed adequately (sufficient coats of material) will have impregnated the conditioned dentin and have sufficient monomer to cover the dentin surface and produce a glistening appearance.
    (D) Adhesive is required to bridge the hydrophilic primer layer to the hydrophobic composite layer.

31. (E) Newer dentin bonding systems combine two of the three components, requiring only two steps rather than three.
    (A) Conditioning is always required for smear layer removal and dentin demineralization, even if it occurs at the same time as priming events.
    (B) Most current dentin bonding systems already are VLC and do not require mixing.
    (C) Thus far, bonding systems are separate steps, and the materials have not been added directly to the composite resins used with them.
    (D) It is important to apply sufficient materials to impregnate and adequately coat dentin, usually mandating that 2 to 5 coats be applied because the materials have solvents that evaporate.

32. (E) Cast gold is not soluble in APF solutions.
    (A) High-strength ceramics contain silicate phases that are susceptible to etching with APF.
    (B) Hybrid dental composites contain silicate fillers that are susceptible to etching with APF.
    (C) Resin-modified glass ionomers contain aluminosilicate glass filler particles that are susceptible to etching with APF.
    (D) PFM contains a porcelain veneer that is susceptible to etching by APF.

33. (A) Copalite produces a temporary cavity seal that is brittle and incomplete because the film forming resin is hydrophobic and does not wet the hydrophilic surface of dentin very well.
    (B) Dentin bonding systems produce relatively complete sealing.
    (C) Amalgam bonding systems are very similar to dentin bonding systems and produce relatively complete sealing.
    (D) Glass ionomer liner that covers all of the dentin in the cavity preparation will produce a complete seal.
    (E) Bonded composite cements (e.g., used with ceramic crowns) use a dentin bonding system and produce a complete seal of the dentin.

34. (B) Eugenol may diffuse to the pulp and produce a palliative action by mitigating the action of the c-axis nerve fibers.
    (A) Calcium hydroxide that diffuses to the dental pulp stimulates the production of secondary dentin but is not palliative.
    (C) HEMA is a monomer that is a sensitizer and would be irritating to cells if it diffused into the dental pulp.
    (D) BIS-GMA is a monomer that would produce irritation of cells if it could diffuse to the dental pulp.
    (E) 4-META is a monomer that would produce irritation of cells if it could diffuse to the dental pulp.

35. (E) Dentin bonding systems are very thin and provide little or no contribution to thermal insulation.
    (A) Glass ionomer liner is generally used in thick enough layers that it contributes to thermal protection of the pulp.
    (B) Zinc phosphate cement bases are thick and good thermal insulators.
    (C) Polycarboxylate cement bases are thick and good thermal insulators.
    (D) Calcium hydroxide liner is relatively thin but where it is used it still provides some contribution to thermal insulation.

36. (E) Zinc oxide is the major powder reactant in zinc phosphate, polycarboxylate, and ZOE cements.
    (A) Water is a component in polycarboxylate and zinc phosphate cement, but not ZOE.
    (B) Silica is not added to most cements, but rather, is the filler in dental composites.
    (C) Mineral acid (phosphoric acid) is the reactive liquid component in zinc phosphate cements.
    (D) Eugenol is the liquid component in ZOE cements.

37. (B) Chelation of calcium ions on tooth structure by ionized polyacrylic acid side-groups is the principal mechanism of chemical adhesion to tooth structure.
    (A) Aluminum ions are involved in cement hardening but do not participate in bonding to tooth structure.
    (C) Electrostatic attraction to aluminosilicate is a nonsense answer.
    (D) Hydration of set materials does nothing to affect the interfacial bonding.
    (E) Fluoride ion release does not affect interfacial bonding with tooth structure.

38. (B) Increasing the P/L ratio increases the modulus because the powder is reinforcing and makes the final material stiffer.
    (A) Increasing the P/L ratio increases the strength because the powder is reinforcing.
    (C) Increasing the P/L ratio decreases the water absorption, because there is less matrix phase to absorb water.
    (D) Increasing the P/L ratio makes the final cement stiffer and more brittle, reducing the toughness.
    (E) Increasing the P/L ratio decreases the overall solubility by reducing the amount of matrix phase.

39. (D) Compomers are hybrids of glass ionomers and composites that approach composite formulations.
    (A) Compomers involve extensive glass ionomer modification.
    (B) Compomers are hybrids of glass ionomers and composites.
    (C) Compomers are as easy to cure as other composite or VLC glass ionomer compositions.
    (E) Compomers are approximately equal in biocompatibility to glass ionomers and composites.
40. (A) Resin-modified glass ionomers allow the material to be cured to a sufficient hardness to allow finishing and polishing immediately.
    (B) Although mixing of some resin-modified glass ionomers is easier, their advantage is related to early finishing.
    (C) Careful use of any material that produces dentin sealing will eliminate postoperative sensitivity problems.
    (D) Resin-modified glass ionomers are less chemically adherent to tooth structure.
    (E) Resin-modified glass ionomers actually undergo more shrinkage on curing.
41. (E) Glass ionomers are often used for root caries lesions because of the potential advantage of fluoride release in helping to control dental caries.
    (A) Glass ionomers are often used in older adults but only where there is a perceived risk of caries.
    (B) Glass ionomers are generally considered too brittle to survive well in thin, saucer-shaped Class V restorations.
    (C) Glass ionomers may be used for Class II restorations in primary teeth, but they have poor wear resistance and relatively low strength.
    (D) Glass ionomers do not have sufficient wear resistance, adhesion, or fracture strength for Class IV restorations.
42. (A) The particle size of the abrasive is related to the size of the scratch or cut that is produced during abrasion, so larger sized particle pastes produce more rapid abrasion.
    (B) Fluoride in the paste is irrelevant to the abrasive action.
    (C) Cooling water is important to keep the substrate from becoming warm but this is more of a secondary factor under most circumstances for cutting effectiveness.
    (D) Vibration of the paste is not nearly as efficient as rotating motion of a rubber cup.
    (E) Extremely thick paste would decrease the pressure of the abrasive on the substrate but this is more a secondary factor for effectiveness.
43. (E) ZOE is an inflexible impression material.
    (A) Alginate is a flexible impression material as long as it is fully hydrated.
    (B) Polyether is a flexible impression material based on an elastic polymer.
    (C) Polyvinyl siloxane is a flexible impression material based on an elastic polymer.
    (D) Polysulfide is a flexible impression material based on an elastic polymer.

44. (A) Agar-agar hydrocolloid is a reversible physical reaction that simply depends on heat.
    (B) ZOE sets by a chemical reaction between eugenol and zinc oxide.
    (C) Polysulfide sets by a chemical reaction.
    (D) Polyether sets by a chemical reaction.
    (E) Polyvinyl siloxane sets by a chemical reaction.
45. (A) Alginate is manually mixed as a powder and liquid in a flexible bowl.
    (B) ZOE is manually mixed as two pastes on a pad.
    (C) Polyether is mixed as two pastes in an auto-mixing gun or using a machine.
    (D) Silicone is mixed as two pastes on a pad.
    (E) Polysulfide is mixed as two pastes on a pad.
46. (A) Dies are teeth that can be removed from the working cast to more carefully work with indirect restorations being fitted onto them.
    (B) A master cast is the first cast produced for capturing the cavity preparation information and occlusion for the production of indirect restorations.
    (C) Impressions are negatives from which casts or positives are produced.
    (D) Duplicates are secondary casts.
    (E) Models capture all soft and hard tissue information about a patient for reference but not for use in producing indirect restorations.
47. (C) Calcium sulfate dihydrate is the reaction product of water and calcium sulfate hemihydrate.
    (A) Calcium sulfate hemihydrate is gypsum that is only partially reacted with water.
    (B) Calcium sulfate monohydrate does not exist.
    (D) Calcium sulfate trihydrate does not exist.
    (E) Calcium sulfate tetrahydrate does not exist.
48. (B) Gypsum for casts is composed of calcium sulfate hemihydrate.
    (A) Gypsum for casts does not contain aluminosilicate glass.
    (C) Gypsum for casts does not contain calcium carbonate.
    (D) Gypsum for casts does not contain sodium fluoride.
    (E) Gypsum for casts does not contain calcium phosphate.
49. (B) 18 ml is the theoretical amount of water required for complete reaction of 100 g of powder, but additional water must always be added to make a workable mixture.
    (A) 10 ml is too little water to produce the complete reaction of 100 g of powder.
    (C) 24 ml is the amount of water routinely required for mixing 100 g of diestone.
    (D) 32 ml is the amount of water routinely required for mixing 100 g of stone.
    (E) 50 ml is the amount of water routinely required for mixing 100 g of plaster powder.

50. (D) Stone has more efficient powder particle packing and requires less excess water for making a suitable mixture.
    (A) Both plaster and stone are calcium sulfate hemihydrate before reaction and calcium sulfate dihydrate after reaction.
    (B) Color is irrelevant and is simply different to distinguish the materials.
    (C) Both have the same chemical reaction on setting.
    (E) Both have adjustable setting times.
51. (A) Different particle shapes produce different packing efficiencies that affect the amount of excess water required for making a suitable mixture.
    (B) All gypsum products set by the same chemical reaction.
    (C) Powder particles are not porous.
    (D) The viscosity is acceptable as long as there is sufficient water to fill in all the spaces between the particles during the mixing and working stages so that it will flow.
    (E) All of the materials are equally hydroscopic in air.
52. (C) Wax cools from the outside to the inside producing distortions when it shrinks.
    (A) Although wax has a low modulus it is acceptable for die applications.
    (B) Wax adhesion to dies is generally not a problem.
    (D) Waxes are not susceptible to water absorption.
    (E) Generally porosity is not a problem with waxes.
53. (C) Paraffin is the major component of most dental waxes.
    (A) Carnauba wax is a modifier wax that affects the melting point.
    (B) Colorant represents only about 1% of the composition.
    (D) Rosin is a modifier wax that affects the melting point and tackiness.
    (E) Beeswax is a modifier wax that affects the melting point and tackiness.
54. (C) Inlay wax patterns and dies will be invested and then must be removed by pyrolysis from the molds so they should easily burn up into CO_2 and H_2O.
    (A) A high modulus for wax would be a disadvantage because it would interfere with the carvability of the wax patterns.
    (B) All components used to formulate dental waxes are organic materials and they all have high coefficients of thermal expansion, unfortunately.
    (D) The color of a wax is easy to change and irrelevant for the application.
    (E) All components of dental waxes are relatively cheap.
55. (A) Dental investment materials are classified based on the composition of the matrix binding together the filler in the composition (e.g., gypsum bonded investment).
    (B) The amount of water required for mixing is irrelevant for classification.
    (C) The extent of expansion, although important, is not the basis for classification.
    (D) Generally, there is not much of a problem with compatibility that would require special classification of investment materials.
    (E) Investments need some strength to survive the casting procedures, but otherwise strength is not a major consideration for classification of investment materials.

56. (A) All gold crowns can be cast at relatively low temperatures and, therefore, gypsum bonded investment is very suitable.
    (B) Silicate bonded investment is for casting higher melting alloys.
    (C) Phosphate bonded investment is for casting higher melting alloys but could be used for alloys for all gold crowns except that it is more expensive than gypsum bonded investment.
    (D) Magnesia investment is used for more complicated and higher temperature casting procedures.
    (E) Ceramming investment is used for stabilizing the shape of cast porcelains during the subsequent heat treatment to precipitate a partly crystalline phase.
57. (B) 12 karat is (12/24)(100%) = 50% Au.
    (A) 10 karat is (10/24)(100%) = 42% Au.
    (C) 20 karat is (20/24)(100%) = 83% Au.
    (D) 24 karat is (24/24)(100%) = 100% Au.
    (E) 50 karat is impossible.
58. (A) If more than 50% of the atoms are Au (about 75% by weight), then the alloy has good corrosion resistance.
    (B) Cu is added to gold to increase its hardness.
    (C) Ag is added to gold to counteract the effect of Cu producing a more orange color.
    (D) Zn is added in small amounts as a processing aid to suppress oxidation during melting and casting.
    (E) Pd is added in minor amounts to adjust the melting temperature and hardness.
59. (C) Ag is added to gold to counteract the effect of Cu producing a more orange color.
    (A) If more than 50% of the atoms are Au (about 75% by weight), then the alloy has good corrosion resistance.
    (B) Cu is added to gold to increase its hardness.
    (D) Zn is added in small amounts as a processing aid to suppress oxidation during melting and casting.
    (E) Pd is added in minor amounts to adjust the melting temperature and hardness.
60. (D) Chromium oxide film forms instantaneously on exposure to oxygen and creates a tight adherent film that prevents further corrosion (oxidation) of the alloy surface.
    (A) There is no positive effect of chromium oxide on alloy production.
    (B) Chromium oxide films are so thin that light passes through and reflects directly off of the metal surface.
    (C) The surface film of chromium oxide does not affect the modulus of the alloy.
    (D) Chromium oxide is not used as an abrasive in dentistry or dental hygiene.

61. (E) Lithium aluminosilicate glass is a ceramic and is not involved in passivation of metal alloys.
    (A) Stainless steel includes 18% to 28% chromium which produces a chromium oxide film that passivates the alloy.
    (B) Cr-Ni alloys produce a chromium oxide film that passivates the alloy.
    (C) Cr-Co alloys produce a mixed oxide film including chromium oxide that together passivate the alloy.
    (D) Titanium forms a titanium oxide film that passivates the metal.

62. (E) Corrosion resistance depends on the metal alloys being joined and the composition of the filler metal but is not substantially different.
    (A) Soldering involves low temperature filler metal joining and brazing involves high temperature filler metal joining.
    (B) The type of solder is irrelevant except that higher temperature filler metal will be a different composition.
    (C) Fluxing is similar for both operations.
    (D) Acid pretreatment is not required but is often included with the flux.

63. (A) 650 fine refers to the 65% gold content of a gold solder.
    (B) Low gold alloys have no special relationship to soldering.
    (C) Passivation is an adherent corrosion film that prevents further corrosion, and although it may interfere with soldering, it is not directly related to dental solders.
    (D) Welding is different from soldering, because no filler metal is involved in the joining operation.
    (E) Vitrification is the partial melting of ceramic compositions.

64. (D) PFM alloys must melt at higher applications to tolerate high temperatures for porcelain application.
    (A) PFM gold alloys do not have better corrosion resistance.
    (B) PFM gold alloys do not have lower thermal conductivity.
    (C) PFM gold alloys might be slightly whiter in color but generally are not.
    (E) This is wrong because they have higher melting temperatures.

65. (D) Ni is normally not part of Co-Cr restorations.
    (A) Ni is part of normal stainless steel compositions for wires and brackets.
    (B) Ni is normally part of the composition of stainless steel used for crowns for primary teeth.
    (C) Ni is part of Ni-Cr PFM restorations.
    (E) This is wrong because Ni is not contained in Co-Cr alloys.

66. (A) The general incidence of Ni sensitivity for men is 1%.
    (B) 4% incidence is too high for men and too low for women.
    (C) 8% incidence is too high for men and too low for women.
    (D) 11% incidence is typical for women.
    (E) 20% incidence is too high for either women or men.

67. (B) Silica, alumina, and potassium oxide are the main components in dental porcelain.
    (A) Calcium carbonate is not a main component in dental porcelain.
    (C) Zinc oxide and fluoride are not main components in dental porcelain.
    (D) Calcium oxide is not a main component in dental porcelain.
    (E) Calcium oxide, magnesium oxide, and chromium oxide are not main components in dental porcelain.

68. (C) Dental ceramics are brittle and are not capable of much plastic deformation, unfortunately.
    (A) Dental ceramics have excellent color and translucency, and thus, good esthetics.
    (B) Dental ceramics typically have very low coefficients of thermal expansion and therefore are well matched to tooth structure.
    (D) Dental ceramics are thermal and electrical insulators which helps to protect the pulp.
    (E) Dental ceramics have high hardness and resist abrasion and wear very well.

69. (C) Traditional cements all involve mixtures of acidic liquids with basic powders to produce reaction salts to hold the mixture together.
    (A) Many of the cements still are mixed manually.
    (B) All cement reactions are exothermic.
    (D) Most of the materials involve some water in the composition and behave more like a hydrophilic material.
    (E) All dental cements are weaker when set than composite materials.

70. (E) All of the choices involve zinc oxide in the powder of the dental cement.
    (A) ZOE is based on eugenol and zinc oxide.
    (B) EBA modified cements are based on ethoxy benzoic acid and eugenol liquids mixed with zinc oxide powder.
    (C) Zinc phosphate is based on phosphoric acid in water mixed with zinc oxide powder.
    (D) Polycarboxylate cement is based on polyacrylic acid in water mixed with zinc oxide powder.

71. (D) Zinc phosphate cement is very exothermic and requires very careful mixing to control the reaction.
    (A) Polycarboxylate cement gels very quickly, is not very exothermic, and therefore the powder and liquid are mixed very rapidly together.
    (B) Composite resin cement is either mixed as two pastes or VLC as one paste but has not critical mixing requirements.
    (C) Resin-modified glass ionomer cements are not very exothermic and can be mixed very readily.
    (E) Zinc oxide eugenol cement reacts slowly and is not very exothermic, so it can be mixed very quickly.

72. (B) Methyl methacrylate is the major monomer in denture base resin.
    (A) Denture bases contain small amounts of ethyl methacrylate as an internal plasticizer for the polymer which is primarily polymethyl methacrylate.
    (C) BIS-GMS is the major monomer used in restorative resin compositions but not in denture bases.
    (D) UDM is used in many restorative resin compositions but not in denture bases.
    (E) HEMA is used in many dentin bonding primers but not in denture bases.

73. (B) Acrylic resin teeth can be bonded to the denture base whereas porcelain teeth must be provided with gross mechanical retention that is not nearly as good.
    (A) Although porcelain teeth are heavier than acrylic resin ones, this is usually not a problem because patients like the excellent esthetics of the porcelain teeth.
    (C) Acrylic resin wears more than porcelain.
    (D) Neither acrylic resin nor porcelain teeth are difficult to clean.
    (E) Porcelain teeth have better esthetics overall than acrylic resin ones.

74. (A) Tissue conditioners are softened by including alcoholic plasticizers that readily desorb from the conditioner over several days, unfortunately.
    (B) Some materials from saliva may migrate into tissue conditioners but generally do not affect the hardness much.
    (C) Tissue conditioners do not undergo further setting reactions in the mouth.
    (D) Cleaning solutions for denture bases should be simply soap and water, and should not react with the tissue conditioner.
    (E) Although fungal growth can occur along the surfaces of dentures and tissue conditioners, it should not significantly alter the properties of the conditioner.

75. (D) Intraoral digital cameras (coupled with Moire photography) are used to collect intraoral surface information for the main chairside CAD/CAM system (Cerec).
    (A) Micro-tomography is not commercially feasible for CAD/CAM operations.
    (B) Automated contact digital profilometry is a laboratory technique only.
    (C) Laser profilometry is a laboratory technique only.
    (E) Silver coated impressions, which would have to be digitized by some method, are not used.

76. (D) Bridges are very difficult to machine by CAD/CAM techniques because of their complex geometry.
    (A) Inlays are relatively easy to machine by CAD/CAM techniques.
    (B) Onlays are relatively easy to machine by CAD/CAM techniques.
    (C) Crowns can now be machined by CAD/CAM techniques.
    (E) Veneers can be machined by CAD/CAM techniques but there are easier ways to make veneers.

77. (D) Dicor MGC is specifically designed to be a "machinable glass ceramic" with good mechanical properties for a restoration.
    (A) Dental composite is relatively difficult to machine because of its filler particles.
    (B) Dental porcelain can be machined but is relatively weak and prone to fracture.
    (C) Dicor is no longer used for all-ceramic restorations because of poor fracture resistance.
    (E) Gold alloys are difficult to machine because they are relatively soft and smear during cutting operations.

78. (C) Copy milling involves using a master die as a pattern while milling a block of ceramic.
    (A) Secondary dies are produced by pouring gypsum materials.
    (B) Replacements for failed CAD/CAM restorations could employ dental composite, cast gold alloys, or many other things.
    (D) There are no such things as standard sized inlays and onlays.
    (E) Copy-milling does not involve the mass production of denture teeth.

79. (D) Composite cements that are used to bond CAD/CAM restorations are actually much softer and are sites of wear.
    (A) CAD/CAM restorations are relatively wear resistant at interproximal contact areas because they are made of ceramic materials.
    (B) CAD/CAM restorations are relatively wear resistant along occlusal surfaces because they are made of ceramic materials.
    (C) CAD/CAM restorations are relatively wear resistant at marginal ridges because they are made of ceramic materials.
    (D) CAD/CAM restorations are relatively wear resistant at cavosurface inlay margins because they are made of ceramic materials.

80. (A) All dental ceramic materials have poor fatigue fracture resistance.
    (B) Milled ceramic restorations should not undergo color changes with time.
    (C) The composite bonding system undergoes wear but does not appear to fail.
    (D) Ceramic restorations are sufficiently hard to resist food abrasion.
    (E) Ceramic restorations generally have excellent wear resistance.

81. (A) Glass ionomers will most likely cease to exist as a dental material because they have moved closer and closer to becoming dental composites.
    (B) Dental composites will be the major materials used as amalgam replacements.
    (C) CAD/CAM and copy-milled restorations will continue to enjoy success for limited applications such as inlays and onlays but will still be expensive restorations.
    (D) Gold alloy crowns will continue to exist.
    (E) All-ceramic crowns and bridges will grow in use as the materials become even better.

Periodontics

Denise M. Bowen

The demand for periodontal therapy is growing. Although periodontal diseases are prevalent in the United States, they are more limited in severity than previously thought. The vast majority of periodontal needs are related to treating gingivitis and early periodontitis, preventing periodontal disease, and maintaining periodontal health following therapy. All of these services are provided by dental hygienists.

A thorough understanding of periodontics is critical to the process of dental hygiene care. Client assessment, care planning, individualized self care instruction, preventive and nonsurgical periodontal therapy, periodontal maintenance procedures, and reevaluation are all essential components of the dental hygienist's role in periodontics. Although this chapter is based on current knowledge, understanding of periodontal diseases is changing rapidly. New clinical interventions and modalities will evolve as the etiology, risk factors, and pathogenesis of these diseases are clarified further. Dental hygiene practitioners are challenged to keep abreast of these developments.

Basic Features of the Periodontium

A. Periodontium (Fig. 11-1) is composed of
   1. Gingiva
   2. Periodontal ligament
   3. Cementum
   4. Alveolar bone

B. Function of the periodontium is to attach the tooth to the alveolar bone tissues of the mandible and maxilla
C. Changes in the periodontium may be a result of
   1. Morphologic and functional alterations
   2. Changes in the oral environment
   3. Age

Gingiva

Definition

A. Part of the oral masticatory mucosa that surrounds the cervical portion of the teeth and covers the alveolar process of the jaws
   1. Apical border is the mucogingival junction that separates the gingiva from the adjacent lining mucosa
   2. On the palatal surface the gingiva blends into palatal masticatory mucosa
B. Components
   1. Marginal gingiva (unattached or free gingiva)
      a. Unattached cufflike tissue that surrounds the teeth facially, lingually, and interproximally
      b. Parts of marginal gingiva
         (1) Gingival margin—most coronal portion of the gingiva and surrounds the teeth in a scalloped outline; located at or approximately 0.5 mm coronal to the cemento-enamel junction
         (2) Gingival groove—only present in 30% to

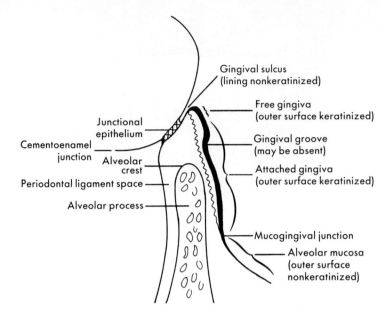

Fig. 11-1 Anatomy of periodontium.

40% of adults; when present, it is located 1 to 1.5 mm apical to the gingival margin

(3) Gingival sulcus—space formed by the tooth and the sulcular epithelium laterally and by the coronal end of the junctional epithelium (base of the sulcus) apically; in absolute periodontal health, almost no gingival sulcus exists; however, a sulcular measurement of 1 to 2 mm facially and lingually and 1 to 3 mm interproximally is considered to be within the range of health

(4) Interdental gingiva—that portion of the gingival margin that occupies the interdental space coronal to the alveolar crest (clinically, it fills the embrasure space beneath the area of tooth contact)

    (a) Interdental gingiva—gingiva consists of two interdental papillae (one facial and one lingual) that are connected by the concave-shaped interdental col

    (b) Col is absent when teeth are not in contact

    (c) Interdental gingiva, like the facial and lingual gingiva, is attached to the tooth by junctional epithelium and connective tissue fibers

2. Attached gingiva

  a. That part of the gingiva that is attached to the underlying periosteum of the alveolar bone and to the cementum by connective tissue fibers and the epithelial attachment

  b. Boundaries

    (1) Apically demarcated by the mucogingival junction (demarcates attached gingiva from alveolar mucosa)

    (2) Coronally demarcated by the base of the gingival sulcus

  c. Width of attached gingiva varies

    (1) Generally widest in facial anterior maxillary areas and narrowest in mandibular premolar facial areas

    (2) Width of attached gingiva is not measured on the palate because it cannot be clinically distinguished from palatal mucosa

3. Changes in width of attached gingiva result from changes at the coronal end; the position of the mucogingival junction remains stationary

Histologic Features

See Chapter 2, section on oral histology.

A. Epithelium

1. Epithelium on the outer surface of marginal and attached gingiva is parakeratinized or keratinized

2. Sulcular epithelium—stratified squamous, nonkeratinized epithelium that is continuous with the oral epithelium; lines the peripheral surface of the sulcus extending to the coronal border of the junctional epithelium

3. Junctional epithelium—stratified squamous, nonkeratinized epithelium that surrounds and attaches to the tooth on one side and attaches on the other side to the gingival connective tissue; new cells

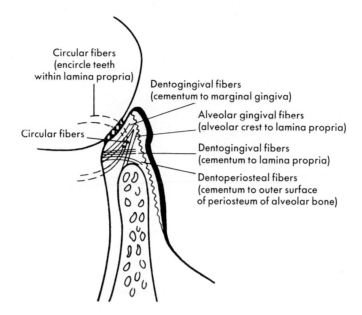

Fig. 11-2   Connective tissue fibers of gingiva. NOTE: Not shown are transseptal fibers that extend from cementum of one tooth through lamina propria to cementum of adjacent tooth (see also Figs. 2-27 and 2-28).

originate from the cells in the apical portion adjacent to the tooth and from the cells in contact with the connective tissue; epithelial cells are shed (desquamation) at the coronal end of the junctional epithelium, which forms the base of the gingival sulcus

    a. Junctional epithelium is more permeable to cells and fluids than is oral epithelium

    b. Serves as the preferred route for the passage of fluid and cells from the connective tissue into the sulcus and for the passage of bacteria and bacterial products from the sulcus into the connective tissue

    c. Is easily penetrated by the periodontal probe; this penetration is increased in inflamed gingiva

    d. Length ranges from 0.25 to 1.35 mm

  4. Epithelial attachment—refers to the basal lamina and hemidesmosomes that connect the junctional epithelium to the tooth surface

  5. Rete pegs—epithelial projections that interweave with the papillary projections of the gingival connective tissue

B. Connective tissue (or lamina propria)—composed of gingival fibers (connective tissue fibers), intercellular ground substance, cells, and vessels and nerves

  1. Gingival fibers—composed of collagen fibers (60% of connective tissue volume) and an elastic fiber system comprised of oxytalin, elaunin, and elastin fibers; fiber bundle groups provide support for marginal gingiva, including the interdental papilla (Fig. 11-2; see also Figs. 2-27 and 2-28)

    a. Circumferential or circular fibers—encircle each tooth separately in a cufflike fashion within the free gingiva

    b. Dentogingival fibers—also called gingivodental fibers; embedded in the cementum; located between the cementoenamel junction and the crest of the alveolar bone; fan outward into the attached and free gingiva; attach gingiva to the tooth apical to the epithelial attachment

    c. Dentoperiosteal fibers—embedded in the same portion of the cementum as the dentogingival fibers, but extend apically *over* the alveolar crest and terminate in the alveolar crest after passing through the lamina propria and the periosteum

    d. Transseptal fibers—embedded in the same portion of the cementum as dentogingival and dentoperiosteal fibers; run a horizontal path from adjacent teeth

    e. Alveologingival fibers—inserted in crest of alveolar process and splay out through lamina propria into the free gingiva

  2. Intercellular ground substance (or matrix)

    a. Gel-like medium that surrounds connective tissue cells

    b. Essential for maintenance of normal function of connective tissue (e.g., transportation of water, electrolytes, nutrients)

c. Composed of water, mucopolysaccharides, and hyaluronic acid
3. Cells
   a. Fibroblasts (predominant cells)
      (1) Produce various types of fibers found in connective tissue
      (2) Instrumental in synthesis of intercellular ground substance
      (3) Wound healing or healing following therapy is regulated by gingival fibroblasts
   b. Other connective tissue cellular components
      (1) Mast cells—participate in the early phase of inflammation
      (2) Macrophages—host defense and repair
      (3) Polymorphonuclear leukocytes—host defense
      (4) Lymphocytes—host defense
      (5) Plasma cells—host defense
4. Vessels and nerves (see section on blood supply to the periodontium)

Normal Clinical Features

A. Color—in light-skinned individuals, pale or coral pink; in dark-skinned individuals, coral pink to brown; color may vary depending on the degree of vascularity, amount of melanin, epithelial keratinization, and thickness of epithelium
B. Texture
   1. Gingival margin—dull, smooth surface
   2. Attached—stippled, "orange peel" surface present on facial surfaces (stippling may not always be present in healthy gingiva)
C. Consistency
   1. Gingival margin—firm and resilient; resists displacement
   2. Attached gingiva—firmly bound to the underlying alveolar bone and cementum
D. Contour and shape
   1. Papillary contour—pointed; papilla fills proximal embrasure space to the contact point
   2. Marginal contour—most coronal edge should form a knifelike edge with a scalloped configuration mesiodistally (follows the cementoenamel junction)
   3. Contour varies with shape and alignment of teeth and with size and position of proximal contacts

Periodontal Ligament

Definition

A. Connective tissue that surrounds the root and connects it with the alveolar bone
B. Is continuous with the connective tissue fibers of the gingiva

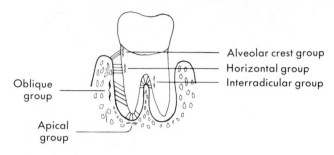

Fig. 11-3 Principal fiber groups of periodontal ligament (see also Fig. 2-27).

C. Contains collagen fibers, which are attached on one side to the alveolar bone and on the other side to the cementum; terminal portions of these fibers, which are embedded into the cementum and alveolar bone, are called Sharpey's fibers
D. Is organized into fiber bundles called principal fiber groups, which are distinguished by their location and direction

Principal Fiber Groups (Fig. 11-3; see also Fig. 2-27)

A. Alveolar crest group—fibers extend from the cementum just below the junctional epithelium and extend obliquely to the alveolar crest
B. Horizontal group—fibers extend at right angles to the long axis of the tooth, from the cementum to the alveolar bone
C. Oblique group—fibers extend from the alveolar bone to the cementum in an apical direction, forming the most numerous fiber group and providing the main support to the tooth; primarily responsible for bearing vertical masticatory stresses
D. Apical group—fibers extend from the alveolar bone to the cementum at the apex of the root
E. Interradicular group—fibers extend from the alveolar bone to the cementum in furcation areas

Functions

A. Physical—attachment of the tooth to the bone, transmission of occlusal forces to the bone, absorption of the impact of occlusal forces, and maintenance of the proper relationship of the gingival tissues to the teeth
B. Formative—participation in formation of cementum and bone and remodeling of the periodontal ligament by activities of connective tissue cells (cementoblasts, fibroblasts, osteoblasts)
C. Resorptive—by activities of connective tissue cells (fibroclasts, osteoclasts, cementoclasts)
D. Nutritive—nutrients carried through blood vessels to the cementum, bone, and gingiva

E. Sensory—proprioceptive and tactile sensitivity provided by innervation to the periodontal ligament

Clinical Considerations

A. Thickness varies from 0.05 to 0.25 mm (mean, 0.2 mm); thickness varies depending on stage of eruption, person's age, and function of a tooth; ligament is thicker in functioning than in nonfunctioning teeth and thicker in areas of tension than in areas of compression; thickest in apical region
B. Periodontal ligament cells can remodel the ligament and adjacent bone when altered forces are applied (e.g., orthodontics)
C. Accidentally exfoliated teeth can be replanted if handling of the torn ligament is minimized before reimplantation

Cementum

See Chapter 2, section on cementum

Definition

A. Calcified mesenchymal tissue that covers the surface of the root
B. Main function is to attach the fibers of the periodontal ligament to the tooth
C. Features
1. Does not contain blood or lymph vessels
2. Has no innervation
3. A mineralized tissue similar to bone
4. Is continuously deposited in the apical area of the root throughout life
D. Two different types (see Fig. 2-25)
1. Acellular—forms in conjunction with root formation and tooth eruption
2. Cellular—forms after the tooth is erupted in the apical one third of the root; contains cementoblasts, inactive cementocytes, fibroblasts from the periodontal ligament, and cementoclasts

Relationship to Enamel (Refer to Fig. 13-2)

A. Cementum overlaps enamel (approximately 60% of all teeth)
B. Cementum and enamel meet (approximately 30% of all teeth)
C. Cementum and enamel do not meet, leaving an area of dentin exposed (approximately 10% of all teeth)

Clinical Considerations

A. Compensates for occlusal wear and continuous eruption by apical deposition of cementum throughout life
B. Protects the root surface from resorption during tooth movement
C. Has a reparative function, which permits reestablish-ment of new connective tissue attachment following certain types of periodontal therapy
D. When enamel and cementum do not meet, cervical hypersensitivity and caries are more likely to develop

Alveolar Process

See Chapter 2, section on alveolar bone, and Fig. 2-26.

Definition

A. Bone that forms and supports the tooth sockets (alveoli)
B. Consists of
1. Alveolar bone proper (or cribriform plate)
   a. Thin layer of compact bone that forms the inner socket wall; numerous perforations are present to permit vascular communication between marrow spaces of cancellous bone and the periodontal ligament; identified on radiographs as the lamina dura
   b. Bundle bone—alveolar bone adjacent to the periodontal ligament (contains Sharpey's fibers)
   c. Alveolar crest—coronal rim of the alveolar bone; generally parallels adjacent cementoenamel junctions; is 1.5 to 2 mm apical to the cementoenamel junction
2. Supporting bone
   a. Surrounds and supports the alveolar bone proper
   b. Composed of two parts
      (1) Compact cortical plates (facial and lingual aspects)
      (2) Spongy or cancellous trabecular bone—located between the cortical plates and alveolar bone proper

Shape, Thickness, and Location

A. Contour of the alveolar bone follows the contour of the cementoenamel junctions and the arrangement of the dentition
B. Shape of the alveolar crest is generally parallel to the cementoenamel junctions of adjacent teeth; is approximately 1.5 to 2 mm apical to the cementoenamel junction
C. Cortical plates generally are thicker in the mandible than in the maxilla
D. Posterior areas—bone generally is thick, and cancellous bone separates the cortical plate from the alveolar bone proper
E. Anterior areas—bone is thin, with little or no cancellous bone separating the cortical plate from the alveolar bone proper
F. Dehiscence—situation in which the marginal alveolar bone is denuded forming a defect extending apical to

the normal level, exposing an abnormal amount of root surface

G. Fenestration—situation in which the margin of the alveolar bone is intact; however, there is an isolated lack of alveolar bone on the root surface (root surface area is covered only by periosteum and overlying gingiva)

Radiographic Features of the Normal Periodontium

A. Alveolar crest—thin, radiopaque line that is continuous with the lamina dura; shape is dependent on
 1. Proximity of adjacent teeth and roots
 2. Level of adjacent cementoenamel junctions
B. Interdental septum—proximal alveolar bone bordered by the alveolar crest
C. Lamina dura—radiographic image of the alveolar bone proper; may or may not be present as a thin radiopaque line surrounding the bone, adjacent to the periodontal ligament
D. Periodontal ligament space—thin radiolucent line surrounding each tooth between the root and adjacent alveolar bone
E. Supporting bone—radiopacity of the trabecular pattern varies depending on the amount, pattern, and/or presence of cancellous and cortical bone
F. Limitations of radiographs
 1. Do not show soft-tissue-to-hard-tissue relationships
 2. Do not show early bone loss
 3. May not show interproximal bony changes accurately
 4. May not show bone changes on facial or lingual surfaces; facial and lingual bony plates may be obscured by roots of teeth
 5. Does not reveal current cellular activity; only reflects past events
 6. Diagnostic value affected by variations in technique

Blood Supply to the Periodontium

A. To the gingiva via supraperiosteal arterioles
 1. Supraperiosteal arterioles are vessels of the periodontal ligament that extend coronally into the gingiva
 2. These arterioles are mainly along the facial and lingual surfaces of the cortical plate
 3. These arterioles emerge from the alveolar crest
B. To the periodontal ligament via inferior and superior alveolar arteries, which reach the periodontal ligament via
 1. Apical vessels
 2. Penetrating vessels from the alveolar bone
 3. Anastomosing (joining) vessels from the gingiva
C. To the alveolar process

 1. To the alveolar bone proper via branches of the apical vessels in the ligaments and vessels in the interdental septum
 2. To the cortical plate via branches of the supraperiosteal arterioles
 3. To cancellous bone via the interdental septum vessels and vessels that also supply the cortical plate and alveolar bone proper

Innervation and Lymphatic Drainage of the Periodontium

Follows pathways similar to those of the vessels supplying blood to the periodontium

Changes Within the Periodontium Associated with Disease

A. Factors that influence periodontal health
 1. Extrinsic etiologic factors—bacterial plaque (primary etiologic factor)
 2. Extrinsic contributing factors
  a. Calculus
  b. Tooth position and anatomy
  c. Condition of dental restorations, permanent or removable prostheses, and/or orthodontic appliances
  d. Oral (functional) habits that create excessive traumatic forces to the periodontium
  e. Food impaction
  f. Mouth breathing
  g. Tobacco use
 3. Intrinsic (systemic) contributing factors
  a. Immunologic defects
  b. Endocrine dysfunctions
  c. Nutritional disorders
  d. Genetically transmitted diseases
  e. Emotional disorders
  f. Drug intake
  g. Hematologic disorders
B. Natural history of periodontal disease
 1. Landmark longitudinal studies conducted by Löe and coworkers examined the course of periodontal disease over a 20 year period in two cohorts: Sri Lankan tea workers who were generally healthy but had never received dental care and did not know of toothbrushing, and students and academicians from Norway who had lifelong dental care and oral self-care education[1-5]
 2. Plaque, calculus, and gingivitis were common conditions in both groups which led to a slow loss of periodontal attachment with increasing age
 3. Periodontal attachment loss progressed at a rate of 0.3 mm per year in Sri Lanka and 0.1 mm per year in

Norway; professional and self care slowed the rate of progression

4. In the Sri Lankan group with no periodontal therapy the following disease patterns were identified:
   a. No progression beyond gingivitis (11%)
   b. Moderate progression of 4 mm attachment loss (81%)
   c. Rapid progression of 9 mm attachment loss (8%)

5. Periodontal disease is most commonly slowly progressive; however, some individuals show no progression even without care; others show rapid progression

6. Because plaque, calculus, and gingival inflammation were present in both cohorts, other risk factors must play a role in progression of periodontal disease

C. Risk factors
1. Periodontal diseases are no longer regarded as infections to which everyone is susceptible
2. Some individuals at greater risk; research is ongoing to identify these individuals or groups
3. Dentally related factors[6]
   a. Sites previously affected by periodontitis are at greatest risk for future loss of attachment
   b. More frequent professional care reduces risk
   c. Missing teeth, mobile teeth, mouth breathing, and areas of food impaction increase the risk of periodontal disease
   d. Increased levels of *Porphyromonas gingivalis, Bacteriodes forsythus, Actinobacillus actinomycetemcomitans,* and *Prevotella intermedia* coupled with factors mentioned above can significantly increase risk of occurrence of periodontitis/attachment loss[7-10]
4. Unchanging subject-related factors
   a. Genetic factors may predispose to periodontal disease; these are most clearly linked to early-onset forms such as localized juvenile periodontitis
   b. Gender differences do not exist for prevalence of attachment loss; however, more severe loss of attachment, deeper probing depths, and recession are more common in males
   c. The relationship of race-ethnicity is unclear; non-Hispanic whites exhibit better periodontal health than either non-Hispanic blacks or Mexican-Americans, but race has been shown to be insignificant when other risk factors are combined and weighted statistically[7,11]
5. Changing subject-related risk factors
   a. Tobacco use is a major environmental risk factor for periodontitis; effects are not only related to local effects in the oral cavity but also to a suppression of the immune system altering host response to periodontal pathogens; pathogens do not differ between smokers and nonsmokers; smokers have greater risk of attachment loss and healing following periodontal therapy is impaired[12]
   b. Chronic alcoholism is a suspected risk factor because of increased bleeding tendencies, poor oral hygiene due to overall neglect, and malnutrition that accompany it[13]
   c. Severity of periodontitis increases with age; it may only be that these effects are related to cumulative effects of past breakdown; good oral hygiene minimizes effect of age; environmental factors affecting the elderly such as changes in diet and nutrition and increases in prescribed medications and systemic diseases may also play a role
   d. Psychosocial factors such as emotional stress can influence immune functions and may influence inflammatory periodontal diseases; evidence strongly suggests that stress is a predisposing factor to acute necrotizing ulcerative gingivitis (ANUG)[14]
   e. Diet and nutrition are important to maintenance of tissue integrity and defense mechanisms; no direct linkages have been made to periodontal disease but the relationship of nutrition to disease susceptibility cannot be ignored; severe vitamin C deficiency has been linked to scurvy and scorbutic gingivitis
   f. Prescription drugs can cause gingival overgrowth; most commonly cited medications include phenytoin (Dilantin), nifedipine (Procardia), and cyclosporin; these drugs can cause noninflammatory hyperplasia or their effects can be exacerbated by bacterial plaque for combined enlargement
   g. Systemic diseases that affect the immune system can exacerbate periodontal degeneration or affect healing following periodontal therapy; these diseases include HIV/AIDS, leukemia, hemophilia, neutropenias, diabetes, Papillon-Lefévre syndrome, Chediak-Higashi syndrome, Wegener granulomatosis, Addison disease, Sjögren's syndrome, Crohn's disease, Sturge-Weber syndrome, Down syndrome, sarcoidosis, and others

6. It is clear that destructive periodontal diseases are a result of a complex relationship between subgingival microflora and nonbacterial risk factors

D. Response of the periodontium to these factors; basic inflammatory response produces
   1. Clinical changes
   2. Histologic changes
   3. Radiographic changes
E. Response within the soft tissue only (gingival inflammation)
   1. Stage I gingivitis, or initial lesion—2 to 4 days following bacterial plaque accumulation
      a. Changes are not clinically visible; subclinical lesion
      b. Histologic changes
         (1) "Widening" of small capillaries (vasodilation)
         (2) Increase in leukocytes, particularly polymorphonuclear leukocytes or neutrophils (PMNs), in the connective tissue, junctional epithelium, and gingival sulcus; PMNs are earliest responders, or the first line of defense in inflammation
         (3) Increase in flow of gingival crevicular fluid into the sulcus
         (4) Inflammatory infiltrate occupies 5% to 10% of the gingival connective tissue where collagen has been lost
   2. Stage II gingivitis, or early lesion—begins 4 to 7 days following bacterial plaque accumulation; may persist for 21 days or longer
      a. Clinical signs of gingivitis appear (erythema and bleeding upon stimulation)
      b. Histologic changes
         (1) Persistence of inflammation from initial lesion
         (2) Leukocyte infiltration into the connective tissue dominated by lymphocytes (75%), macrophages, plasma cells, and mast cells
         (3) Junctional epithelium becomes densely infiltrated with neutrophils and begins to show development of rete pegs
         (4) Destruction of collagen fibers (especially circular and dentogingival) in the infiltrated area; fibroblasts are altered
         (5) Migration of leukocytes into junctional epithelium and gingival sulcus
         (6) Flow of gingival crevicular fluid peaks at 6 to 12 days following clinical signs of gingivitis
         (7) Sulcular lining is ulcerated (allowing bleeding)
   3. Stage III gingivitis, or established (chronic) lesion—time period variable; may persist for months or years without progressing to stage IV (periodontitis)
      a. Clinical changes

(1) Erythema (redness) of the gingiva as a result of proliferation of capillaries (begins in the papillary area) and/or a bluish hue superimposed over the reddened gingiva as a result of congested blood vessels and sluggish blood flow
(2) Bleeding may occur on probing as a result of thinning and/or ulceration of the sulcular epithelium
(3) Color changes begin in the papillary area and gingival margin, and then spread to the attached gingiva
(4) Consistency may be either soft and spongy or firm and leathery; depends on whether destructive changes or reparative changes within the gingiva are dominant
(5) Texture may be either
   (a) Smooth and shiny (destructive, exudative factors dominant) or
   (b) Stippled and nodular (reparative, fibrotic proliferation dominant)
(6) Increase in size of gingiva (enlargement)
(7) Increase in depth of the gingival sulcus—may be caused by enlargement of the gingival tissue *only;* creates a gingival or pseudopocket
   (a) Begins with papillary enlargement
   (b) Extends into margins, producing rounded and bulbous gingival margins
(8) Progression of inflammation
   (a) May remain only within the gingival tissues (gingivitis)
   (b) May extend into the supporting periodontal tissues in stage IV (periodontitis)
   NOTE: Periodontitis must be preceded by gingivitis, but gingivitis does not always progress into periodontitis
b. Histologic changes
   (1) Vascular proliferation and increase in number and predominance of plasma cells, which invade deep into the connective tissue
   (2) Widened intercellular spaces in the junctional epithelium contain lysosomes, lymphocytes, and monocytes
   (3) Junctional epithelium continues to protrude into the connective tissue
   (4) Collagenase actively breaking down connective tissue resulting in continued loss of collagen
   (5) Simultaneous proliferation of collagen fibers and epithelium

(6) Sulcular lining is ulcerated
(7) Bone loss has *not* occurred
F. Stage IV—pathway of inflammation from the gingiva to supporting periodontal tissues (transition from gingivitis to periodontitis), or advanced lesion
1. Generally follows the course of the blood vessels through soft tissues and into the alveolar bone
2. Pattern of inflammatory pathway affects the pattern of bone destruction
3. Initially, inflammation penetrates and destroys gingival fibers near the gingival fiber attachment to the cementum, then spreads
a. Interproximally
(1) Into the bone and periodontal ligament
(2) From the bone to the periodontal ligament
b. Facially and lingually
(1) From the gingiva to the outer periosteum and periodontal ligament
(2) From the periosteum into the bone
G. Formation of the periodontal pocket—persistent, chronic gingivitis may progress to periodontitis, which results in loss of connective tissue attachment, bone destruction, and periodontal pocket formation (see Chapter 13, sections on types of pockets and description of a pocket)
1. Periodontal pocket—pathologic deepening of the gingival sulcus produced by destruction of the supporting tissues and apical migration of the junctional epithelium
2. Classification
a. Suprabony pocket—base of the pocket is coronal to the alveolar crest; also called supracrestal or supraalveolar
b. Infrabony pocket—base of the pocket is apical to the alveolar crest; also called intrabony, intraalveolar, subcrestal
3. Histopathology
a. Gingival epithelium may show evidence of inflammatory changes
(1) Epithelium proliferates into the connective tissue in fingerlike projections
(2) Inflammatory cells are found in the epithelium
(3) Epithelium lining the pocket is ulcerated
(4) Coronal portion of junctional epithelium becomes detached from the root surface as the remaining portion migrates apically
b. Connective tissue changes
(1) Inflammatory cells (lymphocytes, plasma cells, and macrophages) infiltrate the connective tissue
(2) Inflammatory infiltration proceeds through the loose connective tissue along vascular pathways; predominantly B-cell infiltrate
(3) Degeneration of gingival connective tissue fibers; gingival cells release mediators or chemicals which destroy bone
(4) Tissue invasion by periodontal pathogens
c. Changes within the supporting bone as inflammatory processes progress
(1) Osteoclastic cells degenerate mineral content of bone and mononuclear cells degenerate organic matrix of bone
(2) Bone marrow component (fatty tissue) is replaced with inflammatory cell infiltrate, fibroblastic proliferation, and deposition of collagen fibers
(3) Cortical plate of the interdental septum is the first area to be involved (central crestal area where blood and lymph vessels emerge)
(4) Once this central breakthrough has occurred, the supporting bone is destroyed in a lateral direction; bone loss is accompanied by both resorption and formation
H. Common clinical changes associated with periodontitis
1. Similar changes in the gingiva as seen in gingivitis, usually a more chronic appearance
2. Areas of gingival recession
3. Bleeding on probing
4. Periodontal attachment loss
5. True periodontal pockets
6. Loose, extruded, or migrated teeth; diastemas may develop
7. Exudate from the gingival margin in response to pressure
8. Symptoms—generally painless; client may complain of itching gums, loose teeth, food impaction, and bad taste; relief is felt with pressure applied to the gums
I. Radiographic changes associated with periodontitis (usually follow this sequence)
1. Fuzziness and discontinuity of the lamina dura at the proximal aspects of the crest of the interdental septum
2. A wedge-shaped radiolucent area is formed between the mesial or distal aspects of the alveolar crest and the root surface of the involved tooth; also called triangulation
3. Center of the crestal portion of the interdental septum also becomes fuzzy, and faint cup-shaped areas of alveolar crest bone loss appear; bony crater
4. Progression of interdental bone loss
a. Horizontal bone loss—reduction in height of

the interdental septa; however, the crest is parallel to an imaginary line connecting adjacent cementoenamel junctions

b. Angular or vertical bone loss—crest is reduced in a manner that creates angular defects

5. Limitations of radiographs in diagnosis of periodontitis

   a. Radiograph does not reveal minor destructive changes in bone

   b. Involvement of facial and lingual surfaces cannot be seen

   c. Angulation errors can affect radiographic image of alveolar bone

   d. Internal morphology of infrabony craters or defects cannot be seen

   e. As a general rule, bone loss is always greater than the radiograph reveals

J. Periodontal disease activity

1. Refers to the stage(s) of periodontal disease characterized by loss of alveolar bone and connective tissue attachment

2. Implies that the natural history of periodontal disease has periods of active destruction and periods of relative inactivity, although chronic inflammation persists

3. Three theories of periodontal disease activity[15]

   a. Continuous paradigm—implies a slow, constant progression of periodontal degeneration

   b. Random burst theory—implies short periods of destruction followed by periods of no destruction, occurring randomly

   c. Asynchronous multiple burst theory—implies that periodontal disease activity, and resultant destruction, occurs within a specific period of life and is followed by remission

Bacterial Plaque

See Chapter 7, sections on microbiology of the oral cavity and bacterial plaque

A. Definition—dense, noncalcified, highly organized bacterial mass, firmly adherent to the teeth or other hard materials within the mouth; cannot be washed off by salivary or water flow

B. Two categories of bacterial plaque

1. Supragingival

2. Subgingival

C. Stages in supragingival plaque formation

1. Acquired pellicle

   a. Thin, amorphous bacteria-free membranous layer covers the clinical crown; consists of salivary glycoproteins, immunoglobulins, and carbohydrates; functions as protective barrier

   b. Forms on a cleaned tooth within minutes

   c. Within hours, salivary organisms begin to adhere to the surface of the pellicle and are surrounded by a matrix that differs from that of the acquired pellicle

   d. These bacteria and surrounding matrix make up bacterial plaque

2. Bacterial plaque

   a. Heterogeneous, dense, noncalcified bacterial mass that develops on the acquired pellicle; it is a host-associated biofilm[16]

   b. Rate of formation varies from person to person, tooth to tooth, and even in different areas on the same tooth; readily visualized on teeth after 24 to 48 hours without oral hygiene

   c. Shifts in the types of microorganisms occur as plaque ages

      (1) Young plaque is composed of

         (a) Gram-positive cocci (40% to 50%)

         (b) Gram-positive rods (10% to 40%)

         (c) Gram-negative rods (10% to 15%)

         (d) Filaments (4% or less)

      (2) As plaque ages, the percentage of gram-positive organisms decreases (2-week-old plaque is 50% gram positive and 30% gram negative)

      (3) As plaque ages, the number of cocci decreases and the number of filaments (particularly actinomyces) increases

      (4) As plaque ages, aerobic bacteria decrease and anaerobic bacteria increase

   d. Supragingival plaque formation creates an environment that permits the development of subgingival plaque

D. Structure and composition

1. Water (80%)

2. Solids (20%; 95% of which are bacteria)

3. Growth and proliferation of bacteria (not deposition of salivary bacteria) accounts for the increase in plaque bulk with age

4. Different organisms may be found in plaque (cocci, rods, filaments, and spiral forms), and their proportions change with time, diet, and location

5. Extracellular microbial products (e.g., polysaccharides, endotoxins)

6. Host-derived products, such as salivary constituents and immunoglobulins (IgG, IgA)

E. Subgingival plaque

1. Growth, accumulation, and pathogenicity of subgingival plaque is influenced strongly by supragingival plaque, especially in early stages of gingivitis and periodontitis

2. Structure and organization of subgingival plaque

a. Inflammatory changes in the gingival sulcus or periodontal pocket resulting from supragingival plaque modify the relationship between the gingival margin and the tooth surface, creating a protected subgingival area that is bathed by gingival crevicular fluid

b. This environment allows subgingival bacteria to colonize and adhere to other bacteria, the tooth, or the epithelial tissue surrounding the sulcus or pocket

c. Anaerobic bacteria become well established

d. Subgingival plaque may be attached or loosely adherent (epithelium associated)

3. Attached subgingival plaque (also called tooth-associated subgingival plaque)

a. Structure is similar to supragingival plaque

b. Inner layers are dominated by gram-positive rods and cocci, such as *Streptococcus mitis, Streptococcus sanguis, Actinomyces viscosus, Actinomyces naeslundii,* and *Eubacterium* species; gram-negative rods and cocci also are found

c. Apical portions are dominated by gram-negative rods, with some filaments present

d. Associated with calculus formation and root caries[16]

4. Loosely adherent subgingival plaque (also called epithelium—associated or unattached)

a. Extends from gingival margin apical to the junctional epithelium, adjacent to the gingival epithelium or the pocket lumen

b. Primarily gram-negative rods and cocci, as well as motile organisms, filaments, and spirochetes that are not highly organized; predominance of species such as *Porphyromonas gingivalis, Prevotella intermedia,* (both pathogenic) and *Capnocytophaga ochracea* (beneficial)

c. Associated with different forms of periodontitis[16]

5. Bacterial invasion of periodontal tissues

a. Bacteria have been found within diseased periodontal tissues in gingivitis and periodontitis

b. Widened intercellular spaces in the gingival epithelium or pocket lining may allow for penetration of organisms from subgingival bacterial plaque

c. Bacterial invasion may occur, or presence of bacteria within the tissue may be a result of displacement or manipulation rather than actual invasion

6. Bacterial specificity

a. Specific plaque hypothesis—suggests that specific combinations of bacteria cause various forms of periodontal disease; only certain plaque microorganisms are pathogenic

b. Research is further defining the bacterial etiology of destructive periodontal disease[15]

F. Calculus—bacterial plaque that has mineralized (see Chapter 13, section on calculus)

1. Mineralization can begin from 24 to 48 hours or up to 2 weeks after plaque deposition; all plaque does not necessarily calcify

2. Earliest mineralization occurs along the inner surface of the plaque or in attached subgingival plaque

3. Composition

a. Inorganic material (70% to 90%)

b. Remainder is organic material and water

4. Classification

a. Supragingival (supramarginal, salivary)—derives its minerals from saliva

b. Subgingival (submarginal, serumal)—derives its minerals from gingival crevicular fluid

5. Modes of attachment to teeth (see Chapter 13, section on modes of attachment)

a. By acquired pellicle

b. By direct attachment of the calculus matrix to the tooth surface; penetration into cementum

c. By mechanically locking into tooth surface irregularities

6. Effect on the periodontium—because bacterial plaque always covers calculus, it is primarily a bacterial irritant (not mechanical); calculus plays a significant role as a contributing factor in the pathogenesis of periodontal disease; a plaque retentive factor

G. Pathogenic effect on periodontium

1. Bacterial plaque contributes to periodontal breakdown by direct injury to the tissues and by stimulating host-mediated responses that result in tissue injury

2. Direct injury is caused by toxins and enzymes produced by bacteria and by end products of bacterial metabolism

a. Exotoxins are proteins released by organisms, and they cause direct injury to tissues

b. Endotoxins are cellular components of gram-negative bacteria that contribute to the inflammatory process

c. Enzymes, mainly proteases, facilitate bacterial tissue penetration by breaking down structural barriers; collagenase causes dissolution of collagen within the connective tissue; hyaluronidase affects the ground substance within the connective tissue

3. Indirect toxicity results when subgingival bacteria act as antigens and a resultant local immune

reaction occurs; the host response attempts to control the bacterial attack, and some destruction of tissue results by a variety of immunopathologic reactions

H. Host response

1. Host responses play a role in the etiology of inflammatory periodontal infections
2. Inflammatory cells migrate by chemotaxis in response to injury in a localized area and phagocytize bacteria or bacterial components; mast cells, neutrophils (polymorphonuclear leukocytes), macrophages, lymphocytes, and plasma cells are all inflammatory cells that are involved in the host response in periodontal disease
   a. Mast cells—contain histamine in cytoplasm; most important in hypersensitivity reactions of an anaphylactic type
   b. Neutrophils—polymorphonuclear leukocytes (PMNs); circulating white blood cells for phagocytosis and proteolysis; respond first after injury, infection, or irritation; first line of defense in inflammatory periodontal disease; have ingestive enzymes to ingest microorganisms and to neutralize toxic bacterial products
   c. Lymphocytes—monocytes including T cells and B cells; T lymphocytes migrate from the bone marrow to the thymus where they become immunocompetent; B lymphocytes are derived from the liver, spleen, and bone marrow and are involved in humoral immune responses; B cells are identified by their surface immunoglobulins (amino acids); two of these immunoglobulins (IgG and IgM) form antigen-antibody complexes which activate complement
   d. Macrophages—large mononuclear phagocytes that play a direct role in cell-mediated immunity (or delayed hypersensitivity); cellular immunity does not involve antibodies; macrophages and T cells interact to aid the response of B cells by preparing the antigen in the second line of defense in inflammatory periodontal disease
   e. Plasma cells—B cells terminate as plasma cells which produce immunoglobulins and antibodies; they predominate in chronic periodontal lesions
3. Antibodies or immunoglobulins are produced by plasma cells in response to oral bacteria or their by-products
4. Human immunoglobulins are divided into classes and have differing functions
   a. IgG is the most prevalent and acts to neutralize bacterial toxins by enhancing phagocytosis

   b. IgM is produced first after injury and activates the complement system
   c. IgE responds in severe acute allergic reactions
   d. IgD binds to the surface of B lymphocytes and may trigger lymphocyte stimulation
   e. IgA is the principal immunoglobin in exocrine secretions, such as saliva, milk, tears, and respiratory secretions[16]
5. Complement, composed of proteins and glycoproteins, is activated as a consequence of an antigen-antibody (Ag-Ab) reaction; enhances phagocytosis, lysis, or chemotaxis of antibodies by affixing to them
6. Lysosomes are released from phagocytosis of Ag-Ab complexes by PMNs; tissue destruction results
7. Lymphocytes are stimulated by Ag-Ab complexes and lymphokines are produced; lymphokines have both protective and destructive capabilities
8. The bacterial antigen is neutralized by these processes, but tissue destruction occurs concurrently
9. Immune mechanisms serve a protective function but can result in an overreaction or hypersensitivity such as anaphylaxis, cytotoxic reactions, arthus reactions, or cell-mediated immunity (delayed hypersensitivity)

I. Summary—current knowledge of the effect of bacterial plaque on tissues is expanding; however, many questions remain unanswered; to maintain oral health

1. Plaque must be removed or changed in composition from predominantly gram-negative, motile anaerobic bacteria associated with disease to predominantly gram-positive, nonmotile aerobic or facultative bacteria found in periodontal health
2. A balance must be achieved between local factors present and the individual host response

Clinical Assessment of the Periodontium

A. Indices—system for documenting clinical observations to help clients become aware of their present status, demonstrate changes in health over a period of time, and survey large populations for present status and trends in health (see Table 15-3)

1. Periodontal Disease Index (Ramfjord's; PDI)—assesses the prevalence and severity of periodontal disease of individuals or groups by using the following parameters
   a. Gingivitis index—assesses color, form, consistency, and bleeding to determine the presence or absence of inflammation
   b. Calculus index—assesses the presence or absence of calculus and its extent if present

    c. Crevice (sulcus) depth—measurement to determine the distance between the cementoenamel junction and the base of the sulcus (method to assess apical migration of the epithelial attachment)

    d. Plaque criteria (Schick-Ash modification)—assesses presence or absence of plaque and its extent if present

  2. Löe and Silness Gingival Index (GI)—assesses the presence, severity, or absence of gingival inflammation and bleeding; Lobene and associates created the modified GI (MGI) by eliminating the bleeding criteria making it a noninvasive index

  3. Silness and Löe Plaque Index (PI)—assesses the quantity and location of plaque

  4. Muhlemann Sulcus Bleeding Index (BI)—assesses the presence, severity, or absence of bleeding on probing

  5. Eastman Interdental Bleeding Index (Caton and Polson)—assesses the presence or absence of proximal bleeding through stimulation with a wooden wedge

  6. Gingival Bleeding Index (Ainamo and Bay)—assesses presence or absence of bleeding upon gentle probing; expressed as a percentage of sites examined

  7. Gingival Bleeding Index (Carter and Barnes)—assesses presence or absence of interproximal bleeding by using unwaxed dental floss

B. Periodontal documentation

  1. Uses—documentation of existing periodontal status; baseline for future reference

  2. Updated periodically to determine changes in periodontal health

  3. Necessary for care planning

  4. Serves as a guide for the clinician during treatment and evaluation

  5. Serves as a legal document

  6. Serves as a technique for managing risks associated with failure to diagnose and treat periodontal disease

C. Periodontal assessment—complete periodontal documentation should be based on a thorough periodontal assessment, which includes

  1. Description of the gingival tissues, including visual signs of inflammation, such as erythema, edema, enlargement, hyperplasia, fibrosis, or any other changes in color, shape, size, surface texture, or consistency; distribution and severity also should be noted

  2. Findings from examination of the periodontium with a periodontal probe (see Chapter 13), which include[16-18]

    a. Presence of bleeding—widely accepted as an indicator of inflammation; more sensitive than visual signs; however, inflamed sites do not always bleed and bleeding is a poor predictor of attachment loss (only 30%)[15]; results when sulcular lining is ulcerated

    b. Probing depth (also called sulcus/pocket depth)—gives a historical record of past periodontal disease activity; useful in monitoring success of periodontal therapy; important in determining client's ability to maintain health through plaque control; the periodontal probe remains the best diagnostic aid for detecting periodontal pockets and attachment loss; combining bleeding upon probing with pocket depth increases prediction for attachment loss to 70% to 75%[15]

    c. Clinical attachment level—measures from CEJ to attachment; determines amount of apical migration of the junctional epithelium or amount of lost periodontal support to the tooth

    d. Recession—measures from the CEJ to the gingival margin; indicates apical migration of the gingiva

    e. Presence of purulent exudate (suppuration)—in response to lateral digital pressure on the gingival margin or probing; suggests advanced lesion of periodontitis

    f. Adequacy of width of attached gingiva—measures from attachment to mucogingival junction; amount will vary depending on location; adequate zone necessary to withstand mechanical stresses from mastication; if none is present, gingival margin will move with alveolar mucosa

  3. Alternatives to use of standard periodontal probe for periodontal examination

    a. Periodontal screening and recording system (PSR)—designed to provide thorough screening and recording for all clients while saving time in recording aspect of initial exam[19]

      (1) All tooth/implant surfaces are examined individually; however, only the highest score in each sextant is recorded

      (2) Scores range from zero (healthy) to 4 (indicating probing depth greater than 5.5 mm); a specially demarcated probe is used

      (3) Not intended to substitute for or replace full periodontal exams; patients with higher scores in any sextant or with clinical abnormalities must have comprehensive exam

b. Computerized probes[20]
   (1) Increase accuracy by reducing margin of error and standardizing pressure
   (2) Reduce time required for probing and recording; some are voice activated; some provide printouts of probing depths and/or attachment loss (e.g., Florida probe, Toronto automated periodontal probe, VICTOR, Interprobe)
c. Temperature-sensitive probes—measure not only probing depths but also loss of attachment and changes in temperature that may be associated with inflammation[20] (e.g., Perio-Temp)

4. Presence and distribution of bacterial plaque and calculus (may use indices)
5. Condition of tooth proximal contacts—loose or open contacts permit food impaction
6. Degree of pathologic tooth mobility
   a. Grade I—slightly more than normal
   b. Grade II—moderately more than normal
   c. Grade III—severe mobility faciolingually and/or mesiodistally combined with vertical displacement
   d. Pathologic tooth mobility is caused by loss of periodontal support (bone loss); trauma from occlusion; inflammation extending into the periodontal ligament from the gingiva or the apex (abscesses), periodontal surgery (temporarily), hormonal changes associated with pregnancy and sometimes menstruation or use of hormonal contraceptives, pathologic processes of the jaws that destroy the bone and/or roots of teeth (e.g., osteomyelitis or tumors)[16]
   e. Tooth mobility is most commonly assessed by using the blunt ends of the handles of two dental instruments (single-ended); can be measured electronically for objective data (e.g., Periotest)
7. Presence of furcation involvements (see Chapter 4)
   a. Class I—early involvement, in which the probe can enter into the tip of the furcation area; incipient bone loss; may not be visible radiographically
   b. Class II—moderate involvement, in which the probe can enter the furcation but not pass through; partial bone loss; may be visible radiographically
   c. Class III—severe involvement, in which the probe can be passed between the roots; total bone loss; visible radiographically, may or may not be occluded by the gingiva

8. Presence of malocclusion or malposition of teeth
9. Presence and condition of dental restorations and prosthetic appliances; missing teeth; dental implants
10. Presence of overhanging restorations (overhangs)—contributing etiologic factor in periodontal disease attributable to potential for accumulation of bacterial plaque and food impaction
11. Assessment of disease progression by longitudinal comparison of probing depths, attachment levels, and interproximal bone height (radiographic)
12. Interpretation of a satisfactory number of bitewing and periapical radiographs that are of diagnostic quality to assess
    a. Level of alveolar crest in relation to the cementoenamel junction
    b. Interdental bone
    c. Furcation areas
    d. Width of periodontal ligament space
    e. Existing dental restorations and caries
    f. Periapical disease
    g. Length, shape, and position of roots

D. Documentation of oral habits
   1. Bruxing (grinding) or clenching of the teeth
   2. Chewing on fingernails or foreign objects
   3. Smoking habits
   4. Alcohol habits
   5. Movement of the temporomandibular joint (evidenced by crepitus, tenderness, or deviations)

E. Assessment of occlusion—includes
   1. Angle's classification and anterior relationships
   2. Degree of tooth mobility
   3. Excessive wear patterns (facets)
   4. Defective prematurities—isolated occlusal contacts that cause deflection in the pathway of physiologic mandibular movement
   5. Teeth, restorations, or prosthetic appliances that may interfere with normal movements of the mandible
   6. Temporomandibular joint discomfort
   7. Fremitus—vibration of root surfaces as the client "taps" teeth together
   8. Tooth sensitivity to pressure and to hot and cold substances

F. Classification of occlusal trauma (NOTE: There is lack of agreement about the role of occlusal trauma in the etiology and pathogenesis of periodontitis)
   1. Primary occlusal trauma—trauma results from excessive occlusal forces; result could be mobility, excessive wear of a tooth or teeth, sensitivity of involved teeth, or fremitus
   2. Secondary occlusal trauma—supporting periodontium is not normal (some loss of supporting struc-

tures is present); tooth or teeth are not able to withstand even normal occlusal forces, and particularly excessive occlusal forces, without trauma; could result in mobility or sensitivity

G. Additional information obtained through client interview
1. Complete documentation of the client's past and current health status
2. Complete documentation of the client's dental history
3. Client's daily oral hygiene routine
4. Client's attitude toward oral health
5. Client's oral health knowledge level

H. Supplemental diagnostic tests[21]
1. The traditional approach to periodontal diagnosis only measures results of periodontal inflammation and/or destruction; goals for developing newer diagnostic approaches include the ability to detect the presence of disease as early as possible and to predict destruction before it occurs; prognostic devices or tests also would be able to assess the risk of developing disease in the future
2. Validity of a diagnostic test is determined by calculating its sensitivity and specificity
   a. Sensitivity—refers to the probability of a test being positive when a disease is truly present
   b. Specificity—refers to the probability of a test being negative when a disease truly is not present
   c. Predictive value—refers to the probability that a disease will be present when the test is positive, or not present when the test is negative
3. Supplemental diagnostic tests can be used for screening (separating diseased from healthy individuals) or to detect sites or individuals at high risk for progressive disease; the second task is more demanding and has greater value
4. General categories of supplemental diagnostic tests
   a. Detection of substances associated with periodontal pathogens (microbiologic monitoring)
      (1) DNA probes—paper points are inserted into specific site(s) and sent to a laboratory for analysis; lab report returned in 2 weeks specifying levels of eight known periodontal pathogens; general information provided on antibiotic selection (e.g., DMD); high degree of sensitivity and specificity, usually above 90%
      (2) Culturing—plaque samples from specific sites are placed in a vial containing transport medium and sent to a laboratory for analysis; specific percentages of various bacterial species are identified and specific recommendations for antibiotic sensitivity also can be obtained; highly detailed technique required
      (3) Enzyme-linked immunosorbent assay (ELISA)—matches plaque sample DNA and bacterial antigens to periodontal pathogens; used in research rather than practice in the United States; rapid chairside test may be available in future
      (4) Enzymatic tests—immunoassay technology matches the fingerprint of the bacterial antigen to those of selected periodontal pathogens; limited to only three key microorganisms but all have been linked to periodontal destruction; ease of use and immediate chairside results are advantages (e.g., BANA test); highly sensitive and moderately specific
   b. Local measures of host response
      (1) Gingival crevicular fluid (GCF)—levels of enzymes, inflammatory cells/mediators, tissue breakdown products, and microorganisms can be measured to differentiate simple gingival inflammation from higher levels of destructive disease; shows promise for high predictive value; only available for laboratory use at present but shows promise for identifying sites requiring additional therapy before the continued care appointment for periodontal maintenance procedures
      (2) Biochemical tests—chairside tests available to detect collagenase or aspartate aminotransferase with connective tissue breakdown; indicates active gingival inflammation but does not identify the cause (e.g., Periodontal Care Monitoring System, PerioGard)
   c. Serology—blood tests that diagnose neutrophil response and cell surface receptors are used in research on early-onset periodontitis because of known abnormalities in function; not available for widespread clinical application
   d. Digital subtraction radiography—is a computerized image enhancement technique that can detect osseous changes too small to be seen by the eye when comparing two standardized radiographs taken at separate times; software can detect areas of bone loss or gain and color them in different shades; highly sensitive and specific (over 90%); very detailed technique required and cost limits widespread clinical use

Diseases of the Periodontium

Classification of Periodontal Diseases

See Chapter 7, section on inflammatory periodontal diseases.

A. Importance of disease classification
   1. Useful for purposes of diagnosis, prognosis, and care planning
   2. Classifications of periodontal diseases are changing as new information evolves regarding etiology, pathogenicity, and host factors
   3. Useful for legal documentation
B. Current classifications of periodontal diseases[16,22,26]
   1. Gingivitis
      a. Chronic gingivitis (or simple gingivitis)
      b. Necrotizing ulcerative gingivitis (NUG)
      c. Gingivitis associated with systemic disease
         (1) Linear gingival erythema (LGE)
         (2) Scorbutic gingivitis
         (3) Gingivitis associated with hormonal changes
         (4) Gingival enlargement (or overgrowth)
         (5) Miscellaneous gingival changes
         (6) Desquamative gingival changes
   2. Periodontitis
      a. Adult periodontitis (or slowly progressive)
      b. Early-onset periodontitis (aggressive forms)
         (1) Prepubertal periodontitis
         (2) Juvenile periodontitis (localized or generalized)
         (3) Rapidly progressive periodontitis
      c. Necrotizing ulcerative periodontitis (NUP)
      d. Refractory periodontitis (aggressive form)
   3. Trauma from occlusion
   4. Other conditions of the attachment apparatus

Diseases

A. Gingivitis—inflammation of the gingiva
   1. Clinical features (see section on changes in the periodontium associated with disease)
   2. Classification of gingivitis by
      a. Duration
         (1) Acute—sudden onset; short duration; usually some pain or tenderness noted
         (2) Chronic—long duration; painless; may be episodic in progression
      b. Distribution
         (1) Localized—confined to a single tooth or group of teeth
         (2) Generalized—involves entire mouth
         (3) Papillary—involves interdental papilla only
         (4) Marginal—involves gingival margin and papilla
         (5) Diffuse—involves gingival margin, papilla, and attached gingiva
   3. Etiology—most forms are caused primarily by bacterial plaque
   4. Treatment
      a. By clinician—removal of bacterial plaque and calculus deposits and other plaque-retentive factors
      b. By client—daily self care practices for removal of bacterial plaque
B. Subclassifications of gingivitis
   1. Acute or chronic (see previous section)
   2. Necrotizing ulcerative gingivitis (NUG)—inflammatory destructive disease of the gingiva that has a sudden onset with periods of remission and exacerbation; predisposing conditions may be pre-existing (e.g., gingivitis, smoking, period of severe stress, radical change in eating or sleeping habits), acute, chronic, or recurrent
      a. Clinical findings are characterized by crater-like depressions at the crest of the interdental papilla that progress into the marginal gingiva
         (1) Surface of the lesion(s) is covered by a gray, necrotized slough surrounded by an obvious erythematous (red) zone
         (2) Bleeding may be spontaneous and also will occur when necrotic tissue is removed gently
         (3) Initially moderate pain increases as the disease advances
         (4) Fetid odor and increased salivation are present
         (5) Swelling and tenderness of regional lymph nodes (especially submandibular nodes) are present
         (6) Fever and malaise may be present
      b. Radiographic findings—normal unless the disease has not been treated and has led to destruction of supporting structures (necrotizing ulcerative periodontitis)
      c. Etiology—predisposing factors are present, with intermediate-sized spirochetes and *Prevotella intermedia* found within the tissue; however, the primary etiologic factor is uncertain
      d. Treatment
         (1) Debridement for plaque and debris removal—initially by the clinician and daily by the client (may be difficult because of pain); ultrasonic debridement may have some benefit
         (2) Reappoint in 24 to 48 hours to evaluate healing; rapid response in individuals with normal immune function; no response if

immunocompromised; complete thorough scaling, root planing/periodontal debridement at this appointment; pain markedly reduced if healing has begun

(3) Stress recurrent nature of NUG and critical role of self-care practices and frequent continued care visits

(4) Antibiotics may be prescribed if systemic symptoms (lymphadenopathy, fever, etc.) are evident

(5) Soft nutritious diet

(6) Avoidance of spicy foods, alcohol, and smoking

(7) After acute symptoms disappear, gingival tissues may need to be surgically recontoured if destruction resulted in a reverse architecture

3. Gingivitis associated with systemic disease
   a. Linear gingival erythema (LGE)—occurs in individuals infected with the human immunodeficiency virus (HIV) or who have acquired immune deficiency syndrome (AIDS) or other immunocompromising diseases
      (1) Clinical changes—distinct band of severe erythema on marginal gingiva; can be localized or generalized; sometimes punctuated red dots also present on attached gingiva; no ulceration or loss of attachment
      (2) Radiographic changes—none; normal findings
      (3) Etiology—host response to bacterial plaque
      (4) Treatment—scaling and debridement with povidone-iodine irrigation for antimicrobial and topical anesthetic effect; prescription of antifungal agents if candidiasis also present; stress critical importance of thorough self care practices including mechanical removal of bacterial plaque and twice daily 0.12% chlorhexidine rinses, one month reevaluation and continued care recommended for initial interval
   b. Scorbutic gingivitis—classic feature of gingivitis associated with severe ascorbic acid (vitamin C) deficiency; uncommon in industrialized countries
   c. Gingivitis associated with hormonal changes
      (1) Clinical features—clinical signs of gingival inflammation or gingival enlargement; may be marginal or diffuse, localized or generalized; severe cases may progress to pyogenic granuloma (pregnancy tumor)
      (2) Radiographic findings—normal
      (3) Etiology—may be associated with puberty, pregnancy, birth control medication, or steroid therapy; subgingival growth of *Bacteroides*, *Porphyromonas*, or *Prevotella* species; characterized by exaggerated response to bacterial plaque
      (4) Treatment—scaling and debridement for removal of bacterial plaque and calculus deposits; in some cases, modification of hormone therapy or medications

4. Gingival enlargement or overgrowth (also called drug-associated or medication-influenced)
   a. Clinical features—gingival hyperplasia or enlargement; overgrowth of gingival tissues; pseudopockets may be present
   b. Radiographic findings—normal
   c. Etiology—does not require plaque-induced inflammation for development; caused by systemic drug administration (e.g., phenytoin, cyclosporine, nifedipine); bacterial plaque can exaggerate response
   d. Treatment—removal of bacterial plaque and calculus deposits, gingival stimulation and plaque control by client; may require alteration of drug therapy or gingivectomy if severe

5. Miscellaneous gingival changes
   a. Clinical features—includes all other pathologic and physiologic alterations in the gingival tissues; changes include clinical signs of inflammation, atrophy, cyst formation, neoplasia, and degeneration
   b. Radiographic changes—none
   c. Etiology—associated with blood dyscrasias, nutritional deficiencies, tumors, genetic factors, mouth breathing, and diffuse bacterial and viral infections
   d. Treatment—depending on etiology; may require local and/or systemic therapeutic modalities

6. Desquamative gingival changes
   a. Clinical features—characterized by desquamation, or sloughing, of the gingival epithelium, leaving an intensely red surface as a result of vesiculation; may involve all or part of gingiva and other oral mucosal surfaces
   b. Radiographic changes—none
   c. Etiology—a sign rather than a disease entity; may be oral manifestation of dermatologic disorders, erosive lichen planus, bullous pemphigoid, and pemphigus vulgaris
   d. Treatment—requires different types of management, depending on underlying condition; careful examination and history, hemotologic analysis, and/or biopsies may be needed for definitive

diagnosis; local treatment is indicated in all cases; systemic therapy including steroids also may be used

C. Periodontitis
  1. Adult periodontitis—also called slowly progressive; disease resulting from the inflammatory process originating in the gingiva (gingivitis) and extending into the supporting periodontal structures; may have periods of activity and remission
      a. Clinical features (see section on changes in the periodontium associated with disease)
          (1) Early—progression of the gingival inflammation into the deeper periodontal structures and alveolar bone crest, with slight bone loss; with normal gingival contour usual periodontal probing depth is 3 to 4 mm with slight loss of connective tissue attachment and slight loss of alveolar bone; average 2 to 3 mm attachment loss
          (2) Moderate—a more advanced state of the above condition, with increased destruction of the periodontal structures and noticeable loss of bone support, possibly accompanied by an increase in tooth mobility; may be furcation involvement in multirooted teeth; average probing depth of 5 to 6 mm with normal gingival contour; average 4 to 5 mm attachment loss
          (3) Advanced—further progression of periodontitis with major loss of alveolar bone support, usually accompanied by increased tooth mobility; furcation involvement in multirooted teeth is likely; recession is common; average probing depth 7 mm or more with normal gingival contour; average 6 mm or greater attachment loss
      b. Radiographic features (see section on changes in the periodontium associated with disease)
      c. Etiology—host response to bacterial plaque
      d. Treatment—nonsurgical and/or surgical periodontal therapy, followed by periodontal maintenance procedures
  2. Early-onset periodontitis (aggressive or rapidly progressive)[23]
      a. Prepubertal periodontitis—a rare condition
          (1) Clinical features—generalized or localized; affects primary and secondary teeth and begins with eruption of primary teeth; characterized by severe gingival inflammation, rapid bone loss, tooth mobility, and tooth loss
          (2) Radiographic features—localized or generalized bone loss surrounding primary teeth

and partially erupted or recently erupted secondary teeth
          (3) Etiology—unclear at this time; may be related to defective PMNs or mononuclear leukocytes; associated with a subgingival microflora of *Prevotella intermedia, Capnocytophagia sputigena*, and *Eikenella corrodens*[15,16]; may be associated with systemic disease
          (4) Treatment—experimental at this time; referal to specialist indicated
      b. Localized juvenile periodontitis (LJP)—a disease of the periodontium of the permanent dentition that occurs in otherwise healthy young individuals; characterized by rapid loss of connective tissue attachment and alveolar bone
          (1) Localized in early stages, only permanent first molars and incisors are affected
          (2) Epidemiology—onset around puberty; seems to affect females more than males (3:1)
          (3) Etiology—believed to be genetically based; may be inherited as an X-linked dominant trait or an autosomal recessive trait; bacterial plaque with predominantly gram-negative organisms—*Actinobacillus actinomycetemcomitans, Capnocytophaga ochraceus; Prevotella intermedia*, and *Eikenella corrodens*—these organisms have been found within the connective tissue; subgingival plaque is relatively sparse; depressed neutrophil chemotaxis and, to a lesser extent, phagocytosis
          (4) Clinical findings[15]—gingiva around the affected area may appear normal; periodontal probing reveals deep pockets on one or more proximal surfaces of affected teeth; low dental caries rate; rapid rate of attachment loss; rate and severity of destruction is not consistent with relatively sparse plaque and lack of clinical inflammation; often bilaterally symmetric
          (5) Radiographic findings—characterized by severe angular defects, usually bilateral; definitive diagnosis made when at least three sites exhibit greater than or equal to 5-mm attachment loss (with corresponding bony defects)[15]; localized bone loss begins in first molars and incisors
          (6) Treatment—same as adult periodontitis with systemic antibiotic (tetracycline or metronidazole and amoxicillin therapy and

diligent periodontal maintenance procedures)

c. Generalized juvenile periodontitis
   (1) May be related to rapidly progressive periodontitis[15]
   (2) Occurs at an early age (12 to 30 years)
   (3) Neutrophil chemotactic disorder
   (4) Characterized by rapid severe periodontal destruction around most teeth
   (5) Subgingival flora dominated by *Prevotella intermedia* and *Eikenella corrodens*
   (6) Possible sequelae—can see a dramatic decrease in destruction associated with juvenile periodontitis; remission results in slower progression similar to adult periodontitis (called postjuvenile periodontitis)

d. Rapidly progressive periodontitis
   (1) Clinical features—characterized by severe gingival inflammation and rapid loss of connective tissue attachment and alveolar bone
   (2) Epidemiology—occurs in young adults (early 20s to mid 30s)
   (3) Etiology—large percentage of affected persons have depressed neutrophil chemotaxis; associated bacteria include *Porphyromonas gingivalis, Prevotella intermedia, Bacteroides capillus, Eikenella corrodens, Eubacterium brachy, Eubacterium nodatum, Eubacterium timidum, Lactobacillus minitus, Fusobacterium nucleatum,* and *Campylobacter rectus* (formerly *Wolinella recta*)

3. Necrotizing ulcerative periodontitis (NUP)
   a. Occurs in persons who have the human immunodeficiency virus (HIV) or AIDS or other immunocompromising diseases
   b. Characterized by severe soft tissue necrosis and rapid destruction of periodontal attachment and bone; may lead to exposure of alveolar bone and sequestration
   c. Chief complaint may be "jaw pain" or "deep aching pain"
   d. Can be localized or generalized
   e. Treatment requires conventional periodontal therapy with povidine iodine irrigation and pain control; rigorous self-care practices for mechanical plaque removal in conjunction with 0.12% chlorhexidine mouth rinsing and/or judicious use of systemic antibiotics; adjunctive antifungal therapy if indicated; and more frequent maintenance therapy than indicated for persons with adult periodontitis

4. Refractory periodontitis (aggressive form)
   a. Disease in multiple sites in persons who continue to demonstrate attachment loss after apparently appropriate treatment; site(s) continue to be infected by periodontal pathogens
   b. Etiology—refractory clients exhibit elevated levels of *Bacteroides forsythus, Fusobacterium nucleatum, Porphyromonas gingivalis, Streptococcus intermedius, Eubacterium corrodens, Fusobacterium nucleatum,* with or without *Porphyromonas gingivalis*
   c. Treatment—aggressive periodontal therapy with frequent continued care intervals and antibiotic therapy (e.g., metronidazole, Augmentin, ciprofloxacin, doxycycline, clindamycin); cultural analysis of bacterial plaque pathogens may be indicated

5. Pathology associated with occlusion (trauma from occlusion)—tissue injury to the supporting attachment apparatus caused by excessive occlusal forces
   a. Clinical changes (see section on periodontal assessment, documentation of oral habits and assessment of occlusion)
   b. Etiology—most commonly recognized etiologic factor is bruxism
   c. May be associated with disorders of the temporomandibular joints (TMJ)
   d. Treatment—occlusal adjustment or orthodontics if there are signs and symptoms of traumatic occlusion or neuromuscular disturbances; not well justified for treatment of inflammatory periodontal disease, parafunctional habits, or TMJ disorders; occlusal splints may relieve symptoms

6. Other conditions of the attachment apparatus—includes all pathologic processes of the periodontium including infection, abrasion, trauma, and cystic, degenerative, or neoplastic changes

Other Periodontal Conditions

A. Pericoronitis—inflammation of the tissue flap (operculum) surrounding the crown of a partially erupted tooth
   1. Most common in third molar areas
   2. May be acute, subacute, or chronic
   3. Clinical findings if acute
      a. Extremely red, swollen lesion with exudate is present
      b. Area is extremely tender, with pain radiating to the ear, throat, and floor of the mouth
      c. Foul taste in the mouth
      d. Inflammation may progress so that swelling, inability to close the jaw, fever, and malaise may be present; symptoms are less obvious as the situation becomes more chronic

4. Etiology—accumulation of food debris and bacterial growth between the soft tissue flap and tooth; tissue inflammation may be compounded by trauma from the opposing tooth
5. Treatment
   a. Give antibiotics if fever, swelling, or lymphadenopathy is present
   b. Cleanse the area (lavage, debridement, and curettage) and create access for drainage of the exudate
   c. Have the client rinse frequently with warm water; have the client return for continued care after 24 hours
   d. After pain subsides and the infection is controlled, either extract the involved tooth or remove (excise) the soft tissue flap
B. Periodontal (or lateral) abscess—localized, purulent area of inflammation within the periodontal tissue
   1. Clinical findings
      a. Abscess may be in the supporting periodontal tissues on the lateral aspect of the root, which results in a sinus (fistula) opening through the bone extending out to the external surface
      b. Abscess may develop in the soft tissue wall of a deep periodontal pocket, adjacent to a periapical lesion, or following deep scaling/periodontal debridement
      c. Abscess may be acute or chronic
         (1) Acute—extreme pain, sensitivity, mobility, enlarged lymph nodes
            (a) Gingival area is edematous, red, and smooth with a shiny surface
            (b) Exudate may be expressed from the gingival margin on pressure
         (2) Chronic—usually asymptomatic or episodes of dull pain; elevation of the tooth; desire to grind on the tooth (may have acute episodes); usually has a sinus opening onto the gingival mucosa along the root
   2. Radiographic findings (many variations according to the location, stage, and extent of the lesion)—typical appearance is that of a discrete radiolucent area along the lateral aspect of the root
   3. Treatment—debridement and curettage with subgingival saline or chlorhexidine or povidone iodine irrigation; antibiotics if fever, swelling, or lymph node involvement; perioendo therapy combined if related to periapical abscess
C. Dystrophies—pathologic condition caused by abnormal cell biology and physiology
   1. Types
      a. Atrophy—diminished size of the organ or tissue
      b. Hyperplasia—abnormal increase in volume of the tissue or organ caused by the formation and growth of new normal cells
      c. Hypertrophy—increase in size of the tissue or organ caused by an increase in size of its cells; does not occur in gingiva; can occur in periodontal ligaments, cementum, and alveolar bone because of an increase in functional influences
   2. Gingival hyperplasia—overgrowth of gingiva caused by an increase in the fibrous tissue component of the gingiva
      a. Localized "fibroma"—etiology may be unknown or local irritation; treated by surgical removal and elimination of local irritating factors
      b. Generalized gingival fibrous hyperplasia—rare; etiology is unclear
      c. Idiopathic gingival hyperplasia (fibromatosis)—genetic; seems to involve a defect in collagen metabolism; treatment may include surgery; condition tends to recur
      d. Pyogenic granuloma—exaggerated tissue response possibly initiated by minor trauma; if it occurs in pregnant woman, it is called a pregnancy tumor; high incidence of recurrence; most frequently papillary
      e. Medication-induced hyperplasia—hyperplastic reaction of epithelium and connective tissue to phenytoin, nifedipine or cyclosporine; usually with inflammation being a secondary, complicating factor; treatment includes daily, thorough self-care practices with or without surgery (gingivectomy); physician may also try changing the client's drug
   3. Gingival recession (or gingival atrophy)—exposure of the root surface caused by an apical shift in the position of the gingiva
      a. Severity of the recession is determined by the actual position of the gingiva
      b. Recession may be partially clinically visible and partially hidden (covered by inflamed pocket wall); total amount of recession is the sum of the clinical and hidden recession (NOTE: "Recession" documented on periodontal charts is that which is clinically visible only)
      c. *Recession* refers only to the location of the gingiva, not the condition of the gingiva; may have recession of gingiva that is inflamed or noninflamed
      d. Etiology—the following factors have been implicated as possible etiologic factors
         (1) Gingival inflammation
         (2) Faulty toothbrushing (gingival abrasion)
         (3) Tooth position

  (a) In the arch
  (b) Mesiodistal curvature of the tooth
  (4) Location and amount of pull on the margin of the frenum attachment
  (5) Dehiscence
  (6) Increases with age
 e. Clinical significance
  (1) Exposed roots are susceptible to dental caries and abrasion
  (2) Wearing away of cementum on the exposed surface leaves exposed dentin, which may be sensitive to mechanical, chemical, or thermal stimuli
  (3) Interproximal recession creates space for accumulation of bacterial plaque and other debris
 f. Treatment
  (1) Removal of etiologic or contributing factors
  (2) Maintenance of daily thorough oral self-care practices
  (3) Root desensitization if needed
  (4) Gingival graft or periodontal flap surgery may be performed to prevent further recession and loss of attached gingiva

Treatment

Initial Care Plan

A. Collection of data to assess the status of the periodontium (see section on clinical assessment of the periodontium)
B. Formulation of initial care plan based on data collection and assessment
 1. Determination of all etiologic and contributing factors
 2. Removal or control of factors in an organized, logical sequence to include
  a. Plaque removal and control
  b. Pocket reduction or elimination
  c. When possible, removal of contributing factors
 3. Order of treatment will depend on
  a. Severity of the client's periodontal condition
  b. General health status of the client
  c. Client's motivation and cooperation
  d. Prognosis
C. Contributing factors influencing the prognosis
 1. Local factors
  a. Degree of periodontal destruction (amount of attachment lost)
  b. Rate of periodontal destruction (amount of attachment lost per unit of time)
  c. Presence of contributing local factors (e.g., malocclusion, parafunctional habits, position of

teeth in alveoli, malalignment, root proximity, missing teeth)
  d. Quality of restorations present
 2. Systemic factors—client's general health (presence or absence of systemic disease)
 3. Personal considerations
  a. Client's self-care habits, motivation, and willingness to assume responsibility for oral self-care practices
  b. Client's ability to finance specific types of periodontal treatment and restorative/prosthetic needs

Nonsurgical Periodontal Therapy (Also Called Initial Therapy or Phase I Therapy)

A. Principles of nonsurgical periodontal therapy (NSPT)[10,24-27]
 1. Elimination or suppression of pathogenic microorganisms through removal and control of bacterial plaque
 2. Controlling the source of infection and preventing reinfection
 3. Resolution or elimination of inflammation by establishing an environment conducive to health
 4. Consideration of host factors and, if possible, controlling systemic factors
B. Elimination of inflammation and pathogenic microorganisms can be accomplished by
 1. Removing and controlling bacterial plaque and endotoxins
  a. Plaque removal
  b. Plaque control
  c. Scaling/root planing/debridement
  d. Adjunctive use of antimicrobial (chemotherapeutic) agents (e.g., chlorhexidine [Peridex or PerioGard])
 2. Eliminating factors that favor bacterial accumulation
  a. Root surface irregularities
  b. Calculus deposits
  c. Overhanging or poorly contoured restorations
  d. Loose or open proximal contacts
  e. Food impaction
  f. Mouthbreathing
C. The client as a cotherapist
 1. Daily self-care practices performed by the client are important to the success of nonsurgical periodontal therapy
 2. Client must be involved in goal setting, making decisions about treatment and alternatives, and making a commitment to long-term protective oral health behaviors
 3. It is the clinician's responsibility to assist the client in identifying and performing oral self-care prac-

tices and to individualize instructions according to client needs

4. The client's ability to remove and control bacterial plaque also must be considered

D. Components of nonsurgical periodontal therapy[26]

1. Plaque control—involves clinician and client in eliminating and controlling bacterial plaque; long-term success of nonsurgical periodontal therapy depends on adequate bacterial plaque control

2. Oral prophylaxis
   a. Objective is to prevent the initiation of gingivitis and, failing that, to prevent conversion of gingivitis to periodontitis
   b. Performed for clients with healthy periodontium and clients with gingivitis
   c. Procedure includes supragingival and subgingival scaling to remove deposits, followed by selective coronal polishing, if necessary, for plaque and stain removal or for client satisfaction
   d. Scaling refers to supragingival or subgingival calculus removal without intentional removal of tooth surface

3. Therapeutic scaling and root planing[24,26]
   a. Objective is to treat established periodontal disease and to create conditions conducive to health
   b. Rationale includes elimination of bacterial pathogens, endotoxins, calculus, and other irritants from the tooth surface to reduce inflammation, promote tissue regeneration, and create a biologically acceptable root surface
   c. Procedure is technically demanding; a definitive treatment procedure designed to remove cementum or surface dentin that is rough or embedded with calculus, toxins, or microorganisms; usually requires local anesthesia; when performed thoroughly, some unavoidable soft tissue removal occurs
   d. Extremely time consuming, lasting up to 8 hours and requiring several appointments; controversy exists regarding need for extensive cementum removal and possibility of overtreatment
   e. Hand or ultrasonic instruments may be employed for root planing
   f. Scaling and root planing have been shown to be successful in treating gingivitis, incipient periodontitis, and moderate periodontitis; results are less predictable in periodontal pockets over 6 mm in depth or when furcation involvement is present
   g. Root planing is contraindicated in healthy sulcus areas or shallow crevices; has been shown to cause a loss of attachment in crevices less than 3 mm

h. Clinical objectives
   (1) Calculus-free, plaque-free tooth surface
   (2) Smooth, firm root surface free of embedded calculus and bacterial plaque (NOTE: need for root planing should be determined by health status of gingival tissues; a "rough" root without corresponding gingival inflammation is contraindicated for root planing)

4. Periodontal debridement[26]
   a. Defined as treatment of periodontal disease through mechanical removal of tooth and root surface irregularities (including bacterial plaque, clinically detectable calculus, and all plaque retentive factors) only to the extent that adjacent soft tissues are healthy
   b. Removal of calculus is only considered important from the perspective of its plaque retentive nature
   c. Can be supragingival, subgingival, or both
   d. Difference from root planing is in extent of instrumentation; root surface smoothness is not emphasized at the expense of removal of tooth surface; emphasis is on removal of bacterial plaque, its byproducts, and plaque retentive factors only to the extent that soft tissues can return to a healthy state; either technique can be performed with hand or ultrasonic instruments but ultrasonics are advocated for debridement
   e. The trend is toward removal of as little tooth structure as possible; however, all clinically detectable calculus must be removed; root smoothness is not essential for healing, removal of bacterial irritants is the key
   f. Concept is based on the fact that 100% calculus removal is not successful on all root surfaces with any nonsurgical procedure and may not be desirable at the expense of lost tooth structure and dentinal hypersensitivity
   g. A 4- to 6-week reevaluation is critical to determine if clinical judgment regarding extent of debridement was adequate to achieve periodontal health; if unsuccessful, retreatment is indicated
   h. Deplaquing, which includes removal or disruption of bacterial plaque and its toxins subgingivally following completion of periodontal debridement, is recommended at reevaluation and continued care appointments; it is a new concept—not well studied or documented in the literature

5. Elimination of factors affecting bacterial accumulation is essential to successful NSPT

6. Consideration of systemic factors and, if possible, treatment and control; for example
   a. Hormonal—consult endocrinologist
   b. Drug associated—consult physician to change medication
   c. Blood dyscrasia or diabetes—refer to physician for treatment
7. Use of appropriate antimicrobial (chemotherapeutic) agents, if indicated

E. Use of topical antimicrobial agents[25]
1. Indicated for control of supragingival plaque and gingivitis; effectiveness in periodontitis has not been documented; used to augment oral self-care efforts of clients who are only partially effective; also recommended for extensive restorative cases and dental implants; aids healing following periodontal surgery
2. Chlorhexidine
   a. Most effective antimicrobial agent for reducing plaque and gingivitis long-term (55% and 45%, respectively); 0.12% concentration in United States
   b. High substantivity—ability to remain in the mouth for a long duration while releasing active ingredient
   c. Adverse effects—staining, reversible desquamation, poor taste or alteration of taste, increase in supragingival calculus deposits
   d. Approved by the American Dental Association as an antimicrobial and antigingivitis agent (Peridex or PerioGard)
   e. Alcohol content 11.6%; pH 5.5
   f. Twice daily usage favors compliance
3. Stannous fluoride
   a. Antimicrobial mechanism of action appears to be related to the stannous (tin) ion rather than to the fluoride
   b. Short-term and long-term studies have shown mixed results; however, significant reductions in bacterial plaque and gingivitis have been documented; further long-term study is warranted
   c. Most often available in gel form (e.g., Stop, Gel-Kam); 0.4% concentration; no alcohol
   d. Stannous fluoride has low to moderate substantivity; twice daily usage favors compliance
   e. Adverse effects may include taste and tooth staining in some individuals
   f. Stannous fluoride products are accepted by the American Dental Association for their ability to deliver fluoride for anticaries activity but have not been accepted for their bacterial plaque and gingivitis-reducing properties; some also approved for hypersensitivity reduction
4. Phenolic compounds (essential oils)
   a. Approved by the American Dental Association as an antimicrobial and antigingivitis agent (Listerine)
   b. Long-term studies indicate approximately 30% to 35% reduction in plaque and gingivitis
   c. Available products have a high alcohol content (26.9% alcohol; pH 5)
   d. Adverse effects include burning sensation and bitter taste
   e. Twice daily usage favors compliance
5. Sanguinarine
   a. Short-term studies show some reduction in plaque and gingivitis; more effective with combined use of dentifrice and mouthrinse (e.g., Viadent)
   b. Adverse effects include burning sensation and taste
   c. Alcohol content, 11.5%; pH 5.2
6. Prebrushing rinse (sodium benzoate)
   a. Short-term studies show some reduction in plaque, results inconclusive; controlled long-term studies show no beneficial effect in gingivitis (e.g., Plax)
   b. Long-term studies suggest no therapeutic effectiveness
   c. Safety is not a concern; no adverse effects
7. Quaternary ammonium compounds (cetylpyridinium chloride—CPC)
   a. Short term studies show some reduction in bacterial plaque and gingivitis; results inconclusive but therapeutic value is questionable; low substantivity
   b. May have some benefit in reducing halitosis
   c. Adverse reactions include possible slight staining and burning sensation
   d. Well known representatives of this group are Scope, Cepacol, and Oral-B Anti-Bacterial
8. Oxygenating agents
   a. Hydrogen peroxide
      (1) Antiinflammatory properties decrease clinical signs of inflammation, but bacterial pathogens may not be reduced
      (2) Studies do not support long-term use
      (3) Safety questions, such as tissue injury and cocarcinogenicity, have been raised with chronic use of hydrogen peroxide
9. Oxidizing agents (chlorine dioxide)
   a. No therapeutic value but recommended for breath freshening

b. Well known representatives of this group are Oxyfresh and Retard

10. Triclosan
   a. An antibacterial, noncationic agent that has been incorporated in dentifrices in Europe and Canada either in combination with zinc citrate or Gantrex
   b. Studies have shown significant reductions in bacterial plaque and gingivitis greater than control dentifrices and mouthrinses

11. Other—preliminary studies are being conducted on various other agents including but not limited to enzymes, plaque modifiers, and agents affecting bacterial attachment

12. Antibiotics—topical use is of limited value at the present time; development of sustained-release devices offer promise for the future

13. Methods for delivery of antimicrobial agents
   a. Most common methods of delivery for anti-microbials are mouthrinsing and oral irrigation (see next section on delivery of antibiotics)
   b. Mouthrinses deliver agents supragingivally; subgingival penetration is only 0 to 1 mm
   c. Oral irrigation can deliver agent subgingivally; complete plaque removal is not achieved but periodontal pathogens found in loosely adherent plaque can be removed; must be used as an adjunct to mechanical plaque control
   d. Oral irrigation can be accomplished with water or antimicrobial agents; both reduce bleeding and gingivitis but antimicrobials are more effective in removing bacterial plaque; effect on periodontitis is not well documented
   e. Depth of penetration with oral irrigation is related to type of tip used[15]
      (1) Standard jet tip—shallow penetration of 1.8 mm (3 to 6 mm pockets only 44% depth)
      (2) Subgingival (or marginal) tip—90% coverage in pockets of 6 mm or less; decreasing coverage as pocket becomes deeper
      (3) Cannula—75% to 100% coverage if tip reaches base of pocket; safety is a concern for home use
   f. Oral irrigation can have value in conjunction with daily self-care regimen for mechanical plaque removal in treatment of gingivitis or in periodontal maintenance therapy
   g. Professionally-administered oral irrigation has been studied with and without root planing/periodontal debridement; main benefit is from mechanical debridement; a single application of an antimicrobial irrigant has little value because of low substantivity in the periodontal pocket because of presence of serum, proteins, and crevicular fluid

F. Use of systemic antibiotics and other drug therapy
   1. Systemic antibiotics are sometimes used in conjunction with periodontal therapy (surgical or nonsurgical); however, there is no evidence that antibiotics alone arrest periodontal disease
   2. Not recommended for routine treatment of gingivitis or adult periodontitis; problems with drug hypersensitivity, development of resistant strains, and patient adherence limit widespread use
   3. Can be beneficial in treatment of periodontitis in the presence of systemic disease and immunocompromised states, or for aggressive forms such as early-onset periodontitis and refractory periodontitis
   4. Commonly used systemic antibiotics include tetracycline, metronidazole, metronidazole plus amoxicillin, clindamycin, ciprofloxacin, and Augmentin; selection depends on causative bacterial species
   5. Nonsteroidal antiinflammatory drugs (NSAIDs) have been shown to inhibit bone loss in periodontal diseases (e.g., ibuprofen, flurbiprofen)
   6. Local delivery of antibiotics and other drugs
      a. Systems are available for local delivery of antibiotics or antimicrobials to specific subgingival sites (e.g., hollow fibers, gels, collagen film, bioabsorbable material); these methods of local delivery provide for the benefits of antibiotic therapy with greater safety and compliance
      b. Tetracycline fibers have been shown to be effective in nonresponsive sites following initial therapy (e.g., Actisite); effectiveness in initial periodontal therapy less clear; must be removed in the office approximately 10 days after placement
      c. Local delivery offers the advantage of sustained release of a high concentration of the active ingredient to the site of periodontal infection without systemic involvement
      d. Research is being conducted to improve delivery systems (e.g., ease of use, eliminate need for professional removal) and expand therapeutic agents available to include other antibiotics (e.g., metronidazole gel available in Europe), antimicrobials (e.g., chlorhexidine) and nonsteroidal antiinflammatory agents

G. Evaluation of nonsurgical periodontal therapy
   1. Immediate evaluation is accomplished through visual and tactile inspection of tooth surfaces
   2. Healing of tissues for 14 days should be permitted; gingival tissues are then visually reevaluated for response to care

3. Thorough reevaluation 4 to 6 weeks after scaling/root planing/periodontal debridement to determine need for additional therapy (e.g., surgery, antimicrobials, antibiotics)
4. Reevaluation should include
   a. Evaluation of the client's self-care
   b. Updated periodontal assessment
   c. Reassessment of the clinical health of tissues; if areas still show signs of inflammation, the cause should be determined
      (1) Bacterial plaque present—review or supplement self-care
      (2) Deposits of calculus still present—scale, debride, or root plane as needed
      (3) No plaque or calculus noted—check the root surface to determine whether debridement is needed and retreat as indicated
      (4) Pocket depth still moderate to severe—surgical procedures might be warranted
      (5) Inflammation still severe or generalized and etiology and contributing factors cannot be identified—consider physical examination by a physician for a possible systemic risk factor

Gingival Curettage

A. Definition—procedure to remove the ulcerated, chronically inflamed tissue lining a pocket
B. Historical overview
   1. Until recently, gingival curettage was a recommended treatment procedure for areas of gingival inflammation and/or increased probing depths to reduce inflammation and probing depths through shrinkage of tissues and healing by a long junctional epithelium
   2. Studies of gingival curettage almost always have combined this technique with root planing
   3. Research indicates that gingival curettage is ineffective and that root planing alone can, in many cases, reduce inflammation, result in tissue shrinkage, and promote healing of the junctional epithelium
   4. In some states, gingival curettage is a legally permissable procedure for dental hygienists to perform, and many clinicians have received education and training for clinical competence in gingival curettage
C. Current thinking relevant to gingival curettage[15]
   1. Based upon previous research findings, the consensus of most periodontal therapists is that gingival curettage has limited, if any, current application in the treatment of chronic adult periodontitis
   2. If new connective tissue attachment is the goal of a particular periodontal treatment plan, curettage has no justifiable application; healing occurs by means of a longer junctional epithelium and tissue shrinkage
   3. Further research is needed to determine if gingival curettage is appropriate in other cases, including
      a. Treatment of compromised patients
      b. Maintenance debridement of localized sites of recalcitrant periodontitis
      c. Treatment of localized juvenile periodontitis and other types of rapidly progressive or aggressive periodontitis
      d. Cases in which aesthetics are a concern

Additional Clinical Interventions

A. Treatment of occlusal problems
   1. Once diagnosed, occlusal trauma may be treated by
      a. Occlusal adjustment—selective grinding of teeth to equalize the distribution of occlusal forces
      b. Construction of occlusal appliances (e.g., night guard, removable orthodontic appliance) to minimize the effect of destructive forces and/or for minor tooth movement to improve tooth alignment
      c. Splinting of teeth for temporary or permanent stabilization
      d. Restorative dentistry to improve the occlusal plane and replace missing teeth
      e. Orthodontics to correct malocclusion
   2. Limitation of treatment[15]
      a. Occlusal adjustment is recommended only if signs and symptoms of traumatic occlusion and/or neuromuscular disturbances are evident
      b. Research fails to support the use of occlusal adjustment procedures for treatment of inflammatory periodontal disease, parafunctional habits, or TMJ disorders
      c. Orthodontic treatment is not recommended for treatment of periodontitis when there is no strong evidence that malposed teeth strongly correlate with periodontitis
      d. Orthodontic treatment may be useful in cases in which trauma results from malposition of teeth or malocclusion interferes with plaque control or causes mouth breathing, food impaction, etc.
B. Surgical procedures
   1. Rationale
      a. Eliminate active infection
      b. Render the periodontium more cleansable by the client
         (1) Improvement in hard and soft tissue contours
         (2) Pocket elimination or reduction
      c. Replace damaged or destroyed periodontium

(1) Soft tissue replacement (gingival grafts)

(2) Hard tissue replacement (osseous grafts)

d. Surgery is rarely performed solely to remove inflammation or infection, but rather to

(1) Eliminate both hard and soft defects created by disease

(2) Try to restore normal architecture and physiologic function

(3) Try to gain new attachment of the supporting structures

2. Types

a. Gingival curettage—procedure to remove the ulcerated, chronically inflamed tissue lining a pocket (see section on gingival curettage)

b. Gingivectomy—surgical procedure for pocket reduction by complete removal of the soft tissue pocket wall

(1) Indications

(a) Gingival pockets composed of enlarged fibrotic tissue

(b) Correction of severe gingival overgrowth

(2) Contraindications

(a) Reduction of infrabony pockets

(b) Reduction of pockets that extend to or into the alveolar mucosa

c. Periodontal flaps—may be used as a method of surgical curettage (e.g., modified Widman flap) or for pocket elimination by apically repositioning the soft tissue

(1) Advantages (depending on the type of flap)

(a) Better access to achieve thorough scaling and root planing

(b) Thorough removal of the pocket lining

(c) Elimination of pockets

(d) Means to obtain access to the alveolar bone to correct osseous defects

(2) Indications

(a) Probing depths in presence of intrabony defects; probing depths greater than 5 mm after initial therapy; furcation involvements; presence of root anomalies or irregularities

(b) Following unsuccessful nonsurgical periodontal therapy

(c) To enhance cleansibility of areas inaccessible to home care

(d) Need to treat diseased roots subgingivally

(e) In conjunction with other procedures to treat intrabony defects

(f) Progressive attachment loss

(3) Contraindications

(a) If periodontal disease can be treated and controlled by a more conservative approach (nonsurgical periodontal therapy)

(b) In the presence of excessive mobility

(c) Advanced attachment loss; poor prognosis

(d) Inadequate gingiva, poor crown root ratios, or anatomic preclusions

(e) Systemic disorders that contraindicate surgery

(f) Noncompliant client

d. Excisional new attachment procedure (ENAP)—a procedure using internally beveled incision to remove the crevicular lining and junctional epithelium, allowing root preparation

e. Mucogingival surgery

(1) Objectives

(a) Prevent additional loss of keratinized attached gingiva and/or recession

(b) Increase the band of attached gingiva

(c) Root coverage

(2) Indications

(a) Base of the pocket extending apically to the mucogingival junction

(b) Inadequate zone of keratinized attached gingiva (controversy exists about how much is needed)

(c) Frenum pull on the gingiva, causing gingival recession

(d) Localized gingival recession associated with inflammation

(3) Treatment options

(a) Pedicle grafts

(b) Gingival grafts

(c) Gingival augmentation

(d) Partial or full frenectomy

f. Osseous resective surgery

(1) Objectives—removal of alveolar bone to produce a more physiologic architecture or contour; ultimately pocket reduction in one-walled infrabony or vertical defects; also for lengthening the clinical crown for root restoration; goal is to remove minimal amount of bone

(2) Indications—vertical alveolar defects or exostoses requiring reshaping (osteoplasty) or surgical crown lengthening (ostectomy) for access to deep root caries lesions or fractures

g. Regenerative surgery

(1) Objective—promote regeneration of the

connective tissue, periodontal ligament, cementum, and alveolar bone

(2) Indications—two- and three-walled vertical defects, Class II furcation defects, circumferential defects

(3) Two options available

(a) Guided tissue regeneration—involves using a semipermeable membrane between the epithelium and the underlying ligament and bone to prevent rapid downgrowth epithelium which would interfere with connective tissue regrowth after surgical debridement of the defect; nonresorbable (e.g., Goretex) or resorbable (e.g., Guidor or Resolute) membranes are used but the former must be removed 1 to 2 months following surgery

(b) Bone grafts—involve placing bone grafting material into a debrided defect to the level of the uninvolved crest to promote bone healing and regeneration (osseoinduction); the graft stimulates new bone formation and thus new attachment; *autografts* are bone grafts obtained from the same client and *allografts* are processed human cadaver bone that is usually freeze-dried or demineralized

h. Root hemisection or resection

(1) Objective—removal of the crown and/or root to eliminate the involved furcation

(2) Indication—severe furcation involvement that cannot be treated by osseous surgery or regenerative surgery

(3) Two options available

(a) Hemisection—performed on mandibular molars; crown and root is sectioned in half to create two individual roots thus eliminating furcation; sometimes one root must be removed because of instability or severe attachment loss

(b) Root resection—involves removal of one root of a multirooted tooth without sectioning the crown; most often performed on maxillary molars

Sutures

A. Objectives

1. Used to hold soft tissues in place until the healing process has progressed to the point where tissue placement can be self-maintained

2. Stabilizing the soft tissue helps

a. Maintain the blood clot around the wound

b. Protect the wound area during the healing process

B. Desired properties of a suture material

1. Easy to handle

2. Nonallergenic and does not create an environment conducive to bacterial growth

3. Does not shrink after placement

4. Knot holds securely and does not fray

5. Does not easily cut or tear through thin, delicate tissue

6. If absorbable, does so with minimal tissue reaction

C. Types of suture materials

1. Absorbable—gut (from intestines of sheep)

a. Difficult to manipulate

b. Does not hold knot well

c. Tends to harden and cause trauma around the surrounding mucosa

d. Mild inflammatory reaction occurs during the absorption process

2. Nonabsorbable

a. Surgical silk (twisted or braided)

(1) Most widely used material in periodontal surgery

(2) Is a foreign protein and thus is treated by tissues as a foreign body (inflammatory reactions are usually limited if sutures are removed within 7 days)

(3) Braided material tends to trap bacteria within the material

(4) Relatively comfortable and easy to use

b. Surgical cotton and linen—weak material; not used in periodontics

c. Synthetic fibers (polyester, nylon, polypropylene)—strong and well tolerated by tissue, but difficult to knot

D. Procedure for suture removal

1. Gently grasp the knotted end with cotton pliers and pull it away from the tissue

2. Insert the tip of scissors under the suture and cut the suture material that had been in the tissue

3. Gently pull the knotted end so that only suture material that had previously been incorporated within the tissue will pass through the tissue during the removal process

4. Count and record the number of sutures removed and compare this number with the suture placement record

5. Gently cleanse the wound sites (may use an oxygenating agent, warm water, and cotton swabs)

6. Check for bleeding points and control with gauze and pressure

7. Check for and gently remove any calculus or granulation tissue

Periodontal Dressings

A. Rationale for use of a periodontal dressing is to protect the tissues after surgery; no curative properties; it has been demonstrated that wound healing progresses at the same rate with or without a dressing; however, periodontal dressings are sometimes used for the following reasons
   1. Patient comfort, especially if the surgical procedure has left exposed connective tissue or exposed root surfaces
   2. Protection of the wound against trauma (e.g., from sharp, hard food or toothbrush bristles) and prevention of the tongue from constantly rubbing the area
   3. Maintenance of the initial blood clot—dressing may be helpful in preventing the initial blood clot from being dislodged; dressing should be applied only after bleeding has been controlled
   4. Tissue placement—maintains the desired location of the soft tissue flap position (if performed)
B. Desired properties of a dressing material
   1. Soft and flexible to allow for proper adaptation
   2. Reasonable setting time
   3. After setting, should be rigid but not brittle
   4. Smooth dressing surface
C. Types—research is controversial regarding healing properties of eugenol versus noneugenol dressings
   1. Zinc oxide–eugenol dressing—eugenol is added because it has a soothing (obtundent) effect on exposed root surfaces and connective tissue and has antiseptic properties; eugenol may have an irritating effect on bone; firm consistency of this dressing requires some pressure during placement
   2. Zinc oxide–noneugenol dressing—softer dressing than eugenol type; also more pleasant tasting
D. Ingredients
   1. Eugenol type
      a. Powder
         (1) Zinc oxide—slightly astringent and/or antiseptic
         (2) Rosin—filler for strength
         (3) Tannic acid—hemostasis (need for this is questionable)
      b. Liquid
         (1) Eugenol—slightly anesthetic
         (2) Peanut oil—regulates the setting time
   2. Noneugenol type
      a. Paste 1
         (1) Zinc oxide—slightly astringent and/or antiseptic

         (2) Magnesium oxide and oils—regulate the setting time
      b. Paste 2
         (1) Rosin—strength
         (2) Chlorothymol—bacteriostatic
E. Procedure for dressing placement
   1. Explain the process to the patient
   2. Make sure bleeding has ceased
   3. Mix the dressing according to the directions
   4. Gently place the dressing and establish retention in the embrasure spaces
   5. Make sure the dressing does not cover more than the cervical one third of the tooth, does not overextend into the mucobuccal fold, and does not interfere with muscle attachments or with the patient's occlusion
   6. Make sure the surface of the dressing is smooth and well contoured
   7. Evaluate the dressing to ensure that it has not been forced between the soft tissue flap and the underlying tissue or root surface
   8. May place dry foil over the dressing until it has hardened (few hours); foil is then removed (not necessary to use foil)
   9. Give postsurgical instructions to the patient (see section on patient instructions and education)
F. Removal of the periodontal dressing
   1. Remove the dressing within 7 days
   2. Gently tease the edges of the dressing away from the teeth with a curet or cotton/college pliers; be sure that sutures are not embedded in the dressing
   3. After the pack has been removed, gently cleanse the area with *warm* water or dampened cotton tips
   4. Assess tissue healing *but do not probe sulcular areas*
   5. Remove sutures
   6. Gently cleanse the area again with an antimicrobial agent
   7. Evaluate wound healing and determine if the area needs to have a new periodontal dressing

Postoperative Care

Client Instructions and Education

A. Discomfort
   1. Expect discomfort after the anesthesia wears off
   2. Use the prescribed pain medication
   3. Rest and limit physical activities during the first few days to prevent excessive bleeding and promote healing
   4. Use an ice pack to prevent swelling
   5. Eliminate spicy, hot, cold, or hard, sticky foods/

liquids and smoking to limit tissue irritants and protect the dressing

B. Care of the periodontal dressing
1. Do not eat anything for the first few hours until the dressing hardens; may drink cool liquids
2. During the week, pieces of the dressing may chip off; call the office if the area is extremely sensitive, the entire dressing is loose, or the chipped area is irritating the tongue or mucosa

C. Oral hygiene procedures
1. Do not rinse the mouth on the first day because this may disturb the blood clot
2. After the first day, may rinse gently with lukewarm water, a small amount of an antibacterial or antimicrobial rinse
3. Brush and floss nonsurgical areas as usual
4. Gently brush occlusal surfaces of the surgical area
5. Using a soft brush and water, very gently clean the surface of the dressing
6. Brush the tongue
7. Use an antimicrobial agent to help control bacterial plaque (e.g., Peridex or PerioGard)

D. Bleeding
1. Slight seepage of blood during the first few hours is normal
2. Any unusual, persistent bleeding should be reported

Follow-up Visit

A. Client returns approximately 7 days after surgery
B. Dressing and sutures are removed; new dressing may or may not be applied
C. Dentinal hypersensitivity may be experienced; desensitization indicated for dentinal hypersensitivity; desensitization methods may be prescribed (see Chapter 12, section on control of dentinal hypersensitivity)
D. Home care instructions are provided for plaque control
E. Long-term post-operative care requires periodic evaluation (also known as continued care)

Supportive Periodontal Treatment (SPT)

A. An extension of periodontal therapy; also called maintenance therapy or periodontal maintenance procedures (PMP) or continued care
1. Initiated after completion of active periodontal treatment and continued at various intervals
2. Also a mode of therapy for clients who are unable to undergo periodontal surgery because of medical complications or other reasons
B. Objectives of supportive treatment[3,4]
1. To preserve health, comfort, and function of the teeth
2. Long-term control of bacterial plaque

3. Reevaluation of results after active periodontal therapy (nonsurgical or surgical)
4. Reinforcing self-care instructions and encouraging client's long-term protective oral health behaviors
5. Determining need for additional treatment

C. Components of supportive treatment
1. Requires cooperation of client, dental hygienist, dentist, and periodontist
2. Emphasizes scaling/root planing/periodontal debridement, extrinsic stain removal, and reinstruction of client in self-care to maintain attachment levels

D. Periodic reevaluation and assessment
1. Health and dental history review and update
2. Radiographic review
3. Extraoral and intraoral soft tissue examination
4. Dental charting
5. Periodontal assessment and charting
6. Evaluation of client's oral self-care behavior, attitude, and skill

E. Treatment—based on assessment
1. Always includes encouragement of client and oral self-care reinstruction as needed
2. Healthy periodontium—removal of supragingival deposits; no root planing indicated
3. Presence of bleeding/inflammation of the gingiva—treatment depends upon etiology and pocket depth; removal of deposits and contributing factors necessary; possible use of an antimicrobial rinse (e.g., chlorhexidine)
4. Presence of periodontal pockets—scaling and periodontal debridement/root planing followed by reevaluation in 4 to 6 weeks to determine need for adjunctive therapy
5. Frequency of periodontal maintenance procedures must be individualized
   a. Increases when clients have less than optimal oral self-care practices
   b. Longer intervals if client can control bacterial plaque
   c. Goal is to control clinical signs of inflammation and stabilize attachment levels
   d. Frequent intervals (3 months or less) generally necessary for subgingival and supragingival plaque and calculus removal
   e. Generally, the shorter the interval, the greater the long-term success; particularly during healing phase (1 year) after surgery

F. Client adherence (see Chapter 12, section on factors influencing client adherence to preventive regimen)
1. Successful maintenance therapy requires a lifelong commitment from clients for meticulous plaque control and regular supportive treatment visits

2. Because periodontal disease progresses slowly and is painless, it is perceived by clients as nonthreatening

3. Reducing client responsibilities to the minimum that are necessary tends to increase adherence

4. Repeated reinstruction is needed for development of long-term protective health behaviors

5. Evaluation of the client's oral hygiene must be based upon clinical signs of inflammation rather than presence of bacterial plaque alone

6. Clients also must understand the importance of professional periodontal maintenance therapy, particularly in the control of subgingival deposits, because compliance with recommended maintenance intervals has been shown to be poor (ranging from 11% to 45%)

7. Reasons for nonadherence[15]
   a. Personal characteristics—high stress, unstable personal life
   b. Unfavorable dental beliefs
   c. Economics—care is unaffordable, or perceived to be
   d. Lifestyle changes—moves, job changes
   e. Internal health beliefs

G. Instructions for retreatment[15]
   1. Increase in probing depth greater than or equal to 2 mm
   2. Increase in attachment loss greater than or equal to 2 mm
   3. Bleeding on probing that does not respond to periodontal maintenance procedures
   4. Consider severity in determining treatment regimens
   5. If generalized deterioration, systemic complication might be suspected
   6. Retaining questionable teeth is not recommended

Dental Implants[13,28,29]

See Chapter 10, section on dental implants.

A. Definition—artificial replacements of teeth that are permanently affixed into the alveolar bone
   1. Offers an alternative to removable dentures to endentulous or partially edentulous persons
   2. Implants provide a permanent anchor for artificial teeth

B. Materials commonly used for dental implants
   1. Titanium—a metallic element; pure or plasma-sprayed
   2. Hydroxyapatite—plasma-sprayed

C. Two major types of implants[16,27]
   1. Subperiosteal—custom-fabricated framework of metal that is supraalveolar (on top of the bone) but beneath the oral tissues
      a. Posts protrude through tissues to provide anchor for final bridge or denture
      b. Two-step surgery required—initial surgery to deflect soft tissues and make impression of alveolar bone, followed by placement of fabricated implant framework
      c. Use of computerized tomography—could eliminate first step in the future
   2. Endosteal or endosseous (inside bone)
      a. Implant is placed directly into a socket, which has been prepared by a process called *trephining;* uses a series of specially prepared drills and burs
      b. After the bone and soft tissues heal (about 6 months), the final bridge or denture is placed

D. Implant-tissue interface
   1. Controversy exists regarding the implant-tissue interface, although it is agreed that this is the basis of implant success
   2. Epithelial attachment to the implant may be similar to the attachment to a natural tooth (i.e., basal lamina and hemidesmosomes); no periodontal ligament
   3. Perimucosal seal, or biologic seal, is critical to implant retention
   4. Osseointegration—contact established between normal and remodeled bone and the implant surface without the interposition of connective tissue

E. Hygiene protocol and instrumentation[27]
   1. Goals
      a. Maintain health of implant and supporting tissues
      b. Prevent loss of perimucosal seal
      c. Prevent gingivitis and, failing that, prevent conversion of gingivitis to *periimplantitis,* a periodontitis-like disease process that can affect dental implants
         (1) Infectious failure—failing implants with a primarily infectious etiology (microflora characterized by spirochetes and motile rods with a predominance of *Peptostreptococcus* ssp, *Fusobacterium* ssp, and enteric Gram-negative rods)
         (2) Traumatic failure—failing implants with a primarily traumatic etiology (microflora characterized by organisms that are observed in periodontal health)
      d. Provide preventive and maintenance therapy with minimal damage, or surface scratching, to implants
      e. Control bacterial plaque

F. Preventive instrumentation (see Chapter 13 section on plastic instruments for implant care)

1. It is possible that a smooth surface is more conducive to a plaque-free environment and roughening will predispose surface to plaque retention
2. Surface changes in descending order
   a. Ultrasonic/sonic scaling devices—not recommended
   b. Stainless steel, carbon, or titanium-tipped curets —not recommended
   c. Interdental brushes—unitufted brushes or interdental brushes with plastic-coated wire preferred; hand or motorized[27]
   d. Polishing pastes—fine grit or tin oxide (e.g., Abutment Glo or Ora Ti)
   e. Antimicrobials—0.12% chlorhexidine mouth rinse commonly recommended by practitioners
   f. Plastic or Teflon-coated curets that can effectively instrument the subgingival area without changing the implant surface topography are recommended for calculus removal
   g. Plastic periodontal probes are recommended for assessing clinical attachment loss around dental implants if inflammation is present; x-rays also recommended when inflammation is present; no probing necessary if tissue is healthy
G. Sterilization
   1. Affects long-term success or failure of implant—critically important
   2. Autoclaving or chemical sterilization of implant is contraindicated—produces residue
   3. Radio frequency glow discharge (plasma glow) has been shown to leave biomaterial surface uncontaminated and sterile

REFERENCES

1. Löe H, Anerud A, Boysen H: Natural history of periodontal disease in man. Prevalence, severity, and extent of gingival recession. *J Periodontol* 63:489-495, 1992.
2. Löe H, Anerud A, Boysen H, Morrison E: Natural history of periodontal disease in man. Rapid, moderate and no loss of attachment in Sri Lankan laborers 14 to 46 years of age. *J Clin Periodontol* 13:431-440, 1986.
3. Löe H, Anerud A, Boysen, H, Smith MR: Natural history of periodontal disease in man. Study design and baseline data. *J Periodont Res* 13:550-562, 1978a.
4. Löe H, Anerud A, Boysen H, Smith MR: Natural history of periodontal disease in man. Tooth mortality rates before 40 years of age. *J Periodont Res* 13:563-573, 1978b.
5. Löe H, Anerud A, Boysen H, Smith MR: Natural history of periodontal disease in man. The rate of periodontal destruction after 40 years of age. *J Periodontol* 49:607-620, 1978c.
6. Christensson A, et al: Dental plaque and calculus: Risk indicators for their formation. *J Dent Res* 71:1425-1430.
7. Beck JD, et al: Evaluation of oral bacteria as risk indicators for periodontitis in older adults. *J Periodontol* 63:93-99, 1992.
8. Haffajee AD, et al: Factors associated with different responses to periodontal therapy. *J Clin Periodontol* 22:628-636, 1995.
9. Grossi SG, et al: Assessment of risk for periodontal disease. II. Risk indicators for alveolar bone loss. *J Periodontol* 66:23-29, 1995.
10. Wolff L, et al: Bacteria as risk markers for periodontitis. *J Periodontol* 64:498-510, 1994.
11. Brown LJ, et al: Periodontal status in the United States, 1988-1991: Prevalence, extent, and demographic variation. *J Dent Res* 75(Spec Iss):672-683, 1996.
12. American Academy of Periodontology Research, Science and Therapy Committee. Position paper: Tobacco use and the periodontal patient. *J Periodontol* 67:51-56, 1996.
13. Darby ML, Walsh MM: *Dental hygiene theory and practice,* Philadelphia, 1995, WB Saunders.
14. Monteiro da Silva AM, et al: Psychosocial factors in inflammatory periodontal diseases: A review. *J Clin Periodontol* 22:516-526, 1995.
15. American Academy of Periodontology: Proceedings of the world workshop in clinical periodontics, July 23-27, 1989, Princeton, NJ, Chicago, 1989, The Academy.
16. Carranza FA, Newman MG: *Clinical periodontology,* ed 8, Philadelphia, 1996, WB Saunders.
17. Socransky SS, Haffajee AD: The bacterial etiology of destructive periodontal disease: Current concepts. *J Periodontol* 63:322-331, 1992.
18. American Academy of Periodontology Research, Science and Therapy Committee: *Guidelines for periodontal therapy,* Chicago, April 1991, The Academy
19. American Dental Association and American Academy of Periodontology: *Periodontal screening and recording system (PSR) information brochure,* 1993.
20. Goodson JM: Diagnosis of periodontitis by physical measurement: Interpretation from episodic disease hypothesis. *J Periodontol* 63:373-382, 1992.
21. American Academy of Periodontology Research, Science and Therapy Committee: *Diagnosis of periodontal diseases,* Chicago, April 1995, The Academy.
22. American Academy of Periodontology Research, Science and Therapy Committee. *The etiology and pathogenesis of periodontal diseases,* Chicago, November 1992, The Academy.
23. American Academy of Periodontology Research, Science and Therapy Committee: *Periodontal diseases of children and adolescents,* Chicago, April 1991, The Academy.
24. Greenstein G: Periodontal response to mechanical nonsurgical therapy: A review, *J Periodontol* 63:118-130, 1992.
25. American Academy of Periodontology Research, Science and Therapy Committee: *Chemical agents for the control of plaque,* Chicago, April 1994, The Academy.
26. Hodges KO, editor. *Concepts in nonsurgical periodontal therapy,* New York, 1997, Delmar.
27. American Academy of Periodontology. *Periodontal literature reviews,* Chicago, 1996, The Academy.
28. Meffert RM, et al: Dental implants: a review. *J Periodontol* 63:859-870, 1992.
29. American Academy of Periodontology, Committee on Research, Science and Therapy: *Implant maintenance and treatment,* Chicago, April 1995, The Academy.

Review Questions

1 The term *lamina dura* refers to the radiographic image of the
A. Periodontal ligament space
B. Alveolar bone proper
C. Cortical plates
D. Cancellous bone
E. Alveolar crest

2 In acute gingivitis, which is the first inflammatory cell to respond to injury by bacterial plaque?
A. B lymphocytes
B. Plasma cells
C. Neutrophils
D. Lymphokines
E. Macrophages

3 A pseudopocket (or gingival pocket) is formed by the
A. Coronal migration of the gingival margin
B. Coronal migration of the epithelial attachment
C. Apical migration of the gingival margin
D. Apical migration of the epithelial attachment
E. Apically directed resorption of the alveolar crest

4 Periodontal pockets can *BEST* be detected by
A. Radiographic detection
B. The color of the gingival tissues
C. The contour of the gingival margin
D. Probing the sulcular area
E. Noting the presence or absence of bleeding on probing

5 Periodontitis may *BEST* be described as
A. A chronic inflammatory disease with periods of remission and exacerbation
B. A chronic inflammatory disease that usually does not manifest itself clinically before the age of 40
C. A degenerative disease of the periodontium
D. An acute inflammatory disease
E. A chronic inflammatory disease that most often affects the entire dentition equally

6 In cases of periodontitis, the first area to be involved in bone resorption is the
A. Facial and lingual aspects of supporting bone
B. Cribriform plate
C. Cancellous bone
D. Cortical plate of the interdental septum
E. Bone surrounding the apical area of the tooth

7 Which of the following statements about subgingival plaque are true?
A. Its growth and pathogenicity are strongly influenced by supragingival plaque
B. It forms simultaneously and in the same manner as supragingival plaque
C. It consists primarily of aerobic bacteria
D. Bacteria from plaque are not found in diseased periodontal tissues; only bacterial by-products cause destruction
E. Subgingival plaque does not differ from supragingival plaque

8 Sharpey's fibers are
A. Collagen fibers
B. Elastic fibers
C. Gingival fibers
D. Oxytalan fibers
E. Transseptal fibers

9 *Tissue consistency* refers to
A. Thickness
B. Resiliency
C. Texture
D. The location of the margin
E. The presence or absence of stippling

10 All of the following are diagnostic of occlusal trauma *EXCEPT*
A. Wear facets
B. Fremitus
C. Increase in tooth mobility
D. Periodontal pocket formation
E. Increased width of the periodontal ligament space

11 Radiographs will show the
A. Relationships between soft and hard tissue
B. Degree of tooth mobility
C. Extent of all bone loss
D. Presence of calculus
E. None of the above

12 The radiographic findings of gingivitis will demonstrate
A. Vertical bone loss
B. Horizontal bone loss
C. Increase in bone density
D. Change in bone trabeculation
E. Normal bone pattern

13 Which of the following periodontal diseases is characterized by relatively sparse subgingival plaque, onset at the age of puberty, and bilateral angular bone loss in the first molars and incisors?
A. Necrotizing ulcerative gingivitis
B. Rapidly progressive periodontitis
C. Prepubertal periodontitis
D. Localized juvenile periodontitis
E. Refractory periodontitis

14 Which of the following nonsurgical periodontal therapies are appropriate for a client with early periodontitis?
A. Oral prophylaxis
B. Gingival curettage
C. Scaling/periodontal debridement and periodontal maintenance procedures
D. Gingivectomy
E. All of the above

15 Which of the following chemotherapeutic agents has been shown to have a side effect of tooth staining?
A. Sanguinarine
B. Chlorhexidine
C. Hydrogen peroxide
D. Phenolic compound
E. Sodium benzoate

16 The mucogingival junction is located between the
  A. Free gingiva and attached gingiva
  B. Free gingiva and tooth
  C. Attached gingiva and alveolar mucosa
  D. Base of the sulcus and alveolar mucosa
  E. Gingival groove and gingival margin
17 Which tissue(s) has (have) little or no keratinization?
  A. Sulcular epithelium
  B. Attached gingiva
  C. Interdental papilla
  D. Palatal mucosa
  E. Sulcular epithelium and alveolar mucosa
18 The first bacteria to be deposited on the tooth in bacterial plaque formation are
  A. Gram-negative rods
  B. Gram-positive rods
  C. Spirochetes
  D. Gram-positive cocci
  E. Gram-negative cocci
19 The fibers of the attached gingiva are mainly
  A. Collagen
  B. Elastic
  C. Cellulose
  D. Keratinized
  E. Oxytalan
20 Systemic factors are important in the pathogenesis of periodontal disease because
  A. They can be the direct cause of periodontal disease
  B. They have a direct effect on pocket depth
  C. If they are corrected, the periodontal disease can be eliminated
  D. They usually determine the pattern of bone loss
  E. They can intensify the response of the periodontium to the etiologic and local factors
21 The tissue lining of a healthy gingival sulcus consists of
  A. Keratinized epithelium with rete pegs
  B. Keratinized epithelium without rete pegs
  C. Nonkeratinized epithelium with rete pegs
  D. Nonkeratinized epithelium without rete pegs
  E. Parakeratinized epithelium with rete pegs
22 The gingival fibers
  A. Brace the marginal gingiva against the tooth
  B. Help the tooth withstand horizontal forces
  C. Keep the tooth from being forced into the bony socket
  D. Form and resorb cementum
  E. Transmit sensations of occlusal forces applied to the tooth
23 Which of the following is the first *clinical* feature of inflammatory periodontal disease?
  A. Tooth mobility
  B. Drifting of the anterior teeth
  C. Periodontal pocket formation
  D. Gingival recession
  E. Bleeding on probing

24 A cuplike resorptive area at the crest of the alveolar bone is a radiographic finding of
  A. Periodontal abscess
  B. Gingivitis
  C. Occlusal trauma
  D. Acute necrotizing ulcerative gingivitis
  E. Early periodontitis
25 The area within the periodontium *MOST* susceptible to tissue breakdown is the
  A. Free gingiva
  B. Gingival sulcus
  C. Interdental col
  D. Interdental papilla
  E. Attached gingiva
26 The characteristics of gingivitis are
  A. Bone loss, swelling of the soft tissue, apical migration of the epithelial attachment
  B. Swelling of the soft tissue, apical migration of the epithelial attachment, bleeding on probing
  C. Bone loss, apical migration of the epithelial attachment, widening of the periodontal ligament spaces, bleeding on probing
  D. Swelling of the soft tissue, bleeding on probing
  E. Bone loss, swelling of the soft tissue, apical migration of the epithelial attachment, widening of the periodontal ligament space, bleeding on probing
27 Which is *NOT* a contributing factor of periodontal disease?
  A. Open proximal contacts
  B. Diet high in sucrose content
  C. Mouth breathing
  D. Blood dyscrasias
  E. Hormonal imbalance
28 On completion of a client's gingival assessment the hygienist noted that the gingivae are normal in appearance except on the facial area of teeth Nos. 28 and 29. In this area inflammation is noted on the gingival margin. All sulcular readings are between 1 and 3 mm, and the bases of the sulci are at the cementoenamel junctions. The most accurate description would be
  A. Generalized marginal periodontitis
  B. Localized marginal periodontitis
  C. Generalized papillary gingivitis
  D. Localized marginal gingivitis
  E. Localized papillary gingivitis
29 During a periodontal examination a 4-mm pocket is detected on the direct facial surface of tooth No. 19. The gingival margin is located at the cementoenamel junction. What type of pocket is this?
  A. Pseudopocket
  B. Periodontal pocket
  C. Gingival pocket
  D. Combination pseudopocket and periodontal pocket
  E. Combination gingival and periodontal pocket

30 Which situation would be an indication for a gingivectomy?
  A. An edematous, 5-mm pseudopocket
  B. A fibrotic area of free gingiva that covers part of the occlusal surface of tooth No. 32
  C. An infrabony pocket of 6 mm on the distal aspect of tooth No. 30
  D. A fibrotic periodontal pocket that extends into the alveolar mucosa
  E. A localized area of acute necrotizing ulcerative gingivitis

31 The *specific* objective(s) of periodontal pocket elimination is (are) to
  A. Improve the body image of the client and improve the tissue contour
  B. Improve the body image of the client, improve the tissue contour, and remove diseased tissue
  C. Remove diseased tissue
  D. Remove diseased tissue and assist the client in daily plaque control
  E. Improve the body image of the client, improve the tissue contour, remove diseased tissue, assist the client in daily plaque control

32 A pyogenic granuloma
  A. Is also referred to as a pregnancy tumor
  B. Tends to occur frequently in cases of phenytoin hyperplasia
  C. Is usually associated with gingival recession
  D. Is frequently associated with juvenile periodontitis
  E. Is usually treated with antibiotics

33 A gingivectomy is PRIMARILY employed to treat conditions in which
  A. An infrabony pocket is present
  B. The base of the pocket is apical to the mucogingival junction
  C. There is an adequate zone of attached gingiva
  D. The tissues are edematous
  E. There is a gingival recession

34 A mucogingival problem exists when
  A. The base of the pocket extends apically to the mucogingival junction
  B. The base of the pocket is coronal to the mucogingival junction
  C. There is less than 3 mm of attached gingiva
  D. There is less than 5 mm of alveolar mucosa
  E. There is significant bone loss

35 The purpose of placing sutures after periodontal flap surgery is to
  A. Hold the soft tissues in place
  B. Hold the soft tissues in place and protect the wound
  C. Protect the wound and maintain the blood clot
  D. Hold the soft tissues in place and maintain the blood clot
  E. Hold the soft tissue in place, protect the wound, maintain the blood clot, and prevent food impaction into the wound area

36 The advantage of gut sutures is
  A. Their ease of manipulation
  B. They hold the knot well
  C. They do not cause an inflammatory reaction
  D. They dissolve
  E. They do not cause any trauma to the surrounding tissues

37 An advantage of silk braided sutures is that they
  A. Are dissolved by the surrounding tissues
  B. Have antibacterial properties
  C. Are relatively easy to manipulate
  D. Are not treated by the surrounding tissues as a foreign body
  E. Can remain in the tissues for up to 3 weeks without creating an inflammatory reaction

38 The reasons for using a periodontal dressing are to
  A. Minimize the client's discomfort, protect the wound from possible food impaction, and minimize the chance of hemorrhage
  B. Protect the wound from possible food impaction, minimize the chance of hemorrhage, and help protect the teeth against root sensitivity
  C. Help protect the teeth against root sensitivity and help maintain tissue placement
  D. Protect the wound from possible food impaction, minimize the chance of hemorrhage, and help maintain tissue placement
  E. Minimize the client's discomfort, protect the wound from possible food impaction, minimize the chance of hemorrhage, help protect the teeth against root sensitivity and help maintain tissue placement

39 The purpose of using rosin in the periodontal dressing is to
  A. Provide an antibacterial property
  B. Provide a slight anesthetic action
  C. Serve as an astringent
  D. Improve the taste
  E. Act as a filler for strength

40 Following the completion of periodontal therapy, the client should be placed on a continued-care interval of
  A. Every 12 months
  B. Every 6 months
  C. Every 4 months
  D. Every 2 months
  E. No standard time interval

41 Which one of the following is recommended for preventive maintenance with dental implants?
  A. Ultrasonic scaler
  B. Titanium-tipped curet
  C. Chlorhexidine
  D. Coarse polishing paste
  E. Stainless steel curets

42 Dental implants are commonly made of
  A. Titanium
  B. Gold
  C. Aluminum
  D. Teflon
  E. Bonded acrylic resin

43 The single BEST criterion for evaluating the success of periodontal debridement/root planing and oral hygiene 4 to 6 weeks post-treatment is:
  A. All calculus removed
  B. A smooth and glasslike appearance of the root
  C. Lack of accumulation of supra- and submarginal plaque
  D. No evidence of bleeding upon probing
  E. No probing depths greater than 3 mm

44 Which of the following products raises safety concerns with long-term use?
- A. Chlorhexidine
- B. Hydrogen peroxide
- C. Sodium benzoate
- D. Listerine
- E. Triclosan

45 Use of which of the following is *MOST* successful as a means of bacterial plaque control?
- A. Penicillin
- B. Dextranase
- C. Sulfonamides
- D. Tetracycline
- E. Chlorhexidine

46 Nonsteroidal antiinflammatory drugs have which of the following effects in periodontal therapy?
- A. Elimination of inflammation
- B. Inhibiting bone loss
- C. Anesthetic effect
- D. Reducing bleeding
- E. Antimicrobial action

47 Which of the following antibiotics is *NOT* indicated for periodontal therapy?
- A. Erythromycin
- B. Metronidazole
- C. Tetracycline
- D. Augmentin
- E. Ciprofloxacin

48 Which of the following conditions exists when a client demonstrates attachment loss and is infected by periodontal pathogens after appropriate treatment?
- A. Adult periodontitis
- B. Desquamative gingivitis
- C. Linear gingival erythema
- D. Refractory periodontitis
- E. Early onset periodontitis

49 What is the relationship between gingivitis and periodontitis?
- A. Gingivitis will always progress to periodontitis if untreated
- B. Both gingivitis and periodontitis result in attachment loss
- C. Both gingivitis and periodontitis are manifested by alveolar bone loss
- D. Both gingivitis and periodontitis can result in probing depths greater than 3 mm
- E. Periodontitis precedes gingivitis in the periodontal lesion

50 What is the objective/rationale for periodontal debridement/root planing?
- A. To treat established periodontal disease and prevent periodontal disease
- B. To treat established periodontal disease, prevent periodontal disease, and establish conditions conducive to healing of the periodontium
- C. To prevent periodontal disease and eliminate pathogenic microorganisms or shift subgingival microflora toward less harmful microorganisms
- D. To treat established periodontal disease, establish conditions conducive to healing of the periodontium and eliminate pathogenic microorganisms or shift subgingival microflora toward less harmful microorganisms
- E. To treat established periodontal disease, prevent periodontal disease, establish conditions conducive to healing of the periodontium, stimulate regeneration of the alveolar bone, and eliminate pathogenic microorganisms or shift subgingival microflora toward less harmful microorganisms

51 Gingivitis is initiated *MOST* often by:
- A. Malocclusion
- B. A hormonal imbalance
- C. A vitamin deficiency
- D. Microorganisms and their products
- E. Psychosocial factors

52 The incidence of periodontal disease is *MOST* highly correlated with:
- A. Increasing age
- B. Poor oral hygiene
- C. Systemic disease
- D. Poor nutritional status
- E. Occlusal trauma

53 The *MOST* important single factor determining the frequency of continued-care appointments for dental hygiene care is the:
- A. Amount of alveolar bone loss
- B. Prognosis of the case
- C. Amount of calculus present at the reevaluation
- D. Patient motivation
- E. State of health or disease evident at the time of reevaluation

54 A probe reading of 6 mm measures the distance from the:
- A. Marginal ridge to the epithelial attachment
- B. Epithelial attachment to the gingival margin
- C. Alveolar crest to the gingival margin
- D. Cementoenamel junction to the gingival margin
- E. Cementoenamel junction to the epithelial attachment

55 Which of the following is the *MOST* reliable clinical sign of gingival inflammation?
- A. Redness of the gingiva
- B. Loss of stippling
- C. Blunted papillae
- D. Bleeding upon gentle probing
- E. Probing depth

56 Which of the following clinical signs and symptoms is characteristic of necrotizing ulcerative gingivitis?
A. Painless
B. Periodontal pocket formation
C. Ulcerated, crater-like gingival lesions
D. Gingival bleeding
E. Severe erythema

57 Which of the following methods is most successful for prevention of periodontal disease?
A. Regular oral self-care practices and periodontal debridement/root planing
B. Local delivery of antibiotics and periodontal debridement/root planing
C. Regular oral self-care practices and regular oral prophylaxis
D. Regular oral self-care practices, regular oral prophylaxis, and antimicrobial mouthrinses
E. Regular oral self-care practices, periodontal debridement/root planing, and antimicrobial mouthrinses

58 The primary purpose of periodontal debridement is to:
A. Remove all clinically detectable calculus
B. Remove all plaque-retentive factors
C. Remove diseased cementum and calculus
D. Create a smooth tooth surface
E. Restore health of gingival tissues

59 Studies of the natural history of periodontal disease have shown that:
A. Incidence of periodontitis is related to the amount of plaque and calculus present
B. Periodontal therapy and oral self care will slow rate of attachment loss in periodontitis
C. Individuals will progress from gingivitis to periodontitis even without periodontal therapy
D. Periodontal disease is usually rapidly progressive if untreated

60 Which of the following factors increase an individual's risk of attachment loss?
A. Female gender
B. Ethnicity
C. Tobacco use
D. Phenytoin
E. Vitamin C deficiency

Answers and Rationales

1. (B) Alveolar bone proper (or the cribriform plate) is referred to as lamina dura on a radiograph and is seen as a thin radiopaque line outlining the tooth socket.
   (A) The periodontal ligament space is a radiolucent space seen between the root and lamina dura.
   (C) Cortical plates are not identifiable on a full-mouth series of radiographs.
   (D) Cancellous bone is seen as a lacelike radiopaque image (trabecular pattern).
   (E) The alveolar crest is the interproximal extension of the alveolar bone proper.

2. (C) Neutrophils, or polymorphonuclear leukocytes, are the first inflammatory cells to respond in the initial lesion of gingivitis (2 to 4 days after plaque accumulation).
   (A) B lymphocytes predominate (75%) in the early lesion (4 to 7 days minimum after plaque accumulation).
   (B) Plasma cells are characteristic of chronic gingivitis.
   (D) Lymphokines are not inflammatory cells; they are substances produced by antigen-antibody complexes that have both protective and destructive capabilities.
   (E) Macrophages are present in all stages, but they do not predominate initially.

3. (A) The enlargement of the gingival margin coronally (as an inflammatory reaction) is the process that creates a deeper gingival sulcus.
   (B) Coronal migration of the epithelial attachment would constitute a longer epithelial attachment as seen in periodontal regeneration following therapy.
   (C) Apical migration of the gingival margin constitutes recession.
   (D) Apical migration of the epithelial and connective tissue attachment is the formation of a true pocket.
   (E) A pseudopocket does not involve any changes in the bone; the alveolar crest is located at its normal level, whereas it is the gingiva that enlarges to create the pocket depth.

4. (D) Measuring the sulcular areas (by probing) is the most accurate method of assessing the presence or absence of a pocket.
   (A) A radiograph does not illustrate the level of the soft tissues.
   (B) The color of the gingiva may be misleading in that it may appear "normal" even if a periodontal pocket is present.
   (C) The contour of the gingiva can be normal even if a periodontal pocket is present.
   (E) Bleeding on probing may not be readily detected in a chronic, fibrotic situation; it also can occur in normal sulcus depths with inflammation.

5. (A) Periodontitis is usually a long-standing disease that may have episodes of acute inflammatory signs and symptoms.
   (B) Early-onset periodontitis can start in adolescence and even in childhood.
   (C) Periodontitis is an inflammatory and not a degenerative disease.
   (D) The signs and symptoms of periodontitis are not consistent with those of acute inflammation and it is most commonly chronic in nature.
   (E) Periodontitis is "site specific" (i.e., each area of the mouth is affected at a different rate).

6. (D) Following the pathway of inflammation through the periodontal structures, the cortical plate of the interdental septum is the first bony area to be affected by periodontitis.
   (A) The facial and lingual aspects of supporting bone are not the first areas to be involved in bone resorption caused by periodontitis; interdental areas are affected first.
   (B) The cribriform plate is not the first bony area to be affected by periodontitis.
   (C) Cancellous bone is not the first bony area to be affected by periodontitis.
   (E) The bone surrounding the apical area of the tooth is the last area to be affected by periodontitis because the disease migrates apically.

7. (A) Supragingival plaque does influence the growth and pathogenicity of subgingival plaque.
   (B) Supragingival plaque precedes subgingival plaque.
   (C) Subgingival plaque consists primarily of anaerobic bacteria.
   (D) Bacteria from plaque have been found in diseased periodontal tissues.
   (E) Subgingival plaque *does* differ from supragingival plaque.

8. (A) Sharpey's fibers are composed of collagen fibers.
   (B) Elastic fibers are not part of Sharpey's fibers.
   (C) Gingival fibers are coronal to the periodontal ligament and are not part of Sharpey's fibers.
   (D) Oxytalan fibers are immature elastic fibers.
   (E) Transseptal fibers are part of the gingival fiber system.

9. (B) *Consistency* or *resiliency* refers to the response of the tissue to pressure; this response may change as a result of the presence or absence of edema or destruction of the underlying collagen fibers.
   (A) *Tissue consistency* does not refer to thickness of the tissue.
   (C) *Texture* refers to the visual characteristics of the outer surface of the tissue.
   (D) The location of the margin helps describe the overall *contour* or architecture of this gingiva.
   (E) *Stippling* refers to the visual characteristics of the outer surface of the tissue.

10. (D) Periodontal pockets are inflammatory lesions that are not caused by occlusal trauma.
    (A) Wear facets are a symptom of occlusal trauma.
    (B) Fremitus is a symptom of occlusal trauma.
    (C) Increase in tooth mobility is a symptom of occlusal trauma.
    (E) Increased width of the periodontal ligament space is a symptom of occlusal trauma.

11. (E) None of the answers is correct.
    (A) Soft tissue cannot be seen on a radiograph.
    (B) The presence or absence of mobility can be detected only clinically.
    (C) Bone level or loss cannot be accurately determined radiographically because a radiograph cannot present a three-dimensional image.
    (D) Only large, dense pieces of calculus on proximal surfaces can be detected radiographically and then only if the angulation is correct (i.e., no overlap of proximal surfaces of teeth).

12. (E) The changes within the periodontium in cases of gingivitis are confined to the soft tissue.
    (A) Gingivitis does not affect alveolar bone, including vertical bone loss.
    (B) Gingivitis does not affect alveolar bone, including horizontal bone loss.
    (C) Gingivitis does not increase bone density.
    (D) Gingivitis does not change bone trabeculation.

13. (D) Localized juvenile periodontitis is characterized by relatively sparse subgingival plaque, onset at an early age of puberty, and bilateral angular bone loss in permanent first molars and incisors.
    (A) Necrotizing ulcerative gingivitis is associated with poor oral hygiene, ulceration, and pseudomembrane formation without bone loss.
    (B) Rapidly progressive periodontitis is similar to generalized juvenile periodontitis (may be related) and occurs in the early 20s to mid 30s.
    (C) Prepubertal periodontitis occurs before puberty and also affects primary teeth.
    (E) Refractory periodontitis occurs in multiple sites that have previously been treated appropriately and progressed despite treatment efforts.

14. (C) Scaling/periodontal debridement/root planing *and* periodontal maintenance procedures are indicated for nonsurgical treatment of early periodontitis.
    (A) Oral prophylaxis is for healthy periodontium, or conversion of gingivitis to health.
    (B) Gingival curettage is not justified for treatment of slowly progressive periodontitis.
    (D) Gingivectomy is indicated for gingival overgrowth, not bone loss (also see answer A).
    (E) All of these procedures are not indicated for reasons discussed in answers A to D.

15. (B) Although chlorhexidine is shown in long-term studies to reduce plaque by 55% and gingivitis by 45%, it does stain the teeth.
    (A) Sanguinarine does not stain the teeth; side effects are burning sensation and taste.
    (C) Hydrogen peroxide does not stain the teeth; it does, however, raise safety issues with long-term use.
    (D) Phenolic compounds do not stain teeth; side effects are burning sensation and taste.
    (E) Prebrushing rinse does not stain teeth.

16. (C) The attached gingiva and alveolar mucosa meet at the mucogingival junction.
    (A) The gingival groove demarcates the free gingiva and the attached gingiva.
    (B) The gingival margin demarcates the free gingiva and the tooth.
    (D) The space between the base of the sulcus and the alveolar mucosa is occupied by the epithelial attachment and the connective tissue.
    (E) The area between the gingival groove and the gingival margin is the free gingiva.

17. (E) The sulcular epithelium and alveolar mucosa are generally nonkeratinized.
    (A) The alveolar mucosa is also nonkeratinized.
    (B) The epithelial tissues of the attached gingiva are keratinized.
    (C) The sulcular epithelium is also nonkeratinized.
    (D) The palatal mucosa is keratinized on the hard palate.

18. (D) Gram-positive cocci are dominant in the initial formation of bacterial plaque.
    (A) Gram-negative rods are found in older bacterial plaque.
    (B) Gram-positive rods are found in older bacterial plaque.
    (C) Spirochetes are found in older bacterial plaque.
    (D) Gram-negative cocci are found in older bacterial plaque.

19. (A) The gingival fibers are composed of collagen.
    (B) Elastic fibers are predominantly found in the alveolar mucosa.
    (C) No such fibers exist in the gingival tissues.
    (D) This term is descriptive of a certain form of epithelial tissues, not connective tissue fibers.
    (E) Oxytalan fibers are an immature form of elastic fibers.

20. (E) Systemic factors are the so-called contributing factors to the pathogenesis of periodontal disease (i.e., they *cannot* initiate the disease process, but they can affect the severity of the tissue response).
    (A) Systemic factors cannot be the direct cause of periodontal disease.
    (B) Systemic factors do not have a direct effect on pocket depth.
    (C) Systemic factors alone cannot eliminate the periodontal disease.
    (D) Systemic factors do not determine the pattern of bone loss.

21. (D) The lining of a healthy gingival sulcus is composed of nonkeratinized epithelial tissues with no rete pegs present. The presence of rete pegs is indicative of the presence of inflammation.
    (A) Healthy gingival sulcus is lined with nonkeratinized epithelium without rete pegs.
    (B) Healthy gingival sulcus lining is composed of nonkeratinized epithelium.
    (C) Healthy gingival sulcus lining does not have rete pegs.
    (E) Healthy gingival sulcus lining is composed of nonkeratinized epithelium without rete pegs.

22. (A) The function of the gingival fibers is to support the margin of the gingiva against the tooth.
    (B) The periodontal ligament is responsible for withstanding horizontal forces.
    (C) The periodontal ligament is responsible for preventing the tooth from being forced into the bony socket.
    (D) The periodontal ligament is responsible for the formation and resorption of cementum (by cementoblasts and by osteoclasts and cementoclasts).
    (E) The periodontal ligament is responsible for the transmission of sensations of occlusal forces.

23. (E) Bleeding on probing is an early indicator of gingivitis.
    (A) Tooth mobility is indicative of the progression of the disease from gingivitis to periodontitis and is the result of loss of supporting structures of the periodontium.
    (B) Drifting of the anterior teeth indicates the progression of the disease and is a result of loss of supporting structures of the periodontium.
    (C) Periodontal pocket formation is indicative of the progression of the disease from gingivitis to periodontitis.
    (D) Gingival recession is indicative of the progression of the disease.

24. (E) The alveolar area that is initially altered by periodontal disease is the crest of the alveolar bone.
    (A) When a periodontal abscess does affect the alveolar bone, it usually results in a vertical bony defect.
    (B) Gingivitis does not affect the alveolar bone; it is confined to the gingival tissues.
    (C) Occlusal trauma is usually associated with a widened periodontal ligament.
    (D) Occlusal trauma in the absence of bacterial plaque will not cause soft tissue inflammation and will therefore not initiate periodontitis.

25. (C) The interdental col has the thinnest nonkeratinized epithelial layer. Furthermore, it is the most inaccessible area to bacterial plaque removal. Both situations cause this area to be the most susceptible to tissue breakdown and the area where gingival changes are first noticed.
    (A) The free gingiva is not the most susceptible to tissue breakdown.
    (B) The gingival sulcus is susceptible to tissue breakdown; however, the col is most susceptible.
    (D) The interdental papilla is not the most susceptible to tissue breakdown.
    (E) The attached gingiva is not the most susceptible to tissue breakdown.

26. (D) The changes associated with gingivitis are associated only with the soft tissue.
    (A) Bone loss and apical migration of the epithelial attachment are characteristics of periodontitis.
    (B) Apical migration of the epithelial attachment is a characteristic of periodontitis.
    (C) Gingivitis is inflammation that is confined to supracrestal soft tissue and therefore does not influence the width of the periodontal ligament; bone loss is a characteristic of periodontitis.
    (E) Gingivitis is associated only with soft tissue.

27. (B) The presence or absence of sucrose has no effect on the bacteria that are involved in the periodontal disease process.
    (A) Open contacts may result in food impaction and mechanical irritation of the tissues.
    (C) Mouth breathing causes desiccation of the anterior gingival tissues, which results in their irritation.
    (D) Some blood dyscrasias may result in altered cellular and/or humoral immunity, thus rendering the person more susceptible to periodontal disease.
    (E) Hormonal imbalance may intensify the body's immunologic response to bacterial plaque.

28. (D) The inflammation is confined to a limited area of the mouth ("localized"), and the margin is inflamed ("marginal"), which includes papillary inflammation because it is initiated in the papilla and spreads to the margins. Because the bases of all sulci are at their normal location, the disease is still confined only to the soft tissues ("gingivitis").
    (A) The disease is localized and therefore not generalized, marginal periodontitis.
    (B) The disease is localized marginal gingivitis, not periodontitis; no bone loss or attachment loss exists.
    (C) The disease is localized and marginal, not generalized and papillary.
    (E) The disease is marginal gingivitis, not papillary gingivitis; the entire free gingiva is involved.

29. (B) Because the gingival margin is located at the CEJ, the pocket depth is created by the "apical migration of the epithelial attachment" (which is the definition of a true periodontal pocket).
    (A) A pseudopocket is created by the enlargement (coronally) of the gingival margin; the epithelial attachment is still located in its normal position.
    (C) A gingival pocket is a synonym for a pseudopocket.
    (D) The pocket is a periodontal pocket only.
    (E) The pocket is a periodontal pocket only.

30. (B) A gingivectomy is indicated in areas of fibrotic tissues that are forming pseudopockets because total elimination of the excess tissue in this area is necessary but the level of the epithelial attachment does not have to be repositioned.
    (A) This area would most likely respond to thorough scaling and periodontal debridement, and daily plaque removal. No surgical procedure is warranted.
    (C) A gingivectomy is contraindicated in the case of an infrabony pocket.
    (D) A gingivectomy is contraindicated in areas of little or no attached tissue or in cases where the base of the pocket extends into the alveolar mucosa.
    (E) Initially, no surgical procedure should be performed; NUG requires debridement and self care. Once the disease is no longer present, a gingivoplasty (recontouring of the gingival margin) may be needed in severe cases of NUG.

31. (D) The rationale for pocket elimination is to reduce the pocket depth to one that can be adequately cleansed by the client on a daily basis.
    (A) Periodontal disease may or may not have changed the client's appearance; although tissue contours may be improved during periodontal surgery, this is not a specific objective of pocket elimination procedures.
    (B) See A.
    (C) Peridontal pocket elimination may also assist the client in daily plaque control.
    (E) See A.

32. (A) A pyogenic granuloma is an exaggerated tissue response to local irritants, and occurs commonly during hormonal changes, such as those that take place during pregnancy. It is treated by thorough scaling/periodontal debridement/root planing (if needed), and plaque control. If the tissue is fibrotic, a gingivectomy is sometimes warranted.
    (B) A pyogenic granuloma is not related to phenytoin hyperplasia.
    (C) A pyogenic granuloma is not associated with gingival recession pyogenic granuloma is not associated with juvenile periodontitis.
    (E) Pyogenic granulomas are treated by thorough scaling, periodontal debridement/root planing, and plaque control.

33. (C) A gingivectomy results in a loss of attached gingiva. Therefore an adequate amount of attached gingiva must be present before the surgical procedure is done; otherwise the result will be an area with minimal or no attached gingiva.
    (A) A gingivectomy does not provide access to the osseous area, and therefore it is not useful in treating this type of periodontal pocket.
    (B) See C.
    (D) A gingivectomy is most commonly used to treat areas of enlarged, fibrotic pseudopockets.
    (E) Because a gingivectomy results in loss of gingiva, this procedure will only exacerbate the preexisting condition.

34. (A) When this situation exists, all of the keratinized tissue is detached, thus creating a mucogingival problem (i.e., lack of any or an adequate amount of attached gingiva).
    (B) The base of the pocket is normally coronal to the mucogingival junction.
    (C) The minimal zone of attached gingiva is 1 to 2 mm; therefore a 3-mm zone is adequate.
    (D) The width of alveolar mucosa does not determine whether or not a mucogingival problem exists.
    (E) The amount of bone loss does not determine whether or not a mucogingival problem exists.

35. (E) The successful outcome of flap surgery is dependent to a great extent on the maintenance of the correct flap position after surgery, as well as on the wound-healing process. The placement of sutures helps in maintaining the correct flap position as well as allowing wound healing to progress with a minimal amount of trauma.
    (A) In addition to holding the soft tissues in place, sutures protect the wound, maintain the blood clot, and prevent impaction.
    (B) Sutures also maintain the blood clot and prevent food impaction.
    (C) Sutures also hold the soft tisues in place and prevent food impaction.
    (D) Sutures also protect the wound and prevent food impaction.

36. (D) Gut sutures are dissolved by the inflammatory process that occurs in the surrounding tissues.
    (A) Gut sutures are rather difficult to manipulate because they are stiff and break easily.
    (B) Gut sutures, being somewhat stiff, unravel easily.
    (C) An inflammatory reaction does occur around the gut sutures, and in fact it is this process that dissolves the gut sutures.
    (E) Some suture (being a foreign body) will cause some trauma to the surrounding tissues.

37. (C) The silk material makes this type of suture extremely easy to manipulate through the tissues and to knot securely.
    (A) The silk cannot be dissolved.
    (B) The braided sutures readily trap bacteria and often cause bacterial contamination of the surrounding tissues.
    (D) Any type of suture is treated by the body as an antigen (foreign body).
    (E) Sutures should be removed within a week to 10 days. Leaving them in place for longer than this time will continue and possibly exaggerate the inflammatory response surrounding the sutures.

38. (E) Although the routine use of a periodontal dressing following surgery has *not* been shown to enhance the healing *rate* of the tissues, the placement of a dressing does have all of the advantages listed.
    (A) In addition, a periodontal dressing helps protect the teeth against root sensitivity and helps maintain tissue placement.
    (B) In addition, a periodontal dressing minimizes patient discomfort and helps maintain tissue placement.
    (C) In addition, a periodontal dressing minimizes patient discomfort, protects the wound, and minimizes the chance of hemorrhage.
    (D) In addition, a periodontal dressing minimizes patient discomfort and helps protect the teeth against root sensitivity.

39. (E) The purpose of adding rosin to the dressing material is strictly to add strength to the dressing so that it can withstand the normal forces of eating and tongue movement.
    (A) A periodontal dressing does not provide an antibacterial property.
    (B) A periodontal dressing has no anesthetic action.
    (C) A periodontal dressing does not serve as an astringent.
    (D) A periodontal dressing does not improve the taste.

40. (E) The frequency of continued care intervals must be established based on the individual needs of the client; severity of the disease, microbial count, plaque control, general health of the client, etc. There is no set standard of interval for all postoperative periodontal clients.
    (A) A 12-month continued care interval might not be appropriate for some clients.
    (B) A 6-month continued care interval might not be appropriate for some clients.
    (C) A 4-month continued care interval might not be appropriate for some clients.
    (D) A 2-month continued care interval might not be appropriate for some clients.

41. (C) Chlorhexidine is recommended for dental implant preventive maintenance.
    (A) Ultrasonic scalers are contraindicated for use with dental implants.
    (B) Titanium-tipped curets are not recommended for scaling implants.
    (D) Only fine polishing paste is recommended for polishing abutments of dental implants.
    (E) Stainless steel curets also are contraindicated.

42. (A) Dental implants are commonly made of titanium or hydroxyapatite.
    (B) Dental implants are not made of gold.
    (C) Dental implants are not made of aluminum.
    (D) Dental implants are not made of Teflon.
    (E) Dental implants are not made of bonded acrylic resin.

43. (D) At a 4- to 6-week reevaluation, no evidence of bleeding upon gentle probing is the single best evaluative criterion for success of periodontal debridement/root planing because it indicates an absence of inflammation; therefore, the tissues have healed.

    (A) In nonsurgical periodontal therapy, the clinician can only evaluate removal of clinically detectable calculus deposits; it is unlikely that 100% of the calculus is removed from all areas treated.

    (B) Root roughness is not necessarily correlated with disease and root smoothness does not necessarily result in health; removal of bacterial plaque, its products, and retentive factors is most important for attaining health.

    (C) Some supra- and subgingival calculus is commonly found at a 4- to 6-week reevaluation appointment; therefore, localized removal of residual or newly formed deposits is indicated.

    (E) A 4 mm pocket with no inflammation or bleeding in adjacent gingival tissues would be monitored and treated with periodontal maintenance procedures at subsequent continued care intervals; 3 mm probing depths with bleeding would not be successful outcomes at reevaluation.

44. (B) Hydrogen peroxide raises safety concerns with long-term use.

    (A) Chlorhexidine can be safely used long-term; staining is the most common side effect.

    (C) Sodium benzoate raises no safety issues despite the lack of a therapeutic benefit.

    (D) Listerine can be safely used long-term as long as high alcohol content is not a concern (e.g., xerostomia, recovering alcoholics).

    (E) Triclosan raises no safety issues.

45. (E) Chlorhexidine is the most effective antiplaque and antigingivitis agent available.

    (A) Penicillin and other antibiotics are not recommended for plaque control.

    (B) The tin ion in stannous fluoride has some antibacterial effect; however, it is not as effective as chlorhexidine and its ADA seal is for its anticaries benefit.

    (C) Quarternary ammonium compounds have low substantivity; therefore, they are not highly effective as a means of bacterial plaque control.

    (D) Tetracycline and other antibiotics are not recommended for bacterial plaque control, although local delivery of tetracycline fibers can reduce pathogens in periodontal pockets.

46. (B) NSAIDs have been shown to inhibit bone loss in periodontitis.

    (A) Although NSAIDs are antiinflammatory drugs, they have not been clearly documented as effective in reducing gingival inflammation.

    (C) NSAIDs have analgesic effects but not anesthetic effects.

    (D) NSAIDs do not reduce bleeding.

    (E) NSAIDs do not have an antimicrobial action.

47. (A) Erythromycin is not indicated for periodontal therapy; it can be used as a prophylactic antibiotic in patients who are allergic to amoxicillin.

    (B) Metronidazole can be prescribed alone or in conjunction with amoxicillin in treatment of aggressive forms of periodontitis.

    (C) Tetracycline can be prescribed in treatment of juvenile periodontitis.

    (D) Augmentin can be prescribed in treatment of refractory periodontitis.

    (E) Ciprofloxacin can be prescribed in treatment of refractory periodontitis.

48. (D) In refractory periodontitis attachment loss and infection with periodontal pathogens continues even after apparently appropriate treatment and self care.

    (A) Adult periodontitis can be successfully treated with nonsurgical and/or surgical periodontal therapy.

    (B) Desquamative gingivitis is an oral manifestation of underlying systemic disease or condition.

    (C) Linear gingival erythema is a type of gingivitis which occurs in immunocompromised individuals.

    (E) Early onset periodontitis can be successfully treated with conventional periodontal therapy in conjunction with systemic antibiotics, frequent continued care, and sometimes microbiologic monitoring.

49. (D) Both gingivitis and periodontitis can result in probing depths greater than 3 mm but these are pseudopockets in gingivitis and true periodontal pockets with attachment loss in periodontitis.

    (A) Gingivitis can progress to periodontitis if untreated, or it may not depending on the risk factors present and the client's immune response.

    (B) Only periodontitis results in attachment loss, not gingivitis.

    (C) Only periodontitis is manifested by bone loss, not gingivitis.

    (E) Gingivitis precedes periodontitis.

50. (D) Periodontal debridement/root planing is indicated for treatment of periodontal disease and is intended to foster healing of the periodontium by eliminating or reducing periodontal pathogens.

    (A) An oral prophylaxis is performed to prevent periodontal disease.

    (B) See D and A.

    (C) An oral prophylaxis is performed to prevent periodontal disease and to reduce periodontal pathogens or maintain a healthy microflora.

    (E) Periodontal debridement/root planing does not stimulate regeneration of alveolar bone. Also see D and A.

51. (D) Bacterial plaque and its products are the primary etiologic factor in gingivitis.
    (A) Malocclusion does not initiate gingivitis.
    (B) A hormonal imbalance can exaggerate the immune response to bacterial plaque but it does not initiate gingivitis.
    (C) Vitamin C deficiency can contribute to scorbutic gingivitis in severe malnutrition but this condition is rare in industrialized nations.
    (E) Psychosocial factors affect the immune response and, therefore, are risk factors in periodontal disease; however, they do not initiate gingivitis.

52. (B) Poor oral hygiene is most highly correlated with periodontal disease because bacterial plaque and its products are the primary etiology.
    (A) Severity of periodontitis increases with age, possibly due to cumulative effects; however, good oral hygiene minimizes effects of age.
    (C) Systemic diseases are risk factors because they affect the individual's immune response to bacterial plaque but they are not the most highly correlated with incidence of periodontal disease.
    (D) Poor nutritional status affects tissue integrity and defense mechanisms but no direct relationships have been made to periodontal diseases (except scurvy).
    (E) Occlusal trauma is not highly correlated with periodontal disease.

53. (E) Frequency of continued care appointments is decided based upon periodontal status at the time of reevaluation because the goal of periodontal maintenance therapy is to maintain health.
    (A) Amount of alveolar bone loss affects decisions regarding active therapy and prognosis and, although it affects recare intervals, it is not most important.
    (B) Prognosis of the case affects decisions regarding active periodontal therapy.
    (C) Amount of calculus present affects continued care intervals but it is less important than tissue response.
    (D) Client motivation affects oral self-care practices and compliance with continued care recommendations but it is not the most important factor because motivation may or may not result in effective maintenance of periodontal health.

54. (B) Probing depth is measured from the epithelial attachment to the gingival margin.
    (A) The marginal ridge is located on the crown of the tooth and is not used to measure probing depth.
    (C) The epithelial and connective tissue attachment of the gingiva is coronal to the alveolar crest and it is the most apical point of probing depth measurement.
    (D) Recession is measured from the cementoenamel junction apically to the gingival margin; enlargement is measured from the cementoenamel junction coronally to the gingival margin—depending on where the margin of the gingiva is located on the tooth.
    (E) Clinical attachment loss is measured from the cementoenamel junction to the epithelial attachment.

55. (D) Bleeding upon gentle probing is the most reliable clinical sign of gingival inflammation.
    (A) Color of the gingiva also is affected by thickness of the epithelium and connective tissue, vascularity of the tissue, and melanin pigmentation.
    (B) Stippling is not present in all areas of the mouth or in all mouths.
    (C) Contour of the gingiva is affected by position of the teeth and proximal tooth contacts.
    (E) Probing depth is not a sign of gingival inflammation.

56. (C) Necrotizing ulcerative gingivitis (NUG) is characterized by painful, ulcerated, gingival lesions.
    (A) NUG is painful.
    (B) NUG is usually confined to the gingiva and periodontal pockets are not characteristic.
    (D) NUG is accompanied by hemorrhage but bleeding is common in all forms of gingival inflammation.
    (E) NUG can be accompanied by severe erythema but it is not characteristic.

57. (C) Periodontal disease is best prevented by regular oral self-care practices and oral prophylaxis.
    (A) Periodontal debridement/root planing is employed to treat periodontal disease rather than for its prevention.
    (B) Local delivery of antibiotics is a method used for treatment of periodontal disease. Also see A.
    (D) Antimicrobial rinses are used as chemotherapeutic agents for treatment of gingival inflammation rather than for its prevention.
    (E) See C, A, and D.

58. (E) Periodontal debridement is performed to remove all bacterial plaque, byproducts, and plaque retentive factors to the extent needed to restore health of the gingival tissues.
    (A) All clinically detectable calculus must be removed in periodontal debridement but the primary purpose is to restore gingival health.
    (B) See E and A.
    (C) Removal of diseased cementum, calculus, plaque and its products, and creation of a smooth tooth surface is the definition of root planing; periodontal debridement differs in extent of instrumentation and attempts to minimize removal of tooth structure. See E and A.
    (D) Creation of a smooth tooth surface is not the goal of periodontal debridement. Also see C.

59. (B) Studies of untreated Sri Lankan teaworkers and regular dental care attendees from Norway indicate that periodontal therapy and self-care slows rate of attachment loss (0.3 mm and 0.1 mm, respectively).
    (A) Plaque, calculus, and gingival inflammation were common in both untreated and treated groups in studies of the natural history of periodontitis; rate of progression differed rather than incidence of periodontal disease.
    (C) In studies of untreated Sri Lankan teaworkers and regular dental care attendees from Norway, about 10% of cases in both groups never progressed from gingivitis to periodontitis.
    (D) Periodontal disease is most commonly slowly progressive. See C also.

60. (C) Tobacco use increases the incidence and severity of attachment loss in periodontitis.

    (A) Gender differences do not exist for prevalence of attachment loss; however, more severe attachment loss, deeper probing depths and recession are more common in males.

    (B) Ethnicity is not proven to be a risk factor in attachment loss.

    (D) Phenytoin is a risk factor for gingival hyperplasia, not attachment loss.

    (E) Severe vitamin C deficiency results in scorbutic gingivitis, not attachment loss.

Strategies for Oral Health Promotion and Disease Prevention and Control

Linda Rubinstein DeVore   Mary-Catherine Dean

Promotion of oral health and prevention of oral diseases have been the focus of dental hygiene practice since its inception. As an educator and provider of preventive and therapeutic services, the dental hygienist must have a thorough understanding of the strategies and interventions that support prevention-oriented health care. Because much of the success of preventive oral health programs rests with the individual's self-care practices, the dental hygienist focuses considerable attention on ensuring client adherence to appropriate home care regimens. This chapter addresses the dental hygienist's role as a facilitator of client behaviors directed toward health and as a provider of clinical services that are effective for the prevention and control of oral diseases. Topics include the process of care model, educational strategies, client adherence, mechanical and chemical methods of bacterial plaque control, and care of fixed and removable appliances, including dental implant maintenance, fluorides, sealants, desensitization, phase-contrast microscopy, oral cancer self-examination, tobacco use cessation, pulpal vitality testing, and oral exfoliative cytology.

General Considerations

Historical Perspective

A. Dental disease has plagued humankind throughout history
B. Records of every ancient civilization contain descriptions of medications and implements used to prevent the loss of teeth, and evidence of dental caries and periodontal disease has been found in fossilized human skulls of ancient populations
C. Evidence that oral hygiene was practiced in many ancient populations can be found in the earliest written records of civilization
D. The Hindus used frayed sticks to brush their teeth, the Chinese used a chew stick, and the Assyrians and Babylonians wrapped linen strips around their fingers to wipe tooth surfaces clean

Dental Hygiene Process of Care[1]

A. Dental hygiene practice is based on a process of care that involves the steps of assessment, diagnosis, planning, implementation, and evaluation

B. Inherent in the process model is a continuum of care that supports a logical system of determining an individual's health and disease status and selecting appropriate interventions

C. The dental hygiene process is integrated with the individual's comprehensive dental diagnosis and oral care plan

Components of the Process of Care

A. Assessment—systematic collection of data
1. Data collection techniques should be appropriate to the nature of the information sought; data may be collected by interview, questionnaire, observation, measurement, and/or examination
2. Dental hygiene data collection procedures may include
   a. Comprehensive health history
   b. General physical evaluation, including vital signs
   c. Health risk appraisal, including tobacco and alcohol use
   d. Extraoral examination
   e. Intraoral examination
   f. Examination of the teeth, including charting of missing teeth, carious lesions and restorations, occlusal assessment, and deposit assessment
   g. Examination of the periodontium, including sulcus and/or pocket measurement, mobility, loss of attachment, exudate (bleeding, purulence), and soft tissue description (color, tone, architecture, consistency, texture)
   h. Bacterial evaluation using phase-contrast microscopy
   i. Exposure and interpretation of radiographs
   j. Health behavior evaluation, including the current home care practices, adherence, knowledge and skill levels, and psychosocial factors that might influence behaviors and oral habits
   k. Plaque and gingival indices
   l. Intraoral photography
   m. Impressions for study models
   n. Diet diary
   o. Oral exfoliative cytology
   p. Pulpal vitality testing
   q. Bacterial culturing, DNA or RNA probes, antibody and enzyme markers, and gingival crevicular fluid analysis (GCF)
3. Information gathered is always thoroughly documented in the client's permanent record
B. Diagnosis—analysis of data to focus on actual or potential unmet human needs that can be fulfilled through dental hygiene care (Table 12-1)
1. Provides direction for dental hygiene actions
2. Helps focus and individualize dental hygiene care
3. Identifies etiologic factors contributing to human needs deficits
4. Is distinct from the dental diagnosis[1]

C. Planning—identification of current and potential dental hygiene care needs, and specification of a plan to meet these needs
1. Factors contributing to current and potential disease etiology are used to formulate the care plan
2. Goals, scope, and sequence of care are designed based on the analysis of data and dental hygiene diagnosis
3. Client participation in setting goals and designing the care plan increases the potential for success during implementation
4. Clients must be fully informed of the scope and sequence of dental hygiene services, expected outcomes, and limitations

D. Implementation—initiation and completion of activities necessary to meet the assessed needs
1. Activities include preventive and therapeutic services, as well as educational interventions
2. Educational interventions may include bacterial plaque control, diet modifications, use of preventive agents, and tobacco use/smoking cessation strategies
3. Modifications to the initial care plan are made as needed

E. Evaluation—determination of the success of dental hygiene interventions
1. Were the established goals met, partially met, or not met? If not, why?
   a. Was the initial assessment faulty?
   b. Were initial goals possible and realistic?
   c. Did the client receive all services necessary to meet the specified needs?
   d. Did the client demonstrate active participation in implementing the home care plan?
2. Determination is made of the client's continuing care needs
3. Evaluation is based on objective measures (i.e., soft tissue conditions, stability of periodontal attachment levels, no new caries, and effective plaque control)
4. Continued care intervals are determined based on individual client needs, and the client is informed of the rationale for and importance of continued maintenance care
5. Outcomes are documented thoroughly in the client's permanent record

Table 12-1

Assessment Instrument for Planning Dental Hygiene Care

(Circle the criteria that are in deficit for each human need)

Human need definition	Criteria for assessments of deficits	Comments
1) WHOLESOME FACIAL IMAGE: The need to feel satisfied with one's own oral-facial features and breath.	*Client reports dissatisfaction with appearance of:* • teeth • gingiva • facial profile *Client reports dissatisfaction with:* • breath	
2) PROTECTION FROM HEALTH RISKS: The need to avoid medical contraindications related to dental hygiene care.	*Presents with:* • vital signs outside of normal limits • need for prophylactic antibiotics • reported health condition with potential for medical emergency in the oral health care setting.	
3) BIOLOGICALLY SOUND AND FUNCTIONAL DEFINITION: The need to have intact teeth and restorations which defend against harmful microbes, provide for adequate function, and reflect appropriate nutrition/diet.	*Presents with:* • teeth with signs of disease • missing teeth • defective restorations • teeth with abrasion, erosion • teeth with signs of trauma • ill fitting dentures, prostheses	
4) SKIN AND MUCOSA MEMBRANE INTEGRITY OF HEAD AND NECK: The need to have an intact and functioning covering of the person's head & neck area, including the oral/mucosa membranes and periodontium, which defend against harmful microbes; resist injurious substances and trauma; and reflect adequate nutrition.	*Presents with:* • extra/intra-oral swelling or lesion • gingival inflammation • bleeding on probing • pockets >4 mm • attachment loss >4 mm • mucogingival problems • xerostomia	

Dental Hygiene Care Plan: Goals

Goal Evaluation

Table 12-1		
Assessment Instrument for Planning Dental Hygiene Care—cont'd		
Human need definition	**Criteria for assessments of deficits**	**Comments**
5) FREEDOM FROM HEAD AND NECK PAIN The need to be exempt from physical discomfort in the head and neck area	*Clinical reports:* • extra oral pain or sensitivity • intra oral pain or sensitivity	
6) FREEDOM FROM STRESS The need to feel safe and to be free from fear and emotional discomfort in the oral health care environment.	*Client reports fear/anxiety such as:* • fear related to past negative dental experiences • concern about dental hygiene care planned • concern about confidentiality • concern about cost • concern about disease transmission • concern about fluoride toxicity • concern about mercury toxicity • concern about radiation exposure	
7) RESPONSIBILITY FOR ORAL HEALTH: The need for accountability for one's oral health as a result of interaction between one's motivation, physical capability and social environment	*Presents with:* • inadequate oral health behaviors • inadequate parental supervision • no dental exam within the last two years	
8) CONCEPTUALIZATION AND UNDERSTANDING: The need to grasp ideas and abstractions in order to make sound decisions about one's oral health.	*Presents with questions or misconceptions associations with:* • oral disease • rationale for dental hygiene care	
Dental Hygiene Care Plan: Goals		
Goal Evaluation		

Oral Health Education

Basic Concepts

A. Initiation and progression of dental diseases depend on the interaction of host, agent, and environmental factors; thus prevention and control of these diseases require attention to all primary and modifying factors in each category

B. Dental caries and the inflammatory periodontal diseases are complex disease states that require the colonization of bacteria; none will occur in the absence of microbial plaque; thus, control of bacterial plaque is an essential component of any program designed for the prevention of these dental diseases

C. Where once the focus in dentistry was on restorative procedures and surgical interventions, today the emphasis has shifted to preventing disease and maintaining oral health

D. Prevention of dental disease requires the participation of a client with adequate knowledge of the disease process, sufficiently developed skills in implementing oral care procedures, and the motivation to practice preventive procedures over time

E. Many different strategies can be used to facilitate changes in the health behaviors of others; an understanding of the basic concepts underlying educational, motivational, and behavioral theory is necessary to understand the forces influencing a person's oral health practices

F. Educating clients in effective oral care practices follows the process of care model

Process of Care

A. Assessment of current status is based on
1. A thorough clinical examination; medical, dental, behavioral, and psychosocial/cultural history
2. Evaluation of client's current knowledge of dental disease, treatment options, and preventive strategies
3. Self-report of client's current oral care practices, habits, and behaviors that might affect oral health
4. Observation of client's skill and dexterity in plaque control techniques
5. Assessment of client's motivation level, interest, adherence, perceived needs, expectations, wants, health care beliefs, values, and priorities
6. Identification of contingencies that might influence the client's ability to participate in care, complete treatment, and implement effective oral care habits
7. Assessment data may be enhanced by use of a "baseline human needs assessment" (Table 12-1); human need theory explains that need fulfillment dominates human activity and human behavior is motivated by fulfillment of these needs; identification of unmet needs directs the dental hygiene care plan[1]

B. Diagnosis and planning
1. A dental hygiene diagnosis specifies unmet human needs that can be fulfilled through dental hygiene care
2. A comprehensive educational plan is designed cooperatively with the client to include all oral health practices needed for attainment and maintenance of oral health
3. The client must be involved in setting realistic short- and long-term goals
4. Appropriate bacterial plaque control tools, other preventive products, and home care regimens are specified based on the client's individual needs

5. The sequence of interventions must allow for adequate skill building, evaluation, and reinforcement of newly learned skills, and modification of the plan as needed
6. The plan should be based on sound educational and motivational principles, with particular attention to communication skills that facilitate active patient involvement and learning

C. Implementation
1. Centers on providing both a knowledge base and rationale for oral care practices
2. Includes effective skills training with appropriate bacterial plaque control tools in the client's own mouth
3. Demonstration on models (commercial or client's study models) may precede intraoral instruction
4. The hygienist reinforces positive changes and modifies techniques needing improvement
5. The hygienist creates a comfortable, positive, and caring environment for learning
6. The oral care plan is modified as needed
7. The client's progress, including knowledge, adherence, involvement, skills, and clinical changes, are documented in the client's permanent dental record

D. Evaluation
1. Appraisal of changes in the client's behaviors and clinical status as a result of dental hygiene interventions occurs throughout the educational program
2. When positive changes do not occur, the hygienist and the client assess the reasons for lack of progress and modify the plan accordingly
3. If client conditions make the attainment of all goals unlikely, attention should be focused on changing these conditions, whenever possible, reestablishing attainable goals, and planning for additional dental hygiene or dental interventions to enhance the success of the client's oral care practices
4. Outcomes of the educational interventions and continuing needs are documented in the client's permanent record

Sequence in Total Care

A. Bacterial plaque control instructions before instituting any treatment
1. Clients will see positive changes resulting from their actions (limited tissue changes may occur prior to instrumentation for debridement of tooth surfaces)
2. Improved gingival health can result from improved toothbrushing even in the presence of calculus[2]
3. Treatment will progress more efficiently and comfortably in a mouth with less gingival inflammation
4. Client's level of adherence and skill can be considered in the care plan

B. Plaque control instructions throughout dental and dental hygiene care
1. Clients need time for practice
2. Clients need time to go through the stages involved in learning and habituation
3. Evaluation and modifications can occur over time
4. Tissue changes can be effectively demonstrated when treatment and bacterial plaque control are integrated

Stages in Making a Commitment to a New Behavior

See Chapter 16, section on successful client management.

Learning-Ladder or Decision-Making Continuum

A. One approach to achieving the habit of bacterial plaque control is based on the concept that humans learn in a series of sequential steps referred to as the learning-ladder continuum or the decision-making continuum
B. The dental hygienist must first determine the client's entering level on the ladder and then plan for moving up the steps in sequence
C. Steps in the process
1. Unawareness or ignorance—individual lacks information or has incorrect information about the problem (human need deficit in conceptualization and problem-solving)
2. Awareness—individual knows there is or can be a problem but does not act on this knowledge (human need deficit in self-determination and responsibility)
3. Self-interest—individual recognizes the problem and indicates a tentative inclination toward action
4. Involvement—individual's attitudes and feelings are affected, and desire for additional knowledge increases
5. Action—new behaviors directed toward solving the problem are instituted
6. Habit or commitment—new behaviors are practiced over a period of time to become a part of the individual's lifestyle

Learning Domains

A. To be considered successful, disease control education must result in evident behavioral changes; once an individual's learning needs have been assessed, a plan for teaching and learning can be designed
B. Three domains of learning have been classified in hierarchies and are used to specify learning objectives describing behaviors expected of the learner as the result of instruction
1. Cognitive domain—concerned with knowledge outcomes and intellectual abilities and skills; major hierarchical steps are knowledge, comprehension, application, analysis, synthesis, and evaluation
2. Affective domain—concerned with attitudes, interests, appreciation, and modes of interest; major hierarchical steps are receiving, responding, valuing, organization, and characterization
3. Psychomotor domain—concerned with levels of motor skills; major hierarchical steps are perception, set, guided response, mechanism, complex overt response, adaptation, and organization

Instructional Principles

See Chapter 14, Table 14-16 for dental management considerations with individuals who have special needs.
A. A teacher must know how to direct and facilitate learning in order to help people make positive changes in behavior
B. To maximize learning, the following principles can be applied to the design of an educational plan
1. Small step size—present only what the person can assimilate in one session; provide conceptual or factual information when the "need to know" is evident
2. Active participation—provide the time and opportunity for the person to ask questions; offer suggestions and monitor practice of new skills to enhance learning and increase retention
3. Immediate feedback—provide the learner with early and frequent information regarding progress; make suggestions for improvement and use positive reinforcement to support and encourage learning
4. Self-pacing—recognize that each person will progress at a different pace; recognize the learner's needs and establish an instructional pace tailored to each individual
C. Visual aids enhance verbal instructions
1. Use of printed visual aids or videotapes can enhance patient comprehension of oral hygiene instructions
2. Demonstration of bacterial plaque control techniques on models before intraoral demonstration may be helpful
3. Written instructions and illustrated pamphlets reinforce in-office instructions

Human Behavior Principles

A. Values
1. Values form the basis for behaviors
2. Clients come to the dental hygienist with existing values
3. Conflicts between clients' existing values and those that support and enable preventive oral care practices must be recognized and resolved
4. Clients who have value systems that support pre-

ventive health behaviors will adopt new behaviors that fit readily into their existing value system

B. Motivation
1. A desire to fulfill a human need that is in deficit; an inner force that causes a person to act
2. May be internally or externally generated
   a. Internally generated motivation focuses on own perceived needs; generally longer lasting
   b. Extrinsically generated motivation is based on offers of punishment or reward; generally of shorter duration
C. Locus of control[3]
1. Internal locus of control—individuals feel they have control over their own outcomes and that their behavior will make a difference; they are most likely to adopt preventive health behaviors
2. External locus of control—individuals feel outcomes are out of their control and that whatever they do will not affect outcomes; they are less likely to change behaviors and rely more on the dental professional to take care of their problems

Health Belief Model

A. Based on the concept that one's beliefs direct behavior; model is used to explain and predict health behaviors and acceptance of health recommendations; emphasis is placed on *perceived* world of individual, which may differ from objective reality
B. Components
1. Susceptibility—individuals must believe that they are susceptible to a particular disease or condition
2. Severity—individuals must believe that if they get the particular disease or condition, the consequences will be serious
3. Asymptomatic nature of disease—individuals must believe that the disease may be present without their full awareness
4. Behavior change will be beneficial—individuals must believe that there are effective means of preventing or controlling the potential or existing problem and that action on their part will produce positive results
C. Cues to action—once beliefs 1 to 4 are accepted, the individual will act on them when necessary; the stronger the beliefs, the greater the potential that appropriate action will occur

Maslow's Hierarchy of Needs

A. Definition—theory regarding human nature that is used to explain the motivational process; Maslow[4] suggested that inner forces, or needs, drive a person to action; he classified needs in a pyramid according to their importance to the individual, his or her ability

to motivate, and the importance placed on their satisfaction; only when an individual's lower needs are met will the individual become concerned about higher-level needs; once needs are met, they no longer function as motivators

B. Hierarchy of needs
1. Physiologic needs—these survival needs are the most powerful and must be met before any others; they include the components necessary for body homeostasis, such as food, water, oxygen, sleep, temperature regulation, and sex
2. Security and safety needs—these needs are required for protection against physical or psychologic damage and are more cognitive than physiologic in nature; they include shelter, a job for economic self-sufficiency, and a well-organized, stable environment
3. Social needs—once the physiologic and security needs have been met, then the needs for love and social belonging become prime motivators; needs at this level include being accepted and loved, belonging to a group, and having the chance to give and receive friendship and love
4. Esteem or ego needs—two categories of needs exist at this level: one involves feelings of basic worth, such as competence, achievement, mastery, and independence; the other involves gaining the esteem of others and triggers learning and acquiring status, power, and higher-level skills
5. Self-actualization or self-realization needs—needs that drive the individual to reach the very top of his or her field; based on positive actions toward development, growth, and self-enhancement
C. Application—assessment of an individual's level of needs may aid in identification of motivational factors that can be targeted for enhancing behavior change

Factors Influencing Client Adherence to Preventive Regimen

A. Client/clinician interaction
1. The quality of communication between client and hygienist is a critical factor in achieving client adherence to new oral practices
2. Clients must be encouraged to share responsibility for their oral health
3. Authoritarian or autocratic verbal and nonverbal messages from the dental hygienist will be less effective than messages that allow for genuine client involvement and assumption of responsibility
4. The dental hygienist must recognize that old behaviors are hard to change because they generally satisfy needs; new behaviors are adopted slowly
B. Clients' support systems

1. Lifestyle and significant others influence the client's willingness and ability to carry out home care regimens
2. Support systems are important, especially with children and handicapped individuals who must depend on caregivers to carry out home care practices
C. Complexity of therapy
   1. Clients must agree that the time and effort required to practice preventive behaviors are reasonable
   2. Changes in basic lifestyle are harder to achieve than modest modifications to existing behaviors
   3. Cost and product availability affect adherence to home care regimens

Bacterial Plaque Detection

General Considerations

A. Because bacterial plaque is relatively invisible and many tooth surfaces are not easily accessed, teaching clients the skills necessary for disease control can be difficult
B. Agents that make supragingival plaque visible can enhance the teaching-learning process by
   1. Demonstrating a relationship between the presence of supragingival plaque and the clinical signs of disease
   2. Guiding skill development when applied before plaque removal
   3. Allowing evaluation of skill effectiveness when applied after plaque removal
C. Presence of subgingival plaque cannot be demonstrated by the use of disclosing agents
D. Plan for disease control education should include establishing the association between the presence of plaque and clinical signs of disease, such as bleeding
E. Subgingival plaque detection by the client is best managed when there is an understanding of the gingival sulcus and/or pocket and the clinical changes that will occur when bacterial plaque removal is not effective

Disclosing Agents

A. Erythrosin (FD & C Red No. 3 or No. 28)
   1. Available in tablet or solution form; most widely used agent
   2. Tablet form can be dissolved into a solution or chewed to dissolve in the mouth
   3. Tends to stain soft tissues, making postapplication evaluation of the gingiva difficult
B. Fluorescein dye (FD & C Yellow No. 8)
   1. Plaque stained with sodium fluorescein is visible only with the use of a special light source

2. More expensive to use but has the advantage of not interfering with gingival assessment or leaving visible stain on oral tissues
C. Two-tone dyes (FD & C Red No. 3 and Green No. 3)
   1. Combination solution; has the advantage of differentiating mature (stains blue) from new bacterial plaque (stains red)
   2. Discloses bacterial plaque but will not stain gingival tissues
D. Others
   1. Preparations made from iodine, basic fuchsin, merbromin (Mercurochrome), and Bismarck Brown have been used in the past, but are rarely used today
   2. Iodine solutions were a particular problem because they caused severe allergic reactions in sensitive individuals

Application Methods for Disclosing Agents

A. Solutions are applied with a cotton swab; tablets are chewed and swished; client is instructed to rinse and expectorate
B. Agents do not stain plaque-free tooth surfaces unless there is roughness, i.e., decalcification
C. Precautions
   1. Avoid using iodine solutions because they have an unpleasant taste and are associated with a high rate of allergic reactions
   2. Avoid staining restorative materials that may be susceptible to permanent discoloration
   3. Dispense the solution into a disposable cup; do not contaminate the solution by introducing applicators into the container bottle
   4. Erythrosin solutions contain alcohol, which can evaporate over time and alter the concentration of the solution
   5. To avoid staining the lips, apply a light coat of a nonpetroleum-based lubricant
   6. Avoid using before a sealant application
   7. Avoid the potential for staining clothing by providing appropriate protective drapes and using small amounts of solution

Mechanical Plaque Control on Facial, Lingual, and Occlusal Tooth Surfaces

Basic Concepts

A. Products of bacterial plaque metabolism contribute to the initiation of both dental caries and periodontal diseases
B. Mechanical disruption of organized bacterial plaque

colonies, both supra- and subgingivally, is an effective and widely used means of preventing and controlling dental disease

C. Toothbrushing is the most widely used and effective means of controlling bacterial plaque on the facial, lingual, and occlusal surfaces of teeth

D. A wide variety of toothbrush shapes, sizes, and textures are available; new designs are marketed based on manufacturers' claims of superior plaque control capabilities and consumer appeal

E. Brush selection should be based on the client's needs and preferences

F. Special attention to subgingival plaque control in areas deeper than 3 mm is essential; toothbrushes are generally ineffective in depths beyond 3 mm and in furcae; additional tools must be selected

Manual Toothbrushes

A. Description
1. Parts include the handle, head, and shank; the head, or working end, holds clusters of bristles (tufts) in a pattern
2. Design variables
   a. Handle can be in the same plane with the head or offset at an angle
   b. Total length varies, with adult brushes longer than those recommended for children
   c. Tuft placement can be in two to four rows with anywhere from 5 to 12 tufts per row
   d. Brushing planes are even, flat, or uneven
   e. Many newer brushes have bristles of varying lengths, contoured/thick handles, and angled shanks
3. Bristle characteristics
   a. Natural bristles come from hog or boar hairs and are nonuniform in diameter, texture, or durability; hollow bristles may harbor bacteria and absorb water, making them soft and soggy with repeated use
   b. Nylon bristles, or filaments, are manufactured according to specifications that control for uniformity in texture, shape, and size; nonabsorbent nylon bristles are easily cleaned, dry quickly, and are more durable than natural bristles
   c. Relative stiffness—diameter and length of the bristle determine whether the brush will be termed hard, medium, soft, or extra soft
   d. Bristle ends can be cut flat or polished to be rounded at the tip

B. Desirable characteristics—the American Dental Association (ADA) Council on Dental Materials, Instruments, and Equipment recommends many types of toothbrushes; desirable characteristics include the following
1. Conform to individual requirements in size, shape, and texture
2. Be easily and efficiently manipulated
3. Be readily cleaned and aerated
4. Be impervious to moisture
5. Be durable and inexpensive

C. Factors in toothbrush selection—the following factors will influence the recommendation of a particular type and size of toothbrush
1. Oral health status
2. Method of brushing recommended
3. Configuration of hard and soft tissues
4. Patient age, dexterity, and ability to use a brush in an effective and nontraumatic manner
5. Patient preference and motivation

D. Soft, multitufted brushes are generally recommended based on their usefulness in both supra- and subgingival plaque disruption with minimal likelihood of soft and hard tissue trauma

Manual Toothbrushing Methods

Although the Bass, or sulcular, method is widely recognized as the most effective, and therefore, most often recommended method, it is helpful to know about several major techniques. The method selected should disrupt both supra- and subgingival bacterial plaque to the extent possible. The issue of gingival stimulation is of lesser importance than plaque control. Although a horizontal scrub technique is often used, it is not recommended because of potential trauma to hard and soft tissues.

In all of the following methods, the handle is placed parallel to the occlusal plane for posterior (facial and lingual) and anterior facial surfaces, and parallel to the long axis of the tooth (using the toe of the brush) for anterior lingual surfaces. Occlusal surfaces are cleaned with a scrubbing motion.

A. Bass or sulcular brushing method
1. Technique—direct the bristles into the sulcus at a 45 degree angle to the long axis of the tooth; vibrate the bristles in a short back-and-forth motion
2. Advantages—disrupts plaque at and under the gingival margin; good gingival stimulation; widely recognized as an effective plaque control technique

B. Stillman's method
1. Technique—position the bristles on the attached gingiva and direct them apically at a 45 degree angle to the long axis of the tooth; use a firm, gentle vibration with the bristles stationary
2. Advantages—good gingival stimulation

C. Roll method
1. Technique—place the side of the bristles on the

attached gingiva and direct them apically; turn the wrist to roll or sweep the bristles over the gingiva and tooth

   2. Advantages—accesses entire facial and lingual tooth surfaces; often combined with Bass, Charters', or Stillman's method

D. Charters' method

   1. Technique—position the bristle tips toward the occlusal surfaces at a 45 degree angle to the long axis of the tooth; move bristles in a short back-and-forth motion

   2. Advantages—useful with orthodontic appliances, fixed appliances, and following periodontal surgery when sulcular brushing must be avoided to allow wound healing

E. Fones (circular) method

   1. Technique—with upper and lower teeth together, place the bristles perpendicular to the buccal tooth surfaces; use wide circular motion to cover the gingiva and tooth surfaces of both arches; on the lingual, use smaller circles to brush each arch separately

   2. Advantages—easy to learn and execute; can be mastered by children

F. Combination methods

   1. Modified Bass method—combination of the Bass and roll methods

   2. Modified Stillman's method—combination of the Stillman's and roll methods

Powered Toothbrushes

A. General description

   1. Brush head and shank are separate from the handle, which contains the power source

   2. Handles are larger than manual brushes

   3. May receive ADA seal of acceptance after manufacturer submits studies to ADA Council on Dental Materials, Instruments, and Equipment or Council on Scientific Affairs

B. Power source—cordless rechargeable stand plugs into an electrical outlet; when the brush handle is replaced in the stand, the power unit in the handle is recharged; power level is relatively consistent

C. Motion—rapid, short strokes occur in one or a combination of the following basic motions

   1. Head moves to provide elliptic brush strokes

   2. Reciprocating action

   3. Oscillating horizontal and vertical strokes

   4. Rotating tufts of bristles or contrarotary tufts

   5. Vibratory to simulate Bass technique

   6. Some units add sonic vibrations to the mechanical motion of the brush

D. Indications for use

   1. Persons who lack manual dexterity or discipline necessary to master an effective manual toothbrushing technique

   2. Physically and mentally challenged persons (or caregivers)

   3. Persons who prefer purchasing the latest technology and may therefore demonstrate increased adherence

   4. Persons with orthodontic appliances or implants[5]

   5. Persons who prefer a powered toothbrush

   6. Persons with dental stain

Powered Toothbrushing Methods

A. Client variables and manufacturer instructions will determine the need for individualized modifications

B. General principles

   1. Read manufacturer's instructions for use and care

   2. Select soft-bristle brushes to avoid tissue trauma

   3. Select a low-abrasive dentifrice to control the potential for tooth abrasion

   4. Apply a small amount of dentifrice before activating the brush

   5. Position the head and bristles for specific brushing needs and the specific method being used

   6. Hold the brush in one location for a period of time; some powered brushes have time indicators on the handle

   7. Gain access and visibility by retracting the lips and cheeks

   8. Monitor pressure applied to avoid trauma to soft and hard tissues

Comparison of Powered and Manual Toothbrushes

A. Reported effectiveness

   1. Powered brushes compare favorably with manual brushes in their ability to reduce bacterial plaque and gingivitis

   2. Powered brushes have been shown to be more effective than manual brushes for interproximal plaque removal and some powered brushes compare favorably with floss and toothpicks[5,6]

   3. Power brushes were effective in removal of bacterial plaque and control of gingivitis in periodontal maintenance clients[7]

   4. A powered brush with contrarotary tufts has been shown to be twice as effective as manual brushes in subgingival and interproximal plaque removal[8]

   5. Studies have demonstrated that a sonic brush removes extrinsic stains more effectively than manual brushing[9]

B. Powered brushes tend to be easier to use; because the motion is built in, the client has only to properly position the brush head and hold it in place long enough to be effective

Single-tufted Brushes

A. Design—flat or tapered trim
B. Suggested use—to remove bacterial plaque from surfaces not accessible with larger brushes, including areas of crowded or malpositioned teeth, distal surfaces of terminal molars, around pontics, in furcations, and on lingual surfaces of molars; also useful for cleaning fixed orthodontic appliances
C. Technique—position tuft at or just under gingival margin and use a sulcular brushing stroke; placement of tapered angled side against tooth allows for insertion of bristles several millimeters subgingivally

Factors in Toothbrushing Effectiveness

A. Sequence
   1. A methodical, systematic approach will enhance effectiveness
   2. Suggested sequence: begin systematic overlapping strokes at the facial aspect of the maxillary right or left terminal tooth and continue around the arch to the terminal tooth on the opposite side; switch to the lingual aspect and begin working back toward the starting side; use the same pattern for the mandible, then brush the occlusal surfaces
B. Duration
   1. Each time the brush is moved, the time spent in an area should be monitored by counting strokes or seconds
   2. Total manual brushing time of 3 to 5 minutes has been suggested; powered brushes may be used for 2 minutes
C. Frequency
   1. Thorough bacterial plaque removal once a day is the minimum requirement for maintaining periodontal health; it may not, however, be the optimum regimen for some individuals
   2. Frequency should be increased when gingival or periodontal conditions warrant it or when caries risk or activity is high
   3. Brushing removes residual food debris as well as bacterial plaque and is one method for self-application of topical fluoride
D. Skill level
   1. Careful attention should be given to evaluating skill development in all components of brush manipulation, including grasp, placement, activation, wrist movement, and amount of pressure applied
   2. Control of brush placement and motion is essential for effectiveness

Improper Toothbrushing

A. Need to assess
   1. Improper toothbrushing may be a result of a lack of education in proper technique, incorrect application following instruction, or long-established habits
   2. The dental hygienist should plan to evaluate the brushing technique and monitor hard and soft tissue conditions at each continued care visit
   3. Faulty placement, overvigorous motion and/or pressure, and use of a brush with frayed or broken bristles can lead to unwanted consequences
B. Acute consequences—soft tissue injuries such as denuded attached gingiva, lesions that appear punched out and red, and clusters of small ulcerations at the gingival margin
C. Chronic consequences
   1. Soft tissue—loss of gingival tissue or change in contour; malpositioned and/or prominent teeth and an inadequate band of attached gingiva are predisposing factors
   2. Hard tissue—loss of tooth structure and creation of wedge-shaped indentations at the cervical third of the tooth (toothbrush abrasion); malpositioned and/or prominent teeth, toothpastes with highly abrasive formulas, and hard-bristled toothbrushes contribute to the problem

Toothbrush Maintenance

A. Brushes should be rinsed clean after each use, then allowed to air-dry in an upright position
B. Rotating use of more than one brush during 24 hours prolongs brush life
C. Brushes should be replaced when bristles splay or lose resiliency, generally no longer than 3 to 4 months
D. Some brushes have color indicator bristles to monitor replacement time
E. Brushes should be replaced after an illness such as cold or flu or disinfected with a household bleach solution

Controlling Mouth Odors

A. Identifying malodor
   1. Oral malodor (bad breath/halitosis) is a common problem that usually originates in the mouth; systemic causes for oral malodor are less common than intraoral causes
   2. Malodors are produced by microorganisms, usually gram negative, and by smoking
   3. Most common sites for malodor are: posterior area of dorsal surface of the tongue, interdental and subgingival areas, food impaction sites, leaking or overhanging restorations, and dentures

4. Bad breath may be a warning sign of periodontal infections, and is common in necrotizing ulcerative gingivitis (NUG)
5. Individuals often assess their own mouth odors inaccurately; they may be unaware of malodor or may exaggerate severity of odors
6. Most malodors can be eliminated by oral hygiene, including tongue cleaning, possible rinsing with an antimicrobial mouthrinse, and smoking cessation[10]

B. Technique for tongue cleaning
   1. Brushing
      a. With the tongue extended, the brush is placed on the dorsum of the tongue with the tips directed toward the throat; placement is as far posterior as the person can tolerate
      b. Apply light pressure and move the brush forward and out; repeat to cover the entire surface; avoid vigorous scrubbing
   2. Tongue-cleaning devices
      a. Tongue-cleaning devices are available in various designs, but all have some sort of flexible or rigid scraping surface or strip
      b. Device is placed toward the back of the tongue on the dorsal surface, then pulled forward while light pressure is applied

Interdental Bacterial Plaque Control

Basic Concepts

A. Although toothbrushes are effective in removing bacterial plaque from the facial, lingual, and occlusal surfaces of the teeth, they are relatively ineffective on the proximal surfaces
B. Devices designed for access to interproximal surfaces are essential for effective control of bacterial plaque
C. Interdental col area is a protected area that tends to harbor microorganisms that can initiate disease
D. Anatomy of the interdental area is a significant factor in both disease initiation and control
E. Anatomic changes such as loss of papillae and bone, the presence of malpositioned teeth, or tooth loss contribute to interdental bacterial retention

Factors to Consider When Selecting Interdental Cleaning Methods

A. Soft tissue variables include the level of health or disease and the position and architecture of the gingiva and attachment
   1. Type I embrasures are occupied by the interdental papillae

   2. Type II embrasures have slight to moderate recession of the interdental papillae[1]
   3. Type III embrasures have extensive recession or complete loss of interdental papillae[1]
B. Hard tissue variables include tooth position, root anatomy, and the status of restorations and/or prostheses
C. Client variables include the level of manual dexterity, adherence, skill development, and personal preferences

Flosses and Tapes

A. Dental floss is the most frequently recommended device for interdental cleaning of type I embrasures[1]
B. Flossing may precede or follow brushing in a home care regimen
C. As recession increases, as in type II and type III embrasures, the effectiveness of floss decreases; other interdental plaque control aids should be selected[1]
D. Floss type—clinical trials have failed to demonstrate one type as being superior to the other
   1. Unwaxed—unbound filaments spread on the tooth and have more friction for cleaning; filaments hold plaque and debris for easier removal; floss, being less bulky, slips through contacts more easily
   2. Waxed—resists tearing and shredding on faulty restorations or when moved through very tight contacts
   3. Polytetrafluoroethylene (PTFE-type floss)—slides through contacts easily; does not fray; equally effective when compared with waxed floss; may enhance client adherence because of high preference ratings[11]
   4. Tape or ribbon—wider, flatter type of floss covers a broad surface
   5. Variable diameter
      a. Tufted segment combined with floss acts like a brush against proximal surfaces; accesses concavities and irregular surfaces; recommended for type II embrasures
      b. Stiffened end can be threaded under fixed bridge pontics and orthodontic bands
   6. Braided nylon—for use with dental implants
      a. Has a stiff nylon end for threading under implant prostheses
      b. May be rinsed and dried for reuse[1]

Flossing Technique

A. Floss length —varies with the holding technique; 10 to 15 inches when forming a loop; 12 to 24 inches when wrapping around fingers
B. Holding technique

1. Ends may be tied together to form a loop, wrapped around the middle fingers, or tucked into the palm
2. With equal tension in both hands, grasp with both thumbs or the thumb and forefinger for use on the maxilla or with both forefingers for use on the mandible; leave ½- to 1-inch length between fingers

C. Insertion
1. Approach the embrasure space obliquely and ease the floss past the contact with a back-and-forth motion
2. Snapping through the contact can cause tissue injury

D. Adaptation and stroke
1. Position the fingers so that the floss wraps securely against the proximal surface and forms a C shape against the tooth
2. Slide beneath the gingival margin and move in an apicocoronal direction several times

Improper Flossing

A. Acute consequences—snapping through contacts, failure to curve the floss against proximal surfaces, and application of excessive pressure can result in floss cuts of the interdental papillae
B. Chronic consequences
1. Soft tissue—excessive pressure applied submarginally can be destructive to the attachment fibers
2. Hard tissue—repeated heavy sawing movements in a faciolingual direction can abrade proximal tooth structure

Flossing Aids

A. Types of aids
1. Floss holders
   a. General description—double-pronged plastic device onto which the floss is threaded and held, forming a span between the prongs
   b. Technique—prepared holder is positioned for insertion, then adapted and activated in much the same manner as hand-held floss; special care should be taken not to snap the floss through contacts
   c. Indications for use—when an individual lacks the dexterity to floss properly, when tooth position or restorations prevent passing floss through contact areas, and client preference
2. Floss threaders
   a. General description—firm, flexible, blunt ended devices for moving floss through closed contacts or under pontics; a variety of designs are available
   b. Technique—position the floss in the threader with even lengths on each side; pass the threader

through the embrasure from the buccal to the lingual aspect, leaving sufficient length on the buccal aspect; remove the threader and use the floss in a normal manner

Interdental Brushes

A. General description
1. Soft nylon filaments are twisted onto a stainless steel wire to form either a tapered or nontapered small brush; wire may be plastic coated for use around dental implants
2. Some brushes must be used with a special handle; others have wires long enough to use as handles
3. Provide excellent access to root concavities, furcation areas, and proximal surfaces where papillae do not fill interdental spaces as in type II and type III embrasures[1]

B. Technique
1. Choose a brush of appropriate size, moisten the filaments, insert interproximally, and use an in-and-out motion from the buccal to the lingual aspect and from the lingual to the buccal aspect
2. Brushes may be aimed into furcation areas in a similar manner
3. Filaments compress when moving through constricted areas and flare out to adapt to larger spaces
4. Access into interproximal pockets may be achieved with careful vertical placement and movement

C. Precautions
1. Avoid forcing through tight, tissue-filled areas because serious trauma can result
2. Unless properly adapted and activated, the stainless steel wire can puncture tissue
3. Discard the tip when filaments lose their original shape

D. Indications for use—when access permits, for disrupting plaque from root concavities, proximal surfaces, and furcation areas, for delivery of antimicrobial agents

Specialized Bacterial Plaque Control Devices

Gauze Strips

A. Suggested use—on proximal surfaces when large diastemas are present, teeth are isolated, or there is no adjacent tooth; type II embrasures[1]
B. Technique—use one 1-inch width of bandage gauze cut into a 6-inch length and folded the long way into thirds; adapt to the open proximal surface and move back and forth several times
C. Limitations—no subgingival plaque disruption

Knitting Yarn

A. Suggested use—on proximal surfaces with type II embrasures, diastemas, and isolated teeth
B. Technique—use synthetic yarn, not wool; wrap in a C shape against the tooth and move it up and down like floss
C. Limitations—no subgingival access; seldom used as a variety of flosses and interdental brushes are available

Pipe Cleaners

A. Suggested use—to remove bacterial plaque from exposed furcation areas and open interdental areas (see Chapter 4 on furca anatomy)
B. Technique—cut the pipe cleaner to a manageable length, approximately 2 inches; attempt to round off the sharp wire edges and adapt the end to the space; move back and forth several times
C. Precautions—if not properly adapted, pipe wire can cause trauma to soft tissues
D. Limitations—less effective than interdental brushes, but cost may be lower than other aids

Powered Interdental Cleaning Device

A. Design—new powered interdental cleaning device (Braun Oral-B Interclean); a Hytrel filament extrudes and rotates on interproximal surfaces
B. Technique—requires only one hand to operate; tip is aimed into the interproximal space
C. Suggested use—alternative to hand held floss; limited short-term studies have demonstrated safety and effectiveness in removal of interproximal plaque, reduction of gingival inflammation and bleeding on probing[17]

Wooden Devices

A. Toothpicks
   1. Suggested use—for proximal surfaces and concavities, furcation areas, type II embrasures, and just under the gingival margin; also useful around fixed orthodontic bands[1]
   2. Technique—round toothpicks can be used alone in some areas or inserted into special holders (periodontal aids) angulated to enhance access; moisten the tip and adapt it to the surface to be cleaned; subgingivally (submarginally) use a 45-degree angle to the tooth; move in and out several times for interproximal surfaces and follow the tooth contour on facial or lingual surfaces
   3. Precautions—rigid pointed tips can cause injury if forced into tight tissue areas; over time papillae will abrade if toothpicks are used improperly
B. Interdental wedges
   1. Suggested use—for proximal surfaces or just under the gingival margin; triangular in cross sections; should be used interproximally only when there is adequate space for insertion, e.g., type II embrasures[1]
   2. Technique—moisten the tip, position the flat base of the triangle at the gingival border, insert with the tip angled slightly toward the occlusal, and move the wedge in and out with moderate pressure against the surface
   3. Precautions—to avoid gingival splinters, discard tips as soon as splaying occurs; using a fulcrum increases control and reduces the risk of inserting with too much pressure; repeated insertion with tip perpendicular to long axis of tooth may cause blunting of interdental papillae

Special Tips

A. Rubber tip
   1. Suggested uses—for proximal surfaces, in exposed furcations, and under gingival margins; authors differ on the rubber tip's ability to remove plaque; may be used to maintain interproximal gingival contours or recontour papillae following periodontal surgery[5]
   2. Technique
      a. Bacterial plaque removal—trace gingival margin with tip aimed into sulcus
      b. Contouring gingivae—place but do not force the tip into the interdental contour with the tip angled occlusally, press the side of the tip against the gingiva, and use a firm rotary motion to apply intermittent pressure
   3. Precaution—insertion perpendicular to the long axis of the tooth can result in flattened interdental papillae
B. Plastic tip
   1. Suggested use—for open furcation and interdental areas
   2. Technique—similar to that with the rubber tip
   3. Precautions—hard, rigid tip does not adapt easily and can cause discomfort and trauma

Dentifrices

Basic Concepts

A. Definition—substance used with a toothbrush on accessible tooth surfaces; available in gel, paste, or powder form
B. Purposes
   1. Cosmetic—tooth surfaces are cleaned and polished; breath is freshened
   2. Cosmetic-therapeutic—certain   nondrug   sub-

stances augment the efficiency of the brush in the removal of plaque, debris, and stain

  3. Therapeutic—vehicle for transporting biologically active ingredients to the tooth and its environment; fluoride dentifrices inhibit tooth demineralization

C. Basic ingredients

  1. Detergents—lower surface tension to loosen debris and stains; provide the foaming characteristic
  2. Cleaning and polishing agents—abrasives that help remove stain, plaque, and debris from tooth surfaces and give a luster to the tooth surface; should provide maximal cleaning benefit with minimal abrasion
  3. Humectants—retain moisture to ensure a chemically and physically stable product
  4. Binding agents—prevent separation by increasing the consistency of the mixture of liquid and solid ingredients
  5. Flavoring and sweetening agents—provide a pleasant and refreshing flavor and aftertaste and cover unpleasant flavors
  6. Coloring agents—contribute to the product's attractiveness and desirability
  7. Preservatives—prevent bacterial growth and prolong shelf life

Therapeutic Ingredients

A. Definition—biologically active ingredients that produce a beneficial effect on either the hard or soft tissues; dentifrices claiming therapeutic effects are eligible for acceptance by the ADA Council on Scientific Affairs, formerly the Council on Dental Therapeutics; updated lists from ADA should be consulted at least annually

B. Fluoride agents—substantial data exist to show that approved fluoride dentifrices reduce the incidence of caries; fluorides currently used in dentifrices are sodium fluoride, sodium monofluorophosphate, and stabilized stannous fluoride

C. Plaque-inhibiting agents—research has been and continues to be done on the formulation of dentifrices with agents that will reduce plaque formation and gingivitis; examples include sanguinaria, chlorhexidine, lactoperoxidase, triclosan, zinc, and stabilized stannous fluoride

D. Desensitizing agents—fluoride agents have been claimed to have desensitizing properties and are contained in specialized dentifrices (e.g., stannous fluoride); nonfluoride agents commonly used in desensitizing dentifrices include strontium chloride, potassium nitrate, and sodium citrate

E. Tartar control agents—interfere with the calcium-phosphate bond in the calculus matrix, thus allowing easier removal of soft calculus during toothbrushing; effective only on formation of supragingival calculus on enamel surfaces

  1. Pyrophosphate system—pyrophosphate has a negative charge, attracts positively charged calcium ions, and interferes with calculus formation
  2. Zinc system—zinc has a positive charge, attracts negatively charged phosphate ions, and interferes with calculus formation

F. Whitening agents—several dentifrices are marketed for their ability to remove stains; several whitening dentifrices have low abrasive levels; may be effective for maintenance of cosmetic restorations

G. Baking soda—manufacturers claim benefits from addition of baking soda or baking soda and peroxide to dentifrices; therapeutic benefits have not been demonstrated in controlled clinical trials

Guidelines for Dentifrice Selection

A. Products selected should carry the American Dental Association (ADA) seal; acceptance ensures that adequate evidence of safety and efficacy has been demonstrated in controlled clinical trials, that advertising claims comply with ADA standards for accuracy and truthfulness, and that the fluoride will be bioavailable when the dentifrice is used

B. All ADA accepted dentifrices have safe levels of abrasiveness

C. Dentifrices containing fluoride are granted acceptance based on their caries-reduction properties

D. Tartar control dentifrices contain fluoride; those that carry the ADA seal have gained acceptance for the proven efficacy of the fluoride mechanism, not for their tartar control properties, which have not been shown to have a therapeutic value in the prevention and control of periodontal disease

E. Desensitizing dentifrices that carry the ADA seal have gained acceptance for proven efficacy in the control of dentinal hypersensitivity

F. Dentifrices that claim therapeutic benefits other than dental caries reduction (from fluoride) or control of hypersensitivity have not been awarded the ADA seal for such claimed benefits

Guidelines for Dentifrice Use[13]

A. Daily use of fluoride dentifrice should be recommended for all individuals, regardless of caries risk, because these products promote tooth remineralization

B. Young children (under age 6) should be supervised when using fluoride dentifrice

  1. Use of a small pea-sized amount of a toothpaste or

gel containing no more than 1100 ppm fluoride is recommended

2. Swallowing should be avoided
3. Dental fluorosis has been associated with use of more than a pea sized amount of toothpaste by young children living in fluoridated communities[14]

Oral Irrigation

Basic Concepts

Oral irrigation can be a valuable adjunct in helping to maintain oral cleanliness and health; oral irrigating devices force a steady or pulsating stream of water over the gingival tissue and teeth with the goal of removing unattached debris and reducing the concentration of bacteria and cellular end products that may be present; irrigators are also used to deliver antimicrobial agents supra- and subgingivally

Home Irrigation

A. Suggested use
  1. Before brushing and flossing to remove debris or retained food particles or after to deliver antimicrobials
  2. Debridement of recessed areas of fixed prosthetic or orthodontic appliances; around implants
  3. Flushing of periodontal pockets with a controlled, low-intensity pulsated stream of water
B. General description—types of irrigators
  1. Hand syringes—blunt tip, side port cannula; requires high level of dexterity and motivation; not recommended for most clients
  2. Power-driven device—unit with a water reservoir; plugs into an electrical outlet to create a pulsating jet of water; water pressure is regulated by an adjustable dial
  3. Water pressure-driven devices—attaches directly to the water faucet to deliver a constant stream of water; pressure is controlled by regulating the faucet
  4. Tips—standard jet tip or flexible subgingival tip; tips with side or end port design show similar effectiveness
C. Technique for use of powered irrigators
  1. Adjust the water stream to low pressure setting
  2. Lean over the washbasin
  3. Direct the tip interproximally at a right angle (90°) to the tooth surfaces; the stream should move in a horizontal direction through the gingival embrasure
  4. Soft tips designed for subgingival access may be angled into the sulcus

D. Addition of antimicrobial agents—studies document efficacy beyond use of irrigating devices with water alone
  1. Ciancio and coworkers[15,16] demonstrated that plaque and bleeding index scores were significantly reduced with the use of Listerine and the Water Pik when compared with controls
  2. Moderate reduction in total bacterial counts and motile rods were achieved in the Listerine group in the same study
  3. Flemming and coworkers[17] demonstrated efficacy of chlorhexidine (CH) (Peridex) and Water Pik irrigation in reducing gingival inflammation and bleeding on probing when compared with water irrigation, CH rinsing, and toothbrushing controls
  4. Vignarajah and coworkers[18] demonstrated improvement in plaque index, papillary bleeding index, and probeable pocket depths with the use of 0.1% CH and Water Pik irrigation as compared with normal saline irrigation controls
  5. Parsons and coworkers[19] suggested that dilute solutions of sanguinaria delivered supragingivally via an irrigation device reduced established plaque and gingivitis more than manual rinsing with the same product
  6. Boyd and coworkers[20] demonstrated improvement in clinical parameters measured, including plaque index, gingival index, bleeding tendency, loss of attachment, and microbiologic samples of subgingival plaque, with use of 0.02% stannous fluoride solution and the Water Pik as compared with irrigation using water
  7. Depth of penetration into sulcus is generally limited to approximately 4 mm[21]
  8. No studies demonstrate significant benefits in treating periodontitis; demonstrated benefits are currently limited to other parameters, such as plaque and bleeding indices; gingivitis, and reduction of bleeding on probing
E. Precautions
  1. Clients should be taught the proper use of irrigating devices and monitored for adverse effects
  2. Tissue punctures or reductions in the height of papillae are potential outcomes if the pressure used is too great or application is too long in one area
  3. Transient bacteremias may occur following oral irrigation, particularly when untreated disease is present; patients who are at risk for infective endocarditis should be advised against using these devices
  4. Contraindicated for persons with periodontal abscess or ulcerative lesions

In-Office Irrigation

A. Suggested use
1. As an adjunct to mechanical root debridement
2. Studies on the benefits of in-office irrigation vary widely[22,23]; there is little evidence to support in-office irrigation as a means of enhancing efficacy of scaling and root planing[24]
3. An essential oils mouthrinse demonstrates efficacy as a preprocedural irrigant and rinse when used as an adjunct to prophylactic premedication to reduce bloodborne bacteria following invasive dental procedures (i.e., manual or ultrasonic scaling) in persons at risk for infectious endocarditis[25]
4. Simultaneous antimicrobial irrigation and ultrasonic scaling have demonstrated some enhancement of scaling efficacy[26,27]

B. General description—types of irrigators
1. Hand syringe—blunt tip, side-opening cannula
2. Part of an ultrasonic scaling unit
3. Air-driven handpiece attachment

C. Technique for use
1. Techniques for hand syringe and powered irrigators are essentially the same; pressure must be controlled for both
2. Use adequate suction throughout procedure
3. Fill reservoir or syringe with full strength or diluted antimicrobial solution selected; powered irrigators usually use dilution with equal parts water
4. Bend cannula by using protective sheath
5. Adjust flow rate of powered unit to low setting; settings vary with the viscosity of the solution selected
6. Insert cannula to base of pocket/sulcus and retract 1 mm
7. Release irrigant in all areas to be irrigated
8. Consult manufacturer's directions for cleaning and maintenance of the unit; dispose of cannula in biohazard container for sharp objects

D. Antimicrobial agents
1. Stannous fluoride—1.64% SnF_2; dispense equal parts of 3.28% SnF_2 concentrated gel and distilled water; use fresh mixture for each patient
2. Chlorhexidine digluconate—0.12%; may dilute to .06% concentration
3. Essential oils mouthrinse; may dilute with equal parts water for use in powered irrigator
4. Povidone-iodine, metronidazole, and tetracycline have been used

E. Precautions
1. Use of low pressure prevents gingival tissue trauma
2. Persons who are at risk for infectious endocarditis require prophylactic antibiotic coverage according to American Heart Association recommendations

Disease Control for Individuals With Fixed and/or Removable Prostheses

Basic Concepts

A. Clients wearing fixed and/or removable dental prostheses have unique needs that require specific procedures for maintaining both the prosthesis and the retained natural teeth

B. Terminology[28]
1. Appliance—in dentistry, a general term referring to a device used to provide a function or therapeutic effect
2. Abutment—tooth, root, or implant used for support and retention of either a fixed or removable dental prosthesis
3. Clasp—retains and stabilizes denture by attaching it to the abutment teeth
4. Denture—artificial substitute for missing natural teeth and adjacent tissues
5. Pontic—artificial tooth on a fixed partial denture or isolated tooth on a removable partial denture that replaces the lost natural tooth, restores its function, and usually occupies the space previously occupied by the natural crown
6. Dental prosthesis—replacement for one or more of the teeth or other oral structures, ranging from a single tooth to a complete denture
7. Fixed prosthesis—dental prosthesis firmly attached to natural teeth, roots, or implants usually by a cementing agent; cannot be removed by the client
8. Removable prosthesis—dental prosthesis that can readily be placed in the mouth and removed by the wearer
9. Orthodontic bracket—a small metal attachment fixed to a band that serves as a means of fastening the arch wire to the band
10. Orthodontic band—a thin metal ring that secures orthodontic attachments to a tooth
11. Orthodontic wire—a slender, pliable rod or thread of metal used as a source of force to direct teeth to move in desired directions
12. Implant—a device surgically inserted into the jawbone to be used as a prosthodontic abutment

Fixed Prosthesis Maintenance

A. Fixed prostheses such as fixed bridges and orthodontic bands and wires increase the potential for bacterial plaque and debris retention, making access to proximal surfaces more difficult

B. Home care armamentarium allow wearer to
1. Use floss threaders to move floss beneath pontics and between pontics and abutments

2. Access interdental spaces apical to closed contacts using interdental brushes
3. Move into and/or around orthodontic brackets, bands, and wires with special brushes or toothpicks
4. Adapt to the area between the orthodontic appliances and the gingival margin
   a. Special orthodontic brushes available: three rows wide with trimmed, shorter middle row that fits over bands, brackets, and wires
   b. Two-row brushes that will adapt to the narrow area between bands and brackets and the gingiva

Dental Implant Maintenance

See Chapters 10 and 11, sections on dental implants and Chapter 13, section on plastic instruments for implant care.
A. Osteointegrated implants and superstructures require special home maintenance materials and techniques; clients must learn techniques for bacterial plaque control that prevent damage to the implant material and superstructure
B. Home care armamentarium may include
   1. Soft-bristled, multitufted nylon toothbrushes
   2. Interdental brushes with nylon coating over the metal wire cores; this prevents scratching the implant material, which is usually titanium
   3. Flat and tapered end-tuft brushes
   4. Dental floss
   5. Implant flossing aids—reusable braided nylon filament with hook leader for insertion; flat cotton floss; or floss containing a soft filament brush component
   6. Rubber tip stimulator; wood sticks
   7. Disclosing tablets or liquid; may be most useful during initial plaque control training
   8. Antimicrobial mouth rinse; chlorhexidine used twice a day is the rinse of choice posttreatment, other antimicrobial mouthrinses may be used for long-term treatment
   9. Small amount of ADA-approved gel or fine abrasive toothpaste; abrasive toothpastes must be avoided; tartar control formulas acceptable
   10. Oral irrigators may be used on the lowest setting with the tip directed perpendicular to the long axis of the tooth/implant; water, chlorhexidine .12%, phenolic based, or plant alkaloid mouthrinses may be used
C. Bacterial plaque control skill development
   1. Clients must be shown how to control bacterial plaque on all areas of the implant and superstructure
   2. Sufficient supervised practice will ensure adequate skill development

3. The dental hygienist should monitor bacterial plaque control at each continued care appointment and modify techniques as indicated

Removable Prosthesis Maintenance

A. Clients with removable appliances, including orthodontic retainers, must be educated on the need for conscientious home care without damage to the appliance body or clasps
B. Debris, stain, bacterial plaque, and calculus will collect on removable appliances if they are not routinely cleaned
C. Inadequate cleaning also may contribute to the development of soft tissue lesions underlying the appliance or to carious lesions on abutting tooth surfaces; chronic *Candida albicans* infection may also result
D. Removable prostheses can be maintained by
   1. Brushing with water and a mild detergent or dentifrice after each meal and before retiring
      a. Special denture brushes have two different arrangements of filaments to access both the inner curved surface and the outer and occlusal surfaces
      b. Special clasp brushes have a narrow, tapered cylindric design that can adapt to the inner clasp surface, a prime site for bacterial plaque formation and retention
   2. Immersion in a solvent or detergent solution that chemically loosens or removes stains and deposits; appliance should be brushed following soaking to remove residual debris and chemicals; commonly used agents include: dilute sodium hypoclorite (bleach), alkaline peroxide, vinegar, and various enzymes that render proteins less adhesive; bleach will cause corrosion and is not recommended on appliances with metal
E. Removable appliances should be removed at night and stored in a covered container with water or one of the denture solutions listed above
F. Cleansing procedures
   1. Hold the appliance securely to avoid dropping and breakage
   2. When brushing, hold the appliance over a sink partly filled with water or lined with a cushioning material
   3. Overzealous brushing or the use of a strong abrasive should be avoided; plastic resin material can be scratched or abraded to the extent that denture fit is compromised
   4. Remove denture adhesive material from the appliance and underlying mucosa several times a day
   5. Brush the underlying mucosa at least once a day with a soft toothbrush

6. Solutions used for cleansing or soaking a denture should be renewed for each use

Fluorides

See Chapter 10, subsection on fluoride gels. See Chapter 15, section on measures for preventing and controlling oral diseases.

General Considerations

A. Most effective agent for the prevention and control of dental caries, especially on smooth surfaces
B. Multitherapeutic approach most effective; three categories of administration should be considered
    1. Systemic—community water supplies, institutional water supplies, and dietary supplementation
    2. Professional application
    3. Self-applied dentifrices, rinses, and gels
C. Safe when used in recommended amounts and concentrations, but dental hygienists must be aware of the potential for both acute and chronic adverse effects
    1. Large quantities of fluoride products should not be stored in the home
    2. Institutions that have fluoride programs must handle and store fluoride products properly
    3. Parents must be educated to supervise home use of products containing fluoride by young children to prevent acute toxic reactions or long-term effects (e.g., dental fluorosis)
    4. Products intended for topical application should not be swallowed
    5. If excessive amounts have been ingested, vomiting should be induced immediately with ipecac or manually; calcium solution or milk should be administered to slow absorption rate; emergency medical care should be obtained

Systemic Fluorides

A. Ingestion of optimally fluoridated water (approximately 1 ppm) during tooth formation provides highest percentage of caries reduction
B. Maximum benefits are obtained when provided from onset of tooth development until tooth eruption is complete
C. Children between 6 months and 16 years who drink less than optimally fluoridated water should receive dietary fluoride supplementation (for dosage schedule, see Chapter 15, Measures for Preventing and Controlling Oral Diseases)[13]
D. It is not necessary to provide dietary supplementation for pregnant and lactating women who drink less than optimally fluoridated water
E. The dental hygienist has a key role in educating both parents and children about the value of systemic fluoride and gaining their commitment to follow prescribed fluoride supplementation regimens

Fluoride Agents for Professional Application

A. Neutral sodium fluoride (NaF)
    1. Characteristics—first fluoride used for topical application; available as a powder, aqueous solution, foam, or gel; 2% concentration
    2. Application intervals—series of four applications administered 1 week apart at intervals that coincide with the eruption of primary and permanent teeth; suggested ages are 3, 7, 10, and 13 years; some clinicians may administer NaF applications at 6 month intervals as a substitute for APF when porcelain and/or certain types of composite restorations are present; this method of application has not been substantiated in the literature
    3. Advantages—stable solution in plastic containers; relative absence of taste; does not stain teeth or irritate soft tissues; safe for porcelain crowns and composite restorations
B. Stannous fluoride (SnF_2)
    1. Characteristics—available as a powder in gelatin capsules to make an 8% aqueous solution
    2. Application intervals—single applications at 6-month intervals beginning at age 3 years; more frequent applications are indicated when the caries activity or risk is high
    3. Advantages—application intervals parallel typical recall patterns
    4. Disadvantages/precautions—not stable in solution; must be prepared immediately before application; astringent nature and disagreeable taste compromise client acceptance; if spilled, can stain clothing; pigmentation associated with pellicle, carious lesions, demineralized areas, silicate restorations, and restoration margins; burning or sloughing of gingiva has occurred; stannous ions can cause artifacts on radiographic films (radiographs should be taken before stannous fluoride application)
C. Acidulated phosphate fluoride (APF)
    1. Characteristics—available as aqueous solution, foam gels, and thixotropic gels; 1.23% sodium fluoride with 1 M orthophosphoric acid concentration
    2. Application intervals—every 6 months or more frequently when caries activity or risk is high
    3. Advantages—stable when stored in a plastic container; high level of client acceptance; non-irritating to soft tissues; does not discolor tooth structure; highest documented efficacy; most commonly used in-office treatment
    4. Disadvantages/precautions—may cause etching of

porcelain and some composite restorations; porcelain composite should be protected with petroleum jelly; due to potential to etch porcelain and some composite restorations NaF may be used as an alternative

D. Acidulated phosphate fluoride and stannous fluoride combination solutions

1. Characteristics—available as 0.32% APF and 1.64% SnF_2; to be mixed together as a rinse application; fluoride products in these concentrations have *not* received ADA Council on Scientific Affairs acceptance

2. Application intervals—single application at 6-month continued care intervals; more frequently if indicated

3. Advantages—ease of application, good client acceptance

4. Disadvantages/precautions—lack of ADA approval indicates that there is insufficient clinical evidence to support efficacy

E. Stannous fluoride irrigation solution

1. Characteristics—1.64% SnF_2 viscous solution prepared by dispensing equal amounts of 3.28% SnF_2 and distilled water; must be mixed freshly as needed

2. Application intervals—indicated for use as subgingival irrigation solution after scaling and root planing; may be used in irrigating syringes or power irrigators in the oral healthcare environment

3. Advantages—limited evidence suggests decrease in subgingival motile bacteria and spirochetes after irrigation[29]

4. Disadvantages—strong taste may affect client acceptance; lack of ADA Council on Scientific Affairs acceptance indicates that there is insufficient clinical evidence to support efficacy

Indications for Professional Application

A. Topical fluoride therapy by the dental hygienist is an accepted part of the prevention-oriented care plan

B. Assessment of the client's status and identification of current or potential needs will determine an individualized plan for fluoride therapy

C. In many cases the therapy regimen will include application of both professionally applied and self-applied agents

D. Topical fluoride should be considered for inclusion in the care plan based on the following criteria:[13]

1. For children and adults—APF gels are the treatment of choice at continued care intervals; however, NaF may be used as an alternative when porcelain and/or certain composite restorations are present

2. Caries is evident—a new carious lesion has developed within the last year in a child or within the last 3 years for an adult

3. Fair or poor oral hygiene

4. Decalcification, white spots, or incipiences are present

5. Following root instrumentation, dentin can be exposed and dentinal tubules opened; fluoride application facilitates prevention and/or control of hypersensitive root surfaces that often result

6. Fluoride application reduces the incidence of root caries and dentinal hypersensitivity that are associated with exposed root surfaces resulting from gingival recession

7. Irregular dental visits

8. Inappropriate dietary practices, e.g., frequent sugar intake

9. When xerostomia is present as a result of irradiation to the head and neck, certain medications, and some medical conditions that result in changes in the quality and quantity of saliva; caries destruction occurs rapidly and is generalized when salivary production is minimal; multiple fluoride treatments are used to control the high risk for caries associated with xerostomia

10. Clients wearing orthodontic appliances

Application Principles—General Guidelines

A. Client preparation

1. Explain the indication(s) for the procedure, the steps involved, the time it will take, the need to control saliva and avoid ingestion, and the postapplication restriction of anything by mouth for 30 minutes

2. Position the client to facilitate salivary control and reduce the potential for gagging

B. Tooth surface

1. Rubber cup polishing is not required before topical fluoride therapy[30]

2. Calculus, stains, materia alba, and heavy bacterial plaque should be removed

3. Efficacy of fluoride therapy is not reduced by presence of pellicle or bacterial plaque

Application Methods
Tray Systems

A. Designed to be used with fluoride foam and gels; trays cover all the teeth in an arch, come in a variety of materials, shapes, and sizes, and can be used with or without paper or foam liners; tray systems are not appropriate for solutions because they cannot be adequately retained within tray boundaries

B. Tray examples—most commonly used

1. Disposable styrofoam—available in a variety of

sizes and shapes; soft, pliable, and comfortable; good retention of gel or foam, also available with foam liner; used for professional fluoride application

2. Custom-fitted polyvinyl—used by client for self-application of fluoride gel; provides excellent coverage; must be remade as dentition matures; relatively expensive

C. Factors in tray selection—selection of an appropriate tray is important to the success of the procedure; the following criteria can be used to evaluate tray suitability

  1. Adapts to facial and lingual surfaces without extreme gapping

  2. Achieves complete coverage; depth is sufficient to reach the cervical third of the teeth

  3. Minimizes loss of the agent into the mouth

  4. Comfortable for the client

  5. Reasonable cost

  6. Conducive to infection control

D. Application procedure

  1. Assemble armamentarium—trays, fluoride, a saliva ejection device, gauze squares, and a timer or clock

  2. Protect porcelain and composite restorations with petroleum jelly for APF application, or use NaF

  3. Place a thin ribbon of gel or foam in the tray and spread; to minimize fluoride ingestion, minimize the amount of gel or foam dispensed

  4. Dry each arch; prevents dilution and controls for a potential salivary barrier

  5. Insert tray(s); one or two trays can be inserted at once; tray type, client variables, and clinician preference will influence the method selected

  6. Insert the saliva ejection device; reduce both the potential for ingestion and the incidence of nausea and vomiting

  7. Adapt tray(s); dental hygienist or client can gently press on the trays to close any small anterior gaps that may exist

  8. Have the client apply gentle biting pressure to force gel/foam interproximally

  9. Begin timing; trays are left in position for 4 minutes; 1-minute applications recommended by some manufacturers are not supported by clinical studies

  10. Remove tray(s); if only one tray was inserted initially, insert the second tray at this point; do not allow client to rinse between insertions

  11. Clear excess agent from the mouth; instruct the client to expectorate and/or swab the tongue, teeth, and soft tissues with gauze squares

  12. Provide posttreatment instructions; clients are typically told not to eat, rinse, drink, or smoke for at least 30 minutes; this increases the total time fluoride will be in contact with the teeth

E. Advantages of the tray system

  1. Ease of application—fluoride agent is dispensed once

  2. Time efficient—both arches can be treated at once; preparation time is minimal

  3. Client acceptance level is high—trays are comfortable and do not require that the mouth be kept open for long periods

Paint-on System

When fluoride agents are in solution or clients have a limited number of teeth, or root exposure that a tray fails to cover, the fluoride agents must be applied with a technique that allows for small amounts to be continuously applied to properly prepared tooth surfaces; gels may also be applied with this technique.

A. Components of the application procedure

  1. Assemble the armamentarium—long and short cotton rolls and cotton roll holders, fluoride solution or gel and container, saliva ejection device, applicator (cotton pellets and cotton pliers, or cotton-tipped applicator), gauze squares, timer or clock

  2. Protect porcelain and some composite restorations with petroleum jelly for APF application or use NaF

  3. Isolate the teeth using cotton rolls and a suitable holder; a long curved cotton roll can be placed on the buccal aspect and a short one placed on the lingual aspect until full mouth isolation is achieved; depending on client variables and clinician experience, it may be advisable to treat only one half of the mouth at a time

  4. Insert the saliva ejection device

  5. Dry isolated teeth; use a systematic approach

  6. Begin timing

  7. Apply the prepared fluoride by using a thoroughly moistened applicator; when using a solution swab the teeth continuously for 4 minutes

  8. Remove the cotton rolls and holders

  9. Clear excess solution; use optimal evacuation methods and/or ask the client to expectorate

  10. Do not allow the client to rinse

  11. Provide posttreatment instructions

B. Advantages

  1. Allows selective omission of an area or tooth; solution can be kept from surfaces where fluoride is contraindicated

  2. Allows direct observation of the solution or gel during application; dental hygienist can control the

placement of the solution or gel and evaluate the status of salivary control, thus reducing the potential for ingestion

C. Disadvantages
1. Time consuming—cotton roll placement and adaptation should be precise for good results; each side of the mouth is treated independently for 4 minutes
2. Client discomfort—mouth must remain open and the tongue controlled for a relatively long period of time
3. A dry field must be maintained

Self-Applied Fluorides

A. Provide frequent low doses of fluoride to the tooth surface; important in the process of remineralization of enamel
B. Rinses—available by prescription, except as noted
1. Daily use—low potency/high frequency
   a. 0.05% APF rinse supplement; recommended where both rinse and systemic supplementation are needed; may be used for topical effect only if patient is instructed to expectorate
   b. 0.05% NaF (available over-the-counter)
   c. 0.1% stannous fluoride rinse
2. Weekly use—high potency/low frequency
   a. 0.2% NaF
   b. Most commonly used concentration for school-based fluoride rinse programs
3. Many commercially prepared fluoride rinses contain alcohol and should not be recommended for persons with a history of alcoholism; use alcohol-free rinses with children and individuals who want to avoid exposure to alcohol
4. Fluoride rinses are not recommended for children under 6 years old; swallowing small doses of fluoride over a period of time may lead to dental fluorosis
C. Gels—available by prescription
1. 0.4% SnF_2 (brush-on or tray application)
2. 1.1% NaF (brush-on or tray application)
3. 1.1% APF (tray application)
D. Some studies indicate SnF_2 may be effective for antiplaque properties, antihypersensitivity, and anticaries effects[31,32]

Mouthrinses

A. May have cosmetic and/or therapeutic value
B. Effectiveness of most mouthrinses is limited to dislodging gross debris, temporarily reducing microorganisms, and providing a feeling of freshness
C. Antimicrobial mouthrinses have been shown to alleviate unnecessary surgical treatment of caries, reduce existing plaque, prevent formation of new plaque, selectively inhibit only those bacteria associated with disease, inhibit acid production, and glucan synthesis[13]
D. In the late 1980s, two categories of commercial mouthrinses were approved by the ADA Council on Scientific Affairs. Chlorhexidine gluconate 0.12%, (Peridex) and Listerine and other brand names (phenol-related essential oil compound), gained acceptance for control of both bacterial plaque and gingivitis
1. Chlorhexidine gluconate (Peridex, PerioGard)
   a. Available by prescription only
   b. 0.12% concentration in aqueous solution containing 11.6% alcohol, pH 5.5
   c. Clinical effects are comparable to 0.2% mouth rinse used for many years outside the United States; extensive clinical research documents efficacy
   d. Review of numerous studies[33] establishes chlorhexidine as safe, stable, and because of its substantivity, effective in preventing and controlling bacterial plaque and reducing and inhibiting gingivitis
   e. May cause formation of brownish yellow stain and supragingival calculus
   f. Unpleasant taste may hinder client acceptance
   g. Recommended for short-term use only; ½ oz, 30 second rinse, twice daily for 30 days
   h. Can be used as a preprocedural mouthrinse before aerosol-producing procedures; or, a preprocedural subgingival irrigant
2. Phenol-related essential oils (Listerine and many store brands)
   a. Available without prescription
   b. Contains thymol, menthol, eucalyptol, and methylsalicylate in a hydroalcohol solution, 26.9% alcohol, pH 5.0
   c. Low substantivity
   d. Studies on Listerine document efficacy in inhibition of bacterial plaque and gingivitis[34,35]
   e. Strong taste may hinder client acceptance and adherence to manufacturer's recommendation for a 30-second rinse twice a day
   f. Essential oil mouthrinses, basically the same formula as Listerine, are marketed under many store brand names and accepted by the ADA Council on Scientific Affairs as antiplaque/antigingivitis mouthrinses[36]
   g. Can be used as a preprocedural mouthrinse before aerosol-producing procedures; or a preprocedural subgingival irrigant

E. Recommended as adjuncts though not replacements for mechanical bacterial plaque control

F. Effective on supragingival plaque only, unless delivered subgingivally with irrigators

G. Approved mouthrinses should be considered for clients with the following conditions[37]
   1. Inability to achieve acceptable mechanical bacterial plaque control
   2. Fixed splinting, prostheses, dental implants, and overdentures
   3. Orthodontic appliances
   4. Postperiodontal[38] or other oral surgery
   5. Individuals at high risk for caries
   6. Medication-induced gingival hyperplasia
   7. Immunosuppression
   8. Pre-procedurally to minimize bacteremia

H. Most commercially prepared mouthrinses contain alcohol; other ingredients are water, flavoring, coloring, sweetening agents, and a variety of active ingredients
   1. Antimicrobials to reduce or inhibit microbial activity
   2. Oxygenating agents to debride and release oxygen
   3. Astringents to shrink tissues
   4. Anodynes to alleviate pain
   5. Buffering agents to reduce acidity, dissolve mucinous films, and relieve soft tissue pain
   6. Deodorizing and oxidizing agents to neutralize odors
   7. Fluorides to decrease caries incidence (see section on self-applied fluorides)

I. Manufacturer's claims in media advertising often exaggerate the benefits consumers may receive from mouthrinses

J. Inexpensive mouthrinses may be prepared by the client (not recommended for individuals on a low salt or sodium free diet)
   1. Isotonic (normal) saline solution: ½ teaspoon of salt in 8 ounces of water
   2. Hypertonic saline solution: ½ teaspoon of salt in 4 ounces of water
   3. Sodium bicarbonate solution: ½ teaspoon of sodium bicarbonate ("soda") in 8 ounces of water

K. Use of all mouthrinses should be monitored by both the client and dental hygienist; any adverse effects indicate that use should be evaluated and possibly discontinued

L. Mouthrinses containing quarternary ammonium compounds, zinc and copper salts, sanguinaria,[39] octenidine, and stannous fluoride have been effective in short-term studies and warrant further evaluation[40]

M. Mouthrinses, sprays, or swab sticks contain moisteners and may contain fluoride; recommended to relieve oral symptoms of xerostomia

N. Detergent prebrushing mouthrinses have received widespread consumer attention; studies have failed to document efficacy[23]

O. The dental hygienist should educate clients to be wise consumers of mouthrinses helping clients to recognize their benefits, limitations, and appropriate therapeutic regimens

Dental Sealants

General Considerations

See Chapter 10, section on pit and fissure sealants.

A. Although systemic and topical fluorides provide increased resistance to decay, the pit and fissure surfaces do not benefit to the same degree as smooth surfaces

B. Placement of sealants is a safe and highly effective means of reducing or eliminating the dental caries process occurring in pits and fissures

C. Pits and fissures allow for accumulation and stagnation of fermentable substrates and serve as accumulation sites for acidogenic microorganisms capable of demineralizing tooth tissue

D. Effectiveness of dental sealants in prevention of tooth decay has been clearly demonstrated in a variety of research settings

E. Caries protection approaches 100% when pits and fissures remain completely sealed; numerous clinical trials document efficacy at various levels, depending on methods and duration of study

F. Modern comprehensive primary prevention programs incorporate the complementary use of sealants and fluorides

G. Acid-etched resin sealants
   1. Autopolymerizing (chemically cured)
   2. Visible light cured

Indications for Application

A. Factors to consider
   1. Caries activity risk and pattern
   2. Depth of pits and fissures
   3. Dietary patterns
   4. Current and past fluoride exposure
   5. Ability of client to cooperate during sealant placement
   6. Eruption status

B. Recommendations for sealant placement from NIH Consensus Development Conference[13,41]
   1. Clients or guardians should be made aware of availability of sealants as a primary preventive procedure

2. Individuals who can benefit from sealant application include
    a. Children with newly erupted teeth with pits and fissures
    b. Children whose lifestyle, behavior patterns, physical or emotional development, or lack of fluoride exposure put them at high risk for caries
    c. Children whose teeth have deep pits and fissures
    d. Other persons who desire sealants as a preventive measure to protect pits and fissures
C. Teeth with questionable or incipient carious lesions should be sealed; studies have shown incipient lesions are arrested after sealant placement[41,42]
D. Teeth with fractured, noncarious margins of amalgam restorations can be either repaired or sealed

Contraindications to Sealant Application

A. Client behavior does not allow for the maintenance of the dry field necessary for successful application
B. There is a frank carious lesion on the occlusal surface
C. There is a carious lesion on the proximal surface that necessitates preparation of the occlusal surface
D. Tooth has been previously restored, except as noted in D. above.
E. Tooth is not sufficiently erupted to maintain a dry surface
F. The life expectancy of primary tooth is short

Application Guidelines

A. Mechanical cleansing of enamel
    1. Serves to remove bacterial plaque and surface debris which interfere with the effectiveness of the conditioning agent
    2. Cleansing agent may be a watery slurry of flour or pumice, nonfluoridated, or a commercially prepared fluoridated prophylaxis paste; recent studies have shown that the shear bond strength of acid etched enamel was not significantly different when teeth were prepared with fluoridated or nonfluoridated paste or pumice[42]
    3. Careful rinsing to remove residue is important
B. Isolating
    1. Salivary contamination of etched enamel surfaces is thought to be a major reason for sealant failure
    2. Careful isolation using either a rubber dam or cotton rolls is essential for consistent success
C. Drying
    1. Dry the isolated tooth thoroughly in preparation for application of the conditioner

2. Avoid water contamination if using syringes, which deliver combinations of water and air
D. Conditioning
    1. Acid conditioning to etch the enamel surface is an essential prerequisite to application of the resin material; acid solution removes a layer of enamel and increases the total surface area by rendering the deeper enamel regions porous; these micropores are penetrated by the resin monomer to produce a mechanical lock on polymerization
    2. Phosphoric acid in a concentration of from 30% to 50% is the current etching agent of choice
    3. Conditioning agents are available in either a solution or gel form
        a. Solution should be applied by gently dabbing the enamel surface with a saturated cotton pellet, sponge, or brush; avoid rubbing the surface because it causes a breakdown of the latticelike micropores
        b. Gels are applied with a special applicator, brush, cotton tip, or cotton pellet
        c. Whether gel or solution, it is important to cover all susceptible surfaces and cuspal inclines with etchant[42]
        d. Avoid contact of the etchant with the soft tissue
    4. A 15 to 20 second etch for either the primary or permanent dentition has been shown to be adequate for sealant retention[42]
E. Rinsing the conditioned tooth
    1. Thoroughly rinse the etched enamel surfaces by using a water syringe and high-speed evacuation system; do not let the client swish; the rinsing time may need to be increased to ensure complete removal
    2. Salivary contamination at this point will result in a substantial reduction in bond strength
        a. Do not allow the client to close, rinse, or touch the conditioned surface with the tongue
        b. When cotton rolls and/or absorbent pads are used, change as necessary, being careful to avoid salivary contamination
F. Drying the conditioned tooth
    1. Prepare the tooth for resin application by drying thoroughly with compressed air; completely dry surface is essential
    2. Examine the conditioned surface; properly etched surfaces will appear dull and chalky; repeat the conditioning process when these changes are not seen or salivary contamination occurs
G. Applying the sealant material; all susceptible pits and fissures should be sealed including buccal pits of

mandibular molars and lingual grooves of maxillary molars[13,42]

1. Visible light-cured sealants—prepared sealant is applied to the etched surface; light is then directed as close as possible over the entire sealant for a specified period (see manufacturer's directions)
   a. It is important to deliver at least the minimal amount of light exposure, too little exposure could result in sealant failure
   b. Once set sealant should be wiped with a wet cotton roll or pellet to remove air-inhibited layer of nonpolymerized resin; failure to remove this layer will result in an unpleasant taste
   c. Sealant kits deliver sealant material in a variety of ways; single-unit dose dispensers contain enough sealant for one person; this method will reduce the potential for cross-contamination when used properly
2. Chemical or autopolymerizing sealants—catalyst and sealant are mixed and placed immediately on to the prepared tooth surface with a brush or custom dispenser; working time from mixing to setting is 1 to 3 minutes, it is important not to disturb during polymerization
3. Sealant resin should be allowed to flow into all areas to minimize entrapment of air bubbles
4. Avoid applying excess sealant to the occlusal surface which could alter the client's occlusion or flow beyond the etched surface causing margins to leak and stain

H. Evaluating the results
   1. Examine the placed sealant to determine the adequacy of the bond strength and the absence of voids, underextensions, overextensions, or undercuring
   2. Sealed surface should feel completely smooth
   3. Floss to be sure sealant has not flowed interproximally
   4. Occlusion should be checked with articulating paper; frank high spots should be reduced with a finishing bur or fine stone
   5. Evaluate sealant retention at regular intervals; replace as indicated

Phase-Contrast Microscopy

Use for Disease Control

A. Clinical assessment
   1. Microscopic evaluations of bacterial plaque using phase contrast microscopy are primarily adjuncts to oral hygiene instruction and client motivation
   2. Provides a means of determining characteristic morphotypes; does not differentiate between species or between pathogens and nonpathogens with similar morphotypes[43]
   3. Is *not* a diagnostic tool or accurate monitor of disease activity[43]

B. Client education and motivation
   1. When a microscope is linked with a television screen, clients are able to view a bacterial sample from their own mouths
   2. Because the majority of organisms associated with periodontal disease are highly motile, viewing a bacterial plaque sample is a graphic way of demonstrating the significance and role of bacteria in the disease process

Using the Microscope

A. Slide preparation
   1. Hold slide by its edges to avoid fingerprints
   2. Place a drop of water on slide for each sample site
B. Obtaining the sample
   1. Sample sites are selected based on the goals of the demonstration to depict health or disease
   2. Use a curet to obtain a sample from the most apical portion of the site selected
   3. Remove supragingival deposits first to avoid contaminating the sample with calculus or other supramarginal deposits
   4. Gently disperse the sample into a droplet of water on the slide, overmanipulation may disrupt an original organized colony
   5. Place the coverslip on the slide
C. Mounting the slide
   1. Place the prepared slide onto the microscope stage and secure
   2. Center the specimen over the light coming from below; the stage can be moved horizontally, and/or vertically for viewing
D. Selecting the objective—most systems come with two objects (lenses): 40× and 100×; each requires a different condenser setting; 100× lens must always be used with immersion oil to eliminate optical interference from air; one drop of oil is placed directly on the cover slip; 40× lens must never be used with oil
E. Focusing the sample
   1. Adjust the interpupillary distance; position the eyes about 1 inch from the eyepieces and close or pull the eyepieces apart until a single circular viewing field is seen
   2. Raise the stage until the lens seems to *almost* touch the coverslip
   3. Use the fine-focus adjustment to bring the specimen into sharp focus
F. Viewing the sample

1. Sample can be viewed directly or on a video monitor
2. Scan the slide by adjusting the fine focus with one hand while moving the specimen on the stage with the other hand

Evaluating the Sample

A. Explain the sample to the client
B. It has been suggested that the quantity and type of *motile* bacteria and white blood cells can be used as *relative* indicators of disease and health
C. In health, there is a distinctive relative absence of motile organisms; loosely organized bacterial complexes are present

Use of the Microscope in Keyes' Technique—Rationale

A. Bacterial organizations associated with health are different from those associated with disease
B. Therapy should be directed toward elimination or suppression of bacterial populations not associated with health

Tobacco Use Interventions

General Considerations

A. Although the overall percentage of individuals who smoke is declining in the United States, smokeless tobacco use has been rising among adolescents and young men, and a significant number of adolescents have begun smoking
B. Smoking is a primary risk factor for
   1. Lung cancer
   2. Chronic obstructive lung disease
   3. Heart disease
   4. Other cancers, including oral
   5. Periodontal disease[44]
C. Sales, usage, and public acceptance of smokeless tobacco (chewing tobacco and snuff) are increasing, especially among youth
D. Smokeless tobacco use is associated with oral, laryngeal, and pharyngeal cancer
E. Dental hygienists should assume responsibility for facilitating cessation of all tobacco use by their patients; they should advise nonusers not to start[45]
F. Dental hygienists can take an active role in community and legislative efforts to reduce all tobacco use[45]

Tobacco Use Cessation Interventions

A. Oral healthcare facilities should be smoke free
B. Oral health professionals should strive to quit all tobacco habits
C. Smoking and smokeless tobacco use status of all clients should be assessed and documented in the client's permanent record
D. National Cancer Institute (NCI) program has four components of client/provider interaction[45]
   1. Ask—collect data regarding usage, duration, frequency of habit and previous attempts to stop, and concerns related to cessation
   2. Advise—must advise client to refrain from tobacco use; educate clients about changes in their mouth and health risks; do not make client feel ashamed or guilty
   3. Assist—for those who want to stop, provide verbal encouragement and motivational literature; set a quit date; establish a written contract; clients who need additional assistance with physical withdrawal may need a prescription for FDA-approved pharmacologic agents, e.g., nicotine transdermal patch, nicotine polacrilex (gum); refer to dentist for prescription
   4. Arrange—arrange follow-up visits or phone calls; clients may experience withdrawal and be tempted to resume tobacco use; be supportive and encourage multiple attempts to quit
E. Teenagers should be considered potential smokers and/or smokeless tobacco users; interventions include
   1. Questioning about tobacco use
   2. Education about health risks of tobacco use
   3. Encouragement to resist peer pressure and media messages to start

Oral Cancer Self-Examination

Basic Concepts

A. Many oral cancers are, unfortunately, not detected until they have invaded deep tissues and require radical surgical and/or extensive chemotherapy or irradiation
B. Early detection and early treatment are the best ways to manage oral cancer
C. Whereas all clients can potentially benefit from self-examination skills, it is especially important that the dental hygienist educate individuals considered to be at high risk

Oral Cancer High-Risk Factors

A. Tobacco use
   1. Individuals who smoke are estimated to be two to four times at greater risk than nonsmokers
   2. Those who use snuff and smokeless tobacco are prone to squamous cell carcinomas at or near the site where the material is held
B. Alcohol use

1. There is a positive correlation between alcohol use and the incidence of oral cancer
2. Evidence suggests a cocarcinogenesis of tobacco and alcohol

C. Sun exposure—individuals who work outdoors, especially those with fair complexions, seem to be at higher risk for basal cell tumors of the skin

Examination Technique

Materials Needed

A. Large mirror and adequate light source are essential for self-examination procedures
B. Use of a flashlight, mouth-sized mirror, and gauze or tissue squares enhances access to and visualization of intraoral structures

Systematic Approach

A. Face and neck
    1. Symmetry—one-sided irregularities should be questioned; right and left sides should have the same outline and shape
    2. Skin—remove eyeglasses; check for sores, bumps, and discolorations
    3. Neck—palpate lymph chains for lumps or tender areas
B. Lips and gums
    1. Remove full or partial dentures
    2. Retract the lips to look for sores or color changes
    3. Palpate the lips and run a finger over the gingiva to feel for irregularities, tenderness, or roughened areas
C. Cheek
    1. Retract the right, then the left side to visualize the inner surface; look for red, white, brown, or speckled patches
    2. Palpate for lumps or tenderness
    3. Run a finger over the inside surface to check for rough or raised places
D. Roof of the mouth
    1. Tilt the head back and use a flashlight to increase visualization
    2. Use a mouth-sized mirror to reflect the image in a larger mirror
    3. Look for sores, color changes, etc.; feel for lumps or areas of tenderness
E. Tongue
    1. Extend the tongue and look at the top surface
    2. Using a gauze square or tissue, grasp the tongue and pull it to the right, then the left side
    3. Look for sores, color changes, and irregularities
    4. Feel for lumps, areas of tenderness, or roughened surfaces
F. Floor of the mouth

1. Place the tip of the tongue against the roof of the mouth
2. Look for asymmetry, sores, color changes, etc.
3. With the fingers of one hand under the jaw, use the index finger of the other hand to compress structures
4. Check for lumps, tenderness, or irregularities

Teaching Factors

A. Several demonstrations of the self-assessment procedure will probably be necessary for mastery; pamphlets explaining and demonstrating techniques are extremely helpful
B. Introduce the concept of "normal range" and familiarize the client with what is normal in his or her mouth
C. Provide criteria for determining significant deviations from normal
    1. Sores that fail to heal within 2 weeks
    2. Appearance of white, red, or dark-colored patches
    3. Presence of swellings, lumps, bumps, or growths
D. Reinforce the need for a systematic approach to ensure thoroughness
E. Define the dentist's role in interpreting findings; client should report, not diagnose unusual findings
F. Establish the concept that self-examination is not meant to be a substitute for periodic regular professional evaluation

Control of Dentinal Hypersensitivity

General Considerations

A. Dentinal hypersensitivity is an *abnormal* condition occurring when vital dentin is exposed to the environment of the oral cavity with the result that painful stimuli can reach the pulp and be translated as pain
B. Hypersensitivity symptoms are exacerbated by presence of bacterial plaque and its by-products
C. Treatment of dentinal hypersensitivity is a valuable client service; symptoms cause considerable client discomfort and may interfere with both bacterial plaque control and professional treatment
D. It is important to distinguish the pain reaction caused by dentinal hypersensitivity from pain attributable to other etiology
    1. Rapid onset
    2. Sharp pain
    3. Short duration
    4. Stops upon removal of stimulus

Etiology

A. Primary cause of hypersensitivity is exposed dentin and open dentinal tubules

B. Dentin exposure occurs
1. In 10% of all teeth; during development, the enamel and cementum do not join
2. When cementum is lost through abrasion, erosion, dental caries, or scaling and root-planing procedures
3. When soft tissue is lost because of gingival recession, periodontal surgery, or improper toothbrushing habits
4. With regurgitation of acidic gastric juices by bulimic individuals or prolonged/frequent exposure to foods that are very acidic

Pain Mechanism

A. There is no universally accepted theory of the pain transmission mechanism in dentinal hypersensitivity
B. The most widely accepted theories propose that
1. Lymphatic fluid present in the dentinal tubules transmits stimuli
2. Odontoblasts and their processes act as receptors and transmitters of sensory stimuli
3. Stimuli create movement of tubular fluids, causing nerve endings at the pulpal wall to be stimulated

Pain Stimuli

A. Not all stimuli cause pain; each person has a unique set of stimuli that cause sensitivity
B. Mechanical stimuli include instrumentation, home care devices, eating utensils, and friction from removable prosthetic or orthodontic devices
C. Chemical stimuli include foods high in acid or sugars, plaque end products, and some topical medications
D. Thermal stimuli include foods and liquids at extreme temperatures, cold air, and too-rapid drying of a tooth surface, which causes a concurrent rapid drop in tooth temperature

Desensitizing Agents

A. Modes of action
1. Agents are thought to seal dentinal tubules by either surface precipitation of ions, subsurface incorporation of ions, or stimulation of secondary dentin
2. Goal is to occlude dentinal tubules or alter excitability of sensory nerves
B. Optimal agent characteristics—professionally applied agents should ideally be rapidly acting, nontoxic, easy to apply, and have consistent outcomes and long-term effects

Types of Desensitizing Agents

A. To date, no single agent or form of treatment is effective for all persons

B. Numerous agents have been tried with varying degrees of success; they include
1. Solutions, gels, or pastes of fluoride in varying compounds and percentages, stannous fluoride, calcium hydroxide, strontium chloride, potassium nitrate, sodium citrate, formaldehyde, or potassium or ferric oxalate
2. Adhesive, varnish, or bonding materials
3. Iontophoretic devices—iontophoresis is the application of an electrical current to impregnate tissues with ions from dissolved salts; fluoride iontophoresis is thought to result in increased uptake and penetration of fluoride ions into dentin; efficacy has not been demonstrated in controlled clinical trials

Desensitization Methods

A. Home/self-care regimens
1. Effective bacterial plaque control strategies are critically important in gaining and maintaining control of hypersensitivity
2. Toothpastes containing fluoride have been shown to be effective and contribute to the control of root caries
3. Specially formulated toothpastes containing strontium chloride, potassium nitrate, or sodium citrate
4. Daily use of a fluoride gel or rinse is advisable when the problem is generalized or recurrent
B. Professionally delivered regimens should support and/or make possible home/self-care regimens
1. General guidelines
a. Remove all accretions; involved surface must be free of barriers to the agent
b. Local anesthesia is appropriate when scaling and root planing procedures and/or application of the agent are too painful
c. Isolate the sensitive tooth and control saliva
d. Dry the tooth with cotton pellets or gauze; avoid using the air syringe
e. Apply the agent according to the manufacturer's instructions for the method and time required; pastes are usually burnished in with a wooden point, whereas solutions are bathed on; some clients may experience an acute pain reaction to the agent; immediately remove the agent, wait a few minutes, and then attempt reapplication
f. Remove any excess agent to avoid ingestion
g. Test for change in pain reaction; this will not be possible with anesthetized individuals
h. Plan for future reapplication if desensitization has not occurred
2. Precaution—some agents have very high concentrations of fluoride; to prevent nausea, use good agent application and salivary control techniques

Electrical Pulpal Vitality/Digital Pulp Testing

Basic Concepts

A. Teeth may become nonvital as a result of bacterial invasion of the pulp associated with caries or periodontal disease or from injuries of a physical nature such as mechanical or thermal trauma
B. Any tooth suspected of being nonvital should be tested for pulpal vitality
C. Method that provides qualitative assessment is preferred
D. Use of thermal and percussion tests are helpful to correlate findings with the client's chief complaint
E. Precaution—do not use electrical vitality testing procedures for clients with cardiac pacemakers or other electronic life-support devices

Testing Devices

A. Electrical pulp tester (also known as a vitalometer) and digital pulp tester are instruments that use gradations of electrical current to excite a response in pulpal tissues; pulp testers are either battery-operated portable instruments or have cords that plug into electrical outlets for a direct power source; all testers have rheostats with a scale (e.g., 1 to 10 or 1 to 50) that indicates the relative amount of current being applied; digital pulp testers provide a digital reading
B. Procedure
   1. Armamentarium
      a. Testing device
      b. Cotton rolls
      c. Toothpaste or other conducting medium
   2. Client preparation
      a. Explain the procedure to the client; the minimal stimulation necessary is used to evoke a response
      b. Instruct the client to raise a hand when the slightest warmth or tingling sensation is first felt
      c. To acquaint the client with the type of sensation created and to determine a normal response pattern, first test the teeth adjacent and contralateral to the tooth in question
   3. Obtaining a reading
      a. Isolate and dry the teeth to be tested; this prevents the conduction of current into soft tissues
      b. Apply a small amount of toothpaste, or alternative conductor, to the tester tip
      c. Place the tip on sound tooth structure within the middle third of the crown for a single-rooted tooth and within the middle third of each cusp for a multirooted tooth; a clip resting on the client's lip and attached to the handpiece is necessary to create a closed electric circuit and activate the tester
      d. Avoid contact with restorations and/or soft tissues
      e. Slowly advance the rheostat from zero to increasingly higher numbers until sensation is indicated; rheostat should not be moved above that point for that tooth
   4. Documentation
      a. Two readings should be taken for each tooth tested and the readings averaged
      b. Record for all teeth tested the lowest average reading, the type of testing device and conductor used, and any patient actions or reactions that may have affected results
C. Variables affecting results
   1. Pulpal conditions may vary from early inflammation to complete necrosis; responses vary with each condition; pulp of a test tooth is considered to be degenerating when, compared with a control, much more current is required to gain a response
   2. Metallic restorations conduct electrical charges more rapidly than tooth structure and can produce false readings
   3. Teeth involved in splints or bridges or with proximal restorations may produce false-positive reactions because the circuit can be transferred from adjacent vital teeth
   4. Multirooted teeth may have some combination of vital and nonvital canals and test falsely positive
   5. Pain reactions are influenced by attitudes, age, sex, emotions, fatigue, culture, and medications

Exfoliative Cytology

Definition

A. Suspicious lesions in the mouth require biopsy and microscopic evaluation before a definitive diagnosis can be made
B. Exfoliative cytology is a nonsurgical technique for collecting surface cells of a lesion for microscopic evaluation

Advantages

A. Nonsurgical, noninvasive procedure requiring minimal client preparation and no postoperative care
B. Easily and efficiently implemented in any setting, making it ideal for mass screening or use in remote areas
C. Clinical laboratory and professional personnel costs are relatively low

Disadvantages

A. Lacks precision
   1. Only surface lesions can be evaluated; no matter

how hard the lesion is scraped, only surface (not basal) cells are collected

2. Heavily keratinized lesions will not yield adequate cells for examination

B. May delay definitive treatment
   1. Definitive treatment cannot be decided on smear results alone; valuable time may be lost obtaining and analyzing a biopsy specimen
   2. When clinical evidence clearly suggests a malignant lesion, the more precise biopsy is the first procedure of choice

Procedure[1]

A. Armamentarium
   1. Glass microscope slides
   2. Collection instrument
   3. Fixative
   4. Gauze sponges
   5. Laboratory forms
B. Documentation
   1. Print the client's name and the date on the glass slide
   2. Complete laboratory data forms; information usually includes name and address for client and dentist, lesion history, and clinical description (location, size, color, and consistency)
   3. Record service rendered in client's permanent record
C. Obtaining and preparing the sample
   1. Cleanse the lesion—remove surface debris by irrigating with water or gently wiping with wet gauze
   2. Collect the sample—using a flexible metal spatula or moistened wooden tongue blade, firmly scrape the entire surface of the lesion; move in one direction only
   3. Prepare the glass slide—holding the slide by its edges, evenly spread the sample material across the slide surface
   4. Fix the sample—to prevent cell dehydration, quickly cover the sample surface with a layer of 70% alcohol or apply spray fixative; allow the sample to air-dry in an area protected from airborne contamination
   5. Prepare for transfer to the laboratory

Laboratory Findings

A. Classification categories
   1. Unsatisfactory—specimen is not adequate for diagnosis
   2. Class I. Normal—only normal cells are present
   3. Class II. Atypical—some cellular changes may be present, but there is no suggestion of malignancy
   4. Class III. Intermediate—changes may be suggestive

of malignancy, but findings are not clear-cut; biopsy is recommended

5. Class IV. Suggestive of cancer—cells with malignant characteristics are present; biopsy is mandatory
6. Class V. Positive for cancer—cells are obviously malignant; biopsy is mandatory

B. Follow-up needs
   1. Unsatisfactory—schedule for another smear to be taken
   2. Class III, IV, or V findings—client should be referred for biopsy
   3. Class I or II findings—client should be monitored for healing of the lesion or reevaluated if the lesion fails to resolve; false-negative reports are a possibility; healed lesion is the best reassurance for reports in categories I and II

REFERENCES

1. Darby ML, Walsh MM: *Dental hygiene theory and practice*, Philadelphia, 1995, WB Saunders.
2. Gaare D, et al: Improvement of gingival health by toothbrushing in individuals with large amounts of calculus, *J Clin Periodontol* 17:38, 1990.
3. Rotter JB: *Social learning and clinical psychology*, Englewood Cliffs, NJ, 1954, Prentice Hall.
4. Maslow A: A theory of human motivation, *Psychol Rev* 50:370, 1943.
5. Fedi P, Vernino AR, editors: *The periodontic syllabus*, ed 3, Philadelphia, 1995, Lea & Febiger.
6. Murray PA, Boyd RL, Robertson PB: Effect on periodontal status of rotary electric toothbrushes vs manual toothbrushes during periodontal maintenance: II microbiological results, *J Periodontol* 60:396, 1989.
7. Boyd PA, Murray P, Robertson PB. Effect on periodontal status of rotary electric toothbrushes vs manual toothbrushes during periodontal maintenance: Clinical results, *J Periodontol* 60:390, 1989.
8. Khocht A, Spindel L, Person P: A comparative clinical study of the safety and efficacy of three toothbrushes, *J Periodontol* 63:603, 1992.
9. McInnes C, Johnson B, Emling RC, Yankell SL: Clinical and computer-assisted evaluations of the stain removal ability of the Sonicare™ electronic toothbrush, *J Clin Prev Dent* 5(1):13, 1994.
10. Rosenberg M: Clinical assessment of bad breath: Current concepts, *J Am Dent Assoc* 127:475, 1996.
11. Ciancio SG, Shibly O, Farber GA: Clinical evaluation of the effect of two types of dental floss on plaque and gingival health, *Clin Prev Dent* 14:14, 1992.
12. Gordon JM, Frascella JA, Reardon RC: A clinical study of the safety and efficacy of a novel electric interdental cleaning device, *J Clin Dent* 7(3):70, 1996.
13. ADA Council on Access, Prevention and Interprofessional Relations, Caries Diagnosis & Risk Assessment: A review of preventive strategies and management, *J Am Dent Assoc* 126 (Supplement) 15-245, 1995.

14. Pendrys DG: Risk of fluorosis in a fluoridated population: Implications for the dentist and dental hygienist, *J Am Dent Assoc* 126:1617, 1995.
15. Cinacio SG, Mather MS, Reynolds HS, et al: The effect of oral irrigation with Listerine on plaque and gingivitis and the subgingival microflora, *J Dent Res,* Special Issue 66: 1026, 1987.
16. Ciancio SG, Mather ML, Zambon JJ, et al: Effect of a chemotherapeutic agent delivered by an oral irrigation device on plaque, gingivitis, and subgingival microflora, *J Periodontol* 60:310, 1989.
17. Flemmig T, Newman M, Nachnani S, et al: Chlorhexidine and irrigation in gingivitis: 6 months correlative clinical and microbial findings, *J Dent Res,* Special Issue 68:383, 1989.
18. Vignarajah S, Newman HN, Bulman J: Pulsated jet subgingival irrigation with 0.1% chlorhexidine, simplified oral hygiene and chronic periodontitis, *J Clin Periodontol* 16: 365, 1989.
19. Parsons LG, Thomas LG, Southard LG, et al: Effect of sanguinaria extract on established plaque and gingivitis when supragingivally delivered as a manual rinse or under pressure in an irrigator, *J Clin Periodontol* 14:381, 1987.
20. Boyd RL, Leggott P, Quinn R, et al: Effect of self-administered daily irrigation with 0.02% SnF_2 on periodontal disease activity, *J Clin Periodontol* 12:420, 1985.
21. Eakle WS, Ford C, Boyd RL: Depth of penetration in periodontal pockets with oral irrigation, *J Clin Periodontol* 13: 39, 1985.
22. Greenstein G: Effects of subgingival irrigation on peridontal status, *J Periodontol* 58:827, 1987.
23. Rubinstein-DeVore L: Antimicrobials and oral health, *Semin Dent Hyg* 3:1, 1991.
24. American Academy of Periodontology, Committee on Research, Science and Technology: The role of supra- and subgingival irrigation in the treatment of periodontal disease, Chicago, April, 1995, The Association.
25. Fine DH, et al: Assessing pre-procedural subgingival irrigation and rinsing with an antiseptic mouthrinse to reduce bacteremia, *J Am Dent Assoc,* 127:641, 1996.
26. Taggart JA, Palmer RM, Wilson RF: A clinical and microbiological comparison of the effects of water and 0.02% chlorhexidine as coolants during ultrasonic scaling and root planing, *J Clin Periodontol* 17:32, 1990.
27. Reynolds MA, Lavigne CK, Minah GE, et al: Clinical effects of simultaneous ultrasonic scaling and subgingival irrigation with chlorhexidine. Mediating influence of periodontal probing depth, *J Clin Periodontol* 19:595, 1992.
28. Zwemer TJ. *Boucher's clinical dental terminology,* ed 4, St. Louis, 1993, Mosby.
29. Mazza JE, Newman MG, Sims TN: Chemical and antimicrobial effects of stannous fluoride on periodontitis, *J Clin Periodontol* 8:203, 1981.
30. Ripa LW: Need for prior tooth cleaning when performing a professional topical fluoride application: Review and recommendations for change, *J Am Dent Assoc* 109:281, 1984.
31. Camosci DA, Tinanoff N: Anti-bacterial determinants of stannous fluoride, *J Dent Res* 63:1121, 1984.
32. Leverett DH, McHugh WD, Jensen OE: Effect of daily rinsing with stannous fluoride on plaque and gingivitis, *J Dent Res* 63:1083, 1984.
33. Land NP, Breck MC: Chlorhexidine digluconate—An agent for chemical plaque control and prevention of gingival inflammation, *J Periodont Res* (suppl):74, 1986.
34. DePaola LG, Overholser CD, Meiller TF, et al: Chemotherapeutic inhibition of supragingival dental plaque and gingivitis, *J Clin Periodontol* 16:311, 1989.
35. Gordon JM, Lamster IB, Seigler MC: Efficacy of Listerine antiseptic in inhibiting the development of plaque and gingivitis, *J Clin Periodontol* 12:697, 1985.
36. American Dental Association, Council on Scientific Affairs: Products with the ADA Seal of Acceptance, www.ada.org, 1996.
37. Ciancio SG: Use of mouthrinses for professional indications, *J Clin Periodontol* 15:520, 1988.
38. Sang M, et al: Clinical enhancement of post-periodontal surgical therapy by a 0.12% chlorhexidine gluconate mouthrinse, *J Periodontol* 60:570, 1989.
39. Miller RA, McIver JE, and Gunsolley JC: The effects of sanguinaria extract on plaque retention and gingival health, *J Clin Orthop* 22:304, 1988.
40. Mandel ID: Chemotherapeutic agents for controlling plaque and gingivitis, *J Clin Periodontol* 15:488, 1988.
41. National Institutes of Health Consensus Development Conference: Dental sealants in the prevention of tooth decay, Proceedings, *J Dent Educ* 48(Suppl):2, 1984.
42. Waggoner WF, Siegal M: Pit and fissure sealants application: Updating the technique. *J Am Dent Assoc* 127:351, 1996.
43. American Academy of Periodontology: Proceedings of the world workshop in clinical periodontics, pp 1-27, 1989.
44. Perry DA, Beemsterboer PL, Taggert EJ: *Periodontology for the dental hygienist,* Philadelphia, 1996, WB Saunders.
45. Fried JF: Tobacco use intervention: The role of the dental hygienist, *Dent Hyg News* 5:2, 1992.

SUGGESTED READINGS

American Academy of Periodontology, Committee on Research, Science and Technology: *Chemical agents for the control of plaque,* Chicago, April, 1991, The Association.

Borden PS, Christen AG, McDonald JL, et al: A smoking cessation program for the oral health care practice, *Dent Hyg* 62:339, 1988.

Brough-Muzzin KM, Johnson R, Carr P, et al: The dental hygienist's role in the maintenance of osseointegrated dental implants, *J Dent Hyg* 62:448, 1988.

Chambers DW, Abrams RG: *Dental communication,* Norwalk, Conn, 1986, Appleton-Century-Crofts.

Chung L, Smith SR, Joyston-Bechal S: The effect of using a prebrushing mouthwash (PLAX) in man, *J Clin Periodontol* 19:679, 1992.

Cirincione UK: The safe use of fluorides in dental hygiene practice, *J Dent Hyg* 66:319, 1992.

Darby ML, Walsh MM: *Dental hygiene theory and practice,* Philadelphia, 1995, WB Saunders.

DeBiase CB, *Dental health education: Theory and practice,* Philadelphia, 1991, Lea & Febiger.

Dental hypersensitivity: Current perspectives on diagnosis and treatment, Symposium proceedings, Jersey City, NJ, 1987, Block Drug Co.

Forgas LB, Nilius AM: Assessing periodontal disease activity: The role of bacteriological, immunological, and DNA assays, *J Dent Hyg* 65:188, 1991.

Gulch-Scranton J: Motivational strategies in dental hygiene care, *Semin Dent Hyg* 3:1, 1991.

Harris NO, Christen AG: *Primary preventive dentistry,* ed 4, Norwalk, Conn, 1995, Appleton & Lange.

Hodges KO: Concepts in nonsurgical periodontal therapy, Albany, NY, 1998, Delmar.

Ibsen OAC, Phelan JA: *Oral pathology for the dental hygienist,* ed 2, Philadelphia, 1996, WB Saunders.

Keyes PH, Rams TE: A rationale for management of periodontal diseases: Rapid identification of microbial "therapeutic targets" with phase-contrast microscopy, *J Am Dent Assoc* 106:6, 1983.

Lutins ND, Greco GW, McFall WT: Effectiveness of sodium fluoride on tooth hypersensitivity with and without iontophoresis, *J Periodontol* 55:5, 1984.

Mandel ID, editor: Symposium: An update on antimicrobial mouthrinses: Clinical implications and practical applications, *J Am Dent Assoc,* 125 (supplement), 1994.

Mecklenburg RE, Christen AG, Gerbert B, et al: How to help your patients stop using tobacco: A National Cancer Institute manual for the oral health team. NIH Publication 91-3191, Dec 1990.

Mueller Joseph L, Peterson M: *Dental hygiene process: Diagnosis and care planning,* Albany, NY, 1995, Delmar.

National Fluorides Task Force: A guide to the use of fluorides for the prevention of dental caries, ed 2, Chicago, 1986, American Dental Association.

New Ways to Save Your Teeth? *Consumer Reports:* pp 504-509, August 1989.

Rams TE, Slots J: Local delivery of antimicrobial agents, *Periodontology 2000,* 10:139, 1996.

Swongo PA: The use of topical fluorides to prevent dental caries in adults: A review of the literature, *J Am Dent Assoc* 107:9, 1983.

Tarbet WJ, et al: Home treatment for dentinal hypersensitivity: A comparative study, *J Am Dent Assoc* 105:8, 1982.

Tilliss TS: A closer look at tartar control dentifrices, *J Dent Hyg* 63:364, 1989.

Wei SH, editor: *Clinical uses of fluorides,* Philadelphia, 1985, Lea & Febiger.

Weinstein P, Getz T: *Changing human behavior: Strategies for preventive dentistry,* Chicago, 1978, Science Research Associates.

Wilkins EM: *Clinical practice of the dental hygienist,* ed 7, Philadelphia, 1994, Lea & Febiger.

Wilson MB: *The science and art of basic microscopy,* Bellaire, Tex, 1976, American Society for Medical Technology.

Woodall IR, et al: *Comprehensive dental hygiene care,* ed 4, St Louis, 1993, Mosby.

Yura H, Walsh MB: *The nursing process,* ed 3, New York, 1978, Appleton-Century-Crofts.

Review Questions

1 Powered toothbrushes may be
A. Indicated for individuals who are physically or mentally challenged
B. Effective tools for subgingival plaque control in pocket depths up to 4 mm
C. More traumatic to gingiva and cementum than manual toothbrushes
D. Contraindicated for individuals with mitrovalve prolapse
E. More difficult to use and require increased instruction time

2 Which of the following homecare armamentarium is the *LEAST* effective plaque control tool for a client with dental implants and a fixed prosthesis?
A. Tapered end tuft brush
B. Soft bristled, multitufted nylon toothbrush
C. Rubber tip stimulator
D. Mild abrasive, ADA approved toothpaste
E. Unwaxed dental floss

3 Prevention and control of smooth surface dental caries is *MOST* effectively managed by
A. Biannual dental hygiene continued care (recall)
B. Early radiographic detection
C. Dental sealant application
D. Diet rich in fermentable carbohydrates
E. Fluoride therapy

4 Caries and inflammatory periodontal diseases are complex disease states that require the colonization of bacteria; thus control of bacterial plaque is an essential component of any plan to prevent and control these dental diseases.
A. Both statements are *TRUE.*
B. Both statements are *FALSE.*
C. The first statement is *TRUE,* the second statement is *FALSE.*
D. The first statement is *FALSE,* the second statement is *TRUE.*

5 Acidulated phosphate fluoride (APF)
A. Is an acidic preparation of stannous fluoride
B. Is difficult to use because of its instability in solution
C. Should be applied every 6 months
D. Is not recommended for children
E. Is a commonly recommended OTC fluoride preparation

6 All of the following are indications for use of a topical fluoride application *EXCEPT*
A. High caries incidence
B. Xerostomia
C. Orthodontic appliances
D. Athletic mouthguard
E. Exposed root surfaces

7 Application of a pit and fissure sealant is dependent on all of the following *EXCEPT*
A. Cooperation level of client
B. Client's age
C. Client's plaque removal ability
D. Anatomical characteristics of pits and fissures

8 Visible light cured sealant material
   A. Has a working time of 1 to 3 minutes
   B. Must be wiped off immediately following polymerization
   C. Is prepared in the same manner as chemical or self-cure sealant
   D. Flows more readily into the pits and fissures of the occlusal surface
   E. Has a flexible working time because polymerization occurs only when light is applied

9 Obtaining a bacterial plaque sample for microscopic evaluation requires all of the following *EXCEPT*
   A. Supramarginal plaque removal to minimize the possibility of contamination of the sample
   B. Selection of an appropriate client
   C. Thorough scaling and root planing
   D. Thorough explanation of procedure to the client

10 Which of the following is the *LEAST* likely to elicit a painful response by a client who has exposed root surfaces?
   A. Use of a periodontal aid
   B. Vigorous horizontal toothbrushing
   C. Ice cream
   D. Tooth surface evaluation by a dental explorer
   E. Vitalometer evaluation

11 Interdental cleaning devices
   A. Conform to the anatomy of the proximal tooth surface
   B. May result in loss of interdental papillae
   C. Are selected based on the architecture and position of the gingiva
   D. Compare favorably with toothbrushing for interdental bacterial plaque removal
   E. Require excellent manual dexterity to manipulate

12 What etiologic factor is associated with a high risk of oral cancer?
   A. Excessive fluoride applications
   B. Failure to seek routine dental care
   C. Frequent radiographic exposure
   D. The presence of numerous amalgam restorations
   E. Habitual smoking

13 The results of electrical vitality testing may be affected by all of the following *EXCEPT*
   A. The level of bacterial plaque control achieved
   B. The presence of a full crown on the tooth
   C. The age of the client
   D. The client's mental state
   E. The type of conducting agent used

14 Which of the following is an acute consequence of improper flossing technique?
   A. Eroded tooth structure
   B. Enamel mottling
   C. Dilaceration of the root
   D. Proximal composite fracture
   E. Laceration of the papillae

15 Prevention and control of dental diseases are
   A. The primary goal of client education
   B. Impossible
   C. Achieved by mechanical methods only
   D. The goal of oral cancer self examination
   E. Achieved by topical fluoride application

16 Antimicrobial mouthrinses are indicated for all of the following persons *EXCEPT*
   A. Orthodontic clients
   B. Individuals with poor manual dexterity
   C. Clients exhibiting no loss of attachment and exemplary plaque control
   D. Postsurgical clients
   E. Clients who desire the feeling of fresh breath

17 Commercially prepared mouthrinses commonly contain antimicrobials to reduce or inhibit microbial activity. In addition, they contain oxygenating agents which enhance tissue tone and encourage tissue shrinkage.
   A. Both statements are *TRUE.*
   B. Both statements are *FALSE.*
   C. The first statement is *TRUE,* the second statement is *FALSE.*
   D. The first statement is *FALSE,* the second statement is *TRUE.*

18 During an oral cancer self-examination, all of the following conditions indicate to the client a significant deviation from normal *EXCEPT*
   A. A 2 × 3 mm, round ulceration that has been present for 4 weeks
   B. Bilateral, white keratinized linear elevations on the buccal mucosa at the height of the occlusal table
   C. A white, patchy covering on the left buccal mucosa in the vestibule area, adjacent to No. 19-22 in a patient reporting smokeless tobacco use
   D. A loss of distinction to the vermilion border of the labium inferium

19 During the dental hygiene continued care/maintenance appointment, the dental hygienist and the client set goals and determine the course of action for the appointment. What phase is this in the process of care?
   A. Assessment
   B. Diagnosis
   C. Planning
   D. Implementation
   E. Evaluation

20 Disclosing solution is a useful adjunct for teaching individuals their strengths and weaknesses in bacterial plaque removal. It is especially important for assessing subgingival plaque removal techniques.
   A. Both statements are *TRUE.*
   B. Both statements are *FALSE.*
   C. The first statement is *TRUE,* the second statement is *FALSE.*
   D. The first statement is *FALSE,* the second statement is *TRUE.*

21 The addition of antimicrobials to power oral irrigating devices for home use
   A. Has not been documented in the literature as an effective regimen
   B. Provides benefits beyond those achieved by irrigation with water alone
   C. Is effective in subgingival plaque control beyond 5 mm
   D. Should not be recommended for orthodontic clients
   E. Is not recommended by manufacturers of current irrigators

22 Which of the following statements is *NOT* true about mouth malodor?
   A. Odor is most commonly produced by foods
   B. Most common source for odor is the dorsal surface of the tongue
   C. Can be controlled by good oral hygiene
   D. May be a sign of periodontal disease
   E. May be caused by smoking

23 Dentifrices with whitening agents are marketed for their ability to
   A. Coat the tooth with a whitening veneer
   B. Remove extrinsic stains
   C. Bleach intrinsic stains from within the tooth
   D. Elicit a placebo effect
   E. Diminish the fluoride rich enamel layer due to abrasiveness

24 Use of a fluoride dentifrice is an important part of a preventive care plan because
   A. Fluoride controls extrinsic stains
   B. Fluoride remineralizes tooth surfaces
   C. Fluoride interferes with the calcium-phosphate bond in the calcium matrix
   D. Fluoride dentifrices taste better than all others
   E. Fluoride dentifrices control sensitivity

25 Maslow's theory of human needs suggests that
   A. Values form on the basis of previous behaviors
   B. The outcome of an individuals' behavior is beyond the individuals' control
   C. Inner forces or needs drive an individuals' course of action
   D. Motivation is based on offers of punishment or reward
   E. New behaviors will be easily adopted if they fit readily into their existing value system

26 A client demonstrating flossing technique and asking questions on how to modify that technique is an example of
   A. Active participation
   B. Attitudinal motivation
   C. Immediate feedback
   D. Self pacing
   E. Small step size

27 Determining that a client is dissatisfied with the appearance of his/her teeth should occur within the _____ phase of the appointment.
   A. Assessment
   B. Planning
   C. Implementation
   D. Evaluation

28 A dental hygienist, who is introducing a new bacterial plaque control regime, must remember that
   A. Dental hygienists know what is best for their clients
   B. His/her recommendation of a product outweighs the client's concerns about cost
   C. Old habits are hard to change
   D. It is the dental hygienist's responsibility to ensure client adherence to the new technique

29 All of the following statements are true regarding neutral sodium fluoride (NaF) *EXCEPT*
   A. NaF application should coincide with the eruption of primary and permanent teeth
   B. Professional NaF application is a 2% concentration
   C. NaF will not damage porcelain crowns or composite restorations
   D. NaF is the most common professionally applied fluoride agent
   E. Does not promote staining or discoloration of the teeth

30 Before fluoride applications,
   A. All bacterial plaque must be removed to prevent interference with fluoride uptake by the enamel surface
   B. The teeth should be dry to prevent dilution of the fluoride concentration
   C. Petroleum jelly is applied to protect composite restorations, porcelain, and sealants
   D. Clients should be placed in a semi-supine position

31 Questionable or incipient occlusal carious lesions
   A. Require immediate restoration
   B. Are best treated with topical fluoride application(s)
   C. Are indicated for sealant placement to prevent decay progression
   D. Can be "watched," no treatment is indicated

32 Each of the following statements suggests an appropriate use for the phase contrast microscope *EXCEPT*
   A. Client education aid
   B. Diagnostic tool for periodontal disease
   C. Mechanism for treatment evaluation
   D. Determines the presence of bacteria morphotypes associated with health or disease therapy

33 To be truly a primary preventive procedure, dental sealants should be applied
   A. At the first clinical signs of decalcification
   B. Shortly after tooth eruption
   C. Before the radiographs are exposed
   D. Only to those teeth at high risk for caries
   E. After disease control techniques are mastered

34 Which of the following can be used as an initiator in an autopolymerizing dental sealant?
   A. Ultraviolet light
   B. Cryanoacrylates
   C. BIS GMA
   D. Monomer
   E. Tertiary amines

35 Pulsating oral irrigators are contraindicated
   A. For drug addicts
   B. Before amalgam polishing
   C. For use with a low pressure water stream
   D. For persons at risk for infectious endocarditis (SBE)
   E. For persons with fixed orthodontic appliances

36 Data collection procedures are
   A. The same for all clients
   B. Determined by client conditions
   C. Treatment planned after client education
   D. Performed during the evaluation phase of care
   E. Focused on solving the client's identified problems

37 The self-examination for oral cancer
  A. Is easily mastered after the initial demonstration
  B. Assumes all clients are easily motivated to master this skill
  C. Introduces the concept of "normal range"
  D. Evaluates simply the floor of the mouth, tongue, and buccal mucosa
  E. Relieves clinicians of their role in oral cancer examination

38 When there is a wide variation in the vitalometer readings of a single tooth, the dental hygienist should
  A. Average the readings and record the findings
  B. Review the technique and take an additional reading
  C. Refer the client to an endodontist for further evaluation
  D. Test the tooth using a temperature test
  E. Refer the client to an oral surgeon for tooth extraction

39 The Bass, or sulcular, toothbrushing technique
  A. Requires a high level of dexterity to perform
  B. Incorporates a sweeping motion to remove debris away from the gingival sulcus
  C. Disrupts plaque at and under the gingival margin
  D. Uses a circular vibratory stroke
  E. Directs the toothbrush bristles occlusally at a 45 degree angle

40 Oral irrigating devices have been shown to
  A. Reduce the incidence of refractory periodontitis
  B. Initiate keratinization of sulcular epithelium
  C. Negate the effects of occlusal trauma
  D. Promote healing following periodontal surgery
  E. None of the above

41 Rubber tip stimulators may be recommended for maintaining interproximal gingival contours and removal of interproximal plaque. Plaque removal with a rubber tip is accomplished by directing the tip toward the occlusal/incisal surface and tracing the gingival margin.
  A. Both statements are *TRUE*.
  B. Both statements are *FALSE*.
  C. The first statement is *TRUE*, the second statement is *FALSE*.
  D. The first statement is *FALSE*, the second statement is *TRUE*.

42 A hand-held syringe is an acceptable oral irrigating device for home use by clients with high level dexterity. However, caution must be taken with clients who are at risk for infective endocarditis because a transient bacteremia may occur.
  A. Both statement and reason are correct and related.
  B. Both statements are correct, but *NOT* related.
  C. The statement is correct, but the reason is *NOT*.
  D. The statement is *NOT* correct, but the reason is accurate.
  E. Neither the statement nor the reason is correct.

43 Professional oral irrigation has been suggested for use for all of the following *EXCEPT*
  A. As an adjunct to mechanical root debridement
  B. To flush a periodontal abscessed area
  C. To deliver antimicrobial agents subgingivally
  D. To disrupt subgingival bacterial organization

44 The application of dental sealants is
  A. Limited to the permanent dentition
  B. Contraindicated for traumatized teeth
  C. Not effective for smooth surface caries control
  D. Repeated every year beginning at 6 years of age
  E. Still under evaluation for their efficacy

45 Which statement is *NOT* true about antimicrobial oral irrigation?
  A. May enhance effects of scaling and root planing
  B. Must be done using full-strength antimicrobial mouthrinses
  C. Penetrates periodontal pockets up to 4 mm
  D. Is an effective pre-procedural treatment with essential oils mouthrinse
  E. May be delivered simultaneously with ultrasonic scaling

46 A "Baseline Human Needs Assessment" enhances collection of assessment data by identifying the client's unmet needs. Identification of these needs directs the focus of the dental hygiene diagnosis and care plan.
  A. Both statements are *TRUE*.
  B. Both statements are *FALSE*.
  C. The first statement is *TRUE*, the second statement is *FALSE*.
  D. The first statement is *FALSE*, the second statement is *TRUE*.

47 The health belief model includes all of the following concepts *EXCEPT*:
  A. Individuals must believe they are susceptible to disease
  B. Individuals must believe that changing their behavior will be beneficial
  C. Individuals must believe that active participation in learning new behaviors is important
  D. Individuals must believe that the consequences of a disease are serious
  E. Individuals must believe that disease can be asymptomatic

48 What is the *MOST* important reason for using a fluoride dentifrice?
  A. Good taste
  B. Remineralization
  C. Low abrasiveness
  D. Foaming action
  E. All of the above are equally important reasons

49 Mouthrinses
  A. Are an alternative to mechanical bacterial plaque control
  B. Are effective on both supragingival and subgingival bacterial plaque
  C. Containing antimicrobial agents are important adjuncts in the control of dental disease
  D. Are all approved by the ADA Council on Scientific Affairs for prevention and control of gingivitis

50 Frequent low potency doses of fluoride are important for enamel remineralization; 0.2% sodium fluoride is an example of a low dose, high frequency fluoride agent.
A. Both statements are *TRUE.*
B. Both statements are *FALSE.*
C. The first statement is *TRUE,* the second statement is *FALSE.*
D. The first statement is *FALSE,* the second statement is *TRUE.*

Answers and Rationales

1. (A) Powered toothbrushes are indicated for individuals who are physically or mentally challenged to provide an effective means for plaque removal.
   (B) Powered toothbrushes are ineffective for subgingival plaque removal in pocket depths greater than 3 mm.
   (C) Toothbrush trauma, by either manual or powered toothbrushes, is dependent on bristle stiffness and technique.
   (D) Persons with mitrovalve prolapse can safely use powered toothbrushes.
   (E) Powered toothbrushes tend to be easier to learn to use, because the brush motion is built in.
2. (C) The rubber tip stimulator is only minimally effective at plaque removal.
   (A) End tuft or single-tufted brushes are effective in plaque removal from surfaces not accessible with larger brushes.
   (B) Soft bristled, multitufted nylon toothbrushes are effective in removing plaque from fixed prostheses without causing trauma to the patient or prosthesis.
   (D) ADA-approved toothpastes have safe levels of abrasiveness which will not harm the dental implant.
   (E) Waxed dental floss is effective for removal of plaque on proximal surfaces, including proximal surfaces on dental implants.
3. (E) Research has documented repeatedly that fluoride therapy is the most effective agent for the prevention and control of dental caries, especially on smooth surfaces.
   (A) Continued care two times per year allow the opportunity for plaque control, dietary instruction, and fluoride application, but data have not documented a direct relationship between continued care frequency and caries reduction.
   (B) Radiographs can be taken at regular intervals to determine the occurrence of caries once it has begun.
   (C) Dental sealants are a preventive measure for prevention of dental caries in pits and fissures.
   (D) A diet low in sugar will help prevent the incidence of dental caries, but is not the *MOST* effective means of prevention or caries control.
4. (A) *BOTH STATEMENTS ARE TRUE.* Bacterial organization is necessary for caries and periodontal disease to occur, to prevent and control these diseases disruption of bacteria is necessary.
5. (C) Acidulated phosphate fluoride has been shown to be effective in the prevention and control of dental caries when applied professionally every 6 months.
   (A) The combination of 1.23% sodium fluoride and 1 M orthophosphoric acid results in acidulated phosphate fluoride.
   (B) Acidulated phosphate fluoride is very stable in solution.
   (D) There is no age limit with regard to the application of acidulated phosphate fluoride, adults as well as children receive the benefit of this topically applied fluoride.
   (E) The most common recommended over-the-counter fluoride is 0.05% sodium fluoride.
6. (D) An athletic mouthguard is worn for protection of the teeth during sports.
   (A) Fluoride promotes remineralization of demineralized tooth surfaces.
   (B) Caries destruction occurs rapidly when the quality and quantity of saliva is altered.
   (C) Orthodontic appliances make plaque removal difficult and encourage demineralization of the tooth surface.
   (E) Fluoride therapy contributes to the prevention and control of dentin hypersensitivity and root caries.
7. (C) The client's ability to remove plaque has no direct impact on the client's need for dental sealants to protect the pits and fissures of the occlusal surface.
   (A) If the client is unable to cooperate during sealant placement, salivary contamination can occur and result in sealant failure.
   (B) Sealants are ideally placed immediately following eruption of the tooth.
   (D) Shallow pits and fissures are more readily cleansed and less likely to decay.
8. (E) Because polymerization occurs only when light is applied to sealant material, there is time available for manipulation.
   (A) Self-cure or autopolymerizing sealant has a limited working time of 1 to 3 minutes.
   (B) Wiping off the surface of the sealant removes the unpolymerized layer and reduces the unpleasant taste often experienced by the client.
   (C) Autopolymerizing sealants require the mixing of the sealant material with a catalyst solution for polymerization to take place, unlike the visible light cured sealant which polymerizes when light is applied to the material.
   (D) There is no difference in the flow properties of either self-cure or light activated sealant.

9. (C) A thorough scaling and root planing is not necessary to obtain a plaque sample. Limited supragingival scaling may be needed to prevent contamination of a subgingival sample.

(A) Prior to obtaining a subgingival plaque sample, the supragingival deposits should be removed to prevent contamination of the plaque sample.

(B) It is important to select a client who will benefit from the use of the phase contrast microscope during oral hygiene instruction.

(D) If the client is to benefit from the experience they must understand what is involved in the procedure and how the information is beneficial to them.

10. (A) The use of a wooden toothpick on exposed cementum should have a burnishing effect on the surface and reduce the client's painful response.

(B) Vigorous horizontal brushing may cause further trauma and exposed cementum increasing the likelihood of a pain response.

(C) A sudden temperature change in the mouth can elicit a sensation of pain.

(D) The contact of metal on exposed cementum often causes the client to experience pain.

(E) On a vital tooth, the application of an electrical charge to the exposed dentin surface would result in an uncomfortable or painful response by the client.

11. (C) An interdental cleansing device should be chosen to safely remove plaque. Therefore, it must be designed to allow for the restrictions of the interdental space.

(A) Interdental cleaning devices do not conform to the anatomy of the interproximal space but are designed to fit into it.

(B) When used incorrectly interdental cleaning devices can result in a change in the position of the interdental papilla.

(D) The toothbrush does not adapt well interproximally, therefore interdental devices used correctly are more successful in removing plaque.

(E) The amount of manual dexterity to manipulate an interproximal device depends largely on the device chosen.

12. (E) Smokers are estimated to be two to four times at greater risk than nonsmokers.

(A) Fluoride therapy is not an etiologic factor in oral cancer.

(B) Adherence to an oral prophylaxis schedule is not an etiologic factor in oral cancer.

(C) Adhering to radiographic safety procedures during radiographic exposure minimizes client exposure to unnecessary radiation.

(D) Properly placed amalgam restorations, regardless of the number, are not a factor in oral cancer.

13. (A) The client's plaque control does not influence electrical charges.

(B) Metallic restorations conduct electrical charges more rapidly.

(C) Reactions to pain stimuli may vary with age.

(D) Mental state influences the client's response to pain.

(E) Toothpaste or some type of agent to conduct electrical impulses is necessary for an electrical charge to be conducted.

14. (E) Floss snapped through contacts or poorly adapted to surfaces can cut into papillary tissues.

(A) Erosion is a consequence of chemical assault on the tooth.

(B) Enamel hyperplasia is a developmental disturbance.

(C) Root dilaceration occurs during tooth development.

(D) Floss will not fracture composite material.

15. (A) Client education provides the information and skills necessary for preventive behaviors.

(B) There are a variety of strategies and techniques that have been shown effective in preventing dental disease.

(C) Mechanical interventions are but one means of disease control.

(D) Self-examination skills allow early detection of problems but not necessarily prevention.

(E) Topical fluoride therapy achieves caries reduction but will not prevent periodontal disease.

16. (C) Clients with no loss of attachment and who have exemplary plaque control would most likely not receive a therapeutic benefit from a mouthrinse. They may receive cosmetic value from a mouthrinse.

(A) Orthodontic clients would receive a benefit from the mouthrinse's ability to reduce plaque and gingivitis.

(B) Clients with poor manual dexterity have difficulty achieving acceptable mechanical plaque control.

(D) Postsurgical clients are often limited in the types of mechanical plaque control they may use. Certain mouthrinses offer these clients an alternative method of plaque control.

(E) The flavoring or sweetening agents provide a feeling of freshness following rinsing.

17. (C) The first statement is *TRUE*, the second is *FALSE*. Antimicrobials are a common ingredient in mouthrinses and their role is to inhibit microbial activity. Oxygenating agents are included in mouthrinses to debride and release oxygen. Astringents are responsible for encouraging tissue shrinkage.

18. (B) This lesion is linea alba and is a nonpathologic deviation from normal.

(A) A lesion present for more than 2 weeks warrants further evaluation.

(C) A patchy, white covering found in the vestibular area in conjunction with a habit of smokeless tobacco use requires further evaluation.

(D) Any change in the vermilion border is suspect, particularly if the client has a history of frequent or extended exposure to ultraviolet rays.

19. (C) Determining the course of action and setting goals for treatment are accomplished during the planning phase of care.
    (A) Assessment is the gathering of data to be analyzed and developed into a treatment plan.
    (B) Determining a client's unmet needs is accomplished via the dental hygiene diagnosis.
    (C) The implementation phase occurs when the treatment plan is put into action.
    (D) Evaluation determines the success of the interventions performed during the implementation phase.
20. (C) The first statement is *TRUE,* the second statement is *FALSE.* Disclosing solution will clearly display plaque that is present supragingivally for the client, however, it will not show subgingival plaque.
21. (B) Numerous studies document benefits of adding antimicrobial agents to power irrigators.
    (A) Effectiveness has been documented in the literature.
    (C) The depth of penetration of home irrigators is generally limited to 4 mm.
    (D) This is an effective regime for orthodontic clients.
    (E) Most manufacturers of irrigators have designed the units to accept antimicrobial mouthrinses.
22. (A) Malodors are produced most often in the mouth by bacteria, especially gram negative.
    (B) Bacteria colonize on the dorsal surface of the tongue to produce malodor.
    (C) Good oral hygiene, including tongue cleaning, controls most malodors.
    (D) Bacteria in periodontal pockets produce malodor; malodor is found with necrotizing ulcerative gingivitis (NUG).
    (E) Smoking contributes to mouth malodor.
23. (B) Dentifrices containing whitening agents have been shown to be effective at removing extrinsic stains such as: coffee, tea, wine, tobacco, and chlorhexidine.
    (A) Whitening of the tooth surface is accomplished by removal of stains.
    (C) Intrinsic stain removal cannot be accomplished by a dentifrice.
    (D) See B.
    (E) Dentifrices containing whitening agents do have abrasive qualities, research findings place the abrasivity at a low level when compared with other dentifrices including nonwhitening dentifrices.
24. (B) Fluoride dentifrices are most important because they remineralize tooth surfaces and thus prevent dental caries.
    (A) Taste is of lesser importance than the therapeutic effect of the fluoride.
    (C) All ADA approved toothpastes have safe levels of abrasives.
    (D) Although people seem to enjoy the foaming action of dentifrice, this is of lesser importance than the therapeutic benefit of remineralization.
    (E) All are not equal; remineralization is most important.

25. (C) An individual's actions are driven by needs. Needs or inner forces motivate individuals to meet or satisfy their needs; once a need has been met it no longer serves to motivate the individual.
    (A) According to human behavior principles, values are formed based on previous behaviors.
    (B) Individuals whose behaviors are centered around an external locus of control, feel that they themselves have no influence on the outcome of their behaviors.
    (D) Extrinsically generated motivators are based on offers of punishment or reward.
    (E) When examining values under the human behavior principles, if a behavior fits into an already existing value system, it will easily be adopted.
26. (A) Client demonstration and questioning during plaque control instruction indicates active client participation.
    (B) Attitudes are formed, not motivated.
    (C) Immediate feedback reinforces learning and desired behaviors.
    (D) Self-pacing recognizes that each person will progress at a different pace.
    (E) Small step size is an educational concept that introduces information limited to what can be assimilated in one session.
27. (A) Assessment of the client's current status identifies the client's perceived needs, wants, and expectations.
    (B) Planning of client care focuses on developing a comprehensive treatment plan that meets the client's needs.
    (C) The initiation and completion of the interventions necessary to meet the assessed needs occur during the implementation phase.
    (D) The success of the dental hygiene interventions is determined during evaluation.
28. (C) Changing or breaking old habits is very difficult and requires some time.
    (A) Dental hygienists may know the best plaque removal technique to recommend but they may not know what is best for the client.
    (B) Cost is a major concern for clients and although endorsement of a product by a professional is important to the client, it does not necessarily mean the client can afford the product.
    (D) Adherence is in the hands of the client, although a dental hygienist does have a responsibility to educate the client on the importance of the technique introduced.
29. (D) Acidulated phosphate fluoride (APF) is the most commonly applied in-office fluoride treatment.
    (A) The suggested ages for application of neutral sodium fluoride are: 3, 7, 10, and 13 years; this coincides with the eruption of both primary and permanent dentitions.
    (B) Professional applications of sodium fluoride are given at a 2.0% concentration.
    (C) Because it is a neutral preparation it will not cause etching of the porcelain or composite restorations.
    (E) It does not stain or discolor the teeth.

30. (B) It is best to thoroughly dry the teeth before applying the fluoride to maximize the effectiveness of the fluoride application and prevent dilution of the agent.
    (A) Plaque does not interfere with the application of fluoride. However, it is advisable to instruct the client on proper toothbrushing and flossing techniques and this could be done before fluoride application and would remove plaque simultaneously.
    (C) Petroleum jelly is needed to protect porcelain and composite restorations, but is not necessary for sealants.
    (D) Clients should be placed in a position to prevent swallowing fluoride during the fluoride application, either a supine or upright position would be acceptable.

31. (C) The placement of a sealant has been shown to arrest the caries process of incipient lesions.
    (A) Can best be treated with a sealant, a restoration is not indicated for incipient or questionable caries.
    (B) Topical fluoride treatments are most effective on the smooth surfaces of the teeth.
    (D) If the tooth is "watched," it may progress and become a carious lesion resulting in the need for a restoration.

32. (B) Phase contrast microscopy is a useful tool for motivating clients, but it does not provide information specific enough for diagnosis.
    (A) It is a valuable tool to demonstrate the presence of bacterial plaque to a client.
    (C) Comparing pre-treatment plaque samples to post-treatment plaque samples can determine a change in the subgingival bacterial population.
    (D) The presence or absence of various bacterial morphotypes can distinguish the difference between a healthy and a diseased sample site.

33. (B) Primary preventive measures are designed to prevent disease before initiation. Sealing teeth as soon as they are fully erupted is a primary preventive measure.
    (A) Providing treatment after the clinical signs of incipient disease have been recognized is a secondary preventive measure.
    (C) Sealing for primary prevention can occur before or after the first prophylaxis.
    (D) All molars and premolars are sealed in a primary prevention protocol.
    (E) Disease control techniques, such as brushing, are relatively ineffective for control of pit and fissure caries.

34. (E) Polymerization occurs when a tertiary amine is mixed with the monomer.
    (A) Autopolymerizing systems do not require the use of an ultraviolet light.
    (B) Cryanoacrylates are a plastic material.
    (C) BIS-GMA is the most routinely used sealant resin.
    (D) The unpolymerized resin is called a monomer.

35. (D) Transient bacteremias may occur with oral irrigation. Persons who require antibiotic premedication before dental procedures are best advised not to use an oral irrigating device.
    (A) Irrigators do not endanger the health of a drug addict.
    (B) Amalgams are not altered by oral irrigators.
    (C) A low pressure setting creates an ideal water stream that is both safe and effective.
    (E) Orthodontic brackets and bands are appropriately cleaned with oral irrigators.

36. (B) Data collection procedures are determined by client conditions. For example, the full-denture client will not require periodontal pocket measurements.
    (A) Although certain assessment procedures are indicated for all clients, the range of procedures will differ for each client.
    (C) The plan for client education is based on data collection and analysis.
    (D) Treatment goals and continued care intervals are based on previous assessment and success of implemented interventions.
    (E) Data collection assesses the client's current or potential problems. Interventions are focused on solving the problems.

37. (C) Introducing the "normal range" for oral cancer lets clients see what is normal for them.
    (A) Often mastery of the self-examination takes several demonstrations.
    (B) Clients may be interested in the concept of self-examination; however, this does not mean they will be motivated to perform self-exams.
    (D) Self-examination for oral cancer evaluates all structures of the head and neck.
    (E) The clinician plays a vital role in educating individuals at high risk for oral cancer and also continuing to evaluate these clients for signs and symptoms of oral cancer.

38. (B) Evaluate the technique he/she is using, determine if there have been any errors, retake the reading.
    (A) There may have been a problem with the technique and simply averaging the previous readings may not result in an accurate reading.
    (C) Referrals should be made after accurate data have been collected.
    (D) Temperature tests provide additional information. They may not provide enough information for accurate diagnosis or referral.
    (E) Referral to an oral surgeon is generally the last treatment alternative presented to the client and with such a variation in vitalometer readings further evaluation of the tooth is required.

39. (C) The Bass or sulcular brushing technique is an effective toothbrushing method for the disruption of bacterial plaque at or slightly below the gingival margin. The technique is successful because it directs the bristles into the gingival sulcus.
    (A) Dexterity is an important aspect to this technique but a high level of dexterity is not necessary to adapt the toothbrush bristles at a 45 degree angle to the tooth surface.
    (B) A sweeping motion may be used to modify the technique, but it is generally an accepted component of the Roll method.
    (D) A circular or vibratory stroke is used with the Fones toothbrushing method.
    (E) Toothbrush bristles are directed apically for the Bass/sulcular toothbrushing method.

40. (E) *NONE* of the answers were correct.
    (A) The etiology of refractory periodontitis is multifactorial and its incidence is not affected by oral irrigation.
    (B) Sulcular epithelium is not keratinized.
    (C) Uncorrected trauma from occlusion will continue regardless of the level of oral cleanliness.
    (D) Surgically treated tissues are fragile and should not be disturbed by pressurized irrigating devices.

41. (C) The first statement is *TRUE*, the second statement is *FALSE*. Some practitioners have found that a rubber tip stimulator may be an effective adjunct to maintain gingival contours and remove plaque interproximally. In order for the rubber tip to be effective the tip should be directed apically while tracing the gingival margin.

42. (A) *BOTH* the statement and reason are correct and related. Manipulation of a hand-held irrigating syringe requires a great deal of manual dexterity; regulating the pressure and the force of fluid flowing through the syringe is difficult to control. Irrigating solutions could potentially be forced into surrounding tissues during irrigation creating a transient bacteremia.

43. (B) Irrigating an area of a periodontal abscess could potentially force the spread of infection into the surrounding tissue.
    (A) The use of professional irrigation may be an effective adjunct in the promotion of healing following mechanical root debridement.
    (C) Antimicrobial agents can be administered during professional or at home irrigation.
    (D) The mechanical action of irrigation has been shown to be effective in the disorganization of bacterial colonies in the gingival crevice or pocket.

44. (C) Dental sealants are applied to pit and fissure surfaces.
    (A) Caries control for primary teeth may include the application of dental sealants.
    (B) Trauma to the tooth has an effect on the vitality of the tooth not the caries susceptibility.
    (D) Properly applied sealants can be retained for many years. The need for reapplication is determined by clinical examination of the surfaces sealed and not related to a schedule of applications.
    (E) Numerous research studies have shown sealants to be a safe and effective means of reducing the incidence of pit and fissure caries.

45. (B) Studies show efficacy using dilute chlorhexidine or essential oils mouthrinse in a home irrigating device.
    (A) Studies show limited benefits of irrigation following scaling and root planing.
    (C) With the irrigating tip directed perpendicular to the tooth, penetration of the irrigant may reach 4 mm.
    (D) Pre-procedural irrigation has been shown to reduce bloodborne bacteria following invasive dental procedures.
    (E) Some powered scaling units deliver an antimicrobial agent during scaling.

46. (A) *BOTH* statements are *TRUE*. An initial or baseline human needs assessment identifies needs of a client that have not been fulfilled. Fulfillment of these needs will direct or guide the dental hygiene care plan.

47. (B) Frequent use of fluoride in dentifrice remineralizes tooth surfaces to prevent and control caries.
    (A) Cleaning and polishing agents in dentifrices control stains.
    (C) Tartar control agents, pyrophosphate or zinc, interfere with the calcium-phosphate bond in the calculus matrix.
    (D) All dentifrices have flavoring agents; taste is a matter of personal preference.
    (E) Other ingredients, such as potassium nitrate and strontium chloride are added to control dentinal hypersensitivity.

48. (C) The concept of active participation is not part of the Health Belief Model. It is one of the principles of learning.
    (A) Susceptibility is part of the Health Belief Model.
    (B) Belief that changing one's behavior will be beneficial is one of the four parts of the Health Belief Model.
    (D) Belief that the consequences of a disease are serious is one part of the Health Belief Model.
    (E) Belief that a disease can be asymptomatic is also part of the Health Belief Model. If an individual believes all four components of this model, he/she will be more likely to change behaviors than one who does not ascribe to this model.

532 Mosby's Comprehensive Review of Dental Hygiene

49. (C) Mouthrinses that contain antimicrobial agents such as 0.12% chlorhexidine are adjuncts to mechanical plaque control techniques.
   (A) Mouthrinses are an adjunct and not an alternative to mechanical plaque control.
   (B) Mouthrinses are only effective on supragingival plaque, unless they are delivered through an irrigation system subgingivally and would be effective on subgingival plaque.
   (D) Only Peridex, 0.12% chlorhexidine, Listerine, and various brands with the same active ingredients are approved by the ADA Council on Scientific Affairs for the control of bacterial plaque and gingivitis.

50. (C) The first statement is *TRUE*, the second statement is *FALSE*. It is true that frequent low potency doses of fluoride are important for enamel remineralization, however, 0.2% NaF is an example of a high potency/low frequency fluoride agent.

Instrumentation for Client Assessment and Care

Jill S. Nield-Gehrig Esther M. Wilkins

As a primary healthcare provider, the dental hygienist participates in the client's total oral care, using preventive, educational, and therapeutic methods. The dental hygienist is a cotherapist with the dentist and the client and has responsibility during various phases of care.

Initially, the dental hygienist collects and records data for use in making the dental hygiene, periodontal and dental diagnoses and for formulation of the dental and dental hygiene care plans. The techniques required for preparation of the personal, comprehensive health, and dental histories, the radiographic survey, study casts, photographs, records of extraoral and intraoral conditions observed, and chartings of dental and periodontal findings are all part of the specialized skills of the dental hygienist.

As professional treatment is started, the client participates by learning therapeutic disease control techniques for daily home care. The basic initial care procedures performed by the dental hygienist are difficult and exacting and require a high level of skill. This chapter has as its primary focus the dental hygienist's responsibilities in the use of instruments for assessment and periodontal therapy.

Basic Concepts

A. Selection and use of instruments depend on knowledge of the characteristics of the area of treatment in health

and disease, namely, the anatomic and topographic features of the natural and restored tooth surfaces and the anatomy and histopathology of the periodontium (gingiva, periodontal ligament, cementum, alveolar bone)

B. Periodontal examination and recording of findings provide the data for the diagnosis and care plan, which is the blueprint for instrumentation

C. Ultimate purpose of all care is to create an environment in which the periodontal tissues can first be restored to health and then be maintained in health without the recurrence of disease

D. Success of professional care depends on the control of bacterial plaque; therefore, instruction and supervision in plaque removal procedures for the daily participation by the client precedes, continues simultaneously with, and follows instrumentation by the clinician

Environment of Instrumentation

Types of Pockets

See Chapter 11, section on changes within the periodontium associated with disease.

A. Pocket—diseased sulcus or crevice; it is the presence or absence of disease and the level of attached periodontal fibers on the tooth that distinguish a pocket from a sulcus, not only the depth of the pocket as measured with a probe

B. Gingival pocket—pocket formed by gingival enlargement without change in the attachment level and without destruction of the underlying periodontal tissues
    1. Attachment level—at or above the cementoenamel junction
    2. Tooth pocket wall—enamel
    3. Instrumentation surfaces—enamel
C. Periodontal pocket—pocket formed by destruction of underlying periodontal tissues that resulted in migration of the soft tissue attachment; there may also be enlargement of the gingival tissue
    1. Attachment level—below the cementoenamel junction, along the root surface
    2. Tooth pocket wall—when the gingival margin is above the cementoenamel junction, the tooth wall may be partly enamel and partly cementum
    3. Instrumentation surface—may be cementum or both enamel and cementum
    4. Types of periodontal pockets (Fig. 13-1)
        a. Suprabony—base of the pocket is coronal to the crest of the alveolar bone; all gingival pockets are suprabony because no changes have occurred in the bone level or contour
        b. Intrabony (infrabony)—base of the pocket is below or apical to the crest of the alveolar bone

Description of a Pocket

See Chapter 11, section on changes within the periodontium associated with disease.

A. Description
    1. A pocket is formed by the tooth surface wall and the gingival wall
    2. At the base of the pocket the soft tissue is attached to the tooth by the epithelial attachment, which is the inner layer of cells of the junctional epithelium
    3. Location and nature of subgingival instrumentation are directly related to anatomic and pathologic features of the pocket
B. Gingival wall of the pocket
    1. In health
        a. Lining of the sulcus is called *sulcular epithelium,* which is nonkeratinized stratified squamous epithelium
        b. Sulcular epithelium connects directly with the junctional epithelium
    2. In disease
        a. Lining of the pocket is called *pocket epithelium*
        b. Pocket is characterized by
            (1) Degenerative changes in the epithelium with varying degrees of destruction of the intercellular substance
            (2) Ulceration and proliferation of epithelium with increased rete ridges extending into the connective tissue
            (3) Enlargement, which may be either

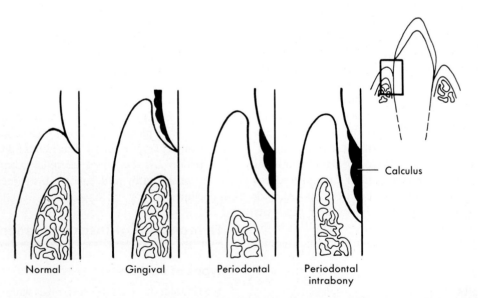

Normal   Gingival   Periodontal   Periodontal intrabony

— Calculus

Fig. 13-1   Types of pockets. (From Wilkins EM: *Clinical practice of the dental hygienist,* ed 7, Baltimore, 1994, Williams & Wilkins.)

(a) Soft, spongy tissue—related to edema and local circulatory stasis
(b) Hard, firm tissue—with long-term chronic inflammation, fibrosis results
C. Junctional epithelium
1. In health—normal junctional epithelium is a collarlike band of stratified squamous epithelium 10 to 20 cells thick near the sulcus and 2 to 3 cells thick at the apical end; it is 0.25 to 1.35 mm long
2. In disease—migration of the junctional epithelium occurs, along with degeneration in the connective tissue under the attachment; as the junctional epithelium proliferates along the root surface, the coronal portion detaches
D. Tooth surface wall of the pocket
1. Gingival pocket—tooth surface wall is enamel; calculus on the subgingival surface is attached to the enamel
2. Periodontal pocket—tooth surface wall may be entirely cementum or partly cementum and partly enamel; calculus is attached to cementum or partly to cementum and partly to enamel
3. Root surface
a. Thickness of cementum
(1) Thickest near apex—may be 150 to 200 μm (0.15 to 0.2 mm)
(2) Thinnest at cervical third—may be 20 to 50 μm (0.02 to 0.05 mm)
b. Causes of surface roughness as detected by a probe or explorer may be
(1) Diseased, altered cementum
(2) Cemental resorption
(3) Calculus

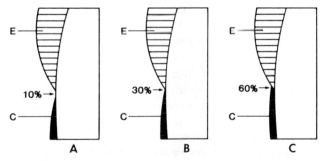

Fig. 13-2   Cementoenamel junction. The possible relationships of the enamel and the cementum at the cementoenamel junction. **A,** The cementum and the enamel do not meet and there is a small zone of dentin exposed in 10% of teeth. **B,** The cementum meets the enamel in approximately 30% of teeth. **C,** The cementum overlaps the enamel in about 60% of teeth. (From Wilkins EM: *Clinical practice of the dental hygienist,* ed 7, Baltimore, 1994, Williams & Wilkins.)

(4) Demineralization or dental caries
(5) Anomalies
(6) Abrasion
(7) Overhanging or deficient filling
(8) Previous instrumentation grooves or scratches
4. Diseased, altered cementum
a. As the junctional epithelium migrates along the root surface, the pocket deepens and the periodontal ligament detaches
b. Cementum is exposed to the pocket environment; the pocket contains many microorganisms in attached and unattached bacterial plaque, bacterial products, sulcus fluid, and white blood cells
c. Cementum is altered, and its physical and chemical properties are changed; bacterial products become incorporated in the surface especially endotoxin, which can interfere with healing of periodontal tissues
d. Calculus subsequently forms on the exposed cementum
(1) Rough surface of calculus harbors many microorganisms of subgingival plaque, which perpetuate inflammation in the pocket wall
(2) The surface of the diseased cementum is removed during instrumentation to create an environment for tissue healing and reattachment
5. Cementoenamel junction (Fig. 13-2)
a. Small zone of dentin between cementum and enamel—5% to 10%
b. Cementum and enamel meet directly—30%
c. Cementum overlaps enamel—60% to 65%

Calculus

See Chapters 7 and 11, sections on bacterial plaque.
A. Definition
1. Calcified or mineralized bacterial plaque
2. Hard tenacious mass that forms on the clinical crowns* of natural teeth and on dentures and other dental prostheses
3. Surface of calculus is very rough and is covered by a layer of bacterial plaque
4. Calculus is designated clinically as light, moderate, or heavy, based on quantity and hardness

---

*The clinical crown is the part of the tooth above the attached periodontal tissues—the part of the tooth where clinical techniques and instrumentation are applied. The clinical root is the part of the tooth to which periodontal fibers are attached.

B. Types, distribution, and shape
   1. Supragingival (supramarginal, salivary)
      a. Located above the gingival margin
      b. Rarely generalized
      c. Most common locations
         (1) Lingual mandibular anterior teeth
         (2) Facial maxillary molars
         (3) Teeth out of occlusion
      d. Subgingival calculus may become supragingival when the pocket wall shrinks and recession occurs
      e. Shape—determined by the anatomy of the teeth, contour of the gingival margin, and pressure of the tongue, lips, and cheeks
         (1) Generally amorphous, bulky
         (2) Gross deposits may form an interproximal bridge between adjacent teeth and/or extend over the margin of the free gingiva
   2. Subgingival (submarginal, serumal)
      a. Located below or beneath the gingival margin
      b. May be generalized or localized; heaviest on proximal surfaces
      c. Extends along the root surface nearly to the bottom of the pocket; the newest, less calcified calculus is at the most apical area, near the soft tissue attachment
      d. Shape—flattened to conform to pressure from the gingival pocket wall; forms of calculus on the tooth surface may include combinations of the following
         (1) Crusty, spiny, or nodular deposits
         (2) Ledge or ringlike formations
         (3) Thin, smooth veneers
         (4) Finger and fernlike formations
         (5) Individual calculus islands
C. Modes of attachment—calculus is more readily removed from some tooth surfaces than others; usually the difficulty is related to the manner in which the calculus is attached; on any one tooth more than one mode of attachment can occur; attachment to hard, smooth enamel is different from attachment to the rough, porous, less hard cemental surface
   1. By an acquired pellicle
      a. Pellicle is a thin, homogeneous, acellular layer that occurs on all exposed tooth surfaces; it appears between the smooth tooth surface and the calculus deposit
      b. Calculus may be removed readily because there is no interlocking or penetration; this is the most common mode of attachment to enamel
   2. By minute irregularities in the tooth surface that permit locking into undercuts
      a. Enamel irregularities—cracks, lamellae, carious defects
      b. Cemental irregularities—tiny spaces left where Sharpey's fibers were detached, resorption lacunae, scaling grooves, cemental tears, or fragmentation
      c. Difficult to detect complete removal because the instrumentation may smooth the surface over an irregularity
   3. By direct attachment of the calcified calculus matrix to the tooth surface
      a. Interlocking of inorganic crystals of the tooth with the mineralizing plaque
      b. During removal distinction between calculus and cementum is difficult
D. Examination and identification of calculus
   1. Supragingival/supramarginal
      a. Direct observation using appropriate procedures of retraction and lighting; mouth mirror is used for indirect lighting and vision
      b. Compressed air—small amounts of calculus may be invisible when wet with saliva; retraction and drying with gentle air stream helps to make the calculus visible
      c. Explorer may be needed for areas not directly observable such as calculus on proximal surfaces (see section on explorers)
   2. Subgingival/submarginal
      a. Visual—calculus within a pocket may be seen just within the edge of the pocket margin; for direct vision the margin may be moved away by a gentle air stream
      b. Transillumination—light through teeth may reveal dark opaque areas; calculus can be confirmed by use of an explorer
      c. Tactile
         (1) Probe will reveal root surface roughness
         (2) Subgingival explorer will adapt to all surfaces to detect calculus or other irregularities before treatment and at the end of treatment to verify completeness of calculus removal and tooth surface smoothness

Principles for Instrumentation

Basic Concepts

A. Each instrument is designed for a particular purpose and is intended to be used for that purpose
B. Effective instrumentation is accomplished by certain general principles of client and clinician positioning; visibility through adequate lighting and retraction of

the client's lips, cheeks, and tongue; and maintenance of a clean field

C. Stability during the application of an instrument depends on the grasp and the finger rest applied; stability is essential for controlled action of the instrument and to prevent trauma to the client

D. Activation of an instrument is accomplished by adaptation, angulation, and stroke

E. Precise familiarity with the specific form, shape, and surface topography of each tooth and the relationship to other teeth in the permanent, mixed, and primary dentitions is essential to the understanding and use of the instruments

Parts of an Instrument

A. Working end—end of the instrument that contacts the tooth or soft tissue to perform the intended function; ends take a variety of shapes; some are sharp, some not sharp; examples include
   1. Blade
      a. Sharp—scaler, curet
      b. Dull—probe; the term *nib* is sometimes used to designate the working end of a nonsharp instrument, particularly in restorative dentistry
   2. Point—explorer
   3. Other—head of a mirror, spatula end

B. Shank—connects the working end with the handle; length, rigidity, and shape are designed to allow proper access of the working end to accomplish the intended instrumentation
   1. Straight—for an area with unrestricted access such as an anterior tooth
   2. Angled or curved—for an area of restricted access such as proximal surfaces of posterior teeth
   3. Lower (terminal) shank—part of the shank next to the working end
   4. Complex shank—curet designed for deep pockets in posterior interdental areas may have a complex shank with several angles

C. Handle—part of the instrument held or grasped during activation of the blade; there are a variety of shapes, weights, sizes, and surface serrations (smooth, ribbed, or knurled)
   1. Types
      a. Single end—with one working end
      b. Double end—may have paired (mirror image) or complementary working ends, one on each end; paired working ends are used for access to proximal surfaces, one for access from the lingual aspect and the opposite for access from the facial aspect
      c. Cone socket—working end and shank are sepa-

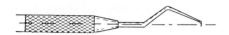

Fig. 13-3 Balanced instrument. Middle of tip (working end) should be centered over long axis of handle. (Modified from Wilkins EM: *Clinical practice of the dental hygienist,* ed 7, Baltimore, 1994, Williams & Wilkins.)

rable from the handle to permit instrument exchanges and replacements
   2. Diameter—small-diameter handles decrease control and increase muscle fatigue; large-diameter handles maximize control and reduce muscle fatigue but restrict movement in treatment areas with restricted access

D. Identification of the working ends of a double-ended instrument
   1. In practice the skilled clinician selects the correct working end by observation
   2. Manufacturers identify each instrument by stamped names and numbers

E. Balance of an instrument—balanced instrument has the working end centered in line with the long axis of the handle (Fig. 13-3)

Instrument Identification

A. Classification by purpose or use
   1. Examination (examples—probe, explorer)
   2. Treatment (examples—scalers, curets)

B. Description on the instrument handle
   1. Design name (may be abbreviated); school or individual originally responsible for the design or development (e.g., TU-17, in which *TU* stands for Tufts University, School of Dental Medicine)
   2. Design number—traditional exact number; often an instrument may be manufactured by different companies but the same number is used (example—Gracey series 1-2, 3-4, etc.)

Stabilization During Instrumentation

The instrumentation grasp and finger rest provide stabilization for instrument control and for prevention of trauma to the patient's teeth and soft tissues.

A. Grasp—manner in which an instrument is held
   1. Modified pen grasp (Fig. 13-4)
      a. Instrument is held by the thumb and index finger at the junction of the instrument shank and handle
      b. Side of pad of the second finger is placed on the shank
         (1) To hold and guide the movement

(2) To prevent the instrument handle from turning

(3) To feel the shank vibrate when the working end encounters roughness on the tooth surface

c. Third (ring) finger is the fulcrum finger

d. Tightness of grasp

(1) Light grasp is needed for increased tactile sensitivity (example—use of an explorer or probe during pocket examination)

(2) Firm grasp is needed during the stroke of a scaler or curet when calculus is being removed

e. Uses—generalized use during all instrumentation except as suggested for the palm grasp

2. Palm grasp

a. Handle of the instrument is held firmly in the palm by cupped index, second, ring, and little fingers

b. Thumb serves as the finger rest

c. Uses—air syringe, rubber dam clamp holder, porte polisher on facial of the anterior surfaces

B. Fulcrum (finger rest)

1. Definitions

a. Fulcrum—support or point of rest on which a lever turns in moving a body

b. Finger rest—support or point of rest of the finger on the tooth surface on which the hand turns in moving an instrument

2. Types of finger rests

a. Conventional intraoral

(1) Placed on a tooth adjacent to the area of instrumentation (Fig. 13-4, note finger numbered 3)

(2) Precaution—the rest is not positioned in line of the stroke to prevent instrument stick of the clinician or the clinician's glove in case of an unexpected movement by the patient

(3) Conventional intraoral finger rest is considered the most desirable because it provides the greatest stability

b. Alternate intraoral—variations of the finger rest may be required for visibility and access; as the rest is moved farther from the work area, less stability may be evident; for example, placing the index finger of the other hand against the alveolar ridge in the area of instrumentation to create a stable platform upon which the fulcrum finger can rest

c. Extraoral fulcrums—in areas of restricted access it may be necessary to use an extraoral fulcrum such as placing the index finger of the other hand against the patient's face to create a stable area for an extraoral rest

3. Pressure applied—pressure on the rest should provide an even balance with the grasp of the instrument and the amount of pressure needed for the particular instrument action; excess pressure decreases stability, tactile sensitivity, and instrument control

4. Objectives—grasp and finger rest

a. Control pressure and length of the stroke

b. Prevent laceration

Adaptation

A. Definition—relationship between the instrument and the surface of the tooth or soft tissue

B. Characteristics

1. Correct adaptation is when the working end of an instrument is positioned to conform to the morphology of the tooth surface

2. Adaptation for line angles

a. Roll the instrument handle between the fingers of the grasp to maintain correct adaptation

b. Only a portion of the blade of a scaler or curet can be used

c. Side of the pointed tip of an explorer is adapted so the sharp tip is held carefully against the tooth (Fig. 13-5)

d. Round, tapered probe adapts readily around a line angle; flat, rectangular probe must be removed and turned for adaptation at a line angle

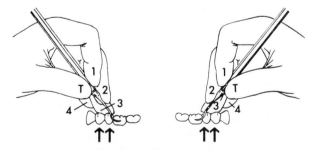

Fig. 13-4 Modified pen grasp. Thumb *(T)* and index finger *(1)* are held opposite each other near junction of handle and shank; second finger *(2)* is placed on shank; ring finger *(3)* is used for rest or fulcrum point. (Modified from Wilkins EM: *Clinical practice of the dental hygienist,* ed 7, Baltimore, 1994, Williams & Wilkins.)

Angulation

A. Definition—angle formed by the working end of an instrument with the surface to which the instrument is applied; each instrument is applied to a tooth surface in a specific manner for optimal action

B. Probe—usual adaptation of a probe is to maintain the

side of the blade on the tooth with the long axis of the blade nearly parallel with the tooth surface

C. Explorer
1. Occlusal surface—tip is held at a right angle to detect occlusal pit or fissure caries
2. Smooth surface
   a. Side of the tip is held against the surface at no more than a 5-degree angle to detect surface irregularities; may require turning or rolling between the fingers depending on type of explorer (see section on explorers)
   b. For a subgingival explorer, a close adaptation and a 5-degree angle prevent unnecessary trauma to the pocket or sulcus soft tissue wall

D. Scalers and curets
1. Working angle between 70 and 80 degrees is formed by the tooth surface and the face of the blade; burnishing of the calculus may result when an angle of less than 45 degrees is applied
2. Insertion of curet for pocket instrumentation—angle closes toward the tooth surface to 5 to 10 degrees

Lateral Pressure

A. Definition—pressure of the instrument against the tooth during activation; described as light, moderate, or heavy
B. Explorers and probe—for the detection instruments, a light touch but with definite contact with the tooth surface is needed for the maximum degree of tactile sensitivity
C. Scalers and curets
1. Placement stroke—light pressure until the instrument is positioned
2. Working stroke
   a. For calculus removal—pressure varies with the type, hardness, and attachment of the deposit; too light a stroke can lead to burnishing the deposit
   b. For root planing—pressure is progressively reduced until a light pressure is used as the root surface becomes smooth

Activation—Strokes

A. Definition—a stroke is an unbroken movement made by an instrument; it is the action of an instrument in the performance of the task for which it was designed; strokes may be identified by their action (movement), by their function, or by their direction
B. Types of strokes by action
1. Pull—scaler removing calculus
2. Push—placement stroke when a curet is being inserted into a subgingival area and positioned for function
3. Combined push and pull—explorer in a walking stroke when the side of the instrument tip is held against the side of the tooth and moved up and down
4. Walking stroke—probe moved up and down touching the bottom of the sulcus or pocket with each down stroke; usually short, accomplished in a circumferential direction
C. Types of strokes by function
1. Assessment stroke (exploratory)—movement of a probe or explorer for examination of a tooth surface
2. Working stroke—movement of a curet to remove calculus from a tooth surface
D. Types of strokes by direction
1. Vertical—parallel with the long axis of the tooth
2. Horizontal—perpendicular to the long axis of the tooth
3. Diagonal or oblique—diagonal to the long axis of the tooth
4. Circular—small (1- to 2-mm diameter) strokes (e.g., for a porte polisher when applying an agent such as desensitizing agent or polishing paste)
5. Circumferential—repetitive vertical or diagonal strokes as the instrument is moved around the tooth

Instrumentation for Examination

Basic Concepts

A. Successful treatment depends on well-developed detection skills for the use of the instruments of examination
1. Before treatment for assessment, analysis, and treatment planning
2. After instrumentation for evaluation of the completeness of treatment
B. Complete examination involves all aspects of the periodontium and the teeth; emphasis on certain parts

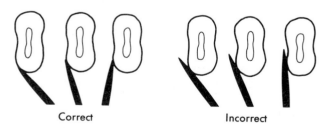

Correct   Incorrect

Fig. 13-5   Adaptation of explorer tip. Side of sharp tip is held carefully against tooth surface; at line angle correct adaptation is maintained by rolling handle between fingers of grasp. (Redrawn from Pattison GL, Pattison AM: *Periodontal instrumentation*, ed 2, Norwalk, Conn, 1992, Appleton & Lange.)

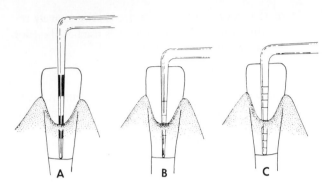

Fig. 13-6 Measurement of same 5 mm pocket with three different probes. **A,** Color coded. **B,** Michigan O. **C,** Williams. (From Wilkins EM: *Clinical practice of the dental hygienist,* ed 7, Baltimore, 1994, Williams & Wilkins.)

with omission of other parts may lead to overlooking items of importance to the total oral health of the client

C. Client preparation based on information from the personal, comprehensive health, and dental histories is essential for safe instrumentation

Essentials for Effective Use of Examination Instruments

A. Accessibility
   1. Client and clinician position
   2. Retraction
   3. Isolation and maintenance of a clean field
B. Visibility
   1. Adequate illumination
   2. Mouth mirror
      a. Purposes
         (1) Indirect vision
         (2) Indirect illumination
         (3) Transillumination
         (4) Retraction of the tongue and cheeks
      b. Technique for use—modified pen grasp with a finger rest positioned to provide stability and to aid in retraction

Probe

A. Characteristics
   1. Straight blade
      a. Shape—slender, rodlike, with a smooth rounded end; may be tapered or straight; round, flat, or rectangular in cross section
      b. Calibrations—millimeter marks at intervals specific for each probe design; some are color coded; examples of markings (Fig. 13-6) include
         (1) Williams—1-2-3-5-7-8-9-10 mm
         (2) Michigan 0—3-6-8 mm
         (3) Color coded—3-6-9-12 mm; 3-6-8-11 mm

   2. Curved blade—noncalibrated furcation probe: curved, narrow, smooth probe with rounded blunt end for investigation of the topography within a furcation area (e.g., Nabers probes)
B. Purposes and uses
   1. Assess the periodontal status and prepare the treatment plan
      a. Aid in classifying the patient's disease as gingivitis or periodontitis by determining probing depth, the level of periodontal attachment, and whether there is bone loss
      b. Determine the extent of inflammation in conjunction with the probing depth and attachment level; bleeding on probing is an early sign of inflammation
   2. Make a sulcus and pocket survey
      a. Examine the shape, topography, and dimensions of sulci and pockets
      b. Measure attachment levels
      c. Measure probing depths
      d. Evaluate the tooth surface pocket wall for calculus and other irregularities
   3. Make a mucogingival examination
      a. Determine the relationship between the gingival margin position, mucogingival junction, and the level of attached periodontal tissue
      b. Measure the width of the attached gingiva
   4. Evaluate bleeding
      a. Identify inflammation if present
      b. Prepare a gingival bleeding index
   5. Determine the consistency of the gingival tissue by gently pressing on the free gingiva
      a. Firm—resists the probe, fibrotic
      b. Spongy—soft, smooth, shiny, edematous
   6. Measure the extent of apparent (visible) gingival recession
   7. Provide a guide to treatment
      a. Gingival characteristics, including probing depth, bleeding, and consistency, provide a basis for patient instruction
      b. Probing depth defines the depth of scaling and root planing
      c. Anatomic configuration of tooth surfaces, shape of calculus deposits, and tooth anomalies and irregularities that complicate instrumentation may be defined by carefully probing before instrumentation
   8. Evaluation of treatment outcomes
      a. Tissue response to the client's self-treatment (therapeutic plaque control)
      b. Tissue response to professional treatment (e.g., scaling, root planing)
      c. Evidence of health determined by the probe

(1) No bleeding on gentle probing
(2) Reduced probing depth
(3) Firm tissue

Techniques for Use

A. Grasp and finger rest for all determinations
   1. Grasp—modified pen
   2. Finger rest—on tooth surface; fulcrum should be located near the area being probed, especially in the same arch, and where possible in the same quadrant
B. Examining pockets
   1. Insertion
     a. Hold the side of the tip against the tooth with a firm but light lateral pressure
     b. Direct the tip toward the gingival margin; gently insert the probe
   2. Activation
     a. Slide the probe along the tooth surface vertically; maintain contact with the tooth at all times
       (1) Gingival pocket—side of the probe is held against the enamel surface
       (2) Periodontal pocket—probe is held against the enamel in the coronal part and then against the root surface as the pocket extends beyond the cementoenamel junction
     b. Evaluate the nature and topography of the tooth surface as the probe passes into the pocket
     c. Interferences—any of the items listed as tooth surface irregularities may be noted; when a protrusion of calculus is felt, the probe should be passed over the surface of the calculus and guided back to the tooth apically
     d. Base of the pocket or sulcus (level of *actual recession*)
       (1) Will feel soft and resilient and offers light to moderate tissue resistance depending on the health of the tissue
       (2) Pressure to use—as little as possible to provide tactile sensitivity to the attached tissue; from 10 to 20 g is usually sufficient
C. Measuring probing depth
   1. Definition—*probing depth* is the distance from the gingival margin to the attachment level
   2. Reading the probe (Fig. 13-6)
     a. With the probe in vertical position and in contact with the attached tissue, count the millimeters that appear above the gingival margin
     b. Subtract the millimeters appearing above the margin from the total number of probe marks of the particular probe being used to obtain the probing depth at that site
     c. When the gingival margin appears between the

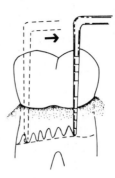

Fig. 13-7 Probe walking stroke. Side of tip of probe is held in contact with tooth. From base of pocket, probe is moved up and down in 1 to 2 mm strokes. Attached periodontal tissue is contacted on each downstroke to identify probing depth in each area. (Redrawn from Wilkins EM: *Clinical practice of the dental hygienist,* ed 7, Baltimore, 1994, Williams & Wilkins.)

probe marks, use the higher number for the final reading
D. Circumferential probe strokes
   1. Pocket is continuous around a tooth, and probing depth will vary considerably on different surfaces; circumferential probing is necessary for a complete evaluation
   2. Maintain the probe in the sulcus or pocket
     a. Proceed to examine the pocket around the tooth
     b. Repeated insertion and removal can cause trauma to the free gingival margin
   3. Walking step (Fig. 13-7)
     a. Hold the probe with a moderate lateral pressure against the tooth
     b. Move the tip up and down in strokes of 1 to 2 mm, gently touching the attachment area on each downstroke while progressing in small 1- to 2-mm steps along the side of the tooth
     c. Observe probe measurements at the gingival margin with each step
E. Adaptation of probe—individual teeth
   1. Insert the probe at the distal line angle of the most posterior tooth of a quadrant; probe in a distal direction, adapting the probe around the line angle; follow the tooth contour across the distal surface, slanting under the contact area as needed to probe across the midline (Fig. 13-8)
   2. Slide the probe back or reinsert at the distal line angle and proceed in a mesial direction, around the mesial line angle, and across the mesial surface to probe across the midline
   3. Proceed to the distal line angle of the next tooth
   4. After probing all aspects of a quadrant from the lingual (or facial) approach, proceed to the distal line angle of the most posterior tooth of the facial (or lingual) aspect

F. Examining furcation areas
   1. Definition—bone loss extends apical to the level where the bifurcation or trifurcation begins and periodontal infection invades the area between and about the roots
   2. Types of furcations—probing of the three general classes may be described as follows

   Class I. Early, or incipient, involvement: probe can enter the furcation area; anatomy of the root surfaces can be felt by moving the probe from side to side, passing over the root, into the tip of the furcation area, and up the other side to the adjacent root

   Class II. Moderate involvement: bone has been destroyed to an extent that allows the probe to enter the furcation area but not to pass through

   Class III. Severe, or advanced, involvement: probe can be passed between the roots through the entire furcation

   Class IV. Same as class III except that the furca is visible clinically because of presence of tissue recession

   3. Anatomic features—probe insertion for furcation detection
      a. Bifurcation (teeth with two roots)
         (1) Mandibular molars—probe midfacial and midlingual aspects
         (2) Maxillary first premolars—probe from mesial and distal aspects, under the contact area
         (3) Primary mandibular molars—probe midfacial and midlingual aspects
      b. Trifurcation (teeth with three roots)
         (1) Maxillary molars—to examine around the palatal root and the two facial roots, probe midfacial, mesial, and distal aspects
         (2) Maxillary primary molars—probe midfacial, mesial, and distal aspects

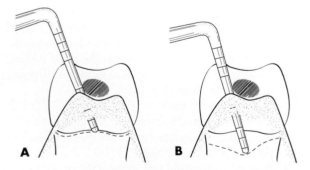

Fig. 13-8 Proximal surface probing. **A,** Probe must be applied more than halfway across from facial to overlap with probing from lingual. **B,** Probe in area of crater formation. Pocket is usually deeper on proximal under contact area than on facial or lingual. (From Wilkins EM: *Clinical practice of the dental hygienist,* ed 7, Baltimore, 1994, Williams & Wilkins.)

4. Furcation accessibility
   a. Apparent gingival recession over the furcation; when the furcation entrance is visible, probing is facilitated
   b. Furcation covered by a soft tissue pocket wall—access with a straight probe may be hampered by firm tissue that resists distention outward when probing to gain access at the facial or lingual division of roots; specially designed, curved Nabers probe may be helpful

G. Measuring clinical attachment level
   1. Definition—*clinical attachment level* refers to the position of the periodontal attached tissue at the base of a sulcus or pocket as measured from a fixed point
   2. Rationale
      a. Probing depth is changeable because of the variability of the position of the gingival margin as inflammation fluctuates
      b. Measuring from a fixed point provides a more significant indication of the level of the attached tissue
      c. More realistic evaluation can be made of the outcome of periodontal therapy and the stability of the tissue attachment during maintenance; when periodontal disease is active, pocket formation can continue and the attachment migrates along the root surface; attachment level changes
   3. Fixed points from which measurement can be made—cementoenamel junction is usually used, or a margin of a permanent metallic restoration; in animal research studies a notch may be made on the tooth; in human research a stent can be made so that the attachment level may be measured for each tooth around the dental arch
   4. Area of apparent (visible) recession
      a. Measure directly from the cementoenamel junction to the attachment level
      b. Scale away calculus if the cementoenamel junction is obliterated
   5. Area where the cementoenamel junction is covered by a soft tissue pocket wall
      a. Scale as necessary to uncover the cementoenamel junction subgingivally
      b. Apply the probe and determine by tactile sensitivity the location of the cementoenamel junction; measure the distance from the gingival margin to the cementoenamel junction
      c. Subtract the distance from the gingival margin to the cementoenamel junction from the total probing depth to obtain the attachment level

H. Amount of attached gingiva (Fig. 13-9)

1. Procedure for measuring the amount of attached gingiva: refer to Figure 13-9
2. When the probing depth is equal to or greater than the amount of total gingiva, there is no attached gingiva; if the probe goes through the mucogingival junction, it means there is mucogingival involvement

I. Bleeding on probing
   1. Rationale
      a. Bleeding on probing is a significant indicator of inflammation and is an earlier clinical sign than the appearance of marginal redness
      b. Bleeding on probing correlates with increases in motile organisms, especially spirochetes, in the pocket
      c. No bleeding on probing is a criterion for healthy tissue
   2. Bleeding indices—several indices have been developed for use in clinical and research evaluation; scores can help to motivate patient cooperation during therapeutic plaque control
   3. Procedure
      a. Insert the probe a few millimeters into the pocket
      b. Slide the probe horizontally along the pocket wall with light pressure
      c. Spongy tissue of a pocket wall will usually bleed

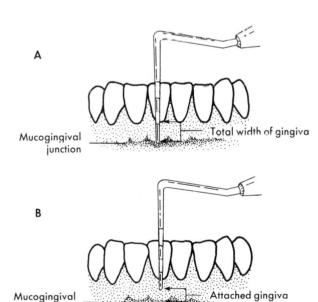

Fig. 13-9 Determining amount of attached gingiva. **A,** On surface of gingiva, measure from gingival margin to mucogingival junction to find total width of gingiva. **B,** Measure probing depth. Width of attached gingiva equals total width of gingiva minus probing depth. (Modified from Nield-Gehrig JS, Houseman GA: *Fundamentals of periodontal instrumentation,* ed 3, Baltimore, 1996, Williams & Wilkins.)

near the orifice; firm chronic pocket linings do not usually bleed until the probe is in the deeper part of the pocket

Probing Factors Summarized

A. Characteristics of a satisfactory technique
   1. Minimal trauma to the tissues and minimal patient discomfort
   2. Time spent is minimal
   3. Findings are consistent; dependable for comparison so that tissue changes may be identified
B. Influence of the severity of the periodontal disease
   1. Tissue resistance—with application of light pressure, the probe is passed to the attached tissue level; diseased tissue offers less resistance, so with increased severity of periodontal disease the probe inserts to a deeper level
   2. Position of the probe tip
      a. Normal tissue—probe is stopped at the base of the sulcus (crevice), which is the coronal part of the junctional epithelium
      b. Gingivitis and early periodontitis—probe tip is within the junctional epithelium
      c. Advanced periodontitis—probe tip may penetrate through the junctional epithelium to reach the attached connective tissue fibers
C. Factors that affect accurate probe determinations
   1. Probe itself
      a. Calibration—must be accurately marked
      b. Thickness—a thinner probe causes less distention of the sulcus or pocket wall
      c. Readability—aided by clear markings, color coding, and technique
   2. Technique—control and stability
      a. Grasp—appropriate for maximal tactile sensitivity
      b. Finger rest always on a firm tooth surface; contributes to uniform application
      c. Placement problems
         (1) Anatomic variations—tooth contours, furcations, contact areas
         (2) Interferences—calculus, anomalies, irregular margins of restorations and others
         (3) Accessibility, visibility
   3. Technique—pressure needed is only enough to detect by tactile means the level of attached tissue, whether that is the junctional epithelium or the deep connective tissue fibers; using a securely placed finger rest, a light pressure of 10 to 20 g should be sufficient

Explorer

A. Characteristics
   1. Flexible, thin wire, round in cross section, with

angulated or straight shank for application of the sharp tip to the tooth surfaces; some are designed primarily for supragingival, others for subgingival instrumentation

2. Design
   a. Single—may be a universal tip or designed for specific application
   b. Paired—mirror images of each other, curved to provide access to contralateral tooth surfaces
3. Shapes—various explorers are available; general shapes with specific examples are as follows
   a. Orban-type explorer (e.g., TU-17, Orban 20)—balanced instrument with a short tip (less than 2 mm) for adaptation to narrow roots and configurations of the subgingival tooth surfaces (see Fig. 13-3); long straight lower shank permits use in deep pockets
   b. Curved No. 3 explorer—single-ended, tapered instrument applicable to varying degrees of depth in pockets depending on the anatomic interferences of tooth contours and flexibility of the soft tissue pocket wall
   c. Pigtail or cow-horn explorers—paired, double ended, designed especially for proximal surfaces; limited to access in 4- to 5-mm pockets because of the wide curvature near the working end
   d. Shepherd's hook—sickle-shaped explorer usually of a thicker wire; useful for supragingival examinations for dental caries and irregular margins of restorations; difficult to adapt for fine determinations on proximal surfaces; not applicable in pockets

B. Purposes and uses
   1. Detect, by tactile sensitivity, the texture and character of tooth surfaces before (for care planning), during, and after treatment to assess the progress and completeness
   2. Examine supragingival tooth surfaces for
      a. Calculus
      b. Decalcified and carious lesions
      c. Defects in margins of restorations and sealants
      d. Anomalies
      e. Other irregularities not apparent on direct observation or that need confirmation by exploring after direct observation
   3. Examine subgingival surfaces for
      a. Calculus
      b. Demineralized and carious lesions
      c. Diseased, altered cementum
      d. Cemental changes that may have resulted from pocket formation
      e. Anomalies
      f. Anatomic grooves, curvatures, furcations, and other configurations where instrumentation may be required
   4. Define the extent of instrumentation for treatment procedures of the tooth surface, including
      a. Scaling and root planing
      b. Finishing of restorations
      c. Removal of overhanging margins
      d. Sealant placement
   5. Evaluate completeness of scaling and root planing by detection of smooth surfaces where instrumentation was performed
   6. Evaluation of tooth surfaces, restorations, and sealants at each continued care appointment (recall)

Techniques for Use

A. Basic instrumentation for all explorers
   1. Consistency of findings—it is important that a routine application that will relay consistent comparative information be used
   2. Grasp—modified pen grasp
   3. Finger rest—a definite finger rest on a tooth surface is necessary
      a. For complete control of the fine, sharp explorer
      b. For uniform tactile sensitivity
B. Supragingival adaptation
   1. Unnecessary exploring should be avoided; with adequate light and a source of air, direct vision or indirect vision with a mouth mirror can provide the necessary information; confirmation with gentle exploration can then be made
   2. Sensitivity—cervical third of the anatomic crown and the root surface apical to the cementoenamel junction are usually the most sensitive to air blasts and the touch of metal instruments
   3. Adapt the side of the explorer tip to the tooth surface with a light but definite lateral pressure
   4. Lead with the tip around line angles by rolling the handle to maintain adaptation of the tip (Fig. 13-5)
   5. Restorations—follow the margins of all restorations around with an explorer to detect irregularities of the margins: overhanging or deficient margins may or may not appear in radiographs depending on the angulation and tooth surface
C. Subgingival adaptation (single explorers No. 3 and No. TU-17)
   1. Hold the side of the sharp tip always against the tooth surface; position with the lower shank (part next to the tip) nearly parallel with the long axis of the tooth
   2. Slide the tip under the margin of the gingiva, down the tooth surface until the base of the pocket is felt with the back of the tip in a manner similar to that described for the probe; calculus and other rough

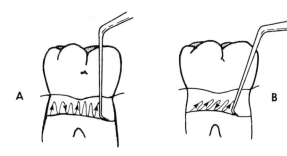

Fig. 13-10 Explorer walking stroke. With side of explorer tip in contact with tooth surface at all times, explorer is moved over surface in vertical walking stroke **(A)** or diagonal or oblique walking stroke **(B)**. Complete exploration of each tooth surface is necessary; therefore groups of strokes are overlapped. (Modified from Wilkins EM: *Clinical practice of the dental hygienist,* ed 7, Baltimore, 1994, Williams & Wilkins.)

areas of the root may be detected by using a light grasp with definite contact to enhance the tactile sensitivity transmitted to the fingers

3. Strokes—vertical or diagonal walking stroke may be used (Fig. 13-10); for a very deep pocket, the root can be divided into two or more sections; great care is taken to overlap the strokes
4. Proximal surfaces
   a. Lead with the tip into the proximal area; do not "back into" an area with the heel of the explorer
   b. As the walking step strokes are continued around a line angle, the instrument handle is rolled between the fingers of the grasp to ensure continued adaptation of the sharp tip
   c. Continue strokes under the contact area to provide careful examination of the entire exposed tooth surface; overlap the strokes from the lingual aspect with those from the facial aspect

Instrumentation for Treatment

Basic Concepts

A. Complete supragingival and subgingival instrumentation for debridement of the teeth, accompanied by the client's therapeutic daily bacterial plaque removal, are specific procedures in the treatment of inflammatory periodontal diseases
B. Basis for personalized client care is *planned* rather than *intuitive* intervention; care plan is determined from the information collected during the initial questioning and clinical examinations
C. Instrumentation requirements will vary with the severity of the disease, attachment levels, probing depths, and the amount and distribution of calculus deposits

Definitions

A. Debridement—removal of all hard and soft deposits from the clinical crowns of the teeth to the extent needed to restore balance between the bacterial flora and the immune responses; the clinical crown being that part of the tooth above the level of attached periodontal fibers
B. Scaling—technique used to accomplish debridement
C. Root planing—care procedure that may follow calculus removal; it is designed to remove rough residual calculus and provide a smooth surface to deter bacterial accumulation
D. Overhang removal—recontouring procedures that correct defective margins of restorations to provide a smooth surface that will not harbor plaque deposits and can be cared for more readily by the patient
E. Gingival curettage—the process of debriding the soft tissue wall of a periodontal pocket to remove inflamed, devitalized, contaminated tissue or foreign material from or next to a lesion; also called closed gingival curettage in contrast with open curettage, a surgical flap procedure
F. Phase I or initial therapy—series of treatment procedures employed to eliminate or at least reduce etiologic and inflammatory factors by therapeutic plaque control instruction and periodontal instrumentation, removal of overhanging fillings, and elimination of other plaque-retaining factors; also included in phase I therapy may be emergency dental care, endodontic requirements, removal of hopeless teeth, caries control, occlusal adjustment, and temporary stabilization
G. Evaluation—after phase I or initial therapy a careful examination is carried out and a *response diagnosis* is made; "response" refers to the changes in the periodontal tissues that show the response to the treatment to that time; for many clients, phase I takes care of the total periodontal treatment needs and phase II is entirely for restorative therapy; for others, phase II includes periodontal surgical treatment; for all clients, the maintenance phase is the third essential phase
H. Maintenance phase—also called continued care, periodontal maintenance therapy (PMT) or supportive periodontal treatment (SPT); the series of appointments for routine examination and additional therapy as required to keep the periodontal tissues healthy without recurrence of disease; maintenance phase is planned immediately following phase I and represents the long-term prevention and control program

Rationale for Periodontal Debridement

A. Arrest the progress of disease
B. Induce positive changes in the subgingival bacterial flora (count and content)

1. Before instrumentation the predominant characteristics of subgingival plaque are anaerobic, gram-negative, motile forms with many spirochetes and rods, very high counts of all microorganisms, and many white blood cells
2. After instrumentation, the total number of microorganisms and white blood cells decreases and there is a shift to a predominance of aerobic, gram-positive, nonmotile, coccoid forms

C. Create an environment that permits the gingival tissue to heal, therefore eliminating inflammation
   1. Convert pocket (disease) to sulcus (health)
      a. Shrinkage of tissue
      b. Reduction of probing depth
   2. Eliminate bleeding
   3. Change quality of tissue from spongy to firm; tissue regeneration
   4. Improve integrity of attachment

D. Make the client's bacterial plaque control procedures more effective

E. Provide initial preparation (tissue conditioning) for complicated periodontal treatments such as surgery
   1. Reduce etiologic and predisposing factors
   2. Permit reevaluation: surgery may be lessened in extent and confined to specific areas or, in certain instances, not needed

F. Prevent recurrence of disease through maintenance, evaluation, and treatment

Rationale for Removal of Overhangs

A. Eliminate irregular surfaces where bacterial plaque can collect
B. Induce positive changes in the microflora of the pocket when the overhang extends subgingivally
C. Encourage resolution of inflammation
D. Facilitate interdental plaque removal and control by the patient

Preparation for Instrumentation

A. Dental hygiene responsibilities for client safety during care
   1. Review the health history and client's records for indications of special needs; prepare for a possible emergency
   2. Observe the client; note signs of stress
   3. Make a blood pressure and pulse determination

B. Dental hygiene responsibilities for prevention of cross-contamination (see Chapter 7, section on clinical application of microbiology in dentistry)
   1. Postpone and reschedule the appointment for a client with a communicable disease or open lesion
   2. Provide methods for lowering the bacterial count of the client's oral surfaces

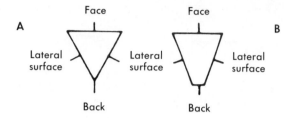

Fig. 13-11 Cross sections of two types of sickle scalers. **A,** Triangular. **B,** Trapezoidal. (Redrawn from Pattison GL, Pattison AM: *Periodontal instrumentation,* ed 2, Norwalk, Conn, 1992, Appleton & Lange.)

   a. Present instruction in bacterial plaque control using a brush, floss, and other aids *before* any instrumentation
   b. Provide a preprocedural antimicrobial mouth rinse for the client to lower microorganisms in aerosols
   3. Prepare all instruments, materials, treatment area, and environmental surfaces for universal infection control
   4. Use personal barriers, including gloves, mask, eye protection, and protective clothing, for prevention of infective material transmission between clinician and client

Hand-Activated Instruments

Scalers

A. Sickle
   1. Description
      a. Two cutting edges, formed by the face and the two lateral surfaces, converge to form the tip of the scaler, which is a sharp point
      b. Lateral surfaces meet to form a sharp, pointed back; some types are made with flattened backs
      c. Cross section—triangular or trapezoidal (Fig. 13-11)
      d. Internal angles of approximately 70 degrees are formed where the lateral surfaces meet the face at the cutting edges
   2. Blade types
      a. Straight sickle—face between the cutting edges is flat
      b. Curved sickle—face between the cutting edges is curved lengthwise
   3. Shank types
      a. Straight shank—primarily for anterior teeth
      b. Modified or contraangle—paired instruments that are mirror images of each other to provide access to the proximal surfaces, particularly of posterior teeth
   4. Uses

a. Primarily for removal of supragingival calculus

b. May be helpful in the removal of gross deposits located just beneath the gingival margin

c. Small sickle blades are especially adaptable beneath the contact area of anterior teeth when the interdental area is triangular and a curet may not be adaptable

5. Flat sides of a sickle cannot be adapted to the curved contours of the teeth

6. Application

a. Angulation—face of the blade is adapted to the tooth surface at an angle of approximately 70 degrees (less than 90 degrees but more than 45 degrees)

b. Stroke—pull stroke may be vertical or oblique

B. Hoe scaler

1. Description

a. Single straight cutting edge beveled at a 45-degree angle to the end of the blade

b. Blade turned at a 99- to 100-degree angle to the shank

c. Shank variously angulated for adaptation of the cutting edge to tooth surfaces; some hoes are paired, double-ended instruments

2. Uses

a. Removal of gross supragingival deposits

b. May be helpful for removal of gross calculus 2 to 3 mm below the gingival margin, provided the tissue is soft and flexible and can easily be displaced by the bulky hoe scaler

3. Contraindications and precautions

a. Lack of adaptability of the wide straight cutting edge to the curved tooth surfaces

b. Difficulty in use on cementum because of the ease of gouging the cemental surface with a sharp corner of the cutting edge; gouging may also occur because it is not possible to apply an even pressure with the whole cutting edge

c. Impossible to reach the base of a pocket because of the size and shape of the blade without over-extension and trauma to the soft tissue pocket wall

4. Application

a. Place the blade under a deposit and use a pull vertical stroke

b. Use a working angulation of approximately 90 degrees

c. Balance the instrument by making a two-point contact (the cutting edge is on the deposit and the side of the shank is held against the crown of the tooth)

d. Primarily for facial and lingual surfaces or on proximal surfaces adjacent to edentulous areas

C. Chisel scaler

1. Description

a. Single straight cutting edge beveled at 45 degrees

b. Blade is continuous with a slightly curved shank

2. Uses

a. Removal of gross supragingival calculus from exposed proximal surfaces of anterior teeth when interdental soft tissue is missing

b. Appropriate for dislodgement of heavy calculus, such as a continuous bridge of calculus across several teeth

3. Precautions

a. Straight cutting edge not readily adaptable to curved tooth surfaces

b. Sharp edges and ends of blade can nick and groove the tooth surface, particularly the cementum

4. Application

a. Apply with a horizontal push stroke

b. Do not direct a push stroke toward the sulcus or pocket to prevent calculus from becoming embedded

D. File scaler

1. Description

a. Multiple cutting edges lined up as a series of hoes on a round, oval, or rectangular base

b. Blades turned at a 90- or 105-degree angle to the shank

c. Shanks are variously angulated similar to the hoes; some are paired and double ended; others are single ended

2. Uses

a. Supplementary instrument used selectively for gross calculus removal

b. Useful for smoothing down overextended or rough amalgam restorations in sites where the file can be effectively applied, such as on certain proximal surfaces or with great care in a cervical area

3. Precautions

a. Blades are straight on a flat base, so are not readily adaptable to curved tooth surfaces

b. Where a tooth surface is rounded, the file blade would have a tangential relationship

c. Where the tooth surface is convex, the file blade would form a bridge over the dip

4. Application

a. Apply with a pull stroke

b. Excessive pressure could lead to gouging

Curets

A. Description

1. Two cutting edges that converge in a round toe on a

curved blade; cutting edge is continuous around the blade (Fig. 13-12)

2. Face—inner surface between the cutting edges; flat in cross section and curved lengthwise
3. Back is rounded, continuous with the lateral surfaces
4. Internal angles of approximately 70 degrees are formed where the lateral surfaces meet the face at the cutting edges
5. Shank is curved, with the shank, handle, and blade in a relatively flat plane in curets designed for anterior instrumentation; for posterior teeth, the shank is contraangled for access

B. Characteristics of a universal curet
1. May be adapted for instrumentation on any tooth surface; with paired mirror-image ends, usually placed on a double-ended handle
2. Both cutting edges are sharpened and used; proper angulation determines the side that fits a given surface to be treated

C. Characteristics of area-specific curets
1. Area-specific curets are designed for specific adaptation to certain teeth and certain surfaces
2. A series of area-specific curets often consists of several paired instruments: for example, the original series of Gracey curets consists of seven pairs
3. Only one cutting edge per blade is used—the longer, outer cutting edge
4. When the lower (terminal) shank is parallel to the tooth surface to be instrumented, the cutting edge will be at the correct angulation for instrumentation
5. Types—certain area-specific curets are available in finishing and rigid types: rigid curets are used to remove moderate calculus deposits; finishing curets are used to remove light calculus deposits and for root planing
6. Design features of the working end
   a. The working end is "offset" at an angle of approximately 60 degrees in relation to the terminal shank, making one cutting edge lower than the other; only the lower cutting edge is used for instrumentation
   b. Area-specific curets are available in instrument designs that have blades that are thinner in width and/or shorter in length than those of the Gracey finishing curets
7. Design features of the instrument shank
   a. Shank length—all area-specific curets have long complex shanks with several angles; area-specific curets for use in pockets 5 mm or more in depth have lower shanks that are several millimeters longer in length than those of Gracey curets
   b. Shank rigidity—curets for use in root planing have flexible shanks; curets for use in removing moderate calculus deposits have rigid shanks

D. Uses
1. Standard instrumentation for subgingival instrumentation—scaling and root planing
2. Recommended for fine supragingival calculus, particularly near the free gingival margin where the triangular back of a scaler could lacerate tissue
3. Useful for obtaining a sample of subgingival plaque to place on a glass slide to observe with a phase microscope

E. Application
1. Angulation—blade is applied so that the face forms

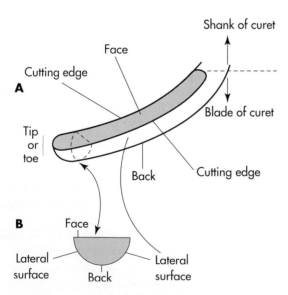

Fig. 13-12 Parts of a curet. **A,** Labeled diagram to show specific parts of curet blade. **B,** Cross section of blade. (Modified from Parr RW, et al: *Subgingival scaling and root planing,* Berkeley, Calif, 1976, Praxis.)

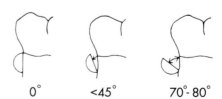

Fig. 13-13 Curet blade in cross section positioned at various angulations against tooth surface: 0 degrees for insertion into pocket, less than 45 degrees ineffective for instrumentation, 70 to 80 degrees used for scaling and root planing. (Redrawn from Pattison GL, Pattison AM: *Periodontal instrumentation,* ed 2, Norwalk, Conn, 1992, Appleton & Lange.)

an angle of approximately 70 degrees with the tooth surface (Fig. 13-13)

2. Strokes—pull stroke only is used, in a vertical or oblique direction
3. Universal curets are used initially to remove as much calculus as possible; smaller curets and the area-specific Graceys are for fine scaling and root planing
4. Design features that make curets the instruments of choice for subgingival instrumentation are
   a. Curved blade that can be adapted to curved tooth surfaces
   b. Rounded, smooth back that permits placement at the base of the pocket without irritation or trauma to soft tissues

Plastic Instruments for Implant Care

A. General description
   1. Special instruments used for dental implants; do not use stainless steel, carbon steel, and ultrasonic instruments on titanium implants; metal instruments may leave scratches on the surface of the implant
      a. Scratches or surface roughness favor bacterial plaque accumulation
      b. Implant's surface coating may be disturbed, thus reducing the biocompatibility of the implant with the surrounding tissues
   2. Instruments used for assessment and calculus removal from implant should be made of a material that is softer than the implant material; plastic instruments most commonly are used; some plastic instruments can be sterilized by autoclave for several cycles; follow manufacturer's instructions for sterilization and reuse
   3. Instruments are available in a variety of designs, some of which have working ends that are similar to conventional periodontal probes, sickle scalers, and universal curets
B. Plastic calibrated probe for assessing dental implants
   1. Peri-implant probing depths are related to the thickness of the mucosa around the implant; deeper probing depths are found in conjunction with a thicker mucosa
   2. Probing around dental implants is controversial; bleeding upon probing is a poor parameter in implants due to the tight marginal cuff around the transmucosal abutment
   3. Considerations
      a. Probing may be invasive because the probe may penetrate through the weakly adherent biologic seal and could introduce bacteria into the peri-implant environment

   b. Accurate probing depths may be difficult to obtain because of the constricted "cervical" area of some implants
   c. Radiographs are more accurate than probe depths for detecting the absence or presence of bone loss around implants
C. Instrumentation for calculus and bacterial plaque removal
   1. Calculus is removed readily from implants because there is no interlocking or penetration of the deposit with the implant surface
   2. Light lateral pressure with a plastic scaler or curet is recommended; care must be taken not to scratch the surface of the implant

Ultrasonic and Sonic Instruments

A. Description
   1. Power-driven instruments used for periodontal debridement; rapid vibrations of the working end of the instrument act to fracture and dislodge calculus from the tooth surface and cleanse the environment within the periodontal pocket
   2. Have a constant stream of water running through the handpiece that exits in a fine spray near the instrument tip
      a. Flow-through design
      b. External adjustable
B. Characteristics of magnetostrictive and piezoelectric ultrasonic instruments
   1. High-frequency electrical energy is converted by the machine into mechanical energy in the form of ultrasonic vibrations; instrument tip vibrations range from 25,000 to 50,000 cycles/second
   2. Heat is produced, which must be dissipated by constant flow of water through the handpiece; antimicrobial solutions may be used instead of water in certain units
C. Characteristics of sonic instruments
   1. Air pressure creates rapid mechanical vibrations; instrument tip vibrations range from 2500 to 7000 cycles/second
   2. No heat generated, so water cooling is not necessary; water coolant is indicated to obtain benefits of water lavage
D. Design features of instrument inserts
   1. Working ends have no cutting edges to cut or tear the tissue; less tissue trauma can result in faster healing rates for ultrasonically or sonically instrumented treatment sites
   2. The entire length of the working end is active; therefore, adaptation is not limited to a single region on the working end

3. Instrument tips are available in a wide variety of designs
   a. Large tips are designed for periodontal debridement of large supragingival calculus deposits and stain removal
   b. Thin tips are designed for periodontal debridement of root surfaces and are significantly smaller than hand-activated curets

E. Uses
   1. Periodontal debridement of bacterial plaque, supra- and subgingival calculus, and endotoxins from root surfaces within 4 to 7 mm pockets
   2. Useful for smoothing down overextended or rough amalgam restorations

F. Contraindications
   1. Client with a communicable disease that can be disseminated by aerosols
   2. Compromised client with outstanding susceptibility to infection that can be transmitted by contaminated water, aerosol, or other means (e.g., debilitated, uncontrolled diabetic, or immunosuppressed individuals)
   3. Client with a cardiac pacemaker; note that some newer pacemakers have built in barriers that make ultrasonic instrumentation safe; check with cardiologist
   4. Young, growing tissue
   5. Primary and newly erupted teeth—danger of heat on the tissues in the large pulp chambers
   6. Subgingival areas where lack of visibility and narrow pockets interfere with proper angulation of the insert tip
   7. Maintenance care clients who are oriented to daily self-care so that only small amounts of calculus accumulate between continued care appointments
   8. Cemental surfaces where ultrasonic scaling can remove tooth surface structure; calculus is harder than cementum
   9. Porcelain jacket crowns that can be fractured by the vibration of the ultrasonic scaler
   10. Titanium implants, unless the ultrasonic instrument is covered with a specially designed plastic sleeve

G. Precautions
   1. Handpiece and working end of ultrasonic instruments must be cooled with constant flow of water to dissipate heat
   2. Aerosols produced may be contaminated with pathogens; use of barriers, surface disinfection, protective clothing, and laminar airflow systems are recommended
   3. Client may experience sensitivity of the teeth

4. Hearing shifts have been reported; effect on the ears of a clinician who frequently uses the ultrasonic or sonic instruments has not been researched

H. Preparation
   1. Clinician, assistant, and client must wear personal protective equipment meeting OSHA Standards
   2. Preprocedural rinse: client should rinse with an antimicrobial solution before the start of procedure to reduce the number of airborne microorganisms in aerosols created by water spray
   3. Monitor the condition of the equipment; replace the insert as soon as it shows signs of wear or damage; thin tips must be replaced more frequently than thicker tips
   4. Inserts and handpiece should be sterilized according to manufacturer's directions; use surface disinfection and barriers on ultrasonic unit

I. Technique for use
   1. Run water through the tubing a full 5 minutes at the start of the day and 3 minutes between clients
   2. Select the appropriate insert for the task at hand; larger tips for heavy supragingival calculus removal; thin tips for light deposits, plaque removal, and endotoxin removal
   3. Use instrument inserts at the lowest frequency power setting at which a particular tip will function properly; manual tuning of the power frequency is recommended when using thin instrument tips; thin tips may damage the root surface if used on a high power setting
   4. Adjust the water spray around the instrument tip to create a light mist or halo effect with no excess dripping of water; insufficient water flow over an ultrasonic tip can result in trauma to the pulp
   5. Position client in supine position with head turned to one side; correct positioning will cause water to pool in the cheek area, minimizing aerosol production
   6. Provide high-volume suction with continual clearance for client comfort and to prevent inhalation of contaminated water spray
   7. Adapt the side of the last several millimeters of the working end to the tooth surface; position with the length of the working end parallel to the long axis of the tooth; avoid direct application of the tip of the working end to the tooth surface
   8. Use a relaxed grasp to apply light stroke pressure; heavy stroke pressure is unnecessary and can damage the tooth surface
   9. Strokes overlap one another in a sweeping- or erasing-type motion; multidirectional strokes

should cover every square millimeter of the root surface

10. To remove heavier deposits, keep the tip in constant motion while making light strokes in a sweeping motion

Steps in a Treatment Appointment

A. Dental hygiene care plan—depends on the extent and severity of periodontal infection, distribution and amount of calculus, probing depths, and characteristics of the soft tissue

1. Single appointment—when it is expected that total scaling can be accomplished in one appointment, supragingival scaling may be completed first, followed by specific finer scaling systematically around each dental arch

2. Planned multiple appointments—when supragingival and subgingival calculus deposits indicate extensive instrumentation, it is recommended that the dentition be divided into quadrant or sextant units for appropriate use of local anesthesia, and instrumentation divided among an appropriate number of appointments

B. Sequence for an individual appointment

1. Client disease control instruction

a. Initial appointment—detailed introduction to instruction

b. Subsequent appointments

(1) Observe the tissue response

(2) Record the gingival bleeding score and/or apply a disclosing agent and record the bacterial plaque score

(3) Reeducate the client as needed to develop client dexterity, motivation, and bacterial control

c. Immediate objectives for plaque check and instruction before instrumentation

(1) Client appreciation of importance of personal care

(2) Removal of bacterial plaque and debris provides preoperative preparation for instrumentation in a clean environment

(3) Removal of bacteria from teeth and mucosal surfaces lessens the contamination of aerosols

(4) Professional time should not be spent removing loose bacteria and debris that are the important visual aids for client instruction and can be removed best by the client

2. Selection of a segment or quadrant for instrumentation

a. Review probing depths and plan strategies

b. Explore to locate calculus and root roughness

3. Administration of an anesthetic

Scaling

Technique Objectives

A. Complete calculus removal

B. Smooth tooth surface

C. Minimal soft tissue trauma

Steps for Calculus Removal

A. Retract; position the mouth mirror

B. Grasp the instrument

1. Use a modified pen grasp

2. Use a light grasp during positioning of the instrument

3. Tighten the grasp for application of lateral pressure and strokes for calculus removal

4. Use the thumb to roll the instrument for adaptation to tooth contours

C. Establish a finger rest

1. Apply the finger rest—select the correct end of a paired instrument

2. Apply the third and little finger together for a firm fulcrum point on a tooth surface

3. Location of the rest

a. Near the site of instrumentation in the same dental arch

b. Precise calculus removal with a carefully controlled stroke becomes increasingly difficult as the finger rest is moved farther away

D. Adjust the grasp-hand-wrist forearm unit

1. Position the middle finger of the instrument grasp close to the third finger on the finger rest to allow the hand to perform as a unit

2. Rationale—hand and arm work together for instrument activation

a. Control of instrument movement—less possibility of slipping

b. Stroke length can be limited to the height of the calculus, which is the correct length of a stroke

E. Adapt the cutting edge

1. Placement stroke—slide the blade lightly over the calculus to the base of the deposit

2. Adapt the blade in keeping with the topography of the tooth surface

3. Position the blade at proper angulation for the working stroke: approximately 70 degrees but not greater than 80 degrees or less than 60 degrees (Fig. 13-13)

F. Apply appropriate lateral pressure

1. Grasp tenses; pressure adapts on the finger rest

2. Nature of calculus deposit or root surface roughness defines the lateral pressure needed

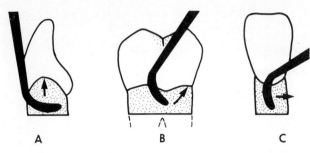

Fig. 13-14 Directions of strokes for scaling and root planing. **A,** Vertical. **B,** Diagonal. **C,** Horizontal. (Modified from Carranza FA, Newman MG: *Glickman's clinical periodontology,* ed 8, Philadelphia, 1996, WB Saunders.)

3. Pressure must be sufficient to prevent burnishing of the deposit, yet light enough to prevent gouging the tooth surface
   a. Burnishing can result from shaving the calculus by layers
   b. Burnished surface may be indistinguishable (when explored) from the tooth surface; calculus removal may be difficult
G. Activation—strokes
   1. Direction—vertical and oblique strokes are most used; horizontal strokes may be applied selectively for otherwise inaccessible areas (see Fig. 13-14)
   2. Pull strokes in a coronal direction are used to prevent particles of calculus from being pushed into the soft tissue
   3. Length—short, smooth, even, controlled strokes for calculus removal; longer lighter strokes for finishing and smoothing the surface
   4. Overlap—strokes should overlap to ensure complete coverage; long, large areas of deposits are treated in sections, from base to crest, with overlapping strokes; also called scaling in "channels" (Fig. 13-15)
   5. Hand-wrist-forearm unit action—strength and control are provided
      a. Movement is initiated at the fulcrum point
      b. Position of the fingers remains constant
      c. Wrist is activated back and forth or up and down (also called "wrist rock")
   6. Completion of stroke
      a. Grasp, finger rest, and lateral pressure are lightened
      b. Blade is returned and positioned for another stroke
   7. Circumferential instrumentation
      a. Calculus surrounding the tooth is removed section by section

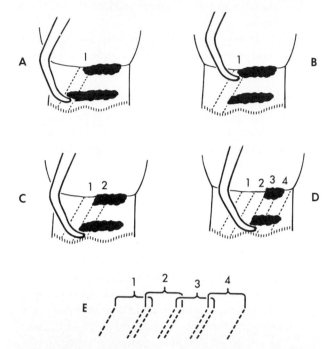

Fig. 13-15 Channel scaling. **A,** Curet inserted to bottom of pocket and positioned in contact with base of calculus deposit. **B,** Calculus removed from first channel. **C,** Curet lowered into pocket to be repositioned for scaling second channel. **D,** Curet in third channel. More than one stroke in each channel is needed to be sure tooth surface is smooth. **E,** Each channel should overlap previous one. (Modified from Parr RW, et al: *Subgingival scaling and root planing,* Berkeley, Calif, 1976, Praxis.)

   b. Blade is adapted at the line angle by rolling the handle between the thumb and fingers of the grasp
   8. Area is checked frequently with a fine explorer to check progress and completion

Applications for Subgingival Scaling

A. Insertion of the instrument (placement stroke)
   1. After selection of the correct end of a double-ended curet and establishment of a definite finger rest, turn the blade for careful insertion into the pocket
   2. Close the face of the blade toward the tooth to insert the blade at an angle of 0 to 10 degrees
   3. Direct the toe under the gingival margin and pass the instrument over the tooth surface or calculus deposit until contact with the tissue attachment is felt; depth can be anticipated by checking the charted probe findings
   4. Adjust the blade to the correct angulation for scaling (approximately 70 degrees)

B. Strokes
  1. Vertical and oblique pull strokes, overlapped
  2. Lateral pressure—light pressure that could burnish the subgingival calculus should be avoided; heavy pressure that can diminish tactile sensitivity and decrease instrument control should also be avoided
  3. Length of strokes—will be determined by the probing depth, the morphology of the tooth surface, and the nature of the deposit being removed; short, smooth, decisive strokes within the confines of the pocket will prevent the need for trauma to the gingival margin by repeated insertion and withdrawal

C. Characteristics of subgingival instrumentation
  1. Accessibility difficult and visibility limited; potential for trauma to soft tissue is greater than with supragingival instrumentation
  2. Keen tactile sensitivity required; most instrumentation will be covered and confined by the soft tissue pocket wall
  3. Adaptation of the curet at the base of the pocket can be difficult
  4. Root surface topography and tooth morphology present problem areas for instrument adaptation, including grooves, concave and convex surfaces, anomalies, narrowing of roots apically, and furcation areas
  5. Probing depths vary around the tooth; pocket narrows near the attachment
  6. Subgingival calculus is harder, more condensed, and more tenacious
    a. Attachment to the tooth is primarily by interlocking in the minute irregularities or by direct apposition, which makes distinction and removal difficult
    b. Irregular deposits occur in nodular, ledge, or smooth veneer forms

Finishing Procedures

A. Technique objectives
  1. Removal of all residual calculus
  2. Bacterial and toxic products debridement
  3. Smooth the tooth surface—no irregularities left when checked with a subgingival explorer
  4. Produce no undue trauma to soft tissue and no grooving of the root surface

B. Technique variations from subgingival scaling
  1. Lateral pressure—as the root surface becomes smoother, the pressure is lightened to prevent grooving; an even light lateral pressure is needed throughout the entire stroke
  2. Strokes

    a. Become longer as the smoothing process is accomplished
    b. Vertical, oblique, and horizontal strokes may be used to prevent or correct grooving
  3. Instrument sharpness—sharp curet is essential

C. Examination for completion of treatment
  1. Tooth surface
    a. Use a fine, sharp, subgingival explorer that can be adapted to the treated surface at the base of each pocket
    b. Adapt the strokes of the explorer in various directions (vertical, oblique, horizontal) to check for minute grooving or roughness of the cemental surface
  2. Gingival tissue
    a. Without intentional curettage, some debridement of the soft tissue lining of the sulcus or pocket occurs
    b. Coincidental or inadvertent curettage is the debridement of a soft tissue pocket wall during scaling by the back or lateral side of the offset cutting edge of the curet

D. Use suction to remove debris from the pocket and to test for residual "tags" of pocket lining tissue

E. Remove tags by direct incision—place the curet cutting edge at the root of the tag and press against the tooth to incise; avoid dulling the cutting edge by not moving the cutting edge over the tooth surface

F. Irrigate to remove particles of calculus; use of an antimicrobial substance may temporarily decrease bacterial count and promote healing; pocket repopulation occurs within a few weeks

G. Apply pressure with a damp sponge to adapt the tissue closely, arrest bleeding, and minimize the size of the blood clot in the pocket

H. Provide oral and/or written instructions for the client's postoperative care

Follow-up Evaluation: Effects of Treatment

Periodontal debridement is an integral part of nonsurgical periodontal therapy. With effective daily bacterial plaque removal by the client, the ultimate goal is to prevent, control, or eliminate periodontal infection.

A. Examine after soft tissue healing
  1. Ten to 14 days for immediate evaluation and to check and review client's bacterial plaque removal methods
  2. Four to 6 weeks for assessing response to healing and determine future needs

B. Expected clinical findings (signs of gingival health)
  1. Improved color, size, shape, and consistency of gingiva
  2. No bleeding on gentle probing

  3. Shrinkage of edematous tissues with reduced probing depths
C. Effect on pocket microorganisms—the subgingival bacterial flora changes remarkably after debridement; before instrumentation, the microorganisms of the diseased pocket are primarily anaerobic, gram-negative, motile forms with many spirochetes; after treatment, the total number of microorganisms decreases, and a shift to a predominance of aerobic, nonmotile, gram-positive organisms with an increase in coccoid forms occurs; such changes cannot be expected to be permanent, and repopulation will occur in the absence of meticulous daily care by the client along with routine professional supervision; delayed healing may be associated with various factors
D. Causes of lack of tissue response
  1. Inflammation from residual deposits or incomplete instrumentation
  2. Inadequate bacterial plaque removal procedures daily by the client: repopulation of the pockets
  3. Delayed healing caused by
    a. Use of alcohol, tobacco, and other drugs
    b. Systemic conditions that interfere such as immunosuppressive diseases, diabetes, or blood disorders
E. Evaluation for continuing care plan
  1. Response diagnosis—revision of original dental hygiene care plan based on the effectiveness of and response to dental hygiene care to date
  2. Needs for additional periodontal therapy—recommendations and consultations after review by dentist
  3. Determination of frequency of appointments for supportive treatment

Dental Stains

Basic Concepts

A. Discolorations of the teeth and restorations occur in three general ways
  1. Stain adhering directly to the tooth surface
  2. Stain contained within calculus and soft deposits
  3. Stain incorporated within the tooth structure
B. Removal of unsightly extrinsic stains may improve the overall appearance, but research has not shown that stain removal directly contributes to periodontal health or to the prevention of dental caries or any oral disease
C. No specific detrimental physical or pathologic effects have been shown to result from the presence of discolorations of the teeth; psychologic influences related to an individual's appearance can be significant with regard to the individual's self-esteem and the response of others
D. Stain removal should be considered a conservative, selective procedure because of potential deleterious effects of stain removal materials and devices on the general health and environment and on the teeth and gingival tissues
E. Decision to include stain removal in an individual treatment plan can best be made after client instruction in procedures for daily bacterial plaque removal and after complete periodontal debridement

Definitions of Types of Stains

A. Identified by location
  1. Intrinsic—stains that occur within the tooth substance
  2. Extrinsic—stains that occur on the external surface of the tooth
B. Identified by sources of the discoloration
  1. Endogenous—stain that originates from within the tooth
    a. Endogenous stains are always intrinsic and frequently are discolorations of the dentin reflecting through the enamel
    b. Examples of sources—drugs, changes in pulp tissue of pulpless teeth, imperfect tooth development
    c. Removal—bleaching techniques or jacket crown to cover the tooth as advised and carried out by the dentist
  2. Exogenous—stain that originates from an external source
    a. Exogenous intrinsic—becomes incorporated into the tooth structure
      (1) Examples of sources—restorative materials, dental caries
      (2) Removal—same as for endogenous intrinsic: by dental bleaching or prosthetic coverage
    b. Exogenous extrinsic—remains on the tooth surface
      (1) Modes of attachment to the tooth
        (a) Contained within bacterial plaque adhering to the tooth surface
        (b) Contained within calculus
        (c) Directly attached to the tooth surface
      (2) Examples of sources of color—drugs, foods, tobacco products, chromogenic bacteria
      (3) Removal—plaque removal by client and scaling, planing, and stain removal procedures by a professional

Rationale for Removal of Extrinsic Stain During Dental Hygiene Therapy

A. Removal of unsightly stains improves appearance
B. Removal of stains contributes to a client's well-being and motivation to adhere to appropriate effective daily bacterial plaque removal for disease prevention

Contraindications and Precautions

The abrasiveness of the agent used, the extent of aerosols produced by a power-driven device, and the integrity of the client's tooth surfaces need particular consideration. The following are some specific cases where stain removal is either contraindicated indefinitely or should be postponed.

A. Immediate evaluation
   1. Client susceptible to bacteremia—because bacteremia can be created during use of a rotating rubber cup polisher, the health history must be prepared initially and reviewed and updated at all appointments; antibiotic prophylaxis is needed by client's susceptible to bacteremia (see Appendix B)
   2. After instrumentation—stain removal is not recommended immediately because the abrasive agent and other constituents of the polishing paste can embed in and irritate the soft tissue pocket lining and hinder the progress of healing; it is recommended that the use of a power-driven rubber cup be withheld until the tissue has healed
   3. Enlarged, inflamed gingival tissue—stain removal is not recommended at any age when the gingiva is enlarged, soft, spongy, and bleeds readily on slight provocation; irritants from the paste can enter the gingival tissue, and the action of the rotating rubber cup can traumatize the gingiva; it is recommended that bacterial plaque control be initiated and stain removal be withheld until the gingiva does not bleed on brushing or probing
B. Factors related to tooth surface—stain removal with an abrasive agent removes the surface layer of tooth structure where the fluoride content is the greatest and most protective; although protection against dental caries is essential for all patients of all ages, the following are special cases where the fluoride of the tooth surface has particular significance and polishing with an abrasive would be contraindicated
   1. Caries-susceptible teeth
      a. Rampant caries; nursing bottle caries; root caries
      b. Radiation therapy to the oral area
      c. Xerostomia from any cause, including medications for systemic conditions
      d. Handicapped persons with limited ability to practice personal bacterial plaque removal and

who have difficulty managing a caries-preventive diet
      e. Areas of demineralization—white spots
   2. Areas of thin or deficient enamel
      a. Amelogenesis imperfecta—enamel in this condition is poorly calcified and partially or completely missing; teeth may be easily abraded
      b. Dentinogenesis imperfecta—enamel may be of normal thickness but may be chipped and lost early through fracturing; attrition may be evident
      c. Enamel erosion
   3. Cemental surfaces—exposed surface near cementoenamel junction has thin cementum or dentin surface that can be abraded or removed with an abrasive agent
   4. Areas of hypersensitivity—application of fluoride is one treatment for tooth sensitivity; protective fluoride must be left undisturbed (see Chapter 12, section on control of dentinal hypersensitivity)
   5. Restored tooth surfaces—gold and other restorations may be scratched by a polishing abrasive
C. Use of power-driven instruments
   1. Aerosol production
      a. Contaminated aerosols present a hazard to the clinician, other dental personnel, and other clients in the oral healthcare environment
      b. Power-driven equipment should not be used for a client with a known communicable condition
   2. Splatter
      a. Protective eye covers are needed for clients and dental team members
      b. Constituents of commercial prophylaxis pastes may include various chemicals that can cause a severe inflammatory response in the eye
   3. Heat production—care must be taken to use a wet polishing agent with minimal pressure and low speed to prevent overheating of a tooth, particularly the pulp tissues of small children

Technique Objectives

A. Client selected for removal of unsightly exogenous extrinsic stains needs instruction in how the stains can be prevented in the future
B. When stain removal is indicated, it should be after plaque control procedures have been supervised and professional scaling and root planing completed
C. Objectives of stain removal are
   1. Remove surface discolorations
   2. Provide minimal removal or abrasion of tooth structure
   3. Minimize trauma to the gingiva

4. Minimize heat production on the tooth surface
5. Leave no damage to restorations

Manual Stain Removal—the Porte Polisher

A. Description
  1. Prophylactic instrument with a thick handle and an adjustable working end designed to hold a wood point at a contraangle
  2. Wood points may be wedge shaped, spoon shaped, or cone shaped to fit various tooth surfaces; orangewood has proved to be the most satisfactory for polishing purposes
B. Technique
  1. Grasp
     a. Modified pen grasp—for all surfaces except maxillary anterior
     b. Palm—for maxillary anterior using the thumb for the fulcrum finger
  2. Activation—strokes
     a. Round—small circles ¹⁄₁₆ to ⅛ inch diameter; apply at the cervical third
     b. Vertical, oblique, and horizontal strokes may be applied to all other surfaces except near the gingival margin, depending on access
     c. Arm and wrist motion is applied with firm pressure and slow, controlled strokes
C. Special uses
  1. Individuals for whom a power-driven instrument cannot be used, such as a person with an active communicable disease; manual procedures can prevent contaminated aerosols
  2. Tooth surfaces that may be inaccessible for a prophylaxis angle, such as
     a. Long proximal surfaces exposed by gingival recession or periodontal surgery
     b. Lingual surfaces of lingually inclined mandibular posterior teeth
     c. Distal surfaces of maxillary molars
  3. Homebound or otherwise bedridden patients where portable power-driven equipment is not available
  4. Application of desensitizing agents
  5. Titanium implant

Power-Driven Stain Removal

A. Description of instruments
  1. Straight handpiece—connected to a power source
  2. Prophylaxis angle—attaches to the handpiece; holds rubber cups and bristle brushes
  3. Attachments
     a. Rubber cups
        (1) Attached by a mandrel or threaded stem, or snap on
        (2) Use—stain removal from tooth surfaces and for polishing restorations
     b. Bristle brushes
        (1) Attached by a mandrel or threaded stem
        (2) Use—stain removal from deep pits and fissures and enamel surfaces away from the gingival margin
        (3) Contraindicated for use on cementum or dentin because of possible grooving and scratching
B. Procedure for use of the rubber cup
  1. Grasp—modified pen grasp to hold the handpiece; position the middle finger pad to provide support; rest the handpiece in the V between the thumb and index finger
  2. Finger rest—establish an intraoral rest on firm teeth (avoid mobile teeth or pontics)
  3. Application of the agent
     a. When stain removal is indicated for a group of teeth, the wet agent may be spread over the teeth first; otherwise dip the rubber cup into the closely held Dappen dish so that application of agent is to individual teeth with stain to be removed
  4. Activate the rubber cup—after applying the grasp and establishing the finger rest, bring the cup almost in contact with the tooth surface before turning on the power
  5. Use the lowest possible speed
  6. Apply the cup to the tooth with a light, intermittent pressure
     a. Edges of the rubber cup should just barely flare
     b. Use continuous motion—avoid holding the cup in a single spot for long to prevent frictional heat
     c. Remember, there is a space in the middle of the cup, so the action on the stain is at the rim
  7. Sequence
     a. From the posterior distal aspect to the mesial aspect; from the cervical aspect to the occlusal aspect
     b. *Apply only where needed to remove stain*
C. Bristle brush
  1. Indications
     a. Selective use—only when the rubber cup cannot accomplish the stain removal
     b. Occlusal pits
        (1) Use a pointed bristle brush
        (2) Recommended during preparations for a pit and fissure sealant (used with fine pumice and water with no additives)
  2. Contraindications
     a. Near the gingival margin where epithelium could easily be denuded

    b. Cemental surfaces—both the bristle brush and the abrasive can remove and groove cementum

  3. Procedure for use

    a. Soak a stiff brush in warm water

    b. Grasp, finger rest, and other techniques are similar to those described above for the rubber cup

D. Airbrasive—airbrasive machine is an air-powered device using air and water pressure to deliver a controlled stream of a specially processed sodium bicarbonate in a slurry to the tooth surface; operation should be precise and controlled and potential damage recognized

  1. Application

    a. Protect client—coverall, hair cover, eye protection, lip lubrication

    b. Protect clinician and assistant—protective barriers for infection control including mask, hair cover, eye protection, and gloves

    c. Preprocedural rinse to lessen contaminated aerosols; have client rinse with antibacterial mouth rinse

    d. Direct the spray in constant motion for only 3 to 5 seconds at any area on the enamel surface; angulate away from gingival margin

    e. Use high-power suction with wide tip

  2. Recommendations and precautions

    a. Avoid use for client with respiratory disease or condition that limits swallowing or breathing and for person with restricted sodium diet

    b. Other contraindications—exposed cementum or dentin, soft spongy gingiva, all nonmetallic restorative materials, and all gold restorations

Postoperative Procedures

A. Remove particles of abrasive at the contact areas by applying dental floss

B. Loosen and remove particles in pockets and sulci by irrigation and aspiration with central suction

C. Provide postoperative instruction

SUGGESTED READING

Nield-Gehrig JS, Houseman GA: *Fundamentals of periodontal instrumentation,* ed 3, Baltimore, 1996, Williams & Wilkins.

Tsutsui PT: Instrumentation theory for professional mechanical oral hygiene care. In Darby ML, Walsh MM, editors, *Dental hygiene theory and practice,* Philadelphia, 1995, WB Saunders, pp 475-534.

Wilkins EM: Clinical practice of the dental hygienist, ed 7, Baltimore, 1994, Williams & Wilkins.

Review Questions

1 The dental hygienist records the following information regarding the facial aspect of tooth #9: probing depth readings of 6-6-6 mm and clinical attachment level readings of 4-4-4 mm. The tissue of tooth #9 evidences a:
A. Normal sulcus
B. Gingival pocket
C. Periodontal pocket
D. Furcation involvement

2 A gingival pocket is a pocket formed by gingival enlargement without change in the attachment level and without destruction of the underlying periodontal tissues. All gingival pockets are intrabony (infrabony) pockets because the base of the pocket is apical to the crest of the alveolar bone.
A. Both statements are *TRUE.*
B. Both statements are *FALSE.*
C. The first statement is *TRUE,* the second statement is *FALSE.*
D. The first statement is *FALSE,* the second statement is *TRUE.*

3 Cementum removal is a necessary and important component of nonsurgical therapy. Elimination of bacterial endotoxins must be accomplished by extensive cementum removal.
A. Both statements are *TRUE.*
B. Both statements are *FALSE.*
C. The first statement is *TRUE,* the second statement is *FALSE.*
D. The first statement is *FALSE,* the second statement is *TRUE.*

4 When adapted appropriately, thin ultrasonic tips provide excellent opportunities for access to root concavities and furcation areas. The fluid lavage produced by ultrasonic instruments will disrupt unattached subgingival bacterial plaque from the sulcus or pocket space.
A. Both statements are *TRUE.*
B. Both statements are *FALSE.*
C. The first statement is *TRUE,* the second statement is *FALSE.*
D. The first statement is *FALSE,* the second statement is *TRUE.*

5 The most efficient means of identifying supragingival calculus is by
A. Visual observation and compressed air
B. Tactile detection with a periodontal probe
C. Tactile detection with an explorer
D. Use of disclosing solution
E. Transillumination

6 An instrument intended for use within a deep pocket on the proximal surface of a posterior tooth would have a/an
A. Straight shank
B. Straight shank with complex shank bends
C. Angled shank with a single shank bend
D. Angled shank with complex shank bends

7 The design characteristics of the shank will influence the use of the instrument. An instrument with a rigid shank is recommended for removal of light, subgingival calculus deposits.
  A. Both statements are *TRUE.*
  B. Both statements are *FALSE.*
  C. The first statement is *TRUE,* the second statement is *FALSE.*
  D. The first statement is *FALSE,* the second statement is *TRUE.*

8 A clinician who is experiencing repetitive strain injuries in the fingers and wrist can reduce muscle fatigue by selecting instruments with
  A. Small-diameter handles with a knurled surface
  B. Large-diameter handles with a knurled surface
  C. Small-diameter handles with a smooth surface
  D. Large-diameter handles with a smooth surface

9 Airbrasive polishers are recommended for use on exposed cementum and dentin surfaces. The use of airbrasive polishers should be avoided for a client with respiratory disease or condition that limits breathing.
  A. Both statements are *TRUE.*
  B. Both statements are *FALSE.*
  C. The first statement is *TRUE,* the second statement is *FALSE.*
  D. The first statement is *FALSE,* the second statement is *TRUE.*

10 In the modified pen grasp, the second finger is positioned with the:
  A. Finger pad on the instrument handle, across from the thumb
  B. Side of the finger resting on a tooth
  C. Finger pad on the instrument shank
  D. Side of the finger against the instrument shank
  E. Finger pad resting on the back of the working end

11 A firm instrument grasp is needed during an instrument stroke when calculus is being removed. A light instrument grasp is needed for increased tactile sensitivity during assessment strokes.
  A. Both statements are *TRUE.*
  B. Both statements are *FALSE.*
  C. The first statement is *TRUE,* the second statement is *FALSE.*
  D. The first statement is *FALSE,* the second statement is *TRUE.*

12 When working in an area of restricted access, the index finger of the nondominant hand against the alveolar ridge in the area of instrumentation is able to provide a stable resting point for the fulcrum finger. The least desirable type of finger rest is an intraoral finger rest on a tooth adjacent to the area of instrumentation.
  A. Both statements are *TRUE.*
  B. Both statements are *FALSE.*
  C. The first statement is *TRUE,* the second statement is *FALSE.*
  D. The first statement is *FALSE,* the second statement is *TRUE.*

13 Adaptation is defined as the angle formed by the working end of an instrument with the tooth surface. Burnishing of a calculus deposit may result when an angle of less than 45 degrees is formed by the tooth surface and the face of the blade.
  A. Both statements are *TRUE.*
  B. Both statements are *FALSE.*
  C. The first statement is *TRUE,* the second statement is *FALSE.*
  D. The first statement is *FALSE,* the second statement is *TRUE.*

14 Correct adaptation is when the working end of an instrument is positioned to conform to the morphology of the tooth surface. When correctly adapted, the entire length of the curet blade will be in contact with the root surface.
  A. Both statements are *TRUE.*
  B. Both statements are *FALSE.*
  C. The first statement is *TRUE,* the second statement is *FALSE.*
  D. The first statement is *FALSE,* the second statement is *TRUE.*

15 When inserting a curet into a periodontal pocket, the angle between the face of the instrument and the tooth surface should be between
  A. 0 and 10 degrees
  B. 35 and 45 degrees
  C. 45 and 90 degrees
  D. 100 and 110 degrees

16 Before initiating a stroke for calculus removal, a _____ -degree angulation should be established between the tooth surface and the instrument face.
  A. 0 to 10
  B. 35 to 45
  C. 70 to 80
  D. 100 to 110

17 An assessment stroke is a type of instrumentation stroke used to remove calculus from tooth surfaces. A walking stroke is accomplished by touching the bottom of the sulcus or pocket with each down stroke of the instrument.
  A. Both statements are *TRUE.*
  B. Both statements are *FALSE.*
  C. The first statement is *TRUE,* the second statement is *FALSE.*
  D. The first statement is *FALSE,* the second statement is *TRUE.*

18 Feather-light pressure should be used when employing assessment strokes with an explorer or periodontal probe. When activating a work stroke with a curet, the clinician should use a firm lateral pressure.
  A. Both statements are *TRUE.*
  B. Both statements are *FALSE.*
  C. The first statement is *TRUE,* the second statement is *FALSE.*
  D. The first statement is *FALSE,* the second statement is *TRUE.*

19 All of the following are purposes and uses of a periodontal probe *EXCEPT:*
- A. Assess the periodontal status
- B. Evaluate restorations and sealants
- C. Make a sulcus and pocket survey
- D. Make a mucogingival examination
- E. Evaluate bleeding

20 When using a Nabers probe to check for furcation involvement on a maxillary molar, the clinician should enter the furcation area from all aspects of the root surface, *EXCEPT* the:
- A. Midfacial aspect
- B. Mesial aspect
- C. Distal aspect
- D. Midlingual aspect

21 The base of a pocket or sulcus will feel hard and offer firm resistance to a periodontal probe. Probing depths may vary considerably on different surfaces of the tooth.
- A. Both statements are *TRUE.*
- B. Both statements are *FALSE.*
- C. The first statement is *TRUE,* the second statement is *FALSE.*
- D. The first statement is *FALSE,* the second statement is *TRUE.*

22 The distance from the gingival margin to the attachment level is the:
- A. Mucogingival border
- B. Probing depth
- C. Clinical attachment level
- D. Width of attached gingiva

23 You are evaluating tooth #30. There is 4 mm of visible tissue recession on the facial aspect. The measurement from the gingival margin to the attachment level is 1 mm on the facial aspect. What is the clinical attachment level on the facial aspect of this tooth?
- A. 1 mm
- B. 2 mm
- C. 3 mm
- D. 4 mm
- E. 5 mm

24 The clinician is evaluating tooth #30. There is 4 mm of visible tissue recession on the facial aspect. The measurement from the gingival margin to the attachment level is 1 mm on the facial aspect. What is the probing depth on the facial aspect of this tooth?
- A. 1 mm
- B. 2 mm
- C. 3 mm
- D. 4 mm
- E. 5 mm

25 When evaluating the col area with a periodontal probe, the clinician should
- A. Position the length of the probe parallel to the CEJ
- B. Position the length of the probe parallel to the long axis of the tooth
- C. Slant the probe so the tip of the probe reaches under the contact area
- D. Use a furcation probe instead of a calibrated periodontal probe

26 Moderate furcation involvement with bone destruction to the extent that a probe can enter the furcation area but not pass through the furcation is classified as
- A. Class I
- B. Class II
- C. Class III
- D. Class IV
- E. Class V

27 Bleeding on probing is a significant indicator of inflammation and is an earlier clinical sign than the appearance of marginal redness. Bleeding on probing correlates with increases in nonmotile organisms in the pocket.
- A. Both statements are *TRUE.*
- B. Both statements are *FALSE.*
- C. The first statement is *TRUE,* the second statement is *FALSE.*
- D. The first statement is *FALSE,* the second statement is *TRUE.*

28 In normal healthy tissue, with application of light pressure, the probe tip is stopped at the coronal part of the junctional epithelium. In advanced periodontitis, the probe tip may penetrate through the junctional epithelium to reach the attached connective tissue fibers.
- A. Both statements are *TRUE.*
- B. Both statements are *FALSE.*
- C. The first statement is *TRUE,* the second statement is *FALSE.*
- D. The first statement is *FALSE,* the second statement is *TRUE.*

29 What is the recommended pressure when using a periodontal probe to assess the clinical attachment level?
- A. 1 to 2 g
- B. 10 to 20 g
- C. 100 to 200 g
- D. 1 to 2 lb
- E. 10 to 20 lb

30 Diseased tissue offers more tissue resistance to the pressure exerted by the clinician with a periodontal probe, so in severe periodontal disease the probe stops in the coronal portion of the junctional epithelium. A probe with a thin working end may insert to a deeper level of the junctional epithelium than a thicker probe.
- A. Both statements are *TRUE.*
- B. Both statements are *FALSE.*
- C. The first statement is *TRUE,* the second statement is *FALSE.*
- D. The first statement is *FALSE,* the second statement is *TRUE.*

31 Bleeding indices have been developed for use in clinical and research evaluation. Bleeding index scores have not been shown to be helpful in motivating client cooperation with bacterial plaque control efforts.
- A. Both statements are *TRUE.*
- B. Both statements are *FALSE.*
- C. The first statement is *TRUE,* the second statement is *FALSE.*
- D. The first statement is *FALSE,* the second statement is *TRUE.*

32 Compressed air and a mouth mirror can be used to detect most supragingival calculus deposits. For subgingival instrumentation, an explorer is used with an assessment stroke to detect calculus deposits.
   A. Both statements are *TRUE.*
   B. Both statements are *FALSE.*
   C. The first statement is *TRUE,* the second statement is *FALSE.*
   D. The first statement is *FALSE,* the second statement is *TRUE.*

33 Adapt the side of the explorer tip to the tooth surface with a light but definite lateral pressure. When exploring around line angles, lead with the heel-third of the tip by rolling the handle to maintain adaptation of the tip.
   A. Both statements are *TRUE.*
   B. Both statements are *FALSE.*
   C. The first statement is *TRUE,* the second statement is *FALSE.*
   D. The first statement is *FALSE,* the second statement is *TRUE.*

34 Which of the following is *NOT* a recommended use for an explorer?
   A. Detection of the texture and character of subgingival tooth surfaces
   B. Removal of endotoxins from the surface of cementum
   C. Evaluation of restorations and sealants at maintenance visits
   D. Examine tooth surfaces for decalcified and carious lesions
   E. Detection of subgingival calculus deposits

35 Before instrumentation the predominant characteristics of subgingival plaque are aerobic, gram positive, nonmotile, coccoid forms of bacteria. After instrumentation the predominant characteristics of subgingival plaque are anaerobic, gram negative, motile forms with many spirochetes and rods.
   A. Both statements are *TRUE.*
   B. Both statements are *FALSE.*
   C. The first statement is *TRUE,* the second statement is *FALSE.*
   D. The first statement is *FALSE,* the second statement is *TRUE.*

36 An overhanging restoration that extends subgingivally can induce negative changes in the microflora of the pocket. Removal of overhanging restorations can facilitate interdental plaque removal and control by the client.
   A. Both statements are *TRUE.*
   B. Both statements are *FALSE.*
   C. The first statement is *TRUE,* the second statement is *FALSE.*
   D. The first statement is *FALSE,* the second statement is *TRUE.*

37 Instructing the client to rinse thoroughly with an antimicrobial mouth rinse *BEFORE* treatment will lower microorganisms in aerosols. Instruction in bacterial plaque control, such as brushing, flossing, or other aids, should be presented *AFTER* instrumentation.
   A. Both statements are *TRUE.*
   B. Both statements are *FALSE.*
   C. The first statement is *TRUE,* the second statement is *FALSE.*
   D. The first statement is *FALSE,* the second statement is *TRUE.*

38 Which instruments are recommended primarily for debridement of dental implants?
   A. Area-specific curets
   B. Plastic instruments
   C. Chisel scalers
   D. Sickle scalers
   E. Universal curets

39 Which instruments are recommended primarily for removal of heavy to moderate supragingival calculus deposits in a posterior sextant?
   A. Area-specific curets
   B. Plastic instruments
   C. Chisel scalers
   D. Sickle scalers
   E. Universal curets

40 Which instruments are recommended primarily for removal of light to moderate subgingival calculus deposits on all tooth surfaces?
   A. Area-specific curets
   B. Plastic instruments
   C. Chisel scalers
   D. Sickle scalers
   E. Universal curets

41 Which instruments are recommended for removal of light calculus deposits located 5 mm beneath the gingival margin?
   A. Area-specific curets
   B. Plastic instruments
   C. Chisel scalers
   D. Sickle scalers
   E. Universal curets

42 An area-specific curet has straight flat blades that are not easily adapted to curved tooth surfaces. The rounded, smooth back of a curet permits placement at the base of the pocket without irritation or trauma.
   A. Both statements are *TRUE.*
   B. Both statements are *FALSE.*
   C. The first statement is *TRUE,* the second statement is *FALSE.*
   D. The first statement is *FALSE,* the second statement is *TRUE.*

43 The treatment area is a deep, 6 mm pocket with light calculus deposits on the cemental surfaces. Which manual instruments would be recommended for use in this treatment area?
   A. Area-specific curets
   B. Plastic instruments
   C. Chisel scalers
   D. Sickle scalers
   E. Universal curets

44 Instruments for use on implant teeth are available in designs that are similar to conventional probes, sickle scalers, and universal curets. Instruments used for assessment and calculus removal of implant teeth should be made of a material that is slightly harder than the implant material.
   A. Both statements are *TRUE.*
   B. Both statements are *FALSE.*
   C. The first statement is *TRUE,* the second statement is *FALSE.*
   D. The first statement is *FALSE,* the second statement is *TRUE.*

45 Calculus is removed readily from implant teeth because there is no interlocking or penetration of the deposit with the implant surface. Stainless steel instruments are recommended for instrumentation of implant teeth.
   A. Both statements are *TRUE.*
   B. Both statements are *FALSE.*
   C. The first statement is *TRUE,* the second statement is *FALSE.*
   D. The first statement is *FALSE,* the second statement is *TRUE.*

46 Ultrasonic/sonic instruments with thin tip design have been shown to be safe and effective in debridement of calculus, plaque, and endotoxins from root surfaces within 4 to 7 mm pockets. Thin ultrasonic tips are only slightly larger than hand-activated curets.
   A. Both statements are *TRUE.*
   B. Both statements are *FALSE.*
   C. The first statement is *TRUE,* the second statement is *FALSE.*
   D. The first statement is *FALSE,* the second statement is *TRUE.*

47 All of the following are advantages of thin ultrasonic tips, *EXCEPT:*
   A. Thin tips are easier to insert beneath tight gingival margins
   B. Thin tips remove more cementum and therefore are more efficient
   C. Thin tips have no cutting edges to cut or tear the tissue resulting in faster healing rates for ultrasonically instrumented treatment areas
   D. The entire length of tip is active; adaptation is not limited to a single region on the tip
   E. The water stream penetrates to the base of the pocket flushing out loose calculus, debris, and unattached plaque

48 Ultrasonically debrided treatment sites have higher levels of bacteria than sites instrumented with hand-activated curets. Both manually-activated and ultrasonic instruments have been shown to accomplish effective periodontal debridement of subgingival root surfaces.
   A. Both statements are *TRUE.*
   B. Both statements are *FALSE.*
   C. The first statement is *TRUE,* the second statement is *FALSE.*
   D. The first statement is *FALSE,* the second statement is *TRUE.*

49 Ultrasonic and sonic instruments produce very low levels of aerosol contamination in the dental operatory. The use of ultrasonic or sonic instruments are recommended for clients with respiratory or pulmonary disease or difficulty in breathing.
   A. Both statements are *TRUE.*
   B. Both statements are *FALSE.*
   C. The first statement is *TRUE,* the second statement is *FALSE.*
   D. The first statement is *FALSE,* the second statement is *TRUE.*

50 Ultrasonic/sonic instruments are used with light stroke pressure. The very end ("point") of the ultrasonic tip should be directly adapted to the tooth surface.
   A. Both statements are *TRUE.*
   B. Both statements are *FALSE.*
   C. The first statement is *TRUE,* the second statement is *FALSE.*
   D. The first statement is *FALSE,* the second statement is *TRUE.*

51 The tip of your area-specific curet breaks during instrumentation. Each of the following steps is appropriate, *EXCEPT* one. Which step is *NOT* recommended?
   A. Isolate the area with gauze or cotton roll
   B. Do not alarm the patient by describing the accident
   C. Dry the area with high velocity suction
   D. Use another curet in a spooning-type motion to examine the sulcus
   E. Make a periapical radiograph of the area

Answers and Rationales

1. (C) The clinical attachment level indicates the position of the periodontal attached tissue at the base of the sulcus or pocket as measured from a fixed point. Because the clinical attachment level is 4-4-4 mm, this tooth evidences a periodontal pocket.
   (A) A normal sulcus has a measurement of 1 to 2 mm facially and lingually, and 1 to 3 mm on proximal surface.
   (B) A gingival pocket is formed by gingival enlargement without change in the attachment level and without destruction of the underlying periodontal tissues.
   (D) Tooth #9 is a single-rooted tooth.
2. (C) All gingival pockets are suprabony because no changes have occurred in the bone level or contour. The base of a gingival pocket is coronal to the crest of the alveolar bone because there is no destruction of the underlying periodontal tissues.
3. (B) Endotoxins are not absorbed very far into the cementum; (the cementum itself is not altered by the presence of endotoxins). Endotoxins are easily removed from the surface of the cementum. Cementum removal is not necessary and is damaging to the periodontium.

4. (A) Modern tips are significantly smaller than manually-activated curets. They are easier to insert beneath the gingival margin and adapt to root concavities. Water from the instrument tip penetrates to the base of the pocket and flushes calculus debris, blood, bacteria, and plaque from the treatment site.

5. (A) Supragingival calculus is easily detected by visual observation using appropriate procedures of retraction, lighting, and mirror for indirect vision. Drying tooth surfaces with a gentle air stream helps to make supragingival calculus visible.

   (B) & (C) Visual detection is faster and easier than tactile detection of supragingival calculus.

   (D) Disclosing solutions are used for the detection of bacterial plaque.

   (E) Transillumination is not considered a major method in the detection of supragingival deposits.

6. (D) An angled shank is designed for use in areas of restricted access such as the proximal surfaces of posterior teeth; the angles extend around convex tooth surfaces. A complex shank with several angles would be ideal for use in a deep pocket on a posterior tooth.

   (A) An instrument with a straight shank is designed for an area with unrestricted access such as an anterior tooth.

   (B) An instrument with complex bends (or angles) could not have a straight shank.

   (C) An instrument shank with complex shank bends would be easier to adapt within a pocket of a posterior tooth.

7. (C) An instrument with a rigid shank would not be recommended for removal of light, subgingival deposits. A rigid shank decreases tactile conduction to the clinician's fingers making calculus detection more difficult. Limited tactile information may result in removal of excess cementum from the root surface.

8. (B) Large-diameter handles with a knurled surface texture are easier to hold and control.

   (A) Small-diameter handles require a tighter grip.

   (C) Smooth handles are difficult to control.

   (D) Smooth handles are difficult to control.

9. (D) Airbrasive polishers are contraindicated for use on exposed cementum and dentin surfaces; the cementum or dentin surface can be abraded or removed by the abrasive agent. Airbrasive polishing generates aerosols which could present a hazard for a client with a respiratory disease or condition that limits breathing.

10. (C) The pad of the middle finger rests on the instrument shank so that the clinician will feel the shank vibrate when the working end encounters roughness on the tooth surface.

    (A) The index and second fingers are used to hold the instrument handle.

    (B) The fourth finger is kept with the third finger in the modified pen grasp.

    (D) Placing the side of the finger against the shank will decrease tactile information to the clinician's hand.

    (E) This position would only be possible if the face of the working end were adapted to the tooth surface and would result in ineffective calculus removal.

11. (A) Both statements are true.

12. (C) An intraoral finger rest on a tooth adjacent to the area of instrumentation is the most desirable type of finger rest because it provides the greatest stability.

13. (D) Adaptation is defined as the relationship between the instrument and the surface of the tooth or soft tissue. Angulation is defined as the angle formed by the working end of an instrument with the tooth surface.

14. (C) It is usually possible to adapt only the toe-third of the cutting edge to a root surface.

15. (A) For insertion, the angulation should be between 0 and 10 degrees.

    (B) This angulation could result in trauma to the tissue.

    (C) This is the correct angulation for calculus removal.

    (D) This angulation would result in trauma to the tissue.

16. (C) For calculus removal, the angulation should be between 70 and 80 degrees.

    (A) This is the correct angulation for insertion.

    (B) This angulation might burnish the calculus deposit.

    (D) This angulation would result in trauma to the tissue.

17. (D) Assessment strokes are used to detect calculus deposits or other plaque retentive factors on the tooth surface.

18. (A) Both statements are true.

19. (B) An explorer is used to evaluate restorations and sealants at each recall follow-up.

    (A) Periodontal probes are used to determine probing depth and clinical attachment level.

    (C) Periodontal probes are used to examine the shape, topography, and dimensions of sulci and pockets.

    (D) Periodontal probes are used to determine the relationship between the gingival margin position, mucogingival junction, and the probing depth.

    (E) Periodontal probes are used to identify bleeding on probing, an early sign of inflammation.

20. (D) Maxillary molars have a palatal root so no assessment can be made from the mid-lingual aspect.

    (A), (B), (C) A trifurcated tooth should be accessed around the palatal root and the two facial roots by probing the mid-facial, mesial, and distal aspects.

21. (D) The base of a pocket or sulcus will feel soft and resilient and offers light to moderate resistance to a periodontal probe depending on the health of the tissue.

22. (B) The probing depth is the distance from the gingival margin to the attachment level.
    (A) The mucogingival junction demarcates the attached gingiva from alveolar mucosa.
    (C) The clinical attachment level refers to the position of the periodontal attached tissue at the base of a sulcus or pocket as measured from a fixed point.
    (D) The width of attached gingiva equals the total width of the gingiva minus the probing depth.

23. (E) The clinical attachment level refers to the position of the periodontal attached tissue at the base of a sulcus or pocket as measured from a fixed point, usually the CEJ. In this case, the distance from the CEJ to the base of the pocket is 4 mm plus 1 mm, for a total of 5 mm.
    (A) One millimeter would be the clinical attachment level *only if* the gingival margin is at the CEJ.
    (B) & (C) The clinical attachment level is the distance from the CEJ to the base of the sulcus or pocket.
    (D) Four mm is the amount of visible tissue recession; the gingival margin is 4 mm apical to the CEJ.

24. (A) The probing depth is the distance from the gingival margin to the attachment level, or in this case, one millimeter.
    (B) & (C) The probing depth is the distance from the gingival margin to the base of the sulcus or pocket.
    (D) Four mm is the amount of visible tissue recession; the gingival margin is 4 mm apical to the CEJ.
    (E) The clinical attachment level refers to the position of the periodontal attached tissue at the base of a sulcus or pocket as measured from a fixed point, usually the CEJ. In this case, the distance from the CEJ to the base of the pocket is 4 mm plus 1 mm, for a total of 5 mm.

25. (C) The working end should be slanted slightly so that the upper portion touches the contact area and the tip reaches under the contact area.
    (A) This technique would position the length of the probe horizontal to the CEJ. It is not possible to take a measurement in this position.
    (B) This is the correct technique for assessing the other areas of the tooth. This technique is not effective in the col area, however, because the contact area blocks direct access to the col.
    (D) A furcation probe is not used to assess the col area of the tooth.

26. (B) Moderate furcation involvement with bone destruction to the extent that a probe can enter the furcation area but not pass through the furcation is classified as a Class II furcation involvement.
    (A) A Class I is early or incipient furcation involvement.
    (C) A Class III is severe, or advanced involvement; probe can be passed between the roots through the entire furcation.
    (D) A Class IV is the same as class III except that the furca is visible clinically because of the presence of tissue recession.
    (E) There is no classification of furcation that is designated as a Class V.

27. (C) Bleeding on probing correlates with increases in motile organisms, especially spirochetes, in the pocket.

28. (A) Both statements are true.

29. (B) A light pressure of 10 to 20 g is recommended.
    (A) This pressure would not be sufficient.
    (C) This pressure would be excessive.
    (D) This pressure would be very excessive.
    (E) This pressure would be very excessive; light pressure is all that is required.

30. (D) Diseased tissue offers less tissue resistance to the pressure exerted by the clinician with a periodontal probe, so the probe inserts to a deeper level of the junctional epithelium.

31. (C) Bleeding index scores can help to motivate client cooperation with plaque control efforts.

32. (A) Both statements are true.

33. (C) Lead with the explorer tip around line angles by rolling the handle to maintain adaptation of the tip.

34. (B) Although endotoxins are easily removed from cemental surfaces, an explorer would not be an efficient means to deplaque tooth surfaces.
    (A) Explorers are used to detect the texture and character of subgingival tooth surfaces.
    (C) Explorers are used to evaluate restorations and sealants at maintenance visits.
    (D) Explorers are used to examine tooth surfaces for decalcified and carious lesions.
    (E) Explorers are used to detect subgingival calculus deposits.

35. (B) Before instrumentation the predominant characteristics of subgingival plaque are anaerobic, gram-negative, motile forms with many spirochetes and rods, very high counts of all microorganisms, and many white blood cells. After instrumentation the predominant characteristics of subgingival plaque are aerobic, gram-positive, nonmotile, coccoid forms of bacteria.

36. (A) Both statements are true.

37. (C) Instruction in bacterial plaque control, such as brushing, flossing, or other aids, should be presented *before* any instrumentation.

38. (B) Plastic instruments are recommended for debridement of implants because metal instruments may leave scratches on the surface of the implant.
    (A) (C) (D) (E) Metal instruments may leave scratches on the surface of the implant; surface roughness may favor bacterial plaque accumulation.

39. (D) Sickle scalers are recommended primarily for removal of heavy to moderate supragingival calculus deposits in a posterior sextant.
    (A) Area-specific curets are recommended primarily for specific adaptation to certain teeth and certain surfaces.
    (B) Plastic instruments are recommended for debridement of implants because metal instruments may leave scratches on the surface of the implant.
    (C) Chisel scalers are recommended for removal of gross supragingival calculus from exposed proximal surfaces of anterior teeth.
    (E) Universal curets are recommended primarily for removal of light to moderate subgingival calculus deposits on all tooth surfaces.

40. (E) Universal curets are recommended primarily for removal of light to moderate subgingival calculus deposits on all tooth surfaces.
   (A) Area-specific curets are recommended primarily for specific adaptation to certain teeth and certain surfaces.
   (B) Plastic instruments are recommended for debridement of implants because metal instruments may leave scratches on the surface of the implant.
   (C) Chisel scalers are recommended for removal of gross supragingival calculus from exposed proximal surfaces of anterior teeth.
   (D) Sickle scalers are recommended primarily for removal of heavy to moderate supragingival calculus deposits in a posterior sextant.

41. (A) Area-specific curets are recommended for removal of light calculus deposits located within periodontal pockets.
   (B) Plastic instruments are recommended for debridement of implants because metal instruments may leave scratches on the surface of the implant.
   (C) Chisel scalers are recommended for removal of gross supragingival calculus from exposed proximal surfaces of anterior teeth when interdental soft tissue is missing.
   (D) Sickle scalers are recommended primarily for removal of heavy to moderate supragingival calculus deposits in a posterior sextant.
   (E) Universal curets are recommended primarily for removal of light to moderate subgingival calculus deposits on all tooth surfaces.

42. (D) An area-specific curet has a curved blade that is easily adapted to curved tooth surfaces.

43. (A) Area-specific curets are recommended for debridement of a deep, 6-mm pocket with light calculus deposits on the cemental surfaces.
   (B) Plastic instruments are recommended for debridement of dental implants.
   (C) Chisel scalers are designed for supragingival use on exposed proximal surfaces of anterior teeth when interdental soft tissue is missing.
   (D) Sickle scalers are designed for use on supragingival tooth surfaces; the straight, flat blades are not readily adaptable to curved subgingival surfaces.
   (E) Universal curets are recommended primarily for removal of light to moderate subgingival calculus deposits on all tooth surfaces.

44. (C) Instruments used for assessment and calculus removal of implant teeth should be made of a material that is softer than the implant material.

45. (C) Metal instruments may leave scratches on the surface of the implant. Instruments used on implant teeth should be made of a material that is softer than the implant material.

46. (C) Thin ultrasonic tips are significantly smaller than hand-activated curets.

47. (B) Thin tips remove less cementum and therefore provide the most conservative approach to subgingival debridement.

48. (D) Ultrasonically debrided treatment sites have lower levels of bacteria than sites instrumented with manually-activated curets.

49. (B) Ultrasonic and sonic instruments produce a high level of aerosol contamination in the dental operatory. The use of ultrasonic or sonic instruments is contraindicated for clients with respiratory or pulmonary disease or difficulty in breathing.

50. (C) Direct application of the very end of an ultrasonic tip to the tooth surface should be avoided.

51. (C) It is imperative to know that the broken tip has been located and removed from the client's mouth. If high velocity suction is used, it is impossible to know whether the tip was suctioned from the client's mouth.
   (A) (B) (D) (E) Are recommended.

Dental Hygiene Care for Individuals with Special Needs

Beverly Entwistle Isman

Every person is unique with differing abilities and needs. Four out of ten persons treated in the oral healthcare environment may require a modified care plan at some point because of "special needs." These special needs may be transient, such as pregnancy or a broken foot, or lifelong, such as end stage renal disease or mental retardation. With national emphasis on access to care for underserved populations, dental hygienists will be serving increased numbers of persons with special needs in a variety of settings.

Client considerations covered in this chapter primarily relate to specific disabling conditions and medical problems with special considerations for various life stages. The format describing each condition follows a similar pattern, including definition; incidence and prevalence; etiology and diagnostic information; signs, symptoms, and clinical manifestations; general medical treatment; and oral manifestations. Specific dental management considerations are summarized in the last half of the chapter. The contemporary dental hygienist should be familiar with this information.

General Considerations

Life Span Approach to Care

A. Principles of growth, development, and maturation
   1. Growth includes physical and functional maturation
   2. Growth is generally a continuous and orderly process but can be modified by numerous factors (e.g., nutritional deficiencies)
   3. Different parts of the body grow and mature at different rates
   4. Critical periods exist in growth and development
   5. Hormonal changes can alter
      a. Physical stature and function
      b. Mental state and mood
      c. Oral status
   6. During growth and maturation, perceptions of self and self in relation to others change
   7. Health status generally progresses from acute illness to chronic illness
   8. Transition from one life stage to another is gradual and not necessarily based on chronologic age
   9. Biologic aging is not synonymous with chronologic age
   10. Signs of aging can appear at any age
B. U.S. healthcare system (see Chapter 15, section on oral healthcare)
   1. Current system is categorical, with many gaps in services
   2. Need to develop a continuum of services through the life stages to ensure
      a. Universal access
      b. Continuity of care
      c. Comprehensive philosophy of care
      d. System of planned change

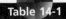

Table 14-1

Life Span Approach to Oral Healthcare

Life stage	General care concerns	Usual oral concerns
Early childhood ↓	Teaching parents/caregiver oral care skills Preventing early occurrence of caries or trauma (protecting developing teeth)	Oral infections Dental development
Childhood	Developing positive dental attitudes and behaviors Teaching self-care skills	Dental caries Gingivitis
Adolescence ↓	Motivating toward self-responsibility for seeking and receiving care Controlling risk factors for disease	Dental caries Gingivitis Dental development
Young adult	Decreasing barriers and integrating oral healthcare into daily schedule	Periodontal diseases
Midlife	Maintaining status and preventing deterioration	Periodontal diseases
Older adult ↓	Motivating to continue preventive care and accept new theories and interventions Decreasing barriers to care	Periodontal diseases Dental caries Oral cancer
Elderly	Maintaining status and function and preventing infections and tooth loss	Periodontal diseases Dental caries Oral cancer Fractures, tooth loss Oral infections

3. Healthcare providers should consider
   a. Heterogeneity of people bearing the same label
   b. Individualized approach to care
4. Oral health needs and approaches to care can differ throughout the life cycle (Table 14-1)

Incidence/Prevalence of Special-Needs Individuals

A. National statistics on incidence and prevalence figures are difficult to compile because of
   1. Unreliable reporting systems
   2. Variable and changing definitions of conditions
   3. Differences between acute versus chronic conditions
   4. Overlap in data when dealing with multiple conditions
B. During 1991-92 about 48.9 million persons (19.4% of the U.S. population) had a disability; 7.9% were children
C. Conditions reported as causing disability in children 17 years and younger are shown in Table 14-2; 1 in 33 babies is born with a structural birth defect
D. Table 14-3 identifies the most common chronic conditions in the elderly population
E. The five most prevalent chronic conditions in the U.S. noninstitutionalized population include sinusitis, arthritis, hypertension, hearing impairment, and heart disease
F. The five most frequently reported chronic conditions that cause work disability and activity limitations in-

Table 14-2

Conditions Reported as Cause of Disability (>2%) among U.S. Children ≤17 Years, 1991-92

Condition	Number	%
Learning disability	1435	29.5
Speech problems	634	13.1
Mental retardation	331	6.8
Asthma	311	6.4
Mental/emotional disorder	305	6.3
Blindness/vision problem	144	3.0
Cerebral palsy	129	2.7
Seizure disorder	128	2.6
Deafness/hearing disorder	116	2.4

Adapted from Table 2, Disabilities among children ≤17 years—United States, 1991-1992, *MMWR* 44(33):609-13, 1995.

clude arthritis, heart disease, spinal curvature/back impairments, impairments of the lower extremities, and diabetes

Dental Hygienist's Role with Special-Needs Individuals

A. Recognize physical, mental, medical, social, and dental needs
B. Communicate with clients and caretakers in a positive, appropriate, nondiscriminatory manner

Table 14-3

Leading Chronic Conditions in the Elderly Population

Noninstitutionalized	Nursing home residents
Arthritis	Arthritis
Hypertension	Heart disease
Hearing impairments	Mental illness
Heart disease	Paralysis

C. Communicate with other professionals and team members to facilitate planning, implementation, and coordination of care

D. Plan, implement, and evaluate community-based and office-based programs

E. Adapt dental hygiene care plans, interventions, and evaluations to meet clients' special needs, considering
  1. Barriers to care
  2. Resources
  3. Personal skills and abilities
  4. Cultural values and beliefs

F. Identify and eliminate potential barriers to care

G. Assess one's own attitudes, values, and commitment to provision of oral health services to these clients

H. Evaluate local, state, regional, and national trends for their potential impact on the provision of oral healthcare

I. Advocate preventive oral health programs, full use of dental hygienists, and development of a sound research base for use in oral health programs

General Definitions

These tend to change frequently and often overlap.

A. *Labeling*—process of classifying people for educational, medical, or financial reasons

B. *Barrier-free environment*—facilities that are physically accessible to everyone

C. *Normalization*—making available patterns and conditions of everyday life that are as close as possible to the norms and patterns of the mainstream of society

D. *Mainstreaming*—integration of people with special needs into community-based programs and services

E. *Access to oral healthcare*—opportunity for each individual to enter into the oral healthcare system and make use of needed services

Goals of Normalization for People with Special Needs

A. Ensure legal and civil rights

B. Guarantee appropriate education for continued learning

C. Increase or maintain social skills and problem-solving abilities

D. Increase employment options and decrease employer discrimination

E. Ensure comprehensive network of community resources

Potential Barriers to Oral Healthcare

A. Accessibility
  1. Financial
    a. One fourth of the elderly population have an inadequate income level; percentages are higher for women, ethnic minorities, and single heads of households
    b. 87% of the elderly's per capita dental expenditures are out-of-pocket; few third-party payment mechanisms exist for this group
    c. Between 65% and 85% of disabled people live near the poverty level
    d. Two thirds of disabled Americans ages 14 to 64 do not work; one fourth have encountered job discrimination because of their disability
    e. People working in sheltered workshops or training centers generally earn less than $2000 per year
    f. Medicaid coverage for oral healthcare is extremely variable across states, often not covering adult care
    g. Medical expenses for many disabled persons consume a major portion of their income
    h. Many special-needs individuals on limited incomes cannot afford standard private practice fees for dental care, have no health insurance, or are underinsured
  2. Transportation/geography
    a. Over 50% of the disabled and elderly population live in urban settings; the remainder live in small rural communities or on farms
    b. Public transportation is often confusing, unaffordable, or nonexistent
    c. Individuals with special needs often rely on others for transportation to dental appointments, thus increasing their dependence and making scheduling difficult
    d. Homebound, hospitalized, or institutionalized persons frequently cannot be transported for care in the community
  3. Physical facilities
    a. Minimum standards for accessibility must be met by dentists according to the Americans with Disabilities Act of 1993
    b. External barriers include parking lots and spaces, walkways, curbs, stairs, narrow doors

and entryways, too-heavy or overpressurized doors, and small-print signs

   c. Internal barriers include narrow passageways or doors, cluttered rooms or hallways, loose rugs or heavy-shag carpets, abrupt changes in floor textures, noncontrasting colors, and bathrooms without grab-bars or other adaptations

B. Psychosocial concerns

   1. Over 50% of Americans express positive attitudes toward the elderly and people with disabilities, yet most really perceive them as different and inferior

   2. Society perceives disabilities, differences, and disease states before recognizing similarities

   3. Feelings of guilt, anxiety, apathy, inadequacy, embarrassment, depression, anger, and resentment about their special needs interfere with attempts to seek care

   4. Fear of or inability to comprehend dental procedures, antisocial or atypical behavior, or overdependency on oral healthcare providers interferes with provision of care

   5. Basic daily needs and activities are often overwhelming and can decrease priorities for oral healthcare

   6. Perception of self-image and worth can affect care planning

C. Provider philosophy/provision of care

   1. The Americans with Disabilities Act requires that public and private dental offices serve persons with disabilities, that treatment is provided on the same basis as for nondisabled persons, and that dentists make reasonable modifications to facilitate access

   2. Despite the Americans with Disabilities Act, surveys indicate that about 20% of dentists are willing to treat persons who are physically or mentally challenged

   3. Reasons given for not treating individuals with special needs include

     a. Inadequate facilities and equipment

     b. Inadequate training (therefore, knowledge and skills)

     c. Not wanting to expose "normal" clients to "special" clients

     d. Inability to collect adequate fees

     e. Additional effort and time required

     f. Personal discomfort about perceived "differences" of special clients

     g. Treatment of medically complex persons increases insurance premiums

D. Communication concerns

   1. Sensory impairments (hearing, visual) limit the ability to transmit and receive communications when scheduling or undergoing oral care or participating in oral health education

   2. Use of technical terminology or inappropriate language level may interfere with understanding

   3. Differences in communication styles (eye contact, physical proximity and contact, formal versus informal pronouns, cultural variations, use of nonverbal cues and verbal language) can impair effective communication

   4. Use of condescending voice tones or language levels closes off communication lines

E. Medical concerns

   1. Situations compromising the provider or client

     a. Inadequate infection control procedures

     b. Inadequate or inaccurate health histories

     c. Inadequate precautions for potential emergencies

     d. Inadequate knowledge of medical conditions and their treatment

   2. Types of treatment/conditions

     a. Medications

     b. Therapies that compromise oral health

     c. Conditions requiring premedication or alteration of treatment

     d. Conditions or situations that contraindicate treatment

     e. Terminal illness or the aging process may change care planning or the prognosis of treatment

     f. Medical problems or disabilities may necessitate provision of care in a setting other than the dental office

F. Mobility/stability concerns

   1. Impaired ambulation or use of assistive devices may hinder access to care

   2. Uncontrolled or sudden movements may interfere with home care or dental hygiene interventions

   3. Uncontrolled or aggressive behavior may endanger the care providers and the client

   4. Spatial disorientation may interfere with client relaxation in the dental chair or performance of oral care procedures

Specific Conditions

See Chapters 6 and 7.

Mental Retardation

A. Definition

   1. Subaverage intellectual functioning originating during the developmental period and associated with impairment in adaptive behavior

   2. Not the same as mental illness

   3. Label represents a highly heterogeneous group of people

B. Incidence—1% to 3% of the population, depending on criteria

C. Categories
   1. Mild (89%)
   2. Moderate (6%)
   3. Severe (3.5%)
   4. Profound (1.5%)
D. Etiology—acquired (12%), inherited (13%), unknown (75%)
   1. Infections and toxemias (rubella, meningitis, lead poisoning)
   2. Trauma, physical or chemical agents (child abuse; fetal alcohol syndrome)
   3. Disorders of metabolism or nutrition (phenylketonuria [PKU])
   4. Gross brain disease (atrophy or neoplasms)
   5. Chromosomal abnormalities (Down syndrome)
   6. Gestational disorders (Rh incompatibility, anoxia, prematurity)
   7. Environmental (lack of stimulation)
E. Signs/symptoms/clinical manifestations
   1. Variable, depending on the etiology
   2. Unusual difficulty in learning and applying what is learned to problems of daily living
   3. Skull or other craniofacial anomalies may exist
      a. Microcephaly—small cranium that restricts brain growth
      b. Hydrocephaly—expansion of the cranium from excessive accumulation of cerebrospinal fluid
      c. Malformation or asymmetry of growth
   4. General developmental delays
   5. Other possible manifestations include motor incoordination, visual and/or hearing disorders, specific learning disabilities, emotional disturbance, medical disabilities, seizure disorders
F. Treatment
   1. Special education services and vocational training
   2. Use of appropriate community resources for identified needs
G. Oral manifestations
   1. Most oral health problems are not inherent to the disability but are related to extrinsic factors (e.g., neglect by caretakers or incoordination leading to poor oral disease control)
   2. DMFS scores comparable to those of the general population, except "decayed" component may be higher because of a lack of professional treatment
   3. Higher prevalence of periodontal conditions, probably related to poor oral hygiene and the lack of regular care
   4. Higher incidence of malocclusion and deviations in tooth eruption is associated with craniofacial syndromes or growth abnormalities
   5. Some instances of enamel dysplasia, more commonly seen in those with severe mental deficiencies

resulting from severe prenatal or perinatal defects or insults
   6. Some instances of physical self-abuse if severely impaired

Fetal Alcohol Syndrome

A. Definition
   1. Fetal alcohol syndrome (FAS)—pattern of malformations caused by maternal alcohol consumption, characterized by prenatal and postnatal growth deficiency, dysmorphic facial features, and central nervous system (CNS) dysfunction
   2. Fetal alcohol effects (FAE)—children who display partial effects of FAS
B. Incidence/prevalence
   1. Incidence of FAS is 1.9 per 1000 live births
   2. FAE occurs 20 times more frequently than FAS
   3. Leading *known* cause of mental retardation in the United States since first recognized in 1973
C. Etiology
   1. Severity of fetal alcohol effects is dose dependent
   2. FAS babies are born to women who are "heavy drinkers" during pregnancy, usually at least 45 drinks per month
   3. Effects related to differences in blood alcohol content and differences in tissue susceptibility
   4. Alcohol affects the cell membrane and cell migration, thus altering organization of embryonic tissue
   5. Brain is most susceptible during third trimester
   6. Metabolic disturbances can retard cell division and growth
D. Signs/symptoms/clinical manifestations
   1. Premature and/or postnatal growth retardation results in short stature, slight build, small head
   2. Craniofacial dysmorphia—short eye openings, short upturned nose, smooth philtrum, flat midface, thin upper lip
   3. Can also have nonspecific abnormalities in any organ system, depending on time of alcohol insult
   4. Wide IQ range, many within the mentally retarded range
   5. May be able to read and write, but with minimal comprehension; also language problems
   6. Poor social judgment and socialization skills
   7. Hyperactivity and short attention span
   8. Heart defects in over 30%
   9. Skeletal and ear disorders
   10. Excessive hairiness at birth
E. Treatment—depends on specific anomalies and organ systems affected
   1. Surgery if indicated for heart or other defects
   2. Infant stimulation programs
   3. Appropriate educational and vocational placements

4. Family counseling since children may be at high risk for physical or sexual abuse and neglect
5. Nutritional and alcohol counseling for family

F. Oral manifestations
1. Majority of children with FAS have oral problems related to tooth eruption, malformations, or malpositioning of teeth (usually Class II or III)
2. May have V-shaped or cleft palate
3. Moderate to severe gingivitis

Down Syndrome

A. Definition/etiology
1. Mental retardation disorder
2. Associated with an anomaly of chromosome 21 (trisomy 21) in all or some body cells

B. Incidence—most common chromosomal abnormality (1 per 800 newborns, but varies with maternal age)

C. Signs/symptoms/clinical manifestations
1. Mental retardation ranging from mild to profound
2. Poor muscular development with hyperflexibility and hypotonia during childhood
3. Short stature with delay in skeletal maturation
4. Short neck and extremities with broad stubby fingers
5. High incidence of congenital heart defects (30% to 50%), language, vision, and hearing problems (>50%), and risk for leukemia and thyroid problems
6. Abnormal craniofacial features
   a. Small brachycephalic skull
   b. Round flat facies
   c. Small nasomaxillary complex
   d. Ocular hypotelorism (eyes closer together)
   e. Epicanthal folds (Fig. 14-1)
   f. Strabismus (convergent eyes)
   g. Simian crease (single transverse palmar crease) (Fig. 14-2)
   h. More susceptible to infection due to poor immune response

D. Treatment
1. Medical care for specific problems
2. Condition can be detected through amniocentesis or chorionic villi sampling
3. Special education

E. Oral manifestations (Fig. 14-3)
1. Relative mandibular prognathism as a result of the small nasomaxillary complex
2. Dry skin and cracking of the lips
3. Fissured tongue
4. Hyperplasia of the adenoids and tonsils
5. Altered salivary gland mechanism (decreased flow)

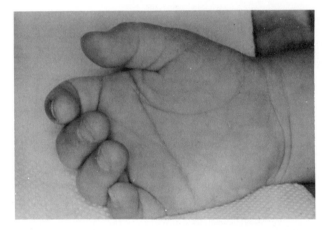

Fig. 14-2 Simian crease, one of the characteristics of Down syndrome.

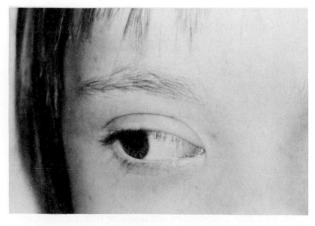

Fig. 14-1 Epicanthal fold, a characteristic of Down syndrome.

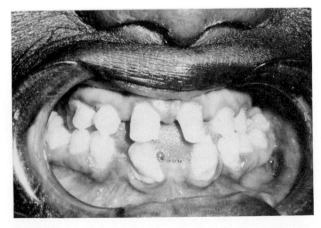

Fig. 14-3 Common oral conditions seen in adult with Down syndrome.

6. Increased susceptibility to severe periodontal disease of early onset, especially in the anterior areas
7. Delayed eruption of teeth
8. Higher incidence of congenitally missing teeth
9. Small tooth crowns with short crown/root ratio
10. Enamel dysplasia
11. Malocclusion—anterior open bite or crossbite, posterior crossbite
12. Attrition

Autism

A. Definition
  1. Developmental disability with specific behavioral and communicative components
  2. Not the same as mental retardation or childhood schizophrenia, as previously thought
B. Incidence/prevalence
  1. Occurs in 15/10,000 births
  2. Four times more common in males
  3. Appears during first 3 years of life
C. Etiology—different theories
  1. Psychogenic theories
  2. Genetic theories
  3. Biochemical deficits theories
  4. Neurophysiologic theories
D. Signs/symptoms/clinical manifestations
  1. Great variability in expression
  2. Extreme aloneness, failure to develop eye contact, not cuddly as infants, failure to develop social relationships or perceive others' feelings
  3. Language disturbances—repetitious speech, pronoun reversals, lack of ability to use gestures; 50% never develop functional speech
  4. Comprehension problems, especially with verbal directions
  5. Obsessiveness about maintaining routines and sameness of the environment (resistance to change)
  6. Eating disturbances
  7. Abnormal response to stimuli; may not respond to pain, or have constant movement and repetitious activity
  8. Intense attachments to objects
  9. May be aggressive or self-abusive
E. Treatment—variety of approaches tried with varying success
  1. Psychotherapy
  2. Behavior therapy
  3. Medications
  4. Special education
  5. Communication therapy

F. Oral manifestations—none directly associated with the syndrome

Specific Learning Disabilities and Attention Deficit Hyperactive Disorder

A. Definition
  1. Deficits in specific areas of learning or impulse control that can cause problems in acquiring new skills
  2. Relates primarily to vision, hearing, language, attention, and touch
B. Incidence/prevalence
  1. Not a distinct group
  2. Much controversy over diagnosis and treatment
  3. Occurs in 5% to 20% of the elementary school population
  4. More common in boys
C. Etiology
  1. Neurologic deficit or neurochemical imbalance
  2. Trauma
  3. Emotional factors
  4. Genetic or familial
  5. Cultural
D. Categories
  1. Areas of central nervous system (CNS) function affected
     a. Input—receiving, recognizing, and decoding messages (e.g., auditory or visual-perceptual problems)
     b. Organization—information storage, integration with other information, and prompt retrieval (e.g., short-term memory problem)
     c. Output—management of movement or utterances (e.g., hyperactivity, apraxia)
E. Signs/symptoms/clinical manifestations
  1. Hyperactivity or hypoactivity
  2. Irritability, impulsiveness, and need for immediate satisfaction
  3. Problems with concentration and memory
  4. Immaturity, clumsiness
  5. Lack of sense of direction, position, or time
  6. Speech and hearing problems
  7. Problems in reading, writing, or math
F. Treatment
  1. Remediation of weakness
  2. Compensation (creating new pathways)
  3. Exploitation of other areas (senses)
  4. Changing the environment
  5. Medications
G. Oral manifestations—none directly associated

Emotional Disturbance/Mental Illness

A. Definition
  1. By psychiatric diagnosis

2. By psychologic tests
3. By self-definition
4. By cultural definition of maladjustment
B. Incidence/prevalence
   1. Of elementary children, 30% have at least mild, subclinical cases (10% need treatment)
   2. At some point in life 1/10 of all adults will need or benefit from some form of mental health intervention
C. Etiology—depends on the type of disturbance
   1. Familial
   2. Life stress (e.g., social, financial, family, abuse)
   3. Depression
   4. Organic
D. Classifications (three common ones)
   1. Psychoneuroses—anxiety, depressive, obsessive, or conversion reactions
   2. Personality disorders—situational or adjustment reactions
   3. Psychoses —schizophrenia
E. Signs/symptoms/clinical manifestations (depend on the type of disorder)
   1. Inner tensions create anxiety, frustration, fears, and impulsive behavior
   2. Examples of behavior
      a. Translation of fears or anxieties into physical symptoms
      b. Regression to earlier forms of behavior
      c. Displays of hostility or aggression
      d. Withdrawal into fantasy (e.g., daydreams)
      e. Fear of failure and criticism
      f. Development of substitute fears, phobias, or compulsions
F. Treatment
   1. Stress management
   2. Psychotherapy
   3. Group therapy
   4. Medications, diet changes, and exercise
G. Oral manifestations
   1. None directly associated
   2. May see intraoral trauma resulting from unusual habits or aggressive behavior
   3. May have xerostomia as a side effect of medications
   4. If compulsive, may have immaculate oral hygiene

Eating Disorders

A. Definition
   1. Anorexia nervosa:
      a. Psychophysiologic condition characterized by suppression and denial of sensation of hunger
      b. May be socially isolated and relatively asexual
      c. Consumption of 300 to 600 calories per day is common
      d. Often come from middle to upper class families with high parental or societal expectations
      e. Perfectionists, competitive, and overachievers
      f. Deny their emaciated appearance
   2. Bulimia
      a. Syndrome involving episodic binge eating and purging
      b. Purging involves self-induced vomiting and use of laxatives, diuretics, or enemas
      c. Often occurs after failed attempts to lose weight through dieting
      d. May be of normal weight
      e. Usually outgoing and sexually active
      f. Calories consumed during binging range from 3,500 to 20,000
      g. Vomiting episodes may last from 5 to 30 minutes
B. Incidence/prevalence
   1. 90% are female
   2. 1/200 white adolescent females
   3. 3% to 20% of college students
   4. Most common age group is 12 to 35 years, but also occurs in the elderly
   5. 27% to 42% of anorectics indulge in bulimia
   6. 9% mortality rate
C. Etiology—multiple interactive causes
   1. Depressive illnesses
   2. Fear of obesity
   3. Endocrine changes at puberty
   4. Feelings of low self-esteem and poor body image
D. Signs and symptoms
   1. Anorexia nervosa
      a. Intense fear of becoming obese; refusal to maintain normal weight
      b. Disturbance of body image
      c. Weight loss of at least 25% of original body weight not caused by any physical illness
      d. Downy growth of body hair
      e. Periods of overactivity
      f. Dry, flaky skin
      g. Lowered blood pressure, body temperature, and pulse
      h. Episodes of bulimia
      i. Complications include cardiac arrhythmia from reduced heart muscle mass and electrolyte imbalance from dehydration
   2. Bulimia
      a. Awareness that eating pattern is abnormal
      b. Depression and self-deprecating thoughts
      c. Repeated attempts to lose weight
      d. Recurrent binging (rapid intake of food in a short period of time), usually high-calorie, easily ingested food
      e. Inconspicuous eating

f. Termination of episodes by abdominal pain, social interruption, or self-induced vomiting

g. Weight fluctuation greater than 10 pounds

h. Dehydration

i. Electrolyte imbalance

j. Gastrointestinal disturbances

E. Treatment

1. Physical stabilization of the seriously compromised patient

2. Psychologic and nutritional counseling

3. Support groups

4. Dental treatment

F. Oral manifestations

1. Esophageal lacerations and chronic sore throat from repeated vomiting

2. Parotid gland swelling and xerostomia

3. Burning sensation of tongue

4. Enamel erosion, dentinal hypersensitivity, and margination of amalgams from acid erosion of vomiting; lingual surfaces of maxillary incisors most often affected

5. Rampant caries from high consumption of sucrose, xerostomia, or dehydration

6. Irritated soft tissues from vomiting, dehydration, and vitamin deficiencies

7. Dentinal hypersensitivity, vitamin deficiencies

Alzheimer's Disease

A. Definition

1. Progressive irreversible brain disorders characterized by intellectual and cognitive disturbance, behavioral changes, and eventually a state of complete dependence

2. A type of senile dementia; probably a cluster of diseases

B. Incidence/prevalence

1. 2 to 4 million cases in the United States

2. Occurs in 5% of persons over age 65, 20% of those over 80

3. Accounts for 50% of all nursing home residents

C. Etiology

1. Unknown

2. Postulated theories

a. Viral agents causing selective cell death

b. Excessive accumulation of toxic agents

c. Gene mutations identified on 3 chromosomes

d. Age-related change in the immune system

e. Impaired synthesis and release of acetylcholine

f. Amyloid deposition toxic to brain cells

D. Signs/symptoms/clinical manifestations: different parts of the brain affected in varying degrees but reflect neuronal degeneration

1. Early

a. Memory loss and inability to concentrate

b. Anxiety, irritability, withdrawal, and petulance

c. Abnormal sleep patterns

d. Motor abnormalities, including exaggerated reflexes and gait disturbances

2. Later

a. Apathy, depression

b. Disorientation and lack of judgment and understanding

c. Incontinence

E. Treatment: no cures yet

1. Medications—a variety are used, but none with significant consistent success

2. Maintenance of current abilities and reality orientation; place in structured, stress-free environment

3. Provisions for ensuring safety and health

4. Support for the family

5. Researching gene therapy

F. Oral manifestations

1. None specific to the condition

2. Disease states usually are a result of neglect, the aging process, or any accompanying chronic illnesses

Seizure Disorders

See Chapter 17, section on seizures and convulsive disorders.

A. Definition

1. Not a disease, but a term used to describe symptoms of recurrent or chronic brain dysfunction

2. Characterized by discrete, recurring behavioral manifestations that include disturbances of balance, sensation, behavior, perception, or consciousness

3. Should not be confused with one-time seizures that result from drug overdoses, brain tumors, or other problems

4. *Seizure* refers to an episode of cerebral dysfunction produced by abnormal, excessive neuronal discharge; not necessarily a recurring condition

5. *Convulsion* refers to a broad range of behavioral manifestations, including seizure activity

6. *Fit* is an outmoded synonym for *convulsion* or *seizure*

7. *Aura* refers to a specific sensation preceding a seizure, lasting from 1 to several seconds and manifested as

a. Numbness, tingling

b. Unusual smell

c. Peculiar sound

d. Feeling of nausea or fear

8. Status epilepticus

a. Continuous convulsion lasting longer than 5 minutes

b. May lead to death

c. Constitutes a medical emergency

B. Incidence/prevalence

1. 4,500,000 cases in the United States

2. Incidence is 0.3% to 0.7% per year; prevalence is 2% of the population

3. Prevalence is highest in childhood

C. Etiology

1. Prenatal

a. Maternal infections

b. Fetal growth abnormalities or prematurity

c. Hormonal imbalances or Rh incompatibility

d. Chromosomal disorders

e. Toxicity or damage from drugs or radiation

f. Genetic influences

2. Perinatal

a. Delivery problems

b. Anoxia

3. Postnatal

a. Degenerative brain disease

b. Injury

c. Tumors

d. Prolonged high fever

e. Parasitic infections

f. Toxic agents (including alcohol and drugs)

4. Unknown

D. Types—can be classified by the origin of the seizure, the etiology, or the type of seizure activity

E. Signs/symptoms/clinical manifestations

1. Generalized tonic-clonic (grand mal)

a. May experience an aura

b. Loss of consciousness

c. Tonic movements (voluntary muscles experience continuous contractions)

d. Clonic movements (intermittent muscular contraction and relaxation)

e. Interruption of respiration and dilation of the pupils

f. Loss of bladder or bowel control

g. Seizure activity usually lasts 1 to 3 minutes

h. Lethargy and disorientation follow the return of consciousness

i. May occur any time during the day or only during sleep

2. Generalized absence (petit mal)

a. Transient loss of consciousness

b. May have minor motor movements of the eyes, head, or extremities

c. Lasts 5 to 30 seconds

d. Person may not be aware of having had a seizure

3. Complex partial (psychomotor)

a. May be preceded by an aura

b. Transient clouding of the consciousness

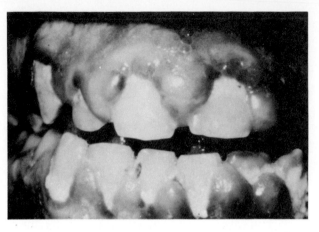

Fig. 14-4 Gingival overgrowth from phenytoin with superimposed inflammation.

c. Behavioral, alterations

d. Purposeless, repetitive, and stereotypic movements or actions

e. Changes in affect or perception

f. May become antisocial

g. Person usually does not remember the incident

4. Mixed

F. Treatment

1. Drug therapy (70% of cases)

a. Complete control is achieved in only about 5% of cases

b. One or more anticonvulsants (e.g., phenytoin [Dilantin], phenobarbital [Luminal], primidone [Mysoline], phensuximide [Milontin], methsuximide [Celontin], trimethadione [Tridione], carbamazepine [Tegretol], acetazolamide [Diamox])

c. Common side effects

(1) Gingival overgrowth (phenytoin)

(2) Drowsiness and headaches

(3) Vision and gait disturbances

(4) Loss of appetite, nausea

(5) Blood dyscrasias

2. Surgery

3. Avoidance of precipitating factors (fatigue, stress, abnormal sensory stimuli, drugs, inadequate medication compliance)

G. Oral manifestations

1. Orofacial trauma—lips, tongue, buccal mucosa, teeth, facial or jaw bones

2. Gingival overgrowth from phenytoin (Fig. 14-4)

a. More marked in anterior regions and facial surfaces

b. Does not occur in edentulous areas

c. Correlated with poor oral hygiene

d. Characteristically pale, pink, and fibrous

e. Creates malpositioning of teeth and compromised aesthetics

f. Superimposed inflammation occurs from food retention or mouth breathing

g. Can sometimes be alleviated through meticulous oral hygiene, surgery, or pressure appliances

Visual Impairment

A. Definition

1. Visual impairment—if after correction visual acuity in the best eye is no better than 20/200 or if central or peripheral vision impairment is present

2. Legally blind—visual acuity of less than 20/200 with correction

B. Incidence/prevalence

1. Severe impairment affects about 6.6 per 1000 persons in the United States

2. Of the legally blind, 50% are over age 60

3. Legally blind persons under age 20 make up 10% of the total

4. About 3% are totally blind

5. Half of the cases of blindness in the United States could have been prevented with proper diagnosis and treatment

6. 70% of adults over age 75 have cataracts

C. Etiology—congenital, perinatal, postnatal, aging

1. Trauma

2. Disease (infections, inflammation, toxicity)

3. Structural or developmental defects

a. Nearsighted

b. Farsighted

c. Astigmatism

4. Retrolental fibroplasia—high concentration of oxygen in the incubators of premature infants causes hemorrhage of retinal blood vessels, scarring, and retinal detachment

5. Macular degeneration (loss of central vision)

6. Retinitis pigmentosa—night blindness and loss of peripheral vision

7. Retinal hemorrhages (e.g., complication of diabetes)

8. Glaucoma—failure of liquid in the eye to drain, resulting in increased pressure, pain, and destruction of the optic nerve

9. Cataracts—clouding and opacity of the lens block light perception (mainly associated with aging or congenital problems)

D. Signs/symptoms/clinical manifestations

1. Wears glasses or contact lenses

2. Awkward ambulation or bumping into objects

3. Eye pain

4. Constant tearing

5. Unusual squinting or blinking

6. Use of a guide dog or cane

7. Deliberate, slow actions

8. Attention to details and orderliness

9. Cloudy or fuzzy vision

10. Problems with glare

11. Double vision

E. Treatment

1. Cataracts—surgery: lens implants, contact lenses, cataract glasses

2. Glaucoma—drugs or surgery

3. Laser treatment

4. Special education—auditory instruction and training in use of tactile senses (Braille)

5. Corrective devices—telescopic or microscopic lenses

6. Adaptive aids—large-print books, nonoptical filters

7. Prevention—use of safety glasses, regular checkups

F. Oral manifestations

1. No particular dental problems

2. Gingivitis if cannot see to monitor

3. Trauma to the orofacial area if the person experiences frequent accidents or falls

Hearing Impairment

A. Definition

1. Hearing impairment—defective but functional hearing

2. Deaf—unable to understand speech, even with the use of an aid

3. Frequency—length of the sound wave (vibrations, or cycles, per second; human range is 16 to 30,000 cps)

4. Intensity—measured in decibels (human range is 1 to 100 dB)

B. Incidence/prevalence

1. There are 28 million deaf and hearing-impaired persons in the United States; 60% of these are age 55 and over

2. Hearing losses are associated with a number of other disabling conditions

a. Cleft palate (90%)

b. Cerebral palsy (20%)

c. Down syndrome (70%)

3. Environmental causes are increasing

C. Classifications—usually by severity of loss, as measured in decibel loss (Table 14-4)

D. Types (Table 14-5)

1. Conductive

a. Injury or disease interferes with organs that conduct sound waves through the outer or middle ear

b. Usually consistent over the entire range of sound

c. Client benefits most from the use of a hearing aid (sound conducted by bone)

d. Speech is soft and low; patient hears own voice louder than that of others

2. Sensorineural

a. Malfunction of organs that perceive sound (the inner ear, the auditory nerve, the auditory center in the brain)

b. Most common cause is the process of aging

c. Involves loss of sensitivity and acuity in one or more frequencies (usually higher frequencies and consonants)

d. If individual wears a hearing aid, sound is conducted by air

e. Speech is loud; person cannot hear own voice

Table 14-4

Hearing Loss and Probable Effects

Classification	Loss (dB)	Hearing without amplification
Normal range	0-15	All speech sounds
Slight loss	15-25	Hears vowel sounds clearly; may miss unvoiced consonant sounds
Mild loss	25-40	Hears only louder-voiced speech sounds
Moderate loss	40-65	Misses most speech at normal conversational level
Severe loss	65-95	Misses all speech at normal conversational level
Profound loss	95+	Hears no speech or other sounds

From Lange BM, Entwistle BM, Lipson LF: *Dental management of the handicapped: approaches for dental auxiliaries,* Philadelphia, 1983, Lea & Febiger.

E. Etiology

1. Prenatal or congenital

a. Genetic defects

b. Infections (rubella accounts for 20% of congenital types), influenza, and syphilis

c. Blood incompatibilities

d. Certain drugs (e.g., thalidomide, streptomycin)

e. Unknown causes (10% to 20% of cases)

f. Environmental noise (over 30% of cases)

2. Acquired

a. Infections (e.g., mumps, measles, poliomyelitis, chronic serous otitis media)

b. Hereditary conditions

c. Trauma

d. Chronic use of certain drugs (e.g., aspirin, streptomycin)

F. Signs/symptoms/clinical manifestations

1. May lip-read or key in on other facial or nonverbal expressions; generally only understand 26% to 40% of what is said this way

2. Speech may be characterized by aberrant modulations, pronunciations, or grammatical structures

3. May use sign language (American Sign Language) or finger spelling (American or manual alphabet)

4. May turn the head to one side if the loss is unilateral

5. Frequently asks people to repeat phrases

6. Person may not acknowledge having a loss

G. Treatment

1. Depends on the person's age at onset and the type and cause of impairment

a. Surgery

b. Hearing aids; cochlear implants and infrared and FM (frequency modulating) devices also being used

c. Education for development of communication skills

d. Direct stimulation of the auditory nerve

Table 14-5

Types of Hearing Problems

Type of problem	Characteristics
Acoustic neurinoma	Benign tumor of the auditory nerve; causes gradual hearing loss, tinnitus, and dizziness
Mastoiditis	Inflammation of the air cells of the mastoid
Ménière's disease	Condition of the inner ear characterized by hearing loss, tinnitus and vertigo
Otitis media	Inflammation of the middle ear
Otosclerosis	Disease characterized by formation of spongy bone in the bone surrounding the inner ear; results in gradual loss of hearing
Presbycusis	Progressive hearing loss that occurs with age
Tinnitus	Sensation of sound in the head (e.g., roaring, hissing, buzzing)

2. Prevention through use of hearing protection devices (e.g., earplugs)

H. Oral manifestations
   1. Not generally seen with hearing impairments unless associated with a syndrome (e.g., rubella syndrome)
   2. Prematurity or rubella may result in enamel dysplasia
   3. Bruxism may be evident

Cleft Lip or Palate

A. Definition—disturbances in embryologic formation resulting in incomplete closure of the lip and/or palatal area
B. Incidence/prevalence
   1. Occurs once in about 550 live births
   2. One of the most common congenital malformations of the face and mouth
C. Classifications of cleft involvement
   1. Tip of the uvula
   2. Bifid uvula
   3. Soft palate (Fig. 14-5)
   4. Soft and hard palates (Fig. 14-6)
   5. Unilateral lip and palate
   6. Bilateral lip and palate
D. Etiology
   1. Most are genetic
   2. Other predisposing factors include maternal nutritional deficiencies, infectious diseases, or smoking
   3. Cleft lip occurs during fetal weeks 4 through 7
   4. Cleft palate occurs during fetal weeks 8 through 12
   5. Vitamin B complex taken in the early stages of pregnancy can help prevent cleft lip
E. Signs/symptoms/associated problems
   1. Oral-facial deformities
   2. Ear disease with resultant hearing loss
   3. Speech difficulties are a major disability caused by
      a. Palatal insufficiency
      b. Missing or malpositioned teeth
      c. Hearing loss
   4. Feeding problems
   5. Predisposition to upper respiratory tract infections
F. Treatment
   1. Surgery—multiple operations at various developmental stages
   2. Taking of impression and insertion of an obturator or other appliance if needed for feeding or speech; need to be remade according to growth pattern
   3. Speech therapy
   4. Antibiotics to prevent infections
   5. Orthodontics
G. Oral manifestations

1. High incidence of missing or maldeveloped teeth in the line of the cleft
2. High incidence of malocclusion resulting from the structural defects
3. Oral motor dysfunction
4. Scar tissue from surgery

Cerebral Palsy

A. Definition—static, nonprogressive neuromuscular condition composed of a series of syndromes that result from damage to the brain
B. Incidence—3/1000 people in the United States, occurring more frequently in males
C. Etiology
   1. Prenatal (genetic or congenitally acquired, e.g., anoxia, infections, Rh incompatibility, metabolic disturbances)
   2. Natal—anoxia, hemorrhage
   3. Postnatal—trauma, infections, neoplasms, anoxia

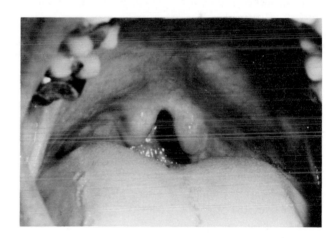

Fig. 14-5   Soft palate cleft.

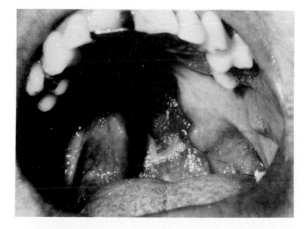

Fig. 14-6   Soft and hard palate cleft.

D. Classification
  1. Motor disorders
    a. Spasticity (50% to 75%)—slight stimulus causes exaggerated muscle contraction
    b. Athetosis (15% to 25%)—muscles contract involuntarily
    c. Ataxia (10%)—muscles respond to a stimulus but cannot complete a contraction
    d. Hypotonia (<10%)—unable to respond to a volitional stimulus
    e. Rigidity(<10%)—increased initial muscle resistance; gives way with little force
    f. Mixed (5% to 10%)—two or more types appearing in the same person
  2. Limbs involved
    a. Monoplegic—one limb
    b. Hemiplegic—both limbs on the same side of the body
    c. Paraplegic—lower limbs
    d. Diplegic—major involvement of the lower limbs, minor involvement of the upper limbs
    e. Quadriplegic—all four limbs
    f. Triplegic—three limbs
E. Signs/symptoms/clinical manifestations (Fig. 14-7)
  1. Characterized by paralysis, weakness, muscle spasms, incoordination, or other aberrations of motor function, especially involving voluntary muscles
  2. Joint immobility and contractures increase with age
  3. Retained primitive reflexes (e.g., asymmetric or symmetric tonic neck reflex)
  4. Other associated conditions
    a. Speech/language disorders (60%)
    b. Hearing disorders (20%)
    c. Visual defects (40%)
    d. Mental retardation (40%)
    e. Seizures (40%)
  5. Wide range of limitation, from mild to totally dependent
F. Treatment
  1. Magnesium sulfate may prevent the disorder in low birthweight babies
  2. Surgery for contractures
  3. Supportive therapies (physical therapy, occupational therapy, speech therapy)
  4. Adaptive equipment (braces, wheelchair, walkers, mouth sticks, augmentative communication devices, voice synthesizers) (Fig. 14-8)
  5. Medications for seizures, muscle relaxation and other manifestations
  6. Special education if needed
G. Oral manifestations—marked variation among individuals

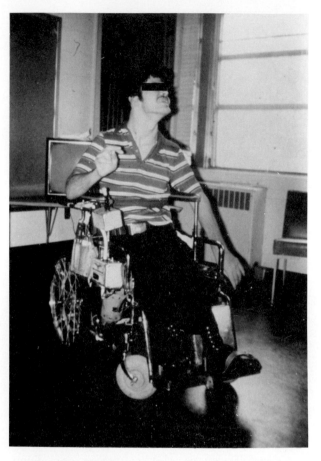

Fig. 14-7 Typical manifestations of cerebral palsy.

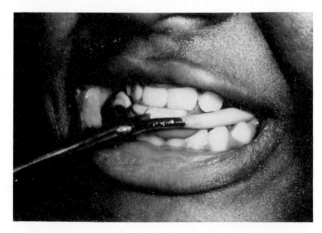

Fig. 14-8 Mouth stick used for typing or grasping.

  1. Higher incidence of bruxism, dental caries, enamel dysplasia, malocclusion, and periodontal problems
  2. Phenytoin-induced gingival overgrowth if this drug is being given
  3. Oral motor dysfunction (e.g., impaired swallowing), mouth breathing

4. Trauma resulting from incoordination and frequent falls
5. Attrition and possible joint disturbances from mouth sticks
6. Dental caries as a result of surgery to control saliva and drooling

Bell's Palsy

A. Definition—paralysis of facial muscles innervated by cranial nerve VII (facial nerve)
B. Incidence/prevalence—most common in adult years
C. Etiology
   1. Unknown
   2. Associated with bacterial and viral infections, trauma from oral extractions, or surgery on the parotid gland
D. Signs/symptoms/clinical manifestations
   1. Abrupt paralysis without preceding pain
   2. Occurs unilaterally
   3. Corner of the mouth droops, causing drooling
   4. Eyelids will not close; the lower eyelid droops; predisposes the eyes to infections
   5. Speech and chewing are difficult
   6. May have spontaneous remission in 2 to 8 weeks or permanent paralysis
E. Treatment
   1. Prednisone therapy
   2. Heat and massage to maintain circulation and muscle tone
   3. Eyedrops or eye shield to prevent infections
   4. Surgery if needed
F. Oral manifestations—oral motor difficulties can cause food retention and the potential for increased caries or gingivitis

Myasthenia Gravis

A. Definition—immunologic neuromuscular disease characterized by variable weakness or fatigue of the striated, voluntary muscles
B. Incidence/prevalence
   1. Onset at any age
   2. If early onset, females affected more often
   3. If late onset, males affected more often
   4. Affects about 1 in 20,000 people
C. Etiology—autoimmune mechanism causing a defect in nerve impulse transmission at the neuromuscular junction
D. Signs/symptoms/clinical manifestations
   1. Affects muscles of the eyes (double vision), facial expression, mastication, and swallowing
   2. Disturbs breathing and speech (weak, muffled voice)
   3. Weakness may increase as the day progresses

4. Precipitated by
   a. Emotional excitement
   b. Surgical procedures
   c. Fatigue/loss of sleep
   d. Infections
   e. Alcoholic intake
5. Myasthenic crisis
   a. Client nonresponsive to drugs
   b. Unable to clear secretions from the throat
   c. Impaired breathing
   d. Double vision
E. Treatment
   1. Medications that block the action of cholinesterase at the myoneural junction (neostigmine [Prostigmin], pyridostigmine [Mestinon], ambenonium [Mytelase])
   2. Radiation therapy or surgical removal of the thymus leads to partial remission
   3. Corticosteroids or adrenocorticotropic hormone (ACTH)
   4. Tracheostomy if needed during the crisis
F. Oral manifestations
   1. Oral motor dysfunction
   2. Retention of food increases susceptibility to dental caries and periodontal problems

Parkinson Disease

A. Definition—progressive disorder of the central nervous system causing loss of postural reflexes, slowness of spontaneous movement, tremors, and muscle rigidity
B. Incidence/prevalence
   1. Develops between ages 40 to 60
   2. Over age 60, 1/100 persons affected
   3. Higher incidence in men (2:1)
C. Etiology
   1. Cause unknown
   2. Imbalance of dopamine and acetylcholine
D. Signs/symptoms/clinical manifestations
   1. Mild, diffuse muscular pain
   2. Tremors of the extremities, occurring mainly at rest
   3. Shuffling, slow gait with the arms held to the side
   4. Slurred, indistinct speech
   5. Staring, masklike facial expression
   6. Excessive salivation or dryness of mouth (side effects of medications)
   7. Intellect not usually affected
   8. Tremors in the lips, tongue, or neck; difficulty in swallowing; can lead to aspiration
   9. Feelings of stiffness and rigidity (particularly of the large joints)
   10. Sensitivity to heat

Table 14-6

Characteristics of Arthritis

	Osteoarthritis	Rheumatoid (adult type)	Rheumatoid (juvenile type)
Incidence/prevalence	16 million in United States; onset at ages 50-70	2 million in United States; onset at ages 20-40; ⅔ are females	250,000 in United States; occurs before age 16
Etiology	Unknown or from trauma, infection, or joint abnormality	Cause unknown; theories include autoimmunity, hereditary or psychosomatic factors, and infection	
Sites affected	Weight-bearing joints (hips, knees, vertebrae)	First affects fingers, hands, and knees; TMJ later	Involves many joints, especially fingers, knees, wrists, vertebrae, and TMJ
Signs/symptoms	Pain, aggravated by temperature changes; joint stiffness after inactivity; develops gradually; swelling rare; does not usually limit range of motion	Fatigue, loss of appetite, low-grade fever, migratory joint pain and swelling, stiffness after periods of inactivity, paresthesia, subcutaneous nodules, joint defmormities, TMJ involvement, muscle atrophy near joints	Joint enlargement, stiffness, and pain; onset is acute with fever, rash, spleen and lymph node enlargement, tachycardia, and limited oral opening

E. Treatment
 1. Medications (see Chapter 8)
  a. Levodopa to alleviate dopamine deficiency, tremors, and rigidity
  b. Side effects—orthostatic hypotension, dizziness
  c. Anticholinergic agents for rigidity
  d. Antispasmodics for tremors
  e. Antihistamines
  f. Analgesics
  g. Sedatives
 2. Physical and occupational therapy
 3. Ongoing clinical trials for new therapies, including fetal brain cell transplants
 4. Surgery
F. Oral manifestations
 1. Impaired oral motor functions and home care skills may increase the incidence of dental caries, periodontal disease, and perioral skin irritation
 2. Side effects of medications (xerostomia) may increase the incidence of dental caries and periodontal disease and negatively affect dental prosthesis retention
 3. Rigidity and tremors can induce orofacial pain, TMJ discomfort, and soft and hard tissue trauma

Arthritis

A. Definition
 1. Term used to describe over 100 disorders causing pain in the joints and connective tissue
 2. Joint inflammation
 3. *Polyarthritis* refers to involvement of many joints
B. Major types (Table 14-6)
 1. Osteoarthritis
 2. Rheumatoid (adult type)
 3. Rheumatoid (juvenile type)
 4. Others include gout, fibromyalgia, ankylosing spondylitis, lupus
C. Incidence/prevalence: common in all age groups (Table 14-6); affects 1 in 7 Americans
D. Etiology
 1. Cause unknown
 2. Theories (Table 14-6)
E. Signs/symptoms/clinical manifestations—these affect various sites in different ways (Table 14-6); most are chronic
F. Treatment
 1. Primarily involves relief of pain and maintenance of function
 2. Medications
  a. Nonsteroidal antiinflammatory drugs (NSAIDs)
  b. Steroids
  c. Gold salts
  d. Antimalaria drugs
 3. Physical therapy and exercise to increase range of motion and prevent deformities
 4. Application of heat or hydrotherapy
 5. Surgery—joint replacement
G. Oral manifestations
 1. Bruxism and occlusal imbalances
 2. Temporomandibular joint (TMJ) pain and limited opening
 3. Masking of inflammation by prolonged steroid therapy

4. Malocclusion occurs in the juvenile type
5. Delayed healing if long-term aspirin therapy is being given
6. Mucosal ulcerations or secondary oral infections (especially of gingiva) if gold salts are being given

Multiple Sclerosis

A. Definition—chronic degenerative disease of the central nervous system where
   1. Myelin is destroyed through the formation of sclerotic tissue called plaque
   2. Nerve impulses to the brain are disrupted or not transmitted
   3. Scattered plaque accumulation causes inflammation and widespread and varied symptoms with periods of exacerbation and remission
B. Incidence/prevalence
   1. 250,000 to 300,000 people affected
   2. Varies geographically; more common in northern climates
   3. More common in women
   4. Onset occurs at any age, but usually between the ages of 20 to 45
C. Etiology
   1. Unknown, but genetic markers recently found
   2. Possibly an autoimmune reaction or associated with viral infections
D. Signs/symptoms
   1. Result from the location of lesions (Table 14-7)
   2. Precipitating factors
      a. Infections
      b. Stress and emotional trauma
      c. Injury
      d. Heavy exercise and fatigue
      e. Pregnancy
      f. Heat
   3. Periods of remission in some; chronic progression in others
   4. Death is usually the result of an infection
   5. Fewer than 50% become nonambulatory
E. Treatment
   1. No current cure; treat symptoms and reduce inflammation
   2. Physical and occupational therapy
   3. Alternating periods of rest and exercise
   4. Medications
      a. ACTH or synthetic steroids
      b. Muscle relaxants
      c. New drugs that slow disease progression are being tested
      d. Anticonvulsants to treat facial pain
   5. Monoclonal antibodies or copolymer 1
   6. Lymphoid radiation and plasmapheresis

Table 14-7

Symptoms Associated with Lesions in the Central Nervous System

Location of lesions	Possible symptoms
Spinal cord	Numbness
	Loss of sensitivity in appendages
	Sensitivity to heat
	Unsteady gait; muscle stiffness
	Loss of strength in the legs
	Impaired eye-hand coordination resulting in difficulty in fine motor movements
Brainstem	Blurred and/or double vision
	Difficulty in swallowing or chewing
	Diminished gag reflex
	Slurred speech
Cerebrum (lesions in the cerebrum usually occur in the latter stages of the disease process)	Disruptions in thinking
	Euphoria
	Depression
	Disruptions in behavior

From Lange BM, Enwistle BM, Lipson LF: *Dental management of the handicapped: approaches for dental auxiliaries,* Philadelphia, 1983, Lea & Febiger.

F. Oral manifestations
   1. Most are the result of poor oral hygiene or the side effects of drugs
      a. Ulcerations
      b. Xerostomia
      c. Gingival overgrowth (phenytoin given for pain)
   2. Facial pain and TMJ dysfunction and pain

Muscular Dystrophies

A. Definition—group of progressive chronic diseases of the skeletal (striated) muscles characterized by the degeneration of muscle cells with replacement by fat or fibrous tissue
B. Incidence/prevalence
   1. Affects 220,000 people in the United States
   2. Two thirds of cases are children
C. Etiology—inherited; defective gene leading to a protein abnormality
D. Types (Table 14-8)
   1. Duchenne
   2. Limb-girdle
   3. Facioscapulohumeral
   4. Myotonic
E. Signs/symptoms/clinical manifestations—varies by site and type (Table 14-8)

Table 14-8

Types and Characteristics of Muscular Dystrophies

	Duchenne	Limb-girdle	Facioscapulohumeral	Myotonic
Onset	Mainly affects boys; occurs before age 10	Occurs later (average age 20); affects both males and females	Males and females equally affected; usually occurs around puberty	Both sexes affected; appears in early adulthood
Severity	Most severe and destructive form	Slower progression in most cases	Least destructive and progresses at slower rate; least common type	Weakening spreads steadily; shortened life span
Etiology	Sex-linked recessive trait with high mutation rate	Autosomal recessive trait	Autosomal dominant trait	Autosomal dominant trait
Sites affected	Pelvis, abdomen, hip, and spine affected first; spreads to trunk, extremities, and myocardium (cranial nerves *not* affected); osteoporosis also noted	Initial weakness in pelvic girdle, then in shoulder	Facial muscles affected first; weakness is asymmetric; progresses to shoulder girdle and upper arm	Weakness of lower legs and arms and facial muscles
Limitations	Becomes confined to wheelchair and bed within a few years of diagnosis; may develop scoliosis, obesity, and cardiopulmonary problems; death usually occurs during adolescence	May be severely disabled by midlife, with decreased life span	May remain in state of indefinite remission, with some people living symptom-free, normal life span	Walking difficult; may be severely disabled; eye cataracts may develop
Signs/symptoms	Clumsiness, frequent falls resulting from precarious balance, toe-walking, weakness of hips, lordosis, cramping of legs and abdomen, Gowers' sign, enlargement of calves, decreased stamina	Begins as pain after exercise; then total muscle involvement	Masklike, wrinkle-free, expressionless facial features; difficulty in closing eyes; muscles above elbow atrophy, below elbow are normal (Popeye effect); difficulty in raising arms	Stiffness, drooping eyelids and jaw, frequent tripping and falling

F. Treatment—goal is to maintain the person's activity and involvement; no cure yet
1. Surgery for contracted tendons
2. Medications
3. Orthopedic devices
4. Nutritional counseling if overweight
5. Physical therapy involves muscle-stretching exercise and use of adaptive aids to
   a. Improve muscle strength
   b. Prevent and correct contractures
   c. Increase efficiency in the activities of daily living
6. Speech therapy if needed
G. Oral manifestations
1. Weakness in the masticatory muscles leads to decreased maxillary biting force
2. Higher incidence of mouth breathing, open bite, and overexpansion of the maxilla
3. In facioscapulohumeral type, the lips appears thick because of involvement of the orbicularis oris muscle
4. Increase in dental disease states if oral hygiene is neglected

Spinal Cord Injuries
A. Definition
1. Fracture, dislocation, hyperextension, compression, or severance of components of the spinal column
2. Occurs most often in the cervical and lumbar curves
3. Cord damage can occur above or below the level of bone injury
B. Incidence/prevalence
1. Affects 150,000 to 200,000 people in the United States
2. About 10,000 new cases per year
3. Seventy percent of patients are below the age of 40; only 15% are female
C. Etiology—acquired injury from accidents
1. Automobile or motorcycle accidents cause 50% of injuries

Table 14-9	
Clinical Manifestations of Spinal Cord Injuries	
Area affected	**Clinical manifestations**

Muscles (limb and trunk)	Innervation and perception to pain and touch disturbed; leads to
	    Muscle atrophy
	    Concerns for safety around varying temperatures
	    Formation of decubitus ulcers (pressure sores) caused by breakdown of tissue from immobilization, bruises, or braces
	    Decreased or absent self-care skills
	    Spasticity and tremors
	    Adaptive equipment required, especially for
	        Wrist stability
	        Pencil grasp
	        Arm movements

Respiration	Intercostal muscles may be paralyzed, resulting in need for diaphragmatic breathing or tracheostomy and total or partial dependence on a respirator

Bowel and bladder	Limited innervation, resulting in incontinence and encopresis or retention
	Can lead to infections, particularly of kidneys
	Autonomic hyperreflexia can occur (medical emergency)
	    Caused by sudden constriction of blood vessels
	    Symptoms—rapid increase in blood pressure (e.g., 280/80), low pulse, pounding headache, skin blotching and sweating above site of injury, cold goose bumps below site of injury

Bones/joints	Contractures from spasticity and immobilization Heterotopic ossifications (bony accumulations) may develop around joints
Metabolism	Regulation of body temperature impaired
Social/emotional status	Problems associated with coping with a debilitating acquired injury May experience stages of shock, denial, anger, depression, mobilization, and coping

    2. Occupational accidents cause 25% of injuries

    3. Sporting accidents cause 18% of injuries

    4. Falls, gunshot wounds, or other trauma cause 7% of injuries

D. Signs/symptoms/clinical manifestations

    1. Depend on the severity and level of injury

    2. Prognosis depends on

        a. First aid measures performed at the site of the accident

        b. Type and level of injury to the spinal cord

    3. *Paraplegia* refers to an injury below the cervical level that results in paralysis of the lower portion of the body

    4. *Quadriplegia* refers to an injury occurring in the cervical region that results in paralysis of all four limbs and the trunk

    5. Most frequent cause of death is kidney stones or infection

    6. Functional limitations and specific manifestations depend on the level of the lesion (Tables 14-9 and 14-10)

E. Treatment

    1. Four phases of rehabilitation

        a. Physical—functional exercises to increase specific skills

        b. Equipment—selection of adaptive equipment to allow for maximum independence

        c. Environment—implementation of structural and other changes in the home and work environment to accommodate the person's limitations

        d. Life—vocational counseling/training and reintegration into daily activities

    2. Team approach required—physician, nurse, occupational therapist, physical therapist, speech therapist, psychologist/counselor, vocational specialist, recreational therapist, dentist, dental hygienist, social worker

    3. Long-term medical management to prevent or control complications such as septicemia, pulmonary embolism, and pneumonia

    4. Ongoing research on spinal cord regeneration

Spina Bifida

A. Definition

    1. Neural tube defect of the spinal column

2. Vertebrae fail to close completely around the spinal cord
B. Incidence/prevalence
   1. Occurs in 1/2000 live births
   2. A major cause of paraplegia in children

C. Etiology—specific cause unknown, but multiple factors, including genetic and environmental factors, are suspected; folic acid supplements taken during pregnancy can prevent this
D. Types (Fig. 14-9)

Table 14-10

Functional Significance of Lesion Levels

Lesion level	Functional expectations for complete lesions
CERVICAL LESIONS	
C-1-3	Respirator dependent; totally dependent
C-4	Incapable of voluntary function in arms, trunk, or legs; poor respiratory reserve; totally dependent
C-5	Can stabilize and rotate neck; has function of rhomboids and deltoids, allowing some shoulder movement, elbow flexion; biceps and brachiocardialis partially innervated
C-6	Can move shoulders well; strong elbow flexion; wrist muscles allow weak closure of hand—can use large-handled, lightweight objects; can sit up in bed with help and roll over; still needs attendant; can drive van with hand controls
C-7	Can lift own body weight; can use hands, which are weak and lack dexterity; can eat independently, with some assistance; confined to wheelchair; can live independently and manage self-care in a wheelchair-accessible environment without attendant
THORACIC LESIONS	
T-1	Independent in bed, self-care (short of lifting weights); lacks trunk stability, respiratory reserve, and trunk fixation of arm prime movers
T-6	Capable of heavy lifting (because of thoracic musculature); increased respiratory reserve; independent transfers, self-application of braces
T-12	Can ambulate with crutches and braces, but still uses wheelchair as primary means of mobility
LUMBAR LESIONS	
L-4	Complete independent in all phases of self-care and ambulation—usually aided by crutches or canes

From Schubert MM, Snow M, Stiefel DJ: DECOD series: Dental management of patients with CNS and neurologic impairment. Spinal cord injury. Seattle, 1989, University of Washington.

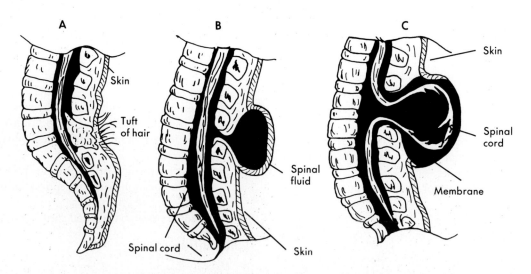

Fig. 14-9 Types of spina bifida. **A,** Spina bifida occulta. **B,** Meningocele. **C,** Meningomyelocele.

1. Spina bifida occulta
   a. Small defect in a vertebra not involving the spinal cord
   b. Often undetected
2. Meningocele—bony defect that allows meninges and cerebrospinal fluid to form a sac protruding from the vertebral column
3. Meningomyelocele—severe defect where the spinal cord also protrudes into the sac

E. Signs/symptoms/clinical manifestations
1. Potential exposure of the nervous system to the external environment results in an increased chance for further damage from trauma or infection
2. Loss of motor function in the lower half of the body
   a. Differential involvement of muscle groups causes muscle imbalance, leading to spinal and limb deformities
   b. Loss of sensation to pain, touch, and temperature creates safety hazards and pressure sores
   c. Loss of bladder and bowel control
   d. Ambulation may be affected, creating a need for orthopedic devices or a wheelchair
3. Deformity of the brain
   a. Most have normal intelligence but experience learning disabilities, especially visual-perceptual problems
   b. Some develop seizure disorders
   c. Sixty-five percent will develop hydrocephalus
      (1) Cerebrospinal fluid accumulates in the ventricles of the brain
      (2) Pressure expands the brain and skull

F. Treatment
1. Surgical correction of the defect
2. Insertion of ventriculoperitoneal or ventriculoatrial shunt if hydrocephalus is present (Fig. 14-10)
3. Orthopedic management through surgery, bracing, and physical therapy
4. Assisted urination or evacuation, catheterization
5. Medications to prevent or treat infections

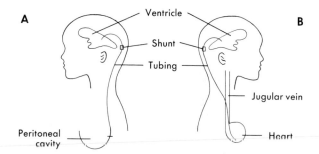

Fig. 14-10 Types of shunts for hydrocephalus. **A,** Ventriculoperitoneal shunt. **B,** Ventriculoatrial shunt.

6. Avoidance of decubitus ulcers
7. Weight control if fairly inactive

G. Oral manifestations—none directly associated

Viral Hepatitis

See Chapter 7, section on infections of the gastrointestinal tract, and Table 7-10.

Acquired Immunodeficiency Syndrome

See Chapter 6, section on acquired immunodeficiency syndrome, and Chapter 7, section on immunodeficiency.

Sexually Transmitted Diseases

See Chapter 7, section on infections of the reproductive and urinary systems.

Tuberculosis

See Chapter 7, section on infections of the respiratory tract, and Table 7-9.

Cystic Fibrosis

A. Definition—inherited disorder of the exocrine glands
B. Incidence/prevalence
   1. Occurs in 1/2000 live births in the United States
   2. Between 2% and 5% of the population are carriers
   3. Males and females equally affected
   4. Most common cause of chronic lung disease in white children
   5. Mean survival now 28.3 years
C. Etiology—autosomal recessive disorder; defect in CF gene on chromosome 7 that results in phenylalanine deletion and problem with chloride ion transport
D. Signs/symptoms/clinical manifestations—include increased viscosity of mucus (obstructs the pancreatic ducts, leading to cyst formation, impaired metabolism, and progressive deterioration)
   1. Accumulation of mucus in the lungs interferes with oxygen exchange
      a. Interferes especially with exhalation, causing a barrel-chested appearance
      b. Air sacs collapse, and infections occur, often leading to suppurative bronchitis, pneumonia, and obstructive emphysema
      c. Clubbing of fingers and toes
      d. Chronic cough
   2. Sweat glands affected, leading to high levels of sodium in the sweat
   3. Salivary glands also affected
   4. Other findings and complications include a small gallbladder, cirrhosis of the liver, diabetes mellitus, and sterility in males
   5. Linear growth and bone development delayed
   6. Death usually occurs in early adulthood

E. Treatment
   1. Antibiotics to eliminate lung infection (tetracycline used in the past)
   2. Aerosol inhalants and various airway clearance methods to maintain lungs as mucus free as possible
   3. Dietary regimen
      a. Reduce total fat with increased calories, protein, and vitamins
      b. Powdered pancreatic enzyme supplements
      c. Regulate salt intake
      d. Other dietary supplements; 5% require insulin
   4. Exercise therapy
   5. General prevention of infections
   6. Gene therapy
   7. Early detection of gene carriers
   8. Possible lung transplant
F. Oral manifestations
   1. Lower dental caries rate and plaque accumulation with increased calculus deposits; probably a result of alterations in saliva and long-term use of antibiotics
   2. Enlargement of the salivary glands
   3. Intrinsic staining of the teeth if tetracycline is administered during the formative years
   4. Mouth breathing if sinuses are occluded

Chronic Obstructive Pulmonary Disease (COPD)

A. Definition
   1. General term for pulmonary disorder characterized by obstruction of airflow during respiration
   2. Consists of two or more disease processes that may coexist
   3. Bronchitis: obstruction caused by narrowing or loss of airways
   4. Emphysema: Loss of elasticity and collapse of over-inflated air sacs; loss of gas exchange surface area; causes obstruction during expiration
B. Incidence/prevalence/etiology
   1. Chronic bronchitis affects 10% to 25% of U.S. adults
   2. More common in males
   3. Most important risk factor is smoking, accounting for 80% to 90% of mortality
   4. Other causes are occupational and environmental pollutants
   5. Can be a hereditary defect in pulmonary tissue or due to severe respiratory illnesses during childhood
C. Signs/symptoms/clinical manifestations
   1. Dyspnea and wheezing on exertion or at rest; orthopnea
   2. Chronic cough, mucus, respiratory infections, and cyanosis in bronchitis

   3. Use accessory muscles of respiration
   4. Chest pain
   5. Advanced complications are heart failure and pulmonary failure
D. Treatment
   1. Eliminate causative factors, e.g., smoking
   2. Use low-flow oxygen and breathing exercises
   3. Medications include β-adrenergic agonists, methylxanthine, chromones, corticosteroids, anticholinergics
   4. Lung transplant
E. Oral manifestations
   1. No associated oral manifestations unless a side effect of the medications

Bronchial Asthma

See Chapter 17, section on respiratory emergencies.
A. Definition
   1. Clinical state of hyperreactivity of the tracheobronchial tree characterized by recurrent paroxysms of dyspnea and wheezing
   2. Results from bronchospasm, bronchial wall edema, inflammation, and hypersecretion by mucous glands
   3. Status asthmaticus—persistent exacerbation of asthma in spite of drug therapy (life threatening)
B. Incidence/prevalence
   1. Twelve million people in the United States
   2. Initial symptoms usually occur in the first 5 years of life
   3. About 50% of affected children become asymptomatic before adulthood
   4. 75% to 85% also have allergies
C. Etiology—unknown, although precipitating factors and their effects are known
   1. Extrinsic factors—dust, mold, pollen, smoke, animal dander, household sprays, smoke, wool, foods, air pollutants, sulfiting agents
   2. Other factors—respiratory tract infections, aspirin and other antiinflammatory drugs, overexertion
D. Signs/symptoms/clinical manifestations
   1. Wheezing, dyspnea, coughing, chest pain, sneezing, sputum production, fatigue
   2. Expiratory phase of breathing is slower and more pronounced
   3. Facial (sinus) pain, conjunctivitis, otitis media
   4. More severe symptoms—syncope, respiratory failure, cyanosis
E. Treatment
   1. Avoid precipitating factors and monitor airflow with a peak flowmeter
   2. Immunotherapy (allergy shots)
   3. Medications—inhaled or oral

a. Bronchodilators such as β-adrenergic agonists to help stop attacks

b. Antiinflammatory agents such as corticosteroids or cromolyn sodium to help prevent attacks

4. Exercise program

F. Oral manifestations

1. β-adrenergic agonists may impair salivary secretions, increasing caries risk

2. Mouthbreathing

3. Candida infections from inhalant use

Congenital Heart Disease

A. Definition

1. Anomalies of heart structure

2. Usually caused during the first 9 weeks in utero

B. Incidence/prevalence

1. Occurs in 0.5% to 0.8% of all live births (25,000 per year)

2. Leading cause of birth defect-related deaths

C. Etiology

1. Generally unknown

2. Genetic (e.g., Down Syndrome)

3. Environmental (maternal)

a. Fetal hypoxia, endocarditis, or immunologic abnormalities

b. Rubella infection (German measles) or other viruses

c. Nutritional deficiencies (especially vitamin deficiencies)

d. Drugs (e.g., lithium, alcohol, cocaine)

e. Radiation

f. Metabolic disorders (PKU or diabetes)

D. Types of malformations

1. Cause initial left-to-right shunting of blood (e.g., atrial-septal defect, ventricular-septal defect, patent ductus arteriosus)

2. Initial right-to-left shunting (e.g., tetralogy of Fallot)—causes significant cyanosis

3. Malformations that obstruct blood flow (e.g., pulmonary stenosis)

E. Signs/symptoms/clinical manifestations

1. Dyspnea, fatigue, weakness (most common symptoms)

2. Cyanosis, dizziness, syncope, or ruddy color, leading to congestive heart failure

3. Clubbing of fingers or toes (Fig. 14-11)

4. Heart murmurs

5. Delayed growth and development

6. Complications—brain abscesses, bacterial endocarditis, congestive heart failure, acute pulmonary edema, bleeding problems

F. Treatment

1. One fourth to one half of infants with these

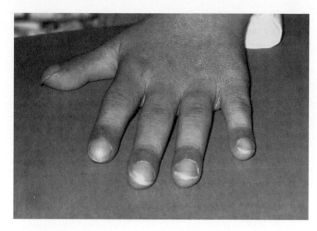

Fig. 14-11 Clubbing of fingers observed in congenital heart disease.

defects require treatment during the first year of life

2. Surgery for others usually between ages 4 and 6

3. Medications

a. Digitalis

b. Anticoagulants

4. Variety of treatments for complications

G. Oral manifestations

1. Bluish mucosa if cyanotic; ruddy color if person has polycythemia

2. Developmental defects of teeth sometimes seen

3. Slight hemorrhaging secondary to trauma if bleeding problems are present

4. May have decreased ability to fight oral infections

Rheumatic Fever and Heart Disease

See Chapter 7, section on infections of the circulatory system, and Appendix B.

Cardiac Arrhythmias

A. Definition

1. Irregular heartbeat manifested as abnormal pulse rates or rhythms

2. Produces alterations in the normal sequence of contractions, leading to inadequate blood flow

3. Produces aberrant electrical depolarization

4. Adversely affects the ventricular rate

B. Etiology

1. Primary cardiovascular disease

2. Pulmonary disorders

3. Autonomic disorders

4. Systemic disorders

5. Side effects of drugs

6. Electrolyte imbalance

C. Types/etiology

1. Bradycardias—slow heart rate (less than 60 beats per minute)
2. Tachycardias—increased heart rate (greater than 100 beats per minute)
3. Isolated ectopic beats—premature impulses resulting in premature atrial beats
4. Preexcitation syndrome
5. Cardiac arrest
D. Signs/symptoms/clinical manifestations
   1. Abnormal pulse
   2. Palpitations
   3. Breathlessness, pallor, fatigue
   4. Syncope or dizziness
   5. Cyanosis
   6. Pain
   7. Cardiac failure
   8. May also be asymptomatic
E. Treatment
   1. Some require no treatment
   2. Antiarrhythmic drugs
   3. Pacemakers; most are demand type—stimulates the heart only when the rhythm deviates from a predetermined norm
   4. Cardioversion through defibrillation
F. Oral manifestations—may have side effects from medications or cyanotic oral tissues

Hypertensive Disease

See Chapter 17, section on vital signs, blood pressure.
A. Definition
   1. Hypertension—more than two elevated readings with average levels of diastolic pressure of 90 mm Hg or greater or systolic pressure of 140 mm Hg or greater for adults age 18 and older
   2. Hypertensive disease—sustained elevation of the diastolic blood pressure, creating an increased workload for the heart and kidney disease
   3. New classification includes high normal and four stages of hypertension
B. Incidence/prevalence
   1. Hypertension affects 60 million people in the United States; more are undiagnosed
   2. About 4% progress to a chronic disease state
   3. Prevalence increases with age and is greater in men and African Americans
C. Etiology
   1. Most are of unknown cause (essential hypertension)
   2. Five percent to 10% are secondary to other conditions such as renal disease or endocrine disorders
   3. Predisposing factors include age, stress, smoking, weight gain, oral contraceptives, or excess salt and fat in the diet

4. Chronic hypertension causes cardiac enlargement and eventually congestive heart failure
D. Signs/symptoms/clinical manifestations
   1. Early—occipital headache, dizziness, tingling of the extremities, vision changes, tinnitis, dyspnea
   2. Advanced—cardiac enlargement, ischemic heart disease, congestive heart failure, renal failure, stroke
E. Treatment (see Chapter 17, section on cardiac emergencies)
   1. Philosophies and therapies vary
   2. Lifestyle changes in terms of stress reduction, avoidance of alcohol and tobacco, diet, and reduction of other risk factors
   3. Drug management with antihypertensives—usually a combination used in a step care approach
      a. Diuretics
      b. Adrenergic-inhibiting agents
      c. Vasodilators
      d. ACE inhibitors
      e. Calcium antagonists
   4. Many side effects and precautions associated with drugs
F. Oral manifestations
   1. Generally no direct oral manifestations
   2. Facial palsy from some drugs
   3. Oral lesions or xerostomia from drugs

Ischemic Heart Disease (Coronary Heart Disease)

A. Definition—coronary atherosclerotic heart disease that is symptomatic
B. Incidence/prevalence
   1. Affects 4 million people in the United States
   2. Leading cause of death after the age of 40 or 50
   3. Incidence and severity increase with age; over 50% who die suddenly have no previous evidence of disease
C. Etiology
   1. Main cause is unknown
   2. Risk factors are the same as for hypertensive disease
   3. Accumulation of lipid plaque inside blood vessels impairs blood flow and thus the oxygen supply to the heart
D. Signs/symptoms/clinical manifestations
   1. Angina pectoris—transient and reversible oxygen deficiency ; classified as stable or unstable
      a. Pain—crushing or paroxysmal, usually less than 10 minutes; often mistaken for indigestion
      b. Sweating, anxiety, pallor, difficulty breathing
      c. Relieved by administration of nitroglycerin or rest
   2. Myocardial infarction—an infarct or necrosis caused by a sudden reduction or arrest of blood flow

a. Pain in the sternum, radiating to the left arm; lasts longer than angina
b. Not relieved by nitroglycerin
c. Same other symptoms as angina, with nausea and vomiting, palpitations, and lowered blood pressure
d. Often leads to sudden death from ventricular fibrillation
E. Treatment (see Chapter 17, section on cardiac emergencies)
   1. Same management as for hypertensive disease
   2. Earlier treatment; 50% wait 2 hours before going to the emergency room
   3. Drug therapy—often in a stepped sequence
      a. Nitroglycerin and other nitrate
      b. β-adrenergic blockers and calcium channel blockers
      c. Aspirin
   4. Coronary artery bypass surgery or coronary angioplasty if indicated
   5. Rest
F. Oral manifestations
   1. None directly associated
   2. Oral lesions or xerostomia may result as a side effect of drugs
   3. Pain may be radiated to the mandible, palate, or tongue

Congestive Heart Failure

A. Definition
   1. Represents a symptom complex that involves failure of one or both ventricles (usually the left ventricle)
   2. Imbalance between the demand placed on the heart and its ability to respond
B. Incidence/prevalence
   1. Most common cause of death in the United States
   2. Prevalence is 1 million persons; incidence is 250,000 cases each year; 5% occur in people younger than age 40
C. Etiology
   1. Underlying causes
      a. Heart valve damage
      b. Obstructive lung disease
      c. Damage to the walls of the heart muscle
   2. Precipitating causes that place an additional demand on the heart
      a. Hypertensive crises
      b. Pulmonary embolism
      c. Arrhythmia
D. Signs/symptoms/clinical manifestations
   1. Dyspnea, irregular breathing pattern, coughing, weakness
   2. Swollen ankles late in the day, pitting edema

3. Cyanosis, anxiety, fear
4. Paleness, sweating, cold skin
E. Treatment (see Chapter 17, section on cardiac emergencies)—depends on type of underlying disease and initial responses to treatment
   1. Rest and limitation of activities
   2. Reduction of weight and other risk factors
   3. Dietary control (limit sodium intake)
   4. Medications
      a. Diuretics (decrease congestion)
      b. Digoxin (increases the force of contractions)
      c. Hydralazine (increases cardiac output)
      d. Prazosin or Captopril (multiple effects)
   5. Heart transplant
F. Oral manifestations
   1. Infections, gingival bleeding, and petechia if have polycythemia

Cerebrovascular Accident (Stroke)

A. Definition—sudden loss of brain function resulting from interference with the blood supply to a portion of the brain
B. Incidence/prevalence
   1. Stroke affects half a million people in the United States; 75% occur in people over age 65
   2. Third leading cause of death in the United States; leading cause of serious disability
   3. Blacks at greater risk than whites
   4. Males at greater risk than females
   5. Likelihood of having a stroke increases with age
C. Etiology
   1. Intracranial hemorrhage
   2. Blockage of vessels by thrombi or emboli (the most common cause)
   3. Vascular insufficiency
   4. Predisposing conditions and risk factors
      a. Cerebral arteriosclerosis
      b. Dehydration
      c. Trauma
      d. Hypertension
      e. Diabetes
      f. Cigarette smoking
D. Signs/symptoms/clinical manifestations—depend on the area of the brain involved and the extent of damage (Table 14-11)
   1. Immediate
      a. Syncope, headache, chills, convulsions, nausea, and vomiting
      b. Changes in the level of consciousness
      c. Transient paresthesias
      d. Mood swing
   2. Residual or chronic
      a. Paralysis—hemiparesis or localized

b. Speech problems and aphasia (reduced capacity for the interpretation and formulation of language)

c. Alterations in reflexes, especially the oral motor reflexes

d. Functional disorders of the bladder or bowel

e. Visual impairments

f. Seizures

E. Treatment (see Chapter 17, section on cerebrovascular accident)

1. Reduce risk factors

2. Surgery if needed

3. Medications

a. Anticoagulant therapy and vasodilators

b. Steroids

4. Physical, occupational, and speech therapy

5. Rehabilitation services or program if needed

F. Oral manifestations

1. Oral motor dysfunction

2. Increased incidence of dental caries or periodontal disease because of oral motor problems and poor oral hygiene

G. Risk reduction: diet, lifestyle, aspirin

Sickle Cell Anemia

A. Definition

1. Defect of hemoglobin that causes red blood cells to become sickle shaped

2. Sickle cell trait—individual shows no symptoms unless experiencing abnormally low concentration of oxygen

3. Sickle cell disease—progressively deteriorating and complex disease with multiple symptoms

B. Incidence/prevalence

1. Found in blacks and other nonwhites; occurs in both sexes

2. Sickle cell anemia found in 15% (1 in 400) of this population; may die before age 40

3. Sickle cell trait found in 9% of this population

4. Babies do not show symptoms until age 6 months

C. Etiology

1. Mutation in the globin gene of hemoglobin

2. Sickle cell trait—individual has half normal hemoglobin and half sickle hemoglobin

3. Sickle cell anemia—individual receives a sickle hemoglobin gene from both parents

4. Sickled cells clog blood vessels

D. Signs/symptoms/clinical manifestations

1. Young children

a. Enlarged spleen, septicemia, and meningitis can develop

b. Swelling of the feet and hands, anemia pallor, tiredness, fever, pneumonia

c. Severe pain crises affecting the extremities

d. Strokes occur in 10% of those affected

2. Children and adolescents

a. Can develop gallstones, enlarged hearts, and lung infarctions

b. Bones degenerate as a result of repeated sickling

c. Delayed growth and late puberty

d. Increased chance for stroke, impaired kidney and liver function with jaundice, and arthritis

e. Continued pain crisis

3. Adulthood

a. Hemorrhage or detached retina in the eye

b. Pain crises—variable in each person

Table 14-11

Functional Limitations in Stroke Victims

Right hemiplegia (L-CVA)	Left hemiplegia (R-CVA)
Language problems	Spatial-perceptual task difficulties—inability to judge distance, size, position, rate of movement, form, and relation of parts to a whole
Decreased *auditory* memory (cannot remember a long series of instructions)	Often thought to be unimpaired because able to speak and understand
Vocabulary problems	Visual field cuts; angles, etc., cannot be perceived
Slow, cautious, disorganized	Patient cannot use mirrors
Anxious	Patient cannot sequence tasks (such as toothbrushing)
	Decreased visual memory (loses place when reading)
	Cannot monitor self (keeps talking even though answered questions already)
	May neglect left side
	Tendency to be impulsive and unaware of deficits. Spatial-perceptual difficulties are easy to miss

From Schubert MM, Snow M, Stiefel DJ: DECOD series: Dental management of patients with CNS and neurologic impairment. Spinal cord injury. Seattle, 1989, University of Washington.

c. Lung and kidney damage, gallstones

d. Leg ulcers and bone changes

e. Infection is a major cause of death and also precipitates crises

4. High altitude, chilling temperatures, stress, psychologic pressures, or infections can precipitate attacks

E. Treatment

1. No cure; treatment is symptomatic and supportive

2. Prevent complications with oral fluids, oxygen, ibuprofen, transcutaneous electrical nerve stimulation for pain

3. Frequent transfusions (every 3 weeks) in some to prevent strokes; Desferal is given to prevent iron toxicity

F. Oral manifestations

1. Sore, painful, and red tongue

2. Loss of taste sensation

3. Osteoporosis

4. Loss of trabecular pattern

5. Mucosal pallor

6. Delayed eruption of teeth

7. Hypoplastic enamel

8. Can have pain in mandible

9. Overbite, overjet

10. Oral infections can lead to osteomyelitis

Cancers

A. Definition—cells that multiply at an abnormally rapid rate, invading and destroying healthy tissue

1. Metastasis—spread of cancer to distant sites

2. Invasion—spread of cancer to local sites

B. Incidence/prevalence

1. Of 240 million Americans alive, more than 4 million will get cancer

2. Each year in the United States over 500,000 people die of cancer; 133 per 100,000 people

3. Only 40% of those who are diagnosed with cancer will live at least 5 years

4. 5-year survival rates for selected cancers (all ages)

a. Breast—83.2%

b. Lung—13.4%

c. Ovarian—44.1%

d. Colorectal—61%

e. Prostate—85.8%

C. Etiology

1. Lifestyle factors account for most of cancer risk and vary by type of cancer; percentages attributable to various factors

a. Diet—35%

b. Tobacco—30%

c. Occupation—4%

d. Alcohol—3%

2. Genetic markers for predisposition continue to be identified

3. Viruses are also associated with certain cancers

4. First stage of cancer development is DNA damage

5. Second stage is latent stage

a. Inhibitors such as certain vitamins and minerals may slow the cancer progress

b. Promoters such as dietary fats may enhance the development of damaged cells

D. Sign/symptoms/clinical manifestations

1. Chronic changes in bowel or bladder habits

2. Sores that do not heal

3. Unusual bleeding or discharge

4. Unaccountable lumps or growths

5. Indigestion or difficulty swallowing

6. Changes in a mole or wart or in the skin

7. Persistent cough

E. Treatment—depends on the type of cancer and stage of disease

1. Early detection through screening tests

2. Surgery usually when tumor is localized

3. Radiation to shrink the tumor

4. Chemotherapy to kill the cells or stop their multiplication; can reach metastasized sites

5. Maintaining protective practices using diet, exercise, sun protection, avoidance of alcohol and tobacco

6. Evolving technologies

a. Immunotherapy

b. Molecular therapy

c. Drugs to destroy new blood vessels that enable cancer invasion

F. Oral manifestations—depend on type of cancer and treatment

1. Oral ulcerations and mucositis

2. Candidiasis

3. Anemia

4. Xerostomia

5. Radiation caries

6. Loss of taste

7. Osteoradionecrosis

8. Tooth sensitivity

9. Muscular dysfunction and trismus

10. Spontaneous gingival bleeding

Leukemias

A. Definition

1. Progressive malignant neoplasms characterized by an overproduction of abnormal leukocytes

2. Abnormal leukocytes displace hematopoietic tissue in the bone marrow, leading to decreased production of platelets, erythrocytes, and normal leukocytes

B. Classification
   1. Chronicity
      a. Acute form (A)—large numbers of immature nonspecific leukocytes are produced
      b. Chronic form (C)—leukocytes are well differentiated and able to mature, but immunologic capacity is decreased
   2. Type of white cell predominating
      a. Myeloid
      b. Lymphoid
      c. Monocytic
C. Incidence/prevalence
   1. Acute type
      a. There are 3 to 4 cases per 100,000 persons in the United States
      b. Complete remission is gained by 85% to 90% using current treatment regimens
   2. Chronic type—rare in children; 10 cases per 18,000 persons over age 75
   3. Seventh leading cause of cancer death in adults; leading cause of cancer death in children
   4. 5-year survival ranges from 11.4% in AML to 68.6% in CLL
D. Etiology
   1. Specific etiology unknown
   2. Predisposing factors—genetic factors, ionizing radiation, chemical agents, exposure to HTLV-1 virus
E. Signs/symptoms/clinical manifestations
   1. Acute form appears suddenly and severely; chronic form is insidious
   2. Fatigue, weakness, pallor, weight loss
   3. Ecchymoses of the skin and nosebleeds
   4. Fever
   5. Headache, nausea, and vomiting
F. Treatment
   1. Chemotherapy with blood transfusions and antibiotics
   2. Irradiation
   3. Bone marrow transplant when indicated
   4. Interferon therapy
G. Oral manifestations
   1. Initial
      a. Leukemic infiltrate of the pulp and gingiva
         (1) Causes pain in teeth
         (2) Enlarged bluish-red, spongy, blunted papilla (Fig. 14-12)
         (3) Ulceration and necrosis
      b. Mucositis, mucosal atrophy, and mucosal pallor
      c. Areas of spontaneous hemorrhage (intermittent oozing) and petechiae
      d. Loss of lamina dura, resorption of alveolar bone, cancellous bone destruction

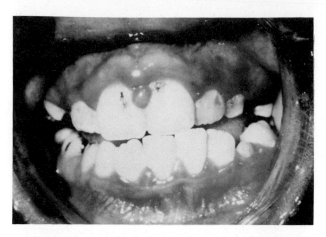

Fig. 14-12   Gingival enlargement in leukemia.

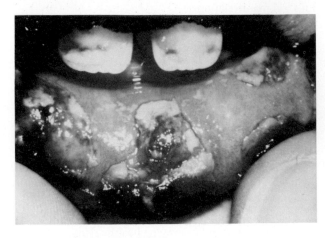

Fig. 14-13   Oral infections in leukemic patient.

   2. Secondary
      a. Mucosal infections (*Candida, Pseudomonas*) and periapical infections (Fig. 14-13)
      b. Acute necrotizing ulcerative gingivitis (ANUG)
      c. Viral infections
      d. Osteomyelitis
   3. Tertiary (treatment effects)
      a. Painful oral ulcerations
      b. Stomatitis
      c. Xerostomia and dental caries
      d. Jaw pain/Bell's palsy
      e. Secondary infections

Hemophilias

See Chapter 6, section on hemophilia.
A. Definition—congenital disorder of the blood-clotting mechanism
B. Incidence/prevalence
   1. Occurs in 1/4000 males in the United States
   2. 80% to 85% have hemophilia A; 10% to 15% have hemophilia B

3. Ninety percent are under age 25
C. Classification
  1. Type
    a. Hemophilia A (factor VIII deficiency)
    b. Hemophilia B (factor IX deficiency)—Christmas disease
    c. Von Willebrand disease (lack of plasma—von Willebrand factor, required for primary hemostasis)
  2. Severity—level of clotting factor (normal level is 50% to 100%)
    a. Severe—have less than 1% of the clotting factor; may bleed spontaneously or from minor trauma
    b. Moderate—have 5% to 25% of the factor present; hemorrhage only with trauma
    c. Mild—have 25% to 50% of the factor present; bleed only after severe injuries and surgery
D. Etiology
  1. Hemophilia A and B
    a. Sex-linked recessive mode of inheritance (female carrier and manifested in males)
    b. High mutation rate
  2. Von Willebrand disease—transmission by the dominant autosomal gene; occurs with equal frequency in both sexes
E. Signs/symptoms/clinical manifestations
  1. Bleeding and bruising from minor cuts or pressure
    a. Ecchymoses and hematomas
    b. Oozing
    c. Intramuscular bleeding causes pain
  2. Hemarthroses—bleeding into the soft tissues of the joints, leading to pain, swelling, and permanent joint contractures
  3. Renal function is impaired; exposure to hepatitis during transfusions
  4. Intracranial hemorrhages can cause seizures or other neurologic disorders
  5. Chronic complications include osteoarthritis, irregular growth, muscular atrophy, and tumor formation
  6. Inhibitor to antihemophilic factor can develop in hemophilia A, making the person resistant to replacement therapy
  7. Complications from bleeds include airway obstruction, intestinal obstruction, and compression of nerves and paralysis
F. Treatment
  1. Factor replacement therapy
    a. Fresh frozen plasma
    b. Cryoprecipitate (factor VIII and fibrinogen)
    c. Concentrates
  2. Amicar or cyclokapian (antifibrinolytics) used to

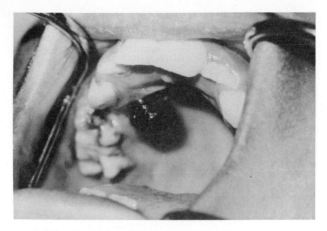

Fig. 14-14   Palatal bleed in hemophiliac patient.

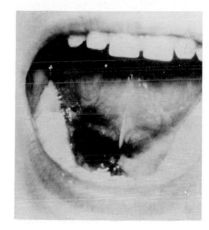

Fig. 14-15   Suction hematoma in hemophiliac patient.

help decrease oral bleeds; needed for periodontal debridement and root planing
  3. Desmopressin acetate used in von Willebrand disease and mild hemophilia
  4. Prevention of bleeds
  5. Joint replacement; antibiotics for invasive procedure
  6. Physical therapy
G. Oral manifestations
  1. Ecchymoses, hematomas, and gingival oozing can be a problem (Fig. 14-14)
  2. Oral trauma is more evident and can be serious (Fig. 14-15)

Diabetes Mellitus

See Chapter 17, section on diabetes mellitus.
A. Definition—hereditary disease of metabolism with
  1. Inadequate production and action of insulin from the pancreas

Table 14-12

Comparison of Type I and Type II Diabetes Mellitus

Characteristic	Insulin-dependent diabetes mellitus	Non–insulin-dependent diabetes mellitus
Age of onset	Usually under 25 years; may appear later	Adulthood, particularly over 40 years; may appear at younger ages
Body weight	Normal or thin	High percent obese at the time of diagnosis
Rate of onset of clinical symptoms	Rapid	Slow/insidious
Severity	Severe	Mild
Diabetic emergency (ketoacidosis)	Common	Rare
Stability	Unstable	Stable
Insulin treatment required	Almost all	Less than 25%
Chronic manifestations	Uncommon before 20 years; prevalent and severe by age 30	Develop slowly with age

From Wilkins EM: *Clinical practice of the dental hygienist,* ed 7, Philadelphia, 1994, Lea & Febiger.

2. Disorders in carbohydrate, protein, and fat metabolism
3. Body cells unable to use glucose, leading to hyperglycemia
4. "Brittle" diabetic person has alternating extremes of hypoglycemia and hyperglycemia

B. Incidence/prevalence
 1. Diabetes mellitus affects 16 million people in the United States, with about 50% as yet undiagnosed
 2. Persons over age 45 constitute four fifths of patients
 3. Third leading cause of death in the United States
 4. Much higher in Hispanics and American Indians

C. Major types (Table 14-12)
 1. Type I, or insulin-dependent
 2. Type II, or non–insulin-dependent
 3. Impaired glucose tolerance—higher than normal levels but not yet diagnostic for diabetes; at risk for atherosclerotic disease
 4. Gestational diabetes—occurs in 2% of pregnant women during second or third trimester; returns to normal after delivery in most cases but 30% to 40% may develop Type II later in life

D. Etiology
 1. Genetic disorder
 2. Destruction of the insulin-producing cells of the pancreas resulting from inflammation, viruses, cancer, or surgery
 3. Secondary to endocrine disorders (e.g., hyperthyroidism)
 4. Iatrogenic disease following the administration of steroids

E. Signs/symptoms/clinical manifestations
 1. Cardinal symptoms are those associated with hyperglycemia (Table 14-13)

Table 14-13

Clinical Manifestations of Diabetes Mellitus

Hyperglycemia	Hypoglycemia
Polydipsia	Early stage
Polyphagia	Diminished cerebral function
Polyuria	Changes in mood
Loss of weight	Decreased spontaneity
Fatigue	Hunger
Headache	Nausea
Blurred vision	More severe hypoglycemia
Nausea and vomiting	Sweating
Tachycardia	Tachycardia
Florid appearance	Piloerection
Hot and dry skin	Increased anxiety
Kussmaul respiration	Bizarre behavior patterns
Mental stupor	Belligerence
Loss of consciousness	Poor judgment
	Uncooperativeness
	Later severe stage
	Unconsciousness
	Seizure activity
	Hypotension
	Hypothermia

From Malamed SF: *Medical emergencies in the dental office,* ed 4, St Louis, 1993, Mosby.

2. An overdose of insulin or inadequate glucose intake to balance the insulin intake can result in insulin shock (hypoglycemia) (Table 14-13)
3. Chronic complications include
 a. Atherosclerosis and other cardiovascular problems
 b. Renal failure

c. Motor, sensory, and autonomic neuropathies

d. Glaucoma and cataracts

e. Associated with increased incidence of large babies, stillbirths, miscarriages, neonatal deaths, and congenital defects

F. Treatment—no known cure

1. Management of acute symptoms
2. Exercise and diet plan (food exchange system)
3. Medications
   a. Insulin therapy (combination of short-, intermediate-, or long-acting insulin)
   b. Oral hypoglycemic agents (sulfonylureas) for type II (Glucotrol), Micronase and Diabinese
   c. New drugs to slow digestion of carbohydrates to decrease rise in blood glucose (Glucophage and Precose)
4. Need to maintain a delicate balance between diet, exercise, and insulin
5. Factors affecting the need for insulin
   a. Food intake
   b. Emotional events
   c. Exercise levels
   d. Infections
6. Gene therapy
7. Education in diabetes self-care
8. Ongoing clinical trials may change regimens

G. Oral manifestations (seen more often in uncontrolled diabetics)

1. Delayed wound healing and inability to manage oral infections (e.g., *Candida* infections), periodontal abscesses
2. Decreased salivary flow may lead to increased caries; may have parotid gland enlargement
3. Predisposition to a rapidly progressing type of periodontal disease in both types of diabetes, even in children and adolescents; magenta hue with edematous glassy tissue, enlarged papilla, mobility, alveolar bone loss
4. Oral infections may undermine blood glucose control
5. Some instances of oral neuropathies such as burning, tingling, and numbness
6. Children with diabetes may have accelerated tooth eruption and enamel hypoplasia

Thyroid Disease

A. Definition

1. Hyperthyroidism (thyrotoxicosis)—excess of thyroid hormones in the bloodstream
2. Graves disease—toxic goiter
3. Hypothyroidism—inadequate thyroid hormones in the bloodstream
   a. Cretinism—childhood onset (congenital)
   b. Myxedema—adult onset (acquired)

B. Incidence/prevalence

1. Hyperthyroidism
   a. Disease is 7 times more common in women, especially being manifested during puberty, pregnancy, or menopause
   b. There are 3 cases per 10,000 adults per year
2. Hypothyroidism
   a. Rare
   b. Myxedema is 5 times more common in females; most common between ages 30 and 60

C. Etiology

1. Hyperthyroidism (Graves disease)
   a. Etiology is unknown
   b. Autoimmune etiology or familial tendency is postulated
2. Hypothyroidism
   a. Disease of the thyroid gland
   b. Myxedema may follow thyroid gland or pituitary gland failure resulting from irradiation, surgery, or excessive antithyroid drug therapy

D. Signs/symptoms/clinical manifestations—results of underproduction or overproduction of thyroid hormone (Table 14-14)

E. Treatment

1. Hyperthyroidism
   a. Antithyroid drugs, radioactive iodine, or iodides; may produce side effects
   b. Surgery
2. Hypothyroidism—daily thyroid supplement

F. Oral manifestations—primarily delayed or accelerated dental development or deterioration of alveolar bone (Table 14-14)

Chemical Dependency

See Chapter 8, section on substance abuse.

A. Definition

1. State of psychic or physical dependence (or both) following administration of a drug on a periodic or continuous basis
2. Drug use: when the effects of a drug can be realized with minimal hazard
3. Drug misuse: when the drug or amount taken make it more dangerous than necessary to produce desired effect
4. Drug abuse: when a person continually misuses any drug or loses control over its use or when it disrupts family, social, or job responsibilities
5. Tolerance: using larger dose levels of a drug to experience the same effects over time
6. Recovery: overcoming physical and psychological dependence, commitment to drug free life

Table 14-14

Clinical Features of Thyroid Disease

HYPOTHYROIDISM		Hyperthyroidism
Cretinism	Myxedema	
Dwarfism and obesity	Obesity	Weight loss
Coarse hair	Hair loss	Fine, friable hair
Eyes set apart	Puffy eyelids	Puffy eyelids
Muscle weakness	Muscle weakness	Exophthalmos
Dry cold skin	Dry cold skin	Tremors
Decreased sweating	Decreased sweating	Warm, moist skin
Cold intolerance	Cold intolerance	Increased sweating
Lethargy	Lethargy	Heat intolerance
Bradycardia	Bradycardia	Hyperactivity
Delayed tooth eruption		Tachycardia
Small jaws and malocculsion		Accelerated tooth eruption
		Large jaws
		Osteoporosis of alveolar bone
		Rapidly developing dental caries and periodontal disease

B. Incidence/prevalence
   1. Several drugs or drug categories cause the most concern: cocaine, heroin, other opiates, marijuana, stimulants, barbiturates and other depressants, hallucinogens (psychedelics), tranquilizers, volatile solvents, and other inhalants
   2. Alcohol is a major problem (see section on chronic alcoholism); 70% of Americans drink at least on a social basis
   3. Other less recognized drugs: coffee, tea, tobacco
   4. Over 217 psychoactive herbs
   5. Nitrous oxide and prescription drug abuse of most concern to dental professionals
   6. Routes of administration: oral ingestion, inhalation, injection, snorting, buccal, suppositories
   7. 37% of U.S. population over age 12 have used illegal drugs at least once in their lives
C. Etiology
   1. Stressful social, psychologic, or economic environments
   2. Peer pressure
   3. Gateway drugs: alcohol, tobacco, marijuana
D. Signs and symptoms—vary with the agent involved and route of administration
   1. Affects autonomic, central, and peripheral nervous system
   2. Drug interactions have additive effects, inhibitory effects, and synergistic effects
   3. Duration of effects ranges from 1 hour to many days
   4. Withdrawal symptoms reported for all drug categories except hallucinogens

5. Possible effects of some drug categories
   a. Narcotics: euphoria, drowsiness, respiratory depression, constricted pupils, nausea
   b. Depressants: slurred speech, disorientation, drunklike behavior
   c. Stimulants: alertness, excitation, euphoria, increased pulse rate and blood pressure, insomnia, loss of appetite
   d. Hallucinogens: illusions and hallucinations, poor perception of time and distance
   e. Marijuana: euphoria, relaxed inhibitions, increased appetite, disoriented behavior
E. Treatment
   1. See Table 14-15; usually a multimodality approach
   2. Abstinence
   3. Educational programs, mentoring and drug-free activities
   4. Confrontational and family-oriented approaches; team also may involve employers and health professionals
   5. "Lifelong recovery" approach
F. Oral manifestations
   1. Oral trauma if engage in aggressive behavior/fights or if have accidents
   2. Xerostomia if become dehydrated
   3. Mucosal lesions and leukoplakia from irritants if smoked or used orally
   4. Increased caries and periodontal disease if oral hygiene neglected or consumes high carbohydrate diet
   5. Exogenous stains

Table 14-15			
An Overview of Drug Treatment Modalities			
DRUG TREATMENT MAY TAKE THE FORM OF			
Supervisory-deterrent approaches	**Medical-distributive approaches**	**Drug-free approaches**	**Crisis intervention approaches**
Incarceration	Maintenance programs	Therapeutic communities	Hot lines
Criminal commitment	Detoxification programs	Self-help societies	Rap centers
Civil commitment	Antagonist programs		Free clinics
	→ Multimodality approaches ←		

From Duncan D, Gold R: *Drugs and the whole person,* New York, 1982, John Wiley & Sons, Inc.

6. Increased risk for oral and esophageal cancer
7. Reduced tolerance to pain
8. Bruxism

Chronic Alcoholism

A. Definition and etiology
   1. Chronic impairment in physical, mental, or social functioning caused by frequent ingestion (more than two drinks per day) of alcohol
   2. Can become dependent on its ingestion and also develop a tolerance to increasing amounts
   3. Genetically transmitted susceptibility to alcoholism
   4. Often induced by a psychiatric disorder or stress
B. Incidence/prevalence
   1. Heavy drinkers make up 7% to 10% of the U.S. population (two or more drinks per day)
   2. Majority are upper middle class
   3. Normal activities are maintained by 95%
   4. Eighty percent are heavy smokers
   5. One of every 12 adult drinkers has an alcohol dependency
   6. 15% of men and 3% of women over age 65 are alcoholics
C. Signs/symptoms/clinical manifestations
   1. Alcoholic breath
   2. Unexplained tremors
   3. Nausea and vomiting, gastrointestinal problems, ulcers
   4. Cutaneous lesions (redness, acne, spider angiomas)
   5. Edema of the eyelids and rest of the body
   6. Nutritional deficiencies (vitamin B, protein, calcium)
D. Long-term complications
   1. Hypertension and other types of heart disease
   2. Increased risk for various types of cancer
   3. Hepatitis, cirrhosis, and hypoglycemia
   4. Interference with the secretion of pancreatic enzymes

5. Altered enzyme functioning and malabsorptive syndromes of the small intestine
6. Irritation of the gastric mucosa leading to bleeding, inflammation, and ulceration
7. Fetal alcohol syndrome (pregnant women)
8. Impotence

E. Treatment
   1. Only about 10% of alcoholics receive treatment
   2. Table 14-15 provides an overview of drug treatment modalities for all types of drug and alcohol dependence
   3. Some alcohol abuse programs involve use of disulfiram (Antabuse), which causes physical discomfort if alcohol is consumed
   4. Dietary modifications
   5. Abstinence is an overriding goal
F. Oral manifestations—increased incidence of
   1. Caries caused by nausea and vomiting, neglected oral hygiene, and xerostomia
   2. Periodontal disease caused by an impaired immune system and the effects on white blood cells
   3. Glossitis and angular cheilitis from nutritional deficiencies
   4. Leukoplakia and oral-pharyngeal cancer
   5. Swelling of the parotid glands leads to decreased salivation and increased caries incidence
   6. Trauma during inebriated states (accidents or fights)
   7. Attrition secondary to bruxism

End Stage Renal Disease

A. Definition
   1. Progressive bilateral deterioration of renal function, resulting in uremia and eventually death
   2. Uremia is the toxic condition produced by retention of urinary constituents in the blood
B. Incidence/prevalence
   1. Affects 8 million people in the United States

    2. Annually, 47,000 die (over 50% are over age 55)

    3. Compromised life unless a successful transplant is performed (about 50% success rate)

    4. About 142,000 people using dialysis in the United States; 90% use hemodialysis

C. Etiology

    1. Infectious diseases (e.g., nephritis, viral and fungal infections)

    2. Hypersensitivity states (e.g., glomerulonephritis)

    3. Developmental defects of the kidneys

    4. Circulatory disturbances (e.g., hypertension, hemorrhages)

    5. Metabolic diseases (e.g., diabetes)

    6. 10% of new cases may be a result of misusing analgesics

D. Signs/symptoms/clinical manifestations

    1. Mental slowness or depression

    2. Swelling and edema

    3. Muscular hyperactivity

    4. Hyperpigmentation of the skin (brownish yellow)

    5. Anorexia and vomiting, diarrhea

    6. Anemia

    7. Possible functional defect in factor VIII protein, leading to hemorrhagic episodes

    8. Hypertension, congestive heart failure

E. Treatment

    1. Potassium regulation

    2. Sodium regulation

    3. Maintenance of water balance (depends on urine output, edema, and weight change)

    4. Protein balance

    5. Acid-base balance—correct acidosis with calcium carbonate (also give vitamin D)

    6. Sedatives and hypnotics to manage neuromuscular complications

    7. Dialysis when other methods alone are not effective

      a. Peritoneal—usually for acute renal failure

        (1) Injection of hypertonic solution into the peritoneal cavity

        (2) Draws out urea and other solutes

        (3) Less costly, easier to perform, but less effective than hemodialysis

        (4) More people using ambulatory type, where continuous dialysis is performed by the patient, with drainage into a bag

      b. Hemodialysis for chronic renal failure

        (1) Creation of an arteriovenous fistula (Fig. 14-16)

        (2) Blood runs from the artery to the dialysis machine, is filtered, and then returned to the vein

        (3) Heparin is added to prevent blood clotting

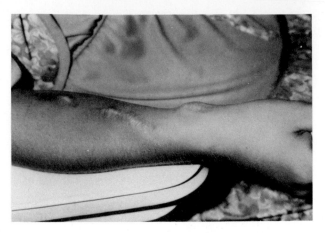

Fig. 14-16 Multiple access sites for arteriovenous shunts for hemodialysis.

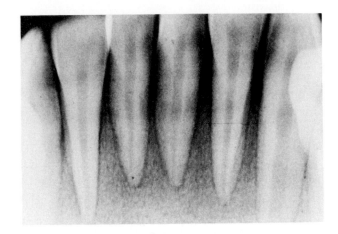

Fig. 14-17 Uremic bone disease in chronic renal failure.

        (4) Patient is at risk for acquiring hepatitis B and non-A non-B from commercial blood products

    8. Kidney transplant—problems with graft rejection and infection; use steroids, antibiotics, and immunosuppressives such as cyclosporine

F. Oral manifestations

    1. Painful oral ulcerations and stomatitis from drugs

    2. Candidiasis or herpetic lesions from immunosuppression

    3. Increased calculus deposits

    4. Anemic mucosa

    5. Oral petechia and hemorrhage

    6. Ground-glass appearance of alveolar bone caused by leaching of calcium (uremic bone disease) (Fig. 14-17)

    7. Bad taste and halitosis from urea in saliva

    8. Enamel hypoplasia (Fig. 14-18)

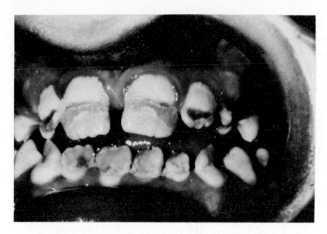

Fig. 14-18 Enamel hypoplasia associated with chronic renal failure.

    9. Immunosuppressed transplant patient may have increased risk for cancer

  10. Gingival hyperplasia from cyclosporine (an immunosuppressant) or nifedipine (a calcium-channel blocker)

Dental Management (Table 14-16)

A. Personal and professional prerequisites

1. Interview in a sensitive manner to gather accurate data; initiate dental hygiene process
2. Analyze and summarize data in oral or written format
3. Use problem-solving skills to develop alternative strategies to manage problems
4. Evaluate client and professional goals and progress for appropriateness and effectiveness
5. Remain current in terms of new conditions, new methods of medical management, and advances in dental and dental hygiene care
6. Apply new knowledge or techniques from other areas to dental management of special clients
7. Apply research principles and techniques to acquire clinical data that serve as the basis for care-planning and decision-making

B. Office management issues

1. Stress a team concept with cooperation among members and coordination of information and activities; dental hygiene procedures may require the help of a dental assistant
2. Identify and anticipate client needs and problems before initiation of care; use of a previsit questionnaire is helpful (see box on p. 616)
3. Obtain informed consent for treatment from the client or an appropriate representative
4. Explain office policies, procedures, and philosophy to the client or guardian before or at the first appointment
5. Determine financial limitations that may affect care planning or payment procedures
   a. Assess additional resources available from other sources (e.g., community organizations)
   b. Attempt to provide flexible payment alternatives
6. If the client is unable to receive care in the office because of physical limitations or geographic distance, determine if care can be provided in a home or community setting with portable equipment
7. If office facilities do not comply with accessibility guidelines, discuss ways to
   a. Make them physically accessible
   b. Accommodate the needs or refer to a provider who can
8. Assure that office layout and environment are not safety or health hazards for some clients
9. Keep scheduling somewhat flexible to allow for transportation or other problems; block appointments are helpful when dealing with groups

C. Medical issues

1. Obtain a health history from the client or caretaker, with supplemental information from other professionals or agency records
2. Update the health history at each visit
3. Because many standard health history forms will be inadequate for the multiple conditions and problems of some clients, ask supplemental questions
4. Obtain specifics regarding medical treatment regimens or other therapies that may affect scheduling or treatment
5. Obtain names, addresses, and phone numbers for all the client's physicians who might provide helpful data (e.g., generalist, cardiologist, orthopedist, endocrinologist) with permission to release information
6. Be particularly alert to the client's physical status during the initial assessment
7. Monitor vital signs as indicated
8. Record all medication information; update at each visit
9. Note any indications or contraindications to treatment or premedication
10. Maintain records of all medical advice, prescriptions, or drugs given
11. If clients refuse to disclose medical information or follow recommended standard procedures for their own protection (e.g., antibiotic premedication), have them sign a statement to that effect for the records

Text continued on p. 616

Table 14-16

Dental Management Considerations for Special-Needs Clients

Condition	Medical issues	Barriers to care	Risk factors	Treatment considerations*	Prevention/education issues
Mental retardation	Syndrome? Associated medical conditions/other disabilities Treatment regimens	Limited financial resources Degree of reliance on others Limited mental ability	Oral motor dysfunction General incoordination Cariogenic foods/reinforcers Self-abuse Resistant behavior	Gagging; radiographs, instrument placement, positioning Mental impairment: communication, cooperation, and stability in chair Limited finances: alternative treatment plans	"Tell, show, do" approach Simple language Frequent repetition and positive reinforcement Involve caretakers Frequent continued care intervals Alternatives for snacks and food reinforcers
Fetal alcohol syndrome	Which organs affected? Heart? Brain? Growth deficiency	Family may be dysfunctional Behavioral problems May have mental disabilities	Attention-deficit disorders Dental malformations	Behavior and attention: short-structured appointments Family problems: assure that follow-up care is understood	Ensure adequate supervision for oral hygiene care Use same methods as for children with learning disabilities or mental retardation
Down syndrome	Heart defects? (antibiotic premedication) Hearing and vision problems? Decreased resistance to infection; frequent respiratory infections	Same as for mental retardation	Same as for mental retardation	Same as for mental retardation plus small oral area: oral access for procedures Hearing/vision disorders: communication	Same as for mental retardation plus stress oral hygiene and supportive periodontal therapy
Autism	No major problems unless self-abusive	Behavior Degree of reliance on others Communication	Eating disorders or fetishes Resistant behavior	Dependence on "routines"; procedure sequencing, desensitization Lack of useful language: communication Learning disabilities/sensitivity to stimuli: communication distractions	Combine verbal and non-verbal communication techniques and positive reinforcers Teach toothbrushing as a "motion" rather than a function Avoid metaphors and complex language structures

Learning disabilities/ADHD	Medications and potential side effects	Depends on type of disability	Depends on disability; Oral motor dysfunction; General incoordination; Hyperactive behavior	Depends on disability; Disorientation/hyperactivity: stability in chair, length of appointments, physical contact	Focus on strengths; Use combination of teaching approaches; Maintain attention through eye contact and physical contact; involve caregiver
Emotional disturbance/mental illness	Medications and potential side effects; Psychologic causes of reported symptoms/diseases, fears	Limited financial resources in some cases; Emotional concerns and fears; Disturbed thought processes	Depends on nature of disturbance; Inadequate diet or strange food practices; Phobias about oral care; Self-abuse; Side effects of medications	Anxiety, fear, aggression: stability in chair, cooperation, communication, safety for patient and clinician	Reality orientation techniques; Possible dietary counseling; Involve caretakers; Positive reinforcement and repetition; Fluoride supplements if xerostomia from medications
Eating disorders	Symptoms; Amount of weight loss; Presence and frequency of bulimia; Medical and psychologic interventions; Eating patterns	Psychologic status; Denial of symptoms; Length of treatment; Compliance with appointments	Eating patterns; Frequent vomiting; Xerostomia; Depression; Life-threatening risk factors: conflict, life crises, major life changes, need for control and approval	Coordinated care: physicians, nutritionist, and psychologist; Carious or eroded teeth: restoration; Anxiety: psychosedation; Pit and fissure sealants if appropriate; Study models to monitor progression of tooth structure loss	Artificial saliva or sugar-free gum for xerostomia; Rinsing with sodium bicarbonate after vomiting rather than using toothbrush; Neutral pH sodium fluoride rinses or stannous fluoride gels used daily; Frequent continued care intervals
Alzheimer's disease	Multiple medical problems; Medications; Reduced bowel and bladder control; Fatigue from abnormal sleep patterns; Wheelchair	Behavior: uncooperative; Finances may be limited by disability and medical problems; Dependence on others	Oral motor dysfunction; Depression or disorientation leading to oral neglect; General motor dysfunction; Potential for injury	Fluctuating moods and disorientation: length of appointments, communication, cooperation, safety; Motor problems: oral access, radiographs, stability in chair; Memory loss: data collection	Use of a mouthguard; Involve caretakers; Involve patient when most lucid and positive; Simple instructions and frequent repetition; Positive reinforcement; Frequent continued care intervals; Prevent oral injury

*Universal precautions for infection control are used at each appointment.

Continued.

Table 14-16

Dental Management Considerations for Special-Needs Clients—cont'd

Condition	Medical issues	Barriers to care	Risk factors	Treatment considerations*	Prevention/ education issues
Seizure disorders	Medications and side effects Seizure information Type of disorder Specific manifestations Presence of aura Frequency/how well controlled General management History of status epilepticus	Disturbance in self-image Transportation if cannot drive Embarrassment	Side effects of medications Potential for orofacial trauma during seizures	Seizure activity: precipitating factors, treatment planning, appointment scheduling, stability in chair, communication; procedures if seizure occurs Tissue overgrowth from phenytoin Prolonged bleeding time from valproic acid	Optimal oral hygiene and frequent continued care intervals to control gingival overgrowth from phenytoin First-aid instructions for oral trauma Positive reinforcement and self-image building
Visual impairment	Degree of impairment? Sensitivity to light Treated versus untreated conditions	Degree of dependence on others Attitudes and stereotypes about disability and toward guide dogs Physical obstacles to or in office	Difficulty monitoring oral status	Sight impairment: appointment scheduling, explanation of procedures, clinician position, communication, positioning of light, mobility in clinic, data collection, noise level Guide dog: role and placement in office	Demonstrate procedures on finger, etc. Precede actions with verbal descriptions Teach toothbrushing in mouth Involve caregiver when necessary Use audio aids or physical models for teaching
Hearing impairment	Degree of impairment? Use interpreter or other assistive devices?	Degree of dependence on others	No specific factors	Hearing impairment: appointment scheduling, explanation of procedures, clinician position, communication, data collection, noise interference, use of hearing aid during appointment	Determine appropriate communication techniques Provide paper and pencil if desired Involve interpreter if needed Watch facial expressions
Cleft lip or palate	Hearing impairment? Upper respiratory tract infections Prosthetic appliances Medications Diet	Fear of healthcare providers Self-image problems	Missing or malaligned teeth Oral motor dysfunction Feeding disorders	Cleft: clear communication, instrument positioning or fulcruming, suctioning and prevention of aspiration Fear: dental procedures, cooperation	Instruct in cleaning any prosthetic aids Involve caretaker when necessary Nutritional counseling if needed

Cerebral palsy	Associated disorders Medications Other therapies Respiration impaired? Presence of primitive reflexes Degree of impairment	Communication Transportation if in wheelchair or cannot drive May have limited financial resources Degree of dependence on others for care Mobility issues if in wheelchair Provider attitudes toward condition Self-image problems	Oral motor dysfunction General motor dysfunction Special diets	Primitive reflexes: patient or clinician position, stability, instrument positioning or fulcruming, oral access, suctioning and amount of water used, protection of airway, radiographs Use of wheelchair: transfers to dental chair, mobility in office, office accessibility	Involve caretakers as appropriate Be patient with slowness of responses and progress Use combination of communication methods Assess need for physical assistance or adaptive aids for home care Frequent continued care Fluoride therapy and antimicrobials if needed Nutritional counseling if needed
Bell palsy	Therapies, especially prednisone Duration of condition Possible surgery to achieve facial symmetry	Language skills Self-image problems	Oral motor dysfunction	Lack of eye closure: protection of eyes (goggles) Oral motor dysfunction: protection of airway	Caution regarding effects of anesthesia Frequent rinsing or toothbrushing for food retention on affected side
Myasthenia gravis	Medications History of radiation therapy or surgery History of myasthenic crises	Communication Patient may hold chin to help during speaking	Oral motor dysfunction	Weakness increases during day: scheduling appointments Oral motor dysfunction/paralysis/impaired breathing: protection of airway, use of rubber dam, suctioning, chair position Weak voice: communication	Frequent continued care intervals to prevent infection Frequent rinsing or toothbrushing for food retention Fluoride therapy or antimicrobials if needed
Parkinson disease	Medications and side effects Rigidity of larger joints Sensitivity to heat	Mobility to and in office Communication Embarrassment about condition	Oral motor dysfunction Side effects of drugs Possible inadequate diet	Tremors: stability, instrumentation, radiographs Sensitivity to heat: temperature of operatory Muscular pain and joint rigidity: chair position, appointment length Slurred speech: communication	Frequent continued care Frequent rinsing and toothbrushing Adaptive equipment or assistance if needed Fluoride therapy or antimicrobials if needed Counseling about side effects of medications

Continued.

Table 14-16

Dental Management Considerations for Special-Needs Clients—cont'd

Condition	Medical issues	Barriers to care	Risk factors	Treatment considerations*	Prevention/ education issues
Arthritis	Medications Degree of impairment Joints affected; pain Joint replacement (premedication may be needed)	Mobility to and in office Limited finances if disabled Weakness or fatigue	General motor impairment Drug-related complications such as prolonged bleeding, adrenal suppression, and bone marrow suppression	Joint pain: chair position, appointment length Limited oral opening: positioning, instrumentation, radiographs, TMJ assessment Joint replacement: antibiotic premedication Long-term aspirin therapy: prolonged bleeding	Adaptive equipment or assistance is needed Counseling about side effects of medications Prevent sources of oral infection
Multiple sclerosis	Medications and side effects Degree of facial pain Degree of impairment Sensitivity to heat	Mobility to and in office, especially if in wheelchair Depression or moodiness Limited finances if disabled	Special diets Side effects of drugs Fine motor coordination problems Oral motor dysfunction Infection Fatigue, stress, and pain	Weakness and numbness: wheelchair transfer, stability, appointment length Oral motor dysfunction: protection of airway Mood changes: communication, acceptance of treatment, cooperation Sensitivity to heat: room temperature Periods of exacerbation/ remission: appointment scheduling	Adaptive equipment or assistance may be needed More frequent rinsing and brushing Assistance in dietary counseling Fluoride therapy or antimicrobials if needed More frequent continued care intervals to prevent infections Refer for TMD assessment
Muscular dystrophies	Medications Other therapies Type and degree of involvement Prognosis Obesity, scoliosis, or cardiopulmonary involvement?	Depends on type Mobility to and in office, especially if in wheelchair Limited financial resources Weakness and possible decreased life span	Oral motor dysfunction General motor weakness and incoordination Dietary inadequacies Mouth breathing	Depends on type and degree of involvement Muscle weakness: stability in chair, wheelchair transfers, radiographs, instrumentation, appointment length Oral motor dysfunction: protection of airway, communication	Frequent continued care More frequent brushing and rinsing Fluoride therapy or antimicrobials if needed Adapted equipment or physical assistance for oral care

Condition					
Spinal injuries	Depends on level of injury Medications Respiratory involvement Decubitus ulcers Incontinence/encopresis Contractures Heterotopic ossifications Body temperature regulation Potential for autonomic hyperreflexia Type of adaptive equipment	Mobility to and in office, especially if in wheelchair or on respirator Limited financial resources Psychosocial concerns/depression Poor self-image	Depends on level of injury Oral motor dysfunction Limited or total dependence on others Special diets	Incoordination: restorative treatment planning and possible emergency care Limited life span: treatment planning, motivation Psychologic state: communication, cooperation Spasticity, tremors: stability Paralysis: mobility, wheelchair transfers, stability in chair, length of appointment, radiographs Impaired respiration/oral motor dysfunction: chair position, use of rubber dam, protection of airway, instrumentation	Adaptive equipment or physical assistance needed Fluoride therapy and antimicrobials if needed Emphasize self-care to degree possible
Spina bifida	Depends on type Similar to spinal injuries Shunt for hydrocephalus (antibiotic premedication) Seizure disorders	Depends on type and degree of impairment Similar to spinal injuries	Similar to spinal injuries, except oral motor dysfunction not apparent	Similar to spinal injuries, although psychologic state not as poor Antibiotic premedication required for clients with shunts	Learning disabilities influence dental health education methods
Viral hepatitis (see Chapter 7)	Type Degree of liver impairment Immunity versus active state versus carrier state Follow-up with physician if status unclear Good history Need for antigen or antibody test to verify carrier state	Weakened state during acute illness	Potential for transmission of virus Potential for abnormal bleeding in cases of significant liver damage Potential for altered drug metabolism Carrier may be asymptomatic High carbohydrate diet	No treatment if active state, careful use of aerosol-producing equipment, e.g., air polisher, air/water syringe, ultrasonic scaler	No specific concerns unless a chronic carrier Isolation of toothbrush from others if a carrier Counseling regarding transmission Discuss blood testing to determine carrier state if unknown Dietary counseling and fluoride therapy while on special diet

Continued.

Table 14-16

Dental Management Considerations for Special-Needs Clients—cont'd

Condition	Medical issues	Barriers to care	Risk factors	Treatment considerations*	Prevention/ education issues
AIDS (see Chapter 7)	Systems involved; Degree of impairment; Consult with physician; Kaposi sarcoma; Treatment regimens; Predisposition to multiple opportunistic infections; Immunosuppression	Finding dentist who will treat; Fear of rejection; Stigmas associated with disease; Decreased motivation/depression; Limited finances if unemployed, underinsured, or uninsured	Oral infections; Debilitated state	Oral infections (e.g., candidiasis): palliation, transmission potential; Kaposi sarcoma: treatment planning; Psychologic state: communication, motivation; Gingivitis should be treated to prevent HIV-periodontitis/necrotizing (ulcerative) periodontitis	Palliative care for oral infections; Increased attention to oral hygiene
Sexually transmitted diseases (see Chapter 7)	Determine status: history of disease, active disease reported or observed, in high-risk group; Treatment regimen and compliance; Follow-up care; Medication sensitivity; Complications from long standing untreated cases	Psychosocial stigma of diseases	Potential for disease transmission	Oral lesions: palliative care	Counseling regarding disease transmission concerns
Tuberculosis (see Chapter 7)	Good history; Treatment regimen (compliance and effectiveness); Appropriate follow-up care; Instances of reinfection	Stigma of condition	Potential for disease transmission; Potential problem if it is multidrug-resistant type of TB	Disease transmission: same as for any infectious disease, especially if not sure if it is active	Counseling regarding disease transmission
Cystic fibrosis	Organ systems affected; Degree of impairment and prognosis; Dietary changes; Treatment regimens	Small stature may cause embarrassment; Prognosis may de-	Decreased resistance to infections; Pulmonary complications compounded	Mucus accumulations/impaired breathing; chair position, appointment scheduling and	Fluoride therapy if dry mouth; Frequent oral care because of mouth

Continued.

Condition					
	Chronic pulmonary disease. Abnormal viscous secretions causing damage to major organs such as lungs, pancreas, and liver	...crease motivation. Finances may be limited	by problems of malabsorption and malnutrition. Recurrent attacks of pneumonia, bronchiectasis	length, coughing, protection of airway, use of rubber dam. Fear of medical situations: cooperation, scheduling. Susceptibility to infections; appointment scheduling. Tetracycline staining; aesthetics, treatment planning	breathing. Coordinate dietary suggestions with other professionals. Artificial saliva because of decreased salivary output
Chronic obstructive pulmonary disease	Single or coexisting conditions. Degree of impairment. Medications or need for oxygen	Portable oxygen. Fear of procedures that impair breathing	Side effects of medications	Impaired respiration: upright position, suctioning and coughing, rubber dam, orthopnea. Medications: avoid those that depress respiration, nitrous is ok, drug interactions	Same as for bronchial asthma
Bronchial asthma	Type and severity of asthma. Frequency and severity of attacks. Precipitating factors. Treatment regimens. History of hospitalizations or status asthmaticus. Instruct patient to bring inhalers if used	Fear of medical/dental environments. Allergens in office	No specific risk factors	Anxiety: possible premedication or relaxation techniques. Medications/precipitating factors: contraindications to prescribing or using certain drugs such as aspirin or β-blockers, appointment scheduling, medical emergency preparedness, eliminate allergens. Have bronchodilator present. Use of local anesthetic without epinephrine or levonordefrin in some cases	Model relaxed, stress-free environment. No specific preventive requirements unless have decreased salivation from medications

Table 14-16

Dental Management Considerations for Special-Needs Clients—cont'd

Condition	Medical issues	Barriers to care	Risk factors	Treatment considerations*	Prevention/ education issues
Congenital heart disease	Type and if repaired Extent of limitations Medications Prognosis Need for antibiotic premedication Physician consult	Financial constraints from medical bills Frequent illness Possibly debilitated state Overprotective attitude of parents	Decreased resistance to infections	Bleeding potential in some cases: treatment planning, need for lab tests, possible referral to specialist Heart condition: antibiotic premedication, stress management protocols, appointment length, chair position	Emphasize danger of intraoral infections in terms of aggravating heart condition Frequent continued care intervals Prevention of infective endocarditis
Rheumatic fever and heart disease	Residual effects of rheumatic fever Physician consult regarding need for antibiotic premedication	No specific barriers	Rheumatic fever Pharyngeal infection with group A streptococci	Heart defects: need for antibiotic premedication Consult with cardiologist Complete as much oral healthcare as possible during the 2-3 hours following the waiting period after the loading dose	Stress oral hygiene to prevent oral infections and self-induced bacteremias Prevention of infective endocarditis
Cardiac arrhythmias	Symptoms Medications and side effects Presence of pacemaker and type	If pacemaker, avoidance of certain electromagnetic equipment	No specific risk factors Development of arrhythmias from cocaine-epinephrine interactions in cocaine abusers	Pacemaker: avoidance of electromagnetic equipment Arrhythmia: stress management protocol, drug precautions, bleeding potential from medications	No specific preventive regimens Artificial saliva substitute if have xerostomia

Condition					
Hypertensive disease	Vital sign monitoring Physician consult or referral Medications and side effects and other treatment regimens Cause: primary or secondary Predisposing or general risk factors Severity, symptoms Possibility of orthostatic hypotension	Anxiety about oral healthcare	Side effects of medications Potential for stroke, myocardial infarction, and renal failure Potential for adverse drug interactions between vasoconstrictors and antihypertensive drugs	Hypertension: stress management protocols, chair position, treatment planning, monitoring vital signs, appointment scheduling, contraindications to treatment Medications: drug interactions, gag reflex, local anesthetics, bleeding potential, pain control	Counseling regarding reducing general risk factors Palliative care for oral infections from medications Fluoride therapy and saliva substitutes for xerostomia Create stress-free environment Prevent postural hypertension
Ischemic heart disease (coronary atherosclerotic heart disease)	Physician consult Angina or myocardial infarction episodes Hospitalizations Medications and side effects Surgery	Possible debilitated state Medical and other expenses Anxiety about dental treatment	Side effects of medications Susceptibility to infections if debilitated	Heart condition: same considerations as for hypertensive disease and preparation for medical emergency, contraindications for treatment if unstable or recent attack (within 6 months) Medications: same as for hypertensive disease; pain control	Palliative care for side effects of medications Counseling regarding decreasing general risk factors Special oral hygiene instructions if hospitalized or bedridden Frequent maintenance visits Create stress-free environment
Congestive heart failure	Same as for severe ischemic or hypertensive heart disease	Mobility	Pulmonary congestion and edema	Prone to nausea and vomiting during oral healthcare Keep client upright in chair	Frequent continued care intervals Create stress-free environment

Continued.

Table 14-16

Dental Management Considerations for Special-Needs Clients—cont'd

Condition	Medical issues	Barriers to care	Risk factors	Treatment considerations*	Prevention/ education issues
Cerebrovascular accident (stroke)	Type of involvement, degree of limitation Seizures? Medications and side effects Other therapies	Communication Accessibility if need adaptive equipment or wheelchair Degree of dependence on others	Oral motor dysfunction Side effects of medications Impaired general motor coordination Dietary inadequacies Transient ischemic attacks Previous stroke, hypertension, cardiac abnormalities, atherosclerosis, diabetes mellitus, elevated blood lipid	Memory impairment: communication, data collection Oral motor dysfunction/paralysis: instrumentation, jaw stability, radiographs, treatment planning Impaired emotional control: cooperation, communication Short morning appointments General paralysis: mobility, possible wheelchair transfers, stability in chair Minimize use of vasoconstrictors	Use combination of teaching approaches Reinforce and repeat instructions Frequent continued care Fluoride therapy or antimicrobial if needed Adaptive aids or supervision for oral care Avoid sensory overload Reorient client to situations Use one-step instructions
Sickle cell anemia	Precipitating factors for crises Symptoms and severity Associated conditions Transfusions? Lab tests needed?	Periods of pain Debilitated condition at times Fear of dental environment Limited financial resources because of medical bills	Susceptibility to infections Low stress tolerance	Sickle cell crises: appointment scheduling, motivation, emergency care only Susceptibility to infections: periodontal maintenance, physician consult for possible antibiotic premedication Reduce patient stress Consultation with physician Avoid medications that depress respiration	Dietary analysis/counseling Dietary counseling Frequent maintenance care because of associated alveolar bone problems and need to control oral infection Involvement of others in care Create a stress-free oral healthcare environment Emphasis on optimal oral healthcare behaviors

Cancers	Parts of body affected, treatment regimens, medications and side effects, potential for bleeding and anemia	Frequent hospitalizations or medical appointments Debilitated states Financial burdens Reliance on others Depression	Side effects of medications Oral infections and ulcerations Metastasis to oral cavity Weakness for self-care	Radiation therapy: pre/post care Prevention and palliative care for oral infections and ulcerations Short appointments and frequent active follow-up Prompt treatment of dental-related infections Need for antibiotic premedication	Fluoride therapy and other antimicrobial rinses Oral hygiene aids Help with oral care if needed Monitor removable appliances Frequent maintenance care Antifungals, saliva substitutes as needed
Leukemias	Type Treatment regimens, frequency Presence of anemia, thrombocytopenia, and infection	Stages of acute disease versus remissions Fear of dental environment	Side effects of chemotherapy or radiation therapy Susceptibility to infections Oral hemorrhage	Bleeding potential: preappointment lab tests, appointment scheduling, physician consult, surgical procedures Susceptibility to infections: periodontal maintenance, antibiotic premedication Ideally, provide invasive care prior to chemotherapy or radiation therapy Acute versus remission stages: treatment planning, appointment scheduling Chemotherapy or radiation therapy: treatment planning Consultation with oncologist	Palliative care for oral lesions Frequent continued care intervals Fluoride program Involvement of others in care program Saliva substitutes Eliminate potential sources of oral infection Meticulous oral hygiene Daily antimicrobial mouth rinses

Continued.

Table 14-16

Dental Management Considerations for Special-Needs Clients—cont'd

Condition	Medical issues	Barriers to care	Risk factors	Treatment considerations*	Prevention/education issues
Hemophilias	Type and severity Frequency and location of bleeds Treatment regimens Joint replacements? Hepatitis? AIDS? Seizures? Inhibitor status Lab tests needed?	Finding dentist who will treat Resources for emergency care	Potential for oral bleeds Potential to acquire hepatitis, cirrhosis, or AIDS associated with frequent clotting factor replacement therapy	Bleeding potential: preappointment lab tests, surgery, physician consult, factor replacement therapy, instrumentation, radiographs, use of rubber dam, suctioning, use of Amicar or Cykokapron Joint replacements: antibiotic premedication Hepatitis carrier: disease transmission procedures AIDS: see management under AIDS	Use of antimicrobial mouthrinses and soft-bristled brush Counseling regarding first aid for oral trauma Frequent continued care intervals
Diabetes mellitus	Type and severity Medication regimens Dietary regimen Complications Hypertension and other heart conditions Frequency of episodes of hypoglycemia or hyperglycemia	Finding dentist who will treat if have chronic complications	Susceptibility to infections (e.g., oral candidiasis) Decreased salivary flow Recalcitrant periodontal disease Slow healing Complications associated with disturbances in vision and kidney function	Insulin/sugar balance: potential for medical emergency; appointment scheduling, stress management protocol Susceptibility to infection: periodontal maintenance, possible antibiotic premedication, treatment planning Associated conditions (see management for each condition)	3-6 month continued care intervals Dietary analysis Fluoride program Need for bacterial plaque control Minimize stress Control of oral infections Prevention of insulin shock or diabetic coma Chemotherapeutic irrigation

Condition					
Thyroid disease	Type and cause Symptoms and severity Medications	No specific barriers Swelling of tongue in hypothyroidism may cause difficulty in speech communication	Abnormal dental development Thyroid crisis is life-threatening	Sensitivity to drugs: treatment planning, postoperative instructions, preparation for medical emergency Mental retardation in some (see management for mental retardation) Abnormal dental development: treatment planning Heat or cold intolerance: room temperature, length of appointment "Thyroid storm" or thyroid crisis precipitated by surgery, infection, trauma, or uncontrolled thyroid disease	Special hygiene instruction if mentally retarded Prevent infection Prevention of thyroid crisis Create a stress-free environment
Chemical dependency	Obtaining adequate history Types of drugs used Symptoms Treatment interventions Potential for drug interactions or overdose Emotional stability during appointment At risk for AIDS, hepatitis	Emotional state Denial of drug problem Demanding requests for use of nitrous oxide or pain medications Disoriented behavior	Neglect personal hygiene Potential for oral trauma Potential link (not documented) to oral cancer Potential drug interaction if local anesthetic with epinephrine is injected into blood vessel	Coordinated care: professional team and family if in treatment program Use of drugs for procedure: restrict Strict guidelines for keeping appointments necessary	Frequent brushing and flossing Teach oral self exams Avoid mouthrinses containing alcohol Topical fluoride program
Chronic alcoholism	Client's perception of severity of problem Symptoms Treatment program Nutritional deficiencies Chronic complications Degree of liver impairment At risk for TB	Potential for no-show appointments or intoxication at appointment	Susceptibility to infection Nutritional deficiencies Nausea and vomiting Potential for oral trauma	Liver impairment and bleeding potential: preappointment lab testing, drug metabolism, instrumentation, treatment planning Inebriated states: emergency care, appointment scheduling, treatment planning, data collection	Nutritional counseling Frequent continued care intervals Fluoride therapy and antimicrobials if needed Frequent soft tissue evaluation for oral cancer Counseling regarding oral trauma Saliva substitute for xerostomia

Continued.

Table 14-16

Dental Management Considerations for Special-Needs Clients—cont'd

Condition	Medical issues	Barriers to care	Risk factors	Treatment considerations*	Prevention/ education issues
				Associated medical problems (see management for each problem) Use only alcohol-free medicaments Recommend alcohol-free mouthrinses	Instill responsibility for oral care
Chronic renal failure	Symptoms and severity Hypertension Dialysis? Transplant? Special diets Need for antibiotic premedication Excretion of drugs Electrolyte and fluid imbalance	Finding dentist who will treat Debilitated condition at times Limited finances Fear of oral healthcare environment	Susceptibility to oral infection Dietary inadequacies Viral hepatitis Gingival hyperplasia from cyclosporine	Hypertension and kidney failure: vital signs, drug interactions, drug metabolism Bleeding tendency: preappointment blood tests, instrumentation, physician consult, hemostatic measures AV fistula: antibiotic premedication, take blood pressure in arm without fistula Dialysis: scheduling, hepatitis precautions Transplants: premedication with steroids or antibiotics, complete all care	3-6 month continued care interval because of increased calculus Prevent infection Palliative care for oral lesions Daily home fluoride therapy Tartar control dentifrices
Pregnancy	Trimester Side effects Nutritional status Rise in progesterone levels Significant changes in the immune response	Frequent sickness Physical comfort Nausea and sensitivity to various odors	Possible dietary inadequacies Vulnerability of fetus during first trimester Increased incidence of gingivitis	Fetal sensitivity: avoidance of drugs, radiographs, elective dental procedures Pressure of fetus on mother: chair position, orthostatic hypotension (turn on left side to alleviate)	Prenatal counseling Meticulous oral hygiene to decrease response to local irritants Education on the relationship between bacterial plaque, hormone level, and periodontal disease

Safest period to provide routine care is second trimester
Short appointments
No routine radiographs

Education on the relationship between caries process and gastric acids from vomiting
Education on care of infant's oral cavity and causes of early childhood caries
Daily home fluoride therapy if episodes of vomiting
Supplemental fluoride drops for nursing infants

PREVISIT QUESTIONNAIRE FOR GATHERING PRELIMINARY DATA ABOUT INDIVIDUALS WITH SPECIAL NEEDS

Name _____ Phone _____

Address _____ Age _____
_____

Name/address of contact person (if different) Phone _____
_____
_____
_____

Physician _____ Specialty _____ Phone _____

Physician _____ Specialty _____ Phone _____

Medical problems/disabling conditions _____

Potential barriers:

　Transportation _____

　Finances _____

　Communication _____

　Psychosocial _____

　Cultural _____

　Medical _____

　Medical/stability _____

　Other _____

Scheduling limitations _____

Other data _____

---

12. Provide both written and verbal instructions for medication regimens or posttreatment suggestions, and health education

13. Develop an office policy for medical situations and emergencies, differentiating between true emergencies and situations that just require common sense and appropriate responses (e.g., myocardial infarction versus a psychomotor seizure)

D. Treatment adaptations

1. Demonstrate understanding and acceptance of conditions or problems to the patient and to caretakers or family

2. Determine which special needs require provider adaptations versus client adaptations

3. Demonstrate empathy, not sympathy

4. Discuss before implementation
   a. Behavioral expectations
   b. Overview of the entire care plan
   c. Procedures that will be performed at that appointment
   d. Approximate time required
   e. Communication techniques to be used during the appointment

5. Introduce clients to the oral healthcare setting gradually by using desensitization, modeling, "show-and-tell," or other methods (Fig. 14-19)

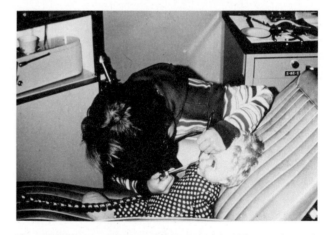

Fig. 14-19 Introducing child to oral healthcare through role playing with doll.

6. Ensure client comfort in the dental chair through frequent assurance, positioning, and supportive measures as needed (e.g., pillows)

7. Explain carefully any need for client restraint for behavioral or stability purposes to ensure the clinician's safety and client's safety while in the chair; Velcro straps similar to seat belts are helpful for stability (Fig. 14-20); need informed consent to use these

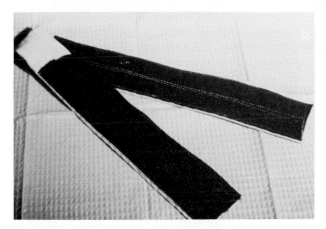

Fig. 14-20 Velcro strap used to provide patient stability in chair.

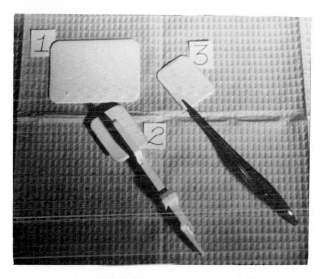

Fig. 14-21 Adaptations for procuring radiographs: *1*, occlusal size film; *2*, Snap-a-Ray; *3*, hemostat.

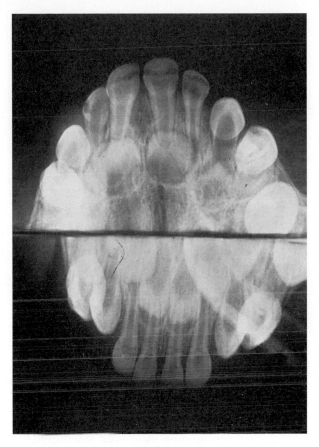

Fig. 14-22 Occlusal film adaptation.

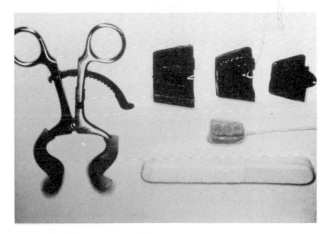

Fig. 14-23 Mouth props are useful for gaining intraoral access and jaw stability.

8. Be aware that adaptations for specific procedures require problem solving and experimentation between the provider, client, and caretaker, if appropriate; Fig. 14-21 and Fig. 14-22 show various adaptations for procuring radiographs; Fig. 14-23 displays a variety of mouth props
9. Discuss mechanisms for wheelchair transfers with each client because preferences and techniques vary
10. Protect the client's airway through use of a rubber dam, adequate suctioning, and other means; this is of paramount importance because of the frequency of impaired oral reflexes

E. Preventive measures
    1. Identify risk factors for oral disease to plan preventive programs that
        a. Maximize positive health behaviors
        b. Eliminate risk factors
        c. Eliminate existing disease
    2. Common risk factors include
        a. Inappropriate nursing and feeding habits (Fig. 14-24)

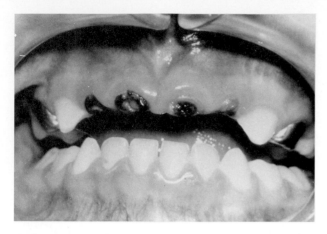

Fig. 14-24 Early childhood caries from inappropriate bottle or breast-feeding.

  b. Nutritionally inadequate diet
  c. Frequent intake of cariogenic foods
  d. Suboptimal fluoride supplementation
  e. Oral motor dysfunction (e.g., hyperactive gag reflex or impaired tongue control)
  f. General motor dysfunction interfering with oral hygiene care
  g. Crisis orientation to care
  h. Preoccupation with one's disability; depression
  i. Previous negative experience with health care
  j. Limited income and education
  k. Different cultural values and beliefs
3. Develop individualized programs to reduce or eliminate the risk factors
4. Consider the person's limitations when recommending home care procedures
  a. Problems with fluoride or antimicrobial rinses or disclosing tablets if the client has oral motor problems
  b. Problems performing the sequence of toothbrushing strokes if the client has memory or general motor impairment
  c. Problems picking up and using a toothbrush and toothpaste if the client has paralysis or control problems
5. Provide anticipatory guidance to parents on milestones and preventive measures at each developmental stage
6. Schedule frequent maintenance care appointments
7. Coordinate preventive efforts in home, school, work place, or oral healthcare setting

SUGGESTED READINGS

Because of constant changes in the incidence and management of the many conditions in this chapter, the author suggests reading articles in professional journals for the most up-to-date information. The following references and self-instructional materials may also prove helpful.

ADHA: Continuing education series on chemical dependence and dental hygiene care; Eating disorder patient: detection and oral care, Chicago, ADHA.

ADHA, ARC, ADH: Prevention and treatment considerations for the dental patient with special needs, Chicago, 1989, ADHA.

CHHIMA: Oral health care guidelines—a series of modules on special patient care, Chicago, ADA.

Darby ML, Walsh MM: *Dental hygiene theory and practice,* Philadelphia, 1995, WB Saunders, pp 751-998.

DECOD Program: Self-instructional series in rehabilitation dentistry, Seattle, University of Washington.

DeBiase CB: *Dental health education. Theory and practice,* Philadelphia, 1991, Lea & Febiger.

Lange BM, Entwistle BM, Lipson LF: *Dental management of the handicapped: Approaches for dental auxiliaries,* Philadelphia, 1983, Lea & Febiger.

Little JW, Falace DA: *Dental management of the medically compromised patient,* ed 5, St Louis, 1996, Mosby.

Malamed SF: *Handbook of medical emergencies in the dental office,* ed 4, St Louis, 1993, Mosby.

McCarthy FM: *Essentials of safe dentistry for the medically compromised patient,* Philadelphia, 1989, WB Saunders.

Rutkauskas JS, editor: Practical considerations in special patient care, *Dent Clin North Am* 38:361, 1994.

Terezhalmy GT, Saunders MJ, editors: Geriatric dentistry, *Dent Clin North Am* 33:1, 1989.

Thomas JE: What is appropriate care for a special patient? *Spec Care Dent* 9:127, 1989.

Wilkins EM: Clinical practice of the dental hygienist, ed 7, Philadelphia, 1994, Lea & Febiger.

Review Questions

Case A: Jerome Hindle

(see the synopsis of this client's history at the top of page 619).

1 The *MOST LIKELY* cause of his inflamed gingival condition is
  A. Bacterial plaque and calculus
  B. Side effects of seizure medications
  C. Side effects of Valium
  D. Necrotizing ulcerative gingivitis
  E. Undetected leukemia

2 Which gingival condition usually is *MOST* characteristic of phenytoin-induced gingival overgrowth (PIGO)?
  A. Bulbous and fibrous interdental papillae
  B. Bulbous and erythematous interdental papillae
  C. Festooned margins
  D. Cratered interdental papillae with exudate
  E. Pink tight gingiva with clefting

SYNOPSIS OF PATIENT HISTORY		
	Age _28_	VITAL SIGNS
	Sex _M_	Blood pressure _N/A_
	Height _N/A_	Pulse rate _N/A_
	Weight _N/A_ lbs _N/A_ kgs	Respiration rate _N/A_
CASE A: _Jerome Hindle_		

1. Under Care of Physician
   Yes No
   [X] [ ] Condition: _cerebral palsy, seizure disorder, mild mental retardation_

2. Hospitalized within the last 5 years
   Yes No
   [X] [ ] Reason: _medication adjustment for uncontrolled seizures_

3. Has or had the following conditions
   wears glasses for severe visual impairment; had surgery for cataracts

4. Current medications
   Dilantin (phenytoin) and Tegretol (carbamazepine) for seizures; Valium (diazepam) for muscle spasms and rigidity

5. Smokes or uses tobacco products
   Yes No
   [ ]   [X]

6. Is pregnant
   Yes No N/A
   [ ]   [ ]   [X]

MEDICAL HISTORY:
He was diagnosed with cerebral palsy (mixed type) as a young child and has received many years of special education, vocational training, along with occupational, physical, and speech therapy.

DENTAL HISTORY:
He received routine dental care as a child, but can't find a dental office where they treat him well and that he can afford. He hasn't been seen in about 2 years. He has some old amalgam restorations.

SOCIAL HISTORY:
He lives in a group home with six other adults and works at a Goodwill Industries sheltered workshop.

CHIEF COMPLAINT:
"I need my teeth cleaned. My gums bleed when I brush. I can't afford to go in very often."

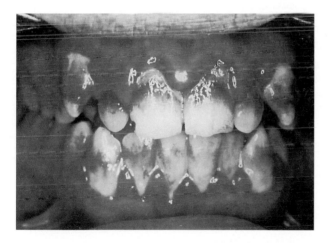

3 When providing toothbrushing instructions to this man, all of the following may be appropriate *EXCEPT* one. Which one is the *EXCEPTION*?
- A. He should use a tartar control toothpaste
- B. He should replace his toothbrush more often
- C. The group home counselor should perform his oral care
- D. He should use a toothpaste with a plaque-inhibiting agent
- E. He should use a toothbrush with a nonslip, enlarged handle

4 If you were providing care to this person, which precaution would *NOT* be appropriate during the appointment?
- A. Frequent suctioning and breaks to swallow
- B. Verbally tell him when you're going to use the air/water syringe
- C. Ask if all seizure medications have been taken as prescribed
- D. Get ready to insert tongue blades between his teeth in case of a seizure
- E. Fulcrum on the labials of the teeth or extraorally

5 Which is the *BEST* way to communicate with this client during the treatment part of the appointment?
- A. Ask him to use sign language
- B. Ask him to write what he wants to say
- C. Ask him questions that require yes/no answers and agree on a hand signal if he has a question or needs a break
- D. Ask him open-ended questions
- E. Tell him to wait until you're done to try to communicate

6 When providing health education, which is the *BEST* approach for his needs and abilities?
- A. Teach toothbrushing using a typodont
- B. Give him a pamphlet to take home
- C. Ask him to assess his progress after his teeth have been professionally cleaned by checking for blood on his toothbrush
- D. Ask him to assess his progress by checking the visual appearance of his gingiva
- E. Ask him to assess his progress by using a disclosing tablet

7 Which of the following probably are *NOT* barriers to dental care for him?
A. Finances
B. Transportation
C. Stability in the dental chair
D. Finding dental staff who are confident in treating him
E. Fear of dental procedures

8 If you were going to select a dental index to use in screening the adults at Goodwill Industries, which one would be *BEST* for assessing oral hygiene status using only a mirror and explorer?
A. OHI-S
B. CPITN
C. PDI
D. defs
E. DMFT

9 Which is the *BEST* radiographic option for this client at an initial examination to determine his needs?
A. Panographic radiograph
B. Two horizontal long bitewings
C. No radiographs
D. Complete radiographic survey
E. Four regular bitewings

10 An office that refuses to schedule an appointment for Jerome "because he has cerebral palsy" is demonstrating which of the following?
A. A legal right of the practitioner based on the client's condition
B. Discrimination according to the Americans with Disabilities Act
C. Discrimination according to the Equal Rights Amendment
D. A personal preference that is not an instance of discrimination
E. An uncommon reaction among primary care dentists in the United States

Case B: Madeline Greenspan

(see the synopsis of this client's history at the top of page 621).

11 The *MOST* likely cause of this client's jaw pain is
A. Dental abscess
B. Periodontal abscess
C. Arthritic involvement of joint
D. Bruxism
E. Undetected multiple sclerosis

12 Any of the following factors may be affecting her need for insulin and, therefore, aggravating her diabetes, *EXCEPT* for one? Which one is the *EXCEPTION*?
A. Depression
B. Food served at the nursing home
C. Periodontal disease
D. Restricted mobility
E. Orofacial pain

13 Diabinese is used for which of the following purposes?
A. An oral hypoglycemic agent
B. An antihistamine
C. An analgesic
D. A diuretic
E. An antidepressant

14 All of the following conditions could present problems when considering treatment options *EXCEPT* for one. Which one is the *EXCEPTION*?
A. Diabetes
B. Limited oral opening
C. Hip replacement
D. Joint deformities in fingers and hands
E. Limited ridge support and number of extractions needed

15 Given her condition, which is the *BEST* radiographic option for this patient at an initial oral examination to determine her needs?
A. Complete radiographic survey
B. Selected periapicals
C. Four bitewings and selected periapicals
D. Panographic radiograph and two bitewings
E. Panographic radiograph

16 What is the *BEST* and most realistic option for oral self-care at this point?
A. More frequent brushing using her current technique
B. Start flossing
C. Antimicrobial rinses
D. Purchase an electric toothbrush
E. Use tartar control toothpaste

17 Which of the following conditions is *NOT* associated with diabetes?
A. Cataracts
B. Delayed healing
C. Rapidly progressing periodontal disease
D. Motor and sensory neuropathies
E. Mucosal bleeding

18 Individuals with all but one of the following conditions may be on a special diet. Which one is the *EXCEPTION*?
A. Cystic fibrosis
B. End stage renal disease
C. Diabetes
D. Mild cardiac arrhythmia
E. Congestive heart failure

19 Secondary hypertension is seen *MOST* often in which one of the following conditions?
A. Cerebral palsy
B. Kidney disease
C. Viral hepatitis
D. Parkinson disease
E. Facioscapulohumoral muscular dystrophy

SYNOPSIS OF PATIENT HISTORY	Age	_72_	VITAL SIGNS	
	Sex	_F_	Blood pressure _N/A_	
	Height	_N/A_	Pulse rate _N/A_	
			Respiration rate _N/A_	
CASE B: _Madeline Greenspan_	Weight	_N/A_ lbs _N/A_ kgs		

1. Under Care of Physician

   Yes [X] No [ ]

   Condition: _Severe rheumatoid arthritis, Type II diabetes_

2. Hospitalized within the last 5 years

   Yes [X] No [ ]

   Reason: _hip replacement_

3. Has or had the following conditions

   severe joint deformities in fingers and hands, uses rolling walker, golfcart, or wheelchair; has glasses, diabetes.

4. Current medications

   Motrin (ibuprofen), Diabinese (chlorpropamide)

5. Smokes or uses tobacco products

   Yes [X] No [ ]

6. Is pregnant

   Yes [ ] No [ ] N/A [X]

MEDICAL HISTORY:

This woman started developing problems in her 50s from adult onset diabetes and also has severe rheumatoid arthritis.

DENTAL HISTORY:

She received regular care throughout her life. She hasn't seen a dentist since her husband died. She has few amalgams and has had some extractions.

SOCIAL HISTORY:

She moved into a nursing home 3 years ago when she became unable to live alone. Her husband died 5 years ago and she has no remaining family.

CHIEF COMPLAINT:

"I have toothaches and pains in my jaw. I can't hold the toothbrush well by myself and my toothbrush is worn out. I can't open my mouth very wide."

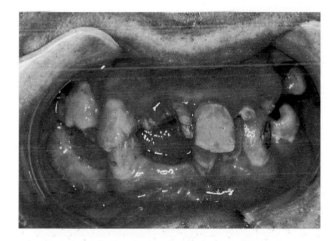

20 If a 200-pound client arrived for an appointment in a wheelchair with his attendant, which one of the following is *NOT* an option for performing a wheelchair transfer to the dental chair?

A. Asking him if he can transfer himself with someone's help

B. Asking the attendant to transfer him

C. Transferring him yourself using a one person transfer technique

D. Ask the dental assistant or dentist to help perform a two person transfer technique

E. Use a transfer board

21 All but one of the following may be a problem for an 85-year-old woman with a vision problem. Which one is the *EXCEPTION?*

A. Glare from the dental light

B. Heavy shag rug in the waiting room

C. Changes in color between the tile floor and the carpet

D. Raised door thresholds

E. Signs on the receptionist's desk

22 When taking a medical history about a seizure disorder, all of the following are critical questions *EXCEPT* one. Which one is the *EXCEPTION?*

A. What medications are you taking and did you take them as prescribed today?

B. Did you bring your medications to the appointment today?

C. What behaviors do you exhibit during a seizure?

D. How long do the seizures last?

E. Do you know when you're going to have a seizure (e.g., experience an aura or other sensation)?

23 All of the following may present problems for a person with Alzheimer's disease. Which one is *LEAST* likely to occur during toothbrushing?
   A. Doesn't brush all areas of the mouth
   B. Cannot follow a recommended sequence
   C. Brushes for the amount of time that is set on an electric timer with a buzzer
   D. Forgetting which is his toothbrush
   E. Wandering from the bathroom into the kitchen and putting the toothbrush into the refrigerator

24 Which of the following is *NOT* an important reason to identify risk factors for oral disease in each client?
   A. To maximize positive health behaviors
   B. To eliminate or reduce risk factors
   C. To eliminate or stabilize oral disease caused by risk factors
   D. To prevent behaviors that may become risk factors
   E. To minimize positive health behaviors

25 Which of the following is a medical emergency?
   A. Acute adrenal insufficiency
   B. A bronchial asthma client who is wheezing
   C. Tremors in an alcoholic
   D. Complete partial (psychomotor) seizure
   E. Tremors in a person with Parkinson disease

26 Which of the following is *NOT* true about osteoporosis?
   A. It is common in postmenopausal females
   B. It is common in young women
   C. Women with reduced estrogen levels are at risk for osteoporosis
   D. Osteoporosis is characterized by loss of bone density
   E. Women with osteoporosis experience more bone fractures

27 Premedication with antibiotics before periodontal debridement to prevent infective endocarditis is recommended for clients with a history of any of the following conditions *EXCEPT* one. Which one is the *EXCEPTION*?
   A. Rheumatic heart disease
   B. Prosthetic heart valves
   C. Myocardial infarction
   D. AV fistula in kidney dialysis patients
   E. Ventriculoatrial shunt for hydrocephalus

28 Chest pain is associated with all *EXCEPT* one of the following conditions. Which one is the *EXCEPTION*?
   A. Emphysema
   B. Angina
   C. Cardiac arrhythmia
   D. Hemophilia A
   E. Chronic obstructive pulmonary disease

Answers and Rationales

Case A. Jerome Hindle

1. (A) Bacterial plaque and calculus are the most likely cause of the inflammation because there is nothing systemic to cause it
   (B) Gingival inflammation is not a side effect of seizure medications
   (C) Gingival inflammation is not a side effect of Valium
   (D) ANUG would present with more blunted and cyanotic papillae
   (E) Leukemia is not generally associated with cerebral palsy

2. (A) Phenytoin-induced gingival overgrowth (PIGO) is characterized by pink fibrous tissue in the interdental spaces and the gingival margins
   (B) Erythema is associated with gingival inflammation, not PIGO without superimposed inflammation
   (C) Festooned margins can occur from a variety of causes
   (D) Cratered papillae are associated with ANUG, not PIGO
   (E) PIGO may show pseudoclefting but the gingiva is bulbous, not tight

3. (C) This client is capable of performing most of his own oral care
   (A) A tartar control toothpaste might reduce calculus buildup, but not necessarily inflammation
   (B) Worn-out toothbrushes will not be effective in removing bacterial plaque
   (D) Toothpaste with a plaque-inhibiting agent may reduce his gingivitis
   (E) Rigidity, contractures, and muscle spasms in cerebral palsy can interfere with effective grasp of the toothbrush

4. (D) Nothing should be forced between the teeth during a seizure
   (A) Frequent suctioning and breaks for swallowing are needed to control secretions
   (B) Use of the air/water syringe can cause an exaggerated startle response
   (C) Always ask if seizure medications have been taken as prescribed
   (E) Fulcruming on the occlusal surfaces sometimes is contraindicated due to bite reflexes and frequent jaw motions

5. (C) This is the best way to elicit information and give this client the most immediate control over communication during the appointment
   (A) Someone with cerebral palsy may not know signing, and the dental hygienist probably won't, so miscommunication is inevitable
   (B) Tremors and spasms interfere with writing, so verbal communication is better
   (D) Speaking in sentences is a prolonged, difficult process for someone with cerebral palsy, so short closed-end questions are best in most cases
   (E) Clients should not have to wait until the end of the appointment to communicate

6. (C) An obvious sign such as blood that is visible on the toothbrush and can be tasted is easiest for him to monitor

    (A) Transference of skills is easier with intraoral teaching

    (B) He may not be able to read well because he has vision problems and also visual motor disturbances from the cerebral palsy

    (D) His visual problem may interfere with seeing evidence of gingivitis intraorally

    (E) Involuntary oral reflexes and drooling make use of disclosing tablets ineffective and inappropriate

7. (E) This client displays no attitudes that would indicate a fear of dental procedures

    (A) Pay rates at sheltered workshops are mostly based on minimum wage scales

    (B) Use of a wheelchair entails finding wheelchair-accessible transportation or waiting for someone to transfer him from his wheelchair to a car and then back to the wheelchair a few times

    (C) Rigidity and spasms can create unstable positioning in the dental chair

    (D) He already has complained about previous dental providers, and many dental providers have not had training or experience in treating persons with developmental disabilities

8. (A) OHI-S was designed to reflect oral hygiene status and calculus in a screening setting using minimal instruments

    (B) CPITN entails use of a probe, good lighting, and good cooperation

    (C) PDI entails use of a probe, good lighting, and good cooperation

    (D) defs is a caries index for children

    (E) DEFT is a caries index for adults

9. (A) A panographic radiograph will show an overview of the entire mouth with minimal cooperation and time

    (B) This is the second best option but may trigger a gag reflex and doesn't show the anterior region

    (C) Some type of radiograph is needed to assess the extent of oral disease

    (D) This patient's involuntary reflexes will make a complete survey with bitewings and periapicals almost impossible

    (E) Four bitewings require more time, will probably trigger his gag reflex, and will not show the anterior region

10. (B) This violates the nondiscrimination requirements of the Americans with Disabilities Act

    (A) The practitioner does not have a legal right to discriminate based solely on a medical label and without seeing the client

    (C) The Equal Rights Amendment does not address the rights of the disabled

    (D) Personal preference in this case is still a case of discrimination

    (E) This reaction tends to be very common in the United States, despite the law

Case B. Madeline Greenspan

11. (C) TMJ involvement is common in severe rheumatoid arthritis

    (A) A dental abscess would generally occur around the tooth, not the joint area

    (B) A periapical abscess would generally occur around the tooth, not the joint area

    (D) Bruxism may cause TMJ pain, but is probably not the primary cause of her jaw pain

    (E) Jaw pain only occurs in some patients with multiple sclerosis, and she would exhibit other symptoms first

12. (B) Individuals with diabetes usually are given carefully planned meals by the dieticians at nursing homes

    (A) Depression can increase need for insulin

    (C) Periodontal disease can increase need for insulin

    (D) Restricted mobility decreases need for insulin

    (E) Orofacial pain can increase need for insulin

13. (A) Diabinese is a common oral hypoglycemic used to increase production of insulin

    (B) There is no need for an antihistamine in this patient

    (C) Aspirin or ibuprofen usually are used as analgesics

    (D) This patient is not on any diuretics

    (E) Although she is depressed, Diabinese is not used as an antidepressant

14. (C) Hip replacement won't usually interfere with treatment options, only the need for oral premedication

    (A) Diabetes can prolong infections and delay wound healing

    (B) Limited oral opening can affect appointment times and ability to insert and remove a removable prosthetic appliance

    (D) Joint deformities and contractures make toothbrushing and ability to grasp removable appliances difficult

    (E) Options for making removable appliances versus maintaining periodontally involved teeth may be limited

15. (E) Given her limited oral opening and your need to visualize the TMJ area, a panographic radiograph is initially indicated

    (A) Her limited opening may preclude a complete radiographic survey

    (B) Periapicals may be accomplished later after an initial treatment plan has been developed

    (C) Limited oral opening will preclude these as a first option

    (D) Bitewings are not very useful for determining periodontal or periapical involvement

16. (C) Given the joint deformities in her hands, antimicrobial rinses would reduce pathogens and gingivitis

    (A) Toothbrushing is difficult given her joint deformities, so her present toothbrushing method is not very effective

    (B) Her joint deformities probably preclude flossing by herself

    (D) Although an electric toothbrush may be beneficial, it is expensive and someone needs to assess if she can hold it and use it effectively

    (E) Tartar control toothpaste may help with calculus, but antimicrobials will be more effective against the inflammation and infection

17. (E) Bleeding disorders are not associated with diabetes
    (A) Cataracts are caused by vascular changes in the eye from the diabetes
    (B) Delayed healing is a common symptom of diabetes
    (C) Infections can progress rapidly and reparative processes are impaired
    (D) Motor and sensory neuropathies are chronic complications in diabetes

18. (D) Mild arrhythmias don't necessitate any dietary modifications
    (A) Cystic fibrosis requires constant monitoring of salt, fat, protein, and caloric intake
    (B) In renal failure, sodium, potassium, water, protein, and maintaining acid-base balance is important
    (C) Glucose intake is crucial in diabetes
    (E) Congestive heart failure requires weight reduction and restriction of sodium

19. (B) Secondary hypertension is common in kidney failure
    (A) Secondary hypertension is not associated with cerebral palsy
    (C) Viral hepatitis affects the liver, not the kidneys
    (D) Orthostatic hypotention occurs in Parkinson disease, not hypertension
    (E) Hypertension is not associated with this type of muscular dystrophy

20. (C) This client is too large for the dental hygienist to perform a transfer alone
    (A) This should be the first question of any patient in a wheelchair
    (B) Personal attendants perform transfers all the time and the patient is probably most comfortable with him doing so
    (D) It is a reasonable expectation that you will need assistance doing most wheelchair transfers
    (E) Transfer boards are sometimes easier to use if the patient has one

21. (C) Changes in color will help this woman identify when there are changes in surfaces
    (A) Glare from the light may further reduce her visual acuity or cause eye pain
    (B) She may trip over a heavy shag rug, especially if she is shuffling her feet
    (D) She can trip over a raised threshold before she sees it
    (E) She may not be able to read directional or other informational signs

22. (B) They don't normally carry their medications to appointments if they have already taken them as prescribed
    (A) Knowing which medications they currently take is important for identifying drug interactions and risk factors for oral problems
    (C) Knowing what behaviors to expect will help in recognizing and managing a seizure, because behaviors vary greatly
    (D) You will need to know the usual duration of seizures to determine if the patient is experiencing status epilepticus
    (E) Sometimes if they feel a seizure occurring you can remove anything that might injure them in the operatory

23. (C) Structuring the setting like this is most apt to assure success
    (A) Attention may drift before all areas of the mouth are brushed
    (B) Remembering sequences is a problem in Alzheimer disease
    (D) Short-term memory is a problem
    (E) Wandering and putting items in strange places is a common problem in Alzheimer disease

24. (E) You should be maximizing these behaviors, not minimizing them
    (A) Maximizing positive behaviors will prevent oral disease
    (B) Eliminating or reducing risk factors will increase oral health
    (C) Identifying the risk factor can help in planning appropriate treatment
    (D) Early identification and counseling about risk factors for disease is an example of primary prevention

25. (A) Acute adrenal insufficiency is a medical emergency
    (B) Wheezing is a characteristic of bronchial asthma and is not an emergency unless the patient goes into status asthmaticus
    (C) Chronic alcoholics generally present with tremors, especially during periods of withdrawal
    (D) Psychomotor seizures generally do not constitute a medical emergency
    (E) Tremors are common in Parkinson disease

26. (B) Osteoporosis is usually not apparent in young women who do not have a systemic medical problem
    (A) Postmenopausal women are at risk for osteoporosis because of reduced estrogen levels
    (C) Decreased estrogen levels lead to osteoporosis
    (D) In osteoporosis the rate at which bone breaks down exceeds the rate at which it is replaced
    (E) Osteoporosis is a common cause of bone fractures and hip replacements in elderly women

27. (C) Myocardial infarction does not require antibiotics because it does not place the patient at risk for bacterial endocarditis
    (A) Rheumatic heart disease may require antibiotic premedication if there is valvular damage
    (B) Prosthetic heart valves require premedication
    (D) Some physicians will prescribe antibiotics for AV fistulas in dialysis patients
    (E) Some physicians will prescribe antibiotics for ventriculoatrial shunts in hydrocephalic patients

28. (D) Joint pain is common in Hemophilia A, not chest pain
    (A) Chest pain in emphysema is from obstructed airways
    (B) Angina produces severe chest pain from cardiovascular disease
    (C) Irregular heart beats can produce chest pain
    (E) In COPD chest pain is from airway obstruction

Community Oral Health Planning and Practice

Pamela Zarkowski

Assessment, planning, diagnosis, implementation, and evaluation—the dental hygiene process of care—are used by the dental hygienist in community oral health practice and program development. Community health extends the role of the dental hygienist from the traditional healthcare setting to the community as a whole. In a sense, the community can be viewed as the client, and the oral care environment is the neighborhood health center, extended care facility, hospital, school, agency, or country.

With increased emphasis on improving public access to oral healthcare, the responsibilities of the dental hygienist to promote oral health in the community take on renewed importance. This chapter focuses on the knowledge and skills necessary for various roles in community oral health. Topics include basic concepts of epidemiology and trends in oral diseases, assessment tools, dental health education strategies, basic statistical and research concepts, evaluation of dental literature, the provision and financing of dental care, and the need for, demand for, and use of dental services.

Basic Concepts

A. Health—"state of well-being with both objective and subjective dimensions that exists on a continuum from maximal wellness to maximal illness. The higher the level of human needs fulfillment, the higher the state of wellness. Health may change along this continuum under the influence of biological, psychological, spiritual, social, and cultural factors that are interrelated and fluctuate over time"[1-3]

B. Public health—science and art of preventing disease, prolonging life, and promoting physical and mental health and efficiency through organized community efforts
  1. Public health is concerned with the aggregate health of a group, a community, a state, a nation, or a group of nations
  2. Public health is people's health
  3. Concerned with four broad areas
    a. Lifestyle, behavior, and culture
    b. The environment
    c. Human biology
    d. The organization of health programs and systems

C. Dental public health—science and art of preventing and controlling oral diseases and promoting oral health through organized community efforts; that form of dental practice that serves the community as a client rather than the individual; concerned with the oral health education of the public, with applied dental research, and with the administration of group oral

Table 15-1

Comparison of Private Dental Practice and Community Oral Health Practice

Private dental practice	Community dental practice
Assessment of client's dental, health, and sociocultural history and oral health status	Survey of community oral health status; situation analysis including assessment of population demographics, mobility, economic resources, and infrastructure
Diagnosis of client's oral health	Analysis of survey data to determine oral health needs
Treatment plan based on diagnosis and client's needs and priorities	Program plan based on data analysis, priorities, and resources available
Treatment plan initiated; primary dentist may coordinate treatment with other providers (e.g., dental hygienists, specialists)	Program operation implemented; personnel will involve a varied group
Payment methods determined	Financing takes place throughout process; may be combination of local, state, and federal funds
Evaluation during treatment, at specific intervals, and/or on completion of treatment	Evaluation/appraisal is ongoing, conducted in terms of effectiveness, efficiency, appropriateness, and adequacy

health care programs, as well as the prevention and control of oral diseases on a community basis
D. Community—not strictly defined by traditional geographic boundaries; as broad as a region of a state or as focused as a nursing home community including administrators, staff, residents, and caretakers
E. Community health—synonymous with public health; full range of health services, environmental and personal, including major activities such as health education of the public and the social context of life as it affects the community; efforts that are organized to promote and restore the health and quality of life of the people
F. Community oral health services are directed toward developing, reinforcing, and enhancing the oral health status of people either as individuals or collectively as groups and communities
G. Comparison of private versus community health (Table 15-1)
H. Criteria for a public health problem
1. A disease or other threat to health is widespread
2. The disease is one that can be prevented, alleviated, or cured
3. Such knowledge is not being applied

Epidemiology

Basic Concepts

A. Epidemiology—study of health and disease in human populations and how these states are influenced by the environment and ways of living; concerned with factors and conditions that determine the occurrence and

distribution of health, disease, defects, disability, and deaths among individuals (Fig. 15-1)
B. Epidemiology, in conjunction with the statistical and research methods used, focuses on comparisons between groups or defined populations
C. Characteristics of epidemiology
1. Groups rather than individuals are studied
2. Disease is multifactorial; host-agent-environment relationship becomes critical
3. A disease state depends on exposure to a specific agent, strength of the agent, susceptibility of the host, and environmental conditions
4. Factors
a. Host: age, race, ethnic background, physiologic state, gender, culture
b. Agent: chemical, microbial, physical or mechanical irritants, parasitic, viral or bacterial
c. Environment: climate or physical environment, food sources, socioeconomic conditions
5. Interaction among factors affects disease or health status
D. Related concepts
1. Acute—beginning abruptly with marked intensity or sharpness, then subsiding after a relatively short period of time
2. Chronic—developing slowly and persisting for a long period of time, often for the remainder of the lifetime of the individual
3. Epidemic—a disease of significantly greater prevalence than normal; more than the expected number of cases; a disease that spreads rapidly through a demographic segment of a population
4. Endemic—continuing problem involving normal

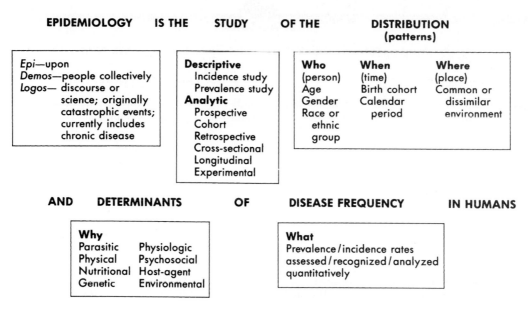

Fig. 15-1 Study of epidemiology

disease prevalence; the expected number of cases; indigenous to a population or geographic area

5. Pandemic—occurring throughout the population of a country, people, or the world
6. Mortality—death
7. Morbidity—disease
8. Rate—a numerical ratio in which the number of actual occurrences appears as the numerator and number of possible occurrences appears as the denominator; often used in compilation of data concerning the prevalence and incidence of events; measure of time is an intrinsic part of the denominator (Table 15-2)

F. Research concepts
1. Research—"continual search for truth using the scientific method"[4]
2. Sample—"a portion of the population that, if properly selected, can provide meaningful information about the entire population; a sample is examined when the researcher has neither the time, money, nor resources to study an entire population"[4]
3. Convenience sample—"used when access to the total population is not feasible; members of the available sample are numbered consecutively, and a table of random sample numbers is used for experimental and control group assignments"[4]
4. Random sample—"a sample composed of subjects who are chosen independently of each other, with known opportunity or probability for inclusion; increases external validity; controls intersubject difference"[4]

5. Nonrandomized sample—"sample that is not randomly selected from a general population, therefore making generalizations to a larger population invalid; intact groups; threatens external validity"[4]
6. Population—"that portion of the universe to which the researcher wants to generalize findings"[4]
7. Table of random numbers—"a table composed of numbers that have been generated by a random technique; used to select a random sample"[4]

Science of Epidemiology

A. Uses of epidemiology
1. Study of patterns among groups
2. Collecting data to describe normal biologic processes
3. Understanding the natural history of disease
4. Testing hypotheses for prevention and control of disease through special studies in populations
5. Planning and evaluating healthcare services
6. Studying of nondisease entities such as suicide or injury
7. Measuring the distribution of diseases in populations
8. Identifying risk factors and determinants of disease
9. Evaluation of intervention and preventive strategies to control disease
10. Evaluating trends in chronic disease and social epidemiology

B. Three classifications of epidemiologic research
1. Descriptive research—"involves description, docu-

	Table 15-2	
	Comparison of Clinical Trials and Epidemiologic Surveys	
	Clinical trial	**Epidemiologic survey**
Populations	Experimental and control groups are specially constituted as representative samples from appropriate populations	Naturally occurring samples of target populations are usually studied
Sample size	Sample sizes are often small, particularly when "treatments" are more complicated	Fairly large sample sizes are employed
Time frame	Trials are conducted over a period of time usually varying from 1 week to 6 months to a couple of years (i.e., caries research), depending on treatment involved, to compare treatment effects	Surveys are usually cross-sectional in design, using only one time period; longitudinal designs are used occasionally
Methods	While assessment methods may be indices, methods used should have acuity and clinical significance	Indices used for assessment establish a disease level of selected populations; these indices should be in general use to enable comparison of data for different populations
Data	Data generated from clinical trials should be applicable for specific hypothesis testing	Data generated from surveys are used to establish underlying etiologic factors and derive possible preventive methods, leading to development of hypotheses to be tested by controlled clinical trials

mentation, analysis, and interpretation of data to evaluate a current event or situation"[1]

a. Incidence—"number of new cases of a specific disease within a defined population over a period of time"[4]

b. Prevalence—"number of persons in a population affected by a condition at any one time"[4]

c. Count—simplest sum of disease; number of cases of disease occurrence

d. Proportion—use of a count with the addition of a denominator to determine prevalence; does not include a time dimension; useful to evaluate prevalence of caries in schoolchildren or tooth loss in adult populations

e. Rate—uses a standardized denominator and includes a time dimension, for example, the number of deaths of newborn infants within first year of life per 1000 births

2. Analytical research—determines the cause of disease or if a causal relationship exists between a factor and a disease

a. Prospective study—planning of the entire study is completed before data are collected and analyzed; population is followed through time to determine which members develop the disease; several hypotheses may be tested at one time

b. Cohort study—individuals are classified into groups according to whether or not they possess a particular characteristic thought to be related to the condition of interest; observations occur over time to see who develops disease or condition

c. Retrospective study (ex post facto study)—decision to carry out an investigation using observations or data that have been collected in the past; data may be incomplete or in a manner not appropriate for study

d. Cross-sectional study—"study of subgroups of individuals in a specific and limited time frame to identify either initially to describe current status or developmental changes in the overall group from the perspective of what is typical in each subgroup"[4]

e. Longitudinal study—"investigation of the same group of individuals over an extended period of time to identify a change or development in that group"[4]

3. Experimental research—used when the etiology of the disease is established and the researcher wishes to determine the effectiveness of altering some factor or factors; deliberate applying or withholding of the supposed cause of a condition and observing the result

C. Distribution and determinants of disease

1. Disease is multifactorial in nature; difficult to identify one particular cause

a. Host risk factors

(1) Immunity to disease/natural resistance
(2) Heredity
(3) Age, gender, race, culture
(4) Physical or morphologic factors
  b. Agent risk factors
(1) Biologic—microbiologic
(2) Chemical—poisons, dosage levels
(3) Physical—environmental exposure
  c. Environment risk factors
(1) Physical—geography and climate
(2) Biologic—animal hosts and vectors
(3) Social—socioeconomic, education, nutrition
2. All factors must be present to be sufficient cause for disease
3. Interplay of these risk factors is ongoing; to affect the disease, attack at the weakest link

Epidemiology of Oral Disease

A. Regional differences in dental caries experience were documented as early as the 1930s in various Native American tribes
1. Surveys of individuals recruited for World War II indicated that severe caries were identified in residents of New England, the Pacific Northwest, and the Great Lakes, with less severity found in individuals from the south, southwest, and mountain states[5]
2. Fluoridation has impacted and somewhat obscured the regional differences
3. Despite a decline in dental caries in children and the improving oral health of adults, regional differences still exist
B. Dental caries in the United States[6]
1. Over the past few decades, a substantial decline in cumulative dental caries experience has been observed among both younger adults and children in the United States
  a. Fluoride is the significant factor for decline
  b. Contributing factors include water fluoridation, the use of fluoride supplements, fluoride dentifrices, and dental sealants
2. The mean decayed, missing and filled surface (DMFS) scores declined among adults aged 18 to 44 years in 1985 compared with individuals of similar age in 1971-74
3. In the 1986-87 National Children's Oral Health Survey, the DMFS score for schoolchildren aged 5 to 17 years of 3.07 was 36% lower than the score of 4.77 observed in 1979-80
4. Although a reported decline, dental caries is widespread
  a. According to the 1986-87 National Children's Oral Health Survey, one half of the 5 to 17-year-olds had experienced dental caries
  b. At age 17, the mean number of decayed and filled surfaces was nearly 8 and only 15.6% of 17-year-olds were caries free
  c. By ages 25 to 29 years, young adults experienced more than 17 DF surfaces
5. Caries patterns have changed showing a greater percent reduction for smooth surface caries, thus there are proportionately fewer smooth surface lesions than pit and fissure lesions on occlusal and faciolingual surfaces.
  a. Most decay on children's permanent teeth occurs in the buccal pits of mandibular molars and lingual grooves of maxillary molars
  b. In 1987 occlusal caries accounted for 58% of the caries observed in children 5 to 17 years of age
  c. In 1987, 88% of the caries in U.S. schoolchildren were found in pit and fissure surfaces and two thirds of the carious or filled surfaces were of the pit and fissure type
6. The NHANES III (Third National Health and Nutrition Examination Survey's [1988-94]) objective was to collect data on the health and nutritional status of the US civilian noninstitutionalized population aged 2 months and older[7]
  a. Oral health component included evaluation of magnitude and relative frequency of selected oral disease; distribution of diseases; describe associated risk factors and document secular trends
  b. Target population included US civilian and noninstitutionalized population in 50 states
  c. Survey yielded weighted estimates for 1988-91 for over 58 million US children and adolescents 1 to 17 years of age
(1) Primary Dentition[6]
    (a) Infants 12 to 23 months, 0.8% were scored positive for early childhood caries
    (b) About 62.1% of children aged 2 to 9 years were caries free in primary dentition
    (c) Similar percentages of females and males were caries free in their primary dentition within every age group
    (d) A higher percentage of white children age 2 to 4 years (85.3%) were caries free in primary dentition than were black children
    (e) Non-Hispanic white children 2 to 4 years of age were more often caries free

in their primary dentition (87.0%) than either non-Hispanic blacks (78.0%) or Mexican-Americans (67.7%)

(f) Both the non-Hispanic white (54.0%) and the non-Hispanic black children (51.4%) aged 5 to 9 were more often caries free in the primary dentition than the Mexican-American children (34.5%)

(g) On the average, children 2 to 9 years of age had 3.1 decayed and filled primary surfaces

(2) Permanent Dentition[6]

(a) About 55% of the children aged 5 to 17 years were caries free

(b) The mean DMFS for children aged 5 to 17 years was 2.5; filled surfaces comprised the largest mean percentage component per individual (78.4%) for children with affected teeth

(c) Males were similar to females

(d) A higher percentage of black children aged 5 to 17 (60.4%) than white children (54.3%) were caries free in their permanent dentition; non-Hispanic black children aged 5 to 17 years had the highest overall percentage of children who were caries free in the permanent dentition as compared with non-Hispanic whites and 51.4% of Mexican-Americans

(e) The mean DMFS was similar for race and race-ethnicity groups; mean percentages of components per person with evidence of dental caries varies—in African Americans on average, more than one third (37.7%) of the DMFS were untreated caries, whereas less than 60% were filled; in contrast, for white persons on average, less than one in five surfaces were decayed (17.2%) and over 80% were filled

(f) Non-Hispanic black and Mexican-American children and adolescents had higher percentages of decayed surfaces and lower percentages of filled surfaces than did non-Hispanic white individuals

(3) Coronal Caries[8]

(a) About 94% of adults in the United States show evidence of past or present coronal caries

(b) In dentate persons, mean number of decayed and filled coronal surfaces per person was 21.5

(c) Dentate females had a lower number of untreated coronal tooth surfaces with caries (1.5), but higher mean number of treated and untreated surfaces per person than males (22.7)

(d) Standardized data for age and gender indicated that dentate non-Hispanic blacks (11.9) and Mexican-Americans (14.1) had half the number of decayed and filed coronal surfaces as non-Hispanic whites (24.3) but more untreated surfaces

(e) Mexican-Americans were most likely to be dentate; had the highest average number of teeth; and had 25% fewer decayed, missed, and filled coronal surfaces (37.6) than non-Hispanic blacks and non-Hispanic whites

(f) Root caries affected 22.5% of the dentate population

(g) Blacks had the most treated and untreated root surfaces with caries (1.6), close to Mexican-Americans (1.4)

(h) Untreated root caries is most common in dentate non-Hispanic blacks (1.5), followed by Mexican-Americans (1.2), with non-Hispanic whites (0.6) having the fewest untreated carious root surfaces

(i) Mean number of root surfaces per person with untreated decay was higher in men (0.9) than women (0.5) and age standardization had no impact on the means

(4) Dental sealants[9]

(a) About 18.5% of US children and youth ages 5 to 17 had one or more sealed permanent teeth

(b) Significantly higher percentage of non-Hispanic whites had sealants in comparison with their non-Hispanic black and Mexican-American counterparts

(c) Molar teeth were most frequently sealed

(d) Only 1.4% of U.S. children aged 2 to 11 years had at least one sealed primary tooth

(e) The prevalence of dental sealants decreased in the US adult population with increasing age, 5.5% of adults ages 18 to 24 years had at least one sealed permanent tooth

(5) Periodontal Status[10]

(a) Over 90% of persons 13 years of age or older had experienced some clinical loss of attachment; only 15% exhibited more severe destruction

(b) Prevalence of moderate and severe loss of attachment and gingival recession increased with age, but prevalence of pockets ≥4 mm or ≥6 mm did not

(c) Prevalence of pockets ≥4 mm in depth was 30%; pockets >6 mm were found in less than 4% of the population

(d) Persons over 45 years of age were estimated to have slightly higher percentages of sites with deep pockets than younger persons

(e) Gingival recession ≥1 mm was 42%; the prevalence of more severe recession >3 mm was 15%

(f) About 63% had some gingival bleeding with the highest among individuals 13 to 17 years of age; among individuals aged 18 years and older, the prevalence of gingival bleeding did not exhibit much variation with age, ranging between 60% and 65%

(g) Females exhibited better periodontal health than males, and non-Hispanic whites exhibited better periodontal health than either non-Hispanic blacks or Mexican-Americans.

(h) Higher prevalence of moderate and deep pockets was found in males than in females; more males (45%) than females (40%) experienced recession

(i) No differences between non-Hispanic whites and non-Hispanic blacks were observed in relation to loss of attachment; the prevalence of loss of attachment ≥1 mm was not different between non-Hispanic whites and Mexican-Americans, both groups demonstrated prevalence of over 90%; higher percentages of sites with loss of attachment ≥3 mm were found among non-Hispanic whites compared with Mexican-Americans, however differences were small

(6) Tooth Retention/Tooth Loss[11]

(a) In 1988-91 89.5% of the population was dentate, and 30.5% had retained all 28 teeth

(b) Mean number of retained teeth was 21.1 for adults and 23.5 for all dentate persons

(c) Most common retained teeth in the mouth were the six anterior mandibular teeth

(d) About 10.5% of the population was edentulous; partial edentulism was more common in the maxilla than in the mandible

(e) Most common missing teeth were the first and second molars

(f) Hispanics had the highest rates of tooth loss

(g) No gender related differences

(7) Denture Use[12]

(a) One in five persons 18 to 74 years of age wears a removable prosthodontic appliance

(b) Removable prosthodontic appliances are worn disproportionately more often by women than by men and less frequently by whites than blacks

(c) Mexican-Americans are less likely to use dentures than either blacks or whites

7. Socioeconomic Status (SES)

a. Includes education, income, occupation, attitudes and values; frequently evaluated as it relates to health-associated characteristics

b. Studies vary; treatment effects in higher SES groups influence DMF scores

c. Powerful determinant of dental caries status

8. Diet is the total oral intake of substances that provide nourishment and/or calories; nutrition is the absorption of nutrients and/or calories (see Chapter 9, section on nutritional counseling)

a. Dietary factors, especially sugar, have an influence on prevalence of dental caries

b. Relationship exists between frequent consumption of fermentable carbohydrate and incidence of dental caries

c. Specific bacteria present in dental plaque ferment dietary carbohydrate to produce organic acids that demineralize tooth structure

d. Plaque bacteria use carbohydrates to produce the sticky gel-like matrix of the plaque

e. Fats and proteins have demonstrated noncariogenic effects
(1) Fats may decrease caries activity by altering surface properties of enamel, reducing sugar solubilization, being toxic to oral bacteria, or simply replacing dietary carbohydrates
(2) Proteins may reduce caries posteruptively by a direct effect on plaque metabolism, by replacement of dietary carbohydrates, or by increasing salivary urea levels
f. Fluoride is an essential nutrient; presence affects decalcification and remineralization process (see Chapter 10, section on fluoride gels, and Chapter 12, section on fluorides)
9. Familial and genetic patterns
a. Familial tendencies for dental caries are reported anecdotally and within the research
b. Studies are not clear whether familial tendencies have a genetic basis or related to familial dietary and behavioral traits
10. Nursing bottle syndrome
a. Studies vary; higher prevalence in specific groups studied; however, a widespread condition
b. Appears more prevalent in low SES-populations or in circumstances where child care is provided by individuals with little education or understanding of disease prevention
C. Periodontal diseases
1. Decline in dental caries has resulted in an increased attention to periodontal diseases by both the public and the oral health professions
2. Gingivitis or periodontitis is almost universally prevalent with over 70% of adults in all countries affected; worldwide data collected in the 1980s indicate the prevalence of severe periodontitis in the range of 7% to 15% in almost all populations, regardless of economic development, oral hygiene, or dental care available[13]
3. Studies indicate that gingivitis of varying severity is a universal finding in children and young adolescents
a. Prevalence of destructive forms of periodontal disease is lower in young individuals than adults
b. Loss of periodontal attachment and supporting bone at one or more sites can be found in 1% to 9% of 5 to 11-year-olds and 1% to 46% of 12 to 15-year-olds
c. Variation in data reported attributed to study design
4. Distinct periodontal infections that can affect young adults include

a. Chronic gingivitis
b. Early-onset periodontitis
c. Necrotizing ulcerative gingivitis/periodontitis
d. Periodontitis associated with systemic diseases
5. Adults[14,15] (see Chapter 11, subsection on Natural History of Periodontal Disease)
a. Findings indicate that a small proportion of individuals experience severe periodontitis; mild gingivitis is common, as is mild to moderate periodontitis; most adults exhibit some loss of bony support and loss of probing attachment while still maintaining a functioning dentition
b. Results of a nationwide survey of the dental health of American adults show gingival bleeding in 43% of working adults and 47% of seniors; 84% of the employed group and 89% of seniors had calculus; 77% of the younger adults and 95% of the older group had at least one site with periodontal attachment loss; average amount of attachment loss was 2 mm in employed adults and 3.2 mm in seniors
c. Periodontal destruction, 4 mm or more of attachment loss, was found in 24% of the employed adults and 68% of the older persons
d. Adults are susceptible to both gingivitis and periodontitis with concomitant attachment loss; gingivitis precedes periodontitis, but a small number of sites with gingivitis later develop periodontitis
e. Difficult to determine prevalence for adult gingivitis because of variance in measurement of different studies; also tendency to pool gingivitis and periodontitis measurements[14]
(1) Data for worldwide prevalence of adult gingivitis vary considerably
(2) Percentage of dental population with gingivitis is high
f. Suggested that most epidemiologic studies severely underestimate adult gingivitis and, to lesser extent, periodontitis
6. It is now recognized that periodontal diseases are manifested as different clinical entities depending on age of onset, severity, teeth affected, rate of progression, and other factors[14]
7. Factors affect the prevalence and severity of periodontal diseases[14]
a. Periodontal disease is inversely correlated to increasing education and increasing family income
b. No real differences in levels of periodontal disease can be detected if groups are balanced for age, gender, or socioeconomic status; differences observed are attributed to oral hygiene status

c. Data suggest greater extent of disease among older than younger persons; prevalence and severity of chronic inflammatory disease increase directly with increasing age; the risk for disease increases for older adults who keep their teeth

d. Prevalence and severity of periodontal disease are higher in rural areas than in urban areas

e. There is a positive relationship between periodontal disease and the level of oral hygiene[14]

(1) Statistically, bacteria in plaque is the primary etiologic factor of periodontal disease

(2) Etiologic role of oral hygiene in periodontitis is similar to sugar in the caries process; more critical among susceptible individuals than the less susceptible

(3) Most forms of gingivitis are direct result of growth and accumulation of oral microorganisms

(4) Difference in periodontal disease levels between peoples of developed and developing countries is attributed to differences in oral hygiene levels

f. No inherent differences between men and women in susceptibility to periodontitis; women do exhibit better oral hygiene practices than men

g. No inherent differences to susceptibility among races or ethnic groups

h. No relationship has been found between nutrition or dietary factors, e.g., deficiency of ascorbic acid and disease; more study is necessary, but increased levels of prevalence and intensity of periodontal disease are found in areas of the world where generalized malnutrition is common

D. Oral cancer

1. Includes cancers of lips, tongue, buccal mucosa, floor of the mouth, and pharynx

2. Occurrence of oral cancer and site distribution within the mouth vary widely in different parts of the world (e.g., carcinoma of buccal mucosa as a result of chewing betel nuts in the Far East)

3. Tobacco use is primary risk factor

4. Oral cancer is two times more prevalent in males, and there are twice as many deaths in males as in females; differences in sites between males and females; affects older men, heavy users of alcohol and tobacco, and individuals exposed to sunlight; males 40 to 65 years of age have highest number of lip and tongue cancers

5. Oral cancer is related to increasing age and exposure to sun

6. Risk factors identified include smoking, alcohol consumption, painful and ill-fitting dentures, chronic inflammation, and use of smokeless tobacco products

E. Cleft lip and palate

1. Genetic and environmental factors significant

2. Approximately 6000 children are born in the United States each year with cleft lip and/or palate

3. The incidence is highest in Asian–Pacific Islanders (particularly Japanese) with approximately 1/500; in whites, 1/700; in African-Americans, 1/2000

4. Epidemiologic correlations indicate

a. More isolated cleft palates appear in girls

b. More facial clefts appear in boys

c. A relation exists between clefts and premature births

d. Infants with clefts are of lower birth weight than the general population of infants

5. Clefts are associated with threatened spontaneous abortion during the first and second trimesters of pregnancy, influenza and fever in the first trimester, and maternal drug consumption during the first trimester (e.g., opiates, penicillin, and salicylates); infectious diseases, nutritional deficiencies, and cigarette smoking

F. Malocclusion

1. Difficult to quantify because of varying cultural perceptions and inability to achieve examiner consistency

2. Decrease in malocclusion associated with increase in use of fluorides

G. Temporomandibular disease

1. Epidemiologic studies vary in focus of measurement; includes signs and symptoms in various population groups

2. Agreement exists that prevalence of conditions, such as pain in joint or masseter muscles with joint movement, mandibular deviations in opening, and joint clicking or crepitus, is high, even among individuals who do not perceive a problem

Indices in Dental Epidemiology

A. Dental index—abbreviated measurement of the amount or condition of disease in a population; graduated numerical scale with defined upper and lower limits designed to facilitate comparison with other populations classified by the same criteria and methods; aids in collection of data

B. Attributes of a good index

1. Validity—measures what it is intended to measure

2. Reliability—measures consistently at different times; reproducibility, stability of measurement

3. Clear, simple, and objective

4. Sensitive to shifts in disease

5. Acceptable to the subjects involved[13]
6. Amenable to statistical analysis
C. Index may assess disease that is a reversible or irreversible condition or combination; therefore, indices are classified as reversible or irreversible
  1. Reversible index—measures conditions that can be reversed (e.g., gingivitis is reversible)
  2. Irreversible index—measures cumulative conditions that cannot be reversed (e.g., dental caries)

D. Common dental indices used in oral health survey (Table 15-3)

Index Selection

A. Index selection is determined by
  1. Type of condition to be assessed; specific to the information of interest
  2. Age of the population to be studied
  3. Purpose of the assessment

Text continued on p. 638

Table 15-3

Common Dental Indices Used in Oral Health Surveys

Dental index	Procedure for use	Interpretation
DENTAL CARIES INDICES		
Decayed-Missing-Filled Teeth Index (DMFT): an irreversible index used to measure past and present caries experience of a population with permanent teeth. *D* indicates a carious tooth; *M* indicates a tooth missing because of caries; *F* indicates a filled tooth The deft index, a variation of the DMFT, is used to measure observable caries experience in primary teeth. The *d* and *f* symbols are the same as in the DMFT. However, *e* indicates need for extraction, and missing teeth are not considered. A tooth that meets the criteria for both *d* and *f* is considered one decayed tooth. The deft does not take into account teeth that have been extracted or exfoliated because of past caries experiences	Count and record the D, M, and F teeth in each member of the sample or population Analyze the scores by using the following formulas: 1. $\text{DMFT count} = \dfrac{\text{Total DMFT}}{\text{Number of people examined}}$ (indicates number of teeth with a history of decay) $\text{deft count} = \dfrac{\text{Total deft}}{\text{Number of children examined}}$ (indicates observable caries experience) 2. $\text{FNM} = \dfrac{F}{\text{Total DMFT}}$ (indicates treatment received for decay [filling needs met]) 3. $\text{Percent of decayed teeth} = \dfrac{D}{\text{Total DMFT}}$ (indicates treatment required for unmet filling needs) 4. $\text{Percent of missing teeth} = \dfrac{M}{\text{Total DMFT}}$ (indicates the number of teeth lost by decay) 5. $\text{Average D, M, or F per individual} = \dfrac{\text{D or M or F}}{\text{Number of people examined}}$	General: indicates cumulative caries experience, total DMF score difficult to determine, specific treatment needs or experiences
Root Caries Index (RCI): a method for reporting root caries that measures the severity of disease and delineates the true intraoral population at risk (the denominator)	Only root surfaces exposed to the oral environment are at risk; the data are recorded as follows: $\dfrac{(R-D)+(R-F)}{(R-D)+(R-F)+(R-N)} \times 100 = RCl$ $R-D$ = Root surface with decay $R-F$ = Root surface that is filled $R-N$ = Root surface that is sound Scoring is relatively straightforward. Four surfaces of the root are evaluated: mesial, distal, facial, and lingual. If multiple type of surfaces are exposed, the most severely affected surface is recorded for the tooth	Rests upon the assumption that gingival recession is a necessary antecedent condition before root caries can develop and that gingival recession must be evident at the time of examination

Modified from Darby ML, Bowen DM: *Research methods for oral health professionals, an introduction*, Pocatello, Id, 1983, Darby and Bowen.

Table 15-3

Common Dental Indices Used in Oral Health Surveys—cont'd

Dental index	Procedure for use	Interpretation
GINGIVITIS INDICES		
Gingival Index (GI): a reversible index based on severity of inflammation and location. Can be used to determine prevalence and severity of gingivitis in epidemiologic surveys as well as individual dentition. GI often used in controlled clinical trial of preventive or therapeutic agents	A score of 0 to 3 assigned to four gingival scoring units: mesial, distal, buccal, and lingual surfaces of teeth. A blunt instrument, such as a periodontal probe, is used to assess bleeding potential. Totaling scores around each tooth yields GI score for area; divide by 4, score for tooth is determined. Totaling all scores and dividing by number of teeth examined provides GI score per person. Can be used on selected or all erupted teeth. Criteria include 0—Normal gingiva 1—Mild inflammation: slight change in color; slight edema; no bleeding on probing 2—Moderate inflammation: redness, edema, and glazing; bleeding on probing 3—Severe inflammation: marked redness and edema, ulceration; tendency to spontaneous bleeding	0.1-1.0: Mild gingivitis 1.1-2.0: Moderate gingivitis 2.1-3.0: Severe gingivitis Difficult to replicate; calibration difficult
Sulcus Bleeding Index (SBI): designed to detect early symptoms of gingivitis; useful in short-term clinical trials	Use maxillary and mandibular anterior teeth; a score is assigned for each of 4 gingival areas/tooth: labial and lingual marginal gingival areas and mesial and distal papillary gingival areas for a total of 64 units; each area probed with blunt periodontal probe (0.5 mm) and observed for 30 seconds SCORES & CRITERIA FOR SULCUS BLEEDING INDEX Scores Criteria 0—Healthy appearance of P and M, no bleeding on sulcus probing 1—Apparently healthy P and M showing no change in color and no swelling, but bleeding from sulcus on probing 2—Bleeding on probing and change of color due to inflammation; no swelling or microscopic edema 3—Bleeding on probing, change in color, and slight edematous swelling 4—Bleeding on probing, change in color, and obvious swelling 5—(1) Bleeding on probing and obvious swelling (2) Bleeding on probing, spontaneous bleeding, change in color, and marked swelling with or without ulceration	Calibration of examiners critical; results reported by frequency of score
PERIODONTAL DISEASE INDICES		
Periodontal Disease Index (PDI): used to measure the presence and severity of periodontal disease; measures reversible and irreversible disease. Used in epidemiologic surveys, longitudinal studies of periodontal disease, and clinical trials of therapeutic or preventive procedures. Gingival index of choice in longitudinal studies of periodontal disease	Six teeth are examined: Nos. 3, 9, 12, 19, 25, and 28. PDI assesses gingivitis, gingival sulcus depth, calculus, plaque, occlusal and incisal attrition mobility, and lack of contact. Criteria used for evaluation of gingiva and gingival crevices are 0—Absence of inflammation 1—Mild to moderate inflammatory gingival changes not extending all around tooth 2—Mild to moderately severe gingivitis extending all around tooth 3—Severe gingivitis, characterized by marked redness, tendency to bleed, and ulceration	Sensitive index. Useful for measuring status of periodontal disease in groups

Continued.

Table 15-3

Common Dental Indices Used in Oral Health Surveys—cont'd

Dental index	Procedure for use	Interpretation
	PERIODONTAL DISEASE INDICES—cont'd	
	4—Gingival crevice in any of 4 measured areas (mesial, distal, facial, lingual) extending apically to cementoenamel junction but not more than 3 mm 5—Gingival crevice in any of 4 measured areas extending apically to cementoenamel junction (3-6 mm) 6—Gingival crevice in any of 4 measured areas extending apically more than 6 mm from cementoenamel junction PDI score is obtained by totaling scores of the teeth and dividing by number of teeth examined*	
Community Periodontal Index of Treatment Needs (CPITN): three indicators of periodontal status are used for this assessment: (a) presence or absence of gingival bleeding, (b) supragingival or subgingival calculus, and (c) periodontal pockets subdivided into shallow (4-5 mm) and deep (6 mm or more) Requires specially designed lightweight probe with a 0.5-mm ball tip bearing a black band between 3.5 and 5.5 mm (list of probes available from World Health Organization)	The mouth is divided into sextants defined by teeth number 1-5, 6-11, 12-16, 17-21, 22-27, and 28-32. Sextant examined only if 2 or more teeth present and not indicated for extraction. For adults 20 years or older use 2, 3, 8, 14, 15, 18, 19, 24, 30, and 31. Two molars in each posterior sextant are paired for recording; if one is missing, no replacement. If no index teeth or tooth present in a sextant qualify for examination, all remaining teeth are examined. For individuals up to age 19 examine teeth numbers 3, 8, 14, 19, 24, and 30. Index tooth probed using probe as sensing instrument to determine pocket depth and detect subgingival calculus. Probe tip inserted gently and depth read against color coding. Six areas on each tooth examined: mesiofacial, midfacial, distofacial, and corresponding lingual sites. One recording made for each sextant, highest score. In epidemiologic surveys, recording based on examination of 2 molars in each posterior sextant and 1 central incisor in each of 2 anterior sextants. Individual screenings, record worst condition around any one of 4 or 6 teeth comprising the sextant	Used as part of the Oral Health Surveys by World Health Organization. Facilitates rapid assessment of mean disease status of a population of various grades of periodontal involvement
	ORAL HYGIENE INDICES	

Simplified Oral Hygiene Index (OHI-S): a reversible index used to measure oral hygiene status. Six teeth—the first fully erupted tooth distal to the second premolar in each quadrant (facial surfaces on maxilla and lingual surfaces on mandible) and maxillary right and mandibular left central incisors (labial surface of each)—are assessed separately for debris and calculus. This assessment yields a DI-S score (debris index—simplified) and a CI-S score (calculus index—simplified)	Surfaces are examined for debris and scored by using DI-S system:
	0—No debris or stain present
	1—Soft debris covering not more than one third of tooth surface being examined or presence of extrinsic stains without debris regardless of surface area covered
	2—Soft debris covering more than one third but not more than two thirds of exposed tooth surfaces
	3—Soft debris covering more than two thirds of exposed tooth surface
	Surfaces are examined for calculus and scored by using the CI-S system:
	0—No calculus present
	1—Supragingival calculus covering not more than one third of exposed tooth surface being examined
		OHI-S:
		  0.0-1.2: Good oral hygiene
		  1.3-3.0: Fair oral hygiene
		  3.1-6.0: Poor oral hygiene
		DI-S or CI-S:
		  0.0-0.6: Good oral hygiene
		  0.7-1.8: Fair oral hygiene
		  1.9-3.0: Poor oral hygiene

Table 15-3

Common Dental Indices Used in Oral Health Surveys—cont'd

Dental index	Procedure for use	Interpretation

ORAL HYGIENE INDICES—cont'd

	2—Supragingival calculus covering more than one third but not more than two thirds of exposed tooth surfaces or presence of individual flecks of subgingival calculus around cervical portion of tooth 3—Supragingival calculus covering more than two thirds of exposed tooth surface or a continuous heavy band of subgingival calculus around cervical portion of tooth	
Plaque Index (PLI): used to assess extent of soft deposits; measures differences in thickness of debris at gingival margin used in conjunction with Gingival Index. Useful in longitudinal studies and clinical trials	Four gingival scoring units: mesial, distal, buccal, lingual; examined by using mouth mirror, dental explorer, air-drying. PII for area is obtained by totaling 4 plaque scores per tooth. If sum of PII scores per tooth is divided by 4, PII score for tooth is obtained. PII score per person is obtained by adding PII scores per tooth and dividing by number of teeth examined. May be obtained for a segment or group of teeth. 0—No plaque in gingival area 1—Film of plaque adhering to free gingival margin and adjacent area of tooth; plaque only noticed by running probe across tooth surface 2—Moderate accumulation of soft deposits within gingival margin and/or on adjacent tooth surface can be seen by naked eye 3—Abundance of soft matter within gingival pocket and/or gingival margin and adjacent tooth surface	
Patient Hygiene Performance (PHP): developed to assess individual's performance in removing debris after toothbrush instruction. Simple to use; can be performed quickly	Teeth disclosed: Six teeth are evaluated: Nos. 3, 8, 14, 19, 24, and 30. Each tooth is divided into 5 areas: 3 longitudinal thirds, distal, middle, and mesial; the middle third is subdivided horizontally into incisal, middle, and gingival thirds. Score per person is obtained by totaling 5 subdivision scores per tooth surface and dividing by number of tooth surfaces examined	

Dental index	Classification	Criteria	Interpretation

DENTAL FLUOROSIS

| *Dean's Classification for Dental Fluorosis:* assigns an individual a score of 0-4 based on second most severely affected tooth | Normal (0) | The enamel presents the usual translucent semi-vitriform type of structure. The surface is smooth, glossy, and usually of a pale, creamy white color | A classification of mild or less is not considered a cosmetic problem; a Community Fluorosis Index (CFI) is assigned based on the mean of all scores of study population |
| | Questionable (0.5) | The enamel discloses slight aberrations from the translucency of normal enamel, ranging from a few white flecks to occasional white spots. This classification is used in those instances where a definite diagnosis of the mildest form of fluorosis is not warranted and a classification of "normal" not justified | |

DEAN'S COMMUNITY FLUOROSIS INDEX SCORES

Range	Significance of scores
0.0-0.4	Negative
0.4-0.6	Borderline
0.6-1.0	Slight
1.0-2.0	Medium
2.0-3.0	Marked
3.0-4.0	Very marked

A CFI score of less than 0.6 is not considered objectionable.

Continued.

Table 15-3

Common Dental Indices Used in Oral Health Surveys—cont'd

Dental index	Classification	Criteria	Interpretation
		DENTAL FLUOROSIS—cont'd	
	Very mild (1)	Small, opaque, paper white areas scattered irregularly over the tooth but not involving as much as approximately 25% of the tooth surface. Frequently included in this classification are teeth showing no more than about 1-2 mm of white opacity at the tip of the summit of the cusps of the premolars or second molars	
	Mild (2)	The white opaque areas in the enamel of the teeth are more extensive but do not involve as much as 50% of the tooth	
	Moderate (3)	All enamel surfaces of the teeth are affected, and surfaces subject to attrition show wear. Brown stain is frequently a disfiguring feature	
	Severe (4)	All enamel surfaces are affected and hypoplasia is so marked that the general form of the tooth may be affected. The major diagnostic sign of this classification is the discrete or confluent pitting. Brown stains are widespread and teeth often present a corroded-like appearance	

B. Examiners should be calibrated or standardized in their use of index criteria
  1. Intrarater reliability—each individual examiner is scoring equivalently time and time again; "extent to which the same investigator remains consistent in scoring techniques when using a data collection instrument"[4]
  2. Interrater reliability—consistency exists between examiners; "degree to which different investigators can obtain the same results when using the data collection instrumentation on a population"[4]

Errors in Assessing Disease

A. Errors in sampling technique
  1. Incorrect sampling technique
  2. Use of nonrandom samples of the target population

3. Nonparticipation of a segment of the target population

B. Errors in collecting, recording, and analyzing data
   1. Variation in assessment; lack of calibration; examiners are not collecting data in a consistent and accurate manner; known or unknown bias
   2. Observations are computed or recorded inaccurately
   3. Data analyzed incompletely or inappropriately

Preventing and Controlling Oral Disease

Public Health Measures

A. Characteristics of a public health measure
   1. Not hazardous to life or function
   2. Effective in reducing or preventing the targeted disease or condition
   3. Easily and efficiently implemented
   4. Potency maintained for a substantial time period
   5. Attainable regardless of socioeconomic status, education, or income
   6. Effective immediately on application
   7. Costs are inexpensive and within the means of the community

B. Examples of public health measures include vaccination programs, water purification, and water fluoridation

Measures for Preventing and Controlling Dental Caries

A. Water fluoridation (see box, Strategies to Implement Fluoridation)
   1. Adjustment of the natural fluoride concentration to about 1 part fluoride to 1 million parts water (1 ppm); range 0.7 to 1.2 ppm depending on mean daily temperature
   2. Most cost-effective and efficient method of bringing the benefits of fluoride to a community
      a. In early studies children reared in a fluoridated-water community showed a 50% to 70% reduction in caries in their permanent dentition when compared with children in a nonfluoridated community; currently, reduction in caries attributed to water fluoridation; incidence of dental caries is reduced by 20% to 40% in the mixed dentition of children (ages 8 to 12) and 15% to 35% in the permanent dentition of adolescents (ages 14 to 17); reduces coronal caries in adults 35%
      b. Costs vary depending on the size of the community and the water system, labor costs, and chemicals used; in large size cities, $0.13 to $0.21;

in medium size cities, $0.18 to $0.75; and in small size cities, $0.77 to $5.48 per person annually
      c. A practical form of preventing caries in communities with established community water systems
      d. Indirect benefits include fewer missing teeth resulting in improved self-image; less complicated restorative procedures; pain reduction, decreased malocclusion
      e. Fluoridated water results in systemic and topical benefits
         (1) Pre-eruption benefits
         (2) Post-eruption benefits include
            (a) Remineralization of incipient caries
            (b) Saliva level is 0.03 to 0.05 ppm
            (c) 25% reduction in posteruptive teeth
   3. Equipment used for community water fluoridation resembles machinery used for adding other materials to water systems

STRATEGIES TO IMPLEMENT FLUORIDATION[16]

1992 Fluoridation Census[17] reports 144 million Americans—55.8% of total U.S. population—are served by drinking water containing optimal or above levels of fluoride

Healthy People 2000 proposes that 75% of the population be served by community water systems providing optimal levels of fluoride

Strategies:
- develop and implement a plan of action to maintain the efficacy of water fluoridation as a proven public health measure
- organize and enlist the support of other state and federal organizations that have an influence in guiding the development of health policies bringing about social change
- effectively translate fluoridation information into languages for all racial and ethnic groups
- develop new and innovative strategies to meet the challenge of fluoridation opponents, past and present
- develop a national clearinghouse for fluoridation materials
- develop a national surveillance system to collect, analyze, and evaluate risk factor data related to fluorides
- support legislation to fund community water fluoridation

From Dyck BC: Community water fluoridation from the past toward the year 2000, *Dent Hyg News* 8:3, 1995.

a. Three types of machinery
   (1) Acid feeders—saturated solution of commercially available fluoride is fed directly into the main water supply at a carefully controlled rate
   (2) Dry feeders—solid material is fed into a dissolving tank at a measured rate by automatic machinery and the concentrated solution is carried to the main water supply
   (3) Saturator—solid material is added to a holding tank containing water in sufficient amounts to create a saturated solution of fluorides that is then fed into the main water supply at a carefully controlled rate
b. Any compound that forms fluoride ions in aqueous solution can be used. Compounds used in fluoridation of water supplies include sodium silicofluoride (solid), sodium fluoride (solid), and hydrofluorosilicic acid (liquid) are most popular; selection depends on number and accessibility of water sources and water quality
c. Fluoridation compatible with other water treatment processes; quality assurance protocol necessary

4. Optimal fluoride levels range from 0.7 ppm to 1.2 ppm depending on the climate; the warmer the climate, the lower the concentration because of increased water consumption; the colder the climate the higher the concentration
5. Communities with excessive amounts of naturally occurring fluoride can use defluoridation equipment; EPA requires defluoridation in areas with >4 ppm
6. Mottled enamel
   a. Chronic endemic form of hypoplasia of dental enamel caused by drinking water with a high naturally occurring fluoride content during the time of tooth formation; defective calcification of teeth giving a white chalky appearance, that may undergo brown discoloration; results from naturally occurring excessive fluoride levels in well water, from children swallowing excessive amounts of fluoride-containing dentifrices, or from inappropriate supplementation with fluoride tablets or fluoride-containing vitamins
   b. Varies from small fine, lacy markings to white specks to severe pitting with heavily stained and friable enamel
   c. Occurs when water with a high fluoride content is ingested during the time of tooth development
   d. Occurs in many parts of the world; a public health problem in East Africa and India
   e. Studies indicate that 7% to 16% of children born and reared in an optimally fluoridated community exhibit mild or very mild dental fluorosis in the permanent dentition
   (1) Mild to moderate fluorosis associated with use of fluoride supplements, especially in higher socioeconomic groups
   (2) Swallowing or overenthusiastic use of fluoridated toothpaste by young children a concern; prudent use advised; a "pea-size" amount on the brush
   (3) Infant formula, especially soybean-based formulas, should be used in moderation in fluoridated communities
   (4) Fruit juices and drinks consumed by children

7. Halo effect
   a. Secondary exposure to fluoridated water in processed foods and beverages
   b. Increased fluoride ingestion from processed foods and beverages is variable and depends on water source
   c. In some nonfluoridated areas, ingestion can be significant

8. Promotion of fluoride
   a. Three methods of implementation
      (1) Administrative decision—a community leader introduces the idea of community water fluoridation through appropriate government channels and the idea is approved by the appropriate governing body, i.e., water board, public services director, mayor, city council
      (2) Initiative petition and/or referendum allowing members of the community to cast a vote for fluoridation of the water supply
      (3) State legislative action—mandate passed by state legislators in some states that requires specified public water supplies to be fluoridated or allows health departments to order public water supplies to be fluoridated under certain conditions
   b. Oral healthcare professionals are responsible for promoting water fluoridation within the community (see box, Strategies to Implement Fluoridation, p. 639)
   c. Public attitudes toward water fluoridation are both positive and negative
      (1) In most instances there is organized opposition to implementation or adoption
      (2) Opponents use arguments such as effectiveness, environmental issues, government overregulation, and suspicion of government programs or officials

(3) Individuals continue to be opposed to water fluoridation; tactics used to oppose fluoridation include

    (a) Associating fluoridation with concerns about health and aging

    (b) Scare tactics that imply water fluoridation causes health hazards such as allergies, cancer, heart disease, increased death rates and Alzheimer disease

    (c) Suggestions that water fluoridation violates an individual's freedom of choice

    (d) Creation of an illusion of scientific controversy where none exists

d. A study conducted by the U.S. Department of Public Health on fluoride evaluated its benefits and risks and concluded the following[17]

    (1) Optimal fluoridation of drinking water is not a detectable cancer risk to humans

    (2) Data available from two studies of the carcinogenicity of fluoride in experimental animals did not report a link between fluoride and cancer

    (3) Additional epidemiologic studies necessary to determine whether an association exists between various levels of fluoride and bone fractures

    (4) Crippling skeletal fluorosis is not a public health problem in the United States

    (5) No support for the use of high doses of fluoride to reduce osteoporosis and related bone fractures

    (6) Chronic low-level exposure to fluoride is not associated with birth defects; no association found with Down syndrome; no effect on organ systems, e.g., gastrointestinal

e. Important for oral healthcare professionals to concentrate their efforts to obtain community support for fluoridation; tactics used to support water fluoridation include

    (1) Knowledge of medical and dental studies that provide the scientific foundation for fluoridation

    (2) Knowledge of the community (e.g., past efforts to either introduce water fluoridation or discontinue water fluoridation)

    (3) Work with all community leaders, community organizations, and members of the community having influence such as newspaper editors or radio or television personalities; collaboration with other health professionals

    (4) Awareness of the methods, tactics, and non-scientific materials used by those opposed to fluoridation

B. Mouthrinse programs, supplementation, and school fluoridators are recommended in areas with suboptimal fluoride

C. School water fluoridation

  1. Reduces dental caries among schoolchildren more than 25%; caries reduction is changing as a result of multiple sources of fluoride ingested[16]

  2. Studies have documented effectiveness; however, not widely implemented

  3. School water is usually fluoridated at 4.5 times the optimum concentration recommended for the community in which the school is located

    a. Increased optimum amount because children drink the water only when school is in session

    b. Uses same basic equipment and materials as used in community programs; monitored by an employee of the school system

  4. Major disadvantage is that children do not receive benefits until they begin school; exposure occurs during school year and school day only, not during summer vacation; some children may choose not to participate

  5. School water fluoridation studies occurred when prevalence of caries in schoolchildren was higher; thus reduction in caries rates was dramatic; although caries rates are declining, there are still groups of children who can benefit from such programs[15]

  6. Several hundred rural schools in the United States and a few schools in Brazil and Thailand practice school water fluoridation

D. Dietary fluoride supplements

  1. Administered at home or as a school-based program

  2. Supplemental forms include tablets, lozenges, drops, liquids, and fluoride-vitamin preparations

  3. Dietary fluoride supplements are available in 0.125, 0.25, and 0.50 mg drops; 0.25, 0.50, and 1.0 mg tablets/lozenges; and 1 mg/5 ml oral rinse supplements

  4. Fluoride dietary supplement use is based on concentration of fluoride in drinking water, weight of the child, available fluoride, and related factors such as cooperation, age, and ability of the child

  5. Fluoride tablets generally are prescribed after a child has a full complement of primary teeth

  6. Tablets contain 1.0 mg of fluoride, although tablets for younger children are available with 0.5 or 0.25 mg (Table 15-4)

	CONCENTRATION OF FLUORIDE IN THE WATER (ppm)		
Age in years	**<0.3 ppm**	**0.3 ppm to 0.6 ppm**	**>0.6 ppm**
6 months-3 yrs	0.25 mg	0	0
3-6 yrs	0.50 mg	0.25 mg	0
6-16 yrs	1.0 mg	0.50 mg	0

Table 15-4

Supplemental Fluoride Dosage Schedule (in mg F per day*) According to Fluoride Concentration of Drinking Water[18]

*2.2 mg NaF contain 1 mg F
From Jakush J: CDT to consider fluoride dosage, *ADA News,* February 21, 1994, p. 16.

a. Tablets contain neutral sodium fluoride (NaF) or acidulated phosphate fluoride (APF)

b. Studies indicate that fluoride tablets taken daily result in a 50% to 80% reduction in caries

c. Tablets and lozenges are chewed, swished, and swallowed

7. No more than 120, 2.2 mg NaF tablets should be prescribed at one time

8. In nonfluoridated areas, fluoride supplements should be prescribed for children from birth to 14 years of age

9. Compliance is essential for successful daily fluoride supplementation

10. School-based dietary fluoride tablet programs

    a. Initial studies demonstrated 30% reduction in dental caries

    b. Initiated at earliest grade, kindergarteners for maximum effectiveness

    c. Provide topical and systemic benefits

    d. Inexpensive and require little time

    e. Nondental personnel can supervise

    f. Require ongoing cooperation of administrators, teachers, parents, and others

    g. School-based dietary fluoride supplement programs were initiated when multiple sources of fluoride were not available; thus, persons in nonfluoridated areas obtain decay preventive benefits from beverages and food products manufactured in fluoridated communities; the need for school-based programs is less compelling but must be considered on a community-by-community basis.[15]

11. Fluoride drops dispensed and measured with a dropper, or

    a. For infants who are formula-fed and who live in a nonfluoridated community

    b. Infants are given fluoride drops with or without vitamins; placed directly in the baby's mouth or added to foods

    c. Effectiveness of fluoride drops and tablets is neither enhanced nor reduced when combined with vitamins; increased client compliance may occur with combined fluoride-vitamin supplements

    d. Dietary supplements not recommended for infants who are breast-fed and reside in optimally fluoridated areas; breast milk contains 0.0004 ppm fluoride

12. Fluoridated salt brings the benefits of systemic fluoride to areas where piped water does not exist

    a. Studies indicate 250 ppm is a suitable concentration

    b. Reduction in caries parallels rates found in communities having water fluoridation

    c. Addition of fluoride to table salt is a feasible way to deliver systemic fluoride, particularly in countries lacking widespread municipal water systems; fluoridated salt has been sold in Switzerland; France and a few countries in Central and South America have introduced fluoridated salt in recent years

    d. Disadvantages include a fixed concentration; difficult to use in areas where naturally occurring fluoride concentrations vary

    e. Concern of salt's role in aggravating hypertension

    f. Never used in the United States or Canada; not appropriate

13. Fluoridated milk also recommended; disadvantages include decrease in amount ingested as child gets older and inability to control dairy production

    a. The addition of fluoride to milk consumed at school has been studied in several countries

    b. Studies have shown protection from caries; however, milk is not an ideal vehicle for fluoride delivery because it only provides a single exposure to fluoride on school days and milk consumption declines with increasing age

E. Topical application of fluorides (see Chapter 10, section on direct preventive/restorative materials, and Chapter 12, section on fluorides)
   1. Professional application of topical fluorides is least cost-effective as a public health measure
   2. Low concentration, frequent use of fluoride, as with fluoridated dentifrices, are more effective
   3. Materials used include sodium fluoride (NaF^-), stannous fluoride (SnF_2), and acidulated phosphate fluoride (APF)
   4. Although not cost-effective as a public health measure, may be appropriate for special-needs groups in specific programs at high risk for caries
F. Fluoride mouthrinses
   1. Studies indicate a 20% to 50% reduction in caries
   2. Most widely used caries-preventive public health method; second to community water fluoridation
   3. Sodium fluoride (NaF) or acidulated phosphate fluoride have been used in mouth rinses; sodium fluoride in a 0.2% concentration is used weekly or in a 0.05% concentration is used daily; equally effective
      a. Sodium fluoride in 0.2% (900 ppm) concentration on a weekly basis or 0.05 NaF (250 ppm) used daily are suitable for school-based public programs
      b. Advantages of the school-based public programs include
         (1) Easy to learn; swished for a minute and expectorated
         (2) Inexpensive in time and resources
         (3) Nondental personnel can supervise
         (4) Appropriate for all grade levels; appears more successful at the elementary grade level
         (5) Note that consent forms are required
   4. A mouthrinse dose is equal to 2 teaspoons (10 ml); 2.25 mg for 0.05% NaF rinses; 9.0 mg fluoride for 0.2% NaF rinses
   5. Mouthrinses have been recommended for individuals in fluoridated and nonfluoridated communities
   6. Special benefits for persons susceptible to caries and other conditions such as xerostomia and root caries; not recommended for any population when a high level of compliance is necessary
   7. Acute fluoride toxicity of child from ingestion of 1 L of 0.2% NaF mouth rinse; ingestion of 1 L of 0.05% NaF mouth rinse leads to nausea and vomiting (see Chapter 17, section on drug-related emergencies and poisoning)
G. Sealant programs (see Chapter 10, section on pit and fissure dental sealants, and Chapter 12, section on dental sealants)
   1. Sealants recommended for all children and teenagers living in fluoridated and nonfluoridated communities
   2. Sealant and fluoride programs are the most beneficial community-based dental disease prevention programs
   3. Reported effectiveness in reducing pit and fissure caries suggests use should be a critical component of disease prevention programs; especially targeted to children with high risk of disease
   4. Use of fluorides in conjunction with sealants recommended so that both smooth surfaces and pit and fissure surfaces benefit
   5. Retention rates are comparable whoever applies sealant; key for retention is a competent operator
   6. Survey of schoolchildren indicates 90% of dental caries occurs in pits and fissures; 10% in smooth surfaces
   7. Efficacy of sealants is well recognized
   8. Third-party payers, although not all, cover sealants; Medicaid funds sealants in a minority of states
   9. Limited resources require that sealant programs use criteria that include dental caries level, availability of care, grade level of targeted group, e.g., second and sixth grades, teeth with deep pits and fissures; place sealant within six months of eruption of first and second molars
   10. Treatment settings may include schools, clinics, daycare facilities, etc.; team approach necessary for screening and treatment; support and cooperation of school administrators, teachers, parents, volunteers necessary
   11. Targeted to groups such as students eligible for free or subsidized lunch programs
   12. Education of the targeted community critical
   13. Based on epidemiologic evidence, sealant programs are justified for children and young adults, but not other age groups
   14. Differences in percent effectiveness, retention, and caries incidence not apparent between studies in fluoridated versus nonfluoridated communities; however, slightly greater benefit for sealants in fluoridated communities

Measures for Preventing and Controlling Periodontal Disease

A. No parallel to water fluoridation for the prevention of periodontal disease exists
B. Research reports indicate that a combination of self-care by individuals on a regular basis and periodic periodontal maintenance therapy leads to improved

gingival health, decreased attachment loss, and maintenance of natural dentition

1. Simple mechanical prophylaxes and instructions in oral hygiene, while sufficient to control gingivitis in children, are insufficient for control of periodontal disease in adults
2. Adults require a maintenance program with removal of bacterial toxins and calculus, root planing, oral hygiene instruction, and client motivation
3. No evidence that controlling gingivitis in children has long-term benefit during adult years
4. Effectiveness of oral health education programs to improve oral hygiene difficult to demonstrate
5. Increasing cultural and commercial emphasis on oral hygiene will continue to influence personal oral health behaviors

C. Community activities should include
1. Public education to emphasize personal oral hygiene and regular professional oral care
2. Support of funding and promotion of research

Measures for Preventing and Controlling Other Oral Diseases and Anomalies

A. Oral cancer
1. Primary prevention technique for cancer does not exist; avoiding known risk factors such as alcohol and tobacco is recommended; decline of cigarette use reported; however, increase in use of smokeless tobacco
2. Periodic visits to the professional oral healthcare setting for examination
3. Secondary prevention or control consists of early detection (screening) and treatment; also oral health education
4. Mass screening for oral cancer is costly; professionals should include oral cancer examinations as part of their prevention routines
5. Public education regarding signs and symptoms of oral cancer is important; self-examination techniques
6. Use of smokeless tobacco a continuing concern; public and individual education necessary to end the habit or not begin
   a. Develop programs and materials to educate the public at risk
   b. Use of health warning labels on products and advertisements
7. Support of research efforts and lobbying strategies

B. Oral clefts
1. Primary prevention technique for cleft lip and palate does not exist
2. Multiple factors are involved with the occurrence of cleft palate; genetic counseling provides a valuable tool for identifying risk factors
3. Programs for treatment of the conditions are available through state children services
4. Dental professionals should be aware of the resources within the community

C. Malocclusion and accidents
1. Oral health education focusing on preventive behaviors
   a. Use of protective devices such as athletic mouth protectors in sports activities (see Chapter 10, section on mouth protectors)
   b. School environment safety programs
2. Habit control
3. Interceptive orthodontics

Steps in Community Planning

General Considerations

A. Community groups vary
1. Planning principles can be applied to all groups
2. Principles are useful for all types of programs
3. Factors to consider include current health system, resources, geography, sociocultural background, socioeconomic status, cultural and political climate

B. Dental hygienist has many roles in community health planning and practice
1. Program planner or initiator
2. Consultant/resource person
3. Service provider
4. Administrator/manager of a particular program/division
5. Researcher
6. Educator and oral health promoter
7. Change agent
8. Consumer advocate
9. Politician

C. Dental public health planning framework
1. Following target population identification
2. Assess the target population
3. Collect and analyze data
4. Determine priorities
5. Develop a program plan
6. Implement plan
7. Education, financing, and evaluation are ongoing concerns during the entire process

Assessment

A. Definition—organized and systematic approach to identify a target group and define the extent and severity of oral health needs present
1. Target group—group of individuals who are the focus of a particular oral health service or program
   a. Health professional may identify the target group

b. Target group with a defined need may contact health professionals
2. Community-oriented primary care (COPC) philosophy of health planning where community identifies its perceived needs and assigns priorities

B. Data collection
1. Important to complete before planning
   a. Identify ongoing oral health programs or projects
   b. Assess oral health status and needs
   c. Develop a community profile of the area where the target population is located
2. Identify ongoing types or programs or projects
   a. Purpose of ongoing programs: provision of oral health services, education, disease prevention, research, or combination
   b. Individuals/groups responsible for the programs and the success within the community
   c. Identify locations or facilities where oral health activities can occur
   d. Identify individuals, special equipment (i.e., mobile vans), facilities, and resources to meet the dental needs of the target population
3. Assess current oral health status and needs
   a. Three methods for obtaining data to document oral health status and needs
      (1) Identify and use an assessment method to obtain specific information related to the proposed project or program
      (2) Coordinate assessment with an agency or group seeking similar information about the identified target population
      (3) Research and collect data accumulated from records available from state or local health agencies, dental or medical programs, and public health or related agencies
   b. Assessment methods
      (1) Baseline data—data collected before program implementation; used for planning and evaluating a program
      (2) Used to identify the extent and severity of need and in determining objectives
      (3) Influenced by the type of information needed
      (4) Assessment methods can be used in combination with each other
      (5) Advantages and disadvantages of assessment methods (Table 15-5)
4. Types of assessment methods
   a. Four types of examinations and inspections
      (1) Type 1—complete examination using a mouth mirror and explorer, adequate illumination, thorough radiographic survey, and when indicated, percussion, pulp vital-

ity tests, transillumination, study models, and laboratory tests; because of the time, expense, and personnel required, seldom used in public health
      (2) Type 2—limited examination using a mouth mirror, explorer, adequate illumination, and posterior bite-wing radiographs (where indicated, periapical radiographs); useful where program may include service to individuals; also helpful in surveys where time and money permit
      (3) Type 3—inspection using a mouth mirror, explorer, and adequate illumination
         (a) Advantages
            [1] Basis for oral health instruction
            [2] Opportunity for establishing rapport and planning motivational strategy
            [3] Provide baseline information on dental needs of target group
         (b) Disadvantages
            [1] Inspection may be relied on as an examination and need for complete assessment might not be perceived
            [2] Inspections of no value unless follow-up occurs
            [3] If inspection occurs in school, parents/guardians not present to observe outcomes
      (4) Type 4—screening with a tongue depressor and available illumination; identifies needs
   b. Survey—common approach used to assess knowledge, oral health status, oral health behavior, values and attitudes
      (1) Can employ various techniques for data collection (e.g., questionnaire, interview, direct observation, indices, records, documents, etc.)
   c. Oral health surveys—surveys to collect information about oral health, disease status and treatment needs for planning or monitoring oral health needs[19]
      (1) Clinical examination
      (2) Review of dental records
      (3) State level data available through Behavioral Risk Factor Surveillance (BRFSS) and Youth Behavior Risk Surveillance System (YRBSS)
      (4) Use of national and state health survey data for comparable group/geographic region
      (5) Special considerations for planning oral health surveys because of characteristics of the primary diseases studied: dental caries and periodontal diseases

Table 15-5

Data Collection Instruments and Applications

Data collection methodology	Instrument	Indications	Advantages	Limitations
Direct observation of events, objects, people	Checklist, content analysis, evaluation forms, camera, tape recorder, videotape, thermometer, sphygmomanometer, rating and ranking scales	1. Used when subject recall may affect accuracy of data collection 2. Used to study behavior 3. Used to study psychomotor activity 4. Used in experimental research	1. Observations can be made as they occur in the "natural" setting 2. Observations can be made of behaviors that might not be reported by respondents	1. Time consuming 2. Difficulty in recording 3. Factors that may interfere with the situation 4. Difficulty in quantification of observations 5. Expensive 6. Observer-respondent interaction
Interview	Interview guide or interview schedule	1. Used for obtaining information on attitudes, beliefs, and opinions 2. Used in a survey 3. Used to gain information on past or present events	1. Flexibility 2. Questions can be clarified and explained 3. Complete data can be collected 4. Subjects do not have to read or write	1. Respondents may be inhibited to respond accurately and truthfully 2. Time consuming 3. Expensive 4. Interviewer may affect the responses
Asking questions	Questionnaire, opinionnaire	1. Used for obtaining information on attitudes, beliefs, and opinions 2. Used to gain information on past events 3. Used when impersonal interactions between researcher and respondent are required	1. Ease of administration 2. Relatively inexpensive 3. Standardization of instructions and questions 4. Economy of time 5. Data can be gathered over a wide geographic area	1. Misinterpretation of questions by respondents 2. Low return may bias results 3. Superficiality of responses 4. Incomplete data collection 5. Honesty of respondent
Survey	Questionnaire, interview, schedule, case study	1. Used for obtaining a broad range of information on the status quo 2. Used to study present conditions 3. Used in planning	1. Data can be gathered to reflect public opinion 2. Vast amount of data can be collected 3. Cross-sectional, generalized statistics can be obtained	1. Superficiality of responses 2. Control of extraneous variables is lacking
Epidemiologic survey	Dental indices	1. Used to study disease patterns in a population 2. Used to evaluate the effectiveness of therapeutic or preventive treatments in a specific geographic area	1. Vast amount of data can be collected 2. Cross-sectional, generalized statistics can be obtained 3. Data are quantifiable	1. Difficulty in determining causation due to complexity of variables 2. Time consuming
Records, documents	Reports of legislative bodies and state or city officials, deeds, wills, appointment records, dental charts, report cards	1. Used to study past events	1. Unbiased in terms of the investigator 2. Inexpensive 3. No subject-investigator interaction 4. Convenience and economy of time	1. Incomplete records 2. Accuracy of records may be unknown

From Darby ML, Bowen DM: *Research methods for oral health professionals: an introduction*, Pocabello, Idaho, 1983, Darby and Bowen.[4]

(a) Disease age related

(b) Significant percentage of the population affected

(c) Dental caries is irreversible; thus data of current status includes both the amount of disease present and previous disease present

(d) Pattern of increase in disease prevalence

(e) Common oral diseases exist in all populations

(f) Extensive documentation on variation of profiles of dental caries exists for population groups with different socioeconomic levels and environmental conditions

(g) Many observations made in standard measurements for each subject[20]

(6) Surveying requires planning, calibration of examiners, and implementation

(7) World Health Organization's suggested format for reporting survey results[20]

(a) Statement of purpose of the survey (or assessment method)

(b) Materials and methods

[1] Description of the area and population surveyed

[2] Types of information collected

[3] Methods of collecting data; year collected

[4] Sampling method

[5] Examiner, personnel, equipment, and physical arrangements

[6] Statistical analysis and computational procedure

[7] Cost analysis

[8] Reliability and reproducibility

(c) Results

(d) Discussion and conclusions

(e) Summary or abstract

C. Development of a community profile

1. Community profile—provides information essential in planning a community health program; general areas for inclusion in the profile are

a. Community overview

(1) Number of individuals in the population

(2) Population distribution by income, age, education, etc.

(3) Geographic location and boundaries

(4) Population setting and density (urban or rural); standard of living

(5) Ethnic background, cultural heritages, languages, customs, behaviors, beliefs

(6) Diet, nutritional levels, nutrition programs

(7) Amount, types, and influence of public services and utilities

(8) Transportation schedules, routes, fares, reliability

(9) Informed consent procedures

(10) Distribution of public and private schools and religious organizations

(11) Extent and type of fluoride therapies

(12) State and local statutes, public health codes, and related administrative rules and regulations

b. Community leadership and organization

(1) Community and financial leaders, liaisons, and councils and their attitudes toward oral health

(2) Community power base for policy formulation

(3) Governance structure (e.g., health council, city government, advisory board, school board, union)

(4) Grassroots individuals with political influence

(5) Educational institutions providing professional education, resources, and support

c. Financing and funding of health services

(1) Budget allocation procedures for dental health programs

(2) Mechanism for requesting the necessary funding

(3) Funding sources (e.g., federal, state, or local funding; individual or third-party payment; private funds, foundations, grants, or endowments)

d. Facilities, resources, and personpower

(1) Location of space and facilities in the community or institution; OSHA standard compliance

(2) Availability and adequacy of equipment

(3) Location of medical centers, clinics, and dental laboratories; ease of access

(4) Number of licensed practicing dentists, dental hygienists, dental assistants, laboratory technicians, medical personnel, or others experienced in working with the target population

(5) May involve identifying a facility or consortium of health professionals, facilities, and resources

2. Rationale for development of a community profile—to understand the environment in which the target population is located

3. Size, location, and type of community dictate the type of information necessary for a community profile

D. Analysis of data
1. Analysis includes organizing, tabulating, and interpreting data
2. Data analysis can range from the simple to the complex
    a. Planner alone tabulates
    b. Statisticians and statistical tests are used
    c. Computers and other technology are used
    d. Must also include a human component that is difficult to quantify, e.g., statistics versus perceptions of need for oral health services
3. Following analysis, needs and priorities can be identified
    a. Target group input is solicited
    b. Community representative and/or advisory groups are consulted
        (1) Advisory groups provide an opportunity for dialogue and support
        (2) Members are determined by the unique characteristics of the project and can include consumers, political and financial leaders, and healthcare professionals
    c. Population groups identified with high-risk oral needs include
        (1) Preschool and school-aged children
        (2) Mentally and physically challenged persons
        (3) Chronically ill and/or medically compromised persons
        (4) Elderly persons
        (5) Expectant mothers
        (6) Low income minority groups

Program Planning

A. Definition—organized response to reduce or eliminate one or more problems; organized effort that includes the objective of reducing or eliminating one or more problems, performance of one or more activities, and utilization of resources
B. Elements of a program plan
1. Identification of program goals and objectives
2. Strategies and specific activities to meet objectives
    a. Sequence of activities
    b. Individuals responsible for each activity
3. Resources required
    a. Location and facilities
    b. Equipment
    c. Personnel
    d. Criteria used to determine resources required
        (1) Appropriateness: most suitable to accomplish the tasks

        (2) Adequacy: the extent or degree to which the resources would complete tasks
        (3) Effectiveness: how capable are the resources at completing the tasks
        (4) Efficiency: the dollar cost and time expended to complete the tasks
4. Timetables and deadlines clearly outlined, with some flexibility
5. Projected costs
6. Program promotion and marketing
7. Identification of possible constraints

C. Goals and objectives
1. For each need prioritized, a goal with related objectives must be determined
    a. Goal—broadly based statement of what changes will occur as a result of the program; provides direction
    b. Objectives—specific statements that describe, in a measurable manner, the desired outcomes from program activities
2. Categories of goals and objectives
    a. Ultimate or long-term
    b. Intermediate
    c. Short-term or immediate (NOTE: Most activities may deal with immediate goals, but intermediate and long-term goals must be considered)
3. Immediate objectives are stated in specific, measurable terms; factors considered
    a. What—identify the condition or situation to be attained
    b. Extent—scope and magnitude of situation or condition to be attained
    c. Who—target group or portion of the community in which attainment is desired
    d. Where—geographic area or physical boundaries of the program
    e. When—time "at or by" which the desired situation or condition is to exist

D. Activities
1. Program activities are the dynamic, energy-using procedures carried out to achieve program objectives; programs might be preventive, educational, treatment oriented, or research oriented
2. To meet objectives, personnel, location, equipment, resources, and costs are determined

E. Promotion
1. Necessary for participation and success of a project
2. Promotion techniques include an advisory committee, liaison groups, television and radio media, printed media, and special-interest publications and programs; smaller programs may use posters, flyers, invitations, newsletter announcements

F. Implementation

1. Process of putting plan into operation
2. Monitoring plan for activities, personnel, equipment, resources, and supplies
3. Feedback mechanism from personnel and participants
4. Ongoing evaluation mechanisms

G. Evaluation
   1. Key element—should take place at all stages
   2. Results of the program are measured against objectives developed during the early planning stages
   3. Assessment method may influence evaluation tool used
   4. Both formal and informal
      a. Systematic and regular evaluation of goals and objectives by using specific measurement instruments; outcome assessment
      b. Quality of program and personnel
      c. Progress and effectiveness of activities; identify problems and solutions to assist in revisions and modifications to meet goals and objectives
      d. Evaluate perceptions and attitudes of recipients of program
      e. Evaluate health status indicator of recipients of program

Implementation

Educational Strategies

A. Health education—provision of health information to people in such a way that they apply it in everyday living; a process with intellectual, psychologic, and social dimensions relating to activities that increase the abilities of people to make informed decisions affecting their personal, family, and community well-being; a process, based on scientific principles, that facilitates learning and behavioral change in both health personnel and consumers; health education and intervention strategies should be based on accepted theories of health behavior; voluntary adaptations of behavior occur

B. Health promotion—any combination of learning opportunities designed to facilitate voluntary adaptations of behavior conducive to health; includes educational, organizational, economic, and environmental

C. Related Concepts
   1. Health continuum—conceptualization of health status as perceived on a continuous scale from optimum health through illness and death
   2. Prevention—dimension of health education that endeavors to endow individuals and groups with the tools and "know-how" to lead a long and productive life

3. Goals of oral health education
   a. Communication
   b. Motivation
   c. Learning
   d. Outcomes

D. Includes both formal and informal activities
   1. Formal activities include the deliberate provision of oral health education designed to elicit specific health promotion or disease prevention behavior (e.g., the curricula of elementary and secondary schools, health professionals conducting in-service workshops and programs, health agencies providing education and service)
   2. Informal activities include the acquisition of oral health-related information that may lead to some specific health promotion or disease prevention behavior; accidental learning (e.g., interaction with colleagues, family, oral healthcare professionals, and the oral healthcare environment)

E. Health education and promotion are an integral part of community activities and may be directed to
   1. Allied health professionals
   2. Elementary and secondary students
   3. Educators
   4. Special population groups and/or caregivers
   5. Adult groups
   6. Institutionalized populations
   7. Other health professionals such as nurses, pharmacists, dietitians

F. Health education topics are not limited to oral hygiene instruction; topics might include
   1. Preventive measures such as fluorides, sealants, mouth protectors, and others and their appropriate use
   2. Dental diseases such as periodontal disease, malocclusion, oral cancer, and risk factors such as tobacco use, diet, systemic diseases, and poor oral self-care behaviors
      a. Assessment, prevention, and treatment
      b. Self-examination techniques
   3. Dental safety and dental emergencies (e.g., what to do if a tooth is avulsed)
   4. Roles of various health professionals and their interrelationships
   5. Care of teeth and prostheses
   6. Careers in dentistry and dental hygiene
   7. Becoming a discriminating dental consumer; oral health products
   8. Effects of tobacco use on the oral environment
   9. Environmental factors affecting oral health, i.e., occupation-related concerns
   10. Prenatal and postnatal oral health issues/parent program/nursing bottle syndrome

11. How to provide oral care for those unable to take care of themselves
12. Oral manifestations of systemic diseases
13. Healthy People 2000 national promotion and disease prevention topics (see box, p. 651)

G. Media—vehicles of communication
   1. Two major categories
      a. Written and audiovisual materials used in teaching individuals or small groups
      b. Mass media
   2. Criteria for selection of media for instruction include[19,21]
      a. Material presented at an opportune time
      b. Material presented at the participants' level of understanding
      c. The size of the participant group conducive to the instructional medium chosen
      d. The audiovisual equipment available and educator familiarity with operation
      e. Environment conducive to use of media, e.g., lighting, seating
   3. Written or audiovisual aids include
      a. Printed materials (e.g., pamphlets, books)
      b. Pictures, charts, posters
      c. Slides, films, videotapes, filmstrips
      d. Board—flannel, bulletin, magnetic
      e. Models, puppets, mobiles
      f. Computer generated media
   4. Mass media
      a. Printed materials
      b. Radio and television (including cable)
      c. Newspaper and magazine
      d. Billboards
      e. Advertisements
   5. General principles for evaluation of media
      a. Specific purpose—arouse interest, give information, develop attitudes
      b. Accuracy and relevancy
      c. Based on scientific principles
      d. Target audience—appropriateness; attractiveness, audience appeal; suitableness
      e. Complexity of information; readability
      f. Physical properties—illustrations, color, continuity, and style

Principles of Learning

See Chapter 12, section on oral health education, and Chapter 16, section on successful client management
A. One learns by doing
B. Without a sufficient stage of readiness, learning is inefficient and may even be harmful
C. Without motivation, there can be no learning at all
D. Responses of the learner must be immediately reinforced

E. For maximum transfer of learning, responses should be learned in the way they are going to be used
F. Individuals' responses will vary according to how they perceive the situation
G. All persons perform based on their physical ability, their background of learning, and the present forces acting on them; individuals must be motivated to learn; individuals possess some basic physical needs and some personal or social needs—desire for recognition, security, response, and new experiences; wants, needs, and motives of the learner should be identified
H. Learners progress in any area of learning only as far as they need to progress to achieve their purposes
I. Learning proceeds much more rapidly and is retained much longer when what is learned possesses meaning, organization, and structure
J. Individuals are more apt to become involved wholeheartedly if they have participated in the selection and planning of the project

Principles of Teaching

A. Identify learner needs and audience level
B. Establish objectives
C. Design learning experiences and methodology based on objectives
D. Plan evaluation

Instruction versus Instructional Objectives

A. Instruction is based on a combination of
   1. Instructional objectives
   2. Learning experiences based on the objectives
   3. Evaluation of learning
B. Instructional objectives are important to successful instruction and learning
   1. Instructional objective—the statement that describes the intended outcome, aim, or product of instruction; what a successful learner is able to do at the end of instruction; expected behavior
      a. Behavior—refers to any overt action displayed by the learner (i.e., visible or audible activity)
      b. Terminal behavior—refers to the behavior the learner can demonstrate when the instructional event ends
      c. Terminal product—refers to the end-product, state, or condition the learner can demonstrate when the instructional event ends
   2. Useful for guiding instruction
C. Components of a good objective include
   1. Performance—an objective always says what a learner is expected to be able to do, using a verb that denotes an observable behavior (e.g., "the client will demonstrate the Bass toothbrushing technique")
   2. Conditions—an objective always describes the im-

HEALTHY PEOPLE 2000 OBJECTIVES RELATED TO ORAL HEALTH[22]

ORAL HEALTH STATUS

- Reduce dental caries so that the proportion of children with one or more caries (in permanent or primary teeth) is no more than 35% among children aged 6 through 8 and no more than 60% among adolescents aged 15
- Reduce untreated dental caries so that the proportion of children with untreated caries (in permanent or primary teeth) is no more than 20% among children aged 6 through 8 and no more than 15% among adolescents aged 15
- Increase to at least 45% the proportion of people aged 35 through 44 who have never lost a permanent tooth due to dental caries or periodontal diseases
- Reduce to no more than 20% the proportion of people aged 65 and older who have lost all of their natural teeth
- Reduce the prevalence of gingivitis among people aged 35 through 44 to no more than 30%
- Reduce destructive periodontal diseases to a prevalence of no more than 15% among people aged 35 through 44
- Reduce deaths resulting from cancer of the oral cavity and pharynx to no more than 10.5 per 100,000 men aged 45 through 74 and 4.1 per 100,000 women aged 45 through 74

RISK REDUCTION OBJECTIVES

- Increase to at least 50% the proportion of children who have received protective sealants on the occlusal (chewing) surfaces of permanent molar teeth
- Increase to at least 75% the proportion of people served by community water systems providing optimal levels of fluoride
- Increase use of professionally or self-administered topical or systemic (dietary) fluorides to at least 85% of people not receiving optimally fluoridated public water
- Increase to at least 75% the proportion of parents and caregivers who use feeding practices that prevent baby bottle tooth decay

SERVICES AND PROTECTION OBJECTIVES

- Increase to at least 90% the proportion of all children entering school programs for the first time who have received an oral health screening, referral, and follow-up for necessary diagnostic, preventive, and treatment services
- Extend to all long-term institutional facilities the requirement that oral examinations and services be provided no later than 90 days after entry into these facilities
- Increase to at least 70% the proportion of people aged 35 and older using the oral healthcare system during each year
- Increase to at least 40 the number of states that have an effective system for recording and referring infants with cleft lips and/or palates to craniofacial anomaly teams
- Extend requirement of the use of effective head, face, eye, and mouth protection to all organizations, agencies, and institutions sponsoring sporting and recreation events that pose risk of injury.

From Healthy People 2000: National Health Promotion and Disease Prevention Objectives, Washington, DC, US Dept of Health and Human Services, Public Health Services, 1990. US Dept of Health and Human Services Publication 017-001-00474.

portant conditions (if any) under which the performance is to occur (e.g., "given a soft-bristled toothbrush, the client will demonstrate the Bass toothbrushing technique")

3. Criterion—whenever possible, an objective describes the criterion of acceptable performance by describing how well the learner must perform to be considered acceptable (e.g., "given a soft-bristled toothbrush, the client will demonstrate the Bass toothbrushing technique and remove all plaque detected by a disclosing agent")
4. Time—whenever possible, an objective identifies the time by which the learner is expected to perform/acquire the behavior (e.g., "given a soft-

bristled toothbrush, the client will demonstrate by January 20 the Bass toothbrushing technique and remove all plaque detected by a disclosing agent)

Health Education Plan Development

A. Health education plan (lesson plan)—organization of topics and learning experiences so that they relate to a central theme or problem; lesson plan should include an organized plan with objectives, activities, materials required, e.g., models, slides, worksheets, paper, and evaluation techniques
B. Objective—provides educators with an organized approach in presenting specific topics and ideas to

achieve stated objectives; vital in dynamic teaching for both student and teacher

C. Rationale—to provide a basic foundation on which teaching and learning can be assessed, planned, implemented, and evaluated

D. Use concept of lesson plan in all health education activities to provide conceptual framework for presentations

Methods of Teaching Instructional Units

A. Lecture—informative talk, prepared beforehand and given before an audience or group
   1. Purposes
      a. Introduce new topics
      b. Present many facts and ideas in a short period of time
      c. Review concepts
      d. Convey information to large numbers of individuals
   2. Advantages
      a. Preparation takes place before presentation
      b. Allows for organization
      c. Integrates diverse materials and pulls various ideas and concepts into an orderly fashion; may use audiovisuals such as slides
      d. Can build on foundation knowledge in subsequent presentations
   3. Disadvantages
      a. No active participation by the learner; stifles creativity
      b. Poor presentation technique may present a barrier to learning
      c. Difficult to monitor student learning

B. Lecture-demonstration—informative talk that presents information supplemented by a demonstration to reinforce learning
   1. Purposes
      a. Introduce information
      b. Demonstrate skills or techniques to supplement information; illustrates visually
   2. Advantages
      a. Sets forth information in a complete format
      b. Allows for concentration of attention and economical use of time
      c. Useful for reinforcing material
      d. May utilize models, slides, videotapes, or other teaching tools
   3. Disadvantages
      a. Difficult for large groups to see a demonstration
      b. Requires careful preparation for success; requires adequate facilities

C. Discussion—group activity in which the student and teacher define a problem and seek a solution or an interaction between teachers and students to promote divergent thinking where closure is not expected
   1. Purposes
      a. Allow interaction among participants
      b. Can include the use of questions by the leader to stimulate interaction
      c. Provide two-way communication between the group leader and members
   2. Advantages
      a. Encourages members to contribute personally to the discussion
      b. Stimulates participants to problem-solve
      c. Participant learns to work within a group setting and accept the group's opinion; development of interpersonal skills
      d. Leader may acquire information about the group that assists in directing the discussion
   3. Disadvantages
      a. Individuals with strong personalities can influence a group
      b. A poor group leader may contribute to the failure of the discussion
      c. Nothing is achieved because discussion goes in many directions without coming to closure
      d. May not be profitable if students do not have appropriate background

D. Discovery learning—uses a less direct questioning format to prod the learner into using logic or common sense to discover ideas or concepts
   1. Purposes
      a. Can build on foundation knowledge
      b. Allows introduction of new concepts
      c. Motivates student to discover "right answer;" several answers may be plausible
   2. Advantages
      a. Learner becomes involved
      b. Requires application of knowledge
   3. Disadvantages
      a. May be interpreted as guessing
      b. Need to guide discussion so that correct information is concluded

E. Brainstorming—group activity in which there is free sharing of ideas generated by unstructured interaction; ideas recorded for future discussion but never analyzed for merit during session
   1. Purpose
      a. Allows for identification of an issue or problem by the group
      b. Encourages application of knowledge
      c. Encourages contribution by all participants with no fear of "wrong answer"
   2. Advantages
      a. Useful for youth and adult groups

b. Encourages creativity
3. a. Group dynamic may be influenced by stronger personalities
   b. Needs to be carefully managed so purpose is not lost
F. Cooperative/collaborative learning activities—occur both in and outside the classroom or learning environment
G. Additional options
1. Field trips
2. Panel discussions/debates
3. Problem solving assignment
4. Symposium reporting
5. Distance learning
6. Computer simulations
7. Library research
8. Independent study

Health Education and Promotion Programs

A. Guidelines
1. Should be characterized by active involvement of the participants
2. Education and intervention, stress skill acquisition and risk-reducing behaviors
3. School setting
   a. Combination of parent, student, school, and community efforts
   b. Reaches significant number of participants
   c. Environment supports learning and reinforcement ideally through an integrated curriculum, not isolated instances
   d. Teachers can serve as role model
   e. Success of programs is enhanced by determining responsible individual(s); involving parents for reinforcement at home; utilizing community resources and personnel, e.g., agencies, oral health professionals; evaluation and revision when appropriate

Evaluation and Research

Statistics in Dental Literature

A. Population—entire group or whole unit to which results of an investigation can be inferred
1. Target population—"all members of a specific group who possess a clearly defined set of characteristics"[4]
2. Sample—"portion of the population, that if properly selected, can provide meaningful information about the entire population; a sample is examined when the researcher has neither the time, money, nor resources to study an entire population"[4]

B. Sampling techniques
1. Random sample—"sample composed of subjects who are chosen independently of each other, with known opportunity or probability for inclusion; increases external validity; controls intersubject differences"[4]
2. Stratified sample—"method of sampling used to represent subgroups proportionately in the sample when they are known to exist in the population"[4]
3. Systematic sample—"sample achieved by drawing every n^{th} subject from a list or file of the total population; considered to be random if the list or file is in random order"[4]
4. Purposive sample—someone with knowledge of population arbitrarily selects sample to represent the population; risk of bias
5. Convenience sample with random assignment—used when access to the total population is not feasible; potential members are numbered consecutively, and a table of random numbers is used for experimental and control group assignments[4]
   a. Experimental group—"sample group in a study that is exposed to the experimental variable under study; a group who receives the independent variable"[4]
   b. Control group—"sample group in an experiment that does not receive the experimental treatment (independent variable) but rather receives a placebo treatment or no treatment at all"[4]

C. Sample size
1. Large sample, if selected properly
   a. Accurately represents the defined population
   b. Increases the precision and accuracy of collected data
   c. Reduces the standard error of the sample mean
2. Small sample
   a. May be necessary depending on the purpose of the research, e.g., a pilot study
   b. When inappropriate for the type of research, may lead to inaccurate conclusions

D. Definitions
1. Research—"continual search for truth using the scientific method;"[4] systematic inquiry leading to discovery or revision of knowledge
2. Scientific method—"methodology used in any type of research involving procedures which increase the likelihood that information gathered will be relevant, reliable, and unbiased; steps of the method include
   a. Identification and statement of the problem
   b. Formulation of a hypothesis
   c. Collection, organization, and analysis of data

d. Formulation of conclusions

e. Verification, rejection or modification of the hypothesis by the list of its consequences in a specific situation"[4]

3. Statistic—"numerical characteristic of a sample derived from the data collected; a characteristic of a sample, identified symbolically with Arabic letters ($\bar{x}$, sd)"[4]

4. Parameter—"characteristic of a population; indicated symbolically by Greek letters (μ, σ)"[4]

5. Variable—"state condition, concept, construct, or event whose value is free to vary, e.g., height, dental caries"[4]

a. Independent variable—"condition of the experiment that is manipulated or controlled by the investigator; the experimental variable; the experimental treatment;"[4] in nonexperimental study it is the factor(s) studied to explain or predict the dependent variable or outcome of interest

b. Dependent variable—"measure thought to change as a result of the presence, absence, or manipulation of the independent variable"[4]

c. Extraneous variables—"uncontrolled variables that are not related to the purpose of the study but may influence the dependent variable and therefore influence the outcome of the study"[4]

Data

A. Data—numbers collected from measurements or counts

1. Continuous data—numerical data capable of being any value along a continuum; measurements made from values (e.g., calculus score, time, or temperature)

2. Discrete data—numerical variables or data that are counted only in terms of whole numbers (e.g., number of clients examined)

B. Scales of measurement—used to measure variables

1. Discrete data

a. Nominal scale—observations fitted into classes or categories (e.g., Republicans/Democrats; male/female; good oral hygiene/poor oral hygiene)

b. Ordinal scale—ranking of characteristics in some empirical order (e.g., ranking students according to grades received; student with highest score is assigned rank of 1, second best, rank of 2, and so on)

2. Continuous data

a. Interval scale—measurement scale characterized by equal intervals along the scale; has no absolute zero (e.g., a Fahrenheit thermometer)

b. Ratio scale—measurement scale characterized by the presence of an absolute zero (e.g., age, weight, and height)

Statistics

A. Statistics—science that describes, summarizes, analyzes, and interprets numerical data for the purpose of making an inference about a population

B. Descriptive statistics—that branch of statistics used to numerically describe and summarize data collected; no attempt is made to generalize research findings beyond the immediate sample unless determined to be a representative sample, then may be generalized

1. Measures of central tendency—used to describe what is typical in the sample group based on the data gathered

a. Mean—sum of the values, divided by the number of items:

$$\bar{x} = \frac{\Sigma x}{N}$$

(1) Incorporates the value of each score
(2) Affected by extreme scores
(3) Interval or ratio statistic

b. Median—point of a distribution with 50% of the scores falling above it and 50% of the scores falling below it; arrange scores of distribution in ascending order of magnitude and locate the midpoint

(1) When the total number of scores is odd, the median is the middle score
(2) When the total number of scores is even, take the two middle scores, sum them, and divide by 2
(3) Median can be a decimal
(4) Not affected by extreme scores
(5) Ordinal statistic

c. Mode—determined by observing the most frequently occurring score in a distribution

(1) Distribution may be unimodal, bimodal, multimodal, or have no mode
(2) Nominal statistic

2. Measures of dispersion—used to describe variability of scores in a distribution

a. Range—the spread between the highest and lowest scores in a distribution

(1) Ordinal statistic
(2) Easily determined
(3) Somewhat unreliable because it is determined by only two scores of the distribution

b. Variance—measure of average deviation or spread of scores around the mean; sum of the squared deviations from the mean divided by N; square root of the variance yields the standard deviation:

$$S_2 = \frac{\Sigma(x - \bar{x})^2}{N}$$

c. Standard deviation—used to analyze descriptively the spread of scores in a distribution; the positive square root of the variance:

$$sd = \sqrt{\frac{\Sigma(x - \bar{x})^2}{N}}$$

(1) The greater the dispersion of scores from the mean of the distribution, the greater will be the standard deviation and variance
(2) Small standard deviation indicates that the distribution of scores is clustered around the mean; large standard deviation indicates that scores are dispersed widely around the mean

C. Correlation—statistical measure for determining the strength of the linear relationship between two or more variables[4]
1. Correlational technique is based on the number of variables to be correlated, the nature of the variable (discrete or continuous), and the scale of measurement (nominal, ordinal, interval, and ratio)
2. Procedure yields a measure called a correlation coefficient, ranging from −1.0 to +1.0; the sign indicates the direction of the correlation, whereas the number indicates the strength of the correlation
3. Types of correlations[4]
   a. Positive correlation—value of one variable increases as the value of the second variable also increases; perfect positive correlation is a +1.0
   b. Negative correlation—inverse relationship between two variables; perfect negative correlation is a −1.0
D. Inferential statistics—that branch of statistics used to infer research findings from the sample to the general population from which the sample was taken; used to generalize results to a larger population of interest[4]
1. Parametric statistical procedures in which the following assumptions are made about population parameters
   a. Data are interval or ratio scaled
   b. Population from which the data are taken is normally distributed
   c. Sample is large and randomized
2. Nonparametric statistics—inferential statistical procedures in which there are fewer assumptions about the population parameters
   a. Data are nominally or ordinally scaled
   b. Population from which the sample is drawn is distribution free; no specific distribution assumed
   c. Sample small
   d. Variables are discrete

Statistical Decision Making[4]

A. Types of hypotheses
1. Hypothesis—proposition, condition, or principle that predicts or indicates a relationship among or behavior of variables under certain conditions
2. Null hypothesis (H_o)—hypothesis that assumes that there are no statistically significant differences between the population groups; hypothesis being tested
3. Research hypothesis or positive hypothesis is stated in terms that express the opinion or prediction of the researcher
4. Failing to accept the null hypothesis means accepting the alternate
B. Type I and type II errors
1. Type I error (alpha, α)—based on statistical results, the researcher rejects the null hypothesis and concludes that a statistically significant difference exists when in fact no true difference is present; rejecting a null hypothesis that is true
2. Type II error (beta; β)—researcher concludes that no statistically significant difference exists and accepts the null hypothesis when in fact a significant difference does exist; accepting a null hypothesis that is false
3. Relationship between two types of testing errors (Fig. 15-2)
C. Statistical significance—"according to the odds established by the alpha level, the obtained result is less likely to be a chance occurrence and more likely the result of the independent variable; does not necessarily mean that data are important, valid, or meaningful"[4]
1. Statistical decision making—tool used by the researcher to aid in the interpretation of findings
2. Statistical decision making is not the sole means by which research findings are interpreted and applied
3. Clinical significance—practical implications of research that may or may not be inherent in research results; findings may have statistical significance without having clinical significance
D. Probability level—"researcher's odds for determining the operation of chance factors in producing the obtained research result; cut-off point for failing to reject

		Null hypothesis is	
		Accepted	Not accepted
Null hypothesis is actually	True	No error	Type I error $(p = \alpha)$
	Not true	Type II error $(p = \beta)$	No error

Fig. 15-2   Type I and type II errors.

or rejecting the null hypothesis; also known as significance level, alpha value, and p-value"[4]

1. p-value—"probability of observing a value of the test statistic equal to or more extreme than its table value"[4]
   a. "Small p-values indicating rare chance occurrences lead to the rejection of the null hypothesis and the assertion of a statistically significant result"[4]
   b. "Large p-values indicate that chance occurrences were likely to have accounted for the result and therefore the null hypothesis should be retained"[4]
2. Maximum p-values typically used on the table of values of the test statistic are 0.10, 0.05, 0.01, and 0.0001
   a. If probability is less than 0.05 ($p < 0.05$), the results obtained are reported as statistically significant
   b. Factor of more than 0.05 ($p > 0.05$) indicates data are not significantly different
   c. Test statistic used depends on the size of the sample, the number of samples, the type of data, and other factors
E. Inferential statistical techniques—parametrics[4]
   1. t-Test for independent samples—inferential statistical analysis of choice for determining if a statistically significant difference exists between two sample groups drawn independently from a population and when only one or two independent variables are tested
      a. Designed for normally distributed, randomly selected data
      b. Data are interval or ratio scaled
      c. Used when sample groups have fewer than 30 observations
   2. t-Test for dependent samples—inferential statistic for determining if a statistically significant difference exists between two samples that are related and when only one independent variable is tested; also known as t-test for correlated samples[4]

   a. Formulas for the test takes into account the fact that two groups are related
   b. More sensitive than the t-test for independent samples because groups are paired, eliminating a possible source of variance
3. Analysis of variance (ANOVA)—inferential statistic used to analyze the effects of two or more independent variables simultaneously within the same research design and to determine interactions among the variables in multiple sample groups[4]
   a. Samples should be randomly and independently selected from normal populations with equal variances
   b. Data must be at least interval or ratio scaled
   c. F ratio—value that results when ANOVA is computed
      (1) Ratio of the variance between the group means over the variance within the groups; determines if the observed differences among the sample means is significant
      (2) Determines if the observed difference among the sample means is large enough to reject the null hypothesis
F. Inferential statistical techniques—nonparametrics
   1. Chi square test (χ^2)—statistical test for determining if a statistically significant difference exists between observed frequencies and expected frequencies; used to analyze discrete, nominally scaled data; has two applications
      a. Used in the single-sample situation to determine whether or not a significant difference exists between the observed number of cases within designated categories and the expected number of cases within designated categories and the expected number predicted in the null hypothesis
      b. Chi square test of the independence of categorical variables is used with two or more samples; allows the testing of hypothesis regarding the interrelationship between and among categorical variables

2. Chi square analysis used primarily to analyze questionnaire data that are discrete and nominally scaled

G. Data presentation

1. Bar graph—a two-dimensional diagram used to pictorially display nominal or ordinally scaled data that are discrete in nature[4]
2. Frequency polygon—a line graph used to represent data that are continuous in nature
3. Histogram—a type of bar graph used to represent interval or ratio scaled variables that are continuous in nature

Evaluating Dental Literature

A. Professional responsibility includes keeping current with new developments
B. Reviewing dental literature is important for the contemporary dental hygienist in the role of clinician, educator, manager, change agent, consumer advocate, and researcher

1. Necessary to study dental literature before and during planning for community programs
2. Dental literature will provide impetus and support for various types of community activities
3. Journal articles serve as a source of current information

C. Reviewing dental literature is a valuable source of continuing education for a professional
D. Scientific writing should be comprehensible for the average reader who is knowledgeable about the general area

Criteria for Reviewing Dental Literature

A. Overall description of the article

1. Title concise and descriptive
2. Author's affiliations and credentials are noted
   a. Researcher has a satisfactory reputation for well-conducted research
   b. Researcher is not affiliated with a commercial firm
3. Article found in a reputable journal
   a. Journal has an editorial review board; refereed
   b. Journal is affiliated with a learned society, professional group, specialty group, or reputable scientific publisher
   c. Journal is not a "popular" magazine sponsored by a cause or published by a commercial firm
   d. Concisely written using a scientific style
4. Data published indicate current knowledge and are not outdated by more recent research

B. Author has qualifications to write the article

1. Author's current or past position supports expertise in a particular area

2. If reporting research results, there is evidence of finances and facilities to support the research

C. References are available for articles

1. References are comprehensive, accurate, and recent
2. Given the topic, there is an appropriate number of current references, although older references may be indicated for historical purposes or because they are considered classic

D. Research problem is clearly, accurately, and completely described

1. Purposes of the study are clearly stated
2. There is a thorough review of the literature
3. Important terms and concepts are defined adequately
4. Hypotheses or objectives are adequate and clearly stated; hypotheses or objectives follow directly from the problem statement

E. Experimental or descriptive research requires a different evaluation and materials and methods section

1. Characteristics of the population sampled are described; allocation of groups outlined if a clinical trial
2. Sampling techniques are described and adequate
3. There is evidence of no bias in selection or assignment of objects or persons in the sample
4. Research design is described; there is control indicated for variables that might influence the results; comparability of experimental and control groups evident
5. Tests and instruments used give reasonable measures of the factors under study
   a. Test and instruments used are valid and reliable
   b. Conditions in which measurements are made are completely described
   c. Duration of study is appropriate
6. All factors needed to test the hypotheses or achieve the objectives are included in the analysis
   a. Statistical tests are described; general-purpose computer programs are specified
   b. Hypotheses are tested through statistical analysis
7. Findings are presented in a clear manner
   a. Data tables and figures are clear and easy to understand
   b. Data are presented in a straightforward manner; authors should report statistical method used and reason for selection
   c. Tables and figures highlighting information within article are presented accurately and are easy to evaluate
8. Discussion highlights significant issues that are the result of the research
   a. Author may speculate on the significance of the findings

b. Strengths and weaknesses of the study are stated
c. Report treatment or study complications
d. Results are related to the current literature
9. Conclusions are supported by the findings

Providing Oral Healthcare

Oral Healthcare Delivery System

A. Definition—resolution of explicit oral health needs through the delivery or provision of oral health services by means of organized and sometimes interdependent activities
B. Oral healthcare delivery system is complex
   1. Structure of the system is related to the manner in which clients and providers get together for the provision of healthcare services
   2. Financing arrangements
   3. Supply and distribution of provider personnel

Diverse Modes of Providing Oral Healthcare in the United States

A. Private sector
   1. Solo practice—dental practice in which there is a single proprietorship by a dentist who may employ dental hygienists, dental assistants, and other appropriate staff
      a. Advantages
         (1) Provider and client flexibility in terms of the availability of services
         (2) Inherent economic incentive to be efficient because of the investment involved
         (3) Provider can accept or refuse clients within acceptable legal parameters
         (4) Provider determines policies and staffing
      b. Disadvantages
         (1) Total responsibility for care of clients lies with one practitioner; may limit times absent from the office
         (2) Limits types of care available to clients
         (3) Quality assurance difficult to monitor
   2. Group practice—dental practice in which dentists, sometimes in association with the members of other health professions, agree formally among themselves on certain arrangements to provide efficient dental services; formally arranged and legally recognized entity that is organized to provide dental care through the services of three or more dentists; sharing the group's expenses and income in a systematic manner; using equipment, records, facilities, and/or personnel in both client care and business management; described as non-solo practice
      a. Advantages
         (1) Dentists in group practices generally enjoy higher levels of income than their solo colleagues; practitioner sustains less stress
         (2) Provides for improved personal freedom because colleagues available to substitute when a dentist is absent; emergency care is available
         (3) Quality may improve because of built-in peer review and consultation
         (4) Fringe benefits are possible because of the number employed within the practice
         (5) Sharing or reduction of management responsibilities
         (6) Potential exists for a variety of specialties to be represented within the practice; more varieties of services can be provided for patients
         (7) Practice grows more quickly; takes advantage of newer technology and marketing strategies
      b. Disadvantages
         (1) Personality conflicts may occur, affecting the practice; philosophy of practice may differ; need to balance personal versus group goals
         (2) Loss of individuality; identity belongs to the group, not the individual practitioner
         (3) More sophisticated and complex systems of management necessary
      c. Prepaid group practice is a group practice that provides dental services on a prepaid basis by some agency (third party)
   3. Closed panel practice—occurs when clients eligible for dental services in a public or private prepayment plan can receive services only at specific facilities by a limited number of dentists (closed panel)
      a. Professional groups have expressed concern about closed-panel groups because clients are denied freedom of choice of dentists
      b. Another argument against the closed panel is related to the quality of care provided, although charges of poor quality cannot be substantiated
   4. Open panel practice—occurs when clients eligible for dental services under a public or private prepayment plan can receive care from any licensed dentist they choose (open panel); any licensed dentist may participate; dentist may accept or refuse any client
   5. Dental department in a hospital
      a. Dental care is provided for special situations,

such as persons requiring general anesthesia or other hospital resources

   b. Routine care for persons with special needs such as individuals with cleft palate repair, trauma to the head and neck region, or specific disease or disability

6. Retail dental clinics—dental care facilities located in retail establishments such as department stores to provide dental services to the public

   a. Department stores view the dental clinic as an additional service for their customers similar to pharmacies or optical departments; combine high visibility, convenient locations, and advertising to attract clients

   b. Most dental practice acts require ownership by a dentist

   c. If state laws allow ownership by nondentists, department stores can own their own clinics and hire dental personnel as salaried employees

   d. Purported to increase access to dental care because of location, hours, flexible appointment scheduling, and marketing techniques

7. Franchise dentistry: system of marketing dental practices under a trade name when permitted by state laws or regulations

   a. Dentists make financial investment and receive benefits of media advertising, national referral system, and financial and management consultation

   b. Located in retail establishments, shopping malls, or freestanding

   c. Extended office hours, convenient locations, and extensive marketing

   d. Advantages include name recognition; discount volume purchasing abilities; management training

   e. Disadvantages include high initial and ongoing costs; dentists relinquish control; ethical considerations related to advertising

8. Corporate dentistry—company owned and operated dental care facility designed to meet the oral health needs of the employees

   a. Provides dental benefits to employees and/or retirees and dependents

   b. Reduces employee absenteeism

   c. Oral healthcare providers are full-time salaried employees of the corporation

B. Public sector

1. Community health centers and migrant health centers—federally funded group practices, primarily medical with a dental component; located in underserved areas to provide services to communities where dental and medical practitioners are not found in adequate numbers

   a. Similar to a well-developed group practice with different financing arrangements

   b. Provide primary medical and dental care; referral services based on income

   c. Centers include neighborhood health centers, family health centers, rural health initiative centers, and migrant health centers

2. US Public Health Service (USPHS)—component of the Department of Health and Human Services

   a. Major responsibilities of the US Public Health Service include health research and the promotion of health through public health efforts

   b. Responsible for dental care provided to American Indians, federal prisoners, Coast Guard personnel, coast and geodetic survey personnel, Merchant Marine personnel, merchant seamen, and individuals suffering from Hansen disease

3. State and local programs—states, counties, and cities have established programs aimed at providing care for indigent populations eligible to receive public welfare

Financing Oral Healthcare

Mechanisms of Payment

A. Barter system—provider and client negotiate payment by exchanging goods or services without using money; still evident in some rural areas; two-party arrangement

B. Fee-for-service—arrangement in which fee scale is developed for a service; charge or payment for performed services; traditional method of billing

1. Declining method of payment

2. Locality-sensitive; 37 million Americans without health insurance

3. Examples of fee for service

   a. Full fee—dentist provides service, client or third party pays fee

   b. Usual, customary, and reasonable fee (UCR)

     (1) Usual—fee most often charged by fee dentist

     (2) Customary—range of fees charged by dentists with similar training and service within a specific and limited geographic area; based on submitted fees

     (3) Reasonable—meets the two previous criteria and is justifiable considering special circumstances, e.g., nature and severity of the condition

   c. Discounted fee—a decreased fee paid by a specifically identified group (students, senior citizens) or by participants in a prepaid group

    d. Copayment—a portion of the cost of each service is paid by the client, the remainder of the fee being covered by the third party or other agency; purpose to discourage overuse

C. Capitation

    1. Fee—a fixed monthly or yearly payment paid to a dentist in a closed panel by a third party based on number of clients assigned for treatment; provider receives the fees whether clients use care or not

    2. Premium—fixed yearly or monthly amount paid to an organization, e.g., prepaid group practice or HMO to provide dental care for individuals participating in the plan

D. Office visits—payment based on each visit

Sources of Payment

A. Two-party system—dentist provides service and client pays with cash, credit card, or check

    1. Postpayment or budget payment plans—mechanisms whereby the client borrows money from a bank to pay dental fees

    2. Client repays the loan with interest to the bank in budgeted amounts

        a. Initially proposed to bring benefits of routine dental care to a large segment of the population

        b. Credit card payment is currently more popular and achieves a similar purpose by allowing postpayment

B. Third-party system

    1. Direct reimbursement—a method of financial assistance; beneficiaries reimbursed by the employer or benefits administrator for any dental expenses or a specified percentage upon presentation of evidence of expenses

    2. Private third-party prepayment plans

        a. Definition—payment for healthcare services by some agency other than the beneficiary of those services (e.g., insurance company, employer)

           (1) Dentist and client are the first and second parties; administrator of the finances is the third party

           (2) Third party may collect premiums, assume financial risk, pay claims, and provide administrative services

           (3) Third party also known as the carrier, insurer, underwriter, or administrative service

           (4) Purchaser of plan can be an organized private group such as a union or employer

        b. Prepayment allows the spread of the financial burden of dental care over a group because

prepayment plans apply to groups of people (e.g., unions, all state employees, etc.)

    c. Reimbursement for prepayment plans is done by the usual, customary, and reasonable (UCR) fee, capitation, discount, or other agreed-upon mechanism

3. Types of prepayment plans

    a. Dental service corporations—legally constituted nonprofit organizations incorporated on a state-by-state basis and sponsored by a constituent dental society to negotiate and administer programs (e.g., Delta Dental Plans)

        (1) Contractual agreement with dentists to provide care to eligible beneficiaries

        (2) Usual and customary fees must be filed with organization

        (3) Dentists accept payment at 90th percentile of fees as payment in full

        (4) Regular fee audits occur

        (5) Inspections of posttreatment clients randomly chosen

        (6) Withholding of a small amount of each payment earmarked to build insurance reserve

    b. Health service corporations—offer limited dental coverage as part of their hospital/surgical/medical policies (e.g., Blue Cross/Blue Shield)

        (1) Recently became interested in dental prepayment

        (2) Use cost control procedures pioneered by other plans

        (3) Establish fee profiles or fee screens for different geographic as a basis for reimbursement

        (4) Active in developing alternative reimbursement plans such as capitation and preferred provider organizations (PPO)

    c. Commercial insurance plans—operate for profit

        (1) Have no obligation to dental health of the community

        (2) Organize levels of reimbursement differently; may use usual, customary, and reasonable fees; table of allowances; fee schedule; capitation; or payment per office visit

        (3) Can be selective about groups to which they offer insurance

        (4) Compete with dental service corporations through promotion and marketing

        (5) Can provide attractive total health package plans to potential purchasers

    d. Prepaid group practice

        (1) Involves large group practices

(2) Contracts to groups of subscribers

(3) Payment mechanisms vary

(4) Less common

c. Health maintenance organization (HMO)—comprehensive prepaid health plan; provides a prescribed range of health services to each individual who has enrolled in the organization in return for a prepaid, fixed, and uniform payment for each person or family unit enrolled; capitation based; emphasis on ambulatory care and reduced hospitalization

(1) Monthly prepayment not related to quantity but to average need for services

(2) Provides medical, dental, and other services; dental services provided by a small proportion

(3) May be open or closed panel

(4) Both dentist and HMO share financial risk

(5) Considered to be a managed care plan

(6) Types of HMO models

(a) Staff model—classic model in which the healthcare plan owns the healthcare facility and pays healthcare providers as employees; enrollees are restricted to the HMO's providers and must see a primary care gatekeeper before referral to a specialist; approximately 10% of HMOs

(b) Group model—variation of staff model; HMO contracts with a single provider to provide care; provider group is managed independently and reimbursed on a capitated basis

(c) Individual practice association—most common type of HMO (65% of all plans); IPAs contract with individual providers or with networks of providers practicing in their own offices; some paid discounted fee-for-service, many capitated; popular because it expands a plan's geographical reach and its enrollees' options

(d) Network model—forms a network of independent provider groups that may be single specialty or subspecialty; paid discounted fee-for-service or capitation; may continue to provide services to private clients

f. Dental capitation

(1) Per capita payment from a defined population

(2) Specific dentists selected; dentist bears risk

(3) Payment made regardless of use

(4) Possibility of underutilization

(5) Possible copayment and maximums

(6) Dentist may bear cost of specialty care

g. Individual practice association (IPA) (also called Independent Practice Association)

(1) Legal entities organized for individual participating dentists to enter into contracts collectively to provide prepaid dental services to enrolled groups

(2) May contract directly with a group purchaser or with insurance carrier

(3) Dentists practice in own offices and also provide care to clients not covered by IPA open panel; dentist can be dropped if fails to abide by rules

(4) Dentists reimbursed for services either on fee-for-service or capitation basis

(5) Dentists assume some financial risk with IPA and employer providing insurance

(6) Considered managed care

h. Preferred provider organization (PPO) also called contract dentist organization (CDO)—practitioners, in combination with an administrator (third party), contract with a purchaser of dental benefits (e.g., employer) to offer services at reduced prices in exchange for faster claims payment and larger client base

(1) Dentists charge fees below those in the community (discounted fee)

(2) Purchaser agrees to promote dental facilities and services to eligible employers

(3) Subscriber has free choice of dentists, but financial incentive to seek care from a contract dentist

(4) Limited dentist membership

(5) Potential for overutilization; dentists agree to utilization review

(6) Marketed as practice builder

(7) Considered to be a managed care plan

i. Exclusive provider arrangement (EPA) occurs when a self-insured employer eliminates the third party and selects its own network of preferred hospitals and healthcare providers and negotiates directly for the services to be provided

(1) Self-insured employer controlled health care plan

(2) Self-insured employer eliminates the "middle man"

(3) Self-insured employer agrees to steer employees to particular hospitals and health

care providers in return for volume discounts on healthcare fees

(4) EPAs reduce costs, allowing for a broader array of benefits

(5) Subscriber has limited choice of healthcare providers

(6) Considered to be a managed care plan

j. Direct reimbursement agreement between an employer and group of employees in which the employer agrees to reimburse the employees for a part of their dental care expenses

(1) Client chooses dentist

(2) Client is responsible for payment to dentist following completion of treatment; receipt is submitted, and employer reimburses based on previously agreed upon terms

(3) Treatment decisions are negotiated between the client and provider

(4) Third party plays no direct role

Managed Care

A. Term refers to the integration of healthcare delivery and financing

1. Arrangements with providers to supply healthcare services to members of the managed care organization

2. Criteria outlined for selection of healthcare providers; providers are designated for members to consult

3. Financial incentives for enrollees to use designated providers; members (or employers) may pay a fixed monthly amount; pay nothing or a small amount for each visit

4. Characterized by internal programs to monitor the amount and quality of services

5. Providers receive compensation in a predetermined form such as salary or fixed amount per program member

6. Combines the traditional role of an insurance company (paying for healthcare) and that of healthcare provider (overseeing and delivering healthcare)

B. Dental managed care has not yet evolved to the extent of managed medical care

1. Major managed dental care entities are PPOs (preferred provider organizations), HMOs (health maintenance organizations) and POs (point of service plans); members can receive care from participating providers in the network or obtain care out of network

2. Private and public sector (Medicaid and Medicare) are examining managed care as a potential general and oral healthcare delivery mechanism

3. Views on managed care vary within the dental professions; dental hygienists may contribute significantly in a managed care model because of the emphasis on prevention and cost-savings; especially in oral healthcare

Public Financing of Care

A. Social Security amendments as of 1965 amended the Social Security Act of 1935 and introduced a plan to remove barriers for obtaining healthcare

1. Title XVIII Medicare—insurance program from trust funds to pay medical bills for insured people

a. All people over 65 are eligible; no income limitations

b. Federal program

c. Dental segment is extremely limited to some inpatient hospital care

d. Two parts—part A, hospital insurance, and part B, voluntary supplemental medical insurance; both have complex service benefits available and require some payment by the patient; dental expenditures have consistently been declining

e. Demand for services for low-income population has increased at a time when available services are declining; proposals for alternative healthcare plans are evident in the current political climate

f. Two coverage options

(1) Traditional fee for service; payments made for services rendered

(2) Enrollment with a managed care group that has entered into a payment agreement with the Medicare program

2. Title XIX Medicaid—assistance program; money from federal, state, and local taxes pays bills for eligible people

a. Certain groups of needy and low-income people are eligible, including the aged, blind, disabled, and members of families with dependent children

b. Federal and state governments form a partnership in financing care; eligibility as well as designated expenditures varies from state to state

c. Dental care not mandatory except for persons under 21 years of age; all states must provide oral health services to Medicaid-eligible children; specified in the Early and Periodic Screening, Diagnosis, and Treatment (EPSDT) program

B. Veteran's Administration (VA) provides some dental care through its hospital system to eligible veterans

C. Treatment for children with craniofacial deformities, cleft lip and palate, and certain other conditions is funded by state and federal money, i.e., Crippled Children's Program

D. Federal government provides financing for dental treatment of children in Headstart, the preschool children development program

E. Military services for personnel and dependents

F. Public Health Service—care financed for defined groups such as prisoners, American Indians, migrant and seasonal farm workers, and homeless

G. Federal block grants, primarily Maternal Child Health (MCH) block grant and Preventive Health and Health Services (PHHS) usually referred to as the Preventive block grant

H. State programs—vary from state to state; care for particular populations; various programs suggested to supplement healthcare costs (e.g., catastrophic health insurance) frequently fail or are modified by state or federal budget concerns

Healthcare Reform

A. Current political environment advocates healthcare reform, e.g., managed competition; although proposals were defeated, concepts are important in discussing modes of improving healthcare delivery

B. Thirty-seven million Americans lack medical insurance, whereas 150 million Americans lack dental insurance; a significant number of Americans are dentally underinsured, and the scope of coverage is declining

C. Proposals include the following elements
1. Two-tier system providing benefits for both the uninsured and underinsured as one tier and a second tier including those already with benefits as a result of their insured status
2. Emphasis is on primary care
3. Individuals with AIDS, cancer, or other preexisting conditions will be eligible for insurance
4. Other aspects proposed include emphasis on promotion of health education and personal responsibility, a healthcare expenditures budget, managed competition, increase in urban and rural clinics, expansion of the National Health Service, and reform in Medicaid and Medicare
5. Dental care a small component of the reform; dental professionals are advocating maximum effectiveness and efficiency through a balance of individual and community and public and private approaches
6. Advantages to universal access to primary oral health services include
   a. Fewer children in pain resulting from oral diseases and fewer school and work absences
   b. Medical complications from oral diseases re-

duced, as well as visits to emergency rooms for care

Need For, Demand For, and Utilization of Dental Services

Definitions

A. Need—normative, usually professional judgment about the amount and kind of health or medical care services required by an individual to attain or maintain some standard level of health; normative need defined as professionally determined
1. Expressed in terms of a population or individual
2. Includes specific items outlined in a client's chart, total professional time needed for treatment, number of professionals required, and total cost for care
3. Perceived need or felt need is defined as determined by the client or the public; can differ from normative need

B. Demand—volume and type of healthcare services that an individual desires to consume at some level of price
1. Effective demand—desire for care and ability to obtain care
2. Potential demand—desire for care and inability to obtain care

C. Utilization—proportion of the population that uses dental services over a period of time; volume and type of services actually consumed

D. Attitude—a pattern of mental views (about healthcare systems, providers or utilization) established because of prior experience; attitudes toward healthcare or health practices may often be changed through communication or education

E. Belief—trust placed in a person, a thing, or a system of healthcare; personal or cultural beliefs about illness, wellness, and healthcare associated values of a person, which may then influence health behaviors

F. Wellness—high level wellness is described as a dynamic process in which the individual is actively engaged in moving toward fulfillment of his or her human needs and potential
1. Changing perceptions of health and wellness from medical model of healthcare that is treatment oriented
2. Prevention orientation examines the relationship of the host, agent, environment, and preventive strategies
3. Health promotion orientation creates an environment that enables individuals to increase control over and improve current and future health status

Health Behavior and Utilization

A. Health belief model (see Chapter 12, section on health belief model) hypothesizes that health-related action depends on simultaneous occurrence of several factors; based on the concept that one's beliefs direct behavior; emphasis is placed on the *perceived* world of the individual, which may differ from an objective reality

B. Utilization patterns for dental care
1. Shift in dental services used has been reported (e.g., there has been an increase in examinations; preventive services, extractions, and dentures show a slight decline)
2. People over 65 are the fastest growing segment of the American population; aging population will influence types of services required
3. Each generation demands a different variety of services, e.g., older populations focus on restoration, prosthesis, and concern for root caries; middle aged need some restorative and periodontal services or orthodontic services
   a. Individuals keeping their teeth longer
   b. Interest in preventive practices
   c. American society's concern for appearance and aesthetics influences demand for restorative options, cosmetic dentistry, orthodontics, periodontal services, and dental implants
4. Age and gender—rise in preschool use of services; peak years are late teenage years and early adulthood; females have more dental visits than males; nonwhites have a lower number of dental visits than whites
5. Tooth retention rates in older adults have resulted in increased utilization of dental services
6. Higher education and income associated with better dental care utilization rates
7. Traditionally utilization of dental care is lower in rural farm and nonfarm communities than in urban areas; overall, however, individuals in rural areas are showing a substantially greater increase in utilization than city dwellers; suburbanites are most frequent users
8. Dental insurance influences the type of services used based on coverage; concerns expressed about insurance companies dictating the care provided based on guidelines for payment; thus demand for services influenced by third-party coverage
9. Race and ethnicity—difficult to determine utilization of dental care because status closely related to socioeconomic status, education, culture, and location[13]
   a. Hispanics and African Americans have experienced limited access opportunities including limited access opportunities including limited dental providers
   b. Data on utilization by American Indians and Alaskan natives are difficult to determine; Native Americans residing on reservations received care through the Indian Health Service of the U.S. Public Health Service; traditionally utilization not high; however, varies from location to location
10. Regional differences in utilization reported in the United States: the south reports the lowest utilization rates, whereas the northeast, midwest, and west are similar

Barriers to Dental Care

A. Barriers not related to cost
1. Lack of need or perception of no need for dental care
2. Pain is associated with dental care
3. Access to care is difficult or impossible
   a. Availability of providers, e.g., office hours, maldistribution of personnel
   b. Types of services required not available because of practitioners' lack of skill or interest
   c. Geographic isolation
   d. Nonambulatory (e.g., homebound)
   e. Confined to an institution
   f. Lack of public transportation
4. Client's time is more valuable than interest in obtaining care
5. Dental personnel are not viewed favorably; not accommodating to special needs

B. Cost-related barriers
1. Services are not affordable; fees are considered too high relative to other life costs
2. Insurance coverage is limited or not available
3. Lost wages are more critical than perceived need for services

C. Social and psychologic barriers
1. Dental care and appearance of teeth are not valued
2. Prior experience has been unpleasant
3. Emotional factors such as fear of dental care

D. Cultural barriers
1. Language—provider does not speak the language
2. Tradition
3. History—no emphasis on dental care
4. Healthcare model of the client
5. Basic cultural beliefs about health, illness, disease

Current and Future Status

A. Approximately 50% to 60% of the population seek care annually[13]
1. Reach those not seeking care and make them aware of available dental care services
2. Caries rates are declining; increasing tooth retention rates

3. Public and profession are focusing on the control and prevention of periodontal disease
4. Emphasis on aesthetics, adult orthodontics, and other emerging dental options, such as dental implants, is broadening treatment options for care
5. Society is more prevention oriented as reflected in the increase in marketing and sale of nonprescription dental products such as dental floss, fluoridated dentrifices, powered toothbrushes, powered interdental cleaners, and mouthrinses
6. Based on disease trends and decline in total tooth loss in elderly; optimism about potential for increased utilization
7. Practitioners must be cautioned not to provide services for which they are not qualified; a litigious minded society demands skilled practitioners and quality services

B. Must be a change in philosophy on the part of dental personnel[23]
   1. Identify those individuals currently not seeking care (e.g., special population groups, low income individuals)
   2. Increase access to and availability of care (e.g., vary office hours, offer care in nontraditional setting, improve payment and financing)
   3. Continue to educate the public; emphasize periodontal disease, as well as caries and other oral conditions and preventive options
   4. Encourage lifelong learning by dental professionals to address changing needs and technologies
   5. Develop strategies to educate health professionals about demographic and ethnic changes in client population groups; educate and sensitize professionals concerning cultural perception of health and disease
   6. Recognize dentistry's changing role; emphasis on diagnostic skills and evaluation
   7. Employ appropriate oral healthcare personnel and recognize the potential and capabilities of all members of the oral healthcare team
   8. Professional education must assess and implement curricular changes to better prepare oral healthcare practitioners for the needs and types of services required to treat all clients according to need

Dental Personnel

A. Types—dentist, dental assistant, dental hygienist, expanded-function dental auxiliary, dental laboratory technician, denturist
B. Patterns of dental school enrollment[24]
   1. Dental schools are reporting an increase in applications; influenced by interest in healthcare professions and dentistry
   2. Since a low of 4001 in 1990-91, the size of the first year class in US dental schools has risen on average 1.2% annually to 4237 in 1995-96
   3. The number of first year female dental students slowly increased from 1324 in 1985-86 to 1498 by 1995-96; the number of male first year dental students dropped by 29.6% from 3519 in 1985-86 to 2479 in 1990-91; male enrollment levels have gradually risen 10.5% to 2739 by 1995-96
   4. According to 1995-96 data, 2706 (63.9%) of the first year US dental school students are white and 1013 (23.9%) are Asian; Asian males (n = 589) outnumber Asian females (n = 434); although generally each ethnic/race category has a greater number of male students relative to female students, the pattern is reversed for African-American students where female students outnumber males (n = 140 and 112 respectively)

C. Studies and subsequent reports have evaluated health education, personpower, and delivery modes
   1. Pew Health Professions Commission reports were profession specific; advocated integration of professions; culturally sensitive care; continued expansion of the scientific bases of health professional schools and innovative collaboration and partnerships[23]
   2. Recommendations for allied health include[23]
      a. Restructuring of missions and organizations of education programs to focus on local community needs
      b. Focus curriculum on multiskilling (training at various appropriate tasks to function in many roles) and interdisciplinary core curricula
      c. Improve articulation and career ladder opportunities
      d. Strengthen linkages with diverse care delivery environments
      e. Improve recruitment of minority, disabled, and disadvantaged students/practitioners
      f. Improve faculty leadership skills and competence in clinical outcomes
      g. Establish innovative collaborations among professional associations
      h. Improve collection, evaluation, and dissemination of data related to allied health education, training, practice, and regulations
   3. Institute of Medicine (IOM) Report on Dental Education[25] addressed concerns and challenges confronting dental education by assessing the status of dental education and developing recommendations for the future
   4. IOM adopted basic policy and strategy principles that included[25]
      a. Oral health is integral to general health

    b. Commitment of dentists and dental hygienists to prevention and primary care should remain vigorous

    c. A focus on health outcomes is essential for dental professionals and schools

    d. Dental education must be scientifically based and encourage an atmosphere of scientific inquiry

    e. Lifelong learning is critical

    f. Qualified dental workforce is critical

    g. In recruitment of students and faculty, designing and implementation of curriculum, conducting research, and providing services, all Americans, regardless of SES must be served

    h. Efforts to reduce widespread disparities in oral health status and access to care should be a priority

  5. IOM proposed 22 recommendations that included oral health status and services, education, research, client care, dental and allied health education; accreditation, and licensure, and the dental workforce[25]

D. Distribution of dentists[13]

  1. Traditionally measured in a population/dentist ratio

  2. Population/dentist ratio not always accurate because of location, population involved, community need, and demand for dental services

  3. Uneven distribution of dentists exists for various reasons

    a. Dentists have freedom to choose their practice location within licensing restrictions

    b. Location of dental schools provides an abundant number in some areas and few in other areas

    c. Popular areas are those with a high demand for services

    d. Rural areas have a lower demand for care

    e. Restrictions in movements from state to state because of licensing requirements

  4. By the year 2000, estimates indicate there will be 1000 active clients per dentist, increased from a 25-year low of 981 clients per dentist predicted for 1989; this results in an improved client to dentist ratio; however, technology has improved the skills and shortened the time required for services provided; dentists will continue to provide services in an efficient and productive manner

E. Trends in distribution of dentists[13]

  1. Dentists will continue to locate in areas of demand and economic opportunity and desirable environments

  2. Dental profession has recognized a need to develop programs to help resolve maldistribution problems

  3. Demographic shifts and resulting demand for services will affect choice of practice setting

F. Supply of dental hygiene, dental assisting, and dental laboratory technology personnel

  1. Dental hygienists, as an organized profession, are seeking alternative avenues to help meet unmet dental needs and improve access to care, develop programs to increase recruitment and retention of members of the profession, improve dental hygiene care to society, and promote higher levels of education within dental hygiene, e.g., baccalaureate and master's degrees and doctoral level preparation

REFERENCES

1. Darby ML, Walsh MM: *Dental hygiene theory and practice,* Philadelphia, 1995, WB Saunders.

2. Yura H, Walsh MM: *The nursing process,* ed 5, Norwalk, Conn., 1988, Appleton & Lange.

3. Fodor JT, Dalis GT: *Health instruction theory and application,* ed 4, Philadelphia, 1989, Lea & Febiger.

4. Darby ML, Bowen DM: *Research methods for oral health professionals: An introduction,* Pocatello, Id, 1983, Darby and Bowen.

5. Ludwig TG, Bibby BG: Geographic variations in the prevalence of dental caries in the United States, *Caries Res* 3:32-43, 1969.

6. Kaste LM, et al: Coronary caries in the primary and permanent dentition of children and adolescents 1-17 years of age. United States 1988-1991, *J Dent Res* 75(Special Issue):631, 1996.

7. Drury TF, et al: An overview of the oral health component of the 1988-1991 National Health and Nutrition Examination Survey (NHANESIII-Phase 1), *J Dent Res* 75(Special Issue): 620, 1996.

8. Winn DM, et al: Coronal and root caries in the dentition of adults in the United States 1988-1991, *J Dent Res* 75(Special Issue):642, 1996.

9. Selwitz RH, et al: The prevalence of dental sealants in the US population, *J Dent Res* 75(Special Issue):652, 1996.

10. Brown LJ, et al: Periodontal status in the United States 1988-1991. Prevalence, extent and demographic variation, *J Dent Res* 75(Special Issue):672, 1996.

11. Marcus SE, et al: Tooth retention and loss in the permanent dentition of adults: United States, 1988-91, *J Dent Res* 75(Special Issue):684, 1996.

12. Redford M, et al: Denture use and technical quality of dental prosthetics among persons 18-74 years of age: United States—1988-91, *J Dent Res* 75(Special Issue):714, 1996.

13. Burt BA, Eklund SA: *Dentistry, dental practice and the community,* Philadelphia, 1992, WB Saunders.

14. Nevins M, et al: Proceedings of the world workshop in clinical periodontics, July 23-27, 1989, Princeton, NJ, Chicago, 1989, American Academy of Periodontology.

15. Burt BA, editor: Proceedings: cost effectiveness of caries prevention in dental public health, May 17-19, 1989, Ann Arbor, Mich *J Public Health Dent* 49:256, 1989.

16. Dyck BC: Community water fluoridation from the past toward the year 2000, *Dent Hyg News* 8:3, 1995.

17. US Department of Health and Human Services: Subcommittee on fluoride of the committee to coordinate environmental health and related programs; Review of fluoride: Benefits and risks, Washington, DC, 1991, US DHHS.

18. Jakush J: CDT to consider fluoride dosage, *ADA News,* February 21, 1994, p 16.

19. Dibiase CB: *Dental health education,* Philadelphia, 1991, Lea & Febiger.

20. World Health Organization: *Oral health surveys—Basic methods,* ed 3, Geneva, 1987, World Health Organization.

21. Greenberg JS: *Health education,* Dubuque, Iowa, Brown, 1989.

22. *Healthy People 2000: National Health Promotion and Disease Prevention Objectives,* Washington, DC, US Department of Health and Human Services, Public Health Services, 1990, US DHHS Publication 017-001-00474.

23. Pew Health Professions Commission. Center for Health Professions: *Critical challenges: Revitalizing the health professions for the twenty-first century,* San Francisco, 1995.

24. American Dental Association: *1995/96 Survey of predoctoral dental educational institutions academic programs enrollment and graduates,* vol 1, 1996, Survey Center.

25. Field MJ, ed: *Institute of Medicine, Dental education at the crossroads—Challenges and change,* Washington, DC, National Academy Press, 1995.

SUGGESTED READINGS

Darby ML, Walsh MM: Cultural diversity and the dental hygiene process. In Darby ML, Walsh MM: *Dental hygiene theory and practice,* Philadelphia, 1995, WB Saunders.

MacDonald LL: Concepts of health and wellness. In Darby ML, Walsh MM: *Dental hygiene theory and practice,* Philadelphia, 1995, WB Saunders.

Rich SK. Behavioral foundations for the dental hygiene process. In Darby ML, Walsh MM: *Dental hygiene theory and practice,* Philadelphia, 1995, WB Saunders.

White BA, et al: A quarter century of changes in oral health in the United States, *J Dent Educ* 59:19, 1995.

Review Questions

1 A media campaign encouraging individuals to visit their dental hygienist and dentist for regular dental checkups and reminding consumers to brush their teeth represents focus on which of the following broad areas of public health?
A. The environment
B. Human biology
C. Lifestyle and behavior
D. The organization of health programs and systems
E. Use of printed or audiovisual techniques

2 Epidemiology focuses on the study of groups and is based on the principle that disease is multifactorial. The broad factors studied as part of epidemiology include
A. Host-agent-environment
B. Ethnic background and physical and mechanical factors
C. Climate and physical environment
D. Agent-host relationship
E. Age, race, and socioeconomic factors

3 A dental hygiene researcher seeks to discover the occurrence of occupational hazards that develop during the careers of dental hygienists. The researcher develops a survey and mails a copy to alumni who graduated from the researcher's alma mater. This type of study is using a
A. Random sample
B. Population sample
C. Convenience sample
D. Table of random numbers
E. Nonrandomized sample

4 The dental hygiene researcher also wishes to determine the occurrence of occupational hazards for this year's graduating class of dental hygienists in the state where the dental hygienist resides. With the graduates' permission, she obtains addresses and plans to survey this year's graduates on a five year cycle for the next 25 years. This type of study is *BEST* described as a
A. Longitudinal study
B. Retrospective study
C. Cross-sectional study
D. Experimental study
E. None of the above

5 On the first day of winter, a dental hygiene researcher attempts to determine the number of health science students afflicted with the flu at a major university. She contacts the student affairs office to determine the number of students reporting absent for the day due to flu. This information would be reported as
A. Incidence
B. Prevalence
C. Count
D. Proportion
E. Rate

6 Dental caries continues to be widespread with caries patterns changing. The *MOST* significant change in caries patterns is
A. A greater percent reduction in smooth surface caries
B. Increase in the pit and fissure caries
C. Dental caries in permanent teeth frequently on buccal pits of mandibular molars and lingual grooves of maxillary molars
D. A and B only
E. A, B, and C

7 Data from the National Health and Nutrition Examination Survey (NHANES III) indicate that non-Hispanic black and Mexican American children and adolescents had higher percentages of decayed surfaces and lower percentages of filled surfaces than did non-Hispanic white individuals. Following the collection of this type of information, the next step in planning a community oral health program targeted at the groups identified should include
   A. Implementing a fluoride rinse program to decrease the development of further caries
   B. Seeking funding to purchase and utilize a mobile dental van to provide treatment in targeted population areas
   C. With community based input, developing a program plan based on data analysis, treatment priorities, and resources available
   D. Seeking financing for dental treatment and oral health education programs
   E. Evaluating the data collection methods used

8 A dental hygienist reviewed recent studies indicating that root caries affects approximately 22.5% of the dentate population. The dental hygienist is planning an oral health education program for a senior citizen center within the community. Based on this information and to assist in planning the program, it is suggested that the dental hygienist
   A. Determine the number of residents with and without their own teeth
   B. Incorporate information about root caries within the presentation
   C. Discuss root caries prevention within the presentation format
   D. Not discuss root caries because 22% is not a significant number of individuals affected by the disease
   E. B and C only

9 In reviewing data about dental sealant use, the following becomes apparent
   A. Molar teeth are the most often sealed
   B. A higher percentage of non-Hispanic whites have benefitted from sealants
   C. Approximately 18.5% of US children between ages 5 and 17 had one or more sealed permanent teeth
   D. A and B only
   E. A, B, and C

10 Periodontal disease continues to be a significant oral health threat. As part of community-based oral health education programs, it is critical to focus periodontal disease prevention strategies primarily with
   A. Adult populations
   B. Adolescent populations
   C. Children
   D. A, B, and C
   E. None of the above

11 A client of a dental hygienist seeks to educate elementary school students about the hazards of tobacco use. The dental hygienist is familiar with the principles of planning an oral health education program. One critical step necessary to contribute to the success of the program is
   A. Discuss with the client his ideas for the smoking cessation program
   B. Talk to the teachers about their feelings on tobacco use
   C. Talk and meet with the school-age children to assess their feelings and habits related to tobacco product use
   D. Talk with the school administration about the effects of tobacco use by school-age children

12 A dental hygienist is a consultant for a local Headstart program. The dental hygienist is collecting data about the dental caries status of the children. An appropriate dental index to use is
   A. DMFT
   B. DMFS
   C. deft
   D. OHI-S
   E. CI-S

13 A dental hygienist is employed by a dental school conducting a clinical trial of a new therapeutic mouthrinse for the inflammation associated with gingivitis. The dental hygienist will use a dental index to gather baseline data and as part of the evaluation of the product through the course of the 2-year study. The dental index that will *MOST* likely be used is the
   A. OHI-S
   B. P1I
   C. GI
   D. SBI
   E. DI-S

14 If the dental school–based study mentioned in item 13 also sought to determine the participants' oral hygiene status and ability to remove debris at the gingival margin, the appropriate index to use is the
   A. OHI-S
   B. P1I
   C. CPITN
   D. PDI
   E. DI-S

15 To prioritize needs and plan appropriate treatment, a dental hygiene class, as part of a community service project, is asked to assess the periodontal health status of a group of recent immigrants relocating within the community. A suitable index to collect appropriate information is the
   A. CPITN
   B. OHI-S
   C. PDI
   D. DMFT
   E. P1I

16 A dental hygienist is concerned about the amount of fluorosis evident in the school-age population within the fluoridated community. The hygienist decides to collect data from school-age children located in different parts of the community, using Dean's Classification for Dental Fluorosis. The mean score for the school children is 1.0. This reflects which of the following?
A. Moderate fluorosis
B. Mild fluorosis
C. Very mild fluorosis
D. Questionable fluorosis
E. Normal

17 The dental hygienist suspects that the cause of the observed fluorosis in the school children is the result of
A. Excessive swallowing of fluoridated toothpaste
B. Excessive fluoride in the water supply
C. Excessive use of dietary fluoride supplements
D. Excess use of topical fluoride treatments
E. None of the above

18 A dental hygienist moves into a community with suboptimal fluoride levels in its water supply. The local health advisory committee, recognizing the value of fluoride, seeks advice on remedying the situation. Which of the following might the dental hygienist recommend?
A. Fluoride mouth rinse program
B. Dietary fluoride supplementation
C. Fluoridating the school water supply
D. A and B
E. A, B, and C

19 The health advisory committee, with community support, decides to fluoridate the three elementary schools located within the community. The optimum amount recommended for the community is 0.7 ppm. Thus, the school fluoridator will provide which of the following amounts of fluoride:
A. 0.7 ppm
B. 1.0 ppm
C. 3.15 ppm
D. 5.2 ppm

20 A dental hygienist is conducting an oral health education program for a Lamaze class of expectant parents. The hygienist reminds the parents that because the local water supply is fluoridated at <0.3 ppm, the recommended supplemental dietary fluoride dosage for the child aged 6 months to 3 years is
A. 0.25 mg
B. 0.50 mg
C. 1.0 mg
D. No fluoride supplement required

21 A school-based fluoride supplement program is characterized by which of the following?
A. Can be initiated at the kindergarten level
B. Provides both topical and systemic benefits
C. Nondental personnel can supervise
D. B and C only
E. A, B, and C

22 Which of the following is the MOST important factor contributing to the success of any fluoride supplementation regimen?
A. The benefits of dietary fluoride supplementation in reducing caries
B. The role of the dental professional in prescribing the supplements
C. Rigorous compliance
D. The age of the children involved
E. B and C only

23 For countries lacking widespread municipal water supplies, which of the following is the MOST feasible method to deliver systemic fluoride?
A. Topical fluoride treatments
B. Dietary fluoride supplementation programs
C. Fluoridated toothpaste
D. Fluoridated salt
E. None of the above

24 A dental hygienist is planning a presentation to the local school board to introduce a fluoride mouthrinse program in the local elementary schools. The options for the fluoride mouthrinse include
A. Sodium fluoride in 0.2% concentration/weekly
B. Sodium fluoride in 0.05% concentration/daily
C. Sodium fluoride in 0.02% concentration/weekly
D. A and B only
E. B and C only

25 A dental hygienist is approached by the local health department as a consultant for a planned pediatric oral healthcare program. The health department recently received a generous monetary grant to provide dental services for low-income families within the community. The MOST beneficial preventive program for dental caries reduction would include
A. Purchasing and distributing toothbrushes for all children
B. Dental sealant and fluoride programs
C. Topical fluoride treatments
D. Employing more dentists and dental hygienists within the community
E. Buying a mobile dental van

26 A dental hygienist, employed by the local health department, received limited funds to conduct a dental sealant program within the community. In selecting the target population for the sealant program, which of the following criteria will be used?
A. Caries rates within the targeted population
B. Eruption pattern and grade levels of children
C. Teeth with deep pits and fissures
D. A and C
E. A, B, and C

27 A dental hygienist is invited to speak to a local community group about preventing periodontal disease. Recognizing that currently there is no parallel to water fluoridation for the prevention of periodontal disease, the dental hygienist will most likely emphasize which of the following principles?
A. The value of self-care strategies including toothbrushing and flossing
B. The use of a specific toothpaste and toothbrush
C. Periodic periodontal maintenance therapy
D. A and C
E. A, B, and C

28 The dental hygienist is asked by the athletic director of a local high school to conduct a seminar on Preventing Problems in the Oral Cavity. Based on the target group, which of the following may be appropriate topics to be reviewed in the presentation?
A. Use of athletic mouthguards
B. Gingivitis
C. Tobacco and smokeless tobacco use
D. A and C
E. A, B, and C

29 With limited financial resources, the dental hygienist seeks to assess quickly a target group's dental needs. Which of the following would provide baseline data on a target population while potentially establishing rapport?
A. Type 1 Inspection
B. Type 2 Inspection
C. Type 3 Inspection
D. Type 4 Inspection
E. None of the above

30 A dental hygienist conducts an in-service for a group of nursing home staff to teach them about caring for the residents' dental prostheses. The dental hygienist demonstrates the technique for cleaning a denture and reviews the important steps in the process. The best method of evaluating the nurses aides' ability to clean a denture is
A. Asking the aide to describe the correct procedure
B. Providing a written examination testing the knowledge of the aides
C. Using a checklist, observe the aides actually cleaning a denture
D. Asking the aides to indicate if they understand the steps for proper denture care
E. Evaluating the dentures following a brushing by the aide

31 A dental hygienist wishes to determine the number of alleged misconduct charges brought against dental hygienists within the legal jurisdiction (state, province). The dental hygienist is interested in writing an article and seeks to get current information quickly and with minimal cost. This best describes which data collection methodology?
A. Interview technique
B. Survey technique
C. Direct observation technique
D. Record assessment technique
E. None of the above

32 As part of a community-based dental project, a dental team seeks to work with the local Hispanic community to develop a dental clinic within the community. As part of the development of the community profile, which of the following are important to include?
A. Location of available space and dental equipment
B. Population characteristics including age, insurance status, education, and income levels
C. School system affiliations
D. Community leaders and formal and informal organization
E. All of the above

33 The community-based program located in the Hispanic community requires input from various facets of the community. Possible sources of target group input include
A. Religious leaders
B. Community leaders
C. Educators
D. Nationally recognized specialists on oral healthcare
E. B, C, and D
F. A, B, and C

34 A oral health program planner has limited resources and personnel to provide services. Many groups within the community have significant dental needs. The planner decides to prioritize groups identified with high risk oral needs. These groups may include
A. Noninsured persons
B. Preschool and school-age children in nonfluoridated areas
C. Chronically ill/medically compromised individuals
D. Low income minority groups
E. All of the above

35 A dental hygienist makes a presentation to a local parent group describing toothpaste selection, over-the-counter mouthrinses and their alcohol content, and the importance of toothbrush selection. The content of this presentation *BEST* describes which of the following health education topics?
A. Dental emergency management
B. Care of teeth
C. Preventive measures
D. Becoming a discriminating dental consumer
E. Prenatal and postnatal oral health issues

36 A dental hygienist conducting an in-service for 20 hospice staff wishes to educate the staff about the effects of radiation on the oral health cavity and possible therapeutic strategies. In selecting audiovisual materials, the dental hygienist should
A. Bring an oral pathology book to show photographs
B. Develop intraoral slides and handouts
C. Describe the oral conditions and strategies
D. Photocopy pictures of postradiation appearance
E. Ask the staff for their observations

37 A dental hygienist is developing a parent information brochure on nursing bottle caries. The dental hygienist selects a cover with a photograph of a primary dentition with severe anterior caries. Which of the following criteria for media does the cover selection reflect?
A. Accuracy
B. Scientifically based
C. Complexity of information
D. Interest arousal
E. Provide information

SITUATION: A dental hygienist conducts an in-service workshop on oral health and related topics for preschool staff that includes teachers and aides. Questions 38-39 refer to the situation.

38 The scenario *BEST* describes which type of community based program?
A. Educational
B. Preventive
C. Treatment
D. Therapeutic
E. Consortium

39 A major emphasis of the program would include which of the following topics?
A. Dental sealant application
B. Baby bottle caries identification
C. Orally safe snacks
D. DMF rates for the target population
E. B and C only

SITUATION: A random sample of Dental Hygiene National Board Scores for the St. Appolonia Dental Hygiene Program reported the following: 98, 92, 75, 76, 86, 87, 87. Questions 40-41 relate to the data presented.

40 What is the mean for the sample?
A. 75.8
B. 78.5
C. 85.8
D. 87.0
E. 88.5

41 What is the median for the National Board Scores based on the data presented?
A. 75.8
B. 85.8
C. 86.8
D. 87.0
E. 23.0

42 In suggesting dietary fluoride supplements for population groups, the oral health professional should be aware of the secondary exposure of fluoride found in processed foods and beverages. The concern for the professional is
A. Fluoride toxicity
B. "Halo effect"
C. Enamel anomalies
D. Enamel pearls

43 A third grade teacher wishes to write a measurable objective for a lesson plan on good oral health practices. The objective written is *The students will appreciate the need not to eat sugary snacks.* Which of the following would be a more suitable objective for the lesson plan?
A. Following the viewing of a videotape, the students will be able to appreciate the need to eat fruits and vegetables
B. Following a discussion about orally safe and unsafe snacks, the students will be able to list three orally safe snacks with 100% accuracy
C. The student will be able to remove all bacterial plaque using the circular scrub method with 100% accuracy
D. Following a discussion, the student will be able to list good nutritional snacks
E. The student will identify the role of sugar in the caries process

44 A dental hygienist speaks to a physical education class at a local high school about the importance of wearing athletic mouth protectors (mouthguards) during sports-related activities. The dental hygienist periodically visits the class unannounced to observe the use of mouthguards by the class. The dental hygienist is seeking to evaluate
A. Instructional criteria
B. Terminal behavior
C. Instructional goals
D. Terminal product
E. Oral health education practices

SCENARIO: Following graduation from a baccalaureate level dental hygiene program, you decide to contract with a nursing home to become the staff dental hygienist. You plan to devote a half day per week to the nursing home staff and residents as a consultant, oral health educator, and service provider. The home purchases portable dental equipment and supplies for you. Assume appropriate financial reimbursement will occur.

45 An appropriate target group for a lecture/demonstration on the care of teeth and dental prosthetic appliances would include
A. Nursing staff
B. Nurses aides
C. Residents with teeth and/or dental prostheses
D. A and B only
E. A, B, and C

46 Bacterial plaque control for residents is noted by the nursing administrator as a high priority. In order to obtain baseline data about plaque levels, which of the following actions is appropriate?
A. No action; the nursing administrator is in charge and has knowledge about bacterial plaque levels in the nursing home residents
B. Assess a sample of dentate residents, using a plaque index
C. Interview the clients about their assessment of bacterial plaque levels within their mouths
D. Read the dental literature about the oral health status of institutionalized elderly
E. Assess bacterial plaque levels of elderly patients within your own private practice within the same age group

47 In order to plan a schedule for providing dental hygiene care, which of the following would be useful?
   A. Identify residents who have or do not have specific dental provider arrangements
   B. Identify clients who can or cannot consent for their own treatment
   C. Determine the daily routine of the nursing home, e.g., meal schedule, social activities, off-site activities
   D. Identify dental insurance or reimbursement capabilities of clients
   E. A, B, C, and D

48 You plan your first client screening session to determine clients' dental and dental hygiene needs. Only one client reports for the screening. You recognize appropriate promotion activities about your services did not occur. Which of the following may have contributed to a full morning scheduled with nursing home residents?
   A. An advertisement in the local newspaper
   B. Pamphlets distributed to eligible residents' rooms, with follow-up visits
   C. Contacting legal guardians of those eligible individuals unable to function appropriately
   D. Posters in the activity room as well as other common meeting areas
   E. All of the above

49 You are invited to discuss career opportunities in the dental hygiene profession with a group of 7th graders. In order to keep their interest, as well as provide the important information, which of the following is the best combination of teaching techniques?
   A. Lecture only
   B. Lecture with slides of dental hygiene professional activities
   C. Question and answer session
   D. Distribute brochures
   E. B and C

50 You are an oral health consultant for Barney's Barnyard Day Care, which is responsible for the care of 200 children, ages 4 to 8 at four sites. The health coordinator wishes to assess the dental status and debris status of the children's oral cavity, and is interested in hiring a dentist and dental hygienist to provide care using portable dentistry equipment. Identify the *BEST* combination of indices to gather the appropriate data?
   A. GI and dfs
   B. dmfs and PlI
   C. dfs and CPITN
   D. dfs and PI
   E. dfs and DI-S

51 In addition to collecting data on the oral health status of teenagers, you want them to visually observe the bacterial plaque in their mouths. You feel that by observing the plaque, the young adults will begin to understand the need for good oral hygiene habits. Which of the following indices would best meet your goals of determining plaque status and provide an opportunity for the teenagers to "observe" plaque?
   A. DMFS and PHP
   B. OHI-S and PHP
   C. DI-S and PlI
   D. PlI and PHP
   E. GI and PlI

52 The organization of topics and learning experiences in a manner that they relate to a central theme or problem *BEST* describes a/an
   A. Terminal behavior
   B. Terminal product
   C. Teaching objective
   D. Lesson plan
   E. Teaching goal

53 To keep the attention of a scout group and encourage learning, a dental hygienist should
   A. Present the unusual
   B. Be enthusiastic
   C. Use few visual aids, they distract
   D. Watch for signs of restlessness
   E. All of the above
   F. A, B, and D only

54 Following graduation from a dental hygiene program, a dental hygienist begins practicing in Colorado. Through newspaper articles she discovers that the community is fluoridated at 7.0 ppm. One of the dental hygienist's clients, the local water quality controller, asks for her suggestion on what should be done about the level of fluoride in the water. What should she suggest?
   A. Citizens should drink bottled water
   B. The city water engineer should install defluoridation equipment
   C. Citizens should be encouraged to drink less water
   D. Dental professionals should discourage the use of fluoride-containing products
   E. None of the above

55 The economically minded individual would be especially pleased to know one of the benefits of water fluoridation is
   A. Improved appearance of the teeth
   B. Less pain and discomfort from decayed teeth
   C. Savings in money spent for dental treatment
   D. Improved retention of teeth

56 A guest lecturer at a parent teacher meeting, an opponent of water fluoridation, informs the audience that water fluoridation is "mass medication." The best counter argument to this comment is:
A. Twelve state Supreme Courts have upheld the legality of water fluoridation
B. Children raised in a community with fluoridated water have lower caries rates than children living in a nonfluoridated community
C. Individuals that oppose all medication in any form are opposed to fluoridation
D. Fluoridation does not treat or cure, it prevents decay
E. None of the above

57 _____ reliability indicates each individual examiner is scoring equivalently time and time again, whereas _____ reliability indicates that consistency exists between examiners.
A. Interrater; intrarater
B. Intrarater; interrater
C. Rater; intrarater
D. Interrater; rater

58 River View Restaurant was the scene of a recent outbreak of food poisoning involving 20 dental hygienists and 40 dentists attending a professional seminar. To determine the cause of the illness, which of the following types of study would be conducted?
A. Longitudinal
B. Prospective
C. Retrospective
D. Cross-sectional
E. Experimental

59 To determine if an oral health education presentation to a group of students has been successful, it is advisable to
A. Ask the teacher for his evaluation of your success
B. Plan the presentation to include an evaluation of the participants' learning based on your objectives
C. Plan the presentation to include an evaluation of your teaching methods
D. Write objectives aimed at the presenter in order to evaluate your success as a teacher
E. None of the above

SCENARIO: Following two years in private practice, you are asked to serve as a dental hygiene consultant/educator for a school within your local school district. You arrange to work with an elementary school (Grades 1-5) to conduct a dental health education pilot project. The school is modern, with approximately two classrooms for each grade. There is one teacher assigned to each classroom and one teacher's aide for each grade with approximately 25 to 30 students per grade. You will be working with the teachers, to assist them in incorporating health education topics into the curriculum and with the students. Your specific role as an educator/consultant is yet to be determined because you want to plan your project using principles of public health planning. Answer questions 60-63 based on the facts presented.

60 Before your first in-service presentation to the teachers, you wish to determine both their cumulative dental experience and their oral hygiene status. You select the DMF for caries status evaluation. The *BEST* index to evaluate the oral hygiene status of this group is the
A. GI
B. PlI
C. PDI
D. CPITN
E. PI

61 In reviewing the data collected, you determine the following:
*The teachers have received a significant amount of dental care and most of the teachers have retained some or all of their teeth
*The teachers' oral hygiene status, based on the index you chose, indicates that their use of appropriate oral hygiene procedures is weak.

To assist the teachers to better understand the value of good oral hygiene, as the dental hygienist you should
A. Recommend that the teachers visit the dentist and have their restorative work evaluated
B. Conduct an in-service program discussing dental caries, periodontal disease and the role of bacterial plaque
C. Distribute toothbrushes and floss to all the teachers
D. Give each teacher a pamphlet about tooth brushing and flossing techniques
E. Show a videotape concerning adult periodontal disease

62 To continue in your role as oral health educator, you decide to assess the oral hygiene status of the students. As a result of your schedule, you sample grades 1, 3, and 6 within the school to determine the children's oral hygiene status, specifically debris. The simplest method to evaluate debris is to use
A. GI
B. PlI
C. OHI-S
D. DI-S
E. CI-S
F. None of the above, observation of intraoral status is recommended

63 As a result of choosing the appropriate index in the above question, you find the mean score for the 180 children that you evaluated is 2.97. The mean scores indicate which of the following?
A. The children evaluated are performing an appropriate level of bacterial plaque removal
B. The children evaluated most likely have poor oral hygiene status and require significant restorative work
C. The majority of children most likely have a significant amount of oral debris present on their teeth
D. Based on the score, the majority of children had little oral debris or stain present on their teeth

64 The presentation of scientifically-based health information in such a way that people incorporate the information into everyday living by making informed decisions affecting their personal, family, and community well-being *BEST* describes
A. Health promotion
B. Dental public health
C. Community dentistry
D. Health education
E. Educational strategies

65 The variable controlled or manipulated in a study is a (an)
A. Population parameter
B. Dependent variable
C. Independent variable
D. Variable
E. Discrete number

66 A dental hygienist is conducting research to determine if one brand of desensitizing toothpaste, No Guts, is better than another brand, No Glory, in reducing tooth sensitivity. Following completion of the research, the dental hygienist's data analysis leads to a decision to reject the null hypothesis when it was actually true. This is best classified as a
A. Type I Error
B. Type II Error
C. Type III Error
D. Research method design error
E. Lack of a control error

67 A pictorial advertisement in a dental hygiene professional journal shows a graph indicating a baseline mean plaque score of 3.1. Following 21 days of normal toothbrushing and the use of the mouthrinse being advertised, data analysis indicated that the mean plaque score was 1.5. No other commentary is offered about the study. In reviewing the information on the mouthrinse advertisement, which of the following can be concluded?
A. There was a statistically significant reduction in plaque scores
B. There appears to be a clinically significant reduction in plaque scores
C. There is both a clinically and statistically significant reduction in mean plaque scores
D. There is neither clinical or statistical significance
E. Toothbrushing and mouthrinse use reduce plaque in a statistically significant manner

68 Dental hygiene students were screening clients in a clinic and making the following judgments: no obvious need for treatment; some treatment needed; substantial amount of treatment needed; treatment needed as soon as possible. Which type of scale of measurement does this *BEST* describe?
A. Ratio
B. Interval
C. Ordinal
D. Nominal
E. Statistical

The following scattergram displays hypothetical scores achieved by a group of candidates on a Dental Hygiene Aptitude Test (DHAT) and the National Dental Hygiene Board examination (NDHB). Use this information to answer questions 70-73.

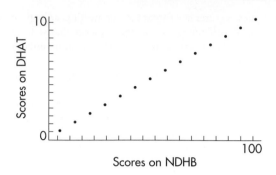

69 The data plotted indicates that the two variables, scores on the DHAT and scores on the NDHB, are
A. Positively correlated
B. Negatively correlated
C. Not correlated
D. Slightly correlated
E. Correlation cannot be determined

70 The correlation coefficient for the data shown would *MOST* likely approximate
A. +1.0
B. −1.0
C. 0
D. −.50
E. Cannot be determined from the data shown

71 One method to decrease examiner variation in assessing and recording observations when conducting a study is to
A. Use a more sensitive index instead of the simple one
B. Have examiners evaluate common subjects, compare results, and come to agreement
C. Have examiners take more time in scoring subjects
D. Increase the number of examiners
E. Rotate the number of examiners

72 In statistical analysis, a *p*-value of 0.0001 denotes findings that are
A. Significantly different
B. Barely significant
C. Very insignificant
D. Very highly insignificant
E. Data are the same—no significance

73 To evaluate the statistical significance of the difference between two means when data meet parametric assumptions, one uses a _____ , whereas to evaluate the expected values versus the observed values of two or more samples when data meet nonparametric assumptions, one uses a _____ . Which combination makes the statement correct?
A. Chi square test, *t*-test
B. Chi square test, *f*-test
C. *t*-Test, chi square test
D. *t*-Test, *f* test
E. Correlation coefficient, chi square test

74 From the consumer's perspective, the advantage(s) of solo practice is/are
A. Provider flexibility in types of services available
B. Provider can control staffing
C. Incentives for practitioners to be efficient
D. A, B, and C
E. A and C

75 A federally funded group practice with both a dental and medical component located in underserved areas with limited healthcare providers *BEST* describes
A. Open panel practice
B. Closed panel practice
C. Community or migrant health centers
D. United States Public Health Service Centers
E. Franchise dental centers

76 The consumer may find a retail dental clinic attractive for which of the following reasons?
A. Convenient locations
B. Significantly lower fees
C. Flexible appointment scheduling
D. A and C
E. A, B, and C

77 Types of fee for service arrangements in various dental benefits programs include
A. Full fee
B. Usual, customary, and reasonable fee (UCR)
C. Discounted fee
D. Copayment
E. All of the above

78 The US Public Health Service (USPHS) is responsible for which of the following
A. Dental care of all Americans
B. Health research and promotion
C. Dental care service for specific groups including Native Americans and federal prisoners
D. A and B
E. B and C

79 A type of prepayment plan that is a legally constituted, nonprofit organization incorporated on a state-by-state basis and sponsored by a constituent dental society to negotiate and administer programs *BEST* describes a
A. Solo private practice
B. Capitation practice
C. Dental service corporation
D. Commercial insurance plan
E. Health maintenance organization

80 The *MOST* common type of health maintenance organization model is the
A. Staff model
B. Group model
C. Individual practice association
D. Network model
E. Capitation model

81 A type of plan in which an administrator (third party) contracts with a purchaser (employer) to offer services at reduced fees in exchange for faster claims and a larger patient base *BEST* describes
A. Health maintenance organization (HMO)
B. Preferred provider organization (PPO)
C. Exclusive provider arrangement (EPA)
D. Commercial insurance plan (indemnity plans)
E. Dental service corporation

82 A type of healthcare system that is characterized by enrollees who are required to use designated providers because of financial incentives, and with internal programs for monitoring the amount and quality of services provided *BEST* describes
A. Commercial insurance plans
B. Dental service corporations
C. Publicly funded insurance plans
D. Managed care
E. None of the above

83 A public assistance program that uses funds from federal, state, and local taxes to pay for care of defined eligible groups of low income individuals and has both a medical and dental component best describes
A. US Public Health Service (USPHS)
B. Medicare (Title XVIII)
C. Medicaid (Title XIX)
D. Veteran's Administration (VA)
E. B and C

84 As part of a local health fair, a team of dental hygienists screens participants and determines that most of the citizens of the community should have a thorough prophylaxis and oral hygiene instruction. This *BEST* describes
A. Need for dental services
B. Demand for dental services
C. Utilization of dental services
D. Attitudes about dental services
E. Beliefs about dental services

85 The emphasis on wellness is characterized by which of the following?
A. A focus on treatment only
B. A preventive orientation that evaluates the relationship among the host, agent, and environment
C. A traditional medical model of healthcare
D. A and C
E. A, B, and C

86 Which of the following statements about utilization of dental services is *NOT* true?
A. Each generation demands a different variety of dental services
B. Age and gender do not play a significant role
C. Higher education and income is associated with better utilization rates
D. Demand for services is influenced by third party coverage
E. Regional differences in utilization exist

87 What barriers to obtaining dental care are *NOT* related to cost?
   A. Limited insurance coverage or insurance not available
   B. Pain associated with dental care
   C. Access to care is difficult
   D. A, B, and C
   E. B and C

88 An individual seeking dental care is unable to locate a provider who speaks the same language. Which of the following categories of barriers to dental care includes this concern?
   A. Cost-related barriers
   B. Non–cost-related barriers
   C. Social barriers
   D. Psychological barriers
   E. Cultural barriers

89 Changes in American society have resulted in a diverse client population seeking oral healthcare. Which of the following is suggested to prepare oral health professionals to meet the needs of the population?
   A. Participate in lifelong learning opportunities
   B. Become familiar with the diversity found within society
   C. Develop a sensitivity to cultural perceptions of health and disease
   D. B and C
   E. A, B, and C

90 The *Healthy People 2000* objectives related to oral health include which of the following?
   A. Reduce dental caries in children
   B. Reduce the prevalence of gingivitis and destructive periodontal diseases
   C. Reduce deaths from cancer of the oral cavity and pharynx
   D. A and B
   E. A, B, and C

91 Applications to dental and dental hygiene programs are increasing in numbers. Increased cultural and gender diversity is evident in the applicant pools.
   A. Both statements are *TRUE*
   B. Both statements are *FALSE*
   C. The first statement is *TRUE,* the second statement is *FALSE*
   D. The first statement is *FALSE,* the second statement is *TRUE*

92 A dental hygiene education program collaborates with other allied health professional programs within a community college to staff a clinic providing preventive oral and healthcare services. Which of the following PEW Health Professions Commission recommendations does this best fulfill?
   A. Improving faculty leadership and skills
   B. Improving career ladder opportunities
   C. Focusing curriculum on interdisciplinary curricula
   D. Restructuring the mission of institution
   E. Improving collection, evaluation and dissemination of educational data

93 The following data were collected by examiners in an oral health survey of 1000 participants randomly selected from the community:
   4000 decayed teeth
   250 extracted teeth
   1000 filled teeth
   The average DMF score for the individuals studied was
   A. 0.052
   B. 0.525
   C. 5.250
   D. 0.005
   E. Cannot be determined

94 An index that measures a stable variable consistently at different times is *BEST* described as
   A. Scientific
   B. Acceptable
   C. Objective
   D. Reliable
   E. Valid

95 Community water fluoridation is an ideal public health measure because of which of the following?
   A. Not hazardous to life or function
   B. Effective in reducing or preventing the targeted disease
   C. Attainable regardless of socioeconomic status, education, or income
   D. A and B only
   E. A, B, and C

96 A patient comments that she believes water fluoridation contributes to an increase in cancer. Which of the following antifluoridationist tactics does this *BEST* describe?
   A. Violation of individual rights
   B. Scare tactics and language related to health
   C. Scare tactics and language related to aging
   D. Creating the appearance of scientific controversy
   E. Misquoting scientific evidence

97 In a recent election, the citizens of the community voted to fluoridate the local water supply system with overwhelming support. Which of the following methods of fluoridation implementation was used?
   A. State legislative action
   B. Referendum
   C. Administrative decision
   D. Water board initiative
   E. Mayoral edict

98 A group of antifluoridationists is seeking to debate the fluoridation issue with local dentists and dental hygienists within the community. To prepare for the debate, which of the following is suggested?
   A. Review fluoridation studies
   B. Become knowledgeable about fluoridation status within the community
   C. Work with local leaders and other influential citizens
   D. Collaborate with other health professionals
   E. All of the above

99 You are asked to speak to a local group of pediatric physicians and nurses in a nonfluoridated community. Which of the following would be a primary recommendation?
A. Fluoride toothpaste will provide adequate fluoride supplementation
B. Dietary fluoride supplements should be prescribed for children from 6 months to 16 years of age
C. Dietary fluoride supplements should be prescribed for children from birth to 5 years of age
D. Fluoride supplements should be prescribed for children before their first visit to the dentist
E. Fluoride supplements are not necessary because of the fluoride content of formulas and juices

Answers and Rationales

1. (C) Encourages changing behavior and prioritizing oral health
   (A) Speaks to physical or nutritional factors
   (B) Genetic and developmental factors affecting disease patterns
   (D) Broader factors affecting oral healthcare delivery
   (E) Describes two categories of media used for public education
2. (A) Lists three factors influencing disease patterns in man
   (B) Specific to host factor
   (C) Specific to environment factor
   (D) Does not include environment as a factor
   (E) Specific to host factor
3. (C) Access to total dental hygiene population may be limited; this example chooses a group that is close and accessible as part of study design and availability of data
   (B) Subjects chosen independently of each other
   (C) Portion of the universe to which findings will be generalized
   (D) Used in choosing a random sample
   (E) Participants not randomly selected, bias may occur
4. (A) Study of a group over an extended period of time
   (B) Investigation uses observations or data previously collected
   (C) Observing and measuring different subgroups of subjects at one point in time in order to study change indirectly
   (D) Etiology established; uses a control group; altering of variable(s) occurs
   (E) Item A is correct
5. (B) Number of persons in a population affected by a condition at only one time
   (A) Number of new cases of a specific disease within a defined population over a period of time
   (C) Summing of a particular disease state or condition
   (D) Uses a count with a denominator to determine prevalence; no time dimension
   (E) Uses a standardized denominator and includes a time dimension

6. (E) Three findings listed in A, B, and C
   (A) Caries reduction in smooth surfaces due to fluoridation; however, not only caries disease pattern evident
   (B) Increase in pit and fissure caries pattern; however, not only caries disease pattern evident
   (C) Buccal pits of mandibular molars and lingual grooves of maxillary molars susceptible to dental caries
   (D) Not all the caries rate patterns noted
7. (C) Development of program plan with priorities is the next step based on data analysis, community input, and resources identified
   (A) Does not address treatment needs
   (B) May have other cost-effective methods to provide prioritized treatment; community may want other options
   (D) Financial support may be one of many priorities developed during program planning
   (E) Data have been collected as part of a major study; planning a program is the next step
8. (E) The target population has to be educated about the prevalence and prevention of root caries
   (A) Epidemiological trends indicate elderly are retaining more teeth
   (B) An important focus for the elderly, but appropriate preventive interventions also critical
   (C) Preventive strategies focused on root caries are important; however, the target population also needs to be informed of their risk factors
   (D) At 22.5%, almost a quarter of the population is affected; an important topic
9. (E) Recently collected data indicate all three findings listed
   (A) Findings reported from NHANES II study
   (B) True when compared with nonHispanic black and Mexican American counterparts
   (C) US children were basis of study
   (D) Excludes third finding
10. (D) All three population groups experience some form of periodontal disease
   (A) Adult population is not the only population group affected by periodontal disease
   (B) Adolescent population is not the sole population group affected by periodontal disease
   (C) Children affected by gingivitis; must be included with other affected age groups
   (E) Not appropriate
11. (C) Input from the target population will assist in developing priorities and strategies and contribute to a successful program
   (A) Client will not be knowledgeable about specific needs of target group
   (B) Teachers provide valuable information, but are not the targeted population
   (D) School administrators can identify resources, but are not the targeted population group

12. (C) deft measures primary dentition; Headstart children are 3 to 4 years of age
    (A) DMFT measures dental caries status of permanent dentition
    (B) DMFS measures dental caries status of surfaces of permanent dentition
    (D) OHI-S measures oral debris and calculus
    (E) CI-S is the calculus portion of OHI-S

13. (C) Measures inflammation levels associated with gingivitis
    (A) Measures oral debris and calculus levels
    (B) Measures bacterial plaque levels
    (D) Measures sulcular bleeding
    (E) Measures oral debris levels

14. (B) Measures extent of soft deposits; thickness of debris at gingival margin
    (A) Measures oral hygiene status; oral debris and calculus
    (C) Measures gingival bleeding, calculus, and periodontal pockets
    (D) Measures presence and severity of periodontal disease
    (E) Oral debris component of the OHI-S

15. (A) CPITN assists in evaluating periodontal disease status and prioritizes needs
    (B) Measures oral debris and calculus levels
    (C) Measures presence and severity of periodontal disease; from gingivitis to bone loss
    (D) Measures dental caries status of permanent teeth
    (E) Measures bacterial plaque levels

16. (C) Findings are characterized as small, opaque, paper white areas scattered over less than 25% of tooth surface
    (A) All enamel surfaces of teeth are affected
    (B) White opaque areas more extensive, but occur on <50% of tooth surface
    (D) Slight aberrations from translucency of normal enamel
    (E) Enamel is smooth, glossy, and a pale creamy color

17. (A) Studies indicate young children may be ingesting excessive toothpaste
    (B) Community water fluoridation is monitored so fluorosis will not occur
    (C) Children in an appropriately fluoridated area would not require dietary supplements
    (D) Dental hygienists and dentists take precautions to prevent excessive ingestion of fluoride

18. (E) A specific assessment of the community resources and the most cost effective method would evaluate A, B, and C as possibilities
    (A) May be an appropriate method based on specific school population needs
    (B) May be appropriate for targeted groups within the community; physician and dental professional involvement needed
    (C) School water systems require evaluation for feasibility
    (D) Excludes consideration of school-based water fluoridators

19. (C) 4.5 ppm × 0.7 = 3.15
    (A) No fluoride has been added
    (B) Optimal for community water fluoridation
    (D) Adding 4.5 ppm to 0.7 ppm is not correct for school water fluoridation

20. (A) Appropriate dose based on water supply and age of child
    (B) Appropriate dose for 3- to 6-year-olds
    (C) Appropriate dose for 6- to 16-year-olds
    (D) False

21. (E) Characterized by A, B, C; early initiation, supervised by teaching staff provides a cost-effective preventive program
    (A) Appropriate beginning at kindergarten
    (B) A value to the school-based fluoride supplement program
    (C) Teachers' aides or parents can be trained to conduct the program
    (D) Excludes grade level

22. (C) Compliance necessary for success; lack of compliance results in failure
    (A) The justification for the program
    (B) The professional needs to be knowledgeable about fluoridation levels within the community
    (D) A factor in prescribing dietary fluoride supplements
    (E) Compliance a key factor in success

23. (D) Salt fluoridation is becoming popular in third world countries
    (A) Dental professionals may not be available or with limited access
    (B) Dependent on organizational structure within a school system; may be lacking
    (C) Availability may be limited or fluoridated toothpaste may be unavailable
    (E) Salt fluoridation is appropriate

24. (D) Equally effective concentrations and regimens
    (A) Appropriate for weekly mouthrinse program
    (B) Appropriate for daily mouthrinse program
    (C) Not appropriate for weekly mouthrinse program
    (E) Includes incorrect weekly dose

25. (B) Provides reduction for smooth and pit and fissure dental caries
    (A) Not the most cost-effective for dental caries reduction
    (C) Useful for smooth surface dental caries reduction
    (D) Not the most cost-effective use of grant money
    (E) Would use a significant amount of funding, may not have resources remaining for staffing and supplies to provide care

26. (E) Criteria for limited funded programs include high-risk populations with deep pit and fissures and teeth recently erupted
    (A) Caries rate is one important consideration
    (B) Age of child and eruption pattern is one consideration
    (C) Teeth with deep pit and fissures are most appropriate
    (D) Does not include appropriate teeth

27. (D) Personal oral hygiene practices with regular maintenance is a useful strategy in preventing periodontal diseases
    (A) One of two important strategies
    (B) Not critical to preventing periodontal diseases
    (C) One of two recommendations for preventing periodontal diseases
    (E) Not an appropriate combination

28. (E) Based on age of group, dental safety, periodontal diseases and tobacco product use are all relevant topics
   (A) One preventive aspect that should be considered
   (B) Gingivitis affects teenagers and should be discussed
   (C) Tobacco and smokeless tobacco use are critical preventive topics
   (D) Missing gingivitis factor
29. (C) Screening is a quick method of assessing a population and an opportunity to build rapport with the study population
   (A) Uses mouth mirror, explorer, illumination and thorough radiographic examination with additional adjunctive tests
   (B) Uses mouth mirror, explorer and adequate illumination and posterior bitewings
   (D) Screening and tongue depressor; available illumination; method of identifying needs
   (E) Not appropriate
30. (C) Demonstration by the aides will indicate if they have acquired the necessary skills
   (A) A verbal recitation of the steps does not indicate the aides can perform the appropriate procedures
   (B) Written examination recalls information, doesn't show skill level
   (D) Does not assess ability to complete task
   (E) Shows outcome; needs to assess aides' ability to perform task
31. (D) Individual board documentation of information about professional misconduct; public record
   (A) Costly and time consuming
   (B) Incurs postage cost; response may be limited or incomplete
   (C) Not applicable to project
   (E) Not appropriate
32. (E) Important to have a complete overview of all aspects of the community as indicated
   (A) Dental equipment and space resources essential, but not enough in itself
   (B) Population profile critical for planning, but not enough in itself
   (C) Collaboration with all levels of leadership within a school system an important aspect, but not enough in itself
   (D) Collaboration with all levels of leadership within a community is an important aspect, but not enough in itself
33. (F) The multilevel leadership within the community provides valuable information and contributes to a successful program
   (A) Religious leadership is one important aspect
   (B) Community leaders serve as a power base and structure; an important aspect
   (C) Educators work with parent and student groups throughout the community
   (D) Not the most critical; unaware of local community needs and characteristics
   (E) Inappropriate combination

34. (E) All groups identified are considered dental high risk
   (A) Lack of financial resources limits access to care
   (B) Children in nonfluoridated areas are at risk for dental caries
   (C) Health status limits accessibility to oral healthcare
   (D) Access to care may be limited due to finances or few providers in geographical areas where minorities reside
35. (D) Topics reviewed assist audience in becoming wise dental consumers
   (A) Topics would include sports related trauma prevention; use of mouthguards
   (B) Techniques for personal oral healthcare practices
   (C) Fluoride therapies and sealant use
   (E) Fluoride supplementation; first dental visit
36. (B) Visual presentation with support materials is appropriate media selection for size of audience and topic
   (A) Difficult for group to see, not as effective as slides
   (B) Descriptions not as effective as photographs/slides
   (D) Photocopy may not be in color; size small
   (E) Audience not skilled to identify conditions and describe
37. (D) A graphic photo of a child's decayed dentition will arouse interest for the pamphlet
   (A) An issue for correctness of material presented; no bias
   (B) Must use state of the art scientific facts
   (C) Reflects readability of printed content
   (D) Overall purpose of pamphlet
38. (A) Providing informative content (education) to assist the staff in planning and implementing activities related to oral health
   (B) Services or education related to bacterial plaque control, fluoride therapies, and dental sealants
   (C) Services including restorative or prosthetic
   (D) Services may be palliative
   (E) Groups of core providers collaborate to provide appropriate referral and services
39. (E) Based on age of children supervised by staff, the topics of baby bottle caries and orally safe snack selection are appropriate
   (A) Preschool children have no permanent teeth
   (B) An oral health condition found in the preschool age group
   (C) Preschool settings providing snack must be aware of orally safe and unsafe snacks and their influence on caries
   (D) DMF relates to permanent dentition; not applicable
40. (C) 601 divided by 7 = 85.8
   (A, B, D, E) Incorrect calculation
41. (D) Score in an array that has an equal number of scores above and below it
   (A, B, C) Incorrect calculation
   (E) Range; 98 − 75 = 23
42. (B) Secondary exposure to fluoridated water from processed foods and beverages
   (A) Overdose of fluoride product
   (C) Developmental disturbances in the enamel
   (D) Enamel pearls are not related to fluoride ingestion

43. (B) Includes condition, performance, and level of acceptability
    (A) Appreciate not a performance or action word; no level of acceptability
    (C) No conditions listed
    (D) No level of acceptability noted
    (E) Only speaks to performance
44. (B) Change in health practices as a result of the instruction
    (A) Level of acceptability
    (C) Broad outcomes anticipated
    (D) Refers to end product, state, or condition learner can demonstrate when instructional event ends
    (E) General topic
45. (E) All three groups would benefit from oral health education
    (A) May or may not be responsive; knowledge is important
    (B) May be required to provide oral healthcare
    (C) Residents, if properly educated, may be able to take care of their own needs
    (D) Excludes residents
46. (B) Discussing target population will provide an accurate picture of conditions found
    (A) Administrator does not have specific knowledge of residents' oral health status
    (C) Gathers residents' opinion of their oral health status
    (D) Provides scientific findings not specific to target group
    (E) Reflects oral health status of noninstitutionalized elderly
47. (E) All information listed is necessary to plan, provide, and be appropriately reimbursed for care
    (A) Residents with providers would not require another provider
    (B) Need to identify individuals and if appropriate, guardians who can provide consent for treatment
    (C) Scheduling will require an understanding of the daily routine of the nursing home
    (D) Identify insured and uninsured for appropriate reimbursement
48. (B) Providing information about the program with personal follow up would market the presentation appropriately
    (A) Residents may not read the newspaper; cost prohibitive
    (C) Only identifies a portion of the nursing home residents
    (D) May or may not be observed; passive marketing; need personal contact with the residents to market the presentation and enhance interest
    (E) Several of the marketing strategies are inappropriate as already mentioned
49. (E) A visual presentation with information presented and opportunity for the audience to ask questions will enhance the presentation
    (A) A presentation with limited dialogue between the speaker and audience; provides information only
    (B) Provides factual information with visual stimulation and reinforcement
    (C) Provides an opportunity for the audience to participate; clarify information
    (D) May not be read, no opportunity to interact with speaker

50. (E) Evaluates decayed and filled surfaces of primary teeth and debris located on the teeth
    (A) Evaluates gingival health at margin; primary dentition decayed and filled surfaces
    (B) Evaluates missing, decayed, and filled surfaces of primary teeth; plaque levels; requires disclosing
    (C) Evaluates decayed and filled primary surfaces and periodontal status
    (D) Evaluates surfaces of primary teeth and periodontal status
51. (D) Both can use a disclosing agent to observe bacterial plaque
    (A) DMFS evaluates dental caries status
    (B) OHI-S visually evaluates debris and calculus
    (C) DI-S is debris portion of OHI-S
    (E) GI evaluates inflammation
52. (A) Indicates behavior that can be demonstrated when instructional event ends
    (B) Refers to end product, state, or condition learner can demonstrate when instructional event ends
    (C) Statement that describes intended outcome
    (D) Organization of experiences based on a topic
    (E) Broad statement of intended outcome of instruction
53. (F) Energetic presentations of a topic in an informative manner will encourage learning and participation
    (A) A suggested method for keeping attention
    (B) Keeps learner attention
    (C) Use many visual aids to reinforce information
    (D) Restlessness may indicate boredom
    (E) Should not include C
54. (B) Defluoridation equipment would reduce the amount of fluoride in the water
    (A) Bottled water may also contain fluoride
    (C) Drinking less water does not reduce the ppm
    (D) Not an appropriate solution
    (E) Incorrect choice
55. (C) Money saved because of lack of need or minimal restorative work required
    (A) Aesthetics, a benefit of fluoridation
    (B) Quality of life, a benefit of fluoridation
    (D) Retained teeth contribute to well-being and improved appearance
56. (D) Fluoridation is not medication; it prevents dental caries
    (A) Does not address mass medication issue
    (B) Speaks to impact on dental caries rates
    (C) A statement related to a philosophy about the use of medication
    (E) Not appropriate
57. (A) Appropriate sequencing of words
    (B) Incorrect sequencing of words
    (C) Rater is not specific, need appropriate preface
    (D) Incorrect sequencing of words

58. (C) Looks to past events or actions; used when variables cannot be directly manipulated
    (A) Studies a cohort from the present to the future; used when variables can be directly manipulated and observed over a long period of time
    (B) Classic method of science where variables are identified, quantified and manipulated so that their effects can be observed and measured under controlled conditions
    (D) Observing and measuring developmentally different groups of subjects at one point in time
    (E) Same as B
59. (B) Evaluation is based on the criteria of acceptability for the learner
    (A) Evaluation looks to learner outcomes
    (C) Evaluation is not one of the teaching methods
    (D) Objectives are written focusing on the learner
    (E) Not appropriate
60. (B) Measures thickness of oral debris at gingival margin
    (A) Measures gingival inflammation
    (C) Assists in prioritizing needs
    (D) Measures periodontal disease
61. (B) Education necessary to provide a foundation on oral health concepts
    (A) Oral health services would be provided on an individual basis
    (C) Without education, teachers may not understand the value of personal oral hygiene or use these items correctly
    (D) Pamphlet is a passive method of presenting information
    (E) Speaks to one of the conditions that may be affecting the teachers
62. (D) Debris portion of the OHI-S; useful with children
    (A) Evaluates gingival inflammation
    (B) Evaluates debris at the gingival margin, requires use of a probe
    (C) Evaluates both debris and calculus
    (E) Calculus portion of the OHI-S
63. (C) Based on the score, the children exhibit a significant amount of oral debris
    (A) High score indicates students are not removing bacterial plaque
    (B) Cannot make a judgment about restorative needs
    (D) Score does not indicate a small amount of oral debris or stain
64. (D) Involves psychological, intellectual, and social dimensions necessary to change behavior
    (A) Any combination of learning opportunities designed to facilitate voluntary adaptations of behavior conducive to health
    (B) Promoting, preventing, and controlling dental diseases through community efforts
    (C) Focus on community-based efforts related to oral diseases
    (E) Range of techniques and tools available to facilitate learning

65. (C) An independent variable is directly controlled or manipulated
    (A) Characteristics of a population are a population parameter
    (B) That variable whose value is thought to change as a result of exposure to the independent variable is a dependent variable
    (D) A characteristic, state, or condition that can vary from subject to subject is a variable
    (E) A number that cannot be subdivided meaningfully is a discrete number
66. (A) Based on statistical results, the researcher rejects the null hypothesis and concludes that a statistically significant difference exists when in fact no true difference is present
    (B) Researcher concludes that no statistically significant difference exists and accepts the null hypothesis when in fact a significant difference exists
    (C) No such error exists
    (D) Specifically describes a Type I error; cannot determine research design error from question
    (E) Appears to have a control; not relevant to question
67. (B) The reduction in the mean plaque score indicates less clinically visible bacterial plaque
    (A) Statistical data were not presented
    (C) Cannot determine because no statistical data were presented
    (D) The reduction in plaque scores indicates a clinically observed difference
    (E) Cannot conclude from the advertisement
68. (C) Ranking of characteristic in some empirical order
    (A) Measurement characterized by the presence of an absolute zero
    (B) Measurement scale characterized by equal intervals along the scale; no absolute zero
    (D) Observations fitted into classes or categories
    (E) Numerical characteristic of a sample derived from sample collected
69. (A) Strong linear relationship; direction and strength indicates a positive correlation
    (B) Value of variable A increases as the value of variable B decreases
    (C) Not true
    (D) Diagram indicates a strong relationship
    (E) Diagram indicates a perfect positive relationship
70. (A) Value indicates a perfect positive relationship
    (B) Value indicates a perfect negative relationship
    (C) Scattergram would be inconsistent in relationship and direction
    (D) Moderate negative correlation
    (E) Can be determined from scattergram

71. (B) Calibrating examiners by examination of a few subjects and comparison of results reduces variation in assessing and recording
    (A) Simple criteria will be sensitive
    (C) Increased time will not necessarily decrease variation. The objective is to use quick-scoring instrument
    (D) Increasing the number of examiners will increase variation
    (E) Rotating examiners will increase chances of less agreement

72. (A) Probability of less than 0.05 indicates that at least two sets of data are significantly different
    (B) Probability of greater than 0.05 indicates that at least two sets of data are not significantly different
    (C) Very insignificant probability would require a greater score than 0.05
    (D) Very highly insignificant probability would require a greater score than 0.05
    (E) The value of p indicates the significance level

73. (C) The t-test, a parametric statistic, determines the significance of the statistical difference between two means; the chi square test, a nonparametric statistic, determines if there is a statistical difference between expected values and observed values
    (A) They are in incorrect order
    (B) The f test is used to compare variances of two or more samples
    (D) Both these tests are used for normally distributed, randomly selected, measured data
    (E) The correlation coefficient determines the strength and direction of the linear relationship between two variables

74. (E) Efficiency will contribute to savings in cost; practitioner can provide a wide range of oral health services
    (A) A characteristic of private practice
    (B) A benefit for the provider
    (C) An advantage for the consumer
    (D) Incorrect selection

75. (C) Similar to group practice; include neighborhood health centers, family centers, and rural initiative centers
    (A) Clients eligible for dental services can receive care from any licensed dentist
    (B) Clients eligible for dental services can receive care only from specific providers
    (D) USPHS provides oral health services for specifically defined groups
    (E) A type of dental practice

76. (D) Location, hours and availability of services are attractive
    (A) Frequently located in retail settings
    (B) Not a characteristic of retail dental clinics
    (C) Hours may parallel retail settings hours
    (E) Incorrect selection

77. (E) All items listed are types of fee for service
    (A) Dentist provides service; client pays fee
    (B) A frequently charged fee common within a specific geographic area
    (C) A decreased fee paid by an identified group, e.g., persons enrolled in a preferred provider organization for healthcare insurance coverage
    (D) A portion of the cost of each service paid by the patient

78. (E) Component of the Department of Health and Human Services with specifically defined responsibilities such as health research and promotion, and the provision of dental care to specific groups
    (A) Not the responsibility of the USPHS
    (B) A responsibility
    (C) Also responsible for Coast Guard personnel, coast and geodetic survey personnel, Merchant Marine personnel, merchant seamen, and individuals suffering from Hansen's disease
    (D) Not appropriate selection

79. (C) Sponsored by a constituent dental society to negotiate and administer programs, e.g., Delta Dental Plans
    (A) Single proprietorship
    (B) Dentist agrees to provide to subscribers certain dental services as specified in the comprehensive plan in return for a per-capita basis per month
    (D) Operate for profit via the collection of premiums to meet the cost of providing dental care
    (E) Comprehensive prepaid plan; provides prescribed range of services for a predetermined fixed payment to subscribers

80. (C) 65% of all plans; popular because of geographic reach and enrollee options
    (A) Classic model where healthcare plan owns facility and pays the providers a salary
    (B) Variation of staff model; HMO contracts with a group practice, partnership, or corporation to provide care; managed independently
    (D) Similar to the IPA; HMO contracts with a network of independent providers who deliver care to subscribers
    (E) Per capita payment where provider receives a fixed sum of money, per capita per month

81. (B) Also called a contract dentists' organization (CDO)
    (A) Comprehensive prepaid plan; provides a range of services to enrollees in return for prepaid amount
    (C) Self-insured employer eliminates the third party and selects its own network of hospitals and healthcare providers; negotiates directly without a third party insurer
    (D) For profit organization; organize levels of reimbursement differently; can be selective in terms of subscribers
    (E) Legally constituted, nonprofit organization incorporated on a state by state basis to administer contracts for dental care

82. (D) Integration of healthcare delivery and financing
    (A) For profit; may provide total healthcare financing package without regard to how care is delivered
    (B) Legally constituted, nonprofit organization incorporated on a state by state basis to administer contracts for dental care
    (C) Medicare is an example
    (E) Not appropriate selection
83. (C) A public assistance program; partnership with federal and state governments
    (A) Health promotion, research, and oral healthcare for defined groups
    (B) Insurance from trust funds to pay medical bills for insured elderly and disabled individuals
    (D) Provides some care for eligible veterans within the hospital system
    (E) Not appropriate
84. (A) Normative, professionally defined estimate of oral health services required
    (B) Volume and type of health services that an individual desires
    (C) Proportion of population that uses dental services
    (D) Pattern of mental views about healthcare influenced by previous experiences
    (E) Personal or cultural views and practices on healthcare
85. (B) A preventive orientation toward attaining and maintaining health
    (A) The current medical model
    (C) Treat illness, little focus on preventing illness
    (D, E) Not appropriate
86. (B) Age and gender influence dental services utilization; youngsters have little control over access; women seek more dental care
    (A) Needs vary based on age and previous dental services
    (C) A true statement
    (D) Third party coverage influences the services sought
    (E) South reports lowest utilization; northeast, midwest, and west are similar
87. (E) Both pain and access are non-cost factors
    (A) A cost related barrier
    (B) A non-cost barrier
    (C) A non-cost barrier related to location, available providers, mobility of the client, and other factors
    (D) Not appropriate selection
88. (E) Language, tradition, and history may be barriers
    (A) Includes fees, insurance, and employment status
    (B) Pain, access, geographic isolation
    (C) Appearance and function of teeth not valued
    (D) Previous unpleasant dental experiences or emotional factors
89. (E) All factors are necessary to assist dental practitioners to meet the needs of the diverse population
    (A) Continuing education provides an opportunity to enhance one's professional skills
    (B) Diversity education important for the professional
    (C) Sensitivity to cultural, ethnic, and racial diversity important for all members of the oral healthcare team
    (D) Not correct

90. (E) Healthy People 2000 has specific objectives within these areas
    (A) Significant reductions in children and adolescents
    (B) Targeting 35 to 44 year old adults
    (C) Targeting both men and women aged 45 to 74
    (D) Not appropriate selection
91. (A) The number of women as well as minority applicants are increasing in both dentistry and dental hygiene
    (B, C, D) Not an appropriate selection
92. (C) Strong emphasis on interdisciplinary education among health professions
    (A) Faculty development and professional growth
    (B) Allied health personnel should have opportunities for professional growth
    (D) Focus on community based healthcare delivery and education
    (E) To assist in developing appropriate curricula and educational focus
93. (C) 5250 divided by 1000 = 5.25
    (A, B, D) Incorrect calculation
94. (D) Consistency of measurement
    (A) Based on accurate, scientific principles
    (B) Client finds use of index acceptable
    (C) Criteria are clearly defined and understandable
    (E) Measures what it is intended to measure
95. (E) Meets all the criteria for a public health measure, other examples, vaccination
    (A) Not harmful to life
    (B) Reduces dental caries rates
    (C) All citizens within a community have access to water supply
    (D) Not appropriate selection
96. (B) Use of words associated with debilitating diseases in order to frighten
    (A) Freedom of choice argument; this was not done in the example
    (C) Argument that fluoridation leads to Alzheimer's disease; this was not done in the example
    (D) Repeating mistruths about fluoridation; this was not done in the example
    (E) Incorrectly citing studies or conclusions; this was not done in the example
97. (B) An opportunity for the community to vote on the issue
    (A) State legislation may mandate fluoridation based on community size
    (C) City council implement community fluoridation
    (D) Local water board or officer implements water fluoridation
    (E) Mayor of community decides to implement water fluoridation

98. (E) Important to prepare comprehensively for a discussion with antifluoridationists
    (A) Historical and current studies are valuable sources of information
    (B) Knowledge about community water supplies and level of fluoride
    (C) Local leaders offer important support and resources; respected within the community
    (D) Collaboration expands community support; identified additional advocates

99. (B) Current recommendation for children in communities with 0.6 ppm or less fluoride in drinking water
    (A) Not recommended as a substitute for supplementation
    (C) Supplementation needed until age 14
    (D) Not the best statement concerning supplementation
    (E) Not true

Practice Management and Career Development Strategies

Sandra Kramer

Achieving and maintaining a successful position as a valued healthcare provider requires not only knowledge and skill in one's profession but also a basic understanding of business management and career development strategies. This chapter is designed to bridge the gap between the educational preparation of the dental hygienist and the reality of the working world. Topics reviewed in this chapter include practice building and management, marketing skills and strategies, employment situations, compensation, job performance, communication techniques, resumé preparation, interviewing, job search strategies and job selection considerations, employment retention and mobility, and personal financial planning. Intentional involvement of the dental hygienist in these concepts should contribute to increased effectiveness as an interdisciplinary team member and personal career satisfaction.

The Dental Hygienist as a Healthcare Provider on the Dental Team

The Team Concept

A. Definition—combined actions with interdependence of the entire staff to promote the unit and efficiency of the group rather than individual interests; "team spirit" is affected by each member
B. Team members

1. Clients
2. Dentists
3. Dental hygienists
4. Dental assistants
5. Receptionists
6. Office managers
7. Dental laboratory technicians
8. Bookkeepers
9. Other healthcare providers

C. Goals
1. High-quality oral healthcare
2. Decentralized management, with each person accepting responsibility and participating in decision making
3. Work simplification
4. Increased efficiency
5. Reduction in work time
6. Increased practice profitability
7. Office harmony and comradery within an enjoyable and supportive environment
8. Job satisfaction for all individuals with achievement of self-esteem and self-actualization
9. Professional growth for each individual

D. Characteristics of an effective work team[1]
1. Group atmosphere is informal, comfortable, relaxed, and supportive, producing a feeling of belonging
2. Flexibility exists to accommodate for change

3. People talk to one another, mostly about the job to be done
4. Job tasks, roles, and functions are well understood and accepted by the staff, with recognition of the special contributions of each individual
5. Staff members respect and value one another
6. Staff members maturely listen to one another and are unafraid to express ideas and opinions; attempts are made to resolve differences, and personnel can accept unresolvable disagreement
7. There is fusion of ideas, energy, and individual expertise
8. Most decisions are reached by consensus, with individuals realizing the importance of a total and united team effort for ultimate benefit to all
9. Criticism is frequent, honest, and relatively comfortable
10. People express their feelings
11. Innovation and change are accepted and are common
12. When action is taken, clear assignments are made and accepted; action is immediate
13. Goals are periodically reevaluated, with adjustments made as needed
14. Leader of the group does not dominate; leadership may shift from person to person

E. Team elements
   1. Interpersonal
      a. Open and frequent communications throughout each day maintain fluid client and procedural activities
      b. Regular staff meetings
         (1) Purposes
             (a) Review goals
             (b) Evaluate progress
             (c) Share updated information
             (d) Air grievances
             (e) Problem-solve and reach agreement on solutions
         (2) Design
             (a) State the purpose of the meeting
             (b) Prepare and distribute the agenda in advance
             (c) Consider agenda items and suggestions from all staff members
             (d) Share discussions among all members; no single person dominates the meeting
             (e) Reach decisions by consensus
             (f) Stay on track; do not stray off of the agenda
             (g) End on a positive, team-building note

c. Includes quality human relations between all office personnel, clients, and members of the professional community
   2. Organizational
      a. Practice philosophy, goals, and objectives are determined by the team and written to direct daily activities
      b. Policy and procedures manuals systematize the practice and clearly familiarize personnel with responsibilities
      c. Staff meetings include organizational and administrative evaluation and control

F. Team building
   1. Definition—synergistic process of developing group goals with motivation and commitment
   2. Technique
      a. Participation of all members
      b. Dissemination of information
      c. Sharing of ideas
      d. Formulation of goals, objectives, and priorities
      e. Critique of plans and anticipation of obstacles
      f. Modification of goals and objectives
      g. Activation of plans
      h. Evaluation of plans
      i. Revisions as needed

Successful Client Management

A. Attitudes toward clients
   1. Client is the most important person in the practice, the purpose for work and for the existence of the dental practice
   2. Client is a member of the "team" and must be included in all decisions about his or her oral care
   3. Each individual is approached as a whole person, including medical, psychologic, and emotional aspects
   4. A variety of value systems exist, all of which are different; intrinsic worth of each individual person is appreciated
   5. Client's personal resources are acknowledged[2]
      a. Level of self-esteem
      b. Experiential background and previous history
      c. Intelligence
      d. Motivation
      e. Values
      f. Socioeconomic level
      g. Ethnicity
      h. Culture
B. Communications[2]
   1. People communicate to satisfy human needs
      a. Need to survive—physiologic
      b. Need for safety and comfort—physical and psychologic security

c. Interpersonal needs—social needs for acceptance, love, and recognition

d. Intrapersonal needs—self-esteem and self actualization

2. Clear and accurate communication between members of the healthcare team and clients is critical to successful client management

   a. Effective communication requires skills in both sending and receiving messages

     (1) Verbal

     (2) Nonverbal

     (3) Written

   b. Oral healthcare appointments often cause increased stress and anxiety partly by

     (1) Oral discomfort, pain, or problems

     (2) Treatments and procedures

     (3) Exclusive behavior of personnel

     (4) Unfamiliar environment

     (5) Fear of the unknown or outcome

     (6) Fear of rejection or criticism

     (7) Embarrassment about health or dental history

3. All communications and behaviors have meaning and result from inner thoughts or feelings

4. Maintain an open, accepting environment by being understanding, permissive, nonjudgmental, and honest

5. Recognize the person as an individual

   a. Call the person by name

   b. Refer to others in the office by name

   c. Be courteous to the person and others who may accompany the person

   d. Respect the person's privacy

   e. Support the person's dignity

   f. Maintain confidentiality

   g. Create an atmosphere of acceptance

   h. Establish rapport by using open-ended interviewing techniques

6. Eliminate barriers created by the oral healthcare environment whenever possible

   a. Be flexible in carrying out routines and policies

   b. Use informed consent

   c. Explain procedures before beginning

   d. Avoid the use of dental jargon that excludes the client

   e. Encourage client participation in discussions and decision making

   f. Create a role for the client as a cotherapist

   g. Value cultural diversity

7. Identify the client's human needs, values, attitudes, and lifestyle and determine priorities for care

   a. Educate the client about the findings

   b. Help the client understand the nature of the findings and accept needed care and consequences

   c. Gain client input to establish priorities together; set goals and priorities with the client

   d. Be nonjudgmental and nonpunitive in your response and behavior; do not "lecture" the client

   e. Build commitment by using client's goals

C. Establishment of a teaching-learning environment[2] (see Chapter 12, section on stages in making a commitment to a new behavior, and Chapter 15, section on implementation)

1. Definitions

   a. Teaching—communication designed to produce learning

   b. Learning—activity by which knowledge, attitudes, and skills are acquired, resulting in behavior change

2. Goals of learning

   a. Acquiring knowledge—cognitive

   b. Developing attitudes—effective

   c. Developing psychomotor skills—conative

3. Principles of the teaching-learning process

   a. Learning occurs best when there is a perceived need or readiness to learn

     (1) Identify the person's motivational readiness

     (2) Identify the person's experiential readiness

     (3) Determine the person's level of adaptation

     (4) Consider the person's level of human needs

     (5) Recognize the signs of learning readiness

       (a) Awareness—person develops awareness of the oral health problem

       (b) Interest—person asks direct questions

       (c) Desire—person seeks information

       (d) Action—person's oral disease condition allows the dental hygienist to intervene through teaching

     (6) Once the need has been recognized by the client and readiness has been determined, develop a plan and facilitate learning

   b. Method of presentation of material influences the person's ability to learn

     (1) Keep information organized, accurate, and brief

     (2) Institute appropriate teaching methods

       (a) Concepts are best taught with discussions and visual aids

       (b) Attitudes are best taught by exploration of feelings, discussion, and an atmosphere of acceptance

       (c) Skills are best taught by illustrations, models, demonstration, return demonstration, feedback, and practice

(3) Encourage persons to ask questions and answer them directly

(4) Provide opportunities for evaluation/self-evaluation

c. Learning is easier when new material is related to what the learner already knows

(1) Assess person's knowledge, attitudes, values regarding the situation or problem

(2) Reinforce the knowledge base, then relate new information to similar, previous experiences

(3) Teach at the person's level of understanding, based on the foundation of the present knowledge

(4) Avoid the use of technical jargon

d. Learning is purposeful—short-term and long-term goals identify desired behavior

(1) Set goals with the client

(2) Criteria for goals

(a) Specific—state exactly what is to be accomplished

(b) Measurable—set a minimum acceptable level of performance

(c) Realistic—must be reasonably achievable

(d) Time frame—set time period for goal attainment

e. Learning is an active process and takes place within the learner

(1) Use a teaching approach that actively involves the learner

(2) Provide opportunities for the person to practice new skills

(3) Encourage self-directed activities

f. Every individual has capabilities and strengths that can help him or her to learn

(1) Identify the client's personal resources

(2) Build on identified strengths

(3) Use personal resources

(4) Try to adapt recommended behavior changes to the person's lifestyle

g. Overall health, outside stresses, and energy will affect the person's ability to learn and perform

h. Learning does not always advance straight ahead—expect plateaus and remissions with a resulting change in needs

(1) Accept the person's feelings regarding lack of progress

(2) Identify progress that has been made

(3) Be patient; do not cause additional stress to the person

(4) Try alternative approaches for achieving goals

(5) Identify short-term goals with which the person can agree

(6) Alter long-term goals if necessary

4. Motivation

a. Definition—process of stimulating a person to assimilate certain concepts or behavior

b. Principles related to dental hygiene approaches

(1) Each person deserves to be cared for as a whole being, as a complex product of life's experiences—be accepting and respectful

(2) Learning is best when information coincides with the client's own attitudes, culture, and value system

(3) A motivated learner assimilates new information more rapidly than a nonmotivated learner

(4) Intrinsic motivation (stimulated from within the learner) is preferable to extrinsic motivation (stimulated from outside the learner)

(a) Identify factors that are essential for the client to have a meaningful achievement

(b) Satisfaction with learning progress promotes additional learning; therefore, design teaching to assist the client in attaining a feeling of meaningful achievement

(c) Encourage the client to participate and be self-directed

(5) Information is learned more readily when it is relevant and meaningful to the person

(a) Help the person interpret why the information is important and how new information will be useful

(b) Relate information by building on the person's foundation of knowledge, experience, attitudes, and feelings

(6) Learning motivated by success or rewards is preferable to learning by failure or punishment

(a) Help the person set realistic goals, focusing on abilities and strengths

(b) Select learning tasks in which the client is likely to succeed

(c) Help the person master or feel successful at each stage of instruction before going on to the next

(d) Accept errors as part of the learning process

(e) Teach tolerance for failure by recalling previous successes

(7) Planned reinforcement is essential for learning
   (a) Identify factors that are stimulants or incentives
   (b) Provide visible reinforcements
   (c) Use repetition as a form of reinforcement (repeated activities become habitual)
      [1] Provide opportunity for the client to practice old and new skills
      [2] Review information previously taught
(8) Evaluation of performance aids in learning
   (a) Purpose
      [1] Measure and interpret results compared with goals set
      [2] Reinforce correct behavior
      [3] Help the learner realize how to change incorrect behavior
      [4] Help the teacher determine adequacy of teaching
   (b) Teacher and learner observe and evaluate together in relation to the desired behavior
   (c) Reasons for a good or poor evaluation require explanation
   (d) Criticism and value judgments must relate to the performance, not the individual

D. Case presentations
1. Definition—process of presenting assessment data to the client along with care options and recommendations to reach agreement on the care plan
2. Elements
   a. Information—share the assessment findings with the client; use charts, dental indices, radiographs, photographs, and study models to give clear and complete explanation
   b. Education—explain the significance of the findings to the client in terms of short- and long-range consequences; ask questions that bring the client into the discussion so you can determine his or her interest and comprehension
   c. Options—present alternative methods of care including benefits, time, risk, and cost for each
   d. Choice—based on the client's understanding of data presented, desires, and perceived needs
   e. Agreement—client and professional concur on a course to follow and who will be responsible for what
3. Case presentations for dental hygiene care
   a. Dental hygienists may be responsible for data collection and presentation of findings and records to the dentist for agreement on care options; dental hygienist then presents the findings and alternatives to the client
   b. Dentist may perform data collection and case presentation and then present the dental hygienist with a prescription for the total dental hygiene care plan as agreed on by the client; in this case the dental hygienist should review the plan with the client before implementation

E. Failure to communicate
1. Dental hygienists play an important role in the continuity of care and must report observations to the dentist, especially alterations in oral health progress
2. Failure or delay in communicating important client findings is considered unethical and can result in a malpractice lawsuit against the dental hygienist
3. Documentation of data without provision of verbal information can also lead to liability; although dental hygienists are not legally allowed to diagnose or plan treatments, the courts believe dental hygienists possess the skill necessary to recognize dental disease and make discriminating professional judgments (see Chapter 18, section on legal relationships in dental hygiene practice)

F. Client noncompliance or nonadherence[3]
1. Definition—lack of client cooperation with recommended oral health
2. Examples
   a. Routine tardy arrival for scheduled appointments
   b. Failure to keep appointments
   c. Unwillingness to have necessary diagnostic tests, such as radiographs
   d. Unwillingness to accept recommended specific procedures or the treatment plan
   e. Unwillingness to accept referrals to specialists
   f. Failure to use medications as instructed
   g. Failure to follow the oral hygiene regimen
3. Significance
   a. Results in compromised oral health
   b. If there is a lawsuit, the decision outcome or amount of settlement may be altered based on patient contributory negligence
4. Managing nonadherence
   a. Recognize it when it happens
   b. Document any instances in the client's records
      (1) Note your explanation of recommended care
      (2) Note observation that instructions are not being followed
      (3) Note the patient's disinclination to follow instructions and the reason

(4) Note your discussion of consequences of not following instructions

  c. Have client sign an informed refusal form

G. Client correspondence

  1. Written communications from the dental hygienist to the client might include

    a. Follow-up to review what was discussed during the appointment

    b. Reinforcement to encourage new skills and behavior

    c. Reminder of the need to schedule an appointment

    d. Personal congratulations, well wishes, or sympathy note

    e. Thank-you notes

  2. Value

    a. Establishes the dental hygienist as an individual within the dental practice

    b. Promotes the practice in general

    c. Promotes the role of the dental hygienist as an educator, client advocate, manager, and change agent

The Dental Hygienist as a Team Member

A. Dental hygienist's role

  1. Contributes knowledge, skills, and experience to the healthcare team

  2. Establishes a mutually cooperative relationship with coworkers to support one another and gain individual daily satisfaction

  3. Develops friendships with colleagues

  4. Establishes and maintains professional behavior with genuine interest in quality client care and the success of the dental practice

B. Dental hygienist's clinical contributions to the practice

  1. Client assessment and data collection

    a. Health history

    b. Dental health history (including fluoride history)

    c. Cultural history

    d. Nutritional/dietary history

    e. Vital signs—body temperature, blood pressure, pulse, and respiration

    f. Extraoral examination

    g. Intraoral examination

    h. Periodontal examination

    i. Dental examination—restorations, dental caries, defects, wear, etc.

    j. Occlusal examination

    k. Myofunctional examination

    l. Bacterial plaque and calculus examination

    m. Diagnostic indicators for periodontal disease, e.g., bacterial culturing, DNA, and gingival crevicular fluid analysis

    n. Radiographic survey

    o. Impressions for study models

    p. Exfoliative cytology

    q. Photography

    r. Intraoral video

  2. Management of information

    a. Charting and record keeping for all of the preceding

    b. Legal evidence

    c. Risk management

  3. Care planning

    a. Establishing priorities with the client

    b. Sequencing of services

    c. Case presentation to the dentist and/or the client

  4. Some dental hygiene interventions (services vary according to state practice acts)

    a. Bacterial plaque control and oral health instruction

    b. Dietary/nutritional counseling

    c. Pain control

      (1) Topical anesthesia

      (2) Local anesthesia

      (3) Nitrous oxide and oxygen analgesia

    d. Scaling and root planing/periodontal debridement

    e. Extrinsic stain removal

    f. Instrument sharpening

    g. Overhanging restoration removal

    h. Amalgam restoration carving and polishing

    i. Fluoride therapy/oral irrigation therapy

    j. Dental sealants

    k. Desensitization of exposed root surfaces

    l. Temporary restoration placement and removal

    m. Periodontal dressing placement and removal

    n. Suture removal

    o. Removable prosthetic appliance care

    p. Cardiopulmonary resuscitation

    q. Constructing mouth protectors

    r. Tobacco cessation intervention

  5. Client evaluation

    a. Repeated data collection

    b. Comparison of data to assess treatment results

    c. Recommendation for further care or continued care interval

C. Integral contributions of the dental hygienist[4]

  1. Assumes responsibility for services rendered with a respectable level of competence

  2. Provides release time for the dentist—performs all procedures legal for dental hygienists, thereby freeing the dentist's time for dental services

  3. Markets oral health services—reports dental needs to clients or treatment that will be needed in the future if restorations deteriorate or the client wishes

to change existing dental conditions (see section on marketing dentistry and dental hygiene)

4. Professional associate of the dentist—participates in case evaluation and care planning for dental hygiene therapy
5. Practice builder—communicates with clients as a professional relations specialist, interpreter, confidante, practice ambassador, and friend
6. Public relations promoter—speaks highly of dental hygiene and dentistry in general when away from the oral healthcare environment
7. Oral disease prevention specialist—educates clients to assume responsibility and care for their own oral health
8. Client advocate—helps clients obtain care via the healthcare system and supports their healthcare decisions
9. Assumes key role in transferring research findings to the consumer

Practice Administration

A. Definition—organization and management of a professional practice; effective practice management benefits clients and staff members alike by serving more people with increased efficiency, saving time and money, reducing pressure and tension, and increasing personal satisfaction
B. Personnel management
   1. Policy manual
      a. Purpose—outlines practice principles
      b. Content
         (1) Practice philosophy
            (a) General attitudes and goals
            (b) Specific objectives
            (c) Issues regarding the success of the practice, standards of care, and satisfaction for all
         (2) Team approach/personnel involvement
         (3) Specific standards of client care for quality assurance and education
         (4) Personnel policies and procedures
         (5) Employment regulations
         (6) Work arrangements
         (7) Guidelines of professional ethics and conduct
         (8) Referrals to specialists
         (9) Office charts, forms, and documentation guidelines
         (10) Appointment administration/fees and financing
         (11) Office safety and emergencies
         (12) Service to the community
   2. Procedures manual
      a. Purpose

(1) Assigns responsibility and describes routines
(2) Provides a job description for each position in the office (clearly defining all aspects of performance), outlines expectations, and serves as a guideline for performance review
b. Contents
   (1) Job titles
   (2) Job summaries—key elements of positions; examples include
      (a) Updating of health histories
      (b) Oral examinations
      (c) Exposing and processing of radiographs
      (d) Oral hygiene instruction
      (e) Scaling, root planing, and extrinsic stain removal (periodontal debridement)
      (f) Application of fluorides and recommending supplemental fluoride therapy; oral irrigation therapy
      (g) Adjunctive services
      (h) Record keeping and documentation
      (i) Scheduling of appointments
   (3) Responsibilities—examples
      (a) Daily routines
         [1] Opening the healthcare setting
         [2] Greeting clients
         [3] Communicating with the dentist and support staff
         [4] Preparing tray setups
         [5] Infection control procedures
         [6] Closing the healthcare setting
      (b) Treatment area maintenance
         [1] Decor for comfort, beauty, and personalization
         [2] Overall organization and cleanliness
         [3] Regular maintenance of the dental equipment
         [4] Care of dental instruments
         [5] Restocking of supplies/inventory control
         [6] Light housekeeping
         [7] Special tasks
   (4) Qualifications—requirements for job applicants
3. See sections on the team concept and dentist–dental hygienist relationship
C. Client management
   1. See section on successful client management
   2. Scheduling of clients[5]—time management is critical to the success of the practice and to quality client care

a. Appointment control—appointment book
   (1) Clearly block out time for staff meetings, lunch hours, days off, holidays, vacations, time away from the office for professional meetings, etc., as far in advance as possible
   (2) Appointment book management systems
      (a) Unlimited future booking—appointments are scheduled as far in advance as is necessary to accommodate all clients; requires careful advance planning for time away from the office
      (b) Restricted appointment booking—limits appointments to a specified time period, such as 1 to 3 months; clients who are not scheduled during this time are placed on a call list and are telephoned when appointments become available
      (c) Waiting list is maintained of clients who need appointments and are available on short notice to fill cancellations
   (3) Appointment book entries (write in pencil)
      (a) Client's name
      (b) Daytime telephone number—identify if it is a work (w) or home (h) number
      (c) Service/type of appointment—R or CC, recall/continued care; NC, new client; Q, quadrant root planing/periodontal debridement
      (d) Length of appointment time/number of time units
      (e) Special instructions—"premedicate," "local anesthesia," "dentist appointment follows"
b. Continued care (recall) health maintenance systems
   (1) Purposes
      (a) Organizes and maintains oral health examinations and periodontal maintenance according to client's needs
      (b) Ensures maximum number of clients receive periodic oral healthcare
   (2) Types
      (a) Advance scheduling—definite future reservation is made, requiring that the appointment book be available 3 to 12 months in advance; clients are reminded by a postcard and/or telephone call approximately 2 weeks before the actual date
      (b) Reminder card—notifies the client by mail that it is time for the health maintenance examinations and requests the client to phone the office to schedule an appointment; assigns responsibility to the client to set up the appointment, and the office maintains cross-reference of who is due
      (c) Telephone reminder—client is contacted by phone, and a definite appointment is scheduled
      (d) Combination—all systems are available within the office with flexibility of choice based on client preferences
   (3) Continued care (recall) references
      (a) Triplicate appointment card—one copy is given to the client, the second one is filed with the client's chart, and the third one becomes a postcard reminder to be mailed before the appointment; can schedule a definite appointment or note it is time for the client to call the office to schedule an appointment
      (b) Tickler file—monthly grouping of cards of clients needing appointments; each card contains a record of previous appointments, what is needed now, and how to best contact and schedule the client
      (c) Alphabetical file—by client name; card lists previous appointments and what is needed next
      (d) Cross-references combine duplicates of the above
c. Client "reclamation"
   (1) Definition—periodic purging of all files to harvest "fugitive" clients to either complete unfinished therapy or return after an extended absence from oral healthcare
   (2) Systems
      (a) Send a card or note stating the date of the last appointment and what needs to be done
      (b) Telephone the client to discuss oral needs and learn client preferences
D. Office management
   1. Treatment area and equipment maintenance
      a. Written guidelines outline required procedures with recommended intervals for best results
      b. Each staff member is assigned appropriate areas of responsibility
   2. Supply and inventory control
      a. Aids office efficiency to maintain an adequate stock and avoid accumulation or waste from excess items

b. Consists of itemized lists of supplies and materials used in the office
(1) Storage location
(2) Purchase information
(a) Item
(b) Cost
(c) Supplier
(d) Quantity
(e) Frequency
(f) Date ordered and date received
(3) Minimum stock for reorder
c. May group items and assign inventory control to different staff members
(1) Receptionist—administrative supplies
(2) Dental assistant—general dental supplies
(3) Dental hygienist—oral hygiene supplies
3. Management information system
a. Computer hardware
b. Computer software
E. Records management
1. Value/purposes
a. Permanent documents provide a "written memory" of what transpired
b. Organization of data collection—should be brief, neat, complete, accurate, and easy to read
c. Evaluation aids for diagnosis
d. Management aids for decision making and care planning
e. Educational aids for client information and instruction
f. Protection of the client regarding general health and discovery of oral diseases
g. Behavior modification tools to establish the patient's goal orientation
h. Enhancement of client confidence in professionals and the practice
i. Communication devices to enhance professionals' mutual case comprehension
j. "Roadmap" for instrumentation guide
k. Regulation of care to identify conditions beyond normal limits or variations from previous conditions
l. "Trend analysis" of data for long-term evaluation and decision making
m. Guidance for consistent, quality therapy
n. Integration for correlation of tissue conditions, oral hygiene, treatment, and responses
o. Third-party justification and satisfaction
p. Accountability for demonstration of responsible care
q. Legal protection to present documentary evidence for defense if necessary
r. Risk management

2. Elements
a. Written client records
(1) Client registration form with administrative information
(2) Health history, including nutritional information
(3) Dental and fluoride history
(4) Dental and periodontal record
(5) Treatment records of assessment findings, diagnosis, and care plan
(6) Treatment records of procedures performed—include who, when, what, where, why, how, and what is needed next
(7) Consent forms to authorize treatment or decline recommended care such as radiographs, premedication, or fluoride therapy
b. Nonwritten records
(1) Photographs
(2) Radiographs
(3) Models
(4) Cephalometric tracings
(5) Intraoral videotapes
(6) Computerized periodontal assessment data

Risk Management

A. Definition—a combination of methods designed to control and/or eliminate situations that can lead to a lawsuit including
1. Loss (risk) identification and evaluation of areas of vulnerability
2. Loss (risk) avoidance or reduction by using preventive measures and providing quality care
3. Loss (risk) financing by purchase of liability insurance
B. Current professional liability environment demonstrates increase in frequency and severity of claims
C. Techniques and tools used in risk management include
1. Good communications
2. Proper protocol
3. Staff training and credentialing
4. Record keeping/documentation
5. Informed consent/informed refusal
6. Accepted standard of care
D. Some reasons for lawsuits
1. Client's expectations are different from services delivered
2. Nonsupportive behavior of dental office personnel
3. Failure to treat
4. Failure to diagnose
5. Failure to take necessary precautions to prevent mechanical injury
6. Failure to identify medically compromised clients

7. Failure to take precautions to protect a medically compromised client

8. Performing a service that is not in the best interest of the client or failure to perform a service that is necessary

9. Failure of treatment, e.g., dental implants

10. Failure to obtain informed consent

E. Informed consent reduces risk by educating client concerning

1. Need for proposed procedure

2. Expected result

3. Known risks and/or limitations of the procedure

4. Risk of *not* doing the procedure

5. Reasonable alternatives

6. Objective standard of care

7. Financial considerations

8. Document discussion, presence of other family members, and outcome

F. Recordkeeping requires notations for all appointments, procedures performed, follow-up instructions, advice for self-care devices and written materials dispensed, referrals and telephone contact with clients or consulting professionals; notations should be

1. Complete

2. Accurate

3. Clear

4. Legible

5. Initialed and dated by provider; corrections and additions initialed and dated by provider

6. Standardized, e.g., abbreviations

7. Confidential

8. Retained forever

G. Dental hygienists' role in risk management

1. Establish responsible professional relationships with clients and dental personnel

2. Use clear, courteous communications to inform and educate clients

3. Provide services that meet the current standard of care

4. Take appropriate precautions when treating clients

5. Use proper protocols

6. Obtain informed consent before client care

7. Record client questions, concerns, and preferences

8. Respect client's time

9. Ease communications between client and dentist

10. Interpret need for client to be seen by dentist in a timely manner

11. Follow proper documentation style in record keeping

12. Avoid criticism of other oral health professionals

13. Ensure that the employment setting has a risk management program

H. Implement a "Risk Management Program"

1. Organize and catalog written materials

2. Create checklist of risk management techniques for office procedure manual

3. Discuss risk management at staff meetings including control methods and role-play client scenarios

I. Dealing with a potential lawsuit (see Chapter 18, section on legal relationships)

1. Contact liability insurance carrier and lawyer immediately for advice

2. Do not alter records

3. Send copies of records, *never* originals, upon signed request

4. Maintain confidentiality

Marketing Dentistry and Dental Hygiene[1]

A. Definition—planning and management of oral health services that benefit clients at a profit to the dental or dental hygiene practice

B. Purpose—to obtain and maintain the desired share of the client population market

C. Strategy

1. Identify target market—groups with similar needs

2. Develop a complete marketing plan to meet and satisfy the desires and needs of the target group

a. Prices/fees

b. Location/convenience

c. Promotion

d. Services

3. Incorporate systems for changes with a step-by-step plan to build the practice

4. All staff members participate in the marketing effort

5. Satisfied clients market dentistry and dental hygiene

D. Goals

1. Goal setting

a. Identify desired situations for the future to guide and direct behavior

b. Involve staff members in discussions

c. Establish step-by-step objectives

d. Review and redefine goals on a regular basis

2. Types

a. Practice organizational goals

b. Procedural goals for staff members

c. Personal goals

E. Practice promotion—all staff members project the desired image for professionals and gain public exposure for the practice

1. Write articles for local newspapers on prevention, oral health, service updates, dental emergencies, evaluation of over-the-counter oral healthcare products, etc.

2. Get a feature article about the practice in the local newspaper

3. Participate in broadcast media (local radio and

television) programming with special interest information, talk shows, community service announcements, etc.

4. Participate in civic, religious, and fraternal group activities (provide opportunities to meet many people at once); be visible

5. Use business contacts within the community client population—distribute your business cards to many

6. Sponsor community projects

7. Participate in community cultural and recreational events

8. Become a public speaker

9. Teach health information and cardiopulmonary resuscitation workshops to consumers and other professionals

10. Become a lifelong student—attend local classes and workshops; earn advanced degrees

11. Meet and cooperate with neighboring health professionals; provide business cards and referral slips

12. Volunteer professional services and demonstrations

13. Perform oral health screenings in schools, health fairs, community and athletic programs, civic groups, and at special events

14. Actively participate in your professional association

15. Participate creatively in the community

16. Use advertising—telephone book, newspaper, radio, and other community media

17. Use mass direct mail—sending oral health education materials, practice brochures, or a newsletter to the client population or the community at large

F. Client satisfaction considerations

1. Offer a wide spectrum of oral healthcare services
   a. Prevention
   b. Maintenance/continued care
   c. Restoration
   d. Cosmetic
   e. Counseling
   f. Reconstruction

2. Provide quality care

3. Provide personalized care—recognize each client as an individual, listen to each one, be responsive, and develop special relationships

4. Be a consumer advocate—stay abreast of consumer trends; counsel clients on use of oral health products on the market

5. Educate people about dentistry and dental hygiene with common language

6. Include alternatives in care planning, explain all the options, and make recommendations; differentiate between what is necessary and what is ideal

7. Maintain fair and reasonable fees

8. Consistently offer dependable care and caring

9. Extend office hours to include early morning, evening, and weekend appointments

10. Appeal to all age ranges—infants through senior citizens (continuum of care)

11. Offer current treatment modalities

12. Allow clients to take responsibility for their own oral health

13. Manage an efficient practice—minimize waiting time

14. Promote positive psychologic attitudes by all staff members

15. Maintain warm, respectful interpersonal relations between staff members and clients

16. Establish a pleasant, comfortable, attractive office decor

17. Offer a variety of financial arrangements

18. Process insurance forms expediently

19. Be prepared for and incorporate changes in the practice as needed

20. Develop and fully utilize staff members

21. Provide strong technical expertise

22. Develop rapport with specialty practices for referrals, coordination of client care, and collaboration

23. Choose a convenient access location with easy parking

24. Provide "give-aways"—toothbrushes and other oral hygiene aids, health education brochures, toys or balloons for children, flowers, etc.

25. Exchange written correspondence with clients—outlines of care plans and copies of letters to other professionals concerning the client's needs and care

26. Send clients personalized thank-you notes, congratulatory notes, special occasion notes, or get well wishes

27. Maintain positive, satisfactory telephone contacts

28. Use follow-up telephone calls after complex treatments and to check on clients

29. Keep clients informed by providing written care plans and briefly explaining procedures before beginning work

30. Quote fees for the care plan and make fair financial arrangements

31. Schedule time realistically

32. Maintain an effective dental health maintenance program to continue dental care on a routine schedule

33. Develop a practice brochure, introducing staff members, the range of services, office hours, financial arrangements, etc.

34. Make accommodations for emergency clients

G. Recognition—express appreciation for staff cooperation daily, note client support and patronage, and recognize referral sources with thank-you notes

H. Evaluation of marketing effectiveness
   1. Internal analysis
      a. Compare gross revenues of the practice—daily, weekly, monthly, and annually
      b. Count clients—maintained and new
      c. Perform an overall financial analysis of the practice
         (1) Budget
         (2) Balance sheet of accounts receivable and accounts payable
         (3) Productivity per hour, day, week, month, and year
      d. Interview all staff members
   2. External analysis
      a. Survey clients by interviews or questionnaires—Are they satisfied? Recommendations for changes?
      b. Survey other community and referral sources—Can any further services be offered?

Dentist-Dental Hygienist Relationship

Employment

A. The Dental Practice Act regulates dental hygiene practice under general, indirect, or direct supervision of a licensed dentist and within specified physical settings: each jurisdiction establishes its own legal guidelines; Colorado recognizes unsupervised dental hygiene practice; California, Michigan, and Wisconsin allow unsupervised dental hygiene practice in some public health settings

B. Financial arrangements between the dentist and dental hygienist are solely the concern of those two individuals and are separate from and not controlled by the dental practice act

C. Employment arrangements
   1. Employer-employee—dental hygienist as an employee, works within the office structure of a dentist (or possibly a dental hygienist in the state of Colorado)
      a. All financial concerns of operating the practice are the responsibility of the employer
      b. Employer pays the employee on an hourly wage, salary, or commission basis, withholding federal, state, and Social Security taxes from the employee's paycheck
      c. Dental hygienist's employer may also be an independent management firm, health maintenance organization, or state, county, or private agency employing individuals for dental offices or other specific work settings
   2. Independent contractor—Internal Revenue Service (IRS) classification of a contractual arrangement between the dentist and self-employed dental hygienist
      a. Dental hygienist provides services to the clients of the dentist, adhering to the dentist's supervision and settings regulated by the state dental practice act
      b. Dental hygienist sets hours, makes appointments, sets fees, collects fees
      c. Financial arrangements for operating the dental hygiene portion of the practice are contracted between the dentist and dental hygienist
      d. No taxes are withheld by the dentist from the dental hygienist's paycheck; dental hygienist pays self-employment (Social Security) tax and files estimated income tax payments
      e. IRS sets rules that establish qualifying criteria for independent contractors; it is illegal for a dentist-employer to arbitrarily "assign" the status of "independent contractor" to a dental hygienist–employee
      f. Independent contractor may hire employees and function as an employer
   3. Unsupervised dental hygiene practice—legal in Colorado
      a. Dental hygienist would provide select services to the public in a separate dental hygiene facility without a dentist's supervision
      b. Dental hygienist would assume all financial responsibility for the practice, would be self-employed, and would function as an employer to the employees of the facility

D. Terms of employment
   1. Permanent—employee service with the employer is secure and of unlimited duration
   2. Temporary—employee service is known to be of limited duration
   3. Probationary—service trial period, usually 1 to 3 months, when employee and employer can evaluate one another and working together; employee may resign or be dismissed immediately for any reason
   4. Full-time—employee works solely in one office the customary number of hours that the facility functions, normally 30 to 40 hours per week
   5. Part-time—employee works less than the full hours of the facility's operation, usually less than 30 hours per week
   6. Job sharing—two or more people share one full-time job by the day, week, month, or year; time can

be split in any fashion agreeable to the job sharers and the employer; salary and benefits are shared proportionally with the time worked

7. Regular hours—coincide with normal office hours
8. Staggered hours—established working hours that fit the life schedule of the employee; hours vary from routine office hours but are stable daily for that employee
9. "Flex" time—employee arrives and leaves work whenever he or she chooses; can change daily

E. Employment rights
1. Non-Discrimination Act, Title VII of the Civil Rights Act of 1964—establishes equal employment opportunity for all during the hiring process and throughout the course of employment; requires fairness and impartiality with regard to race, color, religious belief, gender, national origin, and age
2. Pregnancy Discrimination Act, 1979 amendment to Title VII of the Civil Rights Act of 1964—prohibits discrimination on the basis of pregnancy, childbirth, or related medical conditions; protects women from being fired or refused a job or promotion because of pregnancy; provides that, following maternity leave, the job will be returned with no loss in seniority or fringe benefits
3. Working conditions—each state sets minimum standards for working conditions, including
   a. Hours and days of work
   b. Minimum wage and reports for pay
   c. Employee records
   d. Uniforms and equipment
   e. Meal periods and eating area
   f. Rest periods and rest facilities
   g. Environmental temperature
4. Occupational Safety and Health Standards Board (OSHA)—sets minimum federal requirements for industrial safety
   a. Employer required to furnish safe employment in work place
   b. Required to have accident prevention program, safety training, and scheduled safety inspections
5. Employee Retirement Income Security Act of 1974 (ERISA), a tax statute
   a. Purpose
      (1) Ensures that benefit plan participants know to what they are entitled
      (2) Guarantees that participants receive benefits, even if the business fails
   b. Elements
      (1) Required communications from corporation to employee with a summary of the corporate plan and updates, summary of annual reports, and announcement of plan modifications
      (2) On employee request, the corporation must provide a complete annual report, complete description of the document plan, and full vesting statements of total benefits accrued, nonforfeitable pension benefits, and the earliest date benefits become nonforfeitable

Compensation

A. Methods of remuneration
1. Fixed salary—guaranteed fixed wage for hourly, daily, weekly, or monthly employment
2. Salary plus commission—base salary plus an additional percentage of fees charged for dental hygiene services
3. Commission with guaranteed minimum salary—pays a percentage of fees charged for dental hygiene services, with an ensured minimum wage per day regardless of daily gross production
4. Commission—earnings based on a percentage of fees charged for dental hygiene services
5. Independent contractor—sets and collects all fees and pays overhead costs, with profit fluctuation based on production, collection, and expenses
6. Overtime—usually for hourly wage earners; pays time and a half for all time in excess of the contracted hours per week
7. Compensatory time off ("comp" time)—given for hours worked in excess of the established work week; used in place of overtime pay
8. Profit-sharing bonus—work incentive awarded to employees when profit goals are set and achieved for a specified period; may be calculated monthly, quarterly, or annually
9. Fringe benefits—required and optional services paid by the employer in addition to regular wages (see section on fringe benefits)

B. Negotiating a starting salary
1. Considerations
   a. It is your right to be paid what you are worth
   b. Before interviewing, determine a definite starting salary range that is acceptable to you
   c. Be prepared to discuss salary, including fringe benefits, with facts and a prepared strategy
   d. Think of the employer as the buyer and yourself as the seller; the commodity is your service: personal skills and professional expertise
   e. Unless you participate in negotiating, your salary is often less than it should be; dental practices often expect employees to accept satisfaction of service instead of a reasonable salary

f. First salary offer from the employer is one of the most negotiable points of a new job; do not be too intimidated to make a counteroffer; first offer is usually not final, and employers expect negotiation

g. You have the power to say no to an unacceptable offer

2. Determining factors
   a. Current education, skill level, experience
   b. Office fees, services rendered, daily production
   c. Responsibility for client care and disease recognition
   d. Supply and demand

3. Need to get agreements in writing
   a. Initial probationary period may carry a reduced salary; establish a date for the salary to increase and what the increase will be
   b. Establish intervals for regular salary discussions with expected wage increases

C. Salary increases
1. Usually sporadic and highly subjective for dental hygienists
2. Based on one or more of the following
   a. Responsibility
   b. Seniority
   c. Merit
   d. Production
   e. Cost of living
   f. Educational advancement
   g. Supply and demand
3. Negotiating a raise
   a. Set a definite appointment for the discussion
   b. Be prepared with all the reasons why you deserve a raise, emphasizing your value to the practice, not that you need more money
      (1) List your accomplishments
      (2) Use specific examples
      (3) Present facts and figures
      (4) Be direct and brief
      (5) Show how you have exceeded expectations
   c. Present the specific dollar-figure increase you are seeking with clear justification

D. Payroll
1. Each payroll period includes a written compensation statement identifying gross earnings and itemizing deductions to reach the net amount of the paycheck
2. Required and voluntary deductions are made from the gross compensation to arrive at the net paycheck
   a. Required employee deductions
      (1) Federal income tax withheld, based on declared exemptions
      (2) State income tax withheld, based on declared exemptions
      (3) Federal Insurance Contributions Act (FICA, Social Security), percentage set by the federal government
      (4) State disability insurance (limited to certain states)
      (5) City income tax (limited to certain cities)
   b. Optional employee deductions
      (1) Voluntary contribution to a retirement account
      (2) Professional expenses paid by the employee
      (3) Credit union savings account automatic deposit
3. Employer payroll expenses
   a. Social Security matching funds
   b. Workers' compensation
   c. Federal Unemployment Tax Act
   d. Disability insurance (required by some states)
   e. Pension and profit-sharing plans
   f. Fringe benefits
   g. Bookkeeping and accounting fees

Fringe Benefits[6]

A. Definition—paid services in addition to direct pay
1. Standard part of compensation programs in all sectors of the American economy—private, government, and nonprofit
2. Some are legally required; others are optional
3. Desirable because of the tax advantage of receiving services and benefits from the employer rather than paying for them with posttax paycheck dollars

B. Legally required benefits
1. Social Security—Federal Old Age Survivors' Disability and Hospital Insurance Program includes
   a. Old age benefits—at age 65, provides a tax-free annual family benefit; amount is based on average yearly earnings while working
   b. Survivors' benefits—in case of the employee's death, survivors (including dependent children) may receive a monthly family income
   c. Disability benefits—for some medically caused total disabilities at any age; provides a tax-free monthly income
   d. Hospital insurance—after age 65, covers basic hospitalization, some related care, and at a modest cost to the retiree, supplemental insurance (Medicare) for doctor bills and other medical services
2. Workers compensation—protects the employee from medical expenses and loss of income in the event of injury on the job or job-related disability

   a. Financed entirely by employers via state payroll taxes; rate varies according to job-risk category
   b. Covers all medical expenses
   c. Income benefits vary according to salary level
3. Disability insurance—required in some states to provide benefits for nonoccupational accidents or illnesses
   a. Financing usually combines employer and employee contributions
   b. Disability must be medically certified
   c. Income benefits vary according to salary level
4. Unemployment insurance—provides benefits to individuals involuntarily unemployed
   a. Financed entirely by employers through state and federal unemployment taxes; rate varies based on the employer's past use record
   b. Weekly tax-free payments are made to those eligible
   c. Income benefits vary according to prior earnings
C. Optional fringe benefits ("perks")[7]—depend on office/agency policy; may vary within the setting from employee to employee; flexible program allows employer and employees to design a benefits package with services selected to best suit each individual's needs and lifestyle
1. Paid absences
   a. Sick leave—salary paid during occasional short-term illnesses; usually sick-leave benefits are allowed to accumulate if not used, or unused days are paid at the end of the year as a bonus
   b. Holidays—salary paid for usual, nationally observed holidays
   c. Vacation—salary paid for vacation time off; schedule may vary according to the length of service with the employer; may be able to accumulate unused vacation time; for part-time employees vacation days are prorated (divided proportionally with the work schedule)
   d. Educational level—salary paid for time off to attend educational programs that are work related; may have an annual specified maximum limit; may be given leave without pay
   e. Professional activities—salary paid for time off to attend professional meetings that are work or career related; may have an annual specified maximum limit; may be given leave without pay
   f. Emergency personal leave—paid time off for unexpected events such as a family illness, death, or funeral; jury duty, legal depositions, or court witness appearances; or extreme weather conditions
   g. Maternity leave—time off, usually without pay,

but with the guarantee of job protection on return from the leave; reasonable time limits usually apply
   h. Extended or sabbatical leave—usually leave without pay for a few weeks to several months for the purpose of travel, education, family, or personal needs; job is held during the absence with an agreed-on time of return
2. Insurance benefits
   a. Health insurance—program protects the insured from major medical costs; coverage may be
      (1) Fee-for-service plan where the individual selects the health care provider and submits a bill for payment to the private insurance carrier; usually has a deductible, pays a percentage of costs, excludes some types of care, and has a lifetime dollar value limit on claims per individual
      (2) Health maintenance organization for comprehensive health care services
      (3) Prepaid service plans such as Blue Cross and Blue Shield for service contracts to specific health care providers
      (4) Self-insured plans, which reimburse employees directly for medical expenses without third-party involvement
      (5) Preferred provider organizations, which provide healthcare at a discount to subscribers
   b. Dental insurance—program protects the insured from usual dental expenses; types include
      (1) Schedule plans with specific dollar limits for each dental procedure, usually without a deductible
      (2) Comprehensive plans that reimburse on a "reasonable and customary" basis, with the insurance carrier paying a percentage of the actual charges
   c. Vision insurance—program covers the expenses of eye examinations, eye care, and prescription corrective lenses
   d. Liability (malpractice) insurance—protects the insured against liability for
      (1) Injuries arising out of professional services rendered, including errors, negligence, or omissions
      (2) Injuries from acts or omissions while participating as a member of a professional organization or committee
      (3) Personal injury against claims of slander, libel, defamation of character, false arrest, etc.

(4) Legal fees and court costs paid whether or not the insured is found liable

e. Long-term permanent disability insurance—in the event of severe and/or permanent disability, coverage provides a percentage of the basic wage; usually includes

(1) "Elimination" or waiting period before the policy starts paying benefits, usually 30 days or longer

(2) Benefit period may be a specified number of years, for the length of the disability, until regular retirement benefits begin, or for a lifetime

(3) Partial benefits may be available if the insured is able to return to work on a limited basis

f. Life insurance—provides assistance to building a financial estate for surviving family; basic types include

(1) Term insurance—considered "pure death protection," covering a specific, temporary period; renewal costs increase as the insured ages

(2) Whole life insurance—called "straight," "permanent," or "cash value"; more expensive initially, with costs leveling and the policy building a cash value; may pay dividends or provide borrowing equity

g. Pension plans (see section on retirement)

3. Professional expenses—employer makes direct payment or reimburses for

a. Professional license renewal

b. Protective clothing and eyewear allowance—for purchase and/or maintenance of office attire as required by OSHA

c. Professional education assistance—tuition reimbursement and related expenses, such as books, supplies, equipment, and travel expenses, usually with a specified annual limit; may also include salary for time away from home; educational loan program may provide short- or long-term repayment program or "loan forgiveness" (considered paid) if the employee stays with the employer for an agreed-on period of time

d. Professional activities—reimbursement or payment for registration fees and related travel expenses for participation at meetings related to the field of dental hygiene; usually with a specified annual limit

e. Professional journals and texts—subscriptions and purchase

f. Paid parking, transportation, and/or automobile expenses related to commuting to work

g. Expense account—reimbursement for purchase of items for the office, instruments, forms, equipment, etc.

4. Other benefits

a. Child care expenses

b. Personal legal services

c. Personal financial counseling

d. Notary service

e. Staff functions—meals, parties, and other special events

Employment Agreement/Letter of Intent

A. Definition—written contract describing the terms of employment agreed on by the dental hygienist (employee) and dentist (employer)

B. Functions

1. Clarifies specific details of employment issues for both parties

2. Establishes a stable working relationship

3. May or may not be legally binding

4. Provides psychologic security for both parties

C. Contents

1. Terms of agreement

a. Names of the parties—dental hygienist (employee) and dentist (employer)

b. Job title

c. Date the contract takes effect (employment commencement) and date the contract expires

d. Option of contract renewal

2. Settings and terms of employment

a. Address of oral healthcare setting(s) and name of supervising dentist(s)

b. Agreement of both parties to adhere to the rules and regulations of the state dental practice act

c. Statement of equipment, supplies, and instruments to be provided by the dentist

d. Work arrangement of days of the week or days per month agreed on

e. Workload by hours and scheduling of appointments

f. Overtime to be paid by "comp" time or financial compensation

g. Payment for time not worked, such as holidays, vacation, sick leave, etc.

3. Job description

a. Specific services to be performed

b. Other characteristic duties and responsibilities of the position

c. Opportunities for growth and promotion

4. Compensation

a. Method—hourly, daily salary, commission, or combination

b. Starting remuneration or method of calculation

c. Payroll schedule

d. Increases in remuneration
  (1) Dates of review
  (2) Basis for increase

e. Fringe benefits—listed individually
  (1) Requirements of initial qualification
  (2) Vesting increments
  (3) Accrual techniques

5. Probationary period
  a. Terms and date of probation
  b. Agreement for mutual evaluation at the conclusion of probation
  c. Employment termination options for each party

6. Performance evaluation
  a. Dates for review
  b. Method of evaluation
  c. Criteria for performance success

7. Termination procedures
  a. Advance notice—required length of time
  b. Statement of cause
  c. Employee replacement procedures

8. Signatures of each party with the date

9. Witness signatures (optional)

Job Performance

A. Employment issues affecting job performance[8]
  1. Factors positively influencing dental hygiene employment conditions
    a. Attitudes (self-image) of dental hygienists
    b. Attitudes of dentists
    c. State dental practice acts
    d. Consumer/client awareness and education
    e. Demand for dental hygiene services
    f. Role of the dental hygienist as a practice builder
    g. Role of the dental hygienist as an oral disease prevention specialist
  2. Factors negatively influencing dental hygiene employment conditions
    a. Attitudes (self-image) of dental hygienists
    b. Attitudes of dentists
    c. Dentists' lack of knowledge of full capabilities of dental hygienists
    d. State dental practice acts
    e. Lack of consumer/client awareness and education
    f. Lack of demand for dental hygiene services
    g. Maldistribution and/or overpopulation of dental hygienists
    h. Inflation and/or economic recession
    i. Economic exploitation of dental hygienists
    j. Unfair, financially discriminatory employment practices
    k. Poor practice management by dentists
    l. Lack of business knowledge by dentists
    m. Lack of business knowledge by dental hygienists
    n. Pressure to practice illegally
    o. Overall lack of recognition of the dental hygienist as a professional making valuable contributions as a member of an interdisciplinary healthcare team

B. Job expectations—employer and employee must plan the job together and discuss and agree on minimum performance expectations and results concerning
  1. What is done on the job (basic work responsibilities)
  2. The manner in which it is accomplished (standards of performance)
  3. Why it is done (importance of function)
  4. Skills necessary to perform the job
  5. Goals and limits for achieving expectations

C. Job satisfaction—employment fulfillment is largely dependent on the employee to assert self in using skills and assuming maximum job responsibility leading to professional growth; as one gains competence and respect, job satisfaction follows

D. Performance evaluation
  1. Definition—communication tool based on the agreed-on performance plan; measures work progress and provides constructive feedback; includes criticism and compliments regarding specific elements of employment actions and behavior; should be separate from the salary review
  2. Value
    a. Provides a progress report, recognizes and supports desired behavior, develops strengths, pin points weaknesses, and gives specific direction for change; can give a psychologic boost and rekindle employee interest
    b. Can assist in determining a salary increase
    c. Can be used as a legal tool for dismissal
  3. Frequency
    a. At the completion of the probationary period if the job is new—1 to 3 months after employment commencement
    b. Once or twice a year for continuing employment
  4. Technique
    a. Completion of the office "performance review form" by both the employer and the employee
    b. Meeting of the employer and employee to share, compare, and discuss results of the review form; appraisal should
      (1) Measure progress toward the goal of task and behavior performances
      (2) Compare actual results with the agreed-on plan, citing specific incidents

(3) Praise accomplishments when performance meets or exceeds stated standards

(4) When differences occur, determine the cause, then consider alternatives to facilitate reaching desired outcomes

(5) If corrective action is indicated, state the specific plan with measurable results and gain agreement of both parties

(6) Modify performance standards if indicated and agreed on by both parties

(7) Enhance communications between the employer and employee, giving an opportunity for "coaching" to achieve performance goals, rather than merely "judging" performance

c. Format

(1) Direct statement of behavioral objectives in terms of quality and quantity; standards to achieve a satisfactory performance level

(2) Clear, self-explanatory statements to facilitate both the employer's evaluation of the employee and the employee's self-evaluation

(3) Written document directs the interview and allows for reexamination of all information following the interview

d. Content areas—address all areas of the job description

(1) Participation with the practice and staff as a team member

(2) Knowledge of the dental hygiene field

(3) Treatment procedures and clinical skills

(4) Practice routine with clients

(5) Communication skills with the staff and clients

(6) Dependability to the office and work schedule

(7) Responsibility for the operatory, equipment, and supplies

(8) Work habits

(9) Initiative, leadership, and problem-solving skills

e. Daily verbal feedback—critical to successful performance

(1) Praise good behavior and verbalize the feelings produced

(2) Observe discrepancies, describing specific incidents and the feelings produced

E. Changing performance[6]

1. Planning

a. Describe the performance discrepancy as specifically as possible, listing

(1) Desired standard of performance

(2) Present level of performance

(3) Analysis of performance discrepancy—why is it not satisfactory?

(4) Definition of what needs to be done differently and how it should be properly performed

b. Gain mutual agreement on the desired change; be sure each party is clear

c. Divide changes into small successive steps to progressively implement the ultimate desired result

2. Evaluation

a. Ask for immediate feedback and reinforcement for the new, desired performance

b. Monitor progress, gaining reinforcement often at first, then gradually less often

c. Steadily follow the guidelines for change

d. Be specific in acknowledging how performance is changing

3. Incorporation

a. Strive for high-quality performance

b. Be fair and honest in efforts to change performance

c. Consistently include the desired performance as soon as possible to achieve self-responsibility

F. Job termination

1. Dismissal

a. Clearly understand the grounds for dismissal

(1) Ask for the true, complete picture

(2) Ask for clarification of vague statements

(3) Remember that it is the work performance that is unacceptable, not the person

b. Clarify the severance arrangements

(1) Date of termination

(2) Severance pay

(3) Benefits accrued and due to the employee

c. Behave professionally and with dignity

d. Acknowledge your feelings and mourn the loss

e. Put the terminated job into perspective and enter the job market

(1) Inventory your career goals

(2) Update your resumé

(3) Begin the interviewing process

(4) Move confidently on to the next career stage

2. Resignation

a. Notify your employer of your intentions as soon as possible

b. Do not tell coworkers before notifying your employer

c. Clearly state your grounds for resigning or state that it is time for career advancement

d. Clarify the severance arrangements

(1) Date of termination

  (2) Benefits accrued and due to the employee
  (3) Whether or not the employee plans to find and train a successor
  e. Tie up loose ends
  f. Depart with dignity and behave professionally
G. Changing jobs
  1. Consider the risk of a job change when there is lack of employment satisfaction or growth stagnation on one job
  2. New job should offer new challenges, more responsibility, opportunity for professional growth, and/or increased compensation
  3. Goal is to find a job that offers the best opportunities and become a permanent employee
  4. See section on career mobility

Dentist–Dental Hygienist Communications

A. Overall relationship should be based on adult, professional interdependence
  1. Each respects and recognizes the other's level of competence
  2. Dental hygienist begins a new job by demonstrating knowledge, skills, judgment, and humanistic behavior
  3. Dental hygienist expresses ideas, opinions, and feelings and encourages reciprocal sharing from the dentist
  4. Each assumes responsibility for the treatment rendered and quality client care
B. Dental hygienist's role is that of self-responsibility
  1. State your standards and priorities for all work-related responsibilities
  2. Set limits on what you can effectively and competently accomplish
  3. When you need information or assistance, ask the dentist for input or guidance
  4. Attempt to establish a collaborative model of practice
  5. Welcome criticism from mistakes to enhance your learning and growth
  6. Be cooperative, diplomatic, and friendly
  7. Use an assertive communication style to enhance your effectiveness
  8. Model the behavior you want to receive
C. Disagreement
  1. Conflicts are to be expected, and confrontation should not be avoided
  2. Take the risk to discuss problems assertively and unemotionally
    a. Identify conflict as soon as you recognize it
    b. Discuss issues privately, with diplomacy and tact
    c. Describe the issue first, factually and accurately, then note your feelings

    d. Be ready, and present a solution for the disagreement
    e. Strive for a "win-win" solution for both parties
  3. Ability to deal effectively with conflict increases the dental hygienist's value to the dental practice and wins respect from others

Professional Management

Seeking Employment

A. Resumé
  1. Purpose
    a. Inventories professional qualifications and assets
    b. Is an introduction; creates a first impression
    c. Generates an interview
    d. Can eliminate purposeless interviews
    e. After an interview the resumé becomes a visible reminder of the applicant to the potential employer
  2. Types
    a. Blanket—general resumé for all jobs in the related field
    b. Specific—designed with one particular job in mind
  3. Styles
    a. Descriptive/traditional—lists education, experience, and qualifications in chronologic order; biographic
    b. Functional—states effective accomplishments that support a specific job position; reflects ability
  4. Contents
    a. Personal identification
      (1) Name
      (2) Address
      (3) Telephone number
    b. Job objective
      (1) Statement of the exact job being sought
      (2) May include a brief philosophic statement and professional goals
    c. Professional education applicable to the job objective
      (1) Masters or doctoral degree
      (2) Baccalaureate degree
      (3) Associate degree
      (4) Dental hygiene licensure with license number and special certificates
    d. Professional experience
      (1) New graduates—list special skills and interests from school or jobs in related fields as appropriate

(2) Midcareer professionals—divide experiences into categories such as private practice, teaching, administrative, research, community health, etc.

  e. Professional data—optional

    (1) Professional affiliations

    (2) Community/professional services

    (3) Continuing education courses related to the position sought

    (4) Professional projects

  f. References—optional

    (1) "Available on request" or

    (2) List two sources who speak well of you; include their names, positions, addresses, and telephone numbers

    (3) Notify listed references that they may be contacted

  g. Eliminate unnecessary personal information, such as gender, age, race or color, religion, marital status, children, height, weight, hobbies, etc.

5. Format

  a. Brief—one page

  b. Neat, accurate, typed letter-perfect with correct spelling and grammar

  c. Organized with functional, bold headings to introduce each category

  d. Spaces and wide margins used for easy readability

  e. Original or high-quality photocopy on medium-weight white or ivory bond paper; no carbon copies

B. Cover letter

1. Purpose

  a. Introduces the applicant and the resumé

  b. Highlights important qualifications

2. Content

  a. Introduce yourself courteously and professionally

  b. Tell how you heard of the job or why you like this work environment

  c. Emphasize your qualifications to fit this job

    (1) Demonstrate your understanding of the employer's needs

    (2) Indicate your skills that specifically fit this job

    (3) Demonstrate your interest

  d. Do not repeat yourself in the resumé

  e. State your availability for an interview and your intention to contact the office to schedule an interview

3. Format

  a. Brief and simple—one or two paragraphs

  b. Original, individually typed

  c. Neat, accurate, typed letter-perfect on bond paper with correct spelling and grammar

4. Address the letter to the person of authority and use the person's name and title

5. Sign the cover letter

6. Enclose your resumé

C. Interview[9,10]

1. Types

  a. Information—about the job market and where to look in the field; can use to gather job descriptions

  b. Job search—regarding a specific job being sought

2. Purpose—mutual opportunity of reciprocal information and impressions to evaluate for congruent job objectives

  a. Interviewer appraises the candidate's

    (1) Resumé

    (2) Work qualifications

    (3) Professional philosophy/values

    (4) Behavior/communication skills

    (5) Appearance

  b. Candidate appraises the interviewer and employment situation with regard to

    (1) Job description and responsibility

    (2) Staff members

    (3) Practice philosophy/values

    (4) Office environment

    (5) Working conditions

    (6) Opportunity for job satisfaction, professional growth, challenge, advancement, and responsibility

  c. Fact finding for both parties

  d. Initiation of a relationship between the two parties

3. Styles

  a. Directed

    (1) Follows a specific pattern

    (2) Highly structured format with a checklist of questions

    (3) Usually impersonal and dominated by the interviewer

    (4) Little opportunity for the candidate to initiate questions

  b. Open

    (1) Loosely structured format

    (2) Broad, general questions

    (3) Allows for interaction between the interviewer and candidate

  c. Combination

    (1) Includes both direct and open questions

(2) Opportunity for information exchange between both parties

d. Group interview

(1) Several candidates and one or more interviewer

(2) May begin as or become nondirective, allowing the candidates to conduct the process, while the interviewer does not participate

(3) Expect one candidate to emerge from the others

e. Board interview

(1) One candidate and several interviewers

(2) Each interviewer asks questions in his or her special interest area

4. Obtaining an interview

a. Screening—identify potential acceptable positions; eliminate unacceptable positions

(1) Telephone the office

(2) Ask basic questions about the position

(3) Listen for the office "tune."

b. Make an interview appointment

(1) Set the date, time, and location

(2) Get directions to the office

(3) Ask what is expected to be the length of the interview

(4) Ask who will be the interviewer

5. Preparation

a. Develop self-knowledge—know who you are and what you have to offer

(1) Job qualifications, skill strengths, and weaknesses

(2) Employment expectations

(3) Professional philosophy

(4) Short- and long-range career goals

(5) Personal attributes and philosophy

b. Research the position—limit yourself to job descriptions that meet your goals and suit your practice philosophy

(1) Learn the reputation of the practice, dentist, and employees

(2) Talk to current or previous employees or other dentists

c. Role-play a mock interview

(1) Write possible questions that you may be asked

(2) Present your answers out loud

(3) Write your questions about the position

(4) Present your questions out loud

(5) Ask for a critique from a colleague

(6) Repeat—continuing until you feel, act, and sound informed and professional

d. Imagine the interviewer—plan your approach

(1) Interviewer's position in the office

(2) Interviewer's area of expertise, attitudes, and expectations

(3) Knowledge of job position and dental hygiene skills and services

(4) Personality, disposition, and honesty

(5) Communication skills

(6) Practice philosophy

6. Preliminary interview

a. Introductions

(1) Initial contact, first impressions

(2) Establish rapport

b. Presentation of the candidate's qualifications

(1) Resumé reviewed

(2) Professional philosophy shared

(3) Specific strengths of education and experience stressed

c. Presentation of the position

(1) Job description of specific procedures and the workload

(2) Dental hygienist's general responsibilities, participation with the practice team, and opportunity for professional growth

(3) Description of the office atmosphere and work environment

(4) Philosophy and goals of practice

(5) Compensation

d. Compatibility established between the candidate and position

(1) Candidate's skills and strengths linked with the job description and needs of the practice

(2) Plans made to accommodate for weaknesses in the match

e. Conclusion

(1) Summary of findings

(2) Possible job offer

(3) Plans for a second interview

7. Selection interview/second interview

a. Opportunity for a second look at each other

b. Opportunity for office observation—details and work situation

(1) Dental hygiene operatory

(2) Equipment and instruments

(3) Recordkeeping forms

(4) Office work atmosphere in action

(5) Clientele

c. Opportunity for additional questions between the candidate and employer

d. Discussion of details

(1) Job description

(2) Office policies and procedures

(3) Work schedule

(4) Compensation—starting package and raises

e. Job offer

(1) Starting date

(2) Probationary period

(3) Discussion of an employment agreement or letter of intent

8. Candidate selection criteria

a. Interviewer's subjective feelings about the candidate, the human factor of simply liking another person

b. Overall characteristics of appearance, body language, human relations skills, and verbal communication skills

c. Strength of the candidate's qualifications, performance record, achievements, and success potential

d. Recommendations from references

e. Candidate's attitude—interest, ability, and willingness to do the job

f. Candidate's personality—pleasantness, poise, enthusiasm, intelligence, judgment, maturity, self-confidence, and motivation

9. Strategies

a. Initiate discussion of personally and professionally important issues if they are not covered by the interviewer

b. If the exact job desired does not exist, design it and then promote it to the employer

10. Recommendations for successful interviews

a. Be prompt for a good first impression

b. Attire makes the second impression

(1) Appearance must be professional—present a serious image

(2) Look conservative—wear simple, tasteful attire with soft, blended colors

(3) Avoid distractors such as heavy makeup, elaborate hairstyles, strong or lingering scents, extensive jewelry, and frilly, gaudy, sexy, cute, or overdone dressing

(4) Be neat, clean, fresh, and perfect from head to toe

(5) Dress as though you represent the employer with whom you are interviewing

c. Verbal communications

(1) Address the interviewer by name

(2) Wait for the interviewer to begin the questioning first; follow the interviewer's lead

(3) Listen carefully to each question and answer the actual question asked

(4) Respond to questions with concise answers

(5) Reply to questions with information that demonstrates your knowledge and skills and will establish credibility and trust

(6) Say "I don't know" when you do not know the answer to a question

(7) Be diplomatic and tactful—avoid complaining or negatively judging past experiences, schools, or teachers

(8) State your questions to the interviewer succinctly

(9) Use good grammar and pronunciation; avoid slang and minimize jargon

d. Nonverbal communications and body language

(1) Display your dental hygiene smile

(2) Maintain good posture

(3) Shake hands firmly on meeting the interviewer

(4) Be seated at the direction of the interviewer

(5) Use eye contact throughout the interview

(6) Assume an open, calm body position

(7) Pay attention, demonstrate interest, show eagerness, and take notes if you like

(8) Be human; act as natural as possible

(9) Do not smoke, chew gum, chew fingernails, bite lips, wiggle feet, or display other nervous habits

e. Attitude

(1) Interview the interviewer on a parity basis

(2) Believe in yourself

(3) Heed your own feelings

(4) Be positive and enthusiastic

(5) Be courteous, sincere, and genuine

(6) Be consistent

D. Job search strategies

1. Preparation—focus on yourself

a. Clarify your career goals

(1) Practice philosophy and values

(2) Work objectives related to goals

(3) Compensation needs

b. Identify all your professional skills and personal strengths necessary to achieve your goals

c. Imagine the ideal job situation, and seek or create one that fits this fantasy as closely as possible

d. Know your full value to a dental practice

2. Investigate the job market

a. Research local trends

(1) Job opportunities and growth potential

(2) Job descriptions

(3) Workloads and job sharing

(4) Compensation packages

(5) Job turnovers and layoffs

b. "Shop around" and interview for information
   (1) Learn all the options and make comparisons
   (2) Do not underrate your abilities or undercut a wage
   (3) Choose the best opportunity for you

3. Job sources
   a. Friends, colleagues, and other professional contacts—word of mouth
   b. Verbal or printed announcements at meetings and conferences
   c. Dental hygiene association component employment placement services
   d. Dental society employment placement services
   e. Private healthcare providers' employment placement agencies
   f. Public or county health departments
   g. Dental hygiene school bulletin boards on employment opportunities
   h. Dental hygiene and dental association newsletters, journal job announcements, and professional meetings
   i. Bulletin board job announcements in large office buildings
   j. Contact
      (1) People at offices near where you would like to work
      (2) People mentioned in association newsletters
      (3) Association leaders, authors, speakers, and educators
   k. Employees within the healthcare industry
   l. Canvas
      (1) Local dental association membership directories
      (2) Alumni association membership directories
      (3) Telephone book yellow pages with listings of dentists located near you
   m. Dental supply houses or supply salespersons
   n. Newspaper classified advertisements

E. Job selection considerations[10]
   1. Purpose—candidate compares career needs and desires with what the practice offers
   2. Factors
      a. Overall practice ambience and atmosphere
      b. Practice philosophy, goals, and values
      c. Personnel harmony
      d. Interactions with clients
      e. Quality of care provided
      f. General job description
         (1) Specific job responsibilities
         (2) Variety of services

7. General work conditions
   (1) Workload, scheduling, and hours
   (2) Equipment, instruments, and supplies
      h. Overall role of the dental hygienist—respect and responsibility
      i. Compensation package
         (1) Salary
         (2) Fringe benefits
         (3) Schedule for increases
      j. Opportunity for professional growth
      k. Job security
         (1) Assured client load
         (2) Employee turnover rate
      l. Location of the office, commute time, and parking
      m. Solo or group practice or other
      n. Well-established or new, growing practice
   3. Choose the job that offers the most for you

Career Development

A. Professional stationery and business cards
   1. Purpose
      a. Establish professional identity
      b. Demonstrate personal style
   2. Uses
      a. Exchange of cards at professional introductions
         (1) Job interviews
         (2) Dental professional meetings, conferences, and educational programs
         (3) Nondental professional associations, agencies, and professional contacts
      b. Professional correspondence
      c. Practice promotion
   3. Styles
      a. Engraved business cards
      b. Engraved or printed stationery
      c. Printed memo pads
   4. Design
      a. Name and degrees (B.S., M.S., M.B.A., Ph.D.)
      b. Title
         (1) Registered dental hygienist (R.D.H.)
         (2) Expanded certificate(s)
         (3) Other identifying information such as "oral health specialist" or "oral disease prevention educator"
      c. Home or office address and telephone number
      d. For an office card, may include the dentist's name, such as "in the office of _____, D.D.S."
      e. Select a quality of paper and a design that represent your professional image and abilities
      f. May need more than one card design to represent different affiliations

B. Employment retention

1. Career planning
   a. Definitions
      (1) Career—course or progress of a person's life related to some noteworthy activity or pursuit; total of one's lifework in a chosen field
      (2) Occupation—one's regular or principal business or line of work
      (3) Job—position of employment to gain a livelihood
   b. Career elements
      (1) Continual education to expand knowledge and skills in the field
      (2) Maturation of professional and technical skills
      (3) Responsible contributions for directing the success of patient care or other work objectives and creating a positive work environment
      (4) Participation in the growth of the profession through research, education, politics, organizational leadership, and/or public awareness
      (5) Personal gratification gained through involvement
   c. Goals—short-term objectives that support long-range goals for career development and professional achievement
      (1) Record goals to continually guide direction and contribute to commitment
      (2) Revise goals for growth, advancement, or change
2. Starting a new job—quickly establish, then maintain your "professional personality"
   a. Fill your work role with intelligent, responsible behavior
   b. Use time productively
   c. Demonstrate standards for quality care
   d. Establish a communication style for verbal and written interactions
   e. Mutually with your employer, define performance standards, then meet and surpass your employer's expectations for your performance
   f. Demonstrate your substance
   g. Be consistent
   h. Initially be investigative to learn about this new position and others in the office
   i. Gain respect and build a loyalty base
3. Continuing education—keep current with research developments, new trends in dentistry, and the state of the art of dental hygiene through
   a. Didactic meetings
   b. Clinical workshops
   c. Study groups
   d. Journals, literature, and new and revised texts
   e. Discussions with colleagues
4. Postlicentiate degrees—expand your knowledge and gain additional skills for job retention or career mobility
   a. Baccalaurate degree in dental hygiene
   b. Masters degree in dental hygiene or related area
   c. Doctoral degree
C. Stress and burnout
   1. Definitions
      a. Stress—strain or tension from compulsive pressures; usually diminishes one's resistance
      b. Burnout—combination of physical, emotional, and behavioral changes in an individual as a response to high-intensity or long-duration stress; adaptive capabilities are exceeded
   2. Relationship to dental hygiene[11]
      a. "Giving" role of healthcare providers
      b. Intense interpersonal relations with clients and staff members
      c. Monotonous job tasks
      d. Lack of appreciation (reduced self-esteem)
      e. Being taken for granted (reduced self-worth)
      f. Lack of accomplishment of personal and/or professional goals
      g. Lack of change
   3. Strategies for reducing stress and burnout
      a. Identify when you are experiencing burnout
      b. Identify the causes of stress
         (1) Analyze your feelings to achieve self-awareness of internal issues
         (2) Evaluate your environment and work situation to make external changes
      c. Reprioritize your goals or reevaluate your methods to accomplish reconfirmed goals
      d. Attempt to make changes at work to reduce stress—delegate duties, be creative, or try something new
      e. Modify your behavior to better enjoy the life process
         (1) Take classes to learn assertiveness training, success strategies, communication skills, or time management techniques
         (2) Take good care of your body; get regular sleep, adhere to a physical fitness program, and follow sound nutrition guidelines
         (3) Enjoy recreation
         (4) Try techniques for mind and body relaxation, such as catnaps, slow, deep breathing, stretching, conscious relaxation, meditation, biofeedback, visualization, guided imagery, meditation, yoga, or prayer

(5) Try body relaxation experiences of massage, hot tubs, or saunas

(6) Try new behavior

D. Assertive behavior[6,12]

1. Value—assertive behavior enables one to negotiate mutually satisfactory solutions in a variety of situations with employers, coworkers, clients, and colleagues

2. Definitions

a. Assertive behavior—communicating honestly and openly in a manner that equalizes the parties involved to gain reasonable results; it is personally satisfying and socially effective

b. Passive behavior—submission to others' wants and needs; timidity, usually because of a lack of confidence, fear, or low self-esteem; may lead to frustration and depression

c. Aggressive behavior—attacking, harsh, and demanding; often blaming and harmful to the other party; aimed at domination and humiliation

3. Self concept—assertive behavior is dependent on self-confidence; self-concept can be enhanced by repeated positive thoughts, statements, and images; believe in your right to be treated honestly, with respect, and as a professional

4. Verbal communications

a. Express your thoughts and feelings directly and honestly

b. Use a positive approach in comments you make about yourself without hurting others

c. Take responsibility for your rights

5. Speech patterns[12]

a. Tone and pitch of voice can be intimidating or reassuring; can show weakness or strength

b. Rate of speaking can be paced to include or exclude others; can demonstrate confidence or nervousness

6. Body language[12]—up to two thirds of overall communication is done without speaking; nonverbal messages speak loudly; body language can say something completely opposite from the words being spoken, confusing the listener; nonverbal messages can undermine or support the actual words spoken

a. Gestures—use of the hands can emphasize or distract

b. Eye contact—sets the stage for assertive communication; establishes trust and confidence

c. Facial expression—influences credibility of what is said

d. Habitual mannerisms—can be distracting

e. Laughter—if inappropriate, will subvert communication; may show nervousness or insincerity

f. Posture—stance, demonstrates self-image while sitting, standing, and walking

g. Body movements—can demonstrate discomfort and insincerity and interest

7. Implementing assertive behavior—begin with small steps in assertiveness skills[6]

a. Identify successful assertive behavior you are already using

b. Watch others who are successfully assertive

c. Plan your new assertiveness; imagine, then write an assertive script

(1) Describe the exact thing you want to change; be objective and specific

(2) Express what you think and how you feel about the specific situation

(3) Specify the exact change you desire; work on one thing at a time; request must be reasonable and within the power of the other person to meet

(4) Consequences in the form of rewards and penalties for each party should be spelled out; emphasize the positive consequences; negative consequences must be realistic and believable, not idle threats

d. Practice assertive behavior in front of a mirror, then with a friend

e. Initiate assertive behavior in your speech, eye contact, appearance, body language, and actions

Career Mobility

A. Definitions[13]

1. Allied health personnel—supporting, complementing, and supplementing the professional functions of dentists in the delivery of healthcare to clients

2. Vertical career ladder—moving up the technical ladder from dental assistant to dental hygienist to dentist to dentist in a specialty practice; entry may occur at any of the first three levels

3. Lateral career mobility—combines existing knowledge, skills, and licensure with additional study to qualify for employment in related fields (see D on employment opportunity alternatives to traditional dental hygiene practice)

B. Job changes

1. Periodically review your employment situation, job status, technical skill level, and knowledge

a. Are you satisfied?

b. Are you still experiencing professional growth?

2. Compare your present situation with your stated career goals

a. Are you accomplishing objectives?

b. Is it time to move on?

3. Decide if it is time for a job change

    a. Expand your present employment situation

    b. Switch to a new office in a similar work position

    c. Change to a job that is an alternative to traditional clinical practice with new duties and responsibilities, part time or full time

4. Enhance success at career mobility

    a. Make professional contacts throughout your career

    b. Investigate all possible career options

    c. Plan changes carefully with a clear, thorough idea of what you want to do

    d. Be creative—look for opportunities; redesign your present job or design a new one and sell it to your employer, part time or full time

    e. Be willing to take risks

C. Networks of professional connections

  1. Networking—sharing and extending professional contacts to establish friendships and business relationships; exchanging knowledge and information; advising and developing a professional and moral support system for achievement of goals

  2. Value—professional networks can keep those involved informed of professional developments and apprised of job opportunities, assist in making job changes, and create synergism for participants

  3. Participants

    a. Professional colleagues

    b. Business and professional acquaintances

    c. College classmates and faculty

    d. Present and former coworkers

    e. Friends and relatives

  4. Types

    a. General—all the contacts made during one's professional career

    b. Specific—organized group of professionals meeting on a regular basis to promote growth and development of one another

D. Employment opportunity alternatives to traditional dental hygiene practice—part-time and full-time jobs for dental hygienists are available or may be created in (and are not limited to) the following areas

  1. Private dental practices

    a. Clinical supervision

    b. Administration

    c. Practice management

    d. Service

  2. Dental hygiene schools

    a. Education—didactic and clinical

    b. Administration

    c. Research

    d. Service

  3. Public schools

    a. Oral inspection and disease prevention programs for students and teachers

    b. Nutritional counseling

    c. Sports dentistry

    d. Curriculum development

    e. Teacher in-service education

    f. Research

    g. Client advocacy

  4. Community oral health projects

    a. Prenatal care/infant care

    b. Parents' and children's groups

    c. Senior citizen's groups

    d. Special-needs groups

    e. Research/epidemiological studies

    f. Community-wide needs assessment; program planning, implementation, and evaluation

  5. Consulting and education

    a. Practice management

    b. Designing and teaching continuing education workshops for health professionals

  6. Continuing education business—own and operate

  7. Sports dentistry—mouth protection, education, and planning

    a. Park and recreation departments

    b. Youth teams

    c. Schools

  8. Public and private institutions

    a. Hospitals

    b. Long-term care facilities

    c. Residental care facilities

    d. Hospices

    e. Correctional facilities

  9. Myofunctional therapy

  10. Oral health products industry

    a. Retail representative

    b. Manufacturer's (wholesale) representative

    c. Product marketing

    d. Sales management

    e. Product research and development

    f. Product manufacturing

    g. Professional relations representative

    h. Dental products supply house representative

  11. Insurance industry

    a. Clinician

    b. Dental claims examiner

    c. Marketing and underwriting

    d. Professional relations

    e. Quality assurance

  12. Government service

a. Armed forces
b. Veteran's Administration
c. Public Health Service
d. Indian Health Service
e. State agencies
f. National Institute of Dental Research
13. Health professionals recruiting and placement agency
   a. Own and operate
   b. Associate as personnel consultant
14. Scientific research
   a. National Institute of Dental Research
   b. World Health Organization
   c. University
   d. Business and industry
15. Professional organizations (constituent or American Dental Hygienists' Association [ADHA])
   a. Administration
   b. Management
   c. Research
   d. Service
16. Professional media
   a. Technical or scientific writing and publishing
   b. Educational video production
17. International dental hygiene (see Chapter 1, section on international requirements)

Personal Business Interests

Financial Planning

A. Definition—setting financial goals for the future, taking steps to achieve maximal money management
B. Steps
   1. Evaluate your present financial situation by computing your net worth—the difference between assets (amounts owned) and liabilities (amount owed); include real property, life insurance, stocks, bonds, retirement accounts, household and personal property, and bank accounts; calculate your net worth annually to check progress in reaching your financial goal, then review and update your plan
   2. Set goals for the future, stating specific objectives for short-term accomplishments and long-range goals; plan to spread investments over the years
      a. Set long-range goals, including the desired income at retirement
      b. State other objectives, including income now and in 5 years, then 10 years, etc.; specify investments such as residential property, securities, retirement accounts, education of children, travel, etc.

c. Plan a budget as an effective money management tool; anticipate basic needs and expenses, allocate funds, analyze spending habits, control impulsive buying, and live within income limits; plan for some fun and recreation as well as for emergency expenses; regularly monitor actual expenses as compared with the budget to see if you are on the right track or need to compensate for unexpected bills
d. Keep records—complete and accurate accounting assists with taxes, expense accounts, and forecasting the financial future
e. Establish a credit rating in your own name to facilitate getting loans, a mortgage, or other credit and to function with independence financially; check your credit profile from time to time for accuracy
f. Use credit effectively—for major purchases, spread payments over a long period and pay reasonable finance charges; avoid unnecessary debts, finance charges, and penalties for late payments
g. Pay yourself first—with interest, dividends, and appreciation; begin with small, guaranteed investments; make your money work for you by investigating interest-bearing checking accounts, savings accounts, money market accounts, mutual funds, bonds, certificates of deposit, Treasury bills, etc.; establish a reserve fund for emergencies
h. Purchasing a home is an important major investment, usually the largest single investment of a lifetime; provide your own housing and eliminate paying rent to someone else; financially valuable because it offers safety and security, provides financial leverage as collateral, gains appreciation, and offers a tax advantage
i. Diversify other investments—spread and reduce risks and gain income-producing securities
j. Protect yourself with disability insurance to safeguard your earning power
k. Plan a retirement fund
3. Goals for investments
   a. Preserve capital
   b. Produce income
   c. Provide a tax advantage
   d. Hedge inflation
   e. Show capital growth/appreciation in value
   f. Furnish safety and security
   g. Have liquidity conversion potential
   h. Be maintained management free or with minimal expenses
4. Professional assistance for financial planning

a. Make personal investigations through research, reading, classes, talking with others, studying market indicators, and/or participation in investment clubs

b. Design a carefully planned strategy to achieve financial goals by using the expertise of specialists for help with laws, regulations, intricacies, and refinements
   (1) Banker
   (2) Real estate broker
   (3) Stock broker
   (4) Insurance broker
   (5) Investment advisor
   (6) Accountant
   (7) Lawyer

5. Types of investments—consider how much risk you are willing and able to assume, consider both short- and long-term investments, evaluate income needs now and in the future
   a. Tangibles (hard assets)
      (1) Real estate
      (2) Gold, silver, coins, and gems
      (3) Antiques, art, stamps, rare books, etc.
   b. Intangibles (paper with a guarantee, securities, or liquid assets)
      (1) Banks, savings and loans, or thrifts
         (a) Interest-bearing checking accounts
         (b) Savings accounts
         (c) Money market certificates
         (d) Certificates of deposit
      (2) Government securities
         (a) U.S. Treasury bills
         (b) U.S. Treasury notes and bonds
         (c) U.S. savings bonds
         (d) Federal agency lending programs
         (e) Short-term tax-exempt notes
         (f) Municipal bonds for estates, counties, and municipalities
      (3) Investment firms
         (a) Money market funds
         (b) Stocks
         (c) Corporate bonds
         (d) Mutual funds
         (e) Tax-deferred annuities
         (f) Commodities/financial futures
         (g) Limited partnerships
         (h) Tax shelters
         (i) Trust deeds
         (j) Foreign currency

6. Estate planning
   a. Definition—provides for intentional disposition of possessions and assets on one's death to organize family resources and provide for their future
   b. Value
      (1) Requires careful financial planning and management during one's lifetime
      (2) Intentionally creates, defines, and retains assets of the estate
      (3) Provides for disability
      (4) Plans and provides for retirement
      (5) Can spread family income and ensure prudent money management during one's lifetime
      (6) Trusts can be established to reduce administrative and management costs and protect assets
      (7) Minimizes or avoids taxes imposed on estates and inheritances
      (8) Guarantees financially secure property will be disposed of as one desires
   c. Includes
      (1) Titles of properties
      (2) Insurance
      (3) Pension plans
      (4) Investments
      (5) Management plan
      (6) Disposition of property

Taxes[14]

A. Tax system
   1. Taxes are the largest single item in the budget of the average American; it is worth the additional time and money to be certain one is getting all the possible tax breaks available
   2. One's "tax bracket" is the combined federal and state percentage of taxes paid on the total dollars earned
   3. U.S. tax system is a "marginal progressive" style; it is advantageous to maximize tax deductions to reduce tax liabilities to the lowest tax bracket possible; further, one's tax bracket will help determine the best types of investments for one's financial situation

B. Tax considerations for professionals—in addition to the tax savings available to all taxpayers, professionals are entitled to special tax adjustments, deductions, and credits if these expenses are employment related
   1. Record keeping and substantiation requirements
      a. Calendar of professional activities
      b. Explanation of the professional event, including the date, activity, how it is related and helpful to the job, the sponsor, location, cost, and transportation required

c. Expense record
d. Proof of all expenses, such as receipts, cancelled checks, or credit card vouchers
e. Overall complete, accurate, and permanent
f. Retain federal records for at least 3 years after filing; check for individual state requirements
g. Keep copies of federal and state income tax returns forever
2. Professional activities
a. Meetings of professional organizations
b. Staff meetings
c. Educational programs related to the profession
d. Study groups
e. Employment-seeking expenses for a job change within the same profession
3. Professional expenses are deductible only to the extent that the professional is not reimbursed and can establish his or her right to deduct them
C. Travel and transportation expenses
1. Definitions
a. Travel—ordinary and necessary expenses incurred while away from home (overnight) for the purpose of a professional or job-related activity; deduct as "Employee Business Expense," IRS Form 2106, as an adjustment to income; these include
(1) Fares for airplane, train, bus, etc.
(2) Meals and lodging
(3) Automobile expenses
(4) Related necessary expenses such as telephone calls and laundry
b. Transportation—actual cost of transportation to professional activities not away from home (not overnight); allowable only as an itemized deduction, Schedule A, IRS Form 1040; permits commuting between two jobs on the same day; does not permit basic commuting from home to job and back; these include
(1) Actual automobile expenses
(2) Bus and cab fares
(3) Bridge tolls and parking fees
2. Methods of computation
a. Mileage rate method—multiply the total number of miles driven by the rate allowed by the IRS; instructions for Form 2106 state the rate for each tax year
b. Actual expenses method—compute the ratio of business mileage to total mileage; multiply the ratio times the cost of actual operating expenses (gasoline, oil, repairs, maintenance, licenses, insurance, depreciation or lease payments, loan interest, etc.)

c. Both options require keeping an odometer diary at the beginning and end of each trip; nonprofessional portions are to be excluded from total
3. Calculation of deductible travel
a. If the trip is entirely for professional activities, all expenses are deductible
b. If the trip is primarily professional, with a small portion for personal travel, travel expenses to and from the destination, as well as direct professional expenses, are deductible
c. If the trip is primarily for pleasure, none of the travel expense is deductible, but direct professional expenses at the destination are deductible
4. Travel outside the United States
a. If the trip is entirely professional, all expenses may be deducted
b. If the trip is a combination of professional activities and pleasure, expenses must be divided, with no deduction for the personal portion
c. Limit is two foreign conventions or trips per tax year
d. Substantiation requires a written statement, signed by the attendee, showing the total number of days spent at the convention, the number of hours devoted each day to scheduled professional activities, and an actual program of scheduled activities; a written statement of an officer of the convention is attached with other required statements to the federal tax return
D. Miscellaneous professional expenses—may be deducted only if deductions are itemized; Schedule A, Form 1040
1. Professional education expenses
a. Deducted as ordinary and necessary if they meet express requirements of the employer or the law for retaining professional status and/or licensure; or to maintain or improve skills required in performing the duties of the present profession, including education that leads to a degree
b. If new educational requirements are placed on the present profession, necessary education expenses to meet these stipulations are deductible
c. Expenses for training in a new profession may not be deducted
d. Include tuition, fees for correspondence courses, books, supplies, travel, and transportation costs
e. Proof of attendance may be required
2. Professional uniform expenses
a. Purchase and upkeep costs of work clothes can be deducted if they are specifically required as a condition of employment and are not suitable

for general or everyday wear; must be recognizable as a "uniform"

b. Upkeep includes laundering, dry cleaning, repairs, and alterations

c. Uniform items include dresses, pants and tops, laboratory coats and jackets, clinic shoes, caps, white or support hoisery, protective clothing (such as safety eyeglasses, masks, and gloves), and name tags and pins

3. Other miscellaneous professional expenses

a. Dues to professional organizations

b. Employment-seeking expenses, including agency fees, resumé typing and printing, telephone calls, postage, travel, and transportation expenses

c. Liability (malpractice) insurance premiums

d. Instruments, professional equipment, and supplies

e. Medical examinations required by the employer

f. Subscriptions to professional and trade journals

g. Professional legal expenses

h. Professional license renewal

i. Telephone toll and long-distance calls for professional reasons

E. Retirement accounts

1. Individual Retirement Arrangements (IRAs) are allowed for any person with earned income if there is no participation in another qualified retirement plan by that person or his or her spouse

2. Amount contributed to the IRA is subtracted from the gross income, as an adjustment to income,[11] regardless of whether itemized deductions are made

3. Allowable contributions and interest earned are not taxable during working years; tax is deferred

4. One may not borrow from the IRA before the specified age (59½) without being taxed and penalized

5. See section on retirement

F. Child and dependent care

1. Expenses allowed for children under age 15 or disabled dependents while one is at work or looking for work

2. Credit available is a maximum of 30%, related to the taxpayer's adjusted gross income

G. Tax audits

1. Tax returns are reviewed by agents and computers for errors and omissions, deductions that are beyond the norm relative to a given profession, and other variables

2. Letter of notification indicates specific categories for audit

3. All elements of proof are presented for acceptance of deductions

4. Although all auditors rely on the same reference sources, each may interpret the law slightly differently

5. Repetitive audits for the same items not allowed for 2 years following a clear audit; if an audit finds additional tax liability, the audit can be repeated on that item until the audit is clear; one can be audited every year for a different issue

6. IRS auditors are responsible to both the taxpayer and the government and are charged to be fair

7. Legitimate deductions should not be eliminated to avoid an audit

Retirement

A. Focus on goals

1. Lifestyle, home location, and living conditions

2. Activities, travel, recreation, hobbies, and business involvement

3. Consider your projected living costs and the income required to accommodate your retirement plans; note possible illness or disability

4. Consider your projected income from Social Security, retirement funds, and whole life insurance policies in addition to other investments

5. Write out a plan and review it periodically

B. Tax-deferred retirement accounts

1. Purpose

a. Establish a retirement account

b. Taxes on amounts deposited and interest earned are deferred until withdrawal

c. Reduce the annual adjusted gross income to reduce the income tax debt

2. Types

a. Corporate—may establish a pension plan at the principal's discretion

(1) Requirements—rules set by the corporation

(a) Minimum number of hours per year

(b) Minimum age of employee

(c) May establish a waiting period before the employee can participate in the plan (usually 1 to 3 years)

(d) Vesting schedule options—grants the employee full ownership of monies contributed in his or her name by the corporation

(e) When and if requirements are met, the employee must be included in the plan

(2) Contributions

(a) Maximum allowable is 25% of the annual salary to a maximum of $25,000

(b) Employer contributions (percentage) equal employee contributions

(c) Monies are held in a single corporate account

(d) Lump-sum or regular deposits may be made during the year

(e) Contributions are allowed until April 15 of the following year or the end of the fiscal year

(f) All amounts deposited by the employer are deductible by the employer as a business expense

(3) Termination—employee who leaves employment where there is a retirement plan may take the fund (amount vested) and "roll it over" into an IRA

b. Keogh plan
   (1) Requirements
      (a) Dentist must be self-employed and have a Keogh plan for self
      (b) Employee needs
         [1] Minimum of 3 years continuous employment
         [2] Minimum of 1000 hours per year
         [3] Vesting of 100% is immediate when the above requirements are met
   (2) Contributions
      (a) Maximum allowable is 15% of the annual earned income to a maximum of $7500
      (b) Employer contributions (percentage) equal employee contributions
      (c) Separate account for each plan participant
      (d) Lump-sum or regular deposits may be made during the year
      (e) Contributions allowed until April 15 of the following year or the end of the fiscal year
      (f) All amounts deposited by the employer are deductible by the employer as a business expense
   (3) Termination—employee who leaves employment where there is a Keogh plan may take the fund and "roll it over" into an IRA

c. Individual Retirement Arrangement (IRA)
   (1) Requirements
      (a) Allowable for anyone not included in another retirement account
      (b) Spouse may have a separate IRA account, even if no income
      (c) If one spouse has a qualified retirement plan through employment, neither spouse qualifies for IRA tax deduction

   (2) Contributions
      (a) Maximum allowable is up to 100% of earned income to a maximum of $2000
      (b) For a married couple filing a joint tax return when only one partner earns income, a separate spousal IRA may be established for the nonworking spouse; maximum allowable to both accounts is $2500
      (c) Lump-sum or regular deposits may be made throughout the year
      (d) Contributions are allowed until April 15 of the following year or extended filing of taxes
      (e) All amounts deposited are tax deductible as adjustments to income

3. Termination and withdrawal for all retirement accounts
   a. All accounts may be terminated at any time
   b. Funds must be left on deposit until minimum age 59½, or funds will be taxed and assessed a penalty fee
   c. Withdrawal begins after retirement, age 59½, or disablement
   d. Withdrawal must begin at age 70½, and contributions may continue

4. Mechanisms
   a. Savings account
   b. Mutual funds
   c. Retirement bonds
   d. Retirement annuities
   e. Trust accounts

5. Laws on rules of tax-deferred retirement accounts change frequently; always check for current requirements

Wills[15]

A. Definition—written, legal arrangement for distribution of assets when death occurs

B. Value
   1. Ensures disposal of belongings as one chooses and lets others know of these wishes
   2. Requires that one think about the consequences of one's death and decide what one wants and plan for proper distribution
   3. Protects beneficiaries' rights to receive assets without dispute
   4. Safeguards and ties up all loose ends of financial affairs
   5. Provides for financial and guardian care of minor children
   6. Minimizes expenses of transfers and unnecessary fees

7. Ensures minimum delay in distributing the estate
8. Covers payment of debts of the decedent
9. Provides for tax planning

C. Contents
1. Identifies beneficiaries
2. Identifies all aspects of financial affairs
3. Divides assets
4. Codicil can give away special items

D. Wills are best prepared in consultation with a lawyer to ensure validity and best interests overall

E. Executor duties
1. Carries out provisions of the will
2. Directs financial concerns of the state following death
3. Gathers and preserves property
4. Collects income due
5. Pays bills and taxes
6. Identifies and distributes all remaining assets
7. Provides record keeping to the court

F. Probate—legal process alerting the community of the death, then attending to financial distribution of the estate

REFERENCES

1. Milone CL, Blair WC, Littlefield JE: *Marketing for the dental practice,* Philadelphia, 1982, WB Saunders.
2. Saxton DF, Nugent PM, Pelikan PK: *Mosby's comprehensive review of nursing,* ed 14, St Louis, 1992, Mosby.
3. The Dentists' Insurance Company: Patient noncompliance, TDIC Newsletter 3:3, 1982.
4. Lampner J: Effective career management for hygienists, Los Altos, Calif, 1977, Lange Medical Publications.
5. Schwarzrock S, Jensen J: *Effective dental assisting,* ed 6, Dubuque, Iowa, 1982, Wm C Brown Group.
6. Bower SA, Bower GH: *Asserting yourself,* Reading, Mass, 1976, Addison-Wesley.
7. Jensen J: How to design your agency's employee benefits program, *Grantsmanship Center News,* p 41, Sept-Oct 1979.
8. American Dental Hygienists' Association: Current employment conditions for practice, Annual Report, 1979-1980.
9. Medley HA: *Sweaty palms: the neglected art of being interviewed,* Belmont, Calif, 1978, Wadsworth.
10. Woodall IR: *Legal, ethical, and management aspects of the dental care system,* ed 3, St Louis, 1987, Mosby.
11. Dreyer R: Is burnout inevitable? *Career Dir Dent Hyg* 10(11):1, 1983.
12. Schwimmer LD: *How to ask for a raise without getting fired,* New York, 1980, Harper & Row.
13. Resurreccion RL, Wilson S: A perspective on career mobility in the dental hygiene profession, *J S C Dent Hyg Assoc,* Fall 1980.
14. Kramer S: *Tax guide for allied health professionals,* Oakland, Calif, 1981, Professional Press.
15. Porter S: *Sylvia Porter's new money book,* New York, 1979, Doubleday.

SUGGESTED READINGS

Aiken T: *Legal, ethical and political issues of nursing,* Philadelphia, 1994, FA Davis.

Blanchard K, Johnson S: *The one minute manager,* New York, 1983, William Morrow.

Bloch D: *How to get a good job and keep it,* Chicago, 1994, NTC Publishing Group.

Bloomberg G, Holden M: *The women's job search handbook,* Charlotte, VT, 1991, Williamson.

Byers S: *The executive nurse,* Albany, NY, 1997, Delmar.

Covey S: *The 7 habits of highly effective people,* New York, 1990, Fireside.

Crosby P: *Quality without tears,* New York, 1995, McGraw Hill.

Darby M, Walsh M: *Dental hygiene theory and practice,* Philadelphia, 1995, WB Saunders, ch. 36, 37, 39, 40.

Dellabough R: *The Beardstown ladies stitch-in-time guide to growing your nest egg,* New York, 1996, Hyperion.

Dorio M: *The complete idiot's guide to getting the job you want,* New York, 1995, Alpha Books.

Douglas L: *The effective nurse, leader and manager,* ed 5, St. Louis, 1996, Mosby.

Finkbeiner B: *Practice management for the dental team,* ed 4, St. Louis, 1996, Mosby.

Fisher R, Ury W: *Getting to Yes,* ed 2, New York, 1993, Penguin.

Fuller G: *The workplace survival guide,* Edgewood, NJ, 1996, Prentice Hall.

Good, C: *Resumés for re-entry,* ed 2, Manassas Park, VA, 1993, Impact.

Green P: *Get hired,* Austin, Tex, 1996, Bard.

Harper V, Wood D: *The health professional's job resource guide,* NY, 1994, Wiley.

Harty T, Harty K: *Finding a job after fifty,* Hawthorne, NJ, 1994, Career Press.

Holloway D, Bishop N: *Before you say "I quit,"* New York, 1990, Macmillan.

Hurd D: *The California survival handbook,* Placerville, Calif, 1994, Pro Pen.

Ilich J: *The complete idiot's guide to winning through negotiations,* New York, 1996, Alpha Books.

Ireland S: *The complete idiot's guide to the perfect resume,* New York, 1996, Alpha Books.

King J: *The woman's guide to interviewing and salary negotiation,* ed 2, Franklin Lakes, NJ, 1995, Career Press.

Kramer S: In Darby ML, Walsh MM: *Dental hygiene theory and practice,* Philadelphia, 1995, WB Saunders.

Kraus G: *Health care risk management,* Owings Mills, Md, 1986, Rynd Communications.

Marino K: *Resumés for the health care professional,* New York, 1993, Wiley.

McCormally K: *Cut your taxes,* Washington, DC, 1997, The Kiplinger Washington Editors, Inc.

Morris W: *The dentist's legal advisor,* St. Louis, 1995, Mosby.

Nath R: *Face to face with the IRS,* New York, 1997, Simon and Schuster Macmillan Co.

Ozar D: *Dental ethics at chairside,* St. Louis, 1994, Mosby.

Pollack R: *Dentist's risk management guide,* Chicago, 1990, National Society of Dental Practitioners.

Sullivan M: *Nursing leadership and management,* Springhouse, Pa, 1990, Springhouse Corp.

Weinstein B: *Dental ethics,* Philadelphia, 1993, Lea & Febiger.

Zipperer L: *The health care almanac,* Chicago, 1995, American Medical Association.

Review Questions

1 Each of the following is an essential element for dental hygienists as interdisciplinary team members *EXCEPT* one. Which is the *EXCEPTION?*
A. Team building skills
B. Marketing skills
C. Resumé writing ability
D. Bookkeeping skills
E. Job performance evaluation skills

2 Who is the *MOST* important member on the dental team?
A. Dentist
B. Dental hygienist
C. Receptionist
D. Office manager
E. Client

3 Which of the following would diminish an effective work team?
A. Group atmosphere is informal and supportive
B. People talk with one another, mostly about the job
C. The same organized, systematic approach is followed for each task
D. Job tasks, roles, and functions are well understood for each member
E. People express their feelings

4 Clear communications between members of the healthcare team and clients is critical to successful client management. Effective communication requires skills in receiving messages equal to sending messages.
A. Both statements are *TRUE*
B. Both statements are *FALSE*
C. The first statement is *TRUE* and the second statement is *FALSE*
D. The first statement is *FALSE* and the second statement is *TRUE*

5 The best way to facilitate learning and make it easy includes which of the following?
A. Discuss the fears of the dental office
B. Offer many options and let the client choose which to do
C. Relate new material to what the client already knows
D. Focus education exclusively on the visual
E. Focus education exclusively on the auditory

6 Which of the following applies assessment data to treatment options and recommendations with client discussion to decide on care?
A. Diagnosis
B. Care plan
C. Case presentation
D. Risk management
E. Informed consent

7 Organization and management of a professional practice in order to benefit clients and staff members is called
A. Team building
B. Practice administration
C. Client management
D. Strategic marketing
E. Client reclamation

8 Client noncompliance is defined as lack of client cooperation with recommended oral health practices. It should not be documented on the client record.
A. Both statements are *TRUE*
B. Both statements are *FALSE*
C. The first statement is *TRUE* and the second statement is *FALSE*
D. The first statement is *FALSE* and the second statement is *TRUE*

9 All of the following are elements of the dental hygienist's role in risk management *EXCEPT* one. Which is the *EXCEPTION?*
A. Provide services that meet the current standard of care
B. Use proper protocols
C. Obtain informed consent before client care
D. Interpret need for client to be seen by the dentist
E. Point out incorrect work done by other clinicians

10 Dental hygiene practice is regulated by
A. National dental practice act
B. State dental practice act
C. American Dental Association
D. American Dental Hygienists' Association
E. Dental office policy manual

11 Which of the following types of insurance policies should the dental hygienist purchase?
A. Federal Old Age Survivor's Disability
B. Workers compensation
C. Long-term permanent disability
D. Unemployment insurance
E. Individual retirement

12 Each of the following is an accepted method of payment to dental hygienist employees *EXCEPT* one. Which is the *EXCEPTION?*
A. Hourly rate of pay
B. Daily salary
C. Commission based on production
D. Commission based on collection
E. Salary plus bonus

13 Job expectations are defined by the employer and agreed upon by the employee. The performance evaluation is then completed by the employer based upon the outlined job expectations.
A. Both statements are *TRUE*
B. Both statements are *FALSE*
C. The first statement is *TRUE* and the second statement is *FALSE*
D. The first statement is *FALSE* and the second statement is *TRUE*

14 The dental hygiene professional invests in which of the following in overall career and personal business planning?
   A. Setting financial goals
   B. Organizing estate planning
   C. Performing annual tax planning
   D. Setting retirement goals
   E. All of the above

15 Each of the following is an element in financial planning *EXCEPT* one. Which is the *EXCEPTION*?
   A. Evaluate present financial situation by computing net worth
   B. Set long-term goals
   C. Set short-term goals
   D. Expect employer to provide for retirement
   E. Plan to spread investments over the years

16 What is the largest single financial budget item of the average American?
   A. Retirement
   B. Medical insurance
   C. Disability insurance
   D. Taxes
   E. Liability insurance

17 A written legal arrangement for distribution of assets upon death is called
   A. Keogh plan
   B. IRA
   C. Termination arrangement
   D. Will
   E. Executor

18 A dental hygienist should participate in estate planning, including writing a will. He or she should also participate in a retirement account either provided by the employer or an individual retirement account.
   A. Both statements are *TRUE*
   B. Both statements are *FALSE*
   C. The first statement is *TRUE* and the second statement is *FALSE*
   D. The first statement is *FALSE* and the second statement is *TRUE*

19 When a client requests that the dental hygienist remove brown stains from his teeth, he is expressing which type of communication?
   A. Physiologic
   B. Psychological
   C. Interpersonal
   D. Intrapersonal

20 Each of the following is an element of successful patient management by the dental hygienist *EXCEPT* one. Which is the *EXCEPTION*?
   A. Diagnosis
   B. Attitude
   C. Communications
   D. Case Presentation
   E. Client correspondence

21 Which of the following could be destructive to client communications?
   A. Call the clients and staff members by name
   B. Be courteous to all who are present in the office
   C. Respect the patient's privacy
   D. Share confidentialities
   E. Be nonjudgmental

22 Which of the following should be avoided when teaching new material?
   A. Build on client's current level of knowledge
   B. Use technical terminology
   C. Have client try new techniques during the appointment
   D. Consider the client's attitude toward the problem
   E. Reinforce old information

23 Which of the following is the *MOST* important element in a successful marketing campaign within the dental practice?
   A. Perform oral health screenings in the schools
   B. Adding audiovisual aids for patient education
   C. Writing dental health articles for local newspapers
   D. Volunteer professional services to community clinics
   E. Perform clinical services that result in client satisfaction

Case 1: A recent graduate who is newly licensed begins her first job search. She wishes to interview several practice settings before making a selection.

24 Which of the following would she prepare in anticipation of her interview?
   A. Resumé
   B. Employment contract
   C. Performance evaluation
   D. Letter of intent
   E. Statement of salary and fringe benefit requirements

25 Several written documents will establish guidelines and limits to the work situation and may be provided by prospective employers. The candidate may ask to see all of them in writing *EXCEPT* one. Which of the following would be the *EXCEPTION*?
   A. Dental Practice Act
   B. OSHA Guidelines
   C. Retirement plan
   D. Job description
   E. Performance evaluation

26 The job candidate may gather information about potential jobs in a variety of methods. By which method will she get the best information about issues that concern her?
   A. Request a mission statement of each dental practice to learn the office philosophy
   B. Request a job description for the position of dental hygienist
   C. Allow the dentist to ask all of the questions in order to learn what the office is looking for in an employee
   D. Prepare a variety of questions to ask during the interview to get a broad overview of the office
   E. Ask former employees about the office

27 Which type of interview would be *MOST* advantageous for the candidate?
A. Directed conversational
B. Directed written
C. Group
D. Open conversational
E. Combination

28 As a new graduate dental hygienist, how might the candidate *BEST* prepare for the interview?
A. Ask school instructors for sample questions to ask during the interview
B. Ask employed dental hygienists for sample questions to ask during the interview
C. Write a list of questions to ask during the interview
D. Role play a mock interview
E. Go to the interview with an open mind and be spontaneous

29 One of the potential dental offices asks the interviewing dental hygienist candidate for ways she might market the practice. For a new graduate, which of the following would be evidence of an existing marketing tool listed on a resume?
A. Current participation in community service activities
B. Plans to become a public speaker
C. High academic standing in school
D. Excellent grades in clinical performance in school
E. References from school instructors

30 When should the new graduate begin planning for her retirement?
A. Immediately with her first job
B. After she has been working for at least 5 years
C. After she decides if dental hygiene is the right job for her
D. When she is over age 30
E. When she reaches age 40

Case 2: The recent graduate registered dental hygienist starts her first job. She wants to make a good impression on both the office staff members and the clients.

31 Establishment of a professional approach would include each of the following *EXCEPT* one. Which is the *EXCEPTION*?
A. Fill the role with intelligent, responsible behavior
B. Ask questions to learn about the new position
C. Do things just as they were taught in school
D. Define performance standards and review expectations with the new employer at the outset
E. Establish a consistent communication style for both oral and written interactions

32 Exhibiting which of the following types of behavior will *MOST* benefit the new employee?
A. Assertive
B. Passive
C. Submissive
D. Aggressive
E. Domineering

33 At the end of the initial probationary period, the new employee can expect which of the following?
A. Job satisfaction
B. Mutual evaluation of job performance between dentist and dental hygienist
C. Full vesting in a retirement program
D. Automatic increase in salary
E. Guaranteed permanent job

34 During the first few months at the new job, the best approach for each appointment would be which of the following?
A. Spend time getting to know each client personally
B. Tell each client about your own hobbies and interests
C. Describe your academic success to each patient
D. Let everyone know this is your first job
E. Perform an organized clinical assessment of each client

35 After starting the new job, the dental hygienist wants to establish her "professional personality." Each of the following will be helpful *EXCEPT* one. Which is the *EXCEPTION*?
A. Exhibit responsible behavior
B. Use time productively
C. Define performance standards
D. Change constantly
E. Behave respectfully

36 The new dental hygienist wants to get feedback on how she is performing. Which of the following would provide the desired information?
A. Ask the dentist after each client how she did
B. Ask each client at the end of the appointment if she hurt him
C. Ask the dentist at lunch how she did
D. Ask the receptionist if the clients complain about her
E. Set a time with the dentist for a performance evaluation

37 The new hygienist wants to avoid burnout at the beginning of her new career. Which of the following is *MOST* likely to contribute to burnout?
A. The "giving" role of healthcare workers
B. Professional relations with clients
C. Professional relations with staff members
D. Variation in job tasks
E. Expressed appreciation by clients

Case 3: A dental hygienist with ten years of practice experience is seeking a new job. She updates her resumé and begins to interview.

38 This would be a good time for her to do which of the following?
A. Expect a salary increase with the new job
B. Expect a gain in fringe benefits
C. Review career goals
D. Investigate courses to enhance clinical skills
E. Investigate courses to enhance scientific knowledge

39 The resumé should reflect a balance of the candidate. Listing which of the following would contribute *LEAST* to her resume?
A. Career experience in general and/or periodontal dental practices
B. Continuing education courses completed
C. Personal interests and hobbies
D. Community service activities
E. Activities in professional organizations

40 There are a variety of employment opportunity alternatives to clinical practice that the experienced dental hygienist could consider. Which of the following would *NOT* be a viable alternative?
   A. Teaching in a dental hygiene program
   B. Consulting to dental offices
   C. Sales in the oral health products industry
   D. Dental claims examiner in the insurance industry
   E. Supervision of new dentists in a large dental clinic

41 The dental hygienist decides to "network" to investigate possible job opportunities. Which of the following would yield the *BEST* networking results?
   A. Read newspaper ads
   B. Ask professional colleagues about job opportunities
   C. Read local dental hygiene component newsletter
   D. Read *ADHA Journal of Dental Hygiene* classified ads
   E. Ask friends and relatives about job opportunities

42 The experienced dental hygienist decides to interview in a private general dental practice. Which of the following is the *MOST* important and telling question she can ask of the potential dentist?
   A. What is the salary range you will offer me?
   B. Do you offer fringe benefits?
   C. Can I see your record keeping forms?
   D. Are you open to changes in your dental practice?
   E. Can I see the instruments your dental hygienist uses?

43 A good strategy for an experienced dental hygienist regarding performance evaluation would be which of the following?
   A. Recommend the dentist skip the performance evaluation altogether because as an experienced clinician, she would not need to change or improve
   B. Request an immediate performance evaluation, such as at the end of the first day
   C. Request a 1-month evaluation after probationary period
   D. Request a 6-month evaluation
   E. Request an evaluation at the end of 1 year

Case 4: An experienced dental hygienist has been working at her dental office for five years. She attends a continuing education course and learns new clinical skills, risk management, and better record keeping systems.

44 Regarding the new, advanced clinical skills, how should she handle the new techniques?
   A. Not mention the courses to the dentist and see if he/she notices the changes
   B. Wait for the clients to observe the changes and have them report the changes to the dentist
   C. Tell the dentist of the new skills and request evaluation by the dentist
   D. Write a request for a salary increase based upon the new skills
   E. Ask the receptionist if either the dentist or the clients have mentioned the new skills

45 The communication between the dental hygienist and dentist should model which of the following?
   A. Professional interdependence
   B. Professional independence
   C. Professional counterdependence
   D. Conflict avoidance
   E. Conflict accountability

46 During the seminar in risk management, the dental hygienist learns all of the following regarding dental records are true *EXCEPT* one. Which is the *EXCEPTION*?
   A. Records must be complete
   B. Records must be accurate
   C. Records must be shared with other staff members
   D. Records must be shared with the patient upon request
   E. Records must be initialed and dated by each provider, including the dental assistant

47 What is appropriate behavior for the dental hygienist in a situation where she discovers a potential risk management problem?
   A. Ignore the problem
   B. Tell other dental hygienists of the finding
   C. Criticize the health professional who created the problem
   D. Inform the dentist of the finding
   E. Fix the problem and do not report it to anyone

48 As a result of attending the seminars, the dental hygienist discovers a new and excellent periodontal maintenance record that she would like to use at the dental office. Which of the following would be the best way to incorporate the new chart?
   A. Order it at the seminar, with the invoice billed to the office, and start using it upon its arrival
   B. Order it at the seminar, pay for it herself then request office reimbursement, and start using it upon its arrival
   C. Order it at the seminar, pay for it herself without reimbursement, and start using it upon its arrival
   D. Take a sample back to the office, present it to the dentist, and gain approval of the dentist, then have the office place an order for the forms
   E. Take a sample back to the office, present it to the dentist, and if the dentist does not approve, pay for the forms herself

49 Taking classes to learn new clinical skills and office procedures will help the experienced dental hygienist to avoid which of the following?
   A. Career advancement
   B. Education equity
   C. Burnout
   D. Professional accountability
   E. All of the above

50 After a period of time in the new job, the dental hygienist decides to resign. She should do each of the following *EXCEPT* one. Which of the following is the *EXCEPTION*?
   A. Tell other employees of your decision first, to get their opinions about the possible reaction of the employer
   B. Notify the employer as soon as possible
   C. Clearly state the grounds for resigning
   D. Clarify the severance arrangements
   E. Depart with dignity on appointed date

Answers and Rationales

1. (D) Bookkeeping is not in the realm of the dental hygienist.
   - (A) Team building participation is essential for all personnel for the synergistic process.
   - (B) Marketing knowledge by the dental hygienist helps the practice grow.
   - (C) Resumé writing is necessary for application for new jobs.
   - (E) Job performance evaluation is to be completed by both employer and employee.

2. (E) The patient is the purpose of the work and the reason for the existence of the dental practice.
   - (A) Dentist is a team member.
   - (B) Dental hygienist is a team member.
   - (C) Receptionist is a team member.
   - (D) Office manager is a team member.

3. (C) Flexibility should exist to accommodate individual needs and change.
   - (A) An informal and supportive atmosphere contributes to an effective work team.
   - (B) Talking about the job contributes to an effective work team.
   - (D) Understanding job assignment and descriptions is essential to an effective work team.
   - (E) Expressing feelings and being heard enhance a work team.

4. (A) Both statements are *true*.

5. (C) Client can build on existing knowledge when new material is related.
   - (A) Focusing on emotions does not present new material.
   - (B) Offering many options usually confuses the learner.
   - (D) Educational presentation should address visual, auditory, and kinesthetic.
   - (E) Educational presentation should address visual, auditory, and kinesthetic.

6. (C) Case presentation is the process of presenting data to the client along with options for care so as to reach agreement on the care plan.
   - (A) Diagnosis is naming the disease.
   - (B) Treatment plan is organizing the appointments needed for care.
   - (D) Risk management is controlling situations leading to law suits.
   - (E) Informed consent is a risk reduction technique of client education.

7. (B) Practice administration is defined as organization and management of a professional practice for the benefit of both patients and staff members.
   - (A) Team building is the synergistic process of developing group goals.
   - (C) Client management is one element of practice administration.
   - (D) Strategic marketing is planning for practice growth.
   - (E) Patient reclamation is getting clients to return to the office for care.

8. (C) The definition of noncompliance (nonadherence) is lack of client cooperation with recommended oral health. Noncompliance needs to be documented in order to demonstrate the quality of care being recommended as well as client contribution to impaired health (contributory negligence).

9. (E) Criticizing the work of others may lead to a lawsuit, rather than preventing one, when the care rendered may have been the best possible under the circumstances.
   - (A) Providing current standard of care prevents lawsuits.
   - (B) Following proper protocols prevents lawsuits.
   - (C) Informed consent lowers the risk of lawsuits.
   - (D) The dental hygienist is a client advocate by interpreting the need to be seen by the dentist in a timely manner.

10. (B) Each state's dental practice act regulates dental hygiene practice.
    - (A) There is no national dental regulatory agency.
    - (C) The American Dental Association is not a regulatory agency.
    - (D) The American Dental Hygienists' Association is not a regulatory agency.
    - (E) Each dental office policy manual describes individual office policies.

11. (C) Long-term permanent disability insurance should be purchased in the event of severe or permanent disability. It is not covered by employers.
    - (A) Federal Old Age Survivor's Disability is Social Security and is deducted from the payroll by the employer.
    - (B) Worker compensation protects employees from medical expenses and is financed by employers.
    - (D) Unemployment insurance provides benefits for involuntary unemployment and is deducted from the payroll by employer.
    - (E) Individual retirement is not an insurance coverage but a savings account earmarked for retirement exclusively.

12. (D) Collection is the responsibility of the business manager and should not be an element in the determination of paying another employee.
    - (A) Hourly pay is common for part-time workers.
    - (B) Daily salary is common for part-time workers.
    - (C) Commission based on production is common for dental hygienists' wage determination.
    - (E) Salary plus bonus is a common incentive system of pay.

13. (B) The employer and employee must plan the job together and agree upon minimum performance expectations, *then* the performance evaluation is completed by both the employer and employee for discussion.

14. (E) Each of the elements listed should be part of professional business planning.

15. (D) Employees must accept responsibility for their own retirement. Many employers do not have a retirement plan for themselves or employees.
    (A) The first step in financial planning is evaluation of present situation.
    (B) Setting goals is the second step, beginning with long-term goals.
    (C) Short-term goals establish the steps to achieving long-term goals.
    (E) Gradual, continuous investments over the years will help to achieve the long-term financial goals.
16. (D) Taxes are mandatory and take 20% to over 50% of our earnings, especially when federal and state taxes are combined.
    (A) Retirement accounts, either withheld by employers or voluntary contributions, take less than taxes.
    (B) Medical insurance premiums are less than taxes.
    (C) Disability insurance premiums are less than taxes.
    (E) Liability insurance premiums are less than taxes.
17. (D) A will is a written legal arrangement for assets distribution.
    (A) A Keogh plan is a type of retirement plan.
    (B) An IRA is a type of retirement plan.
    (C) Termination arrangement is a made-up term.
    (E) An executor is the person who administers the will.
18. (A) Estate planning and participation in a retirement plan go hand in hand and should both be included in the dental hygienist's business plan.
19. (C) Interpersonal needs relate to social acceptance.
    (A) Physiologic needs relate to survival.
    (B) Psychologic needs relate to mental security.
    (D) Intrapersonal needs relate to self-actualization.
20. (A) Diagnosis is legally performed by the dentist only.
    (B) Attitude towards patients sets the stage for successful management.
    (C) Clear communications with patients enhance patient management.
    (D) Case presentations by dental hygienists guide management by telling of findings and approaches to care.
    (E) Patient correspondence by the dental hygienist may assist in follow-up and reinforcement.
21. (D) Maintain confidentialities; sharing confidentialities is nonprofessional and could lead to malpractice.
    (A) Using individual names establishes personal communications.
    (B) Courtesy to all enhances comfort in communications.
    (C) Respect for privacy enhances trust in communications.
    (E) Creating an atmosphere of acceptance enhances communications.
22. (B) Use lay terminology; technical terminology can be confusing.
    (A) Begin new information with current knowledge as a base.
    (C) Trying new techniques allows the dental hygienist to assess understanding and skills.
    (D) Clients' attitude will affect their interest in learning new material.
    (E) Positive reinforcement of old information motivates clients to learn new material.

23. (E) Satisfied clients will return to the practice and refer future clients.
    (A) A contribution to the community may not build the practice.
    (B) Audiovisual equipment may contribute slightly to practice growth.
    (C) Published articles may bring in a few new clients.
    (D) A contribution to the community may not build the practice.
24. (A) A resume introduces the candidate and outlines professional qualifications and assets.
    (B) An employment contract describes the terms of employment and can only be written after agreement is reached between the employer and employee.
    (C) Performance evaluation measures work progress and would be designed as a review following a probationary period.
    (D) Letter of intent is the same as an employment contract, which would be designed after agreement is reached between the employer and employee.
    (E) Salary and fringe benefits are negotiable between the employer and employee and should not be predetermined by the candidate.
25. (E) Performance evaluation measures work progress and would be provided as a review following a probationary period.
    (A) Dental Practice Act regulates dental hygiene practice and is a written document provided by each state.
    (B) OSHA, Occupational Safety and Health Standards Boards provide written guidelines outlining minimum federal requirements for employee safety.
    (C) When a dental practice offers a retirement plan to employees, the employer is required to provide a written overview describing the plan rules.
    (D) A job description would include duties of the dental hygienist.
26. (D) The candidate can best appraise the interviewer and employment situation by preparing her own questions and asking them during the interview.
    (A) A mission statement of practice philosophy states a goal only, and does not describe how the work is actually done.
    (B) A job description addresses only one aspect of the employment situation.
    (C) Allowing the interviewer to ask all of the questions eliminates a balanced interview where there is reciprocal sharing to evaluate for congruent job objectives.
    (E) Former employees can provide some information but may be biased against the office.

27. (E) A combination interview includes both direct and open questions and allows for information exchange between both parties.
   (A) A directed conversational interview is highly structured with little chance for questioning by the candidate.
   (B) A directed written interview is highly structured with a checklist of questions and allows for no questions by the candidate.
   (C) Group interviews include several candidates and little opportunity for expression of individual concerns by candidates.
   (D) Open conversational interviews are loosely structured and although they allow for interaction between the parties, the information given by the employer may be too general.

28. (D) Practicing out loud with sample questions and answers is the best way to arrive at the interview rehearsed to act and sound informed and professional.
   (A) Instructors can be helpful to offer a few ideas.
   (B) Employed dental hygienists can be helpful to offer a few ideas.
   (C) A written list of questions is a first step in preparation for an interview.
   (E) Arriving without a plan of specific interview goals limits the potential information and outcome the candidate will receive.

29. (A) Community service provides contacts with the client population market.
   (B) Future possible activities may not come into fruition.
   (C) Academic standing does not indicate participation in a marketing effort.
   (D) Clinical performance does not indicate participation in a marketing effort.
   (E) Positive comments from former instructors may not relate to marketing skills.

30. (A) Begin planning and saving for retirement immediately to build the largest equity possible during the working years.
   (B) Waiting any length of time to begin saving for retirement is too late.
   (C) Saving for retirement should be done with each and every job.
   (D) Beginning at age 30 is too late.
   (E) Beginning at age 40 is too late.

31. (C) Build new skills based on those learned in school. Each office will have a style of its own in which the new graduate employee can enhance school skills.
   (A) Intelligent, responsible behavior demonstrates professionalism.
   (B) Asking questions will guide a professional approach and help to avoid mistakes.
   (D) Having a clear understanding of performance expectations guides a professional approach.
   (E) Developing a consistent communications style is an element of professional behavior.

32. (A) Assertive behavior communicates honestly with others.
   (B) Passive behavior continuously submits to the wants and needs of others.
   (C) Submissive behavior allows one to be controlled by others.
   (D) Aggressive behavior attacks others.
   (E) Domineering behavior tries to control others.

33. (B) A mutual evaluation by both the employer and the employee creates a basis for discussion upon which to determine if employment will continue. Further, it will define any changes requested by either party.
   (A) Job satisfaction does not usually occur during the short probationary period. Rather this is a time of careful consideration and evaluation of the job.
   (C) Qualification for a retirement program does not usually occur until after the probationary period is completed.
   (D) Unless a salary increase was promised to be awarded upon completion of the probationary period, an automatic increase in wage should not be expected. It behooves the employee to discuss this at the time of hire.
   (E) There is no guaranteed permanent job. A cause for dismissal could surprise a complacent employee.

34. (E) A thorough clinical assessment of each client will familiarize the dental hygienist with each case and offer the best care.
   (A) Personal questions do not initiate a professional atmosphere or provide useful clinical information.
   (B) Sharing information about hobbies and interests is not professional and does not provide useful clinical information.
   (C) Sharing academic success takes the focus away from the client.
   (D) Announcing that this is a first job does not instill clients' confidence in the dental hygienist.

35. (D) Being consistent, rather than changing constantly, will enhance professional reliability.
   (A) Responsible behavior indicates professionalism.
   (B) Good time management indicates professionalism.
   (C) Outlining professional standards indicates professional goals.
   (E) Respectful behavior builds professional loyalty.

36. (E) A planned meeting with the employer and employee to share, compare, and describe performance provides time for each to reasonably consider and discuss the dental hygienist's performance.
   (A) Asking after each client when time is limited does not allow for appropriate consideration.
   (B) Asking the client is inappropriate.
   (C) Asking the dentist at lunch may catch the employer off guard and does not allow appropriate consideration.
   (D) The hygienist should not involve the receptionist in performance evaluation.

37. (A) Constantly "giving" drains energy and can cause burnout.
    (B) Keeping relations with clients professional, rather than personal, protects from burnout.
    (C) Keeping relations with staff members professional, rather than personal, protects from burnout.
    (D) Variation, rather than monotonous job tasks, prevents burnout.
    (E) Appreciation raises self-esteem and prevents burnout.
38. (C) Reviewing career goals will set objectives that will guide the new job selection.
    (A) A salary increase may or may not occur, depending on each individual office she interviews.
    (B) A gain in fringe benefits may or may not occur, depending on each individual office she interviews.
    (D) Clinical enhancement should be complete before the job search begins.
    (E) Scientific knowledge should be up to date before the job search begins.
39. (C) Personal interests and hobbies do not contribute to the professional balance on resume.
    (A) Career experience is essential on a resumé.
    (B) Continuing education courses demonstrate an interest in professional growth.
    (D) Community service activities may be professionally related and can contribute to practice marketing.
    (E) Activities in professional organizations reflect an interest in one's career balance and growth.
40. (E) It is not legal for dental hygienists to supervise dentists.
    (A) Teaching dental hygiene is a viable alternative.
    (B) Consulting in dental offices is a viable alternative.
    (C) Sales of oral health products is a viable alternative.
    (D) An insurance dental claims examiner is a viable alternative.
41. (B) Professional colleagues are the best source of published and unpublished job opportunities.
    (A) Many jobs are never advertised in the newspaper.
    (C) Many jobs are not advertised in the component newsletter.
    (D) The *ADHA Journal of Dental Hygiene* classified ads have only a few jobs listed.
    (E) Friends and relatives are unlikely to have knowledge of jobs available in the field of dental hygiene.
42. (D) The experienced dental hygienist will likely have her own contributions to the procedures or administration of dental hygiene care which she will want to incorporate into the practice. Only if the dentist is open to change will she be able to add her ideas to the practice.
    (A) Starting salary can be negotiated or changed soon after employment is begun.
    (B) Fringe benefits can be negotiated or changed soon after employment is begun.
    (C) Record forms are important, but can be changed if they prove to be inadequate to the hygienist.
    (E) Instruments are important, but can be changed if they prove to be inadequate to the hygienist.

43. (C) At the end of one month, the experienced hygienist and the dentist can make a good assessment of one another and how the employee fits into the practice.
    (A) Never eliminate a performance evaluation, both parties can learn from it.
    (B) There is much to learn about any new job and the first day job can be filled with surprises and adjustments, therefore it is generally not good to make a snap judgment about either the employee or the employer.
    (D) Six months is too long to wait for a discussion between the employee and employer.
    (E) One year is too long to wait for a discussion between the employee and employer.
44. (C) The dental hygienist and dentist should work together to encourage and evaluate professional growth by the dental hygienist.
    (A) Keeping secrets will not benefit the professional growth of the dental hygienist.
    (B) The clients may not perceive any change.
    (D) The dentist's acknowledgment of the benefits of the new skills must precede any expectation of salary increase.
    (E) The receptionist should not be involved in discussions of clinical skills of employees.
45. (A) Professional interdependence indicates each respects the other's level of competence.
    (B) Professional independence indicates they do not rely on one another for professional exchange.
    (C) Professional counterdependence indicates they are at odds with one another.
    (D) Conflicts between the two should be resolved, not avoided.
    (E) Conflict accountability is a made-up term.
46. (C) Records are to be kept confidential, and if they contain sensitive information, are not to be shared with the entire staff.
    (A) Completeness is essential.
    (B) Accuracy is essential.
    (D) Clients have a right to their records.
    (E) Each staff member who provides a service to the client must sign and initial, including the dental assistant who may take radiographs or study models.
47. (D) The supervising dentist has the ultimate responsibility for the problem and must be informed.
    (A) Ignoring the problem may contribute to making it worse.
    (B) Telling other coworkers does not inform the responsible party, the dentist.
    (C) Professionals should try to avoid criticism of others.
    (E) Fixing the problem may be helpful, but only with the prior knowledge and agreement of the supervising dentist.

48. (D) This change would represent an example of collaborative decision making between the dental hygienist and the dentist. Periodontal maintenance records are an important element of complete dental records and the dentist, being the professional ultimately responsible for the office documentation and liability, must approve of all forms.

(A, B) The dentist should approve of office forms prior to ordering.

(C) The dentist should approve of office forms prior to ordering and the office should pay for all expenses related to client care.

(E) If the dentist does not approve, the form should not be implemented.

49. (C) Burnout can be reduced by learning new things.

(A) New classes may enhance career advancement.

(B) New classes will build education base or equity.

(D) Professional accountability may be enhanced by new classes.

(E) Burnout (C) is the only one to be avoided.

50. (A) Do not tell coworkers before notifying the employer.

(B) Adequate advance notice allows time to find a replacement employee.

(C) Stating grounds for resigning can be helpful to the office.

(D) Stating severance arrangements protects both the employee and the employer.

(E) Continuous professional behavior until departure is best.

Medical Emergencies

Lynn Utecht

Dental hygienists must prepare to manage any medical emergency that might occur in the oral healthcare environment. Careful observation and questioning during client assessment enables the dental hygienist to identify, prepare, and care for the person who experiences a medical complication. A working knowledge of the principles of first aid, cardiopulmonary resuscitation, and basic life support is essential. Equally important is the ability to measure and record vital signs, recognize signs and symptoms of medical disorders, and prevent further complications through appropriate intervention.

This chapter reviews the basic principles of measuring vital signs and preventing and managing medical emergencies. Periodic review of this knowledge and practice of these skills are necessary to maintain competence in this critical area. A valuable resource is the reference list included at the end of the chapter, which can provide access to pertinent detailed information.

General Considerations

A. Medical emergency
   1. A person who experiences an unforeseen medical

Revision based in part on material by Dr. Marcia K. Brand and Dr. Peggy Reep.

difficulty or difficulties is considered a medical emergency
   2. Medical complications require prompt recognition and action by the dentist and/or dental hygienist to maintain the client's health
B. Dental hygienist's legal responsibility
   1. To provide quality care according to the standards of practice established; standards may include training in medical emergency management and cardiopulmonary resuscitation
   2. Dental hygienist may be held liable if inadequately prepared for a medical emergency within the dental environment according to the standards of care established
   3. To maintain complete records of the medical emergency in the healthcare setting
      a. Complete records describe the onset and management of the emergency, the client's vital signs, type of and response to treatment performed, type and dose of drugs administered; and time treatment is rendered
      b. Complete records serve to document the incident and to protect the oral healthcare team in the event of a legal complication
C. Preventing medical emergencies
   1. Thorough health history reveals conditions that

predispose a client to medical complications; health history is taken at the first appointment and updated at each subsequent appointment

2. Information obtained from the health history is used to modify the client's care plan and reduce the likelihood that the client will experience a medical complication in the oral healthcare setting

3. If more information regarding the client's medical status is needed, the dentist or dental hygienist should consult the physician of record

4. Taking and recording the client's vital signs (generally, blood pressure, body temperature, pulse, respiration rate) provide the dental hygienist with information regarding the client's health status

5. The probability of a stress-induced medical emergency in the oral healthcare environment may be reduced by careful appointment planning, stress management, good client rapport, and/or premedication

D. Preparing for medical emergencies

1. Every healthcare setting should maintain an emergency kit that is accessible to all treatment areas. The dental staff should be familiar with the kit's contents and locale. The kit should include current emergency medications, a positive-pressure oxygen delivery system, a clear face mask, a self-inflating resuscitation bag (Ambu bag), oral airway tubes, a blood pressure measurement device, and other essential items

2. Each member of the dental staff should be currently certified in basic life support and the recognition and management of common medical emergencies

3. Certain states may require dental hygienists to have successfully completed and to be current in basic life support (BLS) for license eligibility

4. Each oral health team member should have delegated responsibilities in event of a medical emergency; periodic staff drills are necessary

Vital Signs

Basic Concepts

A. Vital signs are the numerical values given to blood pressure, body temperature, pulse rate, respiration rate, and body height and weight

B. Vital signs and health history are used to determine a client's ability to undergo oral healthcare

C. Abnormal values and significant findings should be brought to the attention of the dentist, client, and client's physician

D. Vital sign values (blood pressure, body temperature,

pulse rate, respiration rate) should be recorded on the client's chart at each dental visit

E. Dental hygienist should explain the purpose of and method for measuring vital signs to the client before initiating these procedures

Blood Pressure

A. Definition—force exerted by the blood on the walls of the blood vessels during the contraction and relaxation of the heart

1. Systolic pressure—force exerted during ventricular contraction (heartbeat); the highest pressure in the cardiac cycle

2. Diastolic pressure—resting pressure; occurs during ventricular relaxation (heart rest) and is the lowest pressure of the cardiac cycle

3. Pulse pressure—value obtained when the diastolic pressure is subtracted from the systolic pressure

4. Hypertension—sustained, abnormally high blood pressure

5. Hypotension—sustained, abnormally low blood pressure

B. Factors that affect blood pressure values

1. Blood pressure is dependent on the heart's contraction force, peripheral vascular resistance, and vascular volume

2. Blood pressure may increase with age, in response to exercise, stress, or certain medications

C. Normal values for adults and children

1. Client's blood pressure should be measured at each dental visit and recorded on the chart

2. Blood pressure is recorded as millimeters of mercury, with the systolic pressure over the diastolic pressure

$$\frac{\text{Systolic (mm Hg)}}{\text{Diastolic (mm Hg)}}$$

3. Normal systolic values for adults range from 100 to 140 mm Hg

4. Normal diastolic values for adults range from 60 to 90 mm Hg

5. Value of 140 to 160 mm Hg (systolic) over greater than 90 to 95 mm Hg (diastolic) should be rechecked for accuracy

6. A systolic reading greater than 160 and/or diastolic greater than 95 requires medical consultation

7. Normal blood pressure values for children range from about 65 to 140/40 to 70 mm Hg

D. Measuring blood pressure

1. Equipment

a. Sphygmomanometer is used to measure blood pressure; this device consists of an inflatable cuff

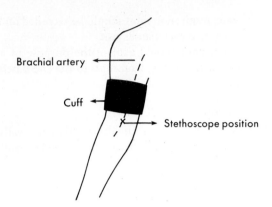

Fig. 17-1 Stethoscope position for blood pressure measurements.

(available in different sizes), a central bulb, and a pressure gauge
b. Width of the cuff should be 20% greater than the diameter of the upper arm (a cuff that is too small will result in an artificially elevated blood pressure)
c. Stethoscope is used to listen to the sounds of the blood as it passes through the brachial artery (Fig. 17-1)
2. Technique—palpatory-auscultatory method
a. Client is seated upright with an arm (palm up) at chest level
b. Cuff is placed snugly around the upper arm so that it is 1 inch above the antecubital fossa; bladder is over the brachial artery
c. Radial artery is palpated, and cuff is inflated until the radial pulse disappears; cuff is then inflated an additional 30 mm Hg
d. Cuff is deflated at a rate of 2 to 3 mm Hg/sec until the radial pulse returns; this value is the palpatory systolic pressure
e. Diaphragm of the stethoscope is placed over the brachial artery; stethoscope earpieces are directed forward
f. Cuff is inflated again to a level 30 mm Hg above the palpatory systolic pressure
g. Cuff is deflated at a rate of 2 to 3 mm Hg/sec
h. Korotkoff sounds (vibrations of an artery under pressure) are heard through the stethoscope; sound intensity decreases as the cuff pressure decreases
i. First sound heard through the stethoscope is the systolic blood pressure
j. Last sound heard is the diastolic blood pressure
k. Blood pressure is recorded as a fraction, systolic/diastolic; measurement should be recorded as measured on the right or left arm

Body Temperature

A. Basic concepts
1. Body temperature should be measured orally in the oral health care setting
2. Body temperature of greater than 99.5° F orally is considered elevated and may suggest the presence of infection or disease
3. Person with an elevated temperature should see the dentist or physician for further evaluation
B. Factors that affect body temperature
1. Body temperature elevation may be caused by exercise, ingesting hot food or drink, or a pathologic condition
2. Body temperature may be decreased due to starvation or shock
3. Body temperature may have diurnal variation
C. Normal values
1. Normal oral temperature for an adult is between 96.0 and 99.5° F (35.5 to 37.5° C). Rectal temperature is approximately 0.5 to 0.7° F (0.27 to 0.38° C) higher than oral. Axillary temperature is 1.0° F less than oral
2. Value greater than 101° F may indicate an active disease process; values greater than 99.5° indicate a fever
D. Measuring body temperature
1. Several different types of thermometers exist; most common are the oral, rectal, and external thermometers; mercury, electronic, and chemical thermometers are available
2. Oral thermometers are contraindicated for small children and unconscious or unstable persons
E. Technique for measuring body temperature with a mercury-column thermometer
1. Thermometer should be shaken until the mercury level is below the mark indicating 96° F
2. If the client has been eating, smoking, or drinking, the temperature should not be measured for 15 minutes
3. Thermometer bulb is placed under the client's tongue for 3 minutes
4. Temperature measurements are given at 0.2 (two tenths) of a degree; record the highest temperature reading
F. Conversion equations
1. $°C = (°F - 32) \times 5/9$
2. $F = (°C \times 9/5) + 32$

Pulse

A. Basic concepts
1. Pulse is the force of the blood through an artery created by the heart's contraction; each contraction creates a wave of blood that can be felt by gently

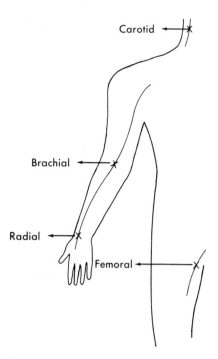

Fig. 17-2 Location of pulse points.

pressing a superficial artery against underlying tissue

2. Pulse is evaluated by rate (fast, slow), rhythm (regular, irregular), and quality (full, thready)
3. Pulse rate is measured as the number of heartbeats per minute

B. Factors that affect the pulse rate
1. Pulse rate may increase because of exercise, certain drugs, anxiety, heat, eating, or disease
2. Pulse rate may decrease because of sleep, certain drugs, fasting, or disease

C. Normal resting heart rate range
1. Adult—60 to 100 beats/minute
2. Infant—100 to 160 beats/minute
3. Child—80 to 120 beats/minute

D. Determining the pulse rate
1. Sites (Fig. 17-2)
   a. Brachial pulse—located on the medial aspect of the antecubital fossa of the elbow
   b. Radial pulse—located on the lateral aspect of the wrist (thumb side) on the ventral surface
   c. Carotid pulse—located in the neck groove, just anterior to the sternocleidomastoid muscle
   d. Femoral pulse—located on the medial aspect of the upper thigh
2. In nonemergency situations the brachial or radial pulse is monitored; in emergency situations the carotid pulse, indicating that blood is flowing to the brain, is monitored. Care is required in carotid

palpation as vagal stimulation may occur, resulting in a decrease in blood pressure and/or syncope. Also, it is of import not to simultaneously palpate the carotid arteries as one or both may be partially occluded

E. Technique for palpating the radial pulse
1. First three fingers are used to locate the radial pulse on the thumb side of the wrist
2. Count the number of beats in 1 minute (pulse rate)
3. Record the pulse rate, rhythm, and quality

Respiration Rate

A. Basic concepts
1. Respiration is the body's inspiration and expiration of air
2. Respiration rate is the number of breaths per minute
3. Evaluate the depth, rhythm, rate, quality, breathing sounds, and client position during respiration

B. Factors that affect respiration
1. Respiration rate may be increased as a result of exercise, pain, certain drugs, anxiety, shock, or disease
2. Respiration rate may be decreased as a result of sleep, certain drugs, or disease

C. Normal respiration rate range
1. Adult—12 to 20 respirations/minute
2. Child—approximately 20 respirations/minute

D. Evaluating respiration
1. After determining the pulse rate, the dental hygienist continues to hold the client's wrist for 60 seconds and counts the number of times the chest rises and falls
2. Record respiration rate, rhythm, depth (shallow, deep), quality (labored, easy), sounds, and patient position (sitting, lying)

Emergency Cardiac Care

Definition

A. Emergency cardiac care (ECC) includes recognition, prevention, reassurance, and the ability to monitor and treat a victim in need of life support; basic life support; advanced cardiac life support; and the transferring of the stabilized victim to a medical care facility for definitive treatment

B. Basic life support (BLS) maintains an individual's heart and lung functions through prompt recognition, intervention, and/or CPR

C. Advanced cardiac life support (ACLS) is BLS with use of additional equipment, an intravenous access, administration of fluids and/or medications, defibrillation, arrhythmia control, and continued care and communication following resuscitation

D. Cardiopulmonary resuscitation (CPR) is a basic life support technique with the goal to provide oxygen to the brain, heart, and other vital organs until definitive medical treatment can be given; CPR requires assessment and basic skills in the areas of airway, breathing, and circulation

E. Emergency medical system (EMS) is a coordinated community system that uses communication, transportation, prevention, education, trained personnel, emergency medical facilities, and other elements in providing emergency medical care

F. "Successful completion" of an American Heart Association (AHA) or other approved course in CPR, BLS, and/or ACLS may be required for dental hygiene licensure in some states

G. Advances in scientific knowledge and clinical research result in frequent changes in ECC technique and protocol; therefore, current literature should be consulted for state-of-the-art information

Basic Concepts

A. ABCs of CPR
  A Airway—assess and establish a clear air passage
  B Breathing—assess and provide respiration through rescue breathing
  C Circulation—assess and provide cardiac support by external cardiac compressions

B. Respiratory arrest is a sudden cessation of breathing

C. Cardiac arrest is a sudden unexpected cessation of the heart and circulation

D. Clinical death is the cessation of the heart and breathing; it may be reversible through life support measures, especially if initiated within 4 to 6 minutes, or it may progress to biologic death

E. Biologic death is permanent cellular damage, particularly of the oxygen-sensitive brain cells, resulting from an inadequate supply of oxygen

Performing CPR

Single-Rescuer CPR

Basic steps for CPR follow. Periodic review and retraining are necessary to remain current. The dental hygienist should consult recent sources for up-to-date protocol.

A. Determining consciousness
  1. Determine the individual's level of consciousness by gently shaking the shoulder and shouting, "Are you OK?"
  2. Activate EMS if the individual does not respond
  3. Carefully turn the victim to a supine position without twisting by rolling the body as an unit; caution is needed if one suspects a back or neck injury

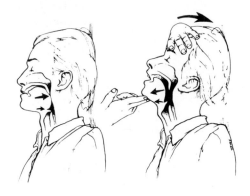

Fig. 17-3 Opening airway with head-tilt/chin-lift technique. (From American Heart Association: *Textbook of advanced cardiac life support,* 1995, The Association.)

B. Opening the airway
  1. The basic technique for opening the airway is head-tilt with anterior displacement of the mandible (chin-lift and, if necessary, jaw-thrust). In the trauma victim with suspected neck injury, the initial step for opening the airway is the chin-lift or jaw-thrust without head-tilt. If the airway remains obstructed, then head-tilt is added slowly and gently until the airway is open* (Fig. 17-3)
  2. Airway technique
    a. Head-tilt is performed by placing one hand (palm) on the forehead of the victim and pressing backward to gently tilt the head back
    b. Chin-lift is achieved by placing the fingers of one hand under the victim's mandible near the chin and raising the chin gently forward. Care is required to not press into the soft tissue and to not use the thumb to lift the chin
    c. Jaw-thrust is used for extra forward displacement of the mandible. It may be the safest method for opening the airway in a victim with a suspected neck injury. To perform the jaw-thrust, use both hands (one on each side), gently grasp the angles of the mandible, and carefully lift to move the jaw forward. The rescuer may need to provide support for the victim's head and avoid head movement

C. Determining breathlessness
  1. Kneel next to victim's shoulders; place your ear next to the mouth and nose to listen and feel for air

---

*From American Heart Association: *Textbook of advanced cardiac life support,* 1995, The Association.

exchange; watch for the chest to rise and fall. Assessment should take 3 to 5 seconds

2. If victim is breathing, monitor vital signs until help arrives
3. If victim is not breathing, immediately begin rescue breathing

D. Performing rescue breathing for an adult
   1. Rescuer position is at victim's shoulders
   2. Open airway or maintain open airway by using the head-tilt/chin-lift (or if neck injury victim, use the jaw-thrust)
   3. Rescue breathing techniques—because disease transmission is a concern, mouth-to-mouth resuscitation should be replaced when possible by ventilation devices such as mouthpieces or resuscitation bags; however, the value of ventilation devices rather than mouth-to-mouth resuscitation in prevention of disease transmission is unknown
      a. Mouth to mask—a transparent mask with mouthpiece and one-way valve may be used for assisted ventilation; technique includes placing the mask around the victim's mouth and nose, placing heel and thumb of each hand on borders of mask to firmly seal margins, grasping the mandible with the index, middle, and ring finger with gentle pressure upward, and ventilating through the mouthpiece
      b. Mouth to mouth uses the rescuer's exhaled air to inflate the victim's lungs. An airtight seal is created by pinching the victim's nostrils closed (use the thumb and index finger of the hand involved in the head-tilt) and by placing your mouth around the victim's mouth after taking a deep breath
      c. Mouth to nose may be needed if it is impossible to ventilate through the victim's mouth. The victim's mouth should be closed. After a deep breath, the rescuer places his or her mouth around the victim's nose and exhales. The rescuer must remove his or her mouth from the nose after each exhalation to allow for the victim to exhale. Periodic opening of the lips may be needed if nasal blockage occurs
      d. Mouth-to-stoma technique is used in a laryngectomy victim with a stoma (opening at the base of the neck connecting to the trachea). Assess for breathing at the stoma site. The rescuer places his or her mouth over the stoma after a breath, exhales, and removes his or her mouth to allow for victim exhalation after each breath
   4. Give two full breaths into the victim's mouth (if mouth to nose or mouth to stoma, use nose or stoma, respectively); check pulse
   5. Watch for chest to rise; allow 1 to 1.5 seconds/breath to provide for chest expansion and to decrease the possibility of gastric distension
   6. Take a breath after each ventilation; assess for adequacy by watching chest rise and fall and by hearing and feeling for air at expiration; adequate volume for an adult is 800 to 1200 ml
   7. If ventilations are unsuccessful, reassess and reposition victim's head; repeat attempt to ventilate
   8. Rescue breathing is performed at 10 to 12 breaths/minute
   9. Monitor vital signs until help arrives

E. Performing rescue breathing for a child—make these modifications
   1. Seal the child's mouthpiece/mouth (and nose) with your mouth, inflate the lungs with less force and volume than with an adult, and give 2 breaths (1 to 1.5 sec/inflation) with a pause between

F. Performing cardiac compressions
   1. Take 5 to 10 seconds to check for carotid pulse
   2. If no pulse, immediately begin cardiac compressions
   3. To perform external cardiac compressions, locate the notch where sternum and ribs meet; place the heel of one hand on the lower ½ of the sternum just superior to the notch
   4. Place the heel of one hand on top of the other hand; fingers may be extended or interlaced
   5. Use both hands to alternately depress the sternum 1½ to 2 inches, then fully release the pressure on the sternum
   6. Compression rate is 80 to 100/minute with a count of "one and, two and, three and, . . . fourteen and, fifteen (administer two breaths), one and . . ."
   7. Continue cycle for a compression:ventilation ratio of 15:2
   8. Administer two breaths after every 15th compression
   9. Check the pulse after 4 cycles and every few minutes thereafter. If there is a pulse, continue rescue breathing. If there is no pulse, continue CPR
   10. To perform cardiac compressions on a child, depress the lower ½ of the sternum about 1 to 1½ inches with the heel of one hand; the compression:ventilation ratio is 5:1 with a rate of 100 compressions/minute
   11. To perform cardiac compressions on an infant, use two or three fingers to depress the midsternum ½ to 1 inch; the compression:ventilation ratio for infant CPR is 5:1 with a rate of 100 to 120 compressions/minute

Two-Rescuer CPR

Two-rescuer CPR uses one rescuer to perform ventilations and one rescuer to perform compressions.

A. Rescuers kneel on opposite sides of the patient: one at the victim's head to perform ventilations, the other at the victim's chest to perform compressions
B. Rescuer performing compressions administers five compressions. On the fifth upstroke, the rescuer providing rescue breathing inflates the victim's lungs. After every fifth compression, a pause in compressions of 1.5 to 2 seconds is allowed for ventilation
C. Count for two-rescuer CPR is "one and, two and, three and, four and, five (breathe), one and, . . ." Compression:ventilation ratio is 5:1 and the compression rate is 80 to 100/minute
D. Rescuers may switch positions, but the CPR cycle should not be interrupted for more than 5 seconds. Pulse should be checked every few minutes and at a rescuer switch
E. The rescuer performing ventilations should monitor the effectiveness of the CPR by assessing the pulse and air exchange

Cricoid Pressure

Cricoid pressure is a technique involving application of backward pressure on the cricoid cartilage to prevent gastric distension and regurgitation during CPR. It should be employed only by healthcare providers trained in the maneuver and during specific circumstances

Basic Life Support in Late Pregnancy

A. Oxygen intake progressively increases during pregnancy (averages 20% to 30% higher) to satisfy the fetus, uterus, and the increased demands on the respiratory and circulatory systems. The functional residual capacity of the lungs is decreased secondary to the upward displacement of the diaphragm. The oxygen reserve is further compromised when the pregnant woman is supine. Also, while supine, the enlarged uterus may compress the abdominal aorta and inferior vena cava, resulting in hypotension and reduced cardiac output by as much as 25%
B. To help alleviate the effects on circulation when a gravid patient is supine (as in CPR), the uterus should be directed toward the left side by placing a folded towel or wedge under the right hip
C. Aspiration is also a concern because of delayed gastric emptying, because the enlarged uterus may compress the stomach, and because of possible decreased tone of the lower part of the esophagus
D. For foreign-body airway obstruction during the last trimester of pregnancy, chest thrusts are recommended rather than abdominal thrusts

Duration of Basic Life Support

BLS should continue until there is effective spontaneous ventilation and circulation; resuscitation efforts have been transferred to another capable of BLS and a physician or emergency medical system arrives and assumes responsibility or the victim is transferred to trained personnel accepting responsibility for emergency medical services; or the rescuer is exhausted and cannot continue

Management of an Obstructed Airway

A. Basic concepts
  1. Obstructed airway occurs when an object prevents an individual from the exchange of air
  2. Foreign-body obstruction may occur when eating, when unconscious (tongue may block pharynx), during resuscitation (aspiration of vomitus or blood), or during other numerous events
B. Recognizing an obstructed airway in a conscious person
  1. In partial airway obstruction with good air exchange the victim can cough forcefully; encourage spontaneous coughing and deep breathing
  2. In partial airway obstruction with poor air exchange the victim has a weak cough, may be cyanotic, makes high pitched noises, and may clutch at the neck; manage as a complete obstruction
  3. Complete airway obstruction is an obstruction in which the victim cannot speak, breathe, or cough and may clutch at the neck
C. Treating an obstructed airway in a conscious person
  1. Determine if the victim has a complete airway obstruction by asking victim to speak; if person can speak, do not interfere with attempts to dislodge the object but remain with person until it is dislodged and/or summon help
  2. Subdiaphragmatic abdominal thrusts (the Heimlich maneuver) are recommended for foreign-body airway obstruction
  3. In a conscious victim who is standing or sitting, the rescuer is positioned behind the victim, wraps an arm around the victim's waist, places the thumb side of the fist between the victim's xiphoid and navel, supports the fist with the other hand, and presses the fist into the victim's abdomen with a brisk upward motion. Each motion should be distinct and repeated until the foreign body is removed or the victim loses consciousness
  4. In an obese or pregnant victim, the rescuer is positioned behind the victim with arms wrapped around the victim's chest. The thumb side of the fist is centered on the midsternum (avoid the xiphoid

and ribs), the other hand is used to support the fist, and backward motions are administered until the foreign body is expelled or the victim loses consciousness

D. Treating an obstructed airway in an unconscious person
   1. Determine unconsciousness, summon help, carefully turn victim on the back by rolling as a unit (caution if suspect neck or back injury), open the airway with head-tilt/chin-lift method (jaw-thrust if neck injury victim), establish breathlessness, and attempt ventilation
   2. If ventilation is unsuccessful, reposition the head, reattempt ventilation, and activate EMS
   3. If ventilation still unsuccessful, kneel astride the victim and perform 6 to 10 abdominal thrusts by placing the heel of one hand just above the victim's navel and well below the xiphoid (the other hand is placed over the first hand) and pressing into the abdomen with distinct upward thrusts
   4. In an obese or pregnant victim, kneel next to the victim and use the hand position for CPR and perform chest thrusts to expel the object
   5. A finger sweep may be performed by opening the victim's mouth with a tongue–jaw lift technique and sweeping the mouth with a finger; the finger sweep is used only on an unconscious victim with a visualized foreign body in the mouth
   6. Open airway with head-tilt/chin-lift maneuver and attempt ventilation. If unsuccessful, repeat sequence of abdominal thrust, finger sweeps, and ventilation attempts
   7. If obstruction is removed, ventilate the lungs twice and continue BLS as indicated
   8. In an infant with a foreign-body obstruction, a combination of back blows and chest thrusts is recommended by the AHA
   9. Do not perform blind finger sweeps in children and infants

Administration of Oxygen

A. Basic concepts
   1. Purpose
      a. Oxygen is essential for most chemical reactions in the body, whereas carbon dioxide is the major waste product of these reactions
      b. Circulatory and respiratory systems transport these gases
      c. During a medical emergency the body's increased need for oxygen or diminished ability to obtain or use oxygen may require administra-

tion of higher concentrations of oxygen than exist in regular air
      d. System for delivering this oxygen to a patient is essential in the management of emergency situations
   2. Indications for oxygen administration include syncope, cardiac problems, and respiratory difficulties (with the exception of hyperventilation)
B. Equipment—portable oxygen unit consists of an oxygen tank (an E cylinder is recommended), tubing, a self-inflating resuscitation bag (Ambu bag), and a clear mask that covers the face and nose
C. Technique for administering oxygen to an unconscious person
   1. Place the person in a supine position and open the airway
   2. Start the oxygen flow from the cylinder, and adjust the rate so that the flow inflates the positive-pressure bag
   3. Secure the mask over the person's face to cover the nose and mouth
   4. Compress the positive-pressure bag once every 3 to 5 seconds to inflate the person's lungs
   5. Observe for chest movement and exhalation
   6. If the person is breathing but breaths appear to be weak or shallow, time the administration of ventilations to support the person's respirations
D. Technique for administering oxygen to a conscious person
   1. Place the person in a supine position, or encourage the person to assume a comfortable position
   2. Disconnect the positive-pressure apparatus (Ambu bag)
   3. Start the oxygen flow from the cylinder, and adjust the rate so that the reservoir bag fills at a rate of approximately 7 to 12 L/minute
   4. Place the clear mask over the person's face to cover the nose and mouth
   5. Allow the person to breathe at his or her own rate
   6. Do not permit the reservoir bag to deflate; monitor the person's breathing and vital signs

Unconsciousness

A. Unconsciousness is inability to respond to stimuli, make purposeful movements, or gain awareness of events taking place
B. Levels of unconsciousness range from syncope (transient, simple fainting) to coma (prolonged, deep unconsciousness)
C. Etiology
   1. Unconsciousness may result from a diminished blood supply to the brain (inadequate cerebral

circulation), altered quality of blood flow to the brain (metabolic disorder), central nervous system disorder, or an emotional disturbance
2. A common cause of unconsciousness in the dental setting is psychogenic factors (fear, anxiety); treatment for this type is aimed at increasing the amount of oxygenated blood received by the brain

D. Preventing loss of consciousness
1. To decrease the probability of a client becoming unconscious, the dental hygienist should perform a thorough health history, evaluate vital signs, and determine the dental stress level for every client
2. Stress reduction, premedication, and/or increased pain control may be of value in treating the anxious client

E. Managing unconsciousness
1. If a person becomes unconscious, the dental hygienist should initiate BLS and summon help. If the client is in the dental chair, the chair back may be lowered to facilitate cerebral blood flow
2. Procedures for emergency management should be initiated immediately, according to the preestablished plan

Managing Other Medical Emergencies

Syncope

A. Syncope is a sudden, transient loss of consciousness
B. Etiology
1. Syncope is caused by decreased cerebral function resulting from impaired circulation or altered metabolism
2. Syncope may result from psychogenic (anxiety, fear) or nonpsychogenic (hypoglycemia, position change, heat) factors

C. Preventing syncope
1. The dental hygienist should obtain a thorough health history to determine prior syncopal episodes, dental stress level, and other pertinent information from each client
2. Anxiety reduction measures may include good client rapport, a low-stress environment, and/or premedication
3. Clients who "feel faint" may be aided by reclining the dental chair to the Trendelenburg position (head lower than legs)

D. Signs and symptoms—three stages of syncope: presyncope, syncope, and postsyncope
1. In presyncope, the person may be subjectively weak and nauseated, with a feeling of malaise; objectively, the dental hygienist may observe pallor and sweating; the attack may be aborted if client reclines

2. The syncope stage is subjectively characterized by flaccid muscles and impaired consciousness; objectively, the victim is pale, the pulse is weak, the breathing is shallow, and the duration is less than 5 minutes
3. In postsyncope, the victim awakes and the blood pressure and pulse rate return to normal; the victim should remain supine and rest for a time sufficient to prevent another episode

E. Managing syncope
1. A person who appears "faint" should be placed in a supine position, and dental or dental hygiene treatment should be discontinued
2. Syncope protocol
   a. Assess and open airway
   b. Determine client's breathing status; if breathing, monitor vital signs and follow BLS as needed; if not breathing, initiate BLS immediately and activate EMS
   c. Keep the client warm
   d. Administer oxygen if possible
   e. Administer a respiratory stimulant, such as an ammonia capsule, if available; gently pass the crushed capsule under the client's nose
   f. Person who has experienced syncope will generally return to consciousness within 5 minutes; when the person regains consciousness, reassure the person that he or she will be fine, and keep the person in the supine position; it is advisable to discontinue dental treatment and make arrangements for the client to be escorted home
   g. If it is likely that the client became unconscious from causes other than simple fainting, medical follow-up may be necessary

Shock

A. Shock may result from diminished blood volume
B. Etiology and pathophysiology—there are five commonly accepted categories, or causes, of shock
1. Hypovolemic shock—caused by inadequate blood volume
2. Anaphylactic shock—caused by an acute allergic reaction
3. Septic shock—caused by an infectious agent
4. Cardiogenic shock—caused by heart failure
5. Neurogenic shock—caused by psychologic or neurologic disorder

C. Signs and symptoms
1. Patient may complain of thirst or restlessness
2. Blood pressure may drop, pulse rate may increase, and skin may be pale and clammy; patient may, in severe cases, go into a coma

Asthma

A. Asthma attacks may be prevented by identifying the client at risk through a thorough health history and reducing stress during dental hygiene care
B. Signs and symptoms of asthma include the onset of an unproductive cough, dyspnea (shortness of breath), anxiety, wheezes, and cyanosis
C. Treatment for an asthma attack
   1. Encourage the person to assume a position that facilitates breathing
   2. Allow the person to administer own prescribed medications (bronchodilators) if available
   3. Administer oxygen
   4. Seek the assistance of the dentist or physician if indicated

Hyperventilation

Hyperventilation is characterized by rapid breathing and is often brought about by pain, anxiety, or drugs; rapid breathing causes an excessive elimination of carbon dioxide, which results in respiratory alkalosis

A. Signs and symptoms of hyperventilation include the patient's subjective report of tingling, giddiness, light-headedness, dizziness, and heart palpitations; dental hygienist may observe rapid respirations and a rapid pulse
B. To assist the hyperventilating person, the dental hygienist should reassure the person that he or she will be all right, loosen tight clothing, and encourage the person to breathe slowly and deeply
C. It may be helpful to have the client breathe into a small paper bag to decrease the oxygen intake; do not administer oxygen

Cardiac Emergencies

See Chapter 14, sections on congenital heart disease, rheumatic fever and heart disease, cardiac dysrhythmias, hypertensive disease, ischemic heart disease, and congestive heart failure.

A. Cardiac emergencies have many causes and require immediate definitive medical treatment; sudden unexpected cessation of cardiac activity is called a cardiac arrest; unless CPR or other ECC is promptly performed and maintains the heart's function, biologic death may result (review section on ECC and other current literature); a cardiac emergency may be caused by accidents (electric shock, drowning, trauma, asphyxiation) or coronary disease, which is the review focus
B. Etiology and pathophysiology—coronary disease and emergencies may result from a change in the heart's function (arrhythmia, hypertrophy, ischemia), blood vessels (atherosclerosis, arteriosclerosis), blood volume (shock, hemorrhage), and/or blood composition (anemia)
C. Prevent cardiac emergencies in the dental setting by identifying persons at risk through a thorough health history, present signs and symptoms, and by prompt referral to a physician; if coronary symptoms develop in the office, then rapid entry into an EMS is indicated
D. Cardiovascular diseases
   1. Hypertension is persistent elevation of blood pressure, which indicates the heart is working harder to supply blood through the arteries; the probability of a stroke, myocardial infarction, congestive heart failure, and/or kidney disease may be increased as a result of a consistently elevated blood pressure
      a. Etiology and pathophysiology
         (1) Primary hypertension comprises approximately 90% of the cases and is of unknown etiology; risk factors include heredity, race, gender, age, diet (high sodium), obesity, stress, nicotine, and lack of exercise
         (2) Secondary hypertension comprises 10% of the high blood pressure cases and has a specific etiology such as kidney disease
      b. Signs and symptoms
         (1) May include headaches, dizziness, or no symptoms
         (2) Consistent, elevated blood pressure readings
      c. Treatment
         (1) The hypertensive person needs referral to a physician; primary hypertension is controlled by reduction of risk factors, medications, and continued medical care; secondary hypertension is controlled by identifying and treating the underlying disease
   2. Angina pectoris
      a. Angina pectoris is a transient (temporary) ischemia (lack of oxygenated blood) of the myocardium (heart muscle) usually manifested by chest pain or discomfort
      b. Signs and symptoms
         (1) Chest pain or discomfort may be described as pressing, crushing, burning, or squeezing; radiate to the shoulders, arms, neck, mandible, or epigastrium; lasting 2 to 15 minutes; be precipitated by exertion; and be accompanied by weakness and shortness of breath
         (2) Dental hygienist may observe labored breathing or sweating of the client
      c. Treatment

(1) Discontinue dental hygiene care and alert dentist and staff

(2) Allow the person to rest; if the person uses nitroglycerin and the prescription is available, he or she may take one nitroglycerin (refer to current literature for protocol)

(3) Administer oxygen

(4) Monitor the client's vital signs

(5) If the pain is relieved by rest and/or nitroglycerin, encourage rest, discontinue the oral health services for that appointment, and recommend further evaluation by a physician

(6) If the pain is not relieved by rest and/or nitroglycerin and the person is uncomfortable for 2 minutes or more, activate the EMS immediately

3. Myocardial infarction

a. Myocardial infarction is a diminished or interrupted supply of oxygenated blood to the heart that causes death (necrosis) of part of the heart muscle, resulting in impaired heart function and diminished cardiac output; if a large area of the heart is affected, the heart may be unable to function and may stop beating

b. Signs and symptoms

(1) A common presentation of a myocardial infarction is chest pain or discomfort that may radiate to the arm, neck, or mandible, lasting for more than 15 to 20 minutes, and is not relieved by nitroglycerin or rest; a myocardial infarction may have various presentations and may include sweating, nausea, shortness of breath, and weakness

(2) The dental hygienist should be aware that in a myocardial infarction, the person may not look "sick" and the pain does not have to be severe

c. Treatment

(1) Discontinue dental hygiene care, alert dentist, and immediately activate the EMS

(2) The person should be in a comfortable position and able to rest

(3) Monitor the person's vital signs, administer oxygen and BLS as needed, and continue support until definitive treatment is available

(4) Person with known cardiac disease who uses nitroglycerin may take one nitroglycerin; pain should be relieved within 3 minutes; if not, suspect impending cardiac arrest (nitroglycerin lowers blood pressure; therefore caution should be used)

4. Congestive heart failure (CHF)

a. Congestive heart failure results when the heart is unable to meet the body's demands; precipitating factors include hypertension, coronary artery disease, congenital and valvular heart disease, toxins, inflammatory disorders, and endocrinopathies

b. Signs and symptoms

(1) The person may complain of weakness, shortness of breath, cough, and swelling

(2) The dental hygienist may note edema, cyanosis, tachycardia, and prominent jugular veins

c. Treatment

(1) A person with congestive heart failure needs continued medical care; the physician of record should be consulted before dental or dental hygiene care

(2) In the dental setting, the person with CHF may feel more comfortable with the dental chair back upright

(3) If the person with CHF has a medical emergency in the dental setting, discontinue dental treatment, allow for a comfortable client position, administer oxygen and BLS as needed, monitor vital signs, alert dentist, and activate the EMS

5. Sudden cardiac death

a. Sudden death is the unexpected cessation of the heart and lungs

b. Etiologies may include coronary artery disease, respiratory arrest, shock, drugs, arrhythmias, accidents, or anaphylaxis

c. Signs and symptoms include unconsciousness; absence of a pulse, blood pressure, and respirations; and/or convulsions

d. Treatment is immediate ECC including BLS, prompt activation of EMS and ACLS, and definitive medical treatment

Allergic Reactions

A. Allergic reactions describe a wide range of the body's physiologic responses caused by hypersensitivity to an allergen

B. Etiology and pathophysiology

1. Allergic responses may be evoked by drugs, pollens, foods, chemicals, insect bites, and other factors

2. When the body contacts these substances, an antigen-antibody reaction causes an inappropriate response of the body's immune system

C. Preventing allergic reactions

1. Thorough health history should reveal a previous

history of allergic reactions to drugs or materials used in dental therapeutics

2. Question the client who has a prior history of an allergic reaction to describe its type and severity

3. Refer the client with a suspected allergy to a physician for evaluation

D. Types

  1. Delayed allergic reactions

    a. Signs and symptoms include skin manifestations (such as erythema, urticaria, angioedema) or respiratory reactions (respiratory distress, wheezing, dyspnea, angioedema)

    b. Treatment

      (1) Delayed reactions may be mild and necessitate no treatment

      (2) If the allergic reaction is severe, the dentist may administer medications (antihistamine, epinephrine) and/or oxygen as needed per client

      (3) If the reaction persists, the client should be accompanied to a physician

  2. Immediate reaction or anaphylaxis

    a. Immediate allergic reactions are characterized by urticaria, nausea, angioedema, and respiratory distress; reaction may progress to cardiovascular collapse; client may have a very rapid, weak pulse, heart palpitations, and may become cyanotic

    b. Treatment

      (1) Anaphylaxis is a life-threatening emergency; immediately activate the EMS and provide BLS until definitive medical treatment is available

      (2) Place the person in a supine position

      (3) Administer oxygen

      (4) Monitor vital signs

      (5) Dentist or physician may administer epinephrine

      (6) Continue BLS as needed

Drug-Related Emergencies and Poisoning

Basic Concepts

A. Drug-related emergencies include allergic response, overdose, psychogenic response (syncope or hyperventilation), idiosyncratic reaction, and/or complications in a person who is chemically dependent

B. Thorough health history should reveal the client's drug allergies, previous adverse reactions, or chemical dependency; these agents and materials and drugs containing these materials must be avoided during dental and dental hygiene care

C. Dental hygienist should be prepared to manage reactions to administration of a local anesthetic or fluoride

Specific Reactions

A. Local anesthesia reactions may be the result of psychogenic or allergic response, toxic overdose, or chemical intoxication

  1. Psychogenic response is usually manifested as syncope or hyperventilation; generally the result of fear of the injection rather than the local anesthesia; these reactions (syncope and hyperventilation) should be managed according to the criteria described in related sections of this chapter

  2. Allergic reactions occur more often with ester-type anesthetics (procaine), are relatively rare, and should be managed by the criteria established under the section on allergic reactions in this chapter

  3. Toxic overdoses of local anesthetic agents may occur as a result of delayed biotransformation or elimination of the agent, excess total dose, or intravascular injection of the agent

    a. Patient who has a toxic overdose may be anxious and confused; may have a rapid pulse and respirations, followed by shock, respiratory arrest, and cardiovascular collapse

    b. Toxic overdose is managed by discontinuing the injection, monitoring vital signs, administering oxygen, activating EMS, and providing BLS as needed

  4. Chemically dependent client

    a. Prevention by identifying the chemically dependent person and adjusting treatment accordingly

    b. If a local anesthetic with epinephrine is injected into the vascular system of a cocaine-intoxicated person, cardiovascular compromise may result necessitating entering the person into the EMS and implementing BCLS as necessary

B. Fluoride poisoning by ingestion may be acute (caused by a single large administration of an agent) or chronic (caused by long-term ingestion)

  1. Acute toxic reactions to fluoride are rare, although fatal fluoride poisoning may be caused by accidental ingestion of large quantities of fluorides, such as those contained in insecticides with sodium fluoride; ingestion of 15 to 30 mg of fluoride per kilogram of body weight may cause death in adults

  2. Some oral healthcare products contain enough fluoride to be hazardous, especially to children; one ounce of topical fluoride gel or one 8-ounce tube of fluoridated tooth paste could be life threatening to a small child

3. Signs of acute fluoride toxicity include nausea, abdominal pain, excessive salivation, vomiting, and diarrhea; in severe cases muscle cramping, bronchospasm, and cardiac arrest may occur
4. Treatment of acute fluoride poisoning
    a. Induce vomiting with ipecac syrup
    b. Monitor vital signs, initiate BLS as needed, and enter the client into a medical care facility for definitive treatment

Bleeding and Hemorrhage

A. Client may have a bleeding problem in the oral healthcare setting because of a dental procedure, accident, or spontaneous bleeding (such as a nosebleed)
B. Persons taking certain types of medications (heparin, coumadin) may be more susceptible to bleeding problems; such persons may be identified by a thorough health history
C. Modifications in the client's medication regimen may be necessary to reduce the likelihood that the person will have a bleeding problem as the result of oral healthcare; physician of record must be consulted before any modifications are suggested
D. Bleeding may be arterial or venous; arterial bleeding is usually more red in color and "spurts" with the contraction of the heart; venous bleeding is darker in color and "oozes"
E. Treatment of hemorrhage usually can be managed by direct pressure on the bleeding area; use sterile gauze to apply pressure
    1. If bleeding is from a dental extraction or surgical site, pack the area with gauze and have the person close until bleeding stops
    2. For nosebleed, apply cold compresses to the nose and apply pressure to the bleeding side; it may also help reduce bleeding if the nostril is gently packed with gauze
    3. If bleeding is severe, watch for signs of shock and activate the EMS

Cerebrovascular Accident (Stroke)

A. Pathophysiology and etiology
    1. Cerebrovascular accident (CVA), or stroke, results when the supply of oxygen to the brain cells is disrupted by ischemia, infarction, or hemorrhage of the cerebral blood vessels
    2. Contributing factors to a CVA include tobacco use, hypertension, diabetes mellitus, and coronary disease
B. Prevention
    1. To decrease the probability of a CVA, regular medical examinations, control of high blood pressure

and diabetes, elimination of tobacco use, and reduction in risk factors are advised
    2. The dental hygienist should perform a thorough health history and evaluate vital signs to help identify persons at risk for a CVA
C. Signs and symptoms
    1. Signals suggestive of a stroke include sudden weakness of one side (hemiparesis), difficulty of speech, temporary loss of vision (especially in one eye), unexplained dizziness, alteration in consciousness, shortness of breath, nausea, severe headache, and/or convulsions
    2. CVA victim may have an elevated blood pressure and cardiac arrhythmias (irregular heartbeats)
D. Treatment
    1. Conscious person
        a. If signs and symptoms of a CVA persist for 30 seconds, discontinue oral healthcare, alert dentist, and activate the EMS
        b. Assist the person in assuming a comfortable position
        c. Monitor the person's vital signs and administer oxygen and BLS as needed
        d. Continue support and monitoring until medical assistance arrives
    2. Unconscious person
        a. Alert the staff and activate the EMS
        b. Monitor vital signs, administer oxygen, initiate BLS as indicated, and continue support until medical assistance arrives

Seizures and Convulsive Disorders

See Chapter 14, section on seizure disorders.
A. Seizures and convulsive disorders are the result of changes in brain function
    1. Seizures are characterized by alterations in consciousness, motor function, and sensory perceptions; usually have a rapid onset and brief duration
    2. Convulsions are involuntary contractions of the voluntary muscles
    3. Epilepsy is a condition characterized by recurrent seizures and convulsions
B. Etiology and pathophysiology
    1. Seizures and convulsions result from a disturbance of the brain's electrical activity
    2. Seizures may be the result of tumors, congenital abnormalities, injuries, drugs, and idiopathic causes
C. Preventing seizures
    1. Thorough health history should identify an individual with a history of seizures or convulsive disorders

2. If a client has a previous history of seizures, determine if medications have been prescribed to control the seizures and if the client has taken the required medication before that appointment
3. Short appointments, scheduled early in the day, may reduce the likelihood that a susceptible person will have a seizure in the oral healthcare setting
4. There is a relative contraindication to the use of nitrous oxide in persons with seizure disorders

D. Types of seizures
   1. Convulsive—generalized tonic-clonic (grand mal) seizure
      a. Signs and symptoms include an aura (change in taste, smell, or sight precedes the seizure), loss of consciousness (a few minutes to hours), an epileptic cry (sudden expulsion of air through glottis), involuntary tonic-clonic muscle contractions, altered breathing, and/or involuntary defecation or urination; after the seizure, the respirations should spontaneously return, the muscles relax, and consciousness returns; victim may have a headache, muscle aches, and be drowsy
   2. Nonconvulsive—absence (petit mal) seizure
      a. Signs and symptoms include a sudden momentary loss of awareness without loss of postural tone, a blank stare, and a duration of several to 90 seconds. Although the individual may twitch, they are usually unaware of the seizure
   3. Complex partial (psychomotor) seizure
      a. Signs and symptoms may include an aura, purposeless movements, loss of awareness, and a duration of a few minutes

E. Treatment
   1. Convulsive seizure in the oral healthcare setting
      a. Lower dental chair and clear area of all sharp and dangerous objects
      b. Make no attempts to restrain the person or place any objects in the mouth
      c. Protect person's head, if needed, by placing a soft item under the head
      d. Assess and establish an airway
      e. Monitor vital signs and initiate BLS and activate EMS if needed
      f. If breathing does not spontaneously return, evaluate for a foreign body (review section on foreign body), associated myocardial infarction, or neck/back injury
      g. If person has pooled secretions, individual may need to be rolled as a unit to his or her side for drainage of the secretions; care required if back or neck injury is suspected
      h. Allow person to rest
      i. After the seizure, arrange for the person to be assisted in leaving the oral healthcare facility, and arrange for medical evaluation
   2. Nonconvulsive seizure in the oral healthcare setting
      a. Closely observe person and clear area of all sharp objects
      b. Monitor vital signs and initiate BLS as needed
      c. Furnish supportive treatment; person may need further evaluation

Diabetes Mellitus

See Chapter 14, section on diabetes mellitus.
A. Diabetes is characterized by elevated levels of blood glucose resulting from an impaired ability to produce or use the hormone insulin
B. Persons with diabetes mellitus will exhibit a number of clinical manifestations of the disease and have an increased susceptibility to infection and diseases of the blood vessels
C. Etiology and pathophysiology
   1. Insulin is normally produced by β-cells of the pancreas
   2. Cells of the body need insulin to take in glucose, and the liver uses insulin to store glucose as glycogen
   3. If glucose and glycogen are unavailable to the body as energy sources, the body must break down other materials for "fuel"
   4. Emergencies related to diabetes may occur as the result of two different situations
      a. Person has too much insulin, resulting in hypoglycemia (low blood sugar)
      b. Person has inadequate insulin, resulting in hyperglycemia (high blood sugar)
D. Types
   1. Type I, or insulin-dependent, diabetes mellitus usually occurs in the young and is more likely to precipitate a diabetic emergency
   2. Type II, or non–insulin-dependent, diabetes mellitus usually occurs in adulthood and rarely results in an emergency situation
E. Preventing diabetic emergencies
   1. Thorough health history is essential to prevent diabetic emergencies in the oral healthcare setting; factors to be determined during the health history include the type and severity of diabetes, medications, and their frequency, duration, and dosage; medical consultation may be necessary
   2. Person whose diabetes is not under control should postpone dental and dental hygiene care except for emergency procedures
   3. Dental hygienist should establish that the client's

medications have been taken according to prescriptions and that the person has eaten meals according to schedule on the day of the appointment

4. Efforts should be made to minimize the client's stress and anxiety

5. Appointments should be scheduled to ensure that the client is rested and that the client's meal and medication schedule is not interrupted; morning appointments are best, 1 to 1.5 hours after breakfast

F. Diabetic emergency—insulin reaction (hypoglycemia or hyperinsulinism)

1. Insulin reaction occurs when there is too much insulin available, with the result that the person's blood glucose is abnormally low (<50 mg/dl); this reaction may occur when the person increases medication, omits a meal, or engages in excessive exercise

2. Signs and symptoms of insulin reaction may occur suddenly and include hunger, headache, pale moist skin, and feelings of dizziness and weakness; person undergoing an insulin reaction will not be thirsty and will have a normal breath odor

3. Treatment for insulin reaction includes the administration of sugar in the form of orange juice, cola, or sugar water; this will usually bring about a rapid recovery; if the person becomes unconscious, seek assistance through the EMS

G. Diabetic emergency/diabetic coma (hyperglycemia, hypoinsulinism ketoacidosis)

1. Diabetic coma occurs when there is insufficient insulin available, with the result that some cells cannot metabolize blood glucose

2. Signs and symptoms of impending diabetic coma in a conscious person include the "classic" signs of polydipsia (excessive thirst), polyuria (excessive urination), polyphagia (excessive hunger), nausea, dry flushed skin, and a "fruity" breath odor, followed by unconsciousness

3. Treatment for a client having symptoms of diabetic coma include discontinuance of oral healthcare, entry into the EMS, and support through BLS if necessary

4. If the dental hygienist has doubts regarding the etiology of a diabetic-related problem, it is advisable to administer a small amount of sugar; because hyperinsulinism is more common than diabetic coma, the administration of sugar will probably improve the person's condition

Acute Adrenal Insufficiency, or Adrenal Crisis

A. Acute adrenal insufficiency (adrenal crisis) occurs when the adrenal gland produces insufficient amounts of cortisol, a glucocorticosteroid that enables the body to respond to stress

B. Dental and dental hygiene care may induce considerable stress for some persons, causing this serious complication

C. Adrenal crisis is a life-threatening situation, and persons having adrenal insufficiency may go into cardiac arrest or shock

D. Etiology and pathophysiology—adrenal gland is unable to produce enough cortisol to enable the body to respond to a stressful situation

E. Signs and symptoms

1. Person undergoing acute adrenal insufficiency may experience confusion, weakness, and abdominal pain

2. Pulse may be rapid and weak; person may develop hypotension, followed by unconsciousness

F. Treatment

1. Alert the staff and enter the person into the EMS

2. Discontinue dental or dental hygiene care

3. Place the person in a supine position

4. Monitor vital signs

5. Administer oxygen

6. Dentist or physician may administer glucocorticosteroid

7. If the person becomes unconscious, BLS may be necessary until definitive treatment is available

Foreign Body in the Eye

A. Having a foreign body in the eye may happen to the dental hygienist, as well as the client, in the oral healthcare environment

B. Safety glasses with side shields should be worn by both the dental hygienist and the client to prevent injury from the splatter of agents or materials during dental hygiene care

C. Foreign material in the eye will usually cause tearing, pain, and blinking

D. Procedure for removing a solid particle from the eye

1. While the person looks down, pull the upper eyelid down over the lower lid

2. If the particle is not removed, turn the lower eyelid down and examine it for irritants

3. If the solid particle is visible and cannot be removed by tearing, remove it with a moistened cotton-tip applicator

4. After the particle is removed, irrigate the eye with an eye cup or with gently running water

5. If the particle cannot be easily removed, refer the person to a physician for prompt treatment; it may be necessary to cover the eye with sterile gauze and adhesive tape to prevent the patient from further damaging the eye by rubbing

E. Procedure for removing a caustic solution from the eye
   1. A chemical solution splashed in the eyes requires immediate copious irrigation with water and prompt evaluation by an ophthalmologist

Managing Dental Emergencies

Dislocated Jaw

A. Dislocated jaw, or mandible, may occur as the result of trauma or forced movement
B. Person with a dislocated jaw cannot return the mandible to a normal position because the head of the condyle is anterior to the articular eminence
C. Patient with a dislocated mandible may have considerable pain and anxiety
D. To return the mandible to its normal position, the dental hygienist should wrap both thumbs in a cloth or towel to protect them and place the thumbs directly on the occlusal surfaces of the mandibular teeth; fingers should be placed under the person's mandible at the curve; to move the mandible back into place, press down and back with the thumbs and pull up and forward with the fingers; mandible should slip into place

Avulsed Tooth

A. Avulsed tooth is a tooth that is forcibly removed from the mouth by trauma
B. Such a tooth should be handled only by the crown
C. Tooth should be rinsed and gently placed into the socket while the person is transported for emergency care
D. If the tooth cannot be placed into the socket, the person should transport the tooth to the oral healthcare setting for emergency treatment in milk or in the vestibule of the mouth; do not allow it to dry out
E. Less preferred transport medium is water
F. Person should receive immediate emergency treatment in the oral healthcare setting

Aspirated Materials

A. Dental materials and instruments may be aspirated during oral healthcare because of the client's position, diminished responses caused by drugs, and diminished "oral awareness" caused by local anesthesia
B. Prevent aspiration of materials through the use of a rubber dam; persons with conditions that predispose them to coughing (COPD) or who may be poor management cases (such as the developmentally disabled) merit careful attention

C. If a client is reclining in the dental chair and aspirates an object into the oropharyngeal area, lower the back of the chair, using gravity to assist the person's efforts to dislodge the object
D. If an object is aspirated into the trachea, activate EMS and manage as partial or complete obstruction
E. If an object that has been swallowed cannot be located, the person must be escorted to seek further medical evaluation

Broken Dental Hygiene Instruments

A. Instrument breakage can be minimized by careful sharpening and frequent inspection
B. If an instrument breaks, stop the procedure immediately and isolate the area where the tip is believed to be located
C. Inform the client of the situation
D. Dry the area and examine it for the tip; if the tip is believed to be in a sulcus or periodontal pocket, use gentle instrumentation to explore the area; take care to avoid pushing the broken tip further into the sulcus
E. If the tip cannot be located, inform the dentist of the situation and use radiographs and transillumination to locate the broken piece
F. Follow-up by a dentist or physician may be necessary

This chapter is only a rough guideline for some but not all of the medical emergencies one may encounter in the dental office. Please consult current textbooks and journals for detailed information as well as the AHA for the recommended protocol and training in BLS, ACLS, and EMS. The following references may be helpful.

SUGGESTED READING

American Heart Association: *Healthcare provider's manual for basic life support,* Dallas, 1994, The Association.
Bennett JD, Dembo JB: Medical emergencies in the dental office, *Dent Clin North Am* 39(3), 1995.
Berkow R, et al: *The Merck manual,* ed 16, Rahway, NJ, 1992, Merck.
Darby ML, Walsh MM: *Dental hygiene theory and practice,* Philadelphia, 1995, WB Saunders.
DeGowin RL: *DeGowin and DeGowin's diagnostic examination,* ed 6, New York, 1994, McGraw-Hill.
Ewald GA, McKenzie CR: *Manual of medical therapeutics,* ed 28, Boston, 1995, Little, Brown.
Hardman JG, et al: *Goodman and Gilman's pharmacological basis of therapeutics,* ed 9, New York, 1995, McGraw-Hill.
Trope M: Clinical management of the avulsed tooth, *Dent Clin North Am* 39(1):93, 1995.

Review Questions

1 Blood pressure may increase because of each of the following *EXCEPT*
   A. Increased age of client
   B. Rest
   C. Exercise
   D. Certain medications

2 The first step in treating an unresponsive person is
   A. Activate the EMS
   B. Open the airway
   C. Perform rescue breathing
   D. Perform cardiac compressions

3 The appropriate depth of chest compressions for a child is
   A. ½ to 1 inch
   B. 1 to 1½ inches
   C. 1½ to 2 inches
   D. 2 to 2½ inches

4 Unconsciousness may be a result of each of the following *EXCEPT*
   A. Inadequate cerebral circulation
   B. Metabolic disorder altering quality of blood flow to the brain
   C. Psychogenic (fear, anxiety)
   D. Hypoglycemia
   E. All of the above may be responsible for loss of consciousness

5 Anaphylactic shock is caused by
   A. Inadequate blood volume
   B. An acute allergic reaction
   C. Heart failure
   D. A psychogenic or neurologic disorder
   E. All of the above may be a cause of anaphylactic shock

6 In addition to the chest pain associated with a myocardial infarction, the victim may experience
   A. Sweating
   B. Nausea
   C. Shortness of breath
   D. Weakness
   E. All of the above

7 Hyperventilation as a response to administration of local anesthetic may manifest by
   A. Increased respiratory rate and respiratory depression
   B. Increased respiratory rate and syncope
   C. Increased respiratory rate, syncope, and respiratory depression
   D. Slow pulse

8 Congestive heart failure may be a result of each of the following *EXCEPT*
   A. Anaphylaxis
   B. Hypertension
   C. Valvular heart disease
   D. Coronary artery disease

9 Cerebrovascular accident results from
   A. Blood clot blocking the cerebral blood vessel
   B. Hemorrhage from the cerebral blood vessel
   C. Low blood sugar
   D. A and B are correct
   E. A and C are correct

10 Signs of acute fluoride toxicity include all of the following *EXCEPT*
   A. Nausea
   B. Abdominal pain
   C. Decreased salivation
   D. Vomiting and diarrhea
   E. All of the above are true

11 The causes for seizures include
   A. Tumors and congenital abnormalities
   B. Tumors and trauma to the head
   C. Tumors, congenital abnormalities, and trauma to the head
   D. Congenital abnormalities, trauma to the head, and drugs
   E. All of the above

SITUATION: A 25-year-old female with a history of diabetes presents for her periodontal maintenance care appointment with the dental hygienist. She reports taking her usual dose of insulin and having a light breakfast. Since it was such a nice morning she walked 12 blocks to her appointment instead of driving. Initially she appears to be feeling fine, but then begins to complain of a headache and dizziness. Questions 12-16 refer to this situation.

12 This client most likely is experiencing
   A. Hyperglycemia
   B. Hypoglycemia
   C. Hyperventilation
   D. Adrenal insufficiency

13 The appropriate treatment is
   A. Administration of insulin based on the client's body weight
   B. Administration of water
   C. Administration of sugar in the form of orange juice or cola
   D. Administration of oxygen

14 How could this client have prevented this adverse reaction?
   A. Eaten a regular breakfast instead of a light breakfast and taken a small dose of insulin
   B. Eaten a regular breakfast instead of a light breakfast and driven to the appointment instead of walking
   C. Taken a smaller dose of insulin and driven to the appointment instead of walking
   D. Taken a smaller dose of insulin, driven to the appointment instead of walking, and made the appointment later in the day
   E. All of the above

15 Other signs and symptoms that would assist in making the correct assessment of this client's situation includes all of the following *EXCEPT*
   A. Pale, moist skin
   B. Confusion
   C. Feeling of weakness
   D. "Fruity" breath odor

16 The client's symptoms are a result of
- A. Too much insulin available
- B. Blood glucose <50 mg/dl
- C. A combination of A and B

17 An avulsed tooth should be
- A. Handled by the crown only and reimplanted as soon as possible
- B. Handled by the crown only, reimplanted as soon as possible, and wrapped in a dry cloth for transportation to emergency care
- C. Handled by the root only and reimplanted as soon as possible
- D. Handled by the root only, reimplanted as soon as possible, and wrapped in a dry cloth for transportation to emergency care

SITUATION: An elderly client arrives for her 3-month continued care appointment. She is on multiple medications but all vital signs are within normal limits and she is eager to begin care. As you begin treatment, an instrument tip breaks off in her mouth. Questions 18-21 refer to this situation.

18 Aspiration of materials is preventable by
- A. Not working on developmentally disabled persons
- B. Use of a rubber dam
- C. Stopping client's medications prior to procedures
- D. Working on clients in the upright position

19 The initial treatment for a broken instrument tip is
- A. Radiograph of the suspected location
- B. Use gentle instrumentation to explore the suspected location if in the sulcus
- C. Immediate consultation with the dentist
- D. Use high powered suction to dislodge the tip

20 In this case it would be BEST to
- A. Inform the client of the situation
- B. Proceed as if nothing is wrong so the client does not become alarmed
- C. Have the client swish and spit

21 Efforts to minimize instrument breakage include all the following EXCEPT
- A. Frequent inspection of all instruments
- B. Disposal of instruments deemed too thin to withstand the stress of instrumentation
- C. Careful sharpening
- D. Disposal of an instrument after it has been sharpened 5 times

22 The force exerted during a ventricular contraction (heartbeat) is known as
- A. Pulse pressure
- B. Diastolic pressure
- C. Systolic pressure

23 An oral temperature reading may be inaccurate if the client has recently been
- A. Eating
- B. Drinking
- C. Smoking
- D. Any of the above

24 In an emergency situation involving an adult, a pulse rate should be determined by palpating the
- A. Carotid artery
- B. Femoral artery
- C. Brachial artery
- D. Radial artery

25 Biological death is permanent cellular damage and will occur if CPR is not initiated within
- A. 1 to 2 minutes
- B. 2 to 4 minutes
- C. 4 to 6 minutes
- D. 6 to 8 minutes

26 External cardiac compressions on a child are performed by placing the heel of one hand on the
- A. Xiphoid process
- B. Lower half of the sternum
- C. Upper half of the sternum
- D. Any of the above is appropriate

27 Compression:ventilation ratio for one-rescuer CPR on an adult is
- A. 15:2
- B. 15:1
- C. 5:2
- D. 5:1

28 A person with partial airway obstruction but good air exchange should
- A. Lie down on his back
- B. Be treated with the Heimlich maneuver
- C. Be treated with sharp back blows
- D. Be encouraged to cough and breathe deeply

29 Syncope may be avoided by each of the following EXCEPT
- A. Placing the person in Trendelenburg position
- B. Obtaining a good health history
- C. Creating a low-stress environment
- D. Giving each client a glucose-containing snack

30 Hypertension increases the risk of all the following EXCEPT
- A. Diabetes
- B. Stroke
- C. Myocardial infarction
- D. Congestive heart failure
- E. Kidney disease

SITUATION: A 59-year-old man with a history of high blood pressure complains of a little pain in the chest. His blood pressure is 145/95 and pulse rate is 95. Within a few minutes he begins to sweat and have labored breathing and now complains of a squeezing sensation in the chest. The client has his medications with him including hydrochlorothiazide, nitroglycerin, and nifedipine. Questions 31-33 refer to this situation.

31 This man may be experiencing which of the following?
- A. Hyperventilation and angina pectoris
- B. Congestive heart failure and angina pectoris
- C. Congestive heart failure and myocardial infarction
- D. Angina pectoris and myocardial infarction

32 The dental hygienist should do which of the following?
 A. Discontinue dental hygiene care and alert the dentist and staff; have the man breathe into a small paper bag; allow the man to rest; and monitor his vital signs
 B. Discontinue dental hygiene care and alert the dentist and staff; have the man breathe into a small paper bag; and allow the man to rest
 C. Discontinue dental hygiene care and alert the dentist and staff; allow the man to rest
 D. Discontinue dental hygiene care and alert the dentist and staff; allow the man to rest; administer oxygen; monitor his vital signs

33 This man should be encouraged to
 A. Take his nitroglycerin tablets as he was directed to do by his physician
 B. Take nitroglycerin tablets from the dental office emergency kit
 C. Do nothing but rest

34 When treating a person with a history of a seizure disorder, each of the following is appropriate *EXCEPT*
 A. Administer nitrous oxide to reduce anxiety
 B. Schedule short appointments
 C. Schedule appointments early in the day
 D. All the above are appropriate

35 The preferred transport medium for an avulsed tooth is
 A. Tap water
 B. Under the tongue of the patient
 C. Hydrogen peroxide
 D. Milk

SITUATION: A 25-year-old very nervous man comes in for his annual dental hygiene care appointment. He denies taking any medications and he has no significant past medical problems. His vital signs are as follows: BP 140/90, Pulse 105, respiratory rate 24. Questions 36-37 refer to this situation.

36 Possible causes for these abnormal vital signs include each of the following *EXCEPT*
 A. Ingestion of certain prescription medication
 B. Ingestion of certain "street" drugs
 C. Anxiety
 D. Internal disease process
 E. All the above could be responsible for the abnormal vital signs

37 The first thing that should be done for this person is
 A. Activate the EMS
 B. Alert the dentist about the abnormal vital signs
 C. Have the person relax for a minute and retake the vital signs
 D. Administer oxygen

SITUATION: Your last client of the day is a 64-year-old man with multiple medical problems including diabetes, hypertension, obesity, and past history of a myocardial infarction. As he sits down for his vital signs to be taken, he is markedly short of breath and diaphoretic (sweating). He says he has not been feeling well over the past week and it has been a very stressful morning so he didn't have a chance to take his medications. As you begin taking vital signs he loses consciousness. Questions 38-43 refer to this situation.

38 The appropriate sequence for treating this man is
 A. Establish an airway; determine the level of consciousness; take 5 to 10 seconds to check carotid pulse; begin chest compressions
 B. Take 5 to 10 seconds to check carotid pulse; begin chest compressions; determine the level of consciousness; establish airway
 C. Determine the level of consciousness; establish an airway; take 5 to 10 seconds to check carotid pulse; begin chest compressions
 D. Take 5 to 10 seconds to check carotid pulse; establish an airway; determine the level of consciousness; begin chest compressions

39 If rescue breathing is necessary it should be performed
 A. At a rate of 16 to 20 breaths/minute
 B. With adequate volume of 800 to 1200 ml/breath
 C. At a rate of 20 to 24 breaths/minute

40 This person has no palpable carotid pulse. Cardiac compressions should be initiated by placing the heel of the hand on the
 A. Xiphoid process
 B. Lower half of the sternum
 C. Upper half of the sternum

41 For single-rescuer CPR, the compression rate for this person should be
 A. 60 to 80 compressions/minute
 B. 80 to 100 compressions/minute
 C. 100 to 120 compressions/minute
 D. 120 to 140 compressions/minute

42 Two-rescuer CPR is started once another office staff member responds to the emergency call. Rescue breathing is now performed
 A. At a rate of 5:2 compression:ventilation ratio and after the 5 compressions without a pause in compressions
 B. At a rate of 5:1 compression:ventilation ratio and after the 5 compressions without a pause in compressions
 C. At a rate of 5:2 compression:ventilation ratio and after the 5 compressions with a pause in compressions
 D. At a rate of 5:1 compression:ventilation ratio and after the 5 compressions with a pause in compressions

43 Compression rate for this person with two rescuers should be
 A. 40 to 60 compressions/minute
 B. 60 to 80 compressions/minute
 C. 80 to 100 compressions/minute
 D. 100 to 120 compressions/minute

44 Treating an obstructed airway in an unconscious person can be achieved by
 A. Kneeling astride the victim and performing 6 to 10 abdominal thrusts
 B. Kneeling astride the victim and performing 6 to 10 chest compressions
 C. Performing finger sweeps if the victim is a child

45 Toxic overdose of local anesthetic may occur as a result of all *EXCEPT*
  A. Delayed biotransformation of the agent
  B. Increased elimination of the agent
  C. Excessive dose of the agent
  D. Intravascular injection of the agent

SITUATION: A 15-year-old female arrives for her morning dental hygiene care appointment. She has normal vital signs and is feeling fine as the dental hygiene procedures are begun. The young woman complains of a very strange smell and suddenly she loses consciousness and begins having involuntary muscular contractions. Questions 46-50 refer to this situation.

46 The first thing that should be done is
  A. Lower the dental chair and clear the area of all sharp and dangerous objects
  B. Restrain the person to prevent injury
  C. Place a bite block in the mouth
  D. Administer oxygen

47 This woman is most likely experiencing a (an)
  A. Complex partial seizure
  B. Stroke
  C. Anaphylactic reaction
  D. Grand mal seizure
  E. Diabetic emergency

48 Another associated sign or symptom this woman may experience is
  A. Blank stare
  B. Epileptic cry
  C. Polydipsia
  D. Unilateral weakness

49 If breathing does not spontaneously return
  A. Evaluate for foreign body obstruction
  B. Administer oxygen
  C. Administer nitrous oxide
  D. Allow the person to rest

50 Once the woman regains consciousness she may
  A. Have a headache
  B. Have muscle aches
  C. Be drowsy
  D. All of the above

Answers and Rationales

1. (B) Rest may result in a decrease in blood pressure
   (A) Increased age may cause an increase in blood pressure
   (C) Exercise may cause an increase in blood pressure
   (D) Certain medications may cause an increase in blood pressure
2. (A) The first step is to activate the EMS
   (B) Opening the airway is the second step
   (C) If after opening the airway the victim is not breathing, rescue breathing is performed
   (D) Cardiac compressions are performed after breathing is established or if there is no pulse

3. (B) 1 to 1½ inches is the correct depth for a child
   (A) ½ to 1 inch is the correct depth for an infant
   (C) 1½ to 2 inches is the correct depth for an adult
   (D) Not correct for any population
4. (E) All may be the cause of unconsciousness
   (A), (B), (C), and (D) are correct but incomplete answers
5. (B) An acute allergic reaction to drugs, chemicals, insect bites and other factors may result in anaphylactic shock
   (A) Inadequate blood volume may result in hypovolemic shock
   (C) Heart failure may cause cardiogenic shock
   (D) Psychogenic or neurologic disorders may result in neurogenic shock
   (E) Only (B) is correct
6. (E) All the symptoms may be experienced by a person experiencing a myocardial infarction
   (A), (B), (C), and (D) may be symptoms associated with a myocardial infarction
7. (B) Increased respiratory rate causing an excessive elimination of carbon dioxide, which results in respiratory alkalosis may ultimately cause a syncopal episode
   (A) Respiratory depression is not a sign of hyperventilation
   (C) Same as (A)
   (D) Same as (A) and usually heart palpitations and a rapid pulse are experienced during hyperventilation
8. (A) Anaphylaxis is not a cause of congestive heart failure
   (B), (C), and (D) are all possible precipitating factors for congestive heart failure. Other causes of congestive heart failure may include toxins, inflammatory disorders, and endocrinopathies
9. (D) Both (A) and (B) are correct
   (C) Low blood sugar is not a direct cause for cerebrovascular accidents
   (E) Same as (C)
10. (C) Usually increased salivation will be seen with fluoride toxicity
   (A), (B), and (D) are signs of acute fluoride toxicity. In severe cases, muscle cramping, bronchospasm and cardiac arrest may occur
   (E) Not correct because (C) is not true
11. (E) Tumors, congenital abnormalities, trauma to the head, and drugs may all cause seizure disorders
   (A), (B), (C), and (D) are all correct but incomplete answers to the question
12. (B) This client is experiencing hypoglycemia (insulin reaction)
   (A) Based on the facts given hypoglycemia is most likely instead of hyperglycemia
   (C) Although light-headedness and dizziness can be seen with hyperventilation, the most likely cause of this client's symptoms is hypoglycemia and this should be addressed first
   (D) Signs and symptoms of adrenal insufficiency/crisis include confusion, weakness, and abdominal pain
13. (C) Administration of sugar in the form of orange juice or cola
   (A) This client already has too much insulin
   (B) This client needs a glucose-containing fluid
   (D) This client needs glucose, not oxygen

14. (B) The client could have prevented these symptoms by eating a regular breakfast and not engaging in excessive exercise, both of which tend to result in a lowering of the blood glucose

    (A, C) The client should not alter the prescribed insulin dose because of a dental appointment

    (D, E) Same as (A) and morning appointments are best

15. (D) "Fruity" breath odor is associated with hyperglycemia or ketoacidosis

    (A), (B), and (C) are other signs and symptoms associated with hypoglycemia (insulin reaction)

16. (C) Both (A) and (B) are correct. This client's symptoms are a result of too much insulin available which results in abnormally low blood glucose (<50 mg/dl). This occurs when a person takes too much insulin, omits a regular meal, or engages in excessive exercise.

17. (A) An avulsed tooth should be handled by the crown only and reimplanted as soon as possible

    (B) The tooth should not be transported dry; transport tooth in milk or client's mouth with water as a last resort

    (C) The tooth should not be handled by the root

    (D) Same as (B) and (C)

18. (B) Rubber dam prevents aspiration of materials

    (A) Incorrect answer because aspiration can occur in any person

    (C) It is not advisable to stop medications without consultation with the prescribing physician

    (D) Incorrect answer because aspiration can occur in persons sitting upright

19. (B) If you suspect that the tip is in the sulcus it is advisable to gently explore the area

    (A) If the tip is not removed by gentle exploration, a radiograph may be necessary

    (C) The dentist should be notified if the tip is not found on gentle exploration

    (D) High powered suction is not indicated because the dental hygienist must find the tip to ensure that it has not been aspirated into the client's lung

20. (A) The client should be informed

    (B) See (A); it would be unethical to deceive the client

    (C) This may result in swallowing the tip; also the dental hygienist must find the tip to ensure that it has not been aspirated into the client's lung

21. (D) Instruments should not be disposed of after they have been sharpened a set number of times

    (A) Frequent inspection of instruments is essential

    (B) Instruments should be recycled when the tips have thinned and cannot withstand the stress of instrumentation

    (C) Careful sharpening will prolong the life of the instrument

22. (C) Systolic pressure is the force exerted during ventricular contraction; the highest pressure in the cardiac cycle

    (A) Pulse pressure is the value obtained when the diastolic pressure is subtracted from the systolic pressure

    (B) Diastolic pressure is the resting pressure that occurs during ventricular relaxation

23. (D) Eating, drinking or smoking can alter the oral temperature reading

    (A) See (D)

    (B) See (D)

    (C) See (D)

24. (A) Carotid pulse is important to monitor because it gives an indication of the blood flow to the brain

    (B) Difficult to reach this area due to clothing and it is a greater distance from where rescue breathing and cardiac compressions are performed

    (C) Palpation of the brachial artery is recommended for infants under 1 year of age

    (D) Radial artery may be used in nonemergent situations

25. (C) Permanent cellular damage may occur if CPR is not initiated within 4 to 6 minutes

    (A, B, D) Incorrect answers

26. (B) Lower half of the sternum is the appropriate location for compressions

    (A) Cardiac compressions on the xiphoid process may result in internal injuries

    (C) Not an effective way to perform cardiac compressions

    (D) See (B)

27. (A) Compression:ventilation should be 15:2

    (B, C, D) Incorrect

28. (D) Because this person has good air exchange, no treatment is necessary but the victim should be encouraged to cough and breathe deeply

    (A) Lying down may increase the obstruction and decrease air exchange

    (B, C) No treatment should be rendered because the victim has good air exchange

29. (D) Giving glucose to clients (except those very rare persons suffering from true hypoglycemia) will not abort syncope

    (A) Trendelenburg position may be helpful

    (B) A good health history may help avoid added stresses on an individual

    (C) Low-stress environment will help prevent psychogenic syncope

30. (A) Diabetes is not a result of hypertension

    (B) Stroke may result from hypertension

    (C) Hypertension is a risk factor for myocardial infarction

    (D) Hypertension is a precipitating factor in congestive heart failure

    (E) Kidney disease may be increased as a result of consistently elevated blood pressure

31. (D) Symptoms are most consistent with angina pectoris or myocardial infarction

    (A) Hyperventilation may be associated with heart palpitations but not chest pain

    (B) Congestive heart failure patients complain of weakness, shortness of breath, cough, and swelling, but they usually do not have acute chest pain

    (C) See (B)

32. (D) Treatment should be discontinued and office staff should be alerted, the man should be encouraged to rest while oxygen is administered and vital signs are monitored
    (A) Breathing into a paper bag will decrease oxygen intake which is the opposite of the treatment that should be rendered in this case
    (B) See (D) and (A)
    (C) See (D)
33. (A) If the man has nitroglycerin, he should take it as directed by his physician
    (B) If the man has not been prescribed nitroglycerin by his physician, he should not take it
    (C) See (A)
34. (A) There is a relative contraindication for the use of nitrous oxide in a person with a seizure disorder
    (B, C) Correct answers
    (D) See (A)
35. (B) Of the choices given, under the tongue is the best answer
    (A) Avoid tap water
    (C) Avoid hydrogen peroxide
    (D) Milk can be used if necessary, but saliva in the mouth of the patient is preferred
36. (E) All the responses could be the cause for abnormal vital signs
37. (C) These vital signs are not dangerously elevated so it would be most appropriate to retake them once the person has relaxed for a minute or two
    (A) Not appropriate at this time
    (B) The dentist should be alerted if the vital signs are still abnormal after the second reading
    (D) Oxygen is not indicated at this time
38. (C) Sequence of treatment should be: determine level of consciousness, establish an airway and render rescue breathing if necessary, take 5-10 seconds to check for a carotid pulse, and if no pulse is palpated, begin chest compressions
    (A, B, D) See (C)
39. (B) Volume for an adult should be 800 to 1200 ml/breath
    (A, C) Rescue breathing is performed at 10 to 12 breaths/minute
40. (B) Lower half of sternum is the correct location for cardiac compressions
    (A) Compressions on the xiphoid process increases the risk of internal injuries
    (C) Compressions on the upper half of the sternum are ineffective
41. (B) 80 to 100 compressions/minute is the desired rate
    (A, C, D) Incorrect
42. (D) Two-rescuer CPR is performed at a rate of 5:1 compressions:ventilation and the rescue breathing is given after the fifth compression with a 1.5 to 2 second pause in compressions
    (A, B, C) See (D)
43. (C) Compression rate with two-rescuer CPR is 80 to 100 compressions/minute
    (A) Incorrect
    (B) Incorrect
    (D) Incorrect

44. (A) Abdominal thrusts are most effectively given by kneeling astride the victim
    (B) Only if the victim is obese or pregnant should chest thrusts be performed. This is done by kneeling next to the victim and placing the hands in the same position used to perform CPR
    (C) Do not perform blind finger sweep on a child
45. (B) Decreased elimination of the agent may result in a toxic overdose of local anesthetic
    (A, C, D) May result in toxic overdose
46. (A) Correct answer
    (B) Do not attempt to restrain the person
    (C) Do not attempt to place anything in the person's mouth
    (D) Not appropriate treatment in this case
47. (D) Signs and symptoms are most consistent with grand mal seizure
    (A) Complex partial seizure signs and symptoms include an aura, purposeless movement, loss of awareness, and a duration of a few minutes
    (B) It would be rare for a person this age to have a stroke and the symptoms are not consistent with a stroke
    (C, E) Incorrect
48. (B) Grand mal seizure patients may emit an epileptic cry which is the result of a sudden expulsion of air through the glottis
    (A) Blank stare is associated with petit mal seizures
    (C) Polydipsia (excessive thirst) is associated with hyperglycemia and impending diabetic emergency
    (D) Unilateral weakness is a symptom of a stroke
49. (A) If breathing does not return spontaneously in a person experiencing a seizure, evaluate for foreign body obstruction—especially the tongue
    (B) If the person is not breathing the oxygen will be of no value
    (C) There is a relative contraindication to the use of nitrous-oxide in a seizure patient
    (D) Airway must be established
50. (D) After a seizure, the person may be drowsy and complain of headache and muscle aches
    (A), (B), and (C) are correct

CHAPTER

18

Historical, Professional, Ethical, and Legal Issues

Michele Leonardi Darby

Although formal recognition and training of dental hygienists began at the beginning of the twentieth century, dental practitioners were discussing the value of preventive care and the need for preventive specialists more than 50 years before dental hygiene's inception. The contemporary dental hygienist needs to be aware of the evolution of dental hygiene to appreciate the responsibilities of the present and opportunities of the future. Each dental hygienist has an obligation to join the American Dental Hygienists' Association, which strives to promote the oral health of the public and ensure a preferred future for all dental hygienists. A knowledge of the history of the profession and a working understanding of the structure and purpose of the professional association are essential.

As healthcare providers, dental hygienists are confronted with legal and ethical dilemmas; therefore, the study of ethical theory and principles helps the dental hygienist to develop a moral perspective and practice ethical decision making. A brief overview of the legal system and relevant legal issues serves to alert the dental hygienist to the benefits and liabilities of a professional facing the twenty-first century.

This chapter reviews the history of dental hygiene, describes the structure and function of the American Dental Hygienists' Association and its constituent and component organizations, reviews the principles and theories of ethics to set standards and provide a frame of reference for future ethical decision making, and provides a synopsis of the US legal system and its relationship to the health professional. Together, the topics discussed make the dental hygienist aware of the rights, privileges, and responsibilities of the profession.

History of the Dental Hygiene Profession in the United States

Establishment of a New Profession in Dentistry—1844 to 1924[1]

A. Recognition of the importance of preventive measures in oral health
   1. 1844—editorial discussing the value of oral hygiene measures appeared in *The American Journal of Dental Science*
   2. 1865—Henry S. Chase emphasized the importance of diet for good dental health
   3. 1870—Andrew McLain published a paper entitled "Prophylaxis or Prevention of Dental Decay," which discussed the principles of mouth hygiene and diet
   4. 1879—George A. Mills published a paper that

advocated clean mouths in children and described the use of the explorer

5. 1884—Meyer L. Rhein
   a. Urged dentists to teach their patients to use a toothbrush and waxed floss
   b. Designed a toothbrush for this purpose
   c. Recommended the establishment of oral health programs in the public schools
6. 1890—Charles B. Atkinson defined dental prophylaxis
7. 1894—David D. Smith initiated the first recorded preventive practice
8. 1896—x-rays first used in the detection of dental disease
9. 1897—Robert R. Andrews suggested mandatory oral examinations of all schoolchildren
10. 1901—David D. Smith differentiated between home care and professional dental prophylaxis

B. Identification of a new subspecialty in dentistry
1. 1902—Cyrus M. Wright
   a. Proposed a subspecialty in dentistry to carry out the tedious work of dental prophylaxis
   b. Specifically recommended women for this subspecialty
2. 1902—Thaddeus P. Hyatt
   a. Advocated educating the public in oral hygiene techniques
   b. Proposed that the tasks related to oral prophylaxis and patient education become the responsibility of a new dental specialty
3. 1903—Meyer L. Rhein
   a. Advocated the training of women to perform dental prophylaxes
   b. Named this subspecialty "dental nurse"
   c. Suggested licensure for the new subspecialty
4. 1903—F.W. Low proposed a new profession of "odontocure" to be practiced by women in the private homes of clients
5. 1906—Alfred Civilion Fones
   a. Became a recognized instructor in the technique of oral prophylaxis
   b. Taught his assistant, Irene Newman, to perform oral prophylaxes
   c. Became known as the "father" of dental hygiene
6. 1907—Connecticut dental law was amended to
   a. Limit the duties of unlicensed assistants in dental office
   b. Allow the cleaning of teeth by trained assistants under supervision

C. Concern for children's dental health
1. 1887—Alabama Dental Association resolved that preventive dental education should be
   a. Routinely conducted in all public schools
   b. Provided by experienced dental health lecturers
2. 1914—Bridgeport School Dental Health Plan provided a program of dental health education and preventive services in the public schools, based on the premise that
   a. Dental decay was the most prevalent defect found in schoolchildren
   b. Prevention, not restoration, was the way to control dental disease
3. Dental dispensaries founded to take care of the dental needs of children
   a. 1910—Forsyth Dental Infirmary (Boston, Mass.)
   b. 1910—Rochester Dental Clinic (Rochester, N.Y.)
   c. 1929—Guggenheim Foundation Clinic (New York City)

D. Early dental hygiene programs—1910 to 1925
1. 1910—Ohio College of Dental Surgery
   a. Started a 1-year program to train dental nurses
   b. Discontinued it in 1914 because of opposition from local dentists
2. 1913—Dr. A.C. Fones
   a. Started a training program to supply the Bridgeport School Dental Health Plan with trained dental health personnel
   b. Named the new profession "dental hygiene" because he wanted to stress prevention, not illness
3. 1914—Colorado College of Dental Surgery initiated a dental nurse program that became a dental hygiene program in 1920
4. 1916 to 1925—10 new dental hygiene programs were started
   a. 1916—Columbia University took over the dental hygiene program that had been started by Hunter College during that year
   b. 1916—Rochester Dental Dispensary initiated a dental hygiene program
   c. 1916—Forsyth Dental Infirmary started a training program for dental hygienists
   d. 1918—University of California Dental School began a 1-year program for dental hygienists; changed to a 2-year program in 1924
   e. 1920 to 1925—dental hygiene training programs started at the University of Minnesota, University of Michigan, Temple University, University of Pennsylvania, Northwestern University, and Marquette University

E. Dental hygiene licensure, the first 10 years—1915 to 1925

1. 1915—Connecticut dental statute first outlined the scope of practice of dental hygiene
2. 1915—Massachusetts dental law was amended to include the responsibilities of dental hygienists
3. 1916—New York enacted legislation defining dental hygiene practice
4. 1916—American Dental Association recognized and endorsed licensure for dental hygienists
5. 1917—Connecticut Board of Dental Examiners presented the first dental hygiene license to Irene Newman, the first person trained by Dr. Fones and a graduate of his first class
6. 1922—American Dental Association adopted a model dental hygiene practice act to be used by the remaining states
7. 1917 to 1924—legislation to allow the practice of dental hygiene was adopted in an additional 20 states, as well as in Hawaii and the District of Columbia

Establishment of the American Dental Hygienists' Association

A. State associations
   1. 1914—Connecticut Dental Hygienists' Association
      a. Established by a group of graduates from Dr. Fones' program
      b. Irene Newman elected as the first president
   2. 1920—there were four state associations: California, Connecticut, Massachusetts, and New York
B. Organization of a national association
   1. 1922—organizational meeting held at the annual meeting of the American Dental Association
   2. 1923—first annual meeting of the American Dental Hygienists' Association
      a. Held in Cleveland, Ohio
      b. Forty-six dental hygienists representing 11 states attended
      c. Winifred A. Hart elected the first President of the American Dental Hygienists' Association
   3. 1925—second national meeting, at which the Constitution and Bylaws of the American Dental Hygienists' Association were adopted
   4. 1926—first code of ethics specifying the responsibilities of members was drafted
      a. Adopted as the Principles of Ethics in 1931
      b. Principles of Ethics revised in 1953, 1969, 1974, and 1995 (Code of Ethics)
   5. 1927—*The Journal of the American Dental Hygienists' Association*
      a. Recognized as the official publication of the American Dental Hygienists' Association
      b. Published monthly beginning with its January 1927 issue
      c. Changed to quarterly publication in 1934
      d. Title changed to *Dental Hygiene* in 1972, and monthly publication resumed in 1975
      e. Title changed to *Journal of Dental Hygiene* (JDH) in October 1988 with nine issues per year
   6. 1927—American Dental Hygienists' Association was incorporated as a nonprofit organization
   7. 1927—first continuing education course was offered to dental hygienists by the University of Buffalo
   8. 1928—American Dental Hygienists' Association
      a. Accepted its first official seal
      b. Revised the Constitution and Bylaws to meet requirements of incorporation
   9. 1929—American Dental Hygienists' Association Code of Ethics adopted
   10. 1931—sixteen dental hygiene programs were operating in the United States
   11. 1935—membership in the American Dental Hygienists' Association reached approximately 1000 with 19 constituent associations
   12. 1938—establishment of the Junior American Dental Hygienists' Association, later renamed the Student American Dental Hygienists' Association
   13. 1937—American Dental Hygienists' Association established first House of Delegates

Events Influencing the Development of Dental Hygiene—1918 to 1944[1]

A. National attention on public health
   1. 1918—North Carolina established the first dental division of a state department of health
   2. 1921—Children's Bureau established, which provided
      a. Healthcare for mothers and children
      b. Jobs for dental hygienists in state health departments
   3. 1930—White House Conference produced a Children's Charter that promoted preventive programs for children; conference led to
      a. Children's Fund of Michigan dental program
      b. W.K. Kellogg Foundation's support of pedodontic clinics
      c. Children's National Dental Health Week
B. 1932—American Dental Association established the Committee on Dental Hygiene to
   1. Survey the curricula of all existing dental hygiene programs
   2. Determine the number of graduate dental hygienists
   3. Determine the number of practicing dental hygienists

4. Review requirements of state departments of education

5. Review state dental practice acts

C. 1935—Social Security Act enacted
1. Title V provided for
   a. Maternal and child health services
   b. Preventive services as a part of the health plan
2. Title VI provided for
   a. Public health services
   b. Training of health professionals

D. 1937—American Dental Association established the Council on Dental Education to oversee educational programs in dentistry and dental hygiene

E. 1940—American Dental Hygienists' Association recommended a 2-year course of study for dental hygiene

F. 1941 to 1944
1. World War II
   a. American Dental Hygienists' Association annual sessions discontinued during the war years (1942 to 1945)
   b. Dental hygienists served as civil service employees
   c. Requests from the American Dental Hygienists' Association to commission dental hygienists in the armed forces were denied
2. National Dental Hygiene Association established by African-American dental hygienists

Era of Dental Research—1943 to 1953[1]

A. 1943 to 1949—dental research on fluoride
1. Indicated the effectiveness of fluoride in reducing dental caries
2. Established the need for fluoride rinse programs for preschool children and schoolchildren
3. Involved dental hygienists in
   a. Advocating and educating the public regarding water fluoridation
   b. Topical fluoride demonstration projects
   c. Conducting dental screenings
   d. Public health and school fluoride programs

B. 1946 to 1953—dental care delivery research
1. U.S. Public Health Service initiated projects to determine the effectiveness of the expanded use of auxiliaries in the delivery of dental care to schoolchildren
2. Forsyth Dental Clinic
   a. Initiated a 5-year research project to evaluate the feasibility of dental hygienists restoring primary teeth
   b. Terminated the project in its third year because of the opposition of local dentists

C. 1948—National Institute of Dental Research
1. Established by the National Dental Research Act

2. Involved dental hygienists in water fluoridation, topical application of fluoride, and oral cancer research

D. 1949—four states allowed application of topical fluoride by dental hygienists

Growth of the Profession During the 1940s and 1950s[1]

A. 1944—American Dental Hygienists' Association divided into nine districts with a trustee for each district

B. 1947—American Dental Association Council on Dental Education
1. Required all dental hygiene programs to be no less than 2 years in length
2. Surveyed colleges and universities to determine the transferability of dental hygiene courses
3. Proposed a standard curriculum for all programs
4. Conducted a curriculum survey of all dental hygiene programs; additional curriculum surveys conducted in 1951, 1958, and 1964

C. 1948—American Dental Hygienists' Association established the
1. Position of Executive Secretary
2. Central office in Washington, D.C.

D. 1951—Texas became the last state in the continental United States to grant dental hygiene licensure

E. 1951 to 1952—American Dental Association Council on Dental Education
1. Recommended that dental hygienists receive training in expanded services
2. Began accrediting dental hygiene programs

F. 1952—dental hygienists invited to be a part of the American Association of Dental Schools (AADS)

G. 1953 to 1954—Alaska and Puerto Rico granted dental hygiene licensure, making it possible to be licensed in the 48 states plus Alaska, the District of Columbia, Hawaii, and Puerto Rico

H. 1956 to 1958—American Dental Hygienists' Association
1. Established the Educational Trust Fund (ETF)
2. Reaffirmed that membership would not be denied because of race, creed, or color
3. Requested that all constituents comply with the American Dental Hygienists' Association membership policy
4. Moved the central office to Chicago
5. Instituted the Dental Hygiene Aptitude Test
   a. As a measure of predicting academic success in dental hygiene
   b. As an admission criterion, adopted by most dental hygiene programs from 1958 to 1964
6. Supported the establishment of the National Dental Hygiene Board Examination

7. Sigma Phi Alpha ($\Sigma\Phi A$), dental hygiene honorary society, formed in Detroit at American Association of Dental Schools' Annual Session in 1958

National Interest in the Delivery of Healthcare in the 1950s and 1960s

A. 1952—President's Commission on the Health Needs of the Nation
   1. Studied
      a. Availability of healthcare
      b. Personnel in the health professions
   2. Recommended
      a. Delegation of responsibilities to allied health personnel
      b. That dental care be considered part of comprehensive health care
      c. Fluoridation of all public water supplies
      d. Support for research
B. 1953—establishment of the Department of Health, Education, and Welfare (DHEW) indicated the nation's interest in the general welfare; dental hygienists became involved in programs funded by the DHEW
C. 1953 to 1957—dental hygiene labor study conducted by the U.S. Public Health Service revealed
   1. Thirty-four dental hygiene programs in existence
   2. Approximately 15,000 graduate dental hygienists
D. 1963 to 1968—federally supported programs included
   1. Vocational Education Act of 1963, which
      a. Contributed to the growth of dental hygiene programs
      b. Introduced dental hygiene programs in technical schools and community colleges
   2. Health Professions Educational Assistance Amendments of 1965 provided
      a. Funds to educational programs that increased the number of students accepted
      b. Funds for the renovation of training facilities
      c. Start-up funds for new programs in the health professions
      d. Loans and scholarships for health professionals in training
   3. Allied Health Professions Personnel Training Act of 1966 provided
      a. Capitation grants to dental hygiene programs
      b. Funds for improvement or initiation of new programs
   4. National Advisory Commission on Health Manpower of 1967 identified the need for additional allied health professionals
   5. Health Manpower Act of 1968 provided funds for
      a. Basic education of health professionals
      b. Advanced training of health professionals
      c. Special projects

6. National Institute of Health Research Training Grants in Dental Health of 1968 provided grant funds to dental and dental hygiene faculty for research, teaching, and related activities

Expansion of Dental Hygiene in the 1960s and 1970s[1]

A. 1960 to 1965—graduate programs in dental hygiene initiated at Columbia University, the University of Michigan, and the University of Iowa provided advanced training in
   1. Education, research, and administration for dental hygiene educators
   2. Principles of public health for dental hygienists
B. 1961—American Dental Hygienists' Association adopted proportional representation in the House of Delegates
   1. Allowing each constituent to have 1 delegate for up to 100 members
   2. Plus 1 delegate for each additional 100 members
C. 1962—National Board Dental Hygiene Examination
   1. Developed by the Dental Hygiene Committee of the National Board of Dental Examiners of the American Dental Association
   2. Administered by the American Dental Association's Commission on National Dental Examinations
   3. Recognized by 25 states immediately; recognized later by all United States licensing jurisdictions (49 states, District of Columbia, Puerto Rico, and Virgin Islands) *except* Delaware
   4. Open to graduates of all accredited dental hygiene programs; however, those graduating before 1955 had to pass the examination by 1965 to use it as a criterion for licensure
D. 1963—professional liability insurance offered
E. 1964 to 1970—acceptance of men for
   1. Dental hygiene licensure in all states except Alabama, Indiana, Louisiana, Mississippi, Nebraska, Rhode Island, and Utah
   2. Membership in the American Dental Hygienists' Association and its constituents
F. 1965—survey of dental practice indicated
   1. Employed dental hygienists numbered 15,400
   2. Decline in public health positions for dental hygienists
   3. Most dental hygienists were employed in private practices
G. 1965—Dental Hygiene Educators Conference
   1. Identified the responsibilities of dental hygienists
   2. Identified the competence students must achieve
   3. Established a network of dental hygiene educators

H. 1965—American Dental Hygienists' Association produced the recruitment film *Bright Future*

I. 1967—American Dental Hygienists' Association studied the need for and design of associate, baccalaureate, and master's level dental hygiene programs

J. 1968—administration of Northeast Regional Board Examination

K. 1970—American Dental Hygienists' Association
1. Sponsored the First International Symposium on Dental Hygiene, held in Italy
2. Produced the first "Curriculum Essentials" document for dental hygiene programs
3. Executive Secretary title changed to Executive Director

L. 1970—Community Oral Health Managers instituted by the US Army resulted in
1. Commissioning of baccalaureate-trained dental hygienists as officers
2. Preventive oral health programs for military personnel and dependents

M. 1970—training in expanded auxiliary management (TEAM) demonstration projects were established to determine the feasibility of teaching registered dental hygienists to perform nontraditional services under the supervision of a dentist
1. Registered dental hygienists were taught to
a. Administer anesthesia
b. Cut hard and soft tissue
c. Place restorative materials
2. Studies conducted at the Forsyth Dental Clinic, the University of Pennsylvania, the University of Iowa, and Howard University
3. Studies indicated that graduate dental hygienists could be trained to perform expanded functions successfully
4. Several projects were stopped because of the objections of local dentists

N. 1971—American Dental Hygienists' Association established a Washington office to
1. Monitor legislation of interest to the profession
2. Provide information to lawmakers
3. Represent the views of the association

O. 1971—dental hygienists became involved in dental auxiliary utilization (DAU); demonstration projects in North Carolina, Iowa, Alabama, Kentucky, Florida, Maryland, Missouri, and Ohio

P. 1971—pant uniforms for dental hygienists offered

Q. 1972—*The Journal of the American Dental Hygienists' Association* adopted the title *Dental Hygiene* (presently called the *Journal of Dental Hygiene*)

R. 1973—Commission on Accreditation of Dental and Dental Auxiliary Programs; name later changed to the Commission on Dental Accreditation

1. Established by the American Dental Association
2. Two members on the commission represent dental hygiene

S. 1974—first male delegate to the American Dental Hygienists' Association

T. 1975—first dental hygienist voting member of Maryland State Board of Dental Examiners

U. 1976—American Dental Hygienists' Association publication *Educational Directions* for dental auxiliaries became the second official publication of the American Dental Hygienists' Association (no longer published)

V. 1976—Linda Krol, R.D.H., became the first dental hygienist to own and manage a practice in dental hygiene

W. 1976—establishment of ADHA's legislative network called ACCENT (ACtion CENTral); vehicle to mobilize broad consumer and dental support on professional issues

X. 1977—Alabama, the last state to allow preceptorship, amended its practice act to permit formal training from an accredited dental hygiene program for licensure

Y. 1978—denturists won legislative approval to practice in Arizona, Maine, and Oregon

Z. 1978—American Dental Hygienists' Association
1. Established District XIII and added the Virgin Islands as a constituent
2. Changed the name of the Educational Trust Fund (ETF) to the American Dental Hygienists' Association Foundation
3. Established the Hygienists' Political Action Committee (HY-PAC)

AA. 1979—ended two decades of rapid expansion in dental hygiene education and practice, resulting in
1. Two hundred one dental hygiene programs in operation, the majority in community colleges and technical institutes
2. Dental hygiene programs in 50 states and Puerto Rico
3. Estimated number of licensed dental hygienists reaching 73,500
4. Some expanded services for dental hygienists legalized by 47 states; Expanded Function Dental Auxiliary (EFDA)

Challenges of the 1980s[1]

A. 1980—state legislative activities
1. After a decade of lobbying, 33 states had dental hygienist representation on boards of dental examiners
2. Sunset review process continued in 23 states whereby programs, agencies, and regulatory

boards are reviewed to determine whether they are meeting the public need

3. Continuing education became mandatory for license renewal in 11 states

B. 1980—Federal Trade Commission proposed nullification of state restrictions requiring dental hygienists to work under the supervision of a dentist because this constitutes restraint of trade

C. 1980—American Dental Hygienists' Association approved statement that dental hygienists may own dental hygiene practices

D. 1980—*Horizons,* the newsletter of the American Dental Hygienists' Association
1. Distributed bimonthly to all members of the American Dental Hygienists' Association
2. Funded by Johnson & Johnson
3. No longer published

E. 1981—American Dental Hygienists' Association created the Dental Hygiene Commission for Assurance of Competence to
1. Define competence in dental hygiene
2. Study methods currently used to ensure competence of dental hygienists
3. Dissolved in 1987

F. 1981—American Dental Hygienists' Association
1. Began meeting twice a year
a. House of Delegates meeting and annual session held for the first time in June at Chicago
b. Council meetings held in the fall of each year
2. Established the council structure, incorporating standing committees into six councils
3. Membership reached over 22,000

G. 1981—*RDH* magazine for dental hygienists first published to address the professional, financial, legal, and personal needs of dental hygienists

H. 1981—Consumer-Patient Radiation Health and Safety Act of 1981 proposed common standards for all healthcare providers using ionizing radiation

I. 1982—American Dental Hygienists' Association produced the film *Dental Hygienist: Your Preventive Professional*

J. 1982—Federal Trade Commission's authority to control state-regulated health professions was challenged by the American Medical Association and the American Dental Association

K. 1982—American Dental Hygienists' Association conducts survey of issues, attitudes, perceptions, and preferences of dental hygienists[1]

L. 1983—legislation was inacted in the state of Washington to establish a[2]
1. Dental Hygiene Examining Committee to license dental hygienists

2. Dental Hygiene Practice Act to govern the practice of dental hygiene

M. 1983—International Liaison Committee (ILC) for dental hygiene
1. Held the Ninth International Symposium on Dental Hygiene in Philadelphia
2. Drafted a constitution and bylaws

N. 1983—Dental Hygiene Aptitude Test (DHAT) was discontinued because it no longer was recognized as the best predictor of success in dental hygiene; SAT and ACT scores used as reliable predictors

O. 1984—American Dental Hygienists' Association established a Universal Registry for Continuing Education

P. 1984—Congress reaffirmed the Federal Trade Commission's authority over the health professions; this was viewed as a political victory by the American Dental Hygienists' Association

Q. 1984—legislation was passed in the State of Washington that permitted unsupervised practice of dental hygiene in nursing homes, hospitals, institutional settings, and public health facilities[2,3]

R. 1985—legislation was enacted in Illinois changing dental hygiene practice from general to direct supervision except in cases of nonambulatory patients in long-term care facilities

S. 1986—American Dental Hygienists' Association issued a policy statement from the House of Delegates supporting the baccalaureate degree as the minimum educational requirement for entry into dental hygiene practice

T. 1986—legislation was passed in Colorado permitting unsupervised practice of dental hygiene in all settings (independent practice)
1. A dental hygienist may be the proprietor of a place where supervised or unsupervised dental hygiene practice is performed
2. A dental hygienist may purchase, own, or lease equipment necessary to perform supervised or unsupervised dental hygiene practice
3. Root-planing and radiographic services cannot be performed during unsupervised dental hygiene practice

U. 1986—HMPP #139-Health Manpower Pilot Project of California to study safety and access to care issues related to unsupervised dental hygiene practice[4]
1. Allows dental hygienists to practice unsupervised in nontraditional setting
2. Provides oral health care to underserved populations
3. Sponsored by University of California at Northridge and accepted by California Office of

Statewide Health Planning and Development (OSHPD)

V. 1986—American Dental Hygienists' Association discontinued the following publications: *Educational Directions, Horizons,* and *Legislative Bulletin*

W. 1986—International Dental Hygienists' Federation was founded during the Tenth International Symposium on Dental Hygiene in Oslo, Norway; founding countries of Canada, Japan, Norway, the Netherlands, Sweden, United Kingdom, and United States were joined at this time by Australia, Denmark, and Switzerland

X. 1987—California Dental Association opposed HMPP #139[4]
  1. 1987—filed suit to block continuation of pilot project; court rejected suit
  2. 1989—appealed the court decision and won
  3. 1989—California Office of Statewide Health Planning and Development (OSHPD) filed petition for rehearing; petition was denied; OSHPD appealed to Supreme Court and won the right to continue the project

Y. 1987—*Access,* the newsmagazine of the American Dental Hygienists' Association
  1. Distributed monthly to all members of the American Dental Hygienists' Association
  2. Began as a newsletter and expanded to newsmagazine in 1988
  3. Replaced *Horizons;* published to address current professional news and legislative political activity in dental hygiene

Z. 1987—American Dental Association House of Delegates developed and passed a Policy Statement on Dental Auxiliaries[5] that encouraged dental societies to advocate for
  1. Removal of "general" supervision nationwide from all state practice acts
  2. Use of "direct," "indirect," or "personal" supervision in the language of state practice acts

AA. 1987—American Dental Association and state dental associations cited shortages of dental hygienists to[6]
  1. Justify changing state practice acts to delegate hygienist functions to dental assistants
  2. Establish preceptorship programs to train hygienists in dental offices

BB. 1987—American Dental Hygienists' Association established a committee to study manpower issues

CC. 1987—Georgia Dental Hygienists' Association successfully had a bill passed that requires dental hygiene education programs to be accredited by the ADA Commission on Dental Accreditation rather than Georgia Board of Dentistry[7]

DD. 1987—California Dental Association filed suit against the California Dental Hygienists' Association for violating antitrust laws and conspired to fix salaries by sharing salary information; suit dismissed in 1989 by Los Angeles County Superior Court[7]

EE. 1987—Florida State Board of Dentistry mandated dentists, dental hygienists, and dental assistants to wear gloves for any intraoral procedure on a patient

FF. 1988—*Teamwork,* a journal of the American Dental Association
  1. Distributed to dental hygienists, assistants, technicians, and office managers free of charge
  2. Published bimonthly to create a "team approach" to dental care
  3. Provides members of oral health teams basic information on practice and provision of dental care

GG. 1988—Texas Dental Board successfully changed the rules to eliminate "general" supervision from dental hygiene practice to "direct supervision;" after much opposition, the Texas Board of Dentistry reversed the practice of dental hygiene back to general supervision in 1990

HH. 1988—legislation was enacted in New Mexico that established a Dental Hygiene Advisory Committee of the Board of Dentistry

II. 1988—American Dental Hygienists' Association conducted the Retention and Reentry Study of all practicing and nonpracticing dental hygiene license holders; the study indicated[6]
  1. Nearly 30% of dental hygienists holding active licenses do not practice
  2. No shortage of dental hygienists exists in the United States
  3. Nonpracticing dental hygienists left the profession because of labor issues of salary, benefits, infectious disease control, family responsibilities, and boredom

JJ. 1988—federal government's Occupational Safety and Health Administration mandated infection control guidelines and procedures for health care workers exposed to HBV and HIV

KK. 1989—Georgia Dental Association introduced a bill that would permit preceptor trained hygienists to become licensed in Georgia[8]
  1. House Bill #200 was delayed by House Health and Ecology Committee and defeated in January 1990
  2. Georgia Dental Hygienists' Association and accredited dental hygiene programs in Georgia investigate flexible scheduling of programs to

recruit more individuals into dental hygiene profession

LL. 1989—bill enacted into law in Maryland to allow health occupation boards to take action against healthcare providers who discriminate against person with a positive HIV status[9]

MM. 1989—the document "Standards of Dental Hygiene Conduct and Practice" was implemented in the state of Washington; it is being enforced by the Department of Health

Challenges of the 1990s

A. Preceptorship[10]
  1. Definition—*preceptor* means teacher or instructor
  2. A number of state dental associations and state dental boards are considering the use of preceptor training for education of dental hygienists, endangering the quality of dental hygiene care to the public
  3. Impact of preceptorship training on the practice of dental hygiene:
    a. Compromises client safety
    b. Decrease the quality of preventive oral healthcare
    c. Diminishes value of dental hygiene licensure
    d. Discredits the dental hygienist's role in the delivery of oral healthcare
    e. Impairs the dental hygienist's marketability to future employers
    f. Devalues formal education and formal educational credentials in the profession of dental hygiene
    g. Decreases the quality of nonsurgical periodontal therapy available to the public
    h. Compromises recruitment of individuals into the profession
    i. Creates risk management problems for the employer
    j. Compromises the standard of care
  4. Alabama Dental Hygiene Program (ADHP)
    a. In existence since 1919; only preceptorship program for dental hygiene in the country
    b. Educational segment of program consists of 165 classroom hours of basic science and clinic theory (2 weeks of lectures; 8 days of seminars on weekends)
    c. Dentist is "preceptor" providing on-the-job clinical training in dental office
    d. Program replaces formal dental hygiene education from an accredited academic program
    e. ADHP graduates are *not* eligible to take the National Dental Hygiene Board Examination and therefore can practice only in the State of Alabama
    f. ADHP graduates are *not* eligible for membership in the American Dental Hygienists' Association
    g. Approximately 150 new dental hygienists are trained in Alabama each year via the preceptorship program

B. Recruitment and retention of dental hygienists
  1. American Dental Hygienists' Association recommendations to recruit and retain future dental hygienists[7]
    a. Revision of compensation/benefit plan for practicing dental hygienists to encourage long-term retention in the profession
    b. Establishment of office policies concerning disease transmission and infection control
    c. Support active recruitment financially and through professional activities
    d. Establishment of reciprocity and licensure by credentials to allow licensed dental hygienists interstate practice without being reexamined
    e. Legalization of general supervision nationwide
    f. Legalization of unsupervised practice to provide professional dental hygiene care to underserved and institutionalized populations
  2. American Association of Dental Schools' recommendations for increasing accessibility of dental hygiene programs to recruit future dental hygienists[11]
    a. Foster creative, flexible dental hygiene curricula that can be accredited by the Commission on Dental Accreditation in institutions of higher education
    b. Organize an information network among dental hygiene directors to disseminate information about the development, operation, and evaluation of flexible curricula
    c. Broaden and strengthen the involvement of dental and nondental interest groups in the development of programs
    d. Encourage higher institutional cooperation and flexibility during the development of innovative curricula in dental hygiene programs
    e. Simplify reporting procedures required by the Commission on Dental Accreditation during curriculum changes and reevaluation of programs
  3. Additional recommendations to recruit and retain future dental hygienists
    a. Institutions of higher education offer refresher courses for the inactive dental hygienists to return to practice
    b. Recognize the valuable role of the nondoctor in healthcare settings
    c. Support staff development and educational op-

portunities that enrich the working environment of dental hygienists

    d. Expand formal degree program and continuing education opportunities via telecommunication technology, e.g., distance education

    e. Expand levels of autonomy in dental hygiene practice

C. Dental hygiene regulation and access to care[12]

  1. American Dental Hygienists' Association supports self-regulation for the dental hygiene profession to better meet the needs and demands of the public

  2. ADHA policy does not support federal licensure and regulation for the dental hygiene profession

  3. In Canada, dental hygienists in Ontario, Alberta, British Columbia, and Quebec are self-regulated[13,14]

  4. Dentistry regulating dental hygiene restricts access to care:

    a. A profession that employs and regulates members from another profession limits access to care for the public

    b. The regulating profession determines which consumers will receive services from the supervised profession and under what conditions

  5. Supervision

    a. American Dental Hygienists' Association supports independent/unsupervised practice for the profession of dental hygiene[12]

    b. State dental hygiene practice acts need to be amended to change supervision requirements to general and unsupervised practice for traditional and nontraditional settings

D. Promote national parameters for dental hygiene education and practice

  1. Support national parameters for formal dental hygiene education and practice

  2. Identify and develop biologic, psychosocial, economic, ethical, and dental hygiene theories to guide practice in a uniform manner

  3. Support national standards that justify greater control over program accreditation by the dental hygiene profession; strengthen accreditation policies and procedures that affect dental hygiene

  4. Educate consumers to recognize and understand the dental hygiene profession

  5. Establish baccalaureate degree as minimum entry level for future dental hygiene practice

    a. Curriculum to integrate broad "general" education with "career" education

    b. Prepare dental hygienists for roles of clinician, health promotor/educator, consumer advocate, administrator/manager, change agent, and researcher

  6. Maintain the National Board Dental Hygiene Examination as a standard in all states

  7. Employ national standards of practice in the delivery and evaluation of dental hygiene care

  8. Support expansion of master's and doctoral level education for dental hygienists

  9. Expand the number of dental hygienists with doctoral degrees

  10. Establish the value of all levels of formal dental hygiene education to the public, dental hygiene, and dentistry

E. Advance dental hygiene as a profession

  1. Promote formal recognition of dental hygiene as a discipline distinct from other disciplines

  2. Promote a paradigm for dental hygiene that includes the four central paradigm concepts (clients, environment, health/oral health, and dental hygiene actions) (Fig. 18-1) and that provides a framework for theory development[15,16]

  3. Promote the discipline statement to identify the uniqueness of dental hygiene as a discipline

  4. Promote advanced levels of education within the dental hygiene discipline

  5. Follow a code of ethics that articulates the core values endorsed by all members of the profession

  6. Promote dental hygiene research

  7. Promote dental hygiene practice built upon theory and research

  8. Work to ensure that dental hygiene is regulated by those within the profession of dental hygiene

F. 1992—ADA House of Delegates adopted a series of resolutions to increase dental control over the education, practice, and regulation of dental hygienists and lower existing standards of education and practice:

  1. Resolution 68H asserts that dental hygiene educational programs should be administered solely by a dentist

  2. Resolution 116H asserts that the ADA opposes the use of the terms "diagnosis" and "treatment planning" in the titles of continuing education courses for dental hygienists, as well as any descriptions of these courses that imply that the program content or prior educational level of dental hygienists is sufficient to make the dental hygienists competent to render diagnosis for dental disease or treatment planning for dental patients

  3. Resolution 22H seeks to advance the development of "flexible training programs" for dental hygienists and authorize funds to implement them

  4. Resolution 141H seeks to advance the training of dental assistants to provide limited dental hygiene services

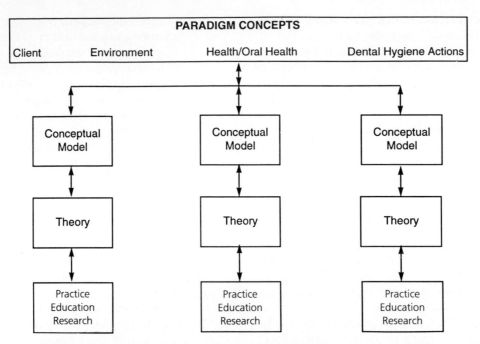

Fig. 18-1 Dental hygiene paradigm and theory development framework. (From Deck S, Nielsen-Thompson N, Walsh M: The ADHA framework for theory development, *J Dent Hyg* 67:166, 1993.)

5. NOTE: The American Association of Dental Examiners expressed its support of ADA Resolutions 116H, 22H, and 141H
G. 1992—The American Dental Hygienists' Association House of Delegates adopted a definition and theoretic paradigm for the professional discipline:

Dental hygiene is the study of preventive oral healthcare, including the management of behaviors, to prevent oral diseases and promote health. The major concepts studied are health/oral health, dental hygiene actions, the client, the environment, their interactions, and the factors that affect them.

H. 1992—Commission on Dental Accreditation of the ADA Revised the Accreditation Standards for Dental Hygiene Education
I. 1992—Occupational Safety and Health Administration (OSHA) Standard for Occupational Exposure to Bloodborne Pathogens became law
J. 1993—American Dental Hygienists' Association launches "Commitment to Responsible Healthcare," a campaign to raise consumer awareness about infection control measures that should be used in all healthcare settings
K. 1993—The First District Court of Appeals in Florida resoundingly upheld the order from Florida Division of Administrative Hearings that revoked the Florida Board of Dentistry rule to approve preceptorship training for dental hygienists
L. 1995—American Dental Hygienists' Association adopts a new Code of Ethics[17]

M. 1996—Establishment of the DHNet which is a web site that provides information on various aspects of dental hygiene; access on the internet by http://jeffline.tju.edu./DHNet
N. 1997—Canadian Dental Hygienists' Association reports that approximately 85% of all dental hygienists in Canada are self-regulated[13]
1. Dental hygienists in the provinces of Alberta, British Columbia, Quebec, and Ontario are self-regulated
2. Dental hygienists in the province of Saskatchewan are working to establish self-regulation

American Dental Hygienists' Association

Purpose of the Organization

A. Constitution, Bylaws, Code of Ethics, and Policy Manual were written, adopted, and may be amended annually by the House of Delegates
1. Constitution of the American Dental Hygienists' Association describes
a. Mission and goals of the organization
b. Composition of its membership
c. Organization structure
d. Governing units
e. Officers
f. Meeting schedule
2. Bylaws are the rules that govern the association
3. Code of Ethics outlines the moral obligations of

each member to the profession and the public; it increases our professional and ethical consciousness and sense of ethical responsibility, it guides our ethical decisions, and it helps the profession achieve its mission

4. Policy Manual describes the association's position on issues confronting the dental hygiene profession[12]

B. Mission of the American Dental Hygienists' Association as stated in the Policy Manual:

To improve the public's total health, the mission of the American Dental Hygienists' Association is to advance the art and science of dental hygiene by ensuring access to quality oral healthcare, increasing the awareness of the cost-effective benefits of prevention, promoting the highest standards of dental hygiene education, licensure, practice, and research, and representing and promoting the interests of dental hygienists.

C. Goals of the American Dental Hygienists' Association as stated in the American Dental Hygienists' Association Policy Manual are to[12]
1. Promote the *dental hygiene* profession as an integral component of interdisciplinary healthcare
2. Promote consumer advocacy in oral healthcare as a part of total health
3. Promote the *dental hygienist* as a primary care provider of preventive and therapeutic services
4. Promote the self-regulation of *dental hygiene* education, licensure, and practice
5. Serve as the authoritative resource on all issues related to *dental hygiene*
6. Promote research relevant to *dental hygiene*
7. Promote membership and participation in the American Dental Hygienists' Association
8. Provide for a viable financial base

D. American Dental Hygienists' Association subscribes to a Code of Ethics, which state the obligations and responsibilities of the membership to[17]
1. Ourselves as individuals
2. Ourselves as professionals
3. Family and friends
4. Clients
5. Colleagues
6. Employees and employers
7. Dental hygiene profession
8. Community and society
9. Scientific investigation

Structure of the American Dental Hygienists' Association

A. Governance of the American Dental Hygienists' Association
1. National level
   a. House of Delegates

(1) Attends to matters of policy
(2) Elects ADHA officers
(3) Establishes councils and standing committees
(4) Is presided over by the Speaker of the House

b. Board of Trustees
(1) Attends to administrative matters, including budget
(2) Appoints and directs Executive Director
(3) Power to exact interim policy
(4) Is presided over by the President

c. Executive Director (Fig. 18-2)
(1) Responsibilities
   (a) Serves under the director of the Board of Trustees
   (b) Principal administrative officer of the Association
   (c) Manages the officers of the Association
(2) Administrative personnel
   (a) ADHA Institute Administrator and Development Director
   (b) Executive Assistant
   (c) Manager of Meeting Planning
   (d) Administrative Associate
(3) Directors
   (a) Assistant Executive Director
   (b) Director of Administration and Special Projects
   (c) Director of Governmental Affairs
   (d) Director of Professional Development
   (e) Director of Member Services
   (f) Director of Communications
   (g) Director of Development

2. District level—12 districts
   a. Established by the House of Delegates
   b. Incorporates a number of constituents
   c. Represented by a district trustee who sits on the Board of Trustees and is elected by delegates from the incorporated constituents

3. Constituent level—51 constituents or state/territory associations; one for each state and one for the District of Columbia and Guam
   a. Chartered by the Board of Trustees; each state, commonwealth, federal district, territory, or possession of the United States is eligible to become a constituent of the American Dental Hygienists' Association
   b. Incorporates a number of components
   c. Represented by delegates who sit in the House of Delegates of the American Dental Hygienists' Association

4. Component level—approximately 404 active components or local associations representing the local

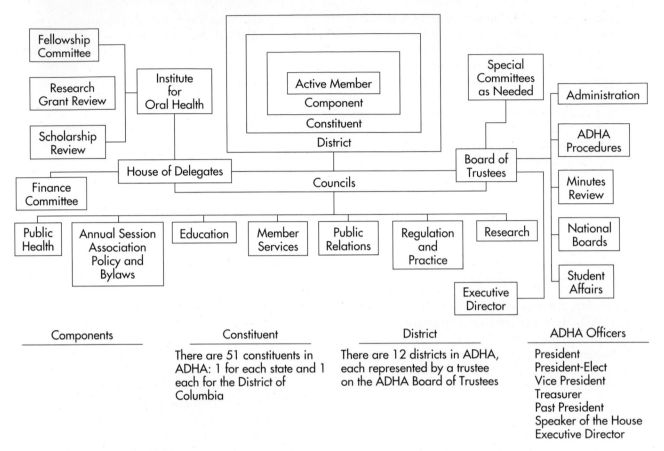

Fig. 18-2 American Dental Hygienists' Association organizational chart. (From American Dental Hygienists' Association, Chicago, 1997, with permission.)

organizational divisions within each state/territory and are not restricted to a specific number, membership, or geographic area
  a. Established by constituent houses of delegates
  b. Not limited to a specific geographic area or designated number
  c. Represented by delegates who sit in the house of delegates of the constituent (state); some constituents have executive boards
B. Representation in the American Dental Hygienists' Association[17]
  1. Classification and privileges of members of the American Dental Hygienists' Association; membership in the American Dental Hygienists' Association requires simultaneous membership in the constituent (state) and component (local) associations
    a. Voting members shall have the right to vote, hold office, and such other privileges as the House of Delegates may determine
      (1) Active member—any dental hygienist who
        (a) Graduates from an accredited dental

hygiene program or is licensed under the provision of a "grandfather" clause
      (b) Is licensed to practice dental hygiene in the United States or its territories
      (c) Agrees to adhere to the Bylaws and Code of Ethics of the American Dental Hygienists' Association
      (d) Agree to hold membership in constituent and component organizations if they exist
    (2) Life member—any active member who
      (a) Has made outstanding contributions to dental hygiene and to the Association
      (b) Is nominated by the Board of Trustees
      (c) Is elected by the House of Delegates or
      (d) Completed the term of office as President of the American Dental Hygienists' Association
    (3) Retired/senior member—any active member who has
      (a) Reached the age of 62

   (b) Been an active member for at least one of the following
     [1] Twenty-five years
     [2] Twenty consecutive years
     [3] Continuously from the date of eligibility
 (4) Members with disabilities—any dental hygienist who
   (a) Has been a voting member
   (b) Is prohibited from being employed due to the person's disability

b. Nonvoting members shall have such privileges as the House of Delegates shall determine, but shall not have the right to vote or hold office
 (1) International member—any licensed dental hygienist who
   (a) Is residing outside the United States under a current license or certificate
   (b) Agrees to adhere to the Bylaws and Code of Ethics of the American Dental Hygienists' Association
 (2) Student member—any student who is
   (a) Enrolled in one of the following programs of study
     [1] Accredited dental hygiene program
     [2] Baccalaureate or graduate degree program that is complementary to a career in dental hygiene
   (b) Recommended by the director or a duly appointed representative of an institution
 (3) Supporting member—any licensed dental hygienist who
   (a) Is not employed in a dental hygiene-related career
   (b) Agrees to adhere to the Bylaws and Code of Ethics of the American Dental Hygienists' Association
   (c) Requires tripartite membership
 (4) Honorary member—any individual who
   (a) Is not a dental hygienist
   (b) Has made outstanding contributions to dental hygiene or dental health
   (c) Has been nominated by the Board of Trustees
   (d) Has been elected by the House of Delegates
 (5) Allied member—any individual who
   (a) Supports the purposes and mission of the association
   (b) Is not otherwise qualified for any other class of membership

 (6) Corporate member—any corporation, institution, or organization that supports the mission of the American Dental Hygienists' Association
2. Officers of the American Dental Hygienists' Association
 a. Elected officers
  (1) Officers assuming a 1-year term as the result of a previous election by the House of Delegates
   (a) President
   (b) Immediate Past President
  (2) Officers elected by the House of Delegates for 1 year
   (a) President-Elect
   (b) Vice-President
  (3) Officers elected by the House of Delegates for 2 years
   (a) Treasurer
   (b) Speaker of the House
  (4) District trustees are elected
   (a) By the delegates of the constituents of their respective districts
   (b) From among the voting delegates of the respective district
   (c) To represent the district on the Board of Trustees
   (d) For a 2-year term
 b. Appointed officer who serves under the direction of the Board of Trustees—Executive Director
3. House of Delegates, consists of members chosen by their respective constituents, is the legislative body of the American Dental Hygienists' Association
 a. Is presided over by the Speaker of the House
 b. Consists of
  (1) Voting members who represent each constituent based on a formula
   (a) One delegate from each constituent plus
   (b) One hundred additional delegates to be allocated among the constituents
   (c) One voting student delegate
  (2) Nonvoting members
   (a) Elected officers of the association
   (b) Appointed officers of the association
   (c) One student delegate from each district
 c. Has the authority to determine the policies to govern the Association
4. Board of Trustees, administrative body of the American Dental Hygienists' Association
 a. Is presided over by the President

  b. Consists of
     (1) Voting members
        (a) President
        (b) President-Elect
        (c) Vice-President
        (d) Treasurer
        (e) Immediate Past President
        (f) District Trustees
     (2) Nonvoting or ex-officio members without vote—Executive Director
  c. Meets at least two times a year
C. American Dental Hygienists' Association policies
  1. Meetings shall be at least twice a year
     a. June meeting shall consist of
        (1) House of Delegates meeting
        (2) Annual session of American Dental Hygienists' Association
        (3) Board of Trustees before and after annual session meetings
     b. Fall meeting shall consist of
        (1) Board of Trustees' meeting
        (2) Councils' meetings
  2. Councils of the American Dental Hygienists' Association
     a. Include
        (1) Council on Annual Session/Association Policy and Bylaws
        (2) Council on Education
        (3) Council on Member Services
        (4) Council on Public Relations
        (5) Council on Regulation and Practice
        (6) Council on Research
        (7) Council on Public Health
     b. Are established by the House of Delegates
     c. Have members and chairs appointed by the President with the approval of the Board of Trustees
  3. Policy Manual of the American Dental Hygienists' Association specifies the association's position on
     a. American Dental Hygienists' Association's mission and goals
     b. Ethics
     c. Licensure
     d. Education
     e. Continuing education
     f. Practice
     g. Public health
     h. Research
     i. Framework on theory development
  4. Official publications of the American Dental Hygienists' Association
     a. *Journal of Dental Hygiene (JDH)*—journal of the American Dental Hygienists' Association; pub-

lished nine times per year; promotes the publication of original research related to the profession, the education, and the practice of dental hygiene
     b. *Access*—American Dental Hygienists' Association newsmagazine; published monthly
     c. *Education Update*—American Dental Hygienists' Association newsletter for educators; published twice a year

Professionalism in Dental Hygiene

Defining a Profession

A. Characteristics of a profession
  1. Special advanced education or preparation
  2. Identifiable membership
  3. Strong service orientation
  4. Promotion of a body of knowledge in the field (e.g., research and theory development)
  5. Autonomy of practice
  6. Self-regulating
  7. Is the recognized authority with societal sanction
  8. Work is primarily intellectual in nature
  9. Adherence to a code of ethics
B. Standards for a profession
  1. Codes of ethics
     a. Ancient codes
        (1) Code of Hammurabi—2100 BC
           (a) First code of ethical standards for business
           (b) Guaranteed justice for all
           (c) Invoked "an eye for an eye" and "a tooth for a tooth"
        (2) Hippocratic Oath—400 BC
           (a) Stated, "Above all, do no harm"
           (b) Protected the rights of the patient
           (c) Admonished physicians to keep the confidence of patients
           (d) Placed the needs of the patient above those of society
           (e) Placed an obligation on physicians to teach the next generation of physicians
        (3) Oath of Maimonides—thirteenth century; admonished physicians
           (a) To do good
           (b) To be sympathetic
           (c) Not to be greedy
     b. Common elements of codes
        (1) Self-imposed
        (2) Set rules governing behavior
        (3) Serve to protect the public
        (4) Strive to enhance the profession

    c. Patient's Bill of Rights
      (1) Focuses on the needs of the client
      (2) Encourages informed choice by the client
      (3) Guarantees quality care to the client
  2. Credentials, type of credentials
    a. Licensure—state regulation of professionals
      (1) Granted by a state agency or board
      (2) Limits practice to
        (a) Responsibilities/behaviors prescribed by law in the state practice act or
        (b) Responsibilities/behaviors delineated by rules and regulations
      (3) Authorizes practice by professionals meeting specified qualifications
    b. Registration—qualified professionals listed in a directory or file
    c. Certification—state or national recognition
      (1) Recognition by a nongovernmental agency (e.g., a professional association)
      (2) Identification of professionals who have met specified qualifications
  3. Accountability—the ability to answer for one's actions; professionals are expected to demonstrate
    a. Competence in skill and knowledge
    b. Adherence to parameters of practice in delivering services
    c. Dedication to the best interests of the client
    d. Integrity in professional activities
    e. Quality client care
    f. Adherence to a professional code of ethics

Ethical Issues in Dental Hygiene

A. Definitions
  1. Ethics
    a. Study of what is right and what is wrong in human conduct
    b. Establishes principles that
      (1) Serve as a guide for conduct and thought
      (2) Are based on theory
      (3) Can be used to justify human conduct
      (4) Can provide a framework for making ethical decisions
  2. Morals
    a. Standards of conduct and thought
    b. Based on ethical and theologic principles
    c. Measure conduct against standards
  3. Mores
    a. Customs of a group
    b. Cultural standards for behavior
    c. Change with time
  4. Values
    a. Beliefs and attitudes
    b. Motivate behavior

    c. Dynamic; may change with time and circumstances
B. Values
  1. Types
    a. Intrinsic—attitudes or beliefs related to the maintenance of life (e.g., valuing healthcare)
    b. Extrinsic—attitudes or beliefs related to alternatives not essential to life (e.g., valuing a specific healthcare provider or agency)
    c. Instrumental—attitudes or beliefs related to a process (e.g., valuing a health lifestyle)
    d. Terminal—attitudes or beliefs related to an outcome or product (e.g., valuing health)
  2. Criteria for adopting values—values are
    a. Freely chosen
    b. Chosen from alternatives
    c. Chosen after consideration
    d. Prized and cherished
    e. Publicly held
    f. Action oriented
    g. Integrated into one's lifestyle
    h. Contribute to one's well-being
  3. Values clarification
    a. Outcome of an activity that
      (1) Leads to an understanding of personal thoughts and actions
      (2) Does not dictate rules, behavior, or thought
      (3) Does not impose or judge the values held by others
    b. Process involves the individual in
      (1) Choosing or identifying his or her own values
      (2) Prizing and affirming his or her own values
      (3) Acting on his or her values
  4. Hierarchy of values—some values are more important than others in motivating action and are therefore considered higher on the scale of values
  5. Values dissonance
    a. Occurs when
      (1) Personally held values are not congruent with
        (a) Those held by the profession
        (b) Those held by others (colleagues, family, clients, supervisors)
      (2) Values come in conflict (e.g., when the value to respect the lifestyle of others conflicts with the value to improve the oral hygiene of the patient)
    b. May result in a change in values
  6. Value judgment—evaluation of the beliefs and behaviors of others based on the values held by self
  7. Origin of values

a. Personal values are influenced and instilled by
  (1) Home and family
  (2) Peers and colleagues
  (3) Professional expectation
  (4) Customs and national mores
  (5) Events and circumstances of life
b. Values accepted by a group are influenced by
  (1) Leaders
  (2) Members
  (3) Time, events, and circumstances

C. Moral reasoning
  1. Characterized by
    a. Cognitive judgment
    b. Independence from prevailing norms, mores, or customs
    c. Philosophic thought rather than behavior
  2. Moral development theory of L. Kohlberg
    a. Assumes that moral development is
      (1) Cognitive—based on thinking and influenced by experience
      (2) Sequential—one stage builds on the previous one
      (3) Hierarchical—each stage is better than the previous one
      (4) Universal—applicable to all persons and cultures
    b. Categorizes moral reasoning into three levels divided into six stages
      (1) Preconventional level—children and adolescents reason at this level
        (a) Stage 1—punishment and obedience orientation; response to punishment or reward; rules are obeyed to avoid punishment
        (b) Stage 2—instrumental relativist orientation; personal interest is paramount, or "I'll scratch your back if you scratch mine"; person conforms to obtain rewards
      (2) Conventional level—most adults reach this level of reasoning
        (a) Stage 3—interpersonal concordance of "good boy–nice girl" orientation; in search of praise and to win approval
        (b) Stage 4—law-and-order orientation; one's duty to maintain social or religious order
      (3) Postconventional level—few adults reach this level of reasoning
        (a) Stage 5—social-contract legalistic orientation; upholding those societal standards that are seen as fair; respect for the rights of others

      (b) Stage 6—universal ethical-principle orientation; guided by principles, not rules and laws; behavior is influenced by conscience

D. Ethical theories—are unchanging, do not change with custom
  1. Criteria that identify an ethical theory; ethical theories
    a. Are systematic approaches to knowledge relevant to ethical thought and action
    b. Make up principles and rules
    c. Assist in decision making
  2. Three major ethical theories
    a. Utilitarian ethics (John Stuart Mill)—focuses on consequences; best possible outcome for the greatest number of people; also known as the "greatest happiness" theory; if one thinks as a utilitarian, one might believe that "the ends justify the means"
      (1) Act utilitarians concentrate on the outcome of a single act under specific circumstances (e.g., tell the client whatever is necessary to achieve a positive outcome)
      (2) Rule utilitarians concentrate on the outcome of types of acts (e.g., in general, tell clients the truth as long as it will not result in harm)
    b. Deontologic ethics (Immanuel Kant)—focuses on the morality of the act rather than the consequence of actions; if one thinks as a deontologist, one might say, "It's the principle of the thing"
      (1) Act deontologists consider the ethical principles involved in an action in light of the circumstances (e.g., do not lie, but you may avoid telling the truth if the whole truth is harmful)
      (2) Rule deontologists concentrate on principles and rules in general as they apply to types of actions (e.g., always tell the whole truth)
    c. Virtue ethics (Aristotle and Plato)—focuses on character traits and excellence of character; following this perspective, one would ask "is this what a virtuous person would do"?
  3. Ethical principles governing professional behavior
    a. Autonomy—the principles of respect for persons; health professional should
      (1) Include the client in the decision regarding care
      (2) Fully inform the client, then allow client to judge for himself
      (3) Obtain informed consent for treatment

(4) Respect the client as an individual

(5) Protect the confidentiality of the client

b. Nonmaleficence—the obligation of nonharm; health professional should

   (1) Above all, do no harm; minimize unavoidable pain

   (2) Prevent harm or the risk of harm

   (3) Consider the risks as well as the benefits of treatment alternatives

   (4) Present the alternative of minimal or no treatment if this is feasible

c. Beneficence—the principle of promoting what is good, kind, and charitable; health professionals should

   (1) Promote well-being or benefit

   (2) Consider whose well-being is being benefited (the client, the family, society, or the health professional)

   (3) Prevent evil or harm

   (4) Consider the costs as well as the benefits of treatment

   (5) Resist being paternalistic whereby the client's autonomy is violated when treatment is dictated; paternalism occurs when the health professional insists on the treatment that he or she believes is best for the client

d. Veracity—the principle of truthfulness and honesty; health professional should

   (1) Be truthful

   (2) Keep promises

   (3) Refrain from deception

   (4) Report known violations of the standard of care by colleagues to the proper authority

e. Justice—epitomized by the "Golden Rule," do unto others as you would have others do unto you; health professional should consider treatment in terms of fairness

   (1) Give others what is due them

   (2) Treat all clients fairly

   (3) Provide access to care for all

   (4) Call attention to situations where clients are treated inequitably

   (5) Distribute healthcare and healthcare resources with equity

E. Ethical decision making—what is an ethical dilemma, and how should decisions be made?

1. Ethical dilemmas

  a. Involve two or more opposing ethical principles that are equally important (e.g., telling the whole truth when doing so will cause harm)

  b. Concern several alternative actions (e.g., lying to spare pain, or telling the truth and causing pain)

  c. Choice of action must be made from several unsatisfactory alternatives (e.g., lying violates the client's autonomy and his or her right to be informed, but telling the truth may hurt the client's chances of recovery)

2. Decisions should be made based on

  a. Ethical theory

  b. Ethical principles and rules (e.g., autonomy, beneficence, etc.)

  c. Relevant facts

  d. Values and values in conflict

  e. Selection from alternatives/options

  f. Justification

F. Ethical issues and public policy

1. Distributive justice—fair allocation of resources involved

  a. Macroallocation of resources based on the needs of the public (e.g., water fluoridation)

  b. Microallocation of resources based on the needs of the individual (e.g., fluoride treatment)

2. Distributive justice or allocation of scarce resources (e.g., who should receive treatment when all cannot be treated?); services may be allocated on the basis of

  a. Equity—all persons receive equal treatment

  b. Need—treatment allocated on the basis of need

  c. Effort—treatment allocated to those who have earned it

  d. Contribution—treatment allocated to those who are making a contribution to society

  e. Merit—treatment allocated to those who are worthy

3. Health policy questions

  a. Should public tax dollars support

    (1) Financial assistance and care of the needy or elderly?

    (2) Financial aid for victims of

      (a) Chronic diseases?

      (b) Acute and devastating diseases?

    (3) Research and experimentation?

      (a) Who should decide what research should be done?

      (b) Who should support research?

  b. What proportion of the national budget should be spent on healthcare?

  c. For whom is healthcare beneficial?

    (1) Public

    (2) Individual

    (3) Healthcare practitioner

  d. Who should decide about treatment?

    (1) Client/legal guardian

    (2) Practitioner

    (3) Third-party payer

    (4) Legislature or Congress (government)

Legal Relationships in Dental Hygiene Practice

Basis of Law in the United States

A. Jurisprudence
1. Defined as philosophy of law
2. Concerns the principles of positive law and legal relations
B. Sources of American law—based on English common law
1. Statutes (statutory law)
   a. Federal statutes or legislation—US Constitution stipulates that all powers not given to the federal government are reserved to the states; these include the authority to
      (1) Police the health and welfare of its citizens (police powers)
      (2) Empower elected or appointed agencies or boards to regulate the practice of the professions, e.g., Board of Dentistry, Board of Dental Hygiene, Board of Medicine
   b. State statutes or legislation—practice acts and rules and regulations governing the practice of selected professions, e.g., dental practice act
2. Judicial decisions (common law)
   a. Unwritten, based on custom
   b. Made by judges or based on previous decisions under the principle of *stare decisis*
C. US legal system is based on adversarial relations
1. No legal action can be initiated between parties or between an agency and an individual without an adversarial relationship or one party injuring the other
2. Constitutionality of a law cannot be tested before its enactment or violation
D. Types of law
1. Criminal law—offense against society punishable by imprisonment, execution, public service, or fine (e.g., a person who practices dentistry or dental hygiene without a license is committing an offense against society)
   a. Types
      (1) Felonies—more serious offenses against individuals or society
      (2) Misdemeanors—less serious crimes
   b. Level of proof required—beyond a reasonable doubt that the jury or judge must be absolutely convinced that the criminal act occurred in order to establish guilt
2. Civil law—concerned with offenses against the legal rights and duties of private persons (e.g., the relationship between an oral health professional and a client is governed by civil law); crime against a person; remedy is usually monetary damages
   a. Contract—conditions of agreement between parties (e.g., once the care plan has been presented and the client has agreed to the fee, a contract is in effect); wills, copyrights, deeds, etc.
   b. Tort—civil wrong or injury committed by one individual against another
      (1) Intentional torts—also may be considered crimes against society and as such fall under both criminal and civil law
         (a) Assault and battery
            [1] Assault—violent verbal attack
            [2] Battery—beating or use of physical force
         (b) Defamation
            [1] Libel—written defamation
            [2] Slander—oral defamation
         (c) Misrepresentation and deceit—deception or misrepresentation with the intention of taking something of value
      (2) Unintentional torts—negligence (also called malpractice)
         (a) Occurs when four conditions exist
            [1] Duty was owed
            [2] Duty was breached
            [3] Damages or injury resulted
            [4] Breach of duty was the direct cause of the injury (proximate cause)
         (b) May result from omission or commission of acts
   c. Level of proof required—preponderance of the evidence means that the jury or judge must be 51% certain that the defendant is guilty or innocent; usual level of proof required in malpractice suits
E. Some legal doctrines
1. Doctrine of Personal Liability—holds every person liable for his or her own negligent conduct even though others also may be negligent
2. Doctrine of the Reasonably Prudent Man—holds a professional person responsible for maintaining the standard of care that is considered reasonable or customary by his or her peers
3. Doctrine of *respondeat superior*—holds an employer liable for the negligent acts of his or her employees that occur while they are carrying out their duties in the general course of employment
4. Doctrine of the Borrowed Servant—holds the supervising physician or dentist liable for the negligent acts of those who are working under his or her supervision, even if he or she is not the employer
5. Doctrine of Corporate Negligence—holds a hospital or healthcare agency liable for negligent acts of its employees or professional staff

6. Doctrine of *res ipsa loquitur* (the thing speaks for itself)—shifts the burden of proof from the plaintiff to the defendant because
   a. That type of injury normally does not occur unless there was negligence (e.g., an infection occurred as the result of unsterile instruments)
   b. Injury was caused by something completely under the control of the defendent (e.g., the instrument slipped)
   c. Injury was not caused by any voluntary action of the plaintiff (e.g., the client did not contribute to the injury)
7. Doctrine of Foreseeability—holds an individual liable for negligent acts or natural consequences that could or should have been foreseen
8. Doctrine of *res judicata*—holds that once the matter has been decided in court, the case cannot be retried
9. Doctrine of *stare decisis*—requires judges to adhere to the precedents of prior decisions; this results in common law or judge-made law
10. Doctrine of *res gestae*—admits pertinent statements made by others (third parties) at the time of the incident as admissible evidence, thereby making an exception to the hearsay rule, which normally excludes statements not made in court
11. Doctrine of Comparative Negligence—compares the negligence of the plaintiff and that of the defendant to determine degrees of failure to exercise due care

Legal Relationships

A. Duties of the healthcare practitioner
   1. Meet all legal requirements associated with practice
   2. Standard of care or due care—professional's duty to
      a. Possess the skill and knowledge expected
      b. Exercise the degree of care a reasonably prudent person would exercise under the same or similar circumstances
   3. Never exceed the scope of practice; when indicated, refer to a specialist who possesses and exercises the standard of care
   4. Duty to render treatment only extends to clients already accepted for care (e.g., a health professional is not required by law to accept any new client)
   5. Duty to continue or complete treatment started within a reasonable time or to arrange alternative sources of treatment for clients already accepted for treatment
   6. Duty to obtain informed consent from responsible

parties (may be a parent or guardian) before treatment; informed consent must be based on
      a. Adequate maturity of the client or guardian
      b. Complete information presented to the client regarding the risks, costs, and benefits of the proposed treatment
   7. Never use experimental procedures or medicaments
   8. Provide adequate client instructions
   9. Charge a reasonable fee
   10. Obtain a reasonable result
   11. Keep accurate records
   12. Maintain client's privacy and confidentiality
   13. Inform client of unexpected occurrences
   14. Employ competent personnel and appropriate levels of supervision
B. Duties of the client
   1. Pay a reasonable fee within a reasonable time
   2. Cooperate in care, e.g., follow instructions, keep appointments
   3. Provide accurate information about health history and status
C. Malpractice—professional negligence
   1. Criteria for malpractice
      a. Health professional owed a duty to the client; relationship between the client and healthcare provider establishes a duty
      b. Duty was breached by the healthcare provider (failure to exercise due care)
      c. Client sustained injury or damage
      d. Injury or damage was the direct result of the breach of duty
   2. Common grounds for malpractice
      a. Poor results when success was guaranteed (e.g., the health professional may have indicated that the results of treatment would be perfect or near perfect)
      b. Failure to exercise proper technique, e.g., in
         (1) Infection control
         (2) Radiographs
         (3) Local anesthesia
      c. Failure to adequately inform the client regarding treatment procedures, outcomes, and risks
      d. Failure to obtain permission-informed consent
         (1) Technical assault—touching or treating without consent (e.g., the health professional treats a child without the parent's consent)
         (2) Breach of confidentiality—divulging private information without consent (e.g., the health professional discusses the case in public using the client's name)
      e. Failure to
         (1) Treat temporomandibular joint disorder

(2) Diagnose periodontal disease or temporo-mandibular joint disorder

(3) Take necessary precautions to prevent mechanical injury

(4) Identify medically compromised clients

(5) Take appropriate precautions to protect a medically compromised client

(6) Identify a drug allergy

f. Other areas of legal vulnerability

(1) No medical emergency protocols

(2) Unqualified staff members

(3) Broken toys/objects in oral healthcare environments

(4) Hazardous sidewalks, parking lots, driveways, steps, etc.

(5) Poor record keeping practices

(6) Lack of adherence to Occupational Safety and Health Administration (OSHA) and Centers for Disease Control and Prevention (CDC) guidelines

(7) Providing care that is beyond one's scope of practice

3. Defense against malpractice

a. Exercise due care, using reasonable skill and care

b. Keep accurate and complete records of each case

c. Contributory negligence by the client relieves the health professional of liability (i.e., the client did not follow instructions or cooperate in care)

d. Statute of limitations—length of time a person legally has to file a suit against another for an alleged injury; length of time varies from state to state and with the type of alleged injury, for example

(1) May be 3 years for a contract action

(2) May be 6 years for a tort action

(3) May start at the time an injury occurs

(4) May start at the time the plaintiff discovers the injury

(5) May start at the time a child reaches the age of maturity

e. Statute of limitations limits the length of time in which a suit may be filed

(1) For adults this is usually 2 years after the injury or damage has been recognized or discovered

(2) For children this is a reasonable period of time after the child reaches the age of maturity

f. Question of proximate cause—if there are possible intervening causes or contributory negligence, these may relieve the health professional from liability

4. Types of damages or redress

a. Nominal damages—monetary compensation for the loss

b. Compensatory damages—actual costs to cover repair or treatment plus general damages to cover pain and suffering

c. Punitive damages—additional monetary compensation to punish the defendant, usually awarded in cases where the professional acted with recklessness or indifference

D. Oral health professionals in court—dental hygienist may be required to appear in court as a witness, as an expert witness, as a defendant, or as a plaintiff

1. Expert witness

a. May testify for either the defendant or the plaintiff

b. Should testify to the professional standard of care

c. Should not advocate or give opinion regarding the guilt or innocence of the defendant

2. Witness may be required to repeat what he or she saw or heard at the time of an incident

a. Report accurately what occurred

b. Should not participate in a "conspiracy of silence"

c. *Always tell the truth*

3. Defendant is best served by

a. Telling the truth

b. Having accurate and complete records of the case

c. Remaining silent on some points—most states allow "privileged communications" to remain confidential

4. Plaintiff is best served by

a. Accurate records

b. Timely action

c. Knowledge of facts

d. Familiarity with legal rights

E. Contractual relationships

1. Contract—promissory agreement between two or more parties that creates, modifies, or destroys a legal relationship; nature of the relationship between the client and health professional becomes contractual when the care plan and fees are agreed on

2. Elements of a contract

a. Mutual assent

b. Promises or consideration

c. Two or more parties

d. Must be a lawful act and not against public policy or law

3. Breach of contract is the unjustified failure to perform the terms of an expressed contract as agreed on

4. Classification of contracts—all are legally binding

a. Expressed
   (1) Are those where the terms are expressly agreed on
   (2) May be oral or written
       (a) Oral contracts are those with the terms verbally agreed on
       (b) Written contracts are those with the terms in writing
b. Implied
   (1) Are those without specific terms, or the terms of the agreement are "understood"
   (2) Agreement made by certain actions on the part of the parties concerned
5. Employment contracts—contractual agreement between an employer and employee regarding terms of employment
   a. Written and signed contract
   b. Includes position description, hours, amount and method of remuneration, benefits, method of evaluation, contract severance, merit raises, and professional advancement

F. Practice arrangements
   1. Partnership—association of two or more persons for the purpose of conducting business
      a. Partners share equally in the profits, expenses, and debts
      b. Partners share equally in liability, one for the other
      c. Partners share equally in liability for acts of employees
      d. Partnership agreement may be verbal or written
      e. Partnerships are dissolved on the loss of any partner
   2. Corporation—single persons or associations of two or more persons for the purpose of conducting business
      a. Members are employees of the corporation
      b. Members are protected from the negligence of the others; only the member involved in the negligence and the corporation are liable
      c. Members of the corporation are not liable for the acts of other employees of the corporation
      d. Articles of incorporation must be written and filed with the state
      e. Corporation continues even if a member is lost
      f. Corporation is subject to regulation by the state
   3. Employee practitioner—a dental hygienist who provides dental hygiene services as an employee in accordance with the state dental hygiene/dental practice act[12]
   4. Independent contractor—a dental hygienist who has a business arrangement consistent with Internal Revenue Service and state requirements, whereby the dental hygienist contracts to provide dental hygiene services in accordance with the state dental hygiene/dental practice act[12]
      a. Receive a fee for service rather than a salary
      b. Are not employees per se; receive no benefits or salary
      c. Independently make judgments and perform techniques to achieve the specified result
   5. Independent practitioner—a dental hygienist who provides dental hygiene services to the public through direct agreement with each client in accordance with the state dental hygiene/dental practice act[12]
      a. May be the proprietor of a place necessary to perform dental hygiene services
      b. May purchase, own, or lease equipment necessary to perform dental hygiene services

Regulation of the Practice of Dental Hygiene

A. Practice acts versus rules and regulations[2,18,19]
   1. The practice of a licensed profession is governed in each legal jurisdiction by
      a. A practice act (statute)—enacted into law by state legislatures; defines the practitioner's relationship with the public
      b. Rules and regulations—written, adopted, and promulgated by the state agency or board that regulates the profession and defines the scope of practice
   2. The statute and rules and regulations governing a profession are used to define how the profession is regulated
   3. The statute always takes precedence over the rules and regulations during the governing of a profession
   4. Rules and regulations may not conflict with the statute
   5. In most states the profession of dental hygiene is regulated by dental practice acts and boards of dentistry (also known as boards of dental examiners)
   6. In general, state dental practice acts including rules and regulations
      a. Provide for a board of dental examiners empowered to regulate the practice of dentistry and dental hygiene within the state
      b. Set criteria for licensure and the renewal thereof
         (1) Educational requirements
         (2) Competence examination and procedures thereof
         (3) Licensure by endorsement requirements (if applicable)
      c. Set grounds for revocation of a license

d. Specify duties permitted by the respective professions
   (1) Duties permitted may be listed; these are called list regulations
   (2) Duties permitted may be left open to interpretation by the supervising professional; these are called open regulations
e. Specify supervision requirements for dental hygienists and dental assistants

B. Boards of dental examiners[18,19]
   1. Are appointed or elected officials who are
      a. Dentists
      b. Dental hygienist representatives
      c. Consumer representatives in many states
      d. Others such as dental assistants or denturists
   2. Regulate application for licensure
   3. Implement mechanisms for measuring competence of prospective registrants (e.g., licensing examinations or boards)
   4. Implement mechanisms for investigating complaints made against practitioners
   5. Are empowered to grant and revoke licenses
   6. Draft laws pertaining to dentistry and dental hygiene, which must be enacted by state legislatures
   7. Design the rules and regulations pertaining to the practice of dentistry and dental hygiene that augment the practice acts
   8. Monitor educational standards in dental hygiene education programs
   9. Issue licenses and monitor completion of related documentation, e.g., mandatory continuing education requirements

C. Boards of dental hygiene examiners
   1. The state of Washington regulates dental hygiene practice through a Dental Hygiene Examining Committee
      a. Established in 1983
      b. Serves the same function as a board of dental examiners
      c. Is composed of three dental hygienists appointed by the governor
      d. Regulates all matters relating to examinations and licensure of dental hygienists
      e. Determines subject matter and scope of the written and practical examinations
      f. Serves as an advisor to the Secretary of the Department of Health
   2. New Mexico maintains a committee that has complete authority for the regulation of dental hygiene
      a. Established in 1994
      b. Serves the same function as a board of dental examiners
      c. Is composed of five dental hygienists appointed by the governor

D. State dental hygiene committees
   1. Several states maintain dental hygiene committees whose functions are advisory in nature to the state board of dentistry; with the exception of Maryland, dental hygiene committee members usually are not members of the board of dentistry (dental regulatory board)
   2. States that have a state dental hygiene committee:
      a. Arizona, Delaware, Florida, Texas—advisory committee to the dental regulatory board
      b. California—administrative committee of the dental board
      c. Maryland—committee of the dental board

E. Representation on state dental boards[19]
   1. The ratio of dental hygienists to dentists in state licensing and regulatory boards is indicated in Table 18-1
   2. The voting power accorded to dental hygienists is indicated in Table 18-1

F. Definitions of supervision in practice acts[5]
   1. Supervision titles used in various states based on practice acts:
      a. General supervision/assignment—supervision whereby a licensed dentist authorizes the procedures that are being carried out in accordance with the diagnosis and treatment plan but need not be physically present in the dental facility; some states require that the dentist must be able to be contacted for consultation or have a designated dentist to be available
      b. Indirect/close supervision—supervision whereby a licensed dentist authorizes the procedures and remains in the dental facility while the procedures are being performed
      c. Direct/immediate supervision—supervision whereby a licensed dentist diagnoses the condition to be treated, authorizes the procedures to be performed, and remains on the premises while the work is being performed before dismissal of the patient; some states do not require a dentist to approve the work before dismissal of the patient
      d. Personal supervision—supervision whereby a licensed dentist is personally operating on a patient and authorizes the auxiliary to aid treatment by concurrently performing supportive procedures
      e. Unsupervised practice—dental hygiene services may be performed by licensed dental hygienists without the supervision of a licensed dentist
   2. These definitions vary somewhat from jurisdiction to jurisdiction

G. State supervision requirement for dental hygienists[2]
   1. Twenty-two states require the physical presence of a

Table 18-1

Licensee Populations and State Board Representation

State	RDH licensee population	DDS license population	#RDH board members	#DDS state board members	#Consumer board members	Other board members	RDH term of office
AL	2492	1742	1	5	0		5 years
AK	378	538	2	6	1		4 years
AZ	1268	1970	2	6	3		4 years
AR	620	1280	1	6	2		5 years
CA	12075	22501	1	8	4	1 dental assistant	4 years
CO	2488*	4387*	2	4	3		4 years
CT	2929*	2939*	0†	5	0		
DE	485*	365*	1	5	3		3 years
DC	NOT AVAILABLE		1	5	1		3 years
FL	7463*	10004*	2	7	2		4 years
GA	4731*	4714*	1	9	1		5 years
HI	417	908	2	9	2		4 years
ID	420	646	2	6	1		5 years
IL	5058*	9748*	1	8	1		4 years
IN	2109	2778	1	9	1		3 years
IA	912	1588	2	5	2		3 years
KS	823	1225	1	3	1		4 years
KY	1007	2052	1	7	1		4 years
LA	901	2012	1	13	0		5 years
ME	694	616	1	5	1		5 years 4 years
MD	1899	3717	3	9	2		4 years
MA	5108*	6881*	1	6	1	2 dental assistants	5 years
MI	7585*	7932‡	1§	7	2	2 dental assistants	4 years
MN	2985*	3841*	1	5	2	1 dental assistant	4 yeras
MS	498	1098	1§	7	0		4 years
MO	2076*	4236*	1§	5	1		5 years
MT	282	492	1	5 (1 non-voting)	2	1 denturist	5 years
NE	496	1096	2	6	2		5 years
NV	500	573	2§	7	1		3 years
NH	811	806	2	6	1		5 years
NJ	3653	6301	1	8	2	1 attorney	4 years
NM	521	658	5 (2 dh on board, 3 dh on committee)	5 (4 DDS on board, 1 DDS on committee)	2 on board, 1 on RDH committee		5 years

State licensee populations based on 1994 figures
*Reflects total licensees-licensed and residing figures not available
†Connecticut dental hygienists are regulated by the Department of Public Health and Addiction Services.
‡Includes 1,000 dentist specialists
§Dental hygienist member has restricted voting privileges
¶Legislation on governor's desk to add board members
From American Dental Hygienist's Association, Unpublished document titled Dental hygiene legislative activity 1985 to 1995.

Continued.

Table 18-1

Licensee Populations and State Board Representation—cont'd

State	RDH licensee population	DDS license population	#RDH board members	#DDS state board members	#Consumer board members	Other board members	RDH term of office
NY	8972	17508	3	13	3		5 years
NC	2559	2726	1§	6	1		3 years
ND	379*	300	1	5	1		5 years
OH	5523*	7850*	1	5	1		5 years
OK	885	1571	1	8	2		3 years
OR	1708	2100	2	6	1		4 years
PA	5140	8685	1	7	2		6 years
RI	822*	899*	2	7	4		3 years
SC	1141	1507	1§	7	1		6 years
SD	265	352	1	5	1		5 years
TN	2437*	3551*	1	6	0	1 dental assistant	3 years
TX	8664	11000+*	2	10	6		2 years 4 years
UT	270*	1875*	2¶	6¶	1		5 years
VT	429	346	2	5	2		5 years
VA	2058	3614	2	7	1		4 years
WA	3348	3448	3 (RDH exam committee, not attached to board)	12 (dental discipline board)	1 on committee, 2 on board		3 years
WV	685	939	1	5	1		5 years
WI	2839	3424	1	5	2		4 years
WY	174	244	1§	5	0		4 years

dentist during dental hygiene procedures (direct supervision); although Oklahoma officially has direct supervision, the dentist may be absent for 24 hours at a time

2. Thirty-two states do not require that a dentist be physically present during traditional dental hygiene procedures in private practice (general supervision)

3. Eleven states require direct supervision for dental hygiene practice in offices but general supervision or unsupervised practice in hospitals and long-term care facilities

4. Six states permit unsupervised practice with or without dental supervision based on stipulations in practice act: Michigan (Board approved settings), Wisconsin (Public Health Settings), Colorado (all settings), Connecticut (range of settings), Washington State (long-term care settings), California (HMPP Program)

5. Twenty-three states permit dental hygienists to administer local anesthesia (Alaska, Arizona, Arkansas, California, Colorado, Hawaii, Idaho, Kansas, Maine, Minnesota, Missouri, Montana, Nebraska, Nevada, New Mexico, Oklahoma, Oregon, South Carolina, South Dakota, Utah, Vermont, Washington, Wyoming) all states except one (Oregon) require the procedure to be completed under direct supervision

H. Professional licensure
1. Definition—licensing is "the process by which an agency of government grants permission to an individual to engage in a given occupation upon finding that the applicant has attained the minimal degree of competency necessary to be reasonably well protected" (US Department of Health Education and Welfare, 1977)

2. Dentists and dental hygienists are licensed in every state and the District of Columbia; requirements for licensure vary from jurisdiction to jurisdiction

3. States requiring continuing education for dental hygiene license renewal:
   - Alabama—1991
   - Alaska—1991
   - Arkansas—1994
   - Arizona—1995
   - California—1974
   - Connecticut—1987
   - Delaware—1988
   - District of Columbia—1988
   - Florida—1980
   - Georgia—1992
   - Idaho—1994
   - Illinois—1992
   - Indiana—1992
   - Iowa—1979
   - Kansas—1978
   - Kentucky—1978
   - Louisiana—1994
   - Maine—1991
   - Maryland—1992
   - Massachusetts—1982
   - Michigan—1994
   - Minnesota—1969
   - Mississippi—1994
   - Missouri—1994
   - Montana—1993
   - Nebraska—1985
   - Nevada—1985
   - New Hampshire—1988
   - New Jersey—1979
   - New Mexico—1979
   - New York—1997
   - North Carolina—1994
   - North Dakota—1976
   - Ohio—1992
   - Oklahoma—1980
   - Oregon—1988
   - Pennsylvania—1999
   - Rhode Island—1992
   - South Carolina—1994
   - South Dakota—1974
   - Tennessee—1991
   - Texas—1995
   - Utah—1996
   - Vermont—1992
   - Virginia—1995
   - Washington—1991
   - West Virginia—1992

I. State restriction requirements for employment of dental hygienists[2]
   1. Thirteen states allow only two dental hygienists to practice per dentist in an office (Arizona, District of Columbia, Illinois, Kentucky, New Jersey, New Mexico, North Carolina, Oklahoma, Oregon, Texas, Utah, Virginia, Washington)
   2. Ohio is the only state that allows three dental hygienists per dentist to practice in an office
   3. All remaining states have no restrictions on the number of dental hygienists that may be employed per dentist

REFERENCES

1. Motley WE: *History of the American Dental Hygienists' Association:* 1923-1982, Chicago, 1986, The Association.
2. American Dental Hygienists' Association Governmental Affairs Division: *A comparative overview of 51 practice acts,* Legislative Action Packet Series, Chicago, 1993, The Association.
3. Perry DA, Freed JR, Kushman JE: The California demonstration project in independent practice, *J Dent Hyg* 68(3):137-142, 1994.
4. American Dental Association, Council on Dental Education, Commission on Dental Accreditation: *Comprehensive policy statement on dental auxiliaries,* Chicago, 1987, The Association.
5. American Dental Hygienists' Association: ADHA study refutes shortage claims, *Access* 3:5, 1989.
6. American Dental Hygienists' Association: Stateline, *Access* 3:2, 1989.
7. American Dental Hygienists' Association: Stateline, *Access* 3:4, 1989.
8. American Dental Hygienists' Association: Stateline, *Access* 3:5, 1989.
9. American Dental Hygienists' Association: *Preceptorship and the registered dental hygienist,* Chicago, 1993, The Association.
10. Bader J, et al: Task force on innovation in dental hygiene curricula, *J Dent Educ* 53:731, 1989.
11. American Dental Hygienists' Association: *Association policy manual,* Chicago, 1997, The Association.
12. Brownstone E: Canadian Dental Hygienists' Association, personal communication, April 1997.
13. Johnson P: Self-regulation for dental hygienists—the Canadian example, *J Dent Hyg* 63:29, 1989.
14. Darby ML: Theory development and basic research in dental hygiene: Review of the literature and recommendations, American Dental Hygienists' Association document, Chicago, 1990.
15. Deck S, Nielsen-Thompson N, Walsh M: The ADHA framework for theory development, *J Dent Hyg* 67:166, 1993.
16. American Dental Hygienists' Association, *Bylaws—code of ethics,* Chicago, 1995, The Association.
17. American Association of Dental Examiners: *Composite,* Chicago, 1997, The Association.
18. American Dental Hygienists' Association, unpublished document titled Dental hygiene legislative activity 1985-1995, Chicago, 1995.

SUGGESTED READINGS

American Dental Hygienists' Association: *Prospectus for dental hygiene,* Chicago, 1988, The Association.

American Dental Hygienists' Association: *Bylaws—principles of ethics,* Chicago, 1995, The Association.

Darby ML, Walsh MM: *Dental hygiene theory and practice,* Philadelphia, 1995, WB Saunders.

Fales MJ: History of dental hygiene education in the United States, 1913-1975, unpublished dissertation, Ann Arbor, 1975, University of Michigan.

Kerner J, et al: The effect of extended functions legislation on dental hygiene education and practice in California, *Dent Hyg* 61:46, 1987.

Monagle JF: *Risk management: A guide for health care professionals,* Rockville, Md, 1985, Aspen Publications.

Motley WE: *Ethics, jurisprudence, and history for the dental hygienist,* ed 3, Philadelphia, 1983, Lea & Febiger.

Odrich J: Education and regulation: The tangled web, *Dent Hyg* 61:461, 1987.

Pollack BR: *Handbook of dental jurisprudence and risk management,* Littleton, Colo, 1987, PSG Publishing.

Tate PS, Schieling-Wilkes J, Frese P: Practice acts and legislation: An historical perspective, *Dent Hyg* 61:469, 1987.

Weinstein BD: *Dental ethics,* Philadelphia, 1993, Lea & Febiger.

Zarkowski P: Ethical and legal decision making in dental hygiene. In Darby ML, Walsh MM: *Dental hygiene theory and practice,* Philadelphia, 1995, WB Saunders.

Review Questions

1 The members of the dental profession who first suggested the need for a new specialty in dentistry devoted to prevention intended to develop a group of professionals who would
   A. Go on to dental school
   B. Become dentists eventually
   C. Become independent practitioners
   D. Improve the oral health of schoolchildren
   E. Perform services the dentists did not have the expertise to perform

2 The "father" of dental hygiene is considered to be
   A. Dr. A.C. Fones
   B. Dr. T.P. Hyatt
   C. Dr. G.A. Mills
   D. Dr. M.L. Rhein
   E. Dr. D.D. Smith

3 The "father" of dental hygiene really wanted to call practitioners in the new dental specialty
   A. Dental aides
   B. Odontocurists
   C. Dental nurses
   D. Dental hygienists
   E. Subspecialty dentists

4 The first state to license dental hygienists was
   A. Ohio
   B. New York
   C. California
   D. Connecticut
   E. Massachusetts

5 Irene Newman was all of the following *EXCEPT*
   A. Dr. A.C. Fones' assistant
   B. President of the Connecticut Dental Hygienists' Association
   C. The first president of the American Dental Hygienists' Association
   D. The first licensed dental hygienist in the United States
   E. A member of the first dental hygiene class conducted in Bridgeport, Conn.

6 The American Dental Hygienists' Association held its first meeting in
   A. 1913
   B. 1923
   C. 1935
   D. 1941
   E. 1943

7 During World War II dental hygienists working for the armed forces were given the status of
   A. Volunteers
   B. Commissioned officers
   C. Private practitioners
   D. Civil service employees
   E. Noncommissioned officers

8 The Forsyth research project to evaluate the feasibility of dental hygienists performing restorative procedures was terminated because of
   A. Lack of funding
   B. Lack of interest
   C. Opposition of local dentists
   D. Opposition of the federal government
   E. Opposition of the citizens of Massachusetts

9 The first central office of the American Dental Hygienists' Association was established in 1948 in
   A. New York City
   B. Washington, D.C.
   C. Cleveland, Ohio
   D. Chicago, Ill.
   E. Boston, Mass.

10 The last state within the continental United States to grant dental hygiene licensure was
   A. Texas
   B. Maine
   C. Oregon
   D. Virginia
   E. New York

11 Until 1964 one group was excluded from dental hygiene licensure in most states and from membership in the American Dental Hygienists' Association. This group was made up of
A. Men
B. African-Americans
C. Women
D. Native Americans
E. Foreign-trained dental hygienists

12 The office that monitors legislation of interest for the American Dental Hygienists' Association is the
A. Chicago office
B. Central office
C. New York office
D. Washington office
E. Bridgeport office

13 The American Dental Hygienists' Association sponsored the First International Symposium on Dental Hygiene in 1970 in
A. Italy
B. France
C. England
D. The United States
E. Australia

14 The Commission on Accreditation of Dental and Dental Auxiliary Programs (now known as the Commission on Dental Accreditation) was established in 1973 by the
A. American Dental Association
B. Council on Allied Health Education
C. American Dental Hygienists' Association
D. Council on Medical and Dental Education
E. American Association of Dental Schools

15 The last state to allow preceptor training in lieu of formal training was
A. Texas
B. Oregon
C. Alabama
D. Kentucky
E. Massachusetts

16 HY-PAC was initiated in 1978 and stands for
A. Hygiene Policy Advisory Committee
B. Hygiene Planning Alliance Commission
C. Hygiene Pilot Articulation Committee
D. Hygienists' Political Action Committee
E. Hygiene Program Accreditation Committee

17 The first state to pass legislation permitting unsupervised practice of dental hygiene in all settings was
A. California
B. Colorado
C. Maine
D. Oregon
E. Washington

18 By 1997 there were approximately 225 dental hygiene programs in operation; most of these are in
A. Universities
B. Proprietary schools
C. Academic health centers
D. Senior colleges and institutions
E. Community colleges and technical institutions

19 The federal agency that proposed nullification of state restrictions that require dental hygienists to work under the supervision of a dentist was the
A. Federal Trade Commission
B. Council of State Governors
C. National Institutes of Health
D. Department of Health and Human Services
E. Department of Health, Education, and Welfare

20 The official journal of the American Dental Hygienists' Association is called
A. *Directions*
B. *Access*
C. *Dental Hygiene*
D. *The Journal of the American Dental Hygienists' Association*
E. *Journal of Dental Hygiene*

21 The document that describes the mission and goals of the American Dental Hygienists' Association is the
A. Bylaws
B. Charter
C. Constitution
D. Practice Act
E. Code of Ethics

22 The detailed rules for governing the American Dental Hygienists' Association are found in the
A. Bylaws
B. Charter
C. Practice Act
D. Constitution
E. Code of Ethics

23 The mission of the American Dental Hygienists' Association includes all the following *EXCEPT*
A. To improve the public's total health
B. To increase awareness of the cost-effective benefits of prevention
C. To ensure access to quality oral healthcare
D. To increase the membership of the American Dental Hygienists' Association to represent the majority of licensed dental hygienists

24 The Code of Ethics outline the moral obligations of
A. The House of Delegates only
B. The officers of the association only
C. The members of boards of dental examiners
D. Each individual member of the American Dental Hygienists' Association
E. The American Dental Hygienists' Association as an organization

25 The policy-making body of the American Dental Hygienists' Association is the
A. Central Office
B. Executive Board
C. Board of Trustees
D. Washington Office
E. House of Delegates

26 There are two major functional governing bodies of the American Dental Hygienists' Association; one is responsible for policy and the other for administration. They are the
   A. Districts and the components
   B. Constituents and the components
   C. State and local associations
   D. Constituents and the Council of Presidents
   E. House of Delegates and the Board of Trustees

27 The Board of Trustees of the American Dental Hygienists' Association
   A. Is self-perpetuating
   B. Appoints the President
   C. Is the legislative body of the association
   D. Is presided over by the Speaker of the House
   E. Is the administrative body of the Association

28 The House of Delegates of the American Dental Hygienists' Association
   A. Hires the staff
   B. Reports to the Executive Director
   C. Is the legislative body of the association
   D. Is the administrative body of the association
   E. Conducts the business affairs of the association

29 The House of Delegates of the American Dental Hygienists' Association has the responsibility for all of the following *EXCEPT*
   A. The election of the President
   B. Setting the policies of the Association
   C. Approving the budget of the Association
   D. The election of the Speaker of the House
   E. The administrative affairs of the Association

30 In order to be a member of the American Dental Hygienists' Association, a dental hygienist must hold membership at each level, with the *EXCEPTION* of the
   A. Local level
   B. District level
   C. National level
   D. Component level
   E. Constituent level

31 An individual, not a dental hygienist, who has gained recognition for contributions to the art and science of dental hygiene may become a (an)
   A. Allied member of the American Dental Hygienists' Association
   B. Active member of the American Dental Hygienists' Association
   C. Associate member of the American Dental Hygienists' Association
   D. Honorary member of the American Dental Hygienists' Association
   E. Retired member of the American Dental Hygienists' Association

32 The President of the American Dental Hygienists' Association presides over the Board of Trustees and is
   A. Elected by the district trustees
   B. Elected by the House of Delegates
   C. Elected by the general membership
   D. Appointed by the Board of Trustees
   E. Appointed by the Executive Director

33 The Speaker of the House is elected by the House of Delegates and presides over the
   A. District meetings
   B. House of Delegates
   C. Component meetings
   D. Council of Presidents
   E. International Liaison Council

34 Members of the American Dental Hygienists' Association have influence over its policies through
   A. The Washington lobbyist
   B. Trustee representation on the Board of Trustees
   C. A direct or referendum vote on each issue or policy
   D. Delegate representation in the House of Delegates
   E. The state president, who sits on the Council of Presidents

35 The Executive Director is responsible for the day-to-day administrative operation of the American Dental Hygienists' Association and is
   A. Appointed by the President
   B. Elected by the membership
   C. Elected by the House of Delegates
   D. Appointed by the Board of Trustees
   E. Appointed by the Council of Presidents

36 Members of the American Dental Hygienists' Association have representation on the Board of Trustees through the district trustee, who is
   A. Elected by local vote
   B. Appointed by the President
   C. Elected by the membership
   D. Appointed by the Executive Director
   E. Elected by delegates from the constituents

37 An appointed official of the American Dental Hygienists' Association is the
   A. District trustee
   B. Vice-President
   C. President
   D. Secretary
   E. Executive Director

38 The study of moral conduct based on theory is known as
   A. Mores
   B. Ethics
   C. Morals
   D. Values
   E. Value clarification

39 Valuing a healthy lifestyle is an example of attitudes or beliefs that represent
   A. Value judgment
   B. Terminal values
   C. Intrinsic values
   D. Extrinsic values
   E. Instrumental values

40 When personally held values are not congruent with those held by the profession or peers, this may result in
   A. Value judgment
   B. Terminal values
   C. Values dissonance
   D. A hierarchy of values
   E. Values clarification

41 Moral reasoning is characterized by
 A. Mores
 B. Feelings
 C. Behavior
 D. Cognitive judgment
 E. Beliefs and attitudes

42 In Kohlberg's hierarchy of moral development the final, or postconventional, level is reached by
 A. No adults
 B. All adults
 C. Few adults
 D. All adolescents
 E. All adolescents and adults

43 In Kohlberg's hierarchy of moral development, stage 4, the law-and-order orientation, is found in the
 A. Conventional level
 B. Preconventional level
 C. Postconventional level
 D. Preconventional and conventional levels
 E. Conventional and postconventional levels

44 If you say, "The ends justify the means," you are thinking as a
 A. Theorist
 B. Legalist
 C. Utilitarian
 D. Kohlbergian
 E. Deontologist

45 If you say, "It's the principle of the thing," you are thinking as a
 A. Theorist
 B. Legalist
 C. Utilitarian
 D. Kohlbergian
 E. Deontologist

46 A person who concentrates on principles and rules in general as they apply to types or classes of actions is a (an)
 A. Legalist
 B. Act utilitarian
 C. Act deontologist
 D. Rule utilitarian
 E. Rule deontologist

47 The person who focuses on the outcome of a single act under specific circumstances is a (an)
 A. Legalist
 B. Act utilitarian
 C. Rule utilitarian
 D. Act deontologist
 E. Rule deontologist

48 The principle that states, "Above all, do no harm" is the principle of
 A. Justice
 B. Autonomy
 C. Veracity
 D. Beneficence
 E. Nonmaleficence

49 The ethical principle that requires health professionals to fully inform their patients and protect the confidentiality of the patients is the principle of
 A. Justice
 B. Autonomy
 C. Veracity
 D. Beneficence
 E. Nonmaleficence

50 When resources are scarce and treatment is allocated only to those who have earned it, this is an example of distributive justice based on
 A. Need
 B. Merit
 C. Equity
 D. Effort
 E. Contribution

51 Suppose a dental hygienist performs treatment that is not within the legal limits of dental hygiene. Although the client is not injured by the treatment, this can be considered
 A. A civil wrong
 B. A federal crime
 C. A criminal wrong
 D. Both a civil and a criminal wrong
 E. Neither a civil nor a criminal wrong

52 Statutory law includes all *EXCEPT* which of the following
 A. State legislation
 B. Dental practice acts
 C. The US Constitution
 D. Previous court decisions
 E. Amendments to the US Constitution

53 Common law is all *EXCEPT* which of the following
 A. Unwritten
 B. Statutory
 C. Made by judges
 D. Based on custom
 E. Based on previous court decisions

54 A dental professional may be criminally liable if the tort he or she commits is
 A. Accidental
 B. Intentional
 C. Contributory
 D. Unintentional
 E. Caused by negligence

55 The legal area covered by the term *tort* usually applies to
 A. Property
 B. Civil offenses
 C. Practice agreements
 D. Contract agreements
 E. Dental practice acts

56 The act that directly results in an injury, and without which the injury would not have occurred, is known in law as
 A. *Res gestae*
 B. *Stare decisis*
 C. Proximate cause
 D. Breach of contract
 E. *Respondeat superior*

57 Intentionally defaming someone in writing is known as
   A. Libel
   B. Fraud
   C. Assault
   D. Slander
   E. Battery

58 The oral health professional's relationships with individual clients are governed by
   A. Civil law
   B. Common law
   C. Federal law
   D. Criminal law
   E. Military law

59 Suppose a dental hygienist, without the employer's knowledge, uses the office after hours to render preventive services to a friend and the treatment results in injury to the friend. Who would be held liable?
   A. The employer
   B. All three parties
   C. The dental hygienist
   D. The employer and the hygienist
   E. The friend under contributory negligence

60 The application of the Doctrine of *Res ipsa loquitur* places a burden of proof on
   A. The court
   B. The plaintiff
   C. The defendant
   D. The expert witness
   E. Both the plaintiff and the defendant

61 Suppose a dental hygienist is employed by and working for Dr. A., who pays her salary and benefits. She is loaned to Dr. B for a day while Dr. B's hygienist is sick. While working in Dr. B's office, the hygienist cuts a client's tongue. In addition to the hygienist, who would be liable?
   A. Dr. A
   B. Dr. B
   C. Both Dr. A. and Dr. B
   D. Neither Dr. A nor Dr. B
   E. The dental hygienist alone

62 The name given to the principle that states that a case, once tried, cannot be retried for the same offense is
   A. *Res gestae*
   B. *Res judicata*
   C. *Stare decisis*
   D. *Res ipsa loquitur*
   E. Statute of limitations

63 The use of unsterilized instruments renders an oral healthcare professional liable for malpractice
   A. Under all circumstances
   B. If the client contributes to the negligence
   C. If the assistant testifies that the instruments were unsterile
   D. If the client is injured as a result of the unsterilized instruments
   E. If the client sees the oral healthcare professional drop the instrument on the floor

64 A physician or dentist is responsible for the negligent acts of his or her employees
   A. At all times
   B. In the general course of employment
   C. When in the presence of clients
   D. Only when carrying out specific instructions
   E. When the employee acts on his or her own initiative

65 An oral healthcare professional may legally discontinue treatment
   A. By moving out of town
   B. Under no circumstances
   C. By refusing to give further appointments
   D. By refunding any money collected for the treatment
   E. By referring the client to another qualified practitioner

66 The most important question in a malpractice suit is whether the practitioner
   A. Was experienced
   B. Had an assistant
   C. Exercised due care
   D. Had advanced training
   E. Had been in practice for 2 years

67 All *EXCEPT* which of the following must occur in a case of negligence?
   A. The duty is breached
   B. A procedure is omitted
   C. The breach of duty caused the injury
   D. There is injury to the patient
   E. There is a duty owed by the practitioner to the patient

68 In a case of proven contributory negligence the
   A. Court becomes liable
   B. Parents become liable
   C. Client becomes liable
   D. Health professional remains liable
   E. Health professional is relieved of liability

69 The statute of limitations for bringing a malpractice suit against a practitioner because of a negligent act committed against an adult may
   A. Be 1 year
   B. Start at the time an injury is discovered
   C. Be 6 years
   D. Be 10 years
   E. Be 12 years

70 A civil complaint may be made by a client against an oral health professional who performs unauthorized care. Such touching without consent is known as
   A. Fraud
   B. Slander
   C. Battery
   D. Technical assault
   E. Breach of contract

71 In law, an acceptable defense against malpractice is
   A. Good faith
   B. High ethics
   C. Reasonable skill and care
   D. The practitioner's education
   E. The practitioner's reputation

72 In considering the liability of an oral health professional for technical assault, which of the following is *MOST* relevant?
A. There was no charge for the service
B. The treatment performed was exploratory
C. The client benefited from the treatment
D. The client had not consented to the treatment
E. The oral health professional was well trained and skillful

73 Expressed contracts differ from implied contracts in that expressed contracts
A. Are always written
B. Have specified terms
C. Are not legally binding
D. Are general understandings
E. Are in effect for only 1 year

74 If a client is injured because of the negligence of one of two partners
A. Both partners are liable
B. Neither partner is liable
C. Only the partner who caused the injury is liable
D. Everyone, including employees of the partnership, are liable
E. No one is liable because proximate cause cannot be established

75 Dental practice acts regulate the oral health professional's relationship with the
A. State
B. Consumer
C. Professional association
D. Internal Revenue Service (IRS)
E. Federal Trade Commission (FTC)

76 Dental and dental hygiene practice acts are enacted by the
A. Local courts
B. Federal courts
C. State legislatures
D. American Dental Association
E. State boards of dental examiners

77 The practice of dental hygiene is governed in each legal jurisdiction by the Practice Act (statute) and Rules and Regulations. The document that always takes precedence is the
A. Board of Dental Examiners report
B. Contract with the employer
C. Practice Act
D. Rules and Regulations
E. Scope of Practice

78 Supervision whereby a licensed dentist authorizes the procedures that are being carried out in accordance with the dentist's diagnosis and treatment plan but need not be physically present in the dental facility is known as
A. Close or indirect supervision
B. Direct or immediate supervision
C. General supervision
D. Personal supervision
E. Unsupervised practice

79 The National Board Dental Hygiene Examination is recognized by all the United States licensing jurisdictions including all 50 states, the District of Columbia, Puerto Rico, and the Virgin Islands
A. True
B. False

80 Which agency is responsible for the development and administration of the National Board Dental Hygiene Examination?
A. American Dental Hygienists' Association, Commission on National Dental Hygiene Examinations
B. American Dental Association, Commission on Dental Accreditation
C. American Dental Association, Commission on National Dental Examinations
D. Canadian Dental Association
E. State boards of dentistry in each licensing jurisdiction

Answers and Rationales

1. **(D)** Improvement of the oral health of schoolchildren was of major concern to the dental community and the public alike during the latter part of the nineteenth century.
   (A) Going on to dental school was not intended for the subspecialty.
   (B) Becoming dentists was not expected; in fact, women were suggested because it was thought that they would not wish to overstep the bounds of dental hygiene.
   (C) Becoming independent practitioners was not the suggestion of most proponents of the new specialty.
   (E) Dentists had the skill to provide the service but did not wish to take the time.

2. **(A)** Dr. A.C. Fones is known as the "father" of dental hygiene because he named the profession "dental hygiene" and started the first successful training program.
   (B) Dr. T.P. Hyatt proposed a new dental specialty.
   (C) Dr. G.A. Mills described the use of the explorer.
   (D) Dr. M.L. Rhein advocated preventive home care and school programs.
   (E) Dr. D.D. Smith had the first preventive practice.

3. **(D)** "Dental hygienists" was the name given to the new professionals by Dr. Fones because he wanted to stress health, not disease.
   (A) "Dental aide" indicates assistant, not specialist.
   (B) "Odontocurists" was the name suggested by F.W. Low.
   (C) "Dental nurses" was the name suggested by M.L. Rhein.
   (E) "Subspecialty dentists" was a description used by C.M. Wright.

4. **(D)** Connecticut was the first state to license dental hygienists.
   (A) Ohio was the location of the first meeting of the American Dental Hygienists' Association.
   (B) New York was the third state to license dental hygienists.
   (C) California was one of the early states, but not the first.
   (E) Massachusetts was the second state to license dental hygienists.

5. (C) The first president of the American Dental Hygienists' Association was Winifred A. Hart.
   (A) Irene Newman was Dr. A.C. Fones' assistant.
   (B) Irene Newman was the first president of Connecticut Dental Hygienists' Association.
   (D) Irene Newman was the first licensed dental hygienist in the United States.
   (E) Irene Newman was a member of the first dental hygiene class conducted by Dr. Fones.

6. (B) The first meeting of the American Dental Hygienists' Association was held in 1923.
   (A) The year the first class was accepted to Dr. Fones' program was 1913.
   (C) The year that the Social Security Act was signed into law was 1935.
   (D) The United States entered World War II in 1941.
   (E) Fluoride research began in 1943.

7. (D) Dental hygienists served as civil service employees during World War II.
   (A) Some dental hygienists may have been volunteers, but most were employed by the civil service.
   (B) The American Dental Hygienists' Association requested commissioned officer status for dental hygienists to make them comparable to nurses with similar training; this request was denied.
   (C) Dental hygienists were not private practitioners during World War II.
   (E) Dental hygienists did not generally serve as noncommissioned officers during World War II.

8. (C) The opposition of local dentists caused the Forsyth research project to be discontinued.
   (A) The project was not discontinued because of a lack of funds.
   (B) The project was not discontinued because of a lack of interest.
   (D) The project was not discontinued because of opposition by the federal government.
   (E) The project had the support of the citizens of Massachusetts.

9. (B) Washington, D.C., was the site of the first central office of the American Dental Hygienists' Association.
   (A) It was not New York.
   (C) Cleveland was the site of the first American Dental Hygienists' Association meeting.
   (D) Chicago is the current site of the central office.
   (E) Boston was the site of the Forsyth research project.

10. (A) Texas was the last state within the continental United States to license dental hygienists in 1951.
    (B) Maine licensed dental hygienists in 1917.
    (C) Oregon licensed dental hygienists in 1949.
    (D) Virginia licensed dental hygienists in 1950.
    (E) New York licensed dental hygienists in 1916.

11. (A) Men were excluded from dental hygiene licensure until 1964 in most states.
    (B) African-American women were not excluded from licensure.
    (C) Women (as opposed to men) were eligible for licensure.
    (D) Native American women were not excluded from licensure.
    (E) Foreign-trained dental hygienists as a group were not denied licensure.

12. (D) Washington, D.C., is the site of the office that monitors legislation.
    (A) Legislation is not the primary focus of the Chicago office.
    (B) The central office is located in Chicago.
    (C) There has never been an American Dental Hygienists' Association office in New York.
    (E) There has never been an American Dental Hygienists' Association office in Bridgeport, Conn.

13. (A) Italy was the site of the First International Symposium on Dental Hygiene in 1970.
    (B) France has not been a site for a symposium.
    (C) England was the site of a later conference.
    (D) The United States was the site of the Ninth International Symposium on Dental Hygiene.
    (E) Australia was not the site of the first symposium.

14. (A) The American Dental Association established the Commission on Accreditation of Dental and Dental Auxiliary Programs.
    (B) It was not established by the Council on Allied Health Education.
    (C) The American Dental Hygienists' Association has representation on the commission but is not its sponsor.
    (D) There is no "Council on Medical and Dental Education."
    (E) The American Association of Dental Schools did not establish the commission.

15. (C) Alabama was the last state to allow preceptor training.
    (A) Texas did not allow preceptor training.
    (B) Oregon did not allow preceptor training.
    (D) Kentucky did not allow preceptor training.
    (E) Massachusetts did not allow preceptor training.

16. (D) HY-PAC stands for Hygienists' Political Action Committee.
    (A) The "Hygiene Policy Advisory Committee" does not exist.
    (B) The "Hygiene Planning Alliance Commission" does not exist.
    (C) The "Hygiene Pilot Articulation Committee" does not exist.
    (E) The "Hygiene Program Accreditation Committee" does not exist.

17. (B) Colorado passed legislation in 1986 permitting the practice of dental hygiene in all settings.
    (A) Under the Health Manpower Pilot Project #139 of 1986, California allows dental hygienists to practice unsupervised in nontraditional settings.
    (C) In Maine denturists may practice independently.
    (D) In Oregon denturists may practice independently.
    (E) In Washington unsupervised practice of dental hygiene is permitted in nursing homes, hospitals, institutional settings, and public health facilities.

18. (E) Most of the dental hygiene programs are located in community colleges and technical schools.
    (A) Universities are not the site of most dental hygiene programs.
    (B) Proprietary schools are not the site of most dental hygiene programs.
    (C) Academic health centers are not the site of most dental hygiene programs.
    (D) Senior colleges are not the site of most dental hygiene programs.

19. (A) The Federal Trade Commission was the agency that proposed nullification of state restrictions regarding supervision of dental hygienists by dentists.
    (B) The Council of State Governors has produced a report recommending less supervision of licensed professionals.
    (C) The National Institutes of Health have not made any recommendations regarding supervision.
    (D) The Department of Health and Human Services has not made any recommendations regarding supervision.
    (E) The Department of Health, Education, and Welfare did not make any recommendations regarding supervision.

20. (E) *Journal of Dental Hygiene* has been the official title of the journal of the American Dental Hygienists' Association since October 1988.
    (A) *Directions* is not a journal title, but *Educational Directions* was a newsletter of the American Dental Hygienists' Association from 1976 to 1986.
    (B) *Access* has been the newsmagazine of the American Dental Hygienists' Association since 1987.
    (C) *Dental Hygiene* was the official title of the journal of the American Dental Hygienists' Association from 1972 to 1988.
    (D) *The Journal of the American Dental Hygienists' Association* was the official title from 1927 to 1972.

21. (C) The Constitution of the American Dental Hygienists' Association describes the mission and goals of the association.
    (A) The Bylaws are the rules that govern the American Dental Hygienists' Association.
    (B) A Charter applies to constituent associations that receive a Charter from the Board of Trustees.
    (D) A Practice Act refers to state law governing the practice of each dental professional.
    (E) The Code of Ethics governs the moral conduct of the members.

22. (A) The Bylaws of the American Dental Hygienists' Association are the rules that govern the association.
    (B) A Charter applies to constituent associations that receive a Charter from the Board of Trustees.
    (C) A Practice Act refers to state law.
    (D) The Constitution describes the mission and goals.
    (E) The Code of Ethics governs the moral conduct of the members.

23. (D) To increase the membership of the American Dental Hygienists' Association to represent the majority of licensed dental hygienists is not one of the stated missions of the American Dental Hygienists' Association but it is one of the *goals* of the Association.
    (A) To improve the public's total health is part of the mission statement.
    (B) To increase awareness of the cost-effectiveness of prevention is part of the mission statement.
    (C) To ensure access to quality oral healthcare is part of the mission statement.

24. (D) The Code of Ethics outlines the moral obligations of each individual member of the American Dental Hygienists' Association.
    (A) The House of Delegates is governed by the Code of Ethics in the same way that each member of the American Dental Hygienists' Association is governed.
    (B) The officers of the association are not the only members governed by the Code of Ethics.
    (C) The members of boards of dental examiners are not affected by the Code of Ethics of the American Dental Hygienists' Association unless they are dental hygienists.
    (E) The Code of Ethics pertains to individual members, not the organization per se.

25. (E) The House of Delegates is the policy-making body of the American Dental Hygienists' Association.
    (A) The Central Office assists in the administration of the organization.
    (B) The Executive Board is the entire Board of Trustees.
    (C) The Board of Trustees is the administrative body of the association.
    (D) The Washington office is responsible for legislative representation for the association.

26. (E) The House of Delegates and the Board of Trustees are the two major functional bodies of the American Dental Hygienists' Association.
    (A) The districts and the components are regional and state bodies of the American Dental Hygienists' Association.
    (B) The constituents and the components are state and local organizations.
    (C) The state and local associations are also known as the constituent and component associations, respectively.
    (D) The constituents are the state organizations, and there is no "Council of Presidents."

27. (E) The administrative body of the Association is the Board of Trustees.
    (A) The Board of Trustees is not self-perpetuating.
    (B) The President is elected by the House of Delegates.
    (C) The legislative body of the Association is the House of Delegates.
    (D) The Speaker of the House presides over the House of Delegates, whereas the President presides over the Board of Trustees.
28. (C) The legislative body of the Association is the House of Delegates.
    (A) The staff is hired by the Board of Trustees.
    (B) The Executive Director reports to the Board of Trustees.
    (D) The administrative body is the Board of Trustees.
    (E) The Board of Trustees and the Executive Director conduct the business of the Association.
29. (E) The administrative affairs of the Association are not the responsibility of the House of Delegates.
    (A) The President is elected by the House of Delegates.
    (B) The policies of the Association are set by the House of Delegates.
    (C) The House of Delegates approves the budget; the Board of Trustees prepares the budget.
    (D) The House of Delegates elects and is presided over by the Speaker of the House.
30. (B) Separate membership at the district level is not necessary because a District incorporates a number of constituents (states).
    (A) The local level is the same as the component level; components are subdivisions of state associations.
    (C) To be a member of the American Dental Hygienists' Association, a dental hygienist must hold membership at the national level.
    (D) The component level is the local level, and a dental hygienist who wishes to be a member of the American Dental Hygienists' Association must also be a member of this organization if one exists.
    (E) The constituent level is the state level, and a dental hygienist who wishes to be a member of the American Dental Hygienists' Association must also be a member of this organization.
31. (D) An honorary member of the association is one who has gained recognition for contributions to the art and science of dental hygiene but who is not a dental hygienist.
    (A) An allied member is any individual who supports the purposes and mission of the association.
    (B) An active member must be a licensed, graduate dental hygienist.
    (C) An associate member must be a dental hygienist who is practicing outside of the United States.
    (E) A retired member is a dental hygienist who had been an active member of the American Dental Hygienists' Association before retirement.

32. (B) The House of Delegates elects the President.
    (A) The district trustees are not involved with the election of the President.
    (C) The general membership does not vote per se; delegates representing the membership of each constituent sit in the House of Delegates, which elects the President.
    (D) The Board of Trustees is presided over by the President, but it does not elect the President.
    (E) The Executive Director is appointed by the Board of Trustees and does not have the power to appoint the President.
33. (B) The House of Delegates is presided over by the Speaker of the House.
    (A) District meetings are presided over by the district trustee.
    (C) Component meetings are presided over by each president of the components, respectively.
    (D) The "Council of Presidents" does not exist.
    (E) The International Liaison Council does not have a direct relationship with the Speaker of the House of the American Dental Hygienists' Association.
34. (D) Delegate representation in the House of Delegates allows the membership of the American Dental Hygienists' Association to have influence over the policies of the Association.
    (A) The Washington lobbyist provides the Association with a way to have some influence over legislative matters at the national level.
    (B) Trustee representation on the Board of Trustees allows influence over the administrative decisions but not over the policies of the Association.
    (C) Direct or referendum votes do not exist in the American Dental Hygienists' Association.
    (E) The state president has influence over the affairs of the constituent organization only, not over the American Dental Hygienists' Association; there is no "Council of Presidents."
35. (D) The Executive Director is appointed by the Board of Trustees.
    (A) The President appoints council members and chairpersons but does not appoint the Executive Director.
    (B) The membership per se does not vote on national matters.
    (C) The House of Delegates elects the President and other elected officers, but the Executive Director is not an elected officer.
    (E) There is no "Council of Presidents."
36. (E) The district trustee is elected by delegates from the constituents.
    (A) There is no local vote on issues of the American Dental Hygienists' Association.
    (B) The President appoints council members and chairpersons but not the trustees.
    (C) The membership of the American Dental Hygienists' Association votes on component officers and issues but not directly for the trustee.
    (D) The Executive Director does not make appointments.

37. (E) The Executive Director is the appointed official of the American Dental Hygienists' Association.
    (A) The district trustee is elected by and from among the delegates of the respective districts.
    (B) The Vice-President is elected by the House of Delegates.
    (C) The President assumes the presidency as a result of an earlier election by the House of Delegates.
    (D) The Secretary is elected by the House of Delegates.
38. (B) Ethics is the study of moral conduct based on theory.
    (A) Mores are the customs of a group.
    (C) Morals are standards of conduct based on ethical principles.
    (D) Values are beliefs and attitudes that motivate behavior.
    (E) Value clarification is an activity that leads to an understanding of personal thoughts and actions.
39. (E) Valuing a healthy lifestyle is an example of attitudes or beliefs that represent instrumental values (values related to a process).
    (A) Value judgment is the evaluation of the beliefs and behavior of others based on the values held by self.
    (B) Terminal values are attitudes or beliefs related to an outcome or product.
    (C) Intrinsic values are attitudes or beliefs related to the maintenance of life.
    (D) Extrinsic values are attitudes or beliefs related to alternatives not essential to life.
40. (C) Values dissonance occurs when personally held values are not congruent with those held by the profession or peers.
    (A) Value judgment occurs when one evaluates the thoughts or behavior of others based on personally held values.
    (B) Terminal values are attitudes or beliefs related to an outcome or product.
    (D) Hierarchy of values occurs when some values hold more importance than others in motivating action.
    (E) Values clarification occurs as the result of an activity that leads to an understanding of personal thought or actions.
41. (D) Cognitive judgment is a characteristic of moral reasoning and is based on thinking and experience.
    (A) Mores are customs of a group.
    (B) Feelings are unreasoned opinion or belief.
    (C) Behavior is a manner of conducting oneself.
    (E) Beliefs and attitudes constitute values and may not be based on reason or knowledge.
42. (C) Few adults reach the postconventional level of Kohlberg's hierarchy of moral development.
    (A) Not correct; some adults do reach the postconventional level. As the name implies, postconventional is beyond conventional.
    (B) Not correct; only a few adults reach this level.
    (D) Not correct; adolescents very rarely reach this level.
    (E) Not correct; few adults and very, very few adolescents reach this level.

43. (A) The conventional level contains stage 3 and stage 4. Stage 3 is the interpersonal concordance or "good boy–nice girl" stage, and stage 4 is the law-and-order stage.
    (B) The preconventional level contains stage 1 and stage 2. Stage 1 is the punishment and obedience orientation, and stage 2 is the instrument relativist orientation.
    (C) The postconventional level contains stage 5 and stage 6. Stage 5 is the social-contract legalistic orientation, and stage 6 is the universal ethical principle orientation.
    (D) Not correct; stage 4 appears only in the conventional level.
    (E) Not correct; stage 4 appears only in the conventional level.
44. (C) A utilitarian may say, "The ends justify the means" because he or she focuses on outcomes or consequences of actions.
    (A) Theorists produce and study theories; they are not particularly likely to say, "The ends justify the means."
    (B) Legalists view things from the legal standpoint; they are not likely to say, "The ends justify the means."
    (D) Kohlbergians are the followers of the theories of Kohlberg; they are not likely to say, "The ends justify the means."
    (E) Deontologists focus on principles, not consequences; they would say, "It's the principle of the thing" rather than "The ends justify the means."
45. (E) A deontologist focuses on principles, not consequences of actions. He or she may say, "It's the principle of the thing."
    (A) Theorists produce and study theories; they are not particularly likely to say, "It's the principle of the thing."
    (B) Legalists view things from the legal standpoint; they are not particularly likely to say, "It's the principle of the thing."
    (C) Utilitarians focus on the consequences of actions; they would say, "The ends justify the means" rather than "It's the principle of the thing."
    (D) Kohlbergians are the followers of the theories of Kohlberg; they are not particularly likely to say, "It's the principle of the thing."
46. (E) A rule deontologist concentrates on principles and rules in general as they apply to types or classes of actions.
    (A) Legalists concentrate on things from the legal standpoint.
    (B) Act utilitarians concentrate on the outcome of a single act.
    (C) Rule utilitarians concentrate on the outcome of types of acts.
    (D) Act deontologists consider the ethical principles involved in an action in light of the circumstances.
47. (B) An act utilitarian focuses on the outcome of a single act under specific circumstances.
    (A) Legalists focus on the legal point of view.
    (C) Rule utilitarians focus on the outcome of types of acts.
    (D) Act deontologists focus on the ethical principles involved in an action in light of the circumstances.
    (E) Rule deontologists focus on ethical principles and rules in general as they apply to types of actions.

48. (E) The principle of nonmaleficence states, "Above all, do no harm."
    (A) The principle of justice requires fairness.
    (B) The principle of autonomy requires respect for the rights of the patient.
    (C) The principle of veracity requires truthfulness.
    (D) The principle of beneficence requires the promotion of well-being.

49. (B) The principle of autonomy requires health professionals to fully inform their patients and protect their confidentiality.
    (A) The principle of justice requires fairness.
    (C) The principle of veracity requires truthfulness.
    (D) The principle of beneficence requires the promotion of well-being.
    (E) The principle of nonmaleficence states, "Above all, do no harm."

50. (D) Distributive justice based on effort would result in the allocation of treatment only to those who have earned it.
    (A) Allocation of treatment based on need would result in all who are in need receiving treatment.
    (B) Allocation of treatment based on merit would result in only those who are considered worthy of receiving treatment.
    (C) Allocation of treatment based on equity would result in each person having an equal share in or an equal chance of receiving treatment.
    (D) Allocation of treatment based on contribution would result in only those who have contributed to society receiving treatment.

51. (C) A criminal wrong occurs when a dental hygienist performs dental treatment that is not within the legal limits of dental hygiene, even if the patient is not harmed.
    (A) A civil wrong occurs when the dental hygienist is negligent and harms a patient.
    (B) A federal crime is not involved in this case because the law that delineates the limits of practice of dental hygiene is a state law.
    (D) Both a civil and a criminal wrong is not correct since the patient was not injured in this case.
    (E) Not correct; practicing dentistry without a dental license is a criminal wrong.

52. (D) Previous court decisions do not constitute statutory law.
    (A) Statutory law is written law and includes state legislation.
    (B) Dental practice acts are statutory laws.
    (C) The US Constitution is statutory.
    (E) Amendments to the US Constitution are statutory.

53. (B) Statutory law is written and therefore is not common law.
    (A) Common law is unwritten.
    (C) Common law is made by judges.
    (D) Common law is based on custom.
    (E) Common law is based on previous court decisions.

54. (B) An intentional tort may be considered a crime.
    (A) An accidental tort constitutes a civil wrong, not a crime.
    (C) A contributory tort may or may not be considered a civil wrong, but it does not constitute a crime.
    (D) An unintentional tort constitutes a civil wrong, not a crime.
    (E) A tort resulting from negligence is a civil wrong, not a crime.

55. (B) Civil offenses are the legal area usually applicable when using the term *tort*.
    (A) The term *tort* is not used in relation to a property issue.
    (C) The term *tort* is not used in relation to practice agreements.
    (D) The term *tort* is not used in relation to contract agreements.
    (E) The term *tort* is not used in relation to dental practice acts.

56. (C) *Proximate cause* is the legal term used to describe an act that directly results in an injury.
    (A) *Res gestae* admits pertinent statements made by third parties as admissible evidence.
    (B) *Stare decisis* requires judges to adhere to the precedents of prior decisions.
    (D) Breach of contract occurs when one party fails to comply with the terms of the contractual agreement.
    (E) *Respondeat superior* holds an employer liable for the negligent acts of his or her employees.

57. (A) *Libel* is the term used when one is guilty of intentionally defaming someone in writing.
    (B) *Fraud* is the term used in deception or misrepresentation with intent to take something of value from someone.
    (C) *Assault* is the term used for violent physical or verbal attack.
    (D) *Slander* is the term used for intentional verbal defamation of someone's character.
    (E) *Battery* is the term used for beating or use of force.

58. (A) Civil law governs the relationship between dental health professionals and patients.
    (B) Common law pertains to unwritten or judge-made law.
    (C) Federal law pertains to statutes promulgated by the federal government.
    (D) Criminal law pertains to acts against society.
    (E) Military law governs the actions of military personnel.

59. (C) The dental hygienist would be liable because he or she presumably did not use due care, which resulted in injury to the friend.
    (A) The employer would not be liable since he or she did not know that the office was being used.
    (B) All three parties would not be liable because the employer and the friend would not be liable.
    (D) Not correct; the employer was not aware of the incident; therefore the hygienist alone would be liable.
    (E) The friend would not be liable even though there was contributory negligence because a person cannot hold himself or herself liable.

60. (C) *Res ispa loquitur* (the thing speaks for itself) places the burden of proof on the defendant.
    (A) The court must decide the matter of facts but does not bear the burden of proof.
    (B) The plaintiff normally bears the burden of proof, but when "the thing speaks for itself," the burden of proof is shifted to the defendant.
    (D) The expert witness has the responsibility of testifying to the standard of care but does not bear the burden of proof.
    (E) The defendant alone bears the burden of proof in this case.

61. (C) Both Dr. A and Dr. B would be liable in addition to the dental hygienist: Dr. A as a result of being the employer (the Doctrine of *respondant superior* applies) and Dr. B under the Doctrine of the Borrowed Servant.
    (A) Dr. A alone would not be liable because Dr. B also would be liable.
    (B) Dr. B alone would not be liable because Dr. A also would be liable.
    (D) Not correct; both Dr. A and Dr. B would be liable.
    (E) Not correct; both Dr. A and Dr. B would be liable in addition to the dental hygienist.

62. (B) *Res judicata* states that a case once tried cannot be retried for the same offense.
    (A) *Res gestae* admits pertinent statements made by third parties at the time of the accident as admissible in court.
    (C) *Stare decisis* requires judges to adhere to the precedents of prior decisions.
    (D) *Res ipsa loquitur* shifts the burden of proof from the plaintiff to the defendant.
    (E) Statute of limitations is the limit placed on the length of time in which a suit may be initiated.

63. (D) If the client is injured as a result of the use of the unsterilized instruments, the dental professional becomes liable for malpractice.
    (A) Not correct; injury must occur in order for malpractice to exist.
    (B) Not correct; the client would not contribute to the use of unsterilized instruments.
    (C) Not correct; without injury there would be no case.
    (E) Not correct; injury must occur for a malpractice suit to be initiated.

64. (B) A physician or dentist is responsible for the negligent acts of his or her staff in the general course of employment under the Doctrine of *respondeat superior*.
    (A) A physician or dentist is not responsible for the negligent acts of his or her employee at all times.
    (C) The presence of clients has no bearing on the responsibility.
    (D) The responsibility of the physician or dentist is not limited to when the employee is carrying out specific instructions.
    (E) The physician or dentist is not responsible for the negligent acts of his or her employee when the employee acts on his or her own initiative.

65. (E) Referring the client to another qualified practitioner is the only way that a dental professional may legally discontinue treatment.
    (A) Moving out of town does not relieve the professional from responsibility unless he or she refers the client to another professional.
    (B) Not correct; the practitioner may legally refer a client to another professional.
    (C) Refusing to give further appointments is not legal unless some other arrangement can be made for the treatment or the patient has been so uncooperative as to have caused the practitioner to be unable to treat the case (contributory negligence).
    (D) Refunding any money collected for unfinished treatment does not relieve the professional from responsibility, but this should be done when a patient is referred to another qualified professional.

66. (C) The exercise of due care is the most important question in a malpractice suit.
    (A) The practitioner's experience is not as pertinent as due care.
    (B) Having an assistant is not relevant.
    (D) Having advanced training is not as pertinent as due care.
    (E) Having been in practice for 2 years is not relevant.

67. (B) A procedure being omitted is the only condition that is *not* necessary for negligence to occur.
    (A) A duty must be breached for there to be negligence.
    (C) The breach of duty must cause an injury for there to be negligence.
    (D) There must be injury to the patient for there to be negligence.
    (E) There must be a duty owed by the practitioner to the client for there to be negligence.

68. (E) The health professional is relieved of liability in the case of proven contributory negligence.
    (A) The court never becomes liable.
    (B) The parents normally do not become liable.
    (C) The client cannot assume liability because one cannot bring charges against oneself.
    (D) The health professional does not remain liable.

69. (B) The statute of limitations for an adult to bring a malpractice suit may start at the time an injury is discovered.
    (A) The usual statute of limitations is not 1 year.
    (C) The usual statute of limitations is not 6 years.
    (D) The usual statute of limitations is not 10 years.
    (E) The usual statute of limitations is not 12 years.

70. (D) Technical assault is the civil complaint made by a patient against an oral health professional who performs unauthorized treatment.
    (A) Fraud is the criminal charge in the case of deception or misrepresentation with intent to take something of value from someone.
    (B) Slander is the criminal charge in the case of intentional verbal defamation of someone's character.
    (C) Battery is the criminal charge in the case of beating or use of force.
    (E) Breach of contract is the civil complaint made when one party fails to comply with the terms of a contractual agreement.

71. (C) Reasonable skill and care is an acceptable defense against malpractice.
    (A) Good faith cannot prevent malpractice.
    (B) High ethics does not guarantee protection from malpractice.
    (D) The practitioner's education does not guarantee protection from malpractice.
    (E) The practitioner's reputation does not guarantee protection from malpractice.

72. (D) The fact that the patient had not consented to the treatment is the most relevant fact in a case of technical assault.
    (A) The fact that there was no charge for the service is not relevant.
    (B) The fact that treatment was exploratory is not relevant.
    (C) The fact that the patient benefited from the treatment is not relevant.
    (E) The fact that the dental professional was well trained and skillful is not relevant.

73. (B) Expressed contracts have specified terms.
    (A) Expressed contracts may be written or oral.
    (C) Expressed contracts are legally binding.
    (D) Expressed contracts are not general understandings but have specific terms, unlike implied contracts, which have understandings rather than specific terms.
    (E) There are no standard limits as to the length of time an expressed or an implied contract may be in effect; the contract itself usually specifies the length of time it will be in effect.

74. (A) Both partners are liable in a case where a client is injured by one of two partners.
    (B) Not correct; both partners are liable.
    (C) Not correct; this would be true in a corporation but not in a partnership.
    (D) Not correct; only the two partners are liable.
    (E) Not correct; proximate cause has been established, and one of the partners was negligent.

75. (A) The oral health professional's relationship with the state is regulated by the dental practice act.
    (B) The relationship between the oral health professional and the consumer is regulated by contract.
    (C) The relationship between the professional and the professional association is regulated by the terms of membership, the constitution, and the bylaws of the association.
    (D) The relationship between the professional and the IRS is regulated by federal tax laws.
    (E) The relationship between the professional and the FTC is regulated by the antitrust laws.

76. (C) State legislatures enact dental and dental hygiene practice acts.
    (A) Local courts uphold, but do not enact dental and dental hygiene practice acts.
    (B) The federal courts have no relationship to the practice acts.
    (D) The American Dental Association may influence the state boards of dental examiners but does not enact the dental practice acts.
    (E) State boards of dentistry draft the practice acts, which are enacted by the state legislatures.

77. (C) The Practice Act is the law and always takes precedence.
    (A) The Board of Dental Examiners report has no weight of law and does not govern practice.
    (B) The contract with the employer outlines the business arrangement between parties and must not conflict with the law.
    (D) The Rules and Regulations define the duties permitted but must not conflict with the Practice Act, which is the law.
    (E) The scope of practice is the combined duties permitted by the law and defend the rules and regulations.

78. (C) Supervision whereby a licensed dentist authorizes procedures to be carried out in accordance with the dentist's diagnosis and treatment plan but the dentist need not be physically present in the dental facility is known as general supervision.
    (A) Supervision whereby a licensed dentist authorizes the procedures and remains in the dental facility while the procedures are being performed is known as close or indirect supervision.
    (B) Supervision whereby a licensed dentist diagnoses the condition to be treated, authorizes the procedures to be performed, remains on the premises while the work is being performed, and approves work before dismissal of the patient is known as direct or immediate supervision.
    (D) Supervision whereby a licensed dentist is personally operating on a client, and authorizes the auxiliary to aid the dentist's treatment by concurrently performing supportive procedures is known as personal supervision.
    (E) Unsupervised practice means that dental hygiene services may be performed by a licensed dental hygienist without supervision of a licensed dentist.

79. (A) All US licensing jurisdictions recognize the National Board Dental Hygiene Examination; however, "preceptor" graduates of the Alabama Dental Hygiene Program (ADHP) are not eligible to take the examination.

    (B) All jurisdictions in the United States recognize the examination; therefore, this choice was inaccurate.

80. (C) The Commission on National Dental Examinations of the American Dental Association develops and administers the National Board Dental Hygiene Examination. The Commission includes 15 members representing dental schools, dental practice, state dental examining boards, dental hygiene, and the public.

    (A) The American Dental Hygienists' Association does not develop or administer the National Board Dental Hygiene Examination.

    (B) The Commission on Dental Accreditation of the American Dental Association is responsible for educational programs but does not develop or administer the National Board Dental Hygiene Examination.

    (D) The Canadian Dental Association does not develop or administer the National Board Dental Hygiene Examination in the United States; the Canadian Dental Hygienists' Association implemented a Canadian Dental Hygiene Board Examination in 1997.

    (E) State boards of dentistry administer dental hygiene licensure but do not develop or administer the National Board Dental Hygiene Examination.

APPENDIX A

Medical Terminology

Prefixes

a, ab-, abs- From; away; departing from the normal

ad- Addition to; toward; nearness

amb-, ambi- Both; ambidextrous, having the ability to work effectively with either hand

amphi- On both sides

ampho- Both

an- Negative; without or not

ana- Upper, away from

andro- Signifying man

ant-, anti- Against

ante-, antero- Front; before

bili- Pertaining to bile

brady- Slow

brom-, bromo- A stench

broncho- Relating to the bronchi

cac- Bad

cardi-, cardio- Relating to the heart

cata- Down or downward

cervico- Relating to the neck

circa- About

circum- Around

co- With or together

con- Together with

contra- Opposite; against

demi- Half

di- Twice

dia- Through

dialy- To separate

en- In

end-, endo-, ento- Inward; within

ep-, epi- On; in addition to

ex- Out; away from

exo- Without, outside of

extra- Outside of; in addition to

fibro- Relating to fibers

gaster-, gastr-, gastro- Pertaining to the stomach

hemi- Half

hemo- Relating to the blood

hepat-, hepatico-, hepato- Pertaining to the liver

heter-, hetero- Meaning other; relationship to another

homeo- Denoting likeness or resemblance

homo- Denoting sameness

hyal-, hyalo- Transparent

hyper- Above; excessive; beyond

hypo- Below; less than

ideo- Pertaining to mental images

idio- Denoting relationship to one's self or to something separate and distinct

in- Not; in; inside; within; also intensive action

infra- Below

inter- In the midst; between

intra- Within

intro- In or into

iso- Equal or alike

juxta- Of close proximity

karyo- Relating to a cell's nucleus

kypho- Humped

laryngo- Pertaining to the larynx

medi- Middle

myelo- Pertaining to the spinal cord or bone marrow

oari-, oaric- Pertaining to the ovary

omni- All

per- Through; by means of
peri- Around; about
post- Behind or after
postero- Relating to the posterior
pre- Before
pro- Before, in front of
pseudo- False
re- Back; again (contrary)
retro- Backward
semi- Half
steato- Fatty
sub- Under; near
syn- Joined together
trans- Across; over
un- Not; reversal

Suffixes

-able, -ible, -ble The power to be
-ad Toward; in the direction of
-aemia, -emia Pertaining to blood
-age Put in motion; to do
-agra Denoting a seizure, severe pain
-algia Denoting pain
-ase Forms the name of an enzyme
-blast Designates a cell or a structure
-cele Denoting a swelling
-centesis Denoting a puncture
-ectomy A cutting out
-esthesia Denoting sensation
-facient That which makes or causes
-gene, -genesis, -genetic, -genic Denoting production; origin
-gog, -gogue To make flow
-gram A tracing; a mark
-graph A writing; a record
-iasis Denoting a condition or pathologic state
-id Denoting shape or resemblance
-ite Of the nature of
-itis Denoting inflammation
-logia Denoting discourse, science, or study of
-oid Denoting form or resemblance
-oma Denoting a tumor
-osis Denoting any morbid process
-ostomosis, -ostomy, -stomy Denoting an outlet; to furnish with an opening or mouth
-plasty Denoting molding or shaping
-rhagia Denoting a discharge; usually a bleeding
-rhaphy Meaning suturing or stitching
-rhea Meaning a flow or discharge
-scopy Generally an instrument for viewing
-tomy Denoting a cutting operation
-trophy Denoting a relationship to nourishment

Combining Forms

aer-, aero- Denoting air or gas
alge-, algesi-, algo- Relating to pain
allo- Other; differing from the normal
anomalo- Denoting irregularity
arthro- Relating to a joint or joints
brevi- Short
celio- Denoting the abdomen
centro- Center
cheil-, cheilo- Denoting the lip
chol-, chole-, cholo- Relating to bile
chondr-, chondri- Relating to cartilage
chrom-, chromo- Relating to color
cole-, coleo- Denoting a sheath
colp-, colpo- Relating to the vagina
cranio- Relating to the cranium of the skull
crymo-, cryo- Denoting cold
crypt- To hide; a pit
cyano- Dark blue
cyclo- Pertaining to a cycle
cysto- Relating to a sac or cyst
cyto- Denoting a cell
dacryo- Pertaining to the lacrimal glands
dactylo- Relating to digits
dent-, dento- Relating to teeth
derma-, dermat- Relating to the skin
desmo- Relating to a bond or ligament
dextro- Right
diplo- Double; twofold
dorsi-, dorso- Referring to the back
duodeno- Relating to the duodenum
electro- Relating to electricity
encephalo- Denoting the brain
entero- Relating to the intestines
episio- Relating to the vulva
eso- Inward
esthesio- Relating to feeling or sensation
facio- Relating to the face
gangli-, ganglio- Relating to a ganglion
geno- Relating to reproduction
gero-, geronto- Denoting old age
giganto- Huge
gingivo- Relating to the gingiva or gum
gloss-, glosso- Relating to the tongue
gluco- Denoting sweetness
glyco- Relating to sugar
gnath-, gnatho- Denoting the jaw
gon- Denoting a seed
grapho- Denoting writing
hapt-, hapte-, hapto- Relating to touch or a seizure
helo- Relating to a nail or a callus
hist-, histio-, histo- Relating to tissue
holo- Relating to the whole
hydr-, hydro- Denoting water
hygro- Denoting moisture
hyl-, hyle-, hylo- Denoting matter or material
ileo-, ilio- Relating to the ileum
ipsi- Meaning self
irido- Relating to a colored circle
iso- Equal
jejuno- Referring to the jejunum
kerato- Relating to the cornea

kino- Denoting movement
labio- Pertaining to the lips
lacto- Relating to milk
laparo- Pertaining to the loin or flank
latero- Pertaining to the side
leido-, leio- Smooth
leuk-, leuko- Denoting deficiency of color
lip-, lipo- Pertaining to fat
litho- Denoting a calculus
macr-, macro- Large; long
mast-, mastro- Relating to the breast
meg-, mega- Great; large
meli- Sweet
meningo- Denoting membranes; covering the brain and spinal cord
micr-, micro- Small in size or extent
mono- One
morpho- Relating to form
multi- Many
my-, myo- Relating to muscle
myc-, mycet- Denoting a fungus
myringo- Denoting tympani or the eardrum
myx-, myxo- Pertaining to mucus
narco- Denoting stupor
naso- Relating to the nose
necro- Denoting death
neo- New
nephr-, nephro- Denoting the kidney
normo- Normal or usual
oculo- Denoting the eye
odyno- Denoting pain
oleo- Denoting oil
onco- Denoting a swelling or mass
onycho- Relating to the nails
oo- Denoting an egg
opisth-, opistho- Backward
ophthal-, ophthalmo- Pertaining to the eye
optico- Relating to the eye or vision
orchi-, orcho- Relating to the testes
oro- Relating to the mouth
ortho- Straight; right
oscillo- Denoting oscillation
osteo- Relating to the bones
ot-, oto- Denoting an egg
palato- Denoting the palate
patho- Denoting disease
pedia-, pedo- Denoting a child
perineo- A combining form for the region between the anus and scrotum or the vulva
phago- Denoting a relationship to eating
pharyngo- Pertaining to the pharynx
phleb-, phlebo- Denoting the veins
phon-, phono- Denoting sound
phot-, photo- Relating to light
phren- Relating to the mind
picr-, picro- Bitter
pilo- Denoting hair

plasmo- Relating to plasma or the substance of a cell
pneuma-, pneumono-, pneumoto- Denoting air or gas
pod-, podo- Meaning foot
poly- Many
proct-, procto- Denoting the anus and rectum
psych-, psycho- Relating to the mind
ptyalo- Denoting saliva
pubio-, pubo- Denoting the pubic region
pulmo- Denoting the lung
pupillo- Denoting the pupil
pyel-, pyelo- Denoting the pelvis
pyloro- Relating to the pylorus
py-, pyo- Denoting pus
recto- Denoting the rectum
rhin-, rhino- Denoting the nose
rrhagia- Denoting abnormal discharge
salpingo- Denoting a tube, specifically the fallopian tube
schizo- Split
sclero- Denoting hardness
scoto- Relating to darkness
sero- Pertaining to serum
sialo- Relating to saliva or the salivary glands
sidero- Denoting iron
sinistro- Left
somato- Denoting the body
somni- Denoting sleep
spasmo- Denoting a spasm
spermato-, spermo- Denoting sperm
sphero- Denoting a sphere; round
sphygmo- Denoting a pulse
splen-, spleno- Denoting the spleen
staphyl-, staphylo- Resembling a bunch of grapes
steno- Narrow; short
sterco- Denoting feces
steth-, stetho- Relating to the chest
stomato- Denoting the mouth
sym-, syn- With; along
tacho-, tachy- Swift
tarso- Relating to the flat of the foot
terato- Denoting a marvel, prodigy, or monster
thoraco- Relating to the chest
thrombo- Denoting a clot of blood
toxico-, toxo- Denoting poison
tracheo- Denoting the trachea
trichi-, tricho- Denoting hair
ur-, uro-, urono- Relating to urine
varico- Denoting a twisting or swelling
vaso- Denoting a vessel
veno- Denoting a vein
ventri-, ventro- Denoting the abdomen
vertebro- Relating to the vertebra
vesico- Denoting the bladder
viscero- Denoting the organs of the body
vivi- Denoting alive
xantho- Denoting yellow
xero- Denoting dryness

Terminology Frequently Used to Designate Body Parts Or Organs

anus Anal, ano-
arm Brachial, brachio-
blood Hem-, hemat-
chest Thoracic, thorax
ear Auricle, oto-
eye Ocular, oculo-, ophthalmo-
foot Pedal, ped-, -pod
gallbladder Chole-, chol-
head Cephalic, cephalo-
heart Cardium, cardiac, cardio-
intestines Cecum, colon, duodenum, ileum, jejunum
kidney Renal, nephric, nephro-

lip Cheil-
liver Hepatic, hepato-
lungs Pulmonary, pulmonic, pneumo-
mouth Oral, os, stoma, stomat-
muscle Myo-
neck Cervix, cervical, cervico-
penis Penile
rectum Rectal
skin Derma, integumentum
stomach Gastric, gastro-
testicle Orchio-, orchi-, orchido-
urinary bladder Cysti-, cysto-
uterus Hystero-, metra
vagina Vulvo, vaginal

Prevention of Bacterial Endocarditis: Recommendations by the American Heart Association

Adnan S. Dajani

Kathryn A. Taubert

Walter Wilson

Ann F. Bolger

Arnold Bayer

Patricia Ferrieri

Michael H. Gewitz

Stanford T. Shulman

Soraya Nouri

Jane W. Newburger

Cecilia Hutto

Thomas J. Pallasch

Tommy W. Gage

Matthew E. Levison

Georges Peter

Gregory Zuccaro

Objective—To update recommendations issued by the American Heart Association last published in 1990 for the prevention of bacterial endocarditis in individuals at risk for this disease.

From the American Heart Association, Dallas, Tex (Drs Dajani, Taubert, Wilson, Bolger, Bayer, Ferrieri, Gewitz, Shulman, Nouri, Newburger, and Hutto); American Dental Association, Chicago, Ill (Drs Pallasch and Gage); the Infectious Diseases Society of America, Alexandria, Va (Dr Levison); American Academy of Pediatrics, Elk Grove Village, Ill (Dr Peter); and American Society for Gastrointestinal Endoscopy, Manchester, Mass (Dr Zuccaro).

Reprints: Kathryn A. Taubert, PhD, Office of Science and Medicine, American Heart Association, 7272 Greenville Ave, Dallas, TX 75231.

Clinical Cardiology section editors: Bruce Brundage, MD, University of California, Los Angeles, School of Medicine; Margaret A. Winker, MD, Senior Editor, *JAMA*.

*This article is one of a series sponsored by the American Heart Association, and was originally published in JAMA 1997; 277:1794-1801.

Participants—An ad hoc writing group appointed by the American Heart Association for their expertise in endocarditis and treatment with liaison members representing the American Dental Association, the Infectious Diseases Society of America, the American Academy of Pediatrics, and the American Society for Gastrointestinal Endoscopy.

Evidence—The recommendations in this article reflect analyses of relevant literature regarding procedure-related endocarditis, in vitro susceptibility data of pathogens causing endocarditis, results of prophylactic studies in animal models of endocarditis, and retrospective analyses of human endocarditis cases in terms of antibiotic prophylaxis usage patterns and apparent prophylaxis failures. MEDLINE database searches from 1936 through 1996 were done using the root words *endocarditis, bacteremia,* and *antibiotic prophylaxis.* Recommendations in this document fall into evidence level III of the US Preventive Services Task Force categories of evidence.

Consensus Process—The recommendations were formulated by the writing group after specific therapeutic regimens were discussed. The consensus statement was subsequently reviewed by outside experts not affiliated with the writing group and by the Science Advisory and Coordinating Committee of the American Heart Association. These guidelines are meant to aid practitioners but are not intended as the standard of care or as a substitute for clinical judgment.

Conclusions—Major changes in the updated recommendations include the following: (1) emphasis that most cases of endocarditis are not attributable to an invasive procedure; (2) cardiac conditions are stratified into high-, moderate-, and negligible-risk categories based on potential outcome if endocarditis develops; (3) procedures that may cause bacteremia and for which prophylaxis is recommended are more clearly specified; (4) an algorithm was developed to more clearly define when prophylaxis is recommended for patients with mitral valve prolapse; (5) for oral or dental procedures the initial amoxicillin dose is reduced to 2 g, a follow-up antibiotic dose is no longer recommended, erythromycin is no longer recommended for penicillin-allergic individuals, but clindamycin and other alternatives are offered; and (6) for gastrointestinal or genitourinary procedures, the prophylactic regimens have been simplified. These changes were instituted to more clearly define when prophylaxis is or is not recommended, improve practitioner and patient compliance, reduce cost and potential gastrointestinal adverse effects, and approach more uniform worldwide recommendations. (*JAMA* 1997;277: 1794-1801)

ENDOCARDITIS is a life-threatening disease, although it is relatively uncommon. Substantial morbidity and mortality result from this infection, despite improvements in outcome due to advances in antimicrobial therapy and enhanced ability to diagnose and treat complications. Primary prevention of endocarditis whenever possible is therefore very important.

Endocarditis usually develops in individuals with underlying structural cardiac defects who develop bacteremia with organisms likely to cause endocarditis. Bacteremia may occur spontaneously or may complicate a focal infection (e.g., urinary tract infection, pneumonia, or cellulitis). Some surgical and dental procedures and instrumentations involving mucosal surfaces or contaminated tissue cause transient bacteremia that rarely persists for more than 15 minutes. Blood-borne bacteria may lodge on damaged or abnormal heart valves or on the endocardium or the endothelium near anatomic defects,

resulting in bacterial endocarditis or endarteritis. Although bacteremia is common following many invasive procedures, only certain bacteria commonly cause endocarditis. It is not always possible to predict which patients will develop this infection or which particular procedure will be responsible.

There are currently no randomized and carefully controlled human trials in patients with underlying structural heart disease to definitively establish that antibiotic prophylaxis provides protection against development of endocarditis during bacteremia-inducing procedures. Further, most cases of endocarditis are not attributable to an invasive procedure. The following recommendations reflect analyses of relevant literature regarding procedure-related endocarditis, including in vitro susceptibility data of pathogens causing endocarditis, results of prophylactic studies in experimental animal models of endocarditis, and retrospective analyses of human endocarditis cases in terms of antibiotic prophylaxis usage patterns and apparent prophylaxis failures.

The incidence of endocarditis following most procedures in patients with underlying cardiac disease is low. A reasonable approach for endocarditis prophylaxis should consider the following: the degree to which the patient's underlying condition creates a risk of endocarditis; the apparent risk of bacteremia with the procedure (as defined in these recommendations); the potential adverse reactions of the prophylactic antimicrobial agent to be used; and the cost-benefit aspects of the recommended prophylactic regimen. Failure to consider all of these factors may lead to overuse of antimicrobial agents, excessive cost, and risk of adverse drug reactions.

This statement provides guidelines for prevention of bacterial endocarditis. It is not intended as the standard of care or as a substitute for clinical judgment. The current recommendations are an update of those made by the committee in 1990[1] and incorporate new data and include opinions voiced by national and international experts at endocarditis meetings around the world.

Cardiac Conditions

Certain cardiac conditions are associated with endocarditis more often than others.[2] Furthermore, when endocarditis develops in individuals with underlying cardiac conditions, the severity of the disease and the ensuing morbidity can be variable. Prophylaxis is recommended in individuals who have a higher risk for developing endocarditis than the general population and is particularly important for individuals in whom endocardial infection is associated with high morbidity and mortality.

Table 1[2-22] stratifies cardiac conditions into high- and moderate-risk categories primarily on the basis of potential outcome if endocarditis occurs.

Table 1

Cardiac Conditions Associated With Endocarditis[2-22]

Endocarditis Prophylaxis Recommended

High-risk category
  Prosthetic cardiac valves, including bioprosthetic and homograft valves
  Previous bacterial endocarditis
  Complex cyanotic congenital heart disease (e.g., single ventricle states, transposition of the great arteries, tetralogy of Fallot)
  Surgically constructed systemic pulmonary shunts or conduits
Moderate-risk category
  Most other congenital cardiac malformations (other than above and below)
  Acquired valvar dysfunction (e.g., rheumatic heart disease)
  Hypertrophic cardiomyopathy
  Mitral valve prolapse with valvar regurgitation and/or thickened leaflets*

Endocarditis Prophylaxis Not Recommended

Negligible-risk category (no greater risk than the general population)
  Isolated secundum atrial septal defect
  Surgical repair of atrial septal defect, ventricular septal defect, or patent ductus arteriosus (without residua beyond 6 mos)
  Previous coronary artery bypass graft surgery
  Mitral valve prolapse without valvar regurgitation*
  Physiologic, functional, or innocent heart murmurs*
  Previous Kawasaki disease without valvar dysfunction
  Previous rheumatic fever without valvar dysfunction
  Cardiac pacemakers (intravascular and epicardial) and implanted defibrillators

*See text for further details.

High Risk

Individuals at highest risk are those who have prosthetic heart valves, a previous history of endocarditis (even in the absence of other heart disease), complex cyanotic congenital heart disease, or surgically constructed systemic pulmonary shunts or conduits.[2,3] These individuals are at a much higher risk for developing severe endocardial infection that is often associated with high morbidity and mortality.

Moderate Risk

Individuals with certain other underlying cardiac defects are at moderate risk for severe infection.[2-4] Congenital cardiac conditions listed in the moderate-risk category include the following uncorrected conditions: patent ductus arteriosus, ventricular septal defect, primum atrial septal defect, coarctation of the aorta, and bicuspid aortic valve. Acquired valvar dysfunction (e.g., due to rheumatic heart disease or collagen vascular disease) and hypertrophic cardiomyopathy are also moderate-risk conditions.

Mitral valve prolapse (MVP) is common, and the need for prophylaxis for this condition is controversial. Only a small percentage of patients with documented MVP develop complications at any age.[5-7] Mitral valve prolapse represents a spectrum of valvular changes and clinical behavior.[5-7] In view of the controversy surrounding the need for prophylaxis of the individual patient with MVP, a detailed description of the spectrum of MVP is warranted.

Normal mitral valve leaflets close at or below the plane of the mitral annulus. This closure position is controlled by the lengths of the leaflets, their attached chordae and papillary muscles, and the systolic size of the ventricle. The closure position will shift beyond the annular plane toward the left atrium, or prolapse, if the lengths of the valve apparatus, which are constant, become too large for the size of the end-systolic ventricle, which is variable and dynamic. Dehydration and tachycardia are common causes of intermittent MVP. Abnormal motion of normal mitral valves is found on echocardiographic examination in a small percentage of the adult and adolescent ambulatory population. The high prevalence of such motion abnormalities in young adults underscores that MVP is often an abnormality of volume status, adrenergic state, or growth phase and not of valve structure or function. When normal valves prolapse without leaking, as in patients with 1 or more systolic clicks but no murmurs and no Doppler-demonstrated mitral regurgitation, the risk of endocarditis is not increased above that of the normal population.[2,6,7] Antibiotic prophylaxis against bacterial endocarditis is therefore not necessary. This is because it is not the abnormal valve motion but the jet of mitral insufficiency that creates the shear forces and flow abnormalities that increase the likelihood of bacterial adherence on the valve during bacteremia.

Normal mitral valves with normal motion often have minimal leaks detectable by Doppler examination. This does not appear to increase the risk of endocarditis. In contrast, the regurgitation that occurs with structurally normal but prolapsing valves originates from larger regurgitant orifices and creates broader areas of turbulent flow. Patients with prolapsing and leaking mitral valves, evidenced by audible clicks and murmurs of mitral regurgitation or by Doppler-demonstrated mitral insufficiency, should receive prophylactic antibiotics.[7-11] This is supported by formal cost-benefit analysis.[12]

Mitral valve prolapse (MVP) also occurs in the setting of myxomatous degeneration of the mitral valve. This is a progressive disorder that has a spectrum of manifestations.[13,14] The mitral leaflets of these patients appear thickened on the echocardiogram, due to accumulations of proteoglycan deposits.[15] The amount of thickening is variable and may increase with age.[16] There is a range of valve motion in these patients as well: they may prolapse continuously or only with changes in heart rate or volume. Further, when prolapse occurs, it may or may not create valvular insufficiency. In patients of any age, myxomatous mitral valve degeneration with regurgitation is an indication for antibiotic prophylaxis.[11,17,18]

Anterior mitral valve thickening is commonly found in both competent and insufficient myxomatous mitral valves, but its presence increases the likelihood of significant mitral regurgitation.[16] Those with significant regurgitation were older and more likely to be men.[16] Other studies have shown that male sex and age older than 45 years represent increased risk for developing endocarditis.[8,10,11,19] Patients with thickened valves that do not leak on resting examination often develop regurgitation with exercise. These patients with exercise-induced mitral insufficiency have been shown to constitute a higher-risk subset for common complications (syncope, congestive heart failure, progressive regurgitation requiring valve replacement); endocarditis and cerebral embolic events, occurring far less frequently, were not demonstrated to be increased in this small series.[20] Men older than 45 years with MVP, without a consistent systolic murmur, may warrant prophylaxis even in the absence of resting regurgitation.[12,19]

Some experts feel that an audible nonejection click even without a murmur may identify patients with a potential for intermittent regurgitation and therefore a risk of developing endocarditis. While there are insufficient data on this issue, an isolated click may be an indication for more thorough evaluation of valve morphology and function, including Doppler-echocardiographic imaging or auscultation during maneuvers that elicit or augment mitral regurgitation.

While children and adolescents with MVP may have the same symptoms as adults, such as palpitations or syncope, the development of symptoms in childhood is relatively unusual. The vast majority of children with chest pain or fatigue do not have any form of heart disease, including MVP. Careful evaluation is nevertheless required in children who have isolated clinical findings, such as nonejection systolic click, since this may be the only indicator of important mitral valve abnormality requiring prophylaxis.[21] In the most recent series of reports, MVP has emerged as an important underlying diagnosis associated with endocarditis in the pediatric age group.[3,21]

A clinical approach to determination of the need for prophylaxis in individuals with suspected MVP is given in the figure on page 796.[23]

Negligible Risk

Although endocarditis may develop in any individual, including persons with no underlying cardiac defect, the negligible-risk category lists cardiac conditions in which the development of endocarditis is not higher than in the general population. Whereas in pediatric patients innocent heart murmurs may be clearly defined on auscultation, in the adult population other studies such as echocardiography may be necessary to confirm that a murmur is innocent. Individuals with innocent heart murmurs have structurally normal hearts and do not require prophylaxis.

Bacteremia-Producing Procedures

Bacteremias commonly occur during activities of daily living such as routine tooth brushing or chewing. With respect to endocarditis prophylaxis, significant bacteremias are only those caused by organisms commonly associated with endocarditis and attributable to identifiable procedures. The procedures for which prophylaxis is recommended are those known to induce such bacteremias and are discussed below. Invasive procedures performed through surgically scrubbed skin are not likely to produce such bacteremias. Many centers do employ periprocedure prophylaxis for transcatheter insertion of prosthetic devices (septal occluders and vascular coils). However, there are no data to support the use of antibiotics in the procedures. Routine cardiac catheterization and angioplasty do not require such precautions.

Dental and Oral Procedures

Poor dental hygiene and periodontal or periapical infections may produce bacteremia even in the absence of

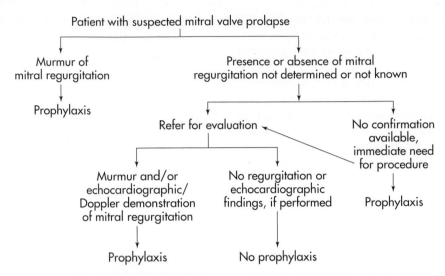

Clinical approach to determination of the need for prophylaxis in patients with suspected mitral valve prolapse. For more details on the role of echocardiography in the diagnosis of mitral valve prolapse, see the text and the 1997 American College of Cardiology/American Heart Association guidelines for the clinical application of echocardiography.[23]

dental procedures. The incidence and magnitude of bacteremias of oral origin are directly proportional to the degree of oral inflammation and infection.[24,25] Individuals who are at risk for developing bacterial endocarditis should establish and maintain the best possible oral health to reduce potential sources of bacterial seeding. Optimal oral health is maintained through regular professional care[24,26,27] and the use of appropriate dental products such as manual and powered toothbrushes, dental floss, and other plaque-removal devices. Oral irrigator or air abrasive polishing devices used inappropriately or in patients with poor oral hygiene have been implicated in producing bacteremia, but the relationship to bacterial endocarditis is unknown.[24,28-31] Home-use devices pose far less risk of bacteremia in a healthy mouth than does ongoing oral inflammation.[24,28-31]

Antiseptic mouth rinses applied immediately prior to dental procedures may reduce the incidence or magnitude of bacteremia.[24] Agents include chlorhexidine hydrochloride and povidone-iodine. Fifteen milliliters of chlorhexidine can be given to all at-risk patients via gentle oral rinsing for about 30 seconds prior to dental treatment; gingival irrigation is not recommended. Sustained or repeated frequent interval use is not indicated as this may result in the selection of resistant microorganisms.[24]

Antibiotic prophylaxis for at-risk patients is recommended for dental and oral procedures likely to cause bacteremia (Table 2[22,24-26,28-31]). In general, prophylaxis is recommended for procedures associated with significant bleeding from hard or soft tissues, periodontal surgery, scaling, and professional teeth cleaning. Similarly, antimicrobial prophylaxis is recommended for tonsillectomy or adenoidectomy. It is recognized that unanticipated bleeding may occur on some occasions. In such an event, data from experimental animal models suggest that antimicrobial prophylaxis administered within 2 hours following the procedure will provide effective prophylaxis.[32] Antibiotics administered more than 4 hours after the procedure probably have no prophylactic benefit. Procedures for which antimicrobial prophylaxis is not recommended are also listed (Table 2).

Edentulous patients may develop bacteremia from ulcers caused by ill-fitting dentures. Denture wearers should be encouraged to have periodic examination or to return to the practitioner if discomfort develops. When new dentures are inserted, it is advisable to have the patient return to the practitioner to correct any problems that could cause mucosal ulceration.

If a series of dental procedures is required, it may be prudent to observe an interval of time between procedures to both reduce the potential for the emergence of resistant organisms and allow repopulation of the mouth with antibiotic susceptible flora. Various studies have suggested an interval of 9[33] to 14[34] days. If possible, a combination of procedures should be planned within the same period of prophylaxis.

Respiratory, Gastrointestinal, and Genitourinary Tract Procedures

Surgical procedures involving the respiratory mucosa may lead to bacteremia; therefore, antimicrobial prophylaxis is recommended (Table 3[35-58]). The use of a rigid

Table 2
Dental Procedures and Endocarditis Prophylaxis[22,24–26,28–31]

Endocarditis Prophylaxis Recommended*

Dental extractions
Periodontal procedures including surgery, scaling and root planing, probing, and recall maintenance
Dental implant placement and reimplantation of avulsed teeth
Endodontic (root canal) instrumentation or surgery only beyond the apex
Subgingival placement of antibiotic fibers or strips
Initial placement of orthodontic bands but not brackets
Intraligamentary local anesthetic injections
Prophylactic cleaning of teeth or implants where bleeding is anticipated

Endocarditis Prophylaxis Not Recommended

Restorative dentistry† (operative and prosthodontic) with or without retraction cord‡
Local anesthetic injections (nonintraligamentary)
Intracanal endodontic treatment; post placement and buildup
Placement of rubber dams
Postoperative suture removal
Placement of removable prosthodontic or orthodontic appliances
Taking of oral impressions
Fluoride treatments
Taking of oral radiographs
Orthodontic appliance adjustment
Shedding of primary teeth

*Prophylaxis is recommended for patients with high- and moderate-risk cardiac conditions.
†This includes restoration of decayed teeth (filling cavities) and replacement of missing teeth.
‡Clinical judgment may indicate antibiotic use in selected circumstances that may create significant bleeding.

bronchoscope may cause mucosal damage, whereas such damage is unlikely with a flexible bronchoscope. Endotracheal intubation per se is not an indication for antibiotic prophylaxis.

The risk of endocarditis as a direct result of an endoscopic procedure is small. Transient bacteremia may occur during or immediately after endoscopy; however, there are few reports of infective endocarditis attributable to endoscopy.[35-43] For most gastrointestinal endoscopic procedures, the rate of bacteremia is 2% to 5%, and the organisms typically identified are unlikely to cause endocarditis.[44,45] The rate of bacteremia does not increase with mucosal biopsy, polypectomy, or sphincterotomy.[46-48] There are no data to indicate that deep biopsy, as may be performed in the rectum or stomach, leads to a higher rate of bacteremia.

Some gastrointestinal procedures are associated with a higher rate of transient bacteremia; for these procedures, antimicrobial prophylaxis is recommended, particularly for patients in the high-risk category (Table 3). Esophageal stricture dilation has been associated with bacteremia rates as high as 45%.[44] However, this number is an average result of several clinical studies in which the rate of bacteremia ranged from 0% to 100%.[49-52] In only one study was the oropharynx the documented source of infection.[52] These studies were performed with differing methods and involved relatively small numbers of patients. Until more data documenting the true rate of bacteremia associated with stricture dilation become available, it is prudent to consider this procedure as one potentially associated with an increased risk of transient bacteremia.

The bacteremia rate associated with sclerotherapy of esophageal varices is approximately 31%.[44] Bacteremia appears to be most associated with increased sclerosant volumes, as can occur with emergency sclerosis for active bleeding, and with relatively longer injection needles. The bacteremia rate is lessened with the use of shorter injection needles and sterile water.[53,54] Endoscopic ligation of varices, or banding, is not associated with increased rates of transient bacteremia.[55]

An obstructed biliary tree, due to benign or malignant disease, may be colonized with a variety of organisms. A prime risk factor for dissemination of infection from an obstructed biliary tree is instrumentation of the obstructed region without provision of adequate drainage. The bacteremia rates for endoscopic retrograde cholangi-

Table 3

Other Procedures and Endocarditis Prophylaxis[35-58]

Endocarditis Prophylaxis Recommended

Respiratory tract
 Tonsillectomy and/or adenoidectomy
 Surgical operations that involve respiratory mucosa
 Bronchoscopy with a rigid bronchoscope
Gastrointestinal tract*
 Sclerotherapy for esophageal varices
 Esophageal stricture dilation
 Endoscopic retrograde cholangiography with biliary obstruction
 Biliary tract surgery
 Surgical operations that involve intestinal mucosa
Genitourinary tract
 Prostatic surgery
 Cystoscopy
 Urethral dilation

Endocarditis Prophylaxis Not Recommended

Respiratory tract
 Endotracheal intubation
 Bronchoscopy with a flexible bronchoscope, with or without biopsy†
 Tympanostomy tube insertion
Gastrointestinal tract
 Transesophageal echocardiography†
 Endoscopy with or without gastrointestinal biopsy†
Genitourinary tract
 Vaginal hysterectomy†
 Vaginal delivery†
 Cesarean section
 In uninfected tissue:
  Urethral catheterization
  Uterine dilatation and curettage
  Therapeutic abortion
  Sterilization procedures
  Insertion or removal of intrauterine devices
Other
 Cardiac catheterization, including balloon angioplasty
 Implanted cardiac pacemakers, implanted defibrillators, and coronary stents
 Incision or biopsy of surgically scrubbed skin
 Circumcision

*Prophylaxis is recommended for high-risk patients; optional for medium-risk patients.
†Prophylaxis is optional for high-risk patients.

ography in the absence of ductal obstruction are approximately equal to most other endoscopic procedures. Prophylaxis should be considered primarily in cases in which biliary obstruction is known or suspected.

In biliary tract surgery, or in any operative procedure that involves the intestinal mucosa, there is a potential for bacteremia with organisms known to cause endocarditis. It is therefore prudent to provide prophylaxis for patients at high risk to develop endocarditis.

Surgery, instrumentation, or diagnostic procedures that involve the genitourinary tract may cause bacteremia. Although the risk that any particular patient will develop endocarditis is low, the genitourinary tract is second only to the oral cavity as a portal of entry for organisms that cause endocarditis. The rate of bacteremia following urinary tract procedures is high in the presence of urinary tract infection (UTI). Sterilization of the urinary tract with antimicrobial therapy in patients with bacteriuria should be attempted prior to elective procedures, including lithotripsy. Results of a preprocedure urine culture will allow the practitioner to choose antibiotics appropriate to the recovered organisms. Procedures for which antimicrobial prophylaxis is or is not recommended are listed in Table 3.

Many procedures involving the urethra and prostatic bed are associated with high rates of bacteremia. The incidence of bacteremia was studied in 300 patients undergoing 1 of 4 different urologic procedures: transurethral resection (TUR) of the prostate, cystoscopy, urethral dilation, and urethral catheterization.[56] Bacteremia was most frequent after TUR of the prostate, occurring in 31% of the patients. In the other procedures, bacteremia occurred in 24% following urethral dilatation, in 17% following cystoscopy, and in 8% following urethral catheterization. Bacteremia was significantly associated with both prostatitis on histological examination of resected prostate and prior UTI following TUR and with prior UTI following urethral dilatation and cystoscopy. Preexisting UTI was the major source of organisms causing the bacteremia following TUR but was the source in only about one third of patients following the other procedures. Enterococci and *Klebsiella* were the most frequent organisms. Although bacteremia due to gram-negative bacilli is unlikely to cause endocarditis unless a prosthetic valve is present, it may nevertheless cause life-threatening sepsis. Therefore, an antimicrobial regimen effective against the infective urinary pathogen, e.g., enteric gram-negative bacilli, in addition to the enterococcus, should be administered before the invasive genitourinary procedures.

Bacteremia follows uncomplicated vaginal delivery in only 1% to 5% of procedures, usually with various types of streptococci[22]; well-documented cases of endocarditis after normal vaginal delivery are uncommon.[57] Therefore, antibiotic prophylaxis for normal vaginal delivery is not

Table 4

Prophylactic Regimens for Dental, Oral, Respiratory Tract, or Esophageal Procedures[1,22,59–61]

Situation	Agent	Regimen*
Standard general prophylaxis	Amoxicillin	Adults: 2.0 g; children: 50 mg/kg orally 1 h before procedure
Unable to take oral medications	Ampicillin	Adults: 2.0 g intramuscularly (IM) or intravenously (IV); children: 50 mg/kg IM or IV within 30 min before procedure
Allergic to penicillin	Clindamycin *or*	Adults: 600 mg; children: 20 mg/kg orally 1 h before procedure
	Cephalexin† or cefadroxil† *or*	Adults: 2.0 g; children; 50 mg/kg orally 1 h before procedure
	Azithromycin or clarithromycin	Adults: 500 mg; children: 15 mg/kg orally 1 h before procedure
Allergic to penicillin and unable to take oral medications	Clindamycin *or*	Adults: 600 mg; children: 20 mg/kg IV within 30 min before procedure
	Cefazolin†	Adults: 1.0 g; children: 25 mg/kg IM or IV within 30 min before procedure

*Total children's dose should not exceed adult dose.
†Cephalosporins should not be used in individuals with immediate-type hypersensitivity reaction (urticaria, angioedema, or anaphylaxis) to penicillins.

recommended. If an unanticipated bacteremia is suspected during vaginal delivery, intravenous antibiotics can be administered at that time. No bacteremia has been detected in studies following cervical biopsy or manipulation of an intrauterine device (IUD) in the absence of obvious infections.[22] Bacteremia following removal of an infected IUD is unresolved[58] but would seem possible and should warrant prophylaxis, as would other genitourinary procedures in the presence of infection.

Prophylactic Regimens

Prophylaxis is most effective when given perioperatively in doses that are sufficient to assure adequate antibiotic concentrations in the serum during and after the procedure. To reduce the likelihood of microbial resistance, it is important that prophylactic antibiotics be used only during the perioperative period. They should be initiated shortly before a procedure and should not be continued for an extended period (no more than 6 to 8 hours). In the case of delayed healing, or of a procedure that involves infected tissue, it may be necessary to provide additional doses of antibiotics for treatment of the established infection.

Practitioners must exercise their own clinical judgment in determining the choice of antibiotics and number of doses that are to be administered in individual cases or special circumstances. Furthermore, because endocarditis may occur in spite of appropriate antibiotic prophylaxis, physicians and dentists should maintain a high index of suspicion regarding any unusual clinical events (such as unexplained fever, night chills, weakness, myalgia, arthralgia, lethargy, or malaise) following dental or other surgical procedures in patients who are at risk for developing bacterial endocarditis.

Regimens for Dental, Oral, Respiratory Tract, or Esophageal Procedures

Streptococcus viridans (α-hemolytic streptococci) is the most common cause of endocarditis following dental or oral procedures, certain upper respiratory tract procedures, bronchoscopy with a rigid bronchoscope, surgical procedures that involve the respiratory mucosa, and esophageal procedures. Prophylaxis should be specifically directed against these organisms. The same regimens are recommended for all these procedures (Table 4[1,22,59–61]). The recommended standard prophylactic regimen for all these procedures is a single dose of oral amoxicillin. The antibiotics amoxicillin, ampicillin, and penicillin V are equally effective in vitro against α-hemolytic streptococci; however, amoxicillin is recommended because it is better absorbed from the gastrointestinal tract and provides higher and more sustained serum levels. Previously the recommended dose was 3.0 g 1 hour before a procedure and then 1.5 g 6 hours after the initial dose.[1] Recent comparisons of 2.0-g and 3.0-g dosing indicate that a 2.0-g dose results in adequate serum levels for several hours and causes less gastrointestinal adverse effects.[59] The newly recommended adult dose is 2.0 g of amoxicillin (pediatric dose is 50 mg/kg not to exceed the adult dose) to be administered 1 hour before the anticipated procedure. A second dose is not necessary, both because of the prolonged serum levels above the minimal inhibitory concentration of most oral streptococci[59] and the prolonged serum inhibitory activity induced by amoxicillin against such strains (6-14 hours).[60] For individuals who are unable to take or unable to absorb oral medications, a parenteral agent may be necessary. Ampicillin sodium is recommended because parenteral amoxicillin is not available in the United States. Individuals who are allergic to penicillins (such as amoxicillin, ampicillin, or penicillin) should be treated with the provided alternative oral regimens. Clindamycin hydrochloride is one recommended alternative. Individuals who can tolerate first-generation cephalosporins (cephalexin or cefadroxil) may receive these agents provided they have not had an immediate, local, or systemic IgE-mediated anaphylactic allergic reaction to penicillin. Azithromycin or clarithromycin are also acceptable alternative agents for the penicillin-allergic individual,[61] although they are more expensive than the other regimens. When parenteral administration is needed in an individual who is allergic to penicillin, clindamycin phosphate is recommended; cefazolin may be used if the individual does not have an immediate type local or systemic anaphylactic hypersensitivity to penicillin. The previous recommendations from this committee listed erythromycin as an alternate agent for the penicillin-allergic patient. Erythromycin is no longer included because of gastrointestinal upset and complicated pharmacokinetics of the various formulations.[62] Practitioners who have successfully used erythromycin for prophylaxis in individual patients may choose to continue with this antibiotic. The regimen is included in our previous recommendations.[1]

Regimens for Genitourinary and Nonesophageal Gastrointestinal Procedures

Bacterial endocarditis that occurs following genitourinary and gastrointestinal tract surgery or instrumentation is most often caused by *Enterococcus faecalis* (enterococci). Although gram-negative bacillary bacteremia may follow these procedures, gram-negative bacilli are only rarely responsible for endocarditis. Thus, antibiotic prophylaxis to prevent endocarditis that occurs following genitourinary or gastrointestinal procedures should be directed primarily against enterococci.

Table 5[1,22] outlines the recommended regimens for prophylaxis for genitourinary or gastrointestinal tract procedures (excluding esophageal procedures). The committee continues to recommend parenteral antibiotics, particularly in high-risk patients. In medium-risk patients requiring prophylaxis, a parenteral (ampicillin) or oral (amoxicillin) regimen is provided. For procedures in which prophylaxis is not routinely recommended, physicians may choose to administer prophylaxis in high-risk patients.

Specific Situations and Circumstances

Patients Already Receiving Antibiotics

Occasionally, a patient may be taking an antibiotic when coming to the physician or dentist. If the patient is taking an antibiotic normally used for endocarditis prophylaxis, it is prudent to select a drug from a different class rather than to increase the dose of the current antibiotic. In particular, antibiotic regimens used to prevent the recurrence of acute rheumatic fever are inadequate for the prevention of bacterial endocarditis. Individuals who take an oral penicillin for secondary prevention of rheumatic fever or for other purposes may have viridans streptococci in their oral cavities that are relatively resistant to penicillin, amoxicillin, or ampicillin. In such cases, the physician or dentist should select clindamycin, azithromycin, or clarithromycin (Table 4) for endocarditis prophylaxis. Because of possible cross-resistance with the cephalosporins, this class of antibiotics should be avoided. If possible, one could delay the procedure until at least 9[33] to 14[34] days after completion of the antibiotic. This will allow the usual oral flora to be reestablished.

Procedures Involving Infected Tissues

Incision and drainage or other procedures involving infected tissues may result in bacteremia with the same organism causing the infection. In individuals at risk for endocarditis (the high- and moderate-risk categories in Table 1), it is advisable to administer antimicrobial prophylaxis before the procedure. Prophylaxis should be directed at the most likely pathogen causing the infection. For non-oral soft tissue infections (cellulitis), or bone and joint infections (osteomyelitis and pyogenic arthritis) an antistaphylococcal penicillin or first-generation cephalosporin is an appropriate choice. For patients who are allergic to penicillins, clindamycin is an acceptable alternative. For those unable to take oral antibiotics or who are known to have methicillin sodium-resistant *Staphylococcus aureus* bacteremia, vancomycin is the regimen of choice. For UTI, agents active against enteric gram-negative bacilli (such as aminoglycosides or third-generation cephalosporins) are advisable.

Patients Who Receive Anticoagulants

Intramuscular injections for endocarditis prophylaxis should be avoided in patients who receive heparin. The use of warfarin sodium is a relative contraindication to intramuscular injections. Intravenous or oral regimens should be used whenever possible.

Table 5		
Prophylactic Regimens for Genitourinary Gastrointestinal (Excluding Esophageal) Procedures[22]		
Situation	**Agents***	**Regiment**
High-risk patients	Ampicillin plus Gentamicin	Adults: ampicillin 2.0 g intramuscularly (IM) or intravenously (IV) plus gentamicin 1.5 mg/kg (not to exceed 120 mg) within 30 min of starting the procedure; 6 h later, ampicillin 1 g IM/IV or amoxicillin 1 g orally
		Children: ampicillin 50 mg/kg IM or IV (not to exceed 2.0 g) plus gentamicin 1.5 mg/kg within 30 min of starting the procedure; 6 h later, ampicillin 25 mg/kg IM/IV or amoxicillin 25 mg/kg orally
High-risk patients allergic to ampicillin/amoxicillin	Vancomycin plus Gentamicin	Adults: vancomycin 1.0 g IV over 1-2 h plus gentamicin 1.5 mg/kg IV/IM (not to exceed 120 mg); complete injection/infusion within 30 min of starting the procedure
		Children: vancomycin 20 mg/kg IV over 1-2 h plus gentamicin 1.5 mg/kg IV/IM; complete injection/infusion within 30 min of starting the procedure
Moderate-risk patients	Amoxicillin or Ampicillin	Adults: amoxicillin 2.0 g orally 1 h before procedure, or ampicillin 2.0 g IM/IV within 30 min of starting the procedure
		Children: amoxicillin 50 mg/kg orally 1 h before procedure, or ampicillin 50 mg/kg IM/IV within 30 min of starting the procedure
Moderate-risk patients allergic to ampicillin/amoxicillin	Vancomycin	Adults: vancomycin 1.0 g IV over 1-2 h; complete infusion within 30 min of starting the procedure
		Children: vancomycin 20 mg/kg IV over 1-2 h; complete infusion within 30 min of starting the procedure

*Total children's dose should not exceed adult dose.
†No second dose of vancomycin or gentamicin is recommended.

Patients Who Undergo Cardiac Surgery

A careful preoperative dental evaluation is recommended so that required dental treatment can be completed before cardiac surgery whenever possible. Such measures may decrease the incidence of late postoperative endocarditis.

Patients who have cardiac conditions that predispose them to endocarditis are at risk for developing bacterial endocarditis when undergoing open heart surgery. Similarly, patients who undergo surgery for placement of prosthetic heart valves or prosthetic intravascular or intracardiac materials are also at risk for the development of bacterial endocarditis. Because the morbidity and mortality of endocarditis in such patients are high, perioperative prophylactic antibiotics are recommended. Endocarditis associated with open heart surgery is most often caused by S. aureus, coagulase-negative staphylococci, or diphtheroids. Streptococci, gram-negative bacteria, and fungi are less common. No single antibiotic regimen is effective against all these organisms. Furthermore, prolonged use of broad-spectrum antibiotics may predispose to superinfection with unusual or resistant microorganisms. Prophylaxis at the time of cardiac surgery should be directed primarily against staphylococci and should be of short duration. First-generation cephalosporins are most often used, but the choice of an antibiotic should be influenced by the antibiotic susceptibility patterns at each hospital. For example, high prevalence of infection by methicillin-resistant S. aureus in a particular inpatient unit should prompt consideration of vancomycin for perioperative prophylaxis. It should be noted, however, that although the majority of nosocomial coagulase-negative staphylococci exhibit the methicillin-resistance phenotype in vitro, endocarditis prophylaxis with first-generation cephalosporins is effective for most patients undergoing cardiac valve surgery.[63] Prophylaxis with the chosen antibiotic should be started immediately before the operative procedure, repeated during prolonged procedures to maintain levels intraoperatively, and continued for no more than 24 hours postoperatively to minimize emergence of resistant microorganisms. The effects of cardiopulmonary bypass and compromised postoperative renal function on antibiotic levels in the serum should be considered and doses timed appropriately before and during the procedure.

Status Following Cardiovascular Procedures

Many reparative cardiac procedures do not modify the patient's long-term risk for infective endocarditis, which continues indefinitely (Table 1). In the case of prosthetic valve replacement, the risk of endocarditis increases postoperatively. In other conditions, such as closure of ventricular septal defect or patent ductus arteriosus without residual leak, the risk of endocarditis diminishes to the level of the general population after a 6-month healing period. Data are insufficient to make recommendations for prophylactic therapy after closure of these lesions by transcatheter devices. There is no evidence that coronary artery bypass graft surgery introduces a risk for endocarditis. Therefore, antibiotic prophylaxis is not needed for individuals who have previously undergone this procedure. Noncoronary vascular grafts may merit antibiotic prophylaxis for the first 6 months after implantation.

There are insufficient data to support recommendations for patients who have had heart transplants. However, such patients are at risk of acquired valvular dysfunction, especially during episodes of rejection. Because of this, and the continuous use of immunosuppression in such patients, most transplant physicians administer prophylaxis according to regimens for the moderate-risk category.

Other Considerations

A case of endocarditis, perceived as result of failure to administer a recommended prophylactic regimen, requires careful analysis. It is important to consider the following factors: (1) the time period between the putatively responsible invasive procedure and the onset of clinical symptoms compatible with endocarditis; (2) the etiologic organism causing endocarditis; (3) the likelihood that the putative invasive procedure resulted in bacteremia; and (4) knowledge by the patient of the presence or severity of the underlying lesion and communication of this information to the treating physician or dentist prior to the procedure. Most cases of procedure-related endocarditis occur with a short incubation period of approximately 2 weeks or less following the procedure.[64] A longer incubation period between the invasive procedure and the onset of symptoms significantly lessens the likelihood that the procedure was the proximate cause of the endocarditis. A national registry established by the American Heart Association in the early 1980s analyzed 52 cases of apparent failures of endocarditis prophylaxis.[65] Only 6 (12%) of the 52 cases had received prophylactic regimens that were currently recommended by the American Heart Association. The vast majority of endocarditis due to oral organisms is not related to dental treatment procedures.[24,27] One recent large-scale, population-based, case-control study, done in 54 Philadelphia area hospitals from 1988 to 1990,

was unable to demonstrate any independent risk for endocarditis attributable to prior dental treatment.[66] In addition, it is unlikely that cases of viridans streptococcal endocarditis would complicate invasive nonesophageal gastrointestinal or genitourinary procedures. Similarly, enterococcal endocarditis would be a very unusual consequence of dental procedures.

The use of prophylactic antibiotics to prevent infection of joint prostheses during potentially bacteremia-inducing procedures is not within the scope of issues addressed by this committee.

The Council on Scientific Affairs of the American Dental Association has approved the manuscript as it relates to dentistry. The American Society for Gastrointestinal Endoscopy has approved the manuscript as it relates to gastroenterology. The authors thank Jeanette Allison for her superb secretarial skills.

REFERENCES

1. Dajani AS, Bisno AL, Chung KJ, et al. Prevention of bacterial endocarditis. *JAMA.* 1990;264:2919-2922.
2. Steckelberg JM, Wilson WR. Risk factors for infective endocarditis. *Infect Dis Clin North Am.* 1993;7:9-19.
3. Saiman L, Prince A, Gersony WM. Pediatric infective endocarditis in the modern era. *J Pediatr.* 1993;122:847-853.
4. Gersony WM, Hayes CJ, Driscoll DJ, et al. Bacterial endocarditis in patients with aortic stenosis, pulmonary stenosis, or ventricular septal defect. *Circulation.* 1993;87(suppl I):121-126.
5. Prabhu SD, O'Rourke RA. Mitral valve prolapse. In: Braunwald E, series ed, Rahimtoola SH, volume ed. *Atlas of Heart Diseases: Valvular Heart Disease: Vol XI.* St Louis: Mosby-Year Book Inc; 1997:10.1-10.18.
6. Boudoulas H, Wooley CF. Mitral valve prolapse. In: Emmanouilides GC, Riemenschneider TA, Allen HD, Gutgesell HP, eds. *Moss and Adams Heart Disease in Infants, Children, and Adolescents Including the Fetus and Young Adult,* 5th ed. Baltimore, Md: Williams & Wilkins; 1995:1063-1086.
7. Carabello BA. Mitral valve disease. *Curr Probl Cardiol.* 1993; 7:423-478.
8. Devereux RB, Hawkins I, Kramer-Fox R, et al. Complications of mitral valve prolapse: disproportionate occurrence in men and older patients. *Am J Med* 1986;81:751-758.
9. Danchin N, Briancon S, Mathieu P, et al. Mitral valve prolapse as a risk factor for infective endocarditis. *Lancet.* 1989;1:743-745.
10. MacMahon SW, Roberts JK, Kramer-Fox R, et al. Mitral valve prolapse and infective endocarditis. *Am Heart J.* 1987;113: 1291-1298.
11. Marks AR, Choong CY, Sanfilippo AJ, Ferre M, Weyman AE. Identification of high-risk and low-risk subgroups of patients with mitral-valve prolapse. *N Engl J Med.* 1989;320: 1031-1036.
12. Devereux RB, Frary CJ, Kramer-Fox R, Roberts RB, Ruchlin HS. Cost-effectiveness of infective endocarditis prophylaxis for mitral valve prolapse with or without a mitral regurgitant murmur. *Am J Cardiol.* 1994;74:1024-1029.

13. Zuppiroli A, Rinaldi M, Kramer-Fox R, Favilli S, Roman MJ, Devereux RB. Natural history of mitral valve prolapse. *Am J Cardiol.* 1995;75:1028-1032.

14. Wooley CF, Baker PB, Kolibash AJ, et al. The floppy, myxomatous mitral valve, mitral valve prolapse, and mitral regurgitation. *Prog Cardiovasc Dis.* 1991;33:397-433.

15. Morales AR, Romanelli R, Boucek RJ, Tate LG, Alvarez RT, Davis JT. Myxoid heart disease: an assessment of extravalvular cardiac pathology in severe mitral valve prolapse. *Hum Pathol.* 1992;23:129-137.

16. Weissman NJ, Pini R, Roman MJ, Kramer-Fox R, Andersen HS, Devereux RB. In vivo mitral valve morphology and motion in mitral valve prolapse. *Am J Cardiol.* 1994;73: 1080-1088.

17. Nishimura RA, McGoon MD, Shub C, et al. Echocardiographically documented mitral-valve prolapse. *N Engl J Med.* 1985;313:1305-1309.

18. McKinsey DS, Ratts TE, Bisno AL. Underlying cardiac lesions in adults with infective endocarditis. *Am J Med.* 1987; 82:681-688.

19. Devereux RB, Kramer-Fox R, Kligfield P. Mitral valve prolapse: causes, clinical manifestations, and management. *Ann Intern Med.* 1989;111:305-317.

20. Stoddard MF, Prince CR, Dillon S, Longaker RA, Morris GT, Liddell NE. Exercise-induced mitral regurgitation is a predictor of morbid events in subjects with mitral valve prolapse. *J Am Coll Cardiol.* 1995;25:693-699.

21. Awadallah SM, Kavey REW, Byrum CJ, Smith FC, Kveselis DA, Blackman MS. The changing pattern of infective endocarditis in childhood. *Am J Cardiol.* 1991;68:90-94.

22. Durack DT. Prevention of infective endocarditis. *N Engl J Med.* 1995;332:38-44.

23. Cheitlin MD, Alpert JS, Armstrong WF, et al. ACC/AHA guidelines for the clinical application of echocardiography: a report of the American College of Cardiology/American Heart Association Task Force on Practice Guidelines (Committee on Clinical Application of Echocardiography). *Circulation.* 1997;95:1686-1744.

24. Pallasch TJ, Slots J. Antibiotic prophylaxis and the medically compromised patient. *Periodontol 2000.* 1996;10: 107-138.

25. Bender IB, Naidorf IJ, Garvey GJ. Bacterial endocarditis: a consideration for physicians and dentists. *J Am Dent Assoc.* 1984;109:415-420.

26. Guntheroth WG. How important are dental procedures as a cause of infective endocarditis? *Am J Cardiol.* 1984;54: 797-801.

27. Kaye D. Prophylaxis for infective endocarditis: an update. *Ann Intern Med.* 1986;104:419-423.

28. Roman AR, App GR. Bacteremia, a result from oral irrigation in subjects with gingivitis. *J Periodontol.* 1971;42: 757-760.

29. Felix JE, Rosen S, App GR. Detection of bacteremia after the use of oral irrigation device on subjects with periodontitis. *J Periodontol.* 1971;42:785-787.

30. Hunter KD, Holborrow DW, Kardos TB, Lee-Knight CT, Ferguson MM. Bacteremia and tissue damage resulting from air polishing. *Br Dent J.* 1989;167:275-277.

31. Berger SA, Weitzman S, Edberg SC, Coreg JI. Bacteremia after use of an oral irrigating device. *Ann Intern Med.* 1974;80:510-511.

32. Berney P, Francioli P. Successful prophylaxis of experimental streptococcal endocarditis with single-dose amoxicillin administered after bacterial challenge. *J Infect Dis.* 1990;161: 281-285.

33. Leviner E, Tzukert AA, Benoliel R, Baram O, Sela MV. Development of resistant oral viridans streptococci after administration of prophylactic antibiotics: time management in the dental treatment of patients susceptible to infective endocarditis. *Oral Surg Oral Med Oral Pathol.* 1987;64:417-420.

34. Simmons NA, Cawson RA, Clark CA, et al. Prophylaxis of infective endocarditis. *Lancet.* 1986;1:1267.

35. Niv Y, Bat L, Motro M. Bacterial endocarditis after Hurst bougiengage in a patient with a benign esophageal stricture and mitral valve prolapse. *Gastrointest Endosc.* 1985;31: 265-267.

36. Rodriguez W, Levine J. Enterococcal endocarditis following flexible sigmoidoscopy. *West J Med.* 1984;140:951-953.

37. Rigilano J, Mahapatra R, Barnhill J, Gutierrez J. Enterococcal endocarditis following sigmoidoscopy and mitral valve prolapse. *Arch Intern Med.* 1984;144:850-851.

38. Pritchard T, Foust R, Cantey R, Leman R. Prosthetic valve endocarditis due to *Cardiobacterium hominis* occurring after upper gastrointestinal endoscopy. *Am J Med.* 1991;90: 516-518.

39. Watanakunakorn C. *Streptococcus bovis* endocarditis associated with villous adenoma following colonoscopy. *Am Heart J.* 1988;116:1115-1116.

40. Baskin G. Prosthetic endocarditis after endoscopic variceal sclerotherapy: a failure of antibiotic prophylaxis. *Am J Gastroenterol.* 1989;84:311-312.

41. Yin T, Dellipiani A. Bacterial endocarditis after Hurst bougiengage in a patient with a benign oesophageal stricture. *Endoscopy.* 1983;15:27-28.

42. Norfleet R. Infectious endocarditis after fiberoptic sigmoidoscopy. *J Clin Gastroenterol.* 1991;13:448-451.

43. Logan R, Hastings J. Bacterial endocarditis: a complication of gastroscopy. *BMJ.* 1988;296:1107.

44. Botoman V, Surawicz C. Bacteremia with gastrointestinal endoscopic procedures. *Gastrointest Endosc.* 1986;32: 342-346.

45. Bryne W, Euler A, Campbell M, Eisenach KD. Bacteremia in children following upper gastrointestinal endoscopy or colonoscopy. *J Pediatr Gastroenterol Nutr.* 1982;1:551-553.

46. Shull H, Greene B, Allen S, et al. Bacteremia with upper gastrointestinal endoscopy. *Ann Intern Med.* 1975;83: 212-214.

47. Low D, Shoenut P, Kennedy J, et al. Prospective assessment of risk of bacteremia with colonoscopy and polypectomy. *Dig Dis Sci.* 1987;32:1239-1243.

48. Low D, Shoenut P, Kennedy J, et al. Risk of bacteremia with endoscopic sphincterotomy. *Can J Surg.* 1987;30:421-423.

49. Raines DR, Branch WC, Anderson DL, et al. The occurrence of bacteremia after oesophageal dilatation and oesophagogastroscopy. *Aust N Z J Med.* 1977;7:22-35.

50. Welsh JD, Griffiths WJ, McKee J, et al. Bacteremia associated with esophageal dilation. *J Clin Gastroenterol.* 1983;5: 109-112.

51. Yin TP, Dellipiana AW. The incidence of bacteremia after outpatient Hurst bougiengage in the management of benign esophageal stricture. *Endoscopy.* 1983;31:265-267.

52. Stephenson PM, Dorrington L, Harris OD, Rao A. Bacteraemia following oesophageal dilatation and oesophagogastroscopy. *Aust N Z J Med.* 1977;7:32-35.

53. Ho H, Zuckerman M, Wassem C. A prospective controlled study of the risk of bacteremia in emergency sclerotherapy of esophageal varices. *Gastroenterology.* 1991;101:1642-1648.

54. Cohen L, Korsten M, Scherl E, et al. Bacteremia after endoscopic injection sclerosis. *Gastrointest Endosc.* 1983;29: 198-200.

55. Tseng C, Green R, Burke S, et al. Bacteremia after endoscopic band ligation of esophageal varices. *Gastrointest Endosc.* 1992;38:336-337.

56. Sullivan N, Sutter V, Mims M, Marsh V, Finegold S. Clinical aspects of bacteremia after manipulation of the genitourinary tract. *J Infect Dis.* 1973;127:49-55.

57. Sugrue D, Blake S, Troy P, MacDonald D. Antibiotic prophylaxis against infective endocarditis after normal delivery: is it necessary? *Br Heart J.* 1980;44:499-502.

58. Child JS. Risks for and prevention of infective endocarditis. In: Child JS, ed. *Cardiology Clinics—Diagnosis and Management of Infective Endocarditis.* Philadelphia, Pa: WB Saunders Co; 1996;14:327-343.

59. Dajani AS, Bawdon RE, Berry MC. Oral amoxicillin as prophylaxis for endocarditis: what is the optimal dose? *Clin Infect Dis.* 1994;18:157-160.

60. Fluckiger U, Franciolo P, Blaser J, Glauser MP, Moreillon P. Role of amoxicillin serum levels for successful prophylaxis of experimental endocarditis due to tolerant streptococci. *J Infect Dis.* 1994;169:397-400.

61. Rouse MS, Steckelberg JM, Brandt CM, Patel R, Miro JM, Wilson WR. Efficacy of azithromycin or clarithromycin for the prophylaxis of viridans streptococcal experimental endocarditis. *Antimicrob Agents Chemother.* In press.

62. Sande MA, Mandell GL. Antimicrobial agents—tetracyclines, chloramphenicol, erythromycin, and miscellaneous antibacterial agents. In: Gilman AG, Rall TW, Nies AS, Taylor P, eds. *Goodman and Gilman's The Pharmacological Basis of Therapeutics,* 8th ed. New York, NY: Pergamon Press Inc; 1990:1117-1145.

63. Bayer AS, Nelson RJ, Slama TG. Current concepts in prevention of prosthetic valve endocarditis. *Chest.* 1990;97: 1203-1207.

64. Starkebaum M, Durack D, Beeson P. The incubation period of subacute bacterial endocarditis. *Yale J Biol Med.* 1977; 50:49-58.

65. Durack DT, Kaplan EL, Bisno AL. Apparent failures of endocarditis prophylaxis: analysis of 52 cases submitted to a national registry. *JAMA.* 1983;250:2318-2322.

66. Strom BL, Abrutyn E, Berlin JA, et al. Prophylactic antibiotics to prevent infective endocarditis? relative risks re-assessed. *J Investig Med.* 1996;44:229. Abstract.

Professional Organizations of Interest to Dental Hygienists

American Association for Dental Research
(Includes dental hygiene researchers)
1619 Duke Street
Alexandria, VA 22314
Phone: (703) 548-0066
Fax: (703) 548-1883
http://www.iadr.com

American Association for Dental Schools
(includes dental hygiene educators)
1625 Massachusetts Ave, N.W., Suite 600
Washington, D.C. 20036-2212
Phone: (202) 667-9433
Fax: (202) 667-0642
http://www.aads.jhu.edu

American Dental Association
211 E. Chicago Ave.
Chicago, IL 60611
Phone: (312) 440-2500
Fax: (312) 440-2800
http://www.ada.org

American Dental Hygienists' Association
444 N. Michigan Ave., Suite 3400
Chicago, IL 60611
Phone: (800) 243-ADHA
http://adha.org

Canadian Dental Hygienists' Association
96 Centre Pointe Drive
Nepean, Ontario
Canada K2G 6B1
Phone: (613) 224-5515
Fax: (613) 224-7283
email: cdha@magi.com

Canadian Dental Association
1815 Alta Vista
Ottawa, Ontario
Canada
Phone: (613) 523-1770
http://www.cda-adc.ca/

Centers for Disease Control and Prevention
1600 Clifton Road NE
Atlanta, GA 30333
Phone: (404) 639-3311
http://www.cdc.gov

FDI World Dental Federation
7 Carlisle Street
London, W1V 5RG
United Kingdom
Phone: +44 (0) 171 935 7852
Fax: +44 (0) 171 486 0183

Hispanic Dental Association
(includes dental hygienists)
188 West Randolph Street
Suite 1811
Chicago, IL 60601
Phone: (312) 577-4013
http://members.aol.com/hdassoc/index.html
email: hdassoc@aol.com

International Association for Dental Research
1619 Duke Street
Alexandria, VA 22314-3406
Phone: (703) 548-0066
Fax: (703) 548-1883
http://www.iadr.com

International Dental Hygienists' Federation
c/o Sue Lloyd
55 Kemble Road
Forrest Hill, London
SE23 2DH United Kingdom

National Center for Dental Hygiene Research
Thomas Jefferson University
College of Allied Health Sciences
130 South 9th Street, 22nd Floor
Philadelphia, PA 19107
http://jeffline.tju.edu/DHNet

National Dental Hygienists' Association
3220 Connecticut Avenue
Washington, D.C., 20008
Phone: (202) 244-6595

Appendix D, the *Simulated National Board Dental Hygiene Examination* parallels the National Board Dental Hygiene Examination in content and question format. This test permits you to experience the reality of the board exam you will soon be taking.

Exam Format
This examination is comprised of two components:
Section One consists of 150 randomly ordered multiple choice questions (i.e., not grouped by subject area)

Section Two (beginning on page 819) consists of 186 case-based questions designed to test your knowledge of all content areas. The forms, radiographs, and clinical photographs needed to answer these questions begin after page 822.

Answers and Rationales for all Simulated National Board Dental Hygiene Examination questions are provided on pages 832-860. We have provided rationales for correct as well as incorrect answers.

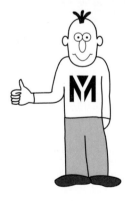

MOSBY WOULD LIKE TO TAKE
THIS OPPORTUNITY TO WISH
YOU GOOD LUCK ON THE
BOARD EXAM!!!

Simulated National Board Dental Hygiene Examination

Patricia Regener Campbell*

Section One

1 Which of the following is *NOT* an example of zoonosis?
   A. Tularemia
   B. Brucellosis
   C. Anthrax
   D. Diphtheria
   E. Toxoplasmosis

2 The treatment for acute fluoride poisoning is to
   A. Have the victim drink milk
   B. Administer charcoal compound to the victim
   C. Induce vomiting in the victim
   D. Have victim drink large quantities of water

3 The administration of oxygen is *NOT* indicated in the treatment of
   A. Asthma
   B. Myocardial infarction
   C. Hyperventilation

4 Which of the following interactions of x-rays and matter results in low energy characteristic radiation produced by outer shell electrons shifting to an inner vacancy?
   A. Compton effect
   B. Photoelectric effect
   C. Thompson scattering
   D. Coherent scattering

5 Craniofacial malformations that might cause malocclusions are seen in all of the following conditions *EXCEPT* one. Which one is this *EXCEPTION*?
   A. Fetal alcohol syndrome
   B. Bell's palsy
   C. Cretinism
   D. Down syndrome
   E. Bilateral lip and palate

6 Which of the following radiographic projections would be *MOST* helpful in imaging the maxillary sinus?
   A. Cephalometric
   B. Lateral oblique mandible
   C. Posterior-anterior skull
   D. Transcranial
   E. Water's projection

SITUATION: A 42-year-old woman on no medications and with no significant past medical history is scheduled with you for comprehensive dental hygiene care. Initially, she has no complaints about her health and her vital signs are within normal limits. After you explain the procedure she will undergo and initiate the dental hygiene intervention, the woman begins to complain of "feeling faint." Questions 7–11 refer to this situation.

7 The initial treatment for this woman should be
   A. Recline the dental chair to the Trendelenburg position
   B. Recheck vital signs to see if they are still normal
   C. Give the woman a sugar-containing drink
   D. Call in the office staff

*Patricia Regener Campbell prepared cases A–O and their associated questions. The remaining test items were prepared by the other contributors.

8 In spite of the above treatment, the woman loses consciousness and is very pale. The next thing that must be done is
A. Place a bite block in the woman's mouth
B. Assess the airway and open the airway if necessary
C. Move the woman from the dental chair to the floor
D. Activate the emergency medical system (EMS)

9 During the loss of consciousness all the following signs may be noted *EXCEPT*
A. Weak pulse
B. Flaccid muscles
C. Shallow respirations
D. "Fruity" breath odor

10 As this woman regains consciousness,
A. Her pulse rate and blood pressure return to normal
B. She should be walked out of the room as soon as possible to avoid recurrence of this event
C. She will feel very sleepy

11 Once this woman states she is feeling fine, she should be
A. Discharged from your care and allowed to go home
B. Transported to the nearest hospital for evaluation
C. Seen by her primary care physician as soon as possible

---

12 The atrioventricular (AV) valve of the heart
A. Has two flaps
B. Is also called the mitral valve
C. Is located between the right atrium and the right ventricle
D. Is located between the left atrium and the left ventricle

13 When an antifungal ointment is applied before a culture, to areas of angular cheilitis, which of the following diagnostic categories is being used?
A. Therapeutic
B. Clinical
C. Laboratory
D. Differential
E. Historical

14 Signs and symptoms of congestive heart failure include each of the following *EXCEPT*
A. Shortness of breath
B. Cough
C. Swelling
D. Prominent jugular veins
E. Low blood sugar

15 Which of the following conditions causes a delay in dental development?
A. Autism
B. Multiple sclerosis
C. Hyperthyroidism
D. Hypothyroidism
E. Spina bifida

16 Which of the following body tissues is the *MOST* radioresistant?
A. Enamel of the teeth
B. Lens of the eye
C. Red bone marrow of the mandible
D. Thyroid gland

17 All of the following muscles move the head *EXCEPT* one. Which one is the *EXCEPTION*?
A. Sternocleidomastoid
B. Brachialis
C. Semispinalis capitis
D. Splenius capitus

18 Which of the following risk factors has been associated with necrotizing ulcerative gingivitis?
A. Leukemia
B. Emotional stress
C. Age
D. Tobacco use
E. Infrequent dental visits

19 A peripheral giant cell granuloma usually arises from the periodontal ligament. Histologically, a practitioner will find
A. Multinucleated giant cells
B. Little or no inflammatory cells
C. Remnants of the enamel or cementum
D. Necrosis of all cells
E. Osteoblasts

20 Most of the carbon dioxide in the blood is carried in the form of
A. Dissolved carbon dioxide
B. Carbaminohemoglobin
C. Carbonic acid and bicarbonate
D. Carboxyhemoglobin

21 The appropriate depth of chest compressions for an adult is
A. ½ to 1 inch
B. 1 to 1½ inches
C. 1½ to 2 inches
D. 2 to 2½ inches

22 Immunity by vaccination is acquired
A. Naturally, active
B. Naturally, passive
C. Artificially, active
D. Artificially, passive

SITUATION: A 6-year-old female arrived for her 6-month dental hygiene care appointment with just one complaint. She feels "itchy" all over and it started about 10 minutes ago when she was outside playing in the grass. Initially, her vital signs are normal except for slight tachycardia. She has some skin lesions that appear to be urticaria and her lower lip is beginning to swell. Within a minute she complains of difficulty breathing and her respiratory rate is elevated. Questions 23–25 refer to this situation.

23 Normal respiratory rate for this child would be
A. 10 to 14 respirations/minute
B. Approximately 16 respirations/minute
C. Approximately 20 respirations/minute

24 This child probably is experiencing a(an)
A. Mild delayed allergic reaction
B. Mild anaphylactic reaction
C. Anaphylactic reaction
D. Skin reaction with hyperventilation

25 This child's condition may progress to
A. Hyperventilation with syncope
B. Cardiovascular collapse
C. Poison ivy
D. Congestive heart failure

---

26 Which of the following is the *GREATEST* contributor of radiation to the population?
A. Consumer and industrial products
B. Healing arts
C. Natural sources
D. Production of nuclear energy

27 The radicular cyst is usually found at the apex of the root and is usually associated with
A. A fistula
B. An unerupted tooth
C. A carious tooth
D. A supernumerary tooth
E. Impacted third molars

28 Which of the following vertebrae are normally fused together?
A. Cervical
B. Thoracic
C. Lumbar
D. Coccygeal

29 What term is used to describe a lesion that is stem-like?
A. Sessile
B. Papule
C. Pedunculated
D. Bulla
E. Lobulated

30 The *PRIMARY* reason for removing subgingival calculus during periodontal debridement is because it
A. Harbors bacterial plaque
B. Acts as a mechanical irritant
C. Degenerates cementum
D. Enters the junctional epithelium

31 Which of the following is *NOT* a bacterial virulence factor?
A. Capsule
B. Endotoxin
C. Kinase
D. Exotoxin
E. Cytokine

32 Osteoarthritis primarily affects
A. Small joints in children
B. Large joints in children
C. Small joints in adults
D. Weight-bearing joints in children
E. Weight-bearing joints in adults

33 Septic shock is usually caused by
A. An infectious agent
B. Heart failure
C. Psychologic disorder
D. Allergic reaction

34 Which of the following methods for delivering antimicrobial agents into a periodontal pocket raises safety concerns for home use?
A. Mouthrinsing twice daily
B. Standard jet irrigation tip
C. Subgingival irrigation tip
D. Cannula

35 The device used to measure blood pressure is called a
A. Sphygomomanometer
B. Stethoscope
C. Korotkoff

36 Different classes of diuretics have activity on various sites in the kidney. Which pair accurately expresses the class of diuretic with its major site of action?

Category	Major Site of Action
A. Carbonic anhydrase inhibitor	Loop of Henle
B. Loop diuretics	Proximal tubules
C. Thiazides	Thick segment of ascending limb
D. Potassium-sparing diuretics	Distal convoluted tubule

37 Which human immunoglobulin is the *MOST* numerous in response to bacterial toxins?
A. IgG
B. IgM
C. IgE

38 Bronchial asthma is characterized by all of the following conditions *EXCEPT* one. Which one is the *EXCEPTION*?
A. Airway obstruction
B. Bronchospasms
C. Airway inflammation
D. Mucous production
E. Airway hyporesponsiveness to stimuli

39 Tissues have the capacity to repair radiation damage to a certain degree. However, some damage cannot be repaired and remains weakened, especially with repeated exposures. What is this phenomenon called?
A. A critical organ
B. Somatic effect
C. Cumulative effect
D. Genetic effect
E. Latent period

40 The corpus luteum is maintained for the first 10 weeks of pregnancy by
A. Human chorionic gonadotropin (hCG)
B. Luteinizing hormone (LH)
C. Estrogen
D. Progesterone

41 The portion of the target bombarded by electrons is called the
A. Copper stem
B. End point
C. Focal spot
D. Focusing cup
E. Tungsten filament

42 Which of the following is *NOT* a treatment for leukemia?
A. Renal surgery
B. Irradiation
C. Chemotherapy with blood transfusions and antibiotics
D. Interferon therapy
E. Bone marrow transplant

SITUATION: A 69-year-old man is a new client to your practice. He states he has a heart condition, but has never had a heart attack. He periodically experiences swelling of the lower legs and is on a medication called digoxin (Lanoxin). He is also on a "water pill." His vital signs are normal but you do notice some edema around the ankle. Questions 43–45 refer to this situation.

43 The *MOST* likely name for this client's "heart condition" is
A. Congestive heart failure
B. Cerebrovascular accident
C. Angina
D. Myocardial infarction

44 The "water pill" he is referring to is probably
A. A beta blocking agent
B. A diuretic agent
C. A calcium channel blocking agent
D. An angiotensin converting enzyme

45 Placing this client in a horizontal position may result in the person
A. Feeling lightheaded
B. Experiencing increased ankle edema
C. Becoming progressively short of breath
D. Breathing more comfortably

---

46 Radiographic diagnosis contributes significantly to the final diagnosis of all of the following *EXCEPT*
A. Internal resorption
B. Odontoma
C. Unerupted supernumerary teeth
D. Impacted third molars
E. Cementoma

47 A periodontal examination conducted on a 48-year-old male reveals probing depths of 5 to 6 mm in proximal surfaces of all posterior teeth, normal gingival contour, radiographic evidence of bone loss, and generalized gingival inflammation. What disease classification is present?
A. Chronic gingivitis
B. Early adult periodontitis
C. Moderate adult periodontitis
D. Advanced adult periodontitis
E. Necrotizing ulcerative periodontitis

48 What is an infection acquired during a hospital stay called?
A. Focal
B. Subclinical
C. Primary
D. Nosocomial
E. Opportunistic

49 A decrease in blood pH (below 7.35) is called
A. Alkalosis
B. Acidosis
C. The Bohr effect
D. The Hering-Breuer reflex

50 An x-ray produced by the slowing down of an accelerating electron as it passes near the nucleus of the target atom is called
A. Bremsstrahlund
B. Characteristic
C. Discrete
D. Particulate

51 Which one of the following is *NOT* considered a variant of normal?
A. Hairy leukoplakia
B. White hairy tongue
C. Fissured tongue
D. Geographic tongue
E. Migratory glossitis

52 The eye has several muscles attached to it. Which extrinsic muscle and cranial nerve that innervates the muscle will rotate the eye toward the midline?

Muscle	Cranial Nerve
A. Superior rectus	Trochlear
B. Inferior rectus	Abducens
C. Medial rectus	Oculomotor
D. Lateral rectus	Abducens

53 External tooth resorption occurs as a result of
A. Dental caries
B. Salivary gland dysfunction
C. Medications
D. Chronic inflammation beginning in the periodontal ligament
E. Use of chemical mouthrinses

54 What oral lesion is observed radiographically as a radiolucent area, in the mandibular anterior region, and occurs most commonly in black females in their 30s; all associated teeth are vital?
A. Cementoblastoma
B. Periapical cemental dysplasia
C. Median mandibular cyst
D. Traumatic bone cyst
E. Odontomas

CASE—MICHAEL DOWD: Questions 55–60 refer to the case history at the top of page 811.

55 Which of the following is the *MOST* important consideration in providing dental care for Michael?
A. Obtaining a complete set of radiographs at the first visit
B. Using oral premedication or nitrous oxide to control behavior
C. Determining the etiology of his behavioral disorder
D. Assuring a safe and structured environment in the dental treatment area during the appointment
E. Teaching him to floss

SYNOPSIS OF PATIENT HISTORY		
	Age	*7*
	Sex	*M*
	Height	*4'1"*
CASE *Michael Dowd*	Weight	*60* lbs / *27* kgs

VITAL SIGNS
Blood pressure *110/60*
Pulse rate *120*
Respiration rate *20*

1. Under Care of Physician
   Yes [X]   No [ ]
   Condition: *Attention deficit hyperactivity disorder*

2. Hospitalized within the last 5 years
   Yes [ ]   No [X]
   Reason: *But has been seen in the emergency room numerous times for minor injuries*

3. Has or had the following conditions
   Hyperactivity, short attention span, learning disability

4. Current medications
   None, but has been on numerous regimens that did not appear to be effective in reducing problematic behavior nor increasing attention span

5. Smokes or uses tobacco products
   Yes [ ]   No [X]

6. Is pregnant
   Yes [ ]   No [ ]   N/A [X]

MEDICAL HISTORY:
Michael was always restless as an infant. When he became ambulatory he did not have impulse control and has had frequent accidents with injuries.

DENTAL HISTORY:
Michael has never seen a dentist because his parents were afraid he wouldn't behave and they could not afford to take him without insurance coverage. They have not noticed any dental problems.

SOCIAL HISTORY:
He has been in 5 different classrooms at 3 schools because of his disruptive behavior and learning disability. The parents are now demanding that the school personnel provide appropriate services for their son in the public school system.

CHIEF COMPLAINT:
Parents would like to have a complete evaluation of his oral health and suggestions for helping him with self-care at home. He is capable of brushing his teeth, but his behavior interferes.

56 All of the following statements are *TRUE* about attention deficit hyperactivity disorder (ADHD) *EXCEPT* one. Which one is the *EXCEPTION?*
   A. ADHD occurs more often in males
   B. ADHD can affect the output areas of central nervous system function
   C. ADHD can cause problems in reading, writing, or math
   D. ADHD can cause problems with concentration and memory
   E. Children with ADHD have a higher incidence of mental retardation

57 Which one of the following oral manifestations are directly associated with ADHD?
   A. Early gingivitis
   B. No oral manifestations are directly associated
   C. Gingival overgrowth from medications
   D. Rampant dental caries
   E. Hypoactive oral reflexes

58 Which one of the following statements is *FALSE?*
   A. Requesting placement in the public school system is an example of the principle of normalization
   B. Michael's diagnosis of attention deficit hyperactivity disorder will enable him to receive special education and support services
   C. The parents do not have a legal right to ask that services be provided in their local school system
   D. Public school buildings have to be physically accessible to children with disabilities
   E. Using the term ADHD is an example of "labeling" for educational purposes

59 Which of the following is *NOT* the dental hygienist's role in relation to Michael's history of minor injuries?
   A. Suggesting that the parents are abusing him
   B. Checking for evidence of past or current oral trauma
   C. Counseling the parents about ways to prevent injuries
   D. Asking the parents to clarify what type of injuries occurred and what caused them.
   E. Asking which of Michael's behaviors put him at risk for injuries

60 If you were planning Michael's first visit to the dental operatory, which one of the following would you *NOT* do?
  A. Place the instrument tray out of his reach
  B. Introduce him to the dental chair and other equipment gradually
  C. Practice touching his face and inside his mouth with the mouth mirror before using the explorer
  D. Give him quick breaks every 5 to 10 minutes
  E. Ask him to sit perfectly still for 30 minutes and then you'll give him a break

61 Professionally administered oral irrigation is
  A. Routinely recommended in nonsurgical periodontal therapy
  B. More effective than periodontal debridement without oral irrigation
  C. Only effective when an antimicrobial is used
  D. Of little value due to low substantivity of irrigating agents in a periodontal pocket

62 Which of the following blood cells is an agranular leukocyte?
  A. Basophil
  B. Thrombocyte
  C. Erythrocyte
  D. Lymphocyte
  E. Platelet

63 Diastolic pressure is
  A. A form of hypertension
  B. The lower reading in the blood pressure
  C. The higher reading in the blood pressure
  D. A form of hypotension

64 Which of the following describes the use of the aluminum filter in the x-ray unit?
  A. Slows down x-ray production
  B. Narrows the beam to a specific diameter
  C. Absorbs excess heat during x-ray production
  D. Removes long wavelengths from the beam

65 If angular cheilitis is treated with an antifungal ointment or cream and the condition clears up, it was *MOST* likely caused by
  A. *Candida albicans*
  B. A bacterial infection
  C. A nutritional deficiency
  D. Cold weather
  E. A denture

66 An example of an infectious disease and possible sequela is
  A. Group A *Streptococcus* and scarlet fever
  B. Lyme disease and arthritis
  C. Hepatitis B and jaundice
  D. Tuberculosis and emphysema
  E. Giardiasis and diarrhea

67 Which *ONE* of the following is *NOT* considered a local sign of inflammation?
  A. Fever
  B. Pain
  C. Swelling
  D. Erythema
  E. Edema

68 Which one of the following muscles of facial expression surrounds the eye in wide sweeping arches?
  A. Obicularis oris
  B. Obicularis oculi
  C. Depressor supercilii
  D. Corrugator supercilii

69 Which of the following blood cells function as phagocytes?
  A. Eosinophils
  B. Neutrophils
  C. Basophils
  D. Lymphocytes
  E. Erythrocytes

70 If you wanted to decrease client radiation exposure, which of the following PIDs (position-indicating devices or cones) would you choose?
  A. 4-inch pointed
  B. 8-inch circular
  C. 12-inch circular
  D. 16-inch circular
  E. 16-inch rectangular

71 An adrenal crisis occurs when the adrenal gland produces an insufficient amount of
  A. Cortisol
  B. Insulin
  C. Oxygen

72 Clubbing of the fingers is *MOST* often seen in
  A. Stroke
  B. Hypertensive disease
  C. AIDS
  D. Congenital heart disease
  E. Cerebral palsy

SITUATION: A woman in her last trimester of pregnancy becomes unresponsive during dental hygiene care. No spontaneous respirations are detected and attempts to ventilate her are unsuccessful. Questions 73–74 refer to this situation.

73 The appropriate treatment for this pregnant woman would be to
  A. Kneel beside the patient and perform abdominal thrusts
  B. Kneel beside the patient and perform chest thrusts
  C. Perform sharp back blows
  D. Administer oxygen

74 Once the pregnant woman regains spontaneous respirations, it is important to
  A. Roll the patient toward her left side to improve circulation by decreasing compression on the aorta by the uterus
  B. Place a towel or wedge under the left hip to increase compression on the aorta by the uterus
  C. Raise the pregnant woman's head at a 20 to 30 degree angle

75 Which of the following cartilages is signet-ring shaped?
  A. Cricoid
  B. Arytenoid
  C. Corniculate
  D. Cuneiform

76 The blood pressure may be artificially elevated if
  A. The client is seated upright while taking the blood pressure
  B. The stethoscope is placed over the brachial artery
  C. The blood pressure cuff is too small
  D. The blood pressure cuff is too large

77 Which of the following cells is associated with hypersensitivity reactions of an anaphylactic type?
  A. Neutrophils
  B. Mast cells
  C. Lymphocytes
  D. Macrophages
  E. Plasma cells

78 Tetracycline fibers are recommended
  A. Instead of periodontal debridement/root planing
  B. For initial therapy of periodontal pockets
  C. In nonresponsive sites following initial therapy
  D. To be used during periodontal flap surgery

79 Which of the following organs is able to tolerate the greatest restriction in blood flow?
  A. Skin
  B. Skeletal muscle
  C. Heart
  D. Brain

80 The abnormal reaction of a person's immune system to a drug is considered a(an)
  A. Side effect
  B. Toxic reaction
  C. Suprainfection
  D. Allergy
  E. Adverse reaction

81 When radiation damage occurs to macromolecules such as DNA by the radiolysis of water to hydrogen peroxide the effect is termed
  A. Direct
  B. Indirect
  C. Primary
  D. Secondary

82 All of the following are etiologic factors for gingival recession EXCEPT
  A. Alveolar bone loss
  B. Tooth position in the arch
  C. Dehiscence
  D. Faulty toothbrushing
  E. Gingival inflammation

83 The larger the crystal size in the emulsion of radiographic film, the less radiation required to produce an image AND the better that image resolution.
  A. Both parts of the statement are correct.
  B. Both parts of the statement are incorrect.
  C. The first part of the statement is correct, the second part is incorrect.
  D. The first part of the statement is incorrect, the second part is correct.

84 Regenerative techniques in periodontal surgery are recommended for
  A. Two- and three-walled vertical defects
  B. One-walled vertical defects
  C. Gingival hyperplasia
  D. Gingival recession
  E. Mucogingival problems

85 Dark stains on radiographic films may result from contamination from all of the following, EXCEPT
  A. Fluoride contamination
  B. Glove powder
  C. Static electricity
  D. Fixer splash before processing
  E. Saliva contamination

86 Chronic liver disease may follow infection with
  A. Hepatitis A and B
  B. Hepatitis A and E
  C. Hepatitis B and E
  D. Hepatitis B and D
  E. Hepatitis D and A

87 Radiopaque structures are easily penetrated by x-rays AND appear light gray to clear on the resultant radiograph.
  A. Both parts of the statement are correct.
  B. Both parts of the statement are incorrect.
  C. The first part of the statement is correct, the second part is incorrect.
  D. The first part of the statement is incorrect, the second part is correct.

88 All of the following conditions are a direct cause of specific oral manifestations EXCEPT one. Which one is the EXCEPTION?
  A. Spina bifida
  B. Bulimia
  C. Sickle cell anemia
  D. Down syndrome
  E. Leukemia

CASE—SHERRY KNOWLES: Questions 89–93 refer to the case study at the top of page 814.

89 All of the following oral manifestations are associated with end stage renal disease or its treatment EXCEPT one. Which one is the EXCEPTION?
  A. Anemic mucosa
  B. Herpes labialis
  C. Supragingival calculus
  D. Ground glass appearance of alveolar bone
  E. Rampant dental caries

90 Which of the following situations is probably NOT an issue when planning a dental appointment for her?
  A. Hypertension
  B. Bleeding tendency
  C. Seizures
  D. Antibiotic premedication
  E. Drug interactions or clearance

SYNOPSIS
OF PATIENT
HISTORY

Age _19_
Sex _F_
Height _5'9"_

VITAL SIGNS
Blood pressure _110/84_
Pulse rate _80_
Respiration rate _15_

Weight _125_ lbs
_56.8_ kgs

CASE _Sherry Knowles—special needs_

---

1. Under Care of Physician
   Yes [X] No [ ]   Condition: _End stage renal disease; hemodialysis_

2. Hospitalized within the last 5 years
   Yes [X] No [ ]   Reason: _Failed kidney transplant_

3. Has or had the following conditions
   Hypertension, headaches

4. Current medications
   Vitamin D, heparin, nifedipine (Procardia)

5. Smokes or uses tobacco products
   Yes [ ] No [X]

6. Is pregnant
   Yes [ ] No [X] N/A [ ]

MEDICAL HISTORY:
This person was born with congenitally deformed kidneys.

DENTAL HISTORY:
She receives sporadic dental care and is very afraid of healthcare providers. She last saw a dentist 1 year ago but that dentist would not treat her because of her complex medical problems and her fear of dentistry.

SOCIAL HISTORY:
She is embarrassed about her small size and that she hasn't yet graduated from high school because of her illness. She wants to go to college to be a social worker.

CHIEF COMPLAINT:
"My mouth is sore from the medications I was taking for my failed transplant and I feel that my gums are growing larger."

---

91 The *MOST* likely reason for the complaint of her "gums growing larger" is
A. Retention of water in her body
B. Accumulation of urea
C. Inflammation
D. Gingival overgrowth from the nifedipine
E. Alveolar bone resorption so the papillae appear larger

92 Hemodialysis places her at *MOST* risk for
A. Hepatitis A
B. Hepatitis A, hepatitis non-A non-B, HIV
C. Tuberculosis
D. Hemophilia
E. HIV and hepatitis A

93 Dental treatment is important to schedule
A. On the day after dialysis
B. Right before dialysis
C. Immediately after dialysis
D. So it coincides with dialysis
E. When heparin is still present in the bloodstream

---

94 Radiographic images that are too light are the result of all of the following, *EXCEPT:*
A. Back of the film packet facing x-ray beam
B. Cold solution temperature
C. Exhausted solutions
D. Overexposure
E. Underdeveloping

95 Sudden momentary loss of awareness without loss of postural tone, a blank stare and a duration of less than 90 seconds *BEST* describes
A. Grand mal seizure
B. Complex partial seizure (psychomotor)
C. Petit mal seizure (absence)
D. Stroke

96 Viruses that persist in the body and cause recurrent disease are called
A. Resistant
B. Cytopathic
C. Opportunistic
D. Oncogenic
E. Latent

97 The precentral gyrus is
A. Involved in muscle control
B. Involved with sensory perception
C. Located in the cerebellum
D. None of the above

98 Manifestations of bulimia include all of the following *EXCEPT* one. Which one is the *EXCEPTION?*
A. Recurrent binging
B. Dehydration
C. Self-induced vomiting
D. Consumption of 300 to 600 calories per day
E. Depression

99 The maleus and incus are
   A. Ear ossicles
   B. Located in the outer ear
   C. Provide a sense of linear acceleration
   D. All of the above

100 Which of the following diagnostic imaging systems uses a conventional x-ray unit and an anatomically adapted charge-coupled device (CCD) sensor to produce an x-ray image on a computer monitor or video screen?
   A. Arthrography
   B. Digital imaging
   C. Magnetic resonance
   D. Nuclear medicine
   E. Sialography

101 If a person is taking a beta-blocking agent (β-adrenergic blocker) such as propranolol (Inderal) or atenolol (Tenormin) it would be unusual for this person to
   A. Demonstrate tachycardia (elevated pulse rate)
   B. Demonstrate increased blood pressure
   C. Exhibit an elevated temperature

102 Measures to prevent coughing and aspiration due to mucus or saliva accumulation or impaired oral reflexes is seen in all of the following EXCEPT one. Which one is the EXCEPTION?
   A. Bronchial asthma
   B. Emphysema
   C. Cystic fibrosis
   D. Parkinson disease
   E. Autism

103 Pathologic tooth mobility can be caused by all of the following EXCEPT
   A. Occlusal trauma
   B. Abscesses
   C. Hormonal changes
   D. Gingival enlargement
   E. Osteomyelitis

104 Endogenous factors influencing the microbial composition of the oral flora include all of the following EXCEPT
   A. pH
   B. Saliva
   C. Diet
   D. Oxygen concentration
   E. Microbial interactions

105 An adult with partial airway obstruction but poor air exchange should
   A. Lie down
   B. Be encouraged to cough and breath deeply
   C. Be treated with sharp back blows
   D. Be treated with the Heimlich maneuver

106 A coin test is used to determine
   A. Film density
   B. Processing errors
   C. Safelight adequacy
   D. Unit output and consistency

107 Internal resorption occurs when
   A. There is pulpal reaction from within the tooth
   B. Stimuli come from the periodontal ligament
   C. There is rapid orthodontic movement
   D. Periapical pathosis occurs first
   E. There is a deep carious lesion

108 The primary cause of a mucocele is
   A. Tumor formation
   B. Inflammation
   C. Obstruction in the duct
   D. Trauma to a minor duct
   E. Blockage at the caruncles

109 A positive tuberculin skin test is an example of which hypersensitivity reaction?
   A. Type I
   B. Type II
   C. Type III
   D. Type IV

110 Which of the following cancers has the BEST 5-year survival rate (all ages included)?
   A. Lung
   B. Breast
   C. Prostate
   D. Ovarian
   E. Colorectal

111 Acid producers which are also aciduric are
   A. Lactobacilli
   B. *Streptococcus mitis*
   C. *Streptococcus sanguis*
   D. *Streptococcus viridans*

112 Clear films result from all of the following, EXCEPT
   A. Placing film in fixer solution first
   B. Nonexposure to x-rays
   C. Accidental white light exposure
   D. Excessive washing

113 The terms soft, firm, semi-firm, and fluid-filled are used to define which ONE of the following
   A. Fissured
   B. Palpation
   C. Papillary
   D. Coalescence
   E. Cyst

114 Which of the following is NOT an oral manifestation of HIV?
   A. Hairy leukoplakia
   B. Candidiasis
   C. Linear gingival erythema
   D. Papillomavirus (warts)
   E. *Pneumocystis carinii*

115 Which drug prescribed for hypertension has been found to cause the LEAST amount of connective tissue proliferation?
   A. Norvasc
   B. Dynacirc
   C. Nifedipine
   D. Procardia
   E. Nitroglycerine

116 Which of the following findings would necessitate retreatment with active periodontal therapy if discovered during a reevaluation at the periodontal maintenance visit?
A. Generalized bacterial plaque
B. Presence of gingival inflammation
C. Gingival recession
D. Localized attachment loss increase of 2 mm
E. Gingival bleeding

117 Which one of the following stages of syphilis is properly matched?
A. Primary—rash
B. Secondary—chancre
C. Primary—gumma
D. Tertiary—rash
E. Tertiary—gumma

118 Which one of the following is *NOT* a characteristic of supernumerary teeth?
A. Most often seen radiographically
B. Usually genetic
C. Can be associated with other syndromes
D. Mesioden is the most common type
E. Never seen in posterior regions

119 Which one of the following statements is *TRUE* regarding the sternohyoid muscle?
A. It is a muscle of facial expression.
B. It is an infrahyoid muscle.
C. It is a circular muscle in cross-section.
D. It has two "bellies."
E. It is a muscle of mastication.

120 Penicillin would be *LEAST* effective when used for which pathogen?
A. Actinomyces
B. Mycoplasma
C. Bacillus
D. Leptospira
E. Treponema

121 Frictional keratosis occurs when
A. There is chewing on an edentulous ridge
B. Client uses mouthrinse
C. There is a malignancy present
D. Client eats a high-fiber diet
E. Client smokes heavily

122 Which one of the following types of periodontal disease is slowly progressive?
A. Localized juvenile periodontitis
B. Adult periodontitis
C. Linear gingival erythema
D. Refractory periodontitis

123 Which of the following is a characteristic of a cardiovascular accident on the *right* side of the brain?
A. Person cannot focus and use a mirror
B. May not be able to remember your name, despite repetitions
C. Has problems phrasing sentences and remembering vocabulary
D. Appears disorganized
E. Exhibits right hemiplegia

124 Hyperplastic candidiasis presents as
A. A removable soft, creamy, white plaque; red and/or bleeding base
B. A raised, white nonremovable plaque
C. A smooth, flat, red lesion on the dorsum of the tongue
D. Cracking or redness around the corners of the mouth

125 The muscles of facial expression are innervated by cranial nerve
A. I
B. III
C. V
D. VII

126 Which of the following cells is associated with cell-mediated immunity?
A. B cells
B. T cells
C. Mast cells
D. Macrophages
E. Neutrophils

127 A radiolucent oval often seen near the apex of the mandibular second premolar that mimics periapical pathology is *MOST LIKELY*
A. Incisive foramen
B. Infraorbital foramen
C. Lingual foramen
D. Mandibular foramen
E. Mental foramen

128 All of the following conditions *EXCEPT* one can result in confinement to a wheelchair to the extent that a transfer to the dental chair may not be feasible or safe. Which one is the *EXCEPTION?*
A. A man with a spinal injury at the C3 level
B. A patient on a respirator
C. A severely debilitated AIDS patient
D. An extremely obese (300+ lbs) man with congestive heart disease
E. A man with a spinal injury at the T6 level

129 Autonomic hyperreflexia is a medical emergency that may occur in persons with
A. Spinal cord injuries
B. Hypothyroidism
C. Hyperthyroidism
D. Cardiac arrhythmias
E. Bronchial asthma

130 PAP is a general acronym for a periapical pathosis associated with a tooth. It may likely be
A. A cyst
B. A periapical granuloma
C. An abscess
D. All of the above
E. B and C only

131 Enamel dysplasia is seen in all of the following conditions *EXCEPT* one. Which one is the *EXCEPTION?*
A. Mental retardation
B. Cerebral palsy
C. Congenital heart disease
D. Sickle cell anemia
E. Muscular dystrophy

132 Which of the following criteria is *MOST* important to determine extent of periodontal destruction in a case of periodontitis?
   A. Tooth mobility
   B. Probing depth
   C. Radiographic evidence of bone loss
   D. Furcation involvement
   E. Attachment loss

133 Retrocuspid papillae would be observed clinically
   A. On the buccal mucosa near the parotid gland
   B. Lingual to the maxillary central incisors
   C. On the gingival margin of the lingual aspect of the mandibular canines
   D. On the floor of the mouth
   E. Posterior dorsal of the tongue

134 Xerostomia is a common oral manifestation accompanying all of the following *EXCEPT* one. Which one is the *EXCEPTION?*
   A. Chronic alcoholism
   B. Diuretic drug therapies
   C. Rheumatic heart disease
   D. Radiation therapy to the head and neck
   E. Uncontrolled diabetes mellitus

135 Which of the following bacteria primarily colonize gingival crevices?
   A. *S. salivarius*
   B. *S. mitior*
   C. *S. milleri*
   D. *S. mutans*
   E. *A. naeslundii*

136 All of the following craniofacial or oral conditions are common in Down syndrome *EXCEPT* one. Which one is the *EXCEPTION?*
   A. Small nasomaxillary complex
   B. Mandibular crowding or malpositioned teeth
   C. Increased susceptibility to periodontal disease
   D. Delayed tooth eruption
   E. Cervical abrasion

137 Black hairy tongue involves elongation of the
   A. Fungiform papillae
   B. Retrocuspid papillae
   C. Foliate papillae
   D. Circumvallate papillae
   E. Filiform papillae

138 Which of the following supplemental diagnostic tests can be used at chairside to immediately detect presence of selected periodontal pathogens in a particular site?
   A. DNA probe
   B. Culturing
   C. ELISA
   D. BANA

139 All of the following statements are true regarding the trigeminal nerve *EXCEPT* one. Which of the following statements is the *EXCEPTION?*
   A. Each of the two divisions sends a small recurrent branch to the dura mater
   B. The cutaneous areas that are supplied by the various divisions comprise the entire face with the exception of a large area at the mandibular angle.
   C. Each division sends fibers to the mucous membranes of the nasal or oral cavity.
   D. The trigeminal nerve arises with a large sensory and a small motor root from the ventral surface of the pons.

140 Which one of the following pairs is correct regarding helminths?
   A. Nematodes—flukes
   B. Nematodes—flatworms
   C. Trematodes—roundworms
   D. Cestodes—tapeworms
   E. Trematodes—flatworms

141 Which *ONE* of the following conditions must have a radiograph to complete the diagnosis?
   A. Supragingival calculus
   B. Torus palatinus
   C. Erupted mesiodens
   D. Retrocuspid papillae
   E. Calcified pulp

142 Use of aspirin is generally contraindicated in all of the following conditions/situations *EXCEPT* one. Which one is the *EXCEPTION?*
   A. Hemophilia A
   B. Rheumatoid arthritis
   C. Bronchial asthma
   D. Persons taking anticoagulants
   E. Chronic alcoholism

143 Which of the following sites is correctly matched with the primary colonizer?
   A. Tongue—*S. sanguis*
   B. Saliva—*S. mutans*
   C. Pit and fissure—*S. milleri*
   D. Root surface—*S. mitior*
   E. Saliva—*S. salivarus*

144 Antibacterial activity of saliva is related to all of the following *EXCEPT*
   A. Flow
   B. Secretory IgA
   C. Lysozyme
   D. Glycoproteins
   E. Interferon

145 The initial response of the body to injury is the process of
   A. Immunity
   B. Infection
   C. Hyperplasia
   D. Inflammation
   E. Hypoplasia

146 During coagulation, the platelet plug is strengthened by a meshwork of insoluble protein fibers known as
   A. Fibrin
   B. Serum
   C. Bradykinin
   D. Prostaglandins

147 Which *ONE* of the following is a progressive condition that may result in early death?
   A. Duchenne muscular dystrophy
   B. Cerebral palsy
   C. Autism
   D. Schizophrenia
   E. Generalized tonic-clonic seizures disorder

148 Scalloping around the root of a tooth, observed radiographically as a radiolucent area may be helpful in diagnosing the
   A. Traumatic bone cyst
   B. Stafne bone cyst
   C. Odontogenic keratocyst
   D. Primordial cyst
   E. Ameloblastoma

149 Which *ONE* of the following is considered an autoimmune disease?
   A. Multiple sclerosis
   B. von Willebrand disease
   C. Sickle cell anemia
   D. Ischemic heart disease
   E. Cystic fibrosis

150 Myasthenic crisis is a medical emergency because
   A. The person's muscles become rigid
   B. The person cannot close the eyelids
   C. The person can experience a seizure
   D. Secretions in the throat can impair breathing
   E. The person might have an angina attack

Section Two

Case A   Illustrations on pages I-2–I-3 refer to this case.

151 A medical consultation with the client's physician is recommended for persons with systemic lupus erythematosus (SLE) for which of the following conditions?
- A. Arthritis
- B. Heart valve pathology
- C. Raynaud's phenomena
- D. Periodontal inflammation

152 If the physician determines that this client should receive antibiotic premedication, what is the proper dosage?
- A. 500 mg amoxicillin 1 hour before the dental/dental hygiene procedure and 250 mg every 6 hours for eight doses
- B. 2 g clindomycin 1 hour before the dental/dental hygiene procedure and 500 mg every 6 hours for eight doses
- C. 2 g amoxicillin orally 1 hour before procedure
- D. 3 g amoxicillin 1 hour before the dental/dental hygiene procedure and 1.5 g 6 hours after the initial dose

153 Because this client has xerostomia, the dental hygienist instructed him to use a fluoridated mouthrinse without alcohol in order to
- A. Prevent an oral fungal infection
- B. Prevent further drying of the tissues
- C. Produce an antimicrobial effect
- D. Avoid alcohol addiction

154 Complete scaling and root planing on this client will be complicated the MOST due to which one of the following factors?
- A. Inadequate oral hygiene
- B. Root sensitivity
- C. Numerous areas of dental caries
- D. Excessive bleeding

155 The cause of this client's xerostomia is most likely which of the following?
- A. Medications
- B. Lupus erythematosis
- C. High blood pressure
- D. Tobacco use

156 The radiopaque areas on the mesial and distal of #4, the distal of #5, and the mesial and distal of #13 are due to which of the following?
- A. Calculus
- B. Dental caries
- C. Enamel pearls
- D. Exostosis

157 According to the American Association of Periodontology, this client's periodontal classification would be which of the following?
- A. Type I
- B. Type II
- C. Type III
- D. Type IV
- E. Type V

158 Which of the following aids would be most helpful to this client in removing supragingival plaque?
- A. Manual soft toothbrush
- B. Dental floss
- C. Interdental stimulator
- D. Rotary toothbrush

159 Which of the following should NOT be used to remove calculus deposits on this client?
- A. Rubber cup
- B. Sonic/ultrasonic scaler
- C. Airbrasive polisher
- D. Water irrigation device

160 Four weeks after initial scaling and root planing on this client, a reevaluation was performed. At this time the client was reprobed and evaluated for home care compliance. There was a decrease in bleeding sites and a decrease in the probing depth in many areas. Which of the following BEST explains the reason for this change?
- A. Normal tissue shrinkage
- B. Better home care techniques
- C. Increase in anaerobic bacteria
- D. Decrease in the disease process

161 What is the radiolucent area at the tip of #29?
- A. Mental foramen
- B. Apical abscess
- C. Exostosis
- D. Cyst

162 The recession along the cervical one third of tooth #21 and 28 is MOST likely due to which of the following?
- A. Improper toothbrushing technique
- B. Heavy calculus deposits
- C. High lateral frenum attachment
- D. Improper flossing technique

163 Which of the following in-office fluoride products should be used on this client?
- A. Sodium fluoride gel or foam (2% concentration)
- B. Stannous fluoride gel (8% concentration)
- C. Acidulated phosphate fluoride gel or foam (1.23% concentration)
- D. Sodium fluoride rinse (0.2% concentration)

164 This client has Class II mobility on tooth #23 and 24. Which of the following BEST describes this classification of tooth mobility?
- A. Barely discernible movement
- B. Combined faciolingual movement totaling 2 mm, and tooth depressable in the socket
- C. Combined faciolingual movement totaling between 2 and 3 mm
- D. Combined faciolingual movement totaling 3 mm or more and/or tooth is depressable in socket

165 Which of the following probes is preferred to detect furcation involvement?
- A. Marquis probe
- B. Williams probe
- C. Michigan-O probe
- D. #2 Nabers probe

Case B Illustrations on pages I-4–I-5 refer to this case.

166 Complications from Sjögren syndrome include all of the following *EXCEPT*
A. Fissured tongue
B. Intraoral yeast infections
C. Burning mucosa
D. Increase in dental caries
E. Enlargement of the salivary gland

167 Which of the following medications taken by the client compounds the xerostomia caused by her Sjögren syndrome?
A. Librax
B. Premarin
C. Prozac
D. Zantac

168 Which type of fluoride should be used on this client?
A. Acidulated phosphate fluoride
B. Neutral sodium fluoride
C. Stannous fluoride
D. Fluoride should not be used on this client

169 Which of the following should this client be encouraged to use as a regular part of her home care regimen?
A. Topical fluoride gel
B. Chlorhexidine mouthwash
C. Fluoride toothpaste
D. Flavored mouthrinses

170 The gingival margin around teeth #22 through 28 can *BEST* be described by which of the following terms?
A. Cratered
B. Clefted
C. Receded
D. Festooned

171 The red scattered papillae that are prominent near the tip of this client's tongue are called
A. Circumvallate papillae
B. Filiform papillae
C. Foliate papillae
D. Fungiform papillae

172 All of the following are important considerations when planning care for this client *EXCEPT*
A. Give client frequent breaks
B. Allow client to exercise her jaw frequently
C. Give frequent sips of water
D. Use air frequently

173 When planning educational services for this client, which *ONE* of the following practices should receive the highest priority?
A. Oral cancer self-examination
B. Home fluoride therapy
C. Flossing techniques
D. Use of saliva substitutes

174 Taking the facts you have learned about this client and her oral conditions, what would be the *BEST* recommended continued care interval for her?
A. 2 months
B. 3 months
C. 4 months
D. 6 months

175 What is the radiolucent area on the mesial surface of #7 in the panogram?
A. Amalgam restoration
B. Gold restoration
C. Composite restoration
D. Dental caries

176 Which of the following instruments should be used to scale the distal of tooth #25?
A. Gracey 1/2 curet
B. Gracey 11/12 curet
C. Gracey 13/14 curet
D. Columbia 13/14 curet

177 While you are polishing this client's teeth using a toothbrush, she asks why you are not using the "electric polisher" like the last dental hygienist. When explaining selective tooth polishing to her, which of the following is *NOT* true of the effects of polishing?
A. Produces a bacteremia
B. Abrades and removes only cementum and dentin
C. May impact polishing into the gingiva
D. Produces heat which can cause pain

178 Which of the following is an additional hazard to the clinician when performing motor-driven rotary or air-abrasive extrinsic stain removal procedures?
A. Heat generated during extrinsic stain removal
B. Removal of surface fluoride
C. Contaminated aerosol produced during extrinsic stain removal
D. Use of highly abrasive polishing agents

Case C Illustrations on pages I-6–I-7 refer to this case.

179 The radiolucent area to the distal of tooth #31 is due to which of the following?
A. Periapical abscess
B. Recent extraction site
C. Possible carcinoma
D. Radicular cyst

180 After the client's implants were placed, she was placed on ampicillin. What additional information should be given to the client regarding this medication?
A. Antibiotics may decrease the effectiveness of the birth control pills
B. Extreme bruising may occur due to the antibiotic
C. Discontinue medication if urticaria occurs
D. A and C

181 When instrumenting around the dental implants, the dental hygienist should do which of the following?
   A. Use Gracey curets to instrument around the dental implants
   B. Use plastic instruments to instrument around the dental implants
   C. Use an ultrasonic scaler to instrument around the dental implants
   D. Use coarse polishing paste

182 Which of the following should be used to probe this client's dental implants?
   A. Plastic probe
   B. Metal probe
   C. The implants should not be probed
   D. Naber's probe

183 Which of the following should *NOT* be recommended to this client to care for her implants at home?
   A. Powered toothbrush
   B. Stainless steel coated wire interproximal brush
   C. Filament floss
   D. End tuft toothbrush

184 The client is concerned about doing all the right things to maintain the area. You advise her that all of the following materials are appropriate to use around her implant *EXCEPT* which one?
   A. Metal
   B. Wood
   C. Nylon
   D. Plastic

185 The type of dental implant that was placed in the client's mouth is which of the following?
   A. Subperiosteal implant
   B. Endosteal (endosseous) implant
   C. Transosteal (transosseous) implant
   D. None of the above

Case D Illustrations on pages I-8–I-9 refer to this case.

186 The initial blood pressure readings on the client at this continued care appointment were as follows: first reading 145/100 mm Hg, second reading 150/110 mm Hg, and third reading 145/95 mm Hg. Which of the following guidelines should be followed for this client?
   A. No unusual precautions related to client management. Recheck blood pressure at regular 6 month continued care visit.
   B. Recheck blood pressure before dental or dental hygiene therapy for three consecutive appointments; if all readings exceed guidelines, seek medical consultation.
   C. Recheck blood pressure in 5 minutes. If still elevated, seek medical consultation before dental or dental hygiene therapy.
   D. Recheck blood pressure in 5 minutes. Immediate medical consultation if still elevated.

187 Of the medications currently taken by this client, which is used to control blood pressure?
   A. Monopril (fosinopril sodium)
   B. Zocor (simvastatin)
   C. Tavist-D

188 The indistinct vermillion border shown in photograph #1 is *MOST* likely a result of which of the following?
   A. Normal aging process
   B. Surgery to correct cleft lip
   C. Frequent herpetic lesions
   D. Sun exposure

189 The black spots on the left border of the mandible are the result of which of the following?
   A. Improper developing technique
   B. Film exposed to light
   C. Improper film handling
   D. Touching the film during processing

190 The dark area on the gingiva to the mesial of #20 is *MOST* likely which of the following?
   A. Melanoma
   B. Amalgam tattoo
   C. Kaposi sarcoma
   D. Hematoma

191 Which of the following aids would be *MOST* helpful to this client in removing interproximal plaque?
   A. Floss
   B. Interdental stimulator
   C. Interproximal brush
   D. Floss aid

192 The hard palate contains several localized areas of inflammation. The cause of this is *MOST* likely which of the following?
   A. *Candida albicans*
   B. Denture stomatitis
   C. Ulcerative stomatitis in-situ
   D. Herpetic lesions

193 What technique should be used to remove the soft deposits on this client's teeth?
   A. Airbrasive polisher
   B. Rubber cup
   C. Toothbrush
   D. Irrigating device

194 What recommendations should be made to the client regarding his angular cheilosis?
   A. Stay out of the sun
   B. Use sunblock
   C. Use a lubricant frequently
   D. Rinse frequently with chlorhexidine mouthrinse

195 One primary concern in planning treatment for this client is
   A. Aspiration of liquids into the sinus
   B. Speech difficulties of the client
   C. Tooth sensitivity to cold
   D. Sinus infections

196 What is the preferred instrument to root plane the distal surface of the mesial root of #30?
   A. Gracey 11/12 curet
   B. Gracey 13/14 curet
   C. Columbia 13/14 curet
   D. Gracey 4R/4L curet

197 The fluoride of choice for in-office therapy is which of the following?
A. Sodium fluoride gel or foam (2% concentration)
B. Acidulated phosphate gel or foam (1.23% concentration)
C. Stannous fluoride gel (8% concentration)
D. Sodium fluoride rinse (0.2% concentration)

198 When cleaning this client's partial in the treatment area, which of the following is *NOT* an acceptable method?
A. Manual scaling with a curet
B. Manual scaling with an ultrasonic instrument
C. Brushing with a denture brush and cleanser
D. Polishing on a dental lathe

| Case E | Illustrations on pages I-10–I-11 refer to this case.

199 Which of the following antibiotics is contraindicated for this pregnant woman?
A. Cephalosporin
B. Clindamycin
C. Penicillin
D. Tetracycline

200 Which of the following is the *BEST* time to perform elective dental restorative procedures on this client?
A. 1st trimester
B. 2nd trimester
C. 3rd trimester
D. None of the above

201 The client asks many questions related to her health and that of her baby. She wants to know when her baby's teeth will begin to develop. Which of the following is correct?
A. 1 to 3 weeks in utero
B. 4 to 5 weeks in utero
C. 6 to 7 weeks in utero
D. 8 to 10 weeks in utero

202 Which of the following *BEST* describes this client's gingival disease?
A. Pregnancy gingivitis
B. Necrotizing ulcerative gingivitis
C. Acute periodontitis
D. Acute/chronic gingivitis

203 The client reports that she does not like milk and does not eat breakfast. All of the following foods *EXCEPT* which one should be recommended to her to increase her intake of calcium?
A. Yogurt
B. Salmon with bones
C. Fresh spinach
D. Cucumbers

204 Which of the following motivational appeals would be *MOST* effective with this client?
A. Concern for her unborn child
B. Concern for her appearance
C. The cost of dental care
D. Pain involved in neglecting her teeth

205 All of the following factors *EXCEPT* which one directly contributed to this woman's present oral condition?
A. Tobacco use
B. Not using dental floss
C. Pregnancy
D. Neglect of dental care

206 Which of the following mouthrinses should be recommended to this client to use while her tissues are healing?
A. Fluoride mouthrinse
B. Alcohol-free mouthrinse
C. Chlorhexidine gluconate mouthrinse
D. Mouthrinse is contraindicated

207 At the initial visit with this client, you begin taking periodontal probe readings and she reports that what you are doing hurts and she wants you to stop. Which of the following procedures would be *BEST* to follow?
A. Tell the client that it is important that you get this information and ask her to try to concentrate harder.
B. Give the client nitrous oxide and oxygen analgesia so you can complete her assessment.
C. Discontinue probing and take readings after the acute stage of the disease has been resolved.
D. Suggest that the client be given local anesthesia so you can complete her assessment.

208 The client tells you that she has smoked cigarettes for a long time and asks if her smoking will affect her baby. All of the following adverse effects can occur in the fetus as a result of the mother's smoking habit *EXCEPT* which one?
A. Low birth weight
B. Premature birth
C. Miscarriage
D. Mental retardation

209 Which of the following terms *BEST* describes the condition of the gingiva on the facial of tooth #10?
A. Acute marginal gingivitis
B. Chronic marginal gingivitis
C. Acute diffuse gingivitis
D. Chronic diffuse gingivitis

210 The contour of the gingival papilla around the mandibular teeth is *BEST* described by which of the following terms.
A. Blunted
B. Bulbous
C. Cratered
D. Rolled

211 When the client returns for the evaluation following her periodontal debridement, you notice that there is gingival bleeding and edema on the mesial and distal of tooth #10. Which of the following is the treatment of choice?
A. Treatment is not necessary
B. Probe periodontal sulcus
C. Take a periapical radiograph
D. Remove residual calculus and bacterial plaque

The following pages contain the forms, radiographs, and clinical photographs that are referred to in Cases A–O presented earlier in Section Two of this simulated board exam. The test items for these fifteen cases are contained in pages 819-831.

Many of the radiographs and clinical photographs used in the following pages have been cropped, reduced, or enlarged to enhance the clarity of the structures or the lesions they represent.

SYNOPSIS OF PATIENT HISTORY

Age __33__
Sex __M__
Height __5'4"__

Weight __165__ lbs
__75__ kgs

CASE *Adult periodontitis*

VITAL SIGNS
Blood pressure __128/88__
Pulse rate __80__
Respiration rate __20__

1. Under Care of Physician
   Yes [X] No [ ]
   Condition: *Systemic lupus erythematosus (SLE)*

2. Hospitalized within the last 5 years
   Yes [ ] No [X]
   Reason: _____

3. Has or had the following conditions
   Lupus, ulcers, Raynaud's phenomena
   _____

4. Current medications
   Plaquenil (hydroxychloroquine), Meticorten (prednisone), Feldene, (piroxicam)
   _____

5. Smokes or uses tobacco products
   Yes [X] No [ ]

6. Is pregnant
   Yes [ ] No [ ] N/A [X]

MEDICAL HISTORY:
The client reports a history of ulcers, frequent headaches, arthritis in his hands and knees, and lupus. He is allergic to codeine.

DENTAL HISTORY:
It has been 5 years since his last dental treatment. He had an examination with a periodontist 6 months ago, because of "loose teeth and pain." He did not seek further treatment at the time due to the expense.

SOCIAL HISTORY:
The client is divorced and works at a convenience store.

CHIEF COMPLAINT:
"My teeth are loose and they hurt."

ADULT CLINICAL EXAMINATION

Current oral hygiene status
Moderate to heavy bacterial plaque. Client reports brushing twice a day but does not floss.

Supplemental oral examination findings
1. *Generalized bleeding upon probing.*
2. *Heavy subgingival calculus and moderate supragingival calculus.*
3. *Class I mobility on #3, 13, 15, 25, and 26. Class II mobility on #23 and 24.*
4. *Xerostomia*
5. *Recession generalized on all mandibular teeth.*

Clinically visible carious lesion
Clinically missing tooth
△ Furcation
▲ "Through and through" furcation

Probe 1: initial probing depth
Probe 2: probing depth 1 month after scaling and root planing

Maxillary — facial

	1	2	3	4	5	6	7	8	9	10	11	12	13	14	15	16
Probe 2	545		534	434	4 4		4		434	4 4	4 4	4 4	4 5	545	659	746	545
Probe 1	556		535	534	333	445	434		434	444	444	445	545	659	957	655

Maxillary — palatal

	1	2	3	4	5	6	7	8	9	10	11	12	13	14	15	16
Probe 1	446		535	435	534	4 4	4 4	4 4	4 4	4 4	4 4	434	434	5 5	557	655
Probe 2	546		434	434	5 5	4 4	4 4	4 4	4 4	4 4	4 4	4 4	444	556	544

Mandibular — lingual

	32	31	30	29	28	27	26	25	24	23	22	21	20	19	18	17
Probe 2	546	545	444	4 4	4 4	4 4	4		4 4	4 4	4 4	4	4 4	445	544	
Probe 1	546	545	444	444	4 4	444	4 4	4 4	435	544	435	434	4 5	556	644	

Mandibular — facial

	32	31	30	29	28	27	26	25	24	23	22	21	20	19	18	17
Probe 1	556	656	646	5 4	4 4	4 5	5 4	4 4	334	436	625	544	434	746	646	
Probe 2	546	646	5 4	4 4	4 4	4 5	5 4	4 4	4 4	4 4	4 4	4 4	4 4	545	546	

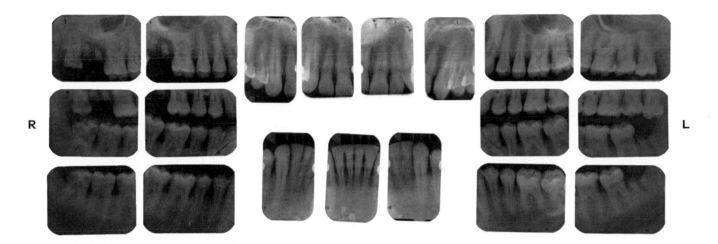

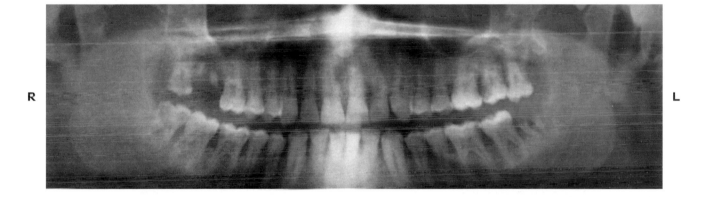

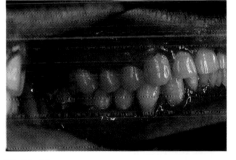

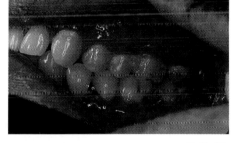

Right side

Left side

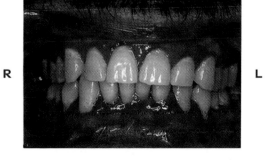

SYNOPSIS OF PATIENT HISTORY

Age __50__
Sex __F__
Height __5'10"__

Weight __180__ lbs
__82__ kgs

CASE _Medically compromised_

VITAL SIGNS
Blood pressure __118/76__
Pulse rate __72__
Respiration rate __16__

1. Under Care of Physician
   Yes [X] No [ ] Condition: _Hiatal hernia_

2. Hospitalized within the last 5 years
   Yes [ ] No [X] Reason: _____

3. Has or had the following conditions
   Lupus erythematosus, rheumatoid arthritis, TMJ disorder

4. Current medications
   Librax (chlordiazepoxide), Zantac (ranitidine hydrochloride), Prozac (fluoxetine hydrochloride), Premarin (conjugated estrogens)

5. Smokes or uses tobacco products
   Yes [ ] No [X]

6. Is pregnant
   Yes [ ] No [X] N/A [ ]

MEDICAL HISTORY:
Client reports a history of Sjögrens syndrome, lupus erythematosus, rheumatoid arthritis, depression, a spastic colon, and hiatal hernia. She had a melanoma removed from her right arm 3 years ago. Her health problems began after her silicone breast implants ruptured.

DENTAL HISTORY:
The client has had extensive dental treatment. Her TMJ becomes sore following dental treatment. She has limited mouth opening since both TMJ disks were surgically removed. She has severe xerostomia and brushes and flosses 2 to 3 times a day.

SOCIAL HISTORY:
She is currently enrolled in college part-time, and is heavily involved in a class action suit against the pharmaceutical company that made her breast implants.

CHIEF COMPLAINT:
"My mouth is dry and I need to have my teeth cleaned."

ADULT CLINICAL EXAMINATION

Current oral hygiene status
Light to moderate bacterial plaque with light calculus and stain

Supplemental oral examination findings
1. Localized areas of bleeding
2. Recession on all facial surfaces

Clinically visible carious lesion
Clinically missing tooth
Furcation
"Through and through" furcation
Probe 1: initial probing depth
Probe 2: probing depth 1 month after scaling and root planing

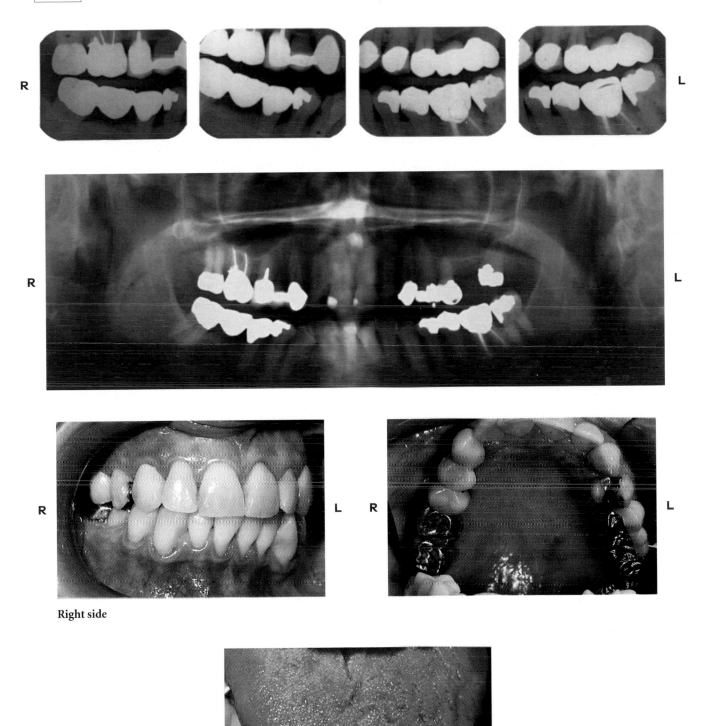

Right side

SYNOPSIS
OF PATIENT
HISTORY

CASE *Dental implants*

Age *17*
Sex *F*
Height *5'4"*

Weight *120* lbs
54.5 kgs

VITAL SIGNS
Blood pressure *110/70*
Pulse rate *85*
Respiration rate *20*

1. Under Care of Physician
   Yes ☐   No ☒   Condition:_____

2. Hospitalized within the last 5 years
   Yes ☐   No ☒   Reason:_____

3. Has or had the following conditions
   Migraine headaches

4. Current medications
   Demulen (ethynodial diacetate with ethinyl estradiol), Imitrex (sumatriptan succinate)

5. Smokes or uses tobacco products
   Yes ☐   No ☒

6. Is pregnant
   Yes ☐   No ☒   N/A ☐

MEDICAL HISTORY:
Migraine headaches occasionally. No other health problems.

DENTAL HISTORY:
Regular dental care. Has never had a carious lesion. Wore orthodontic appliances and retainers for three years. One dental implant was completed a year ago. The second has just been placed.

SOCIAL HISTORY:
She lives with her younger brother and parents. She is a very active teenager and will be going away to college in about 6 months.

CHIEF COMPLAINT:
"It's time for my regular dental checkup."

ADULT CLINICAL EXAMINATION

Current oral hygiene status
Very good home care.

Supplemental oral examination findings
1. No bleeding in any areas.
2. Gingiva healthy

Dental implant

Clinically visible carious lesion

Clinically missing tooth

△ Furcation

▲ "Through and through" furcation

Probe 1: initial probing depth
Probe 2: probing depth 1 month after scaling and root planing

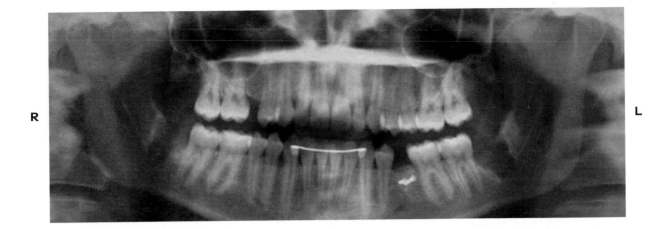

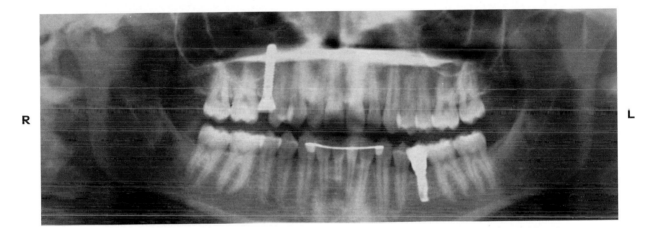

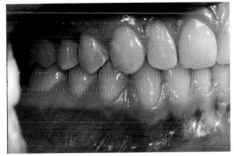

Right side

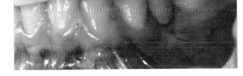

Left side

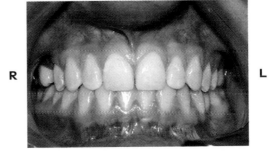

SYNOPSIS
OF PATIENT
HISTORY

CASE *Special needs*

Age _62_
Sex _M_
Height _5'9"_

Weight _178_ lbs
_81_ kgs

VITAL SIGNS
Blood pressure _145/95_
Pulse rate _67_
Respiration rate _20_

1. Under Care of Physician
   Yes [X] No [ ]
   Condition: _Hypertension_

2. Hospitalized within the last 5 years
   Yes [ ] No [X]
   Reason: _____

3. Has or had the following conditions
   Kidney stones, cleft lip and palate
   _____

4. Current medications
   Monopril (fosinopril sodium), Zocor
   (simvastatin), Tavist-D
   _____

5. Smokes or uses tobacco products
   Yes [ ] No [X]

6. Is pregnant
   Yes [ ] No [ ] N/A [X]

MEDICAL HISTORY:
Client has unilateral cleft lip and palate that were surgically corrected when he was a child. He has frequent sinus infections and had a basal cell carcinoma removed from his neck 6 months ago. He is allergic to penicillin.

DENTAL HISTORY:
Client's maxillary anterior teeth were removed while he was in high school because they were malposed and he has worn a removable partial denture since then. He brushes 4 to 5 times daily and uses floss regularly.

SOCIAL HISTORY:
The client is college educated, single, and works as a computer analyst. He is an avid golfer, playing at least 3 times a week.

CHIEF COMPLAINT:
"I have broken a clasp on my partial and I need to have my teeth cleaned."

ADULT CLINICAL EXAMINATION

Probe 2 / Probe 1 (maxillary facial), teeth 1–16:

	1	2	3	4	5	6	7	8	9	10	11	12	13	14	15	16
Probe 2		344	3 4								3 4	4 4	4 4	5 4		
Probe 1		344	3 4								4 5	5 4	5 4	544		

facial

palatal

	1	2	3	4	5	6	7	8	9	10	11	12	13	14	15	16
Probe 1		545	544	4 4	444							4 4	444	446		
Probe 2																

Current oral hygiene status
Moderate bacterial plaque, light stain and calculus.

Supplemental oral examination findings
1. Radiographs were taken one year prior to photographs— tooth #15 and 18 were extracted due to periodontal involvement.
2. Severe recession on all teeth.
3. Bleeding on probing in posterior areas.
4. Class I mobility #23–25.
5. Furcation involvement on #3, 14, 19, 30 and 31.

Mandibular lingual, teeth 32–17:

	32	31	30	29	28	27	26	25	24	23	22	21	20	19	18	17
Probe 2		334	34	5										4	5	
Probe 1		335	334	5	4 4	4 4	4 4	4 4	4 4					4	5	

lingual

facial

	32	31	30	29	28	27	26	25	24	23	22	21	20	19	18	17
Probe 1		546	4	5 3		3 4		4		4 4				4	5	
Probe 2		5 5 4	4											4	5	

Legend:

Clinically visible carious lesion

Clinically missing tooth

△ Furcation

▲ "Through and through" furcation

Probe 1: initial probing depth
Probe 2: probing depth 1 month after scaling and root planing

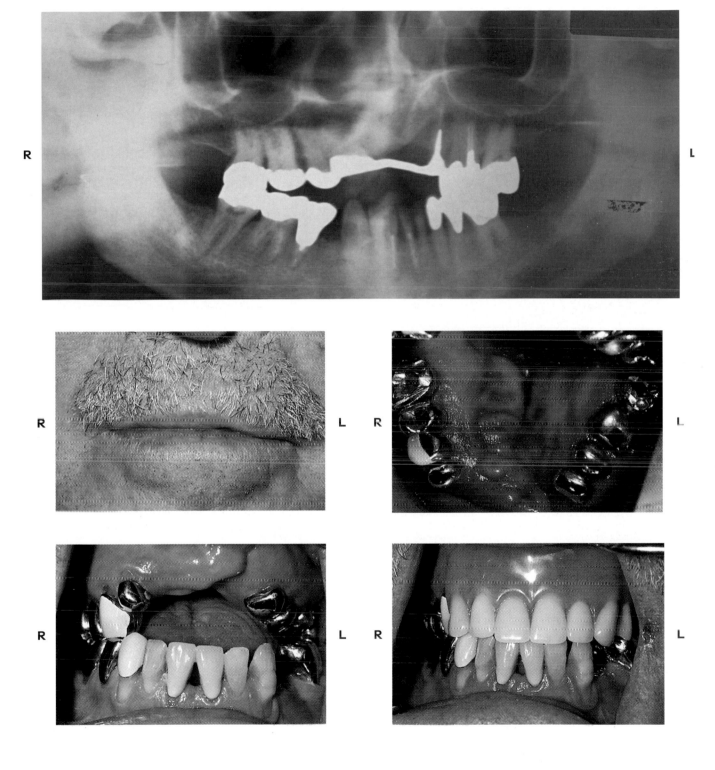

SYNOPSIS OF PATIENT HISTORY

Age _26_
Sex _F_
Height _5'3"_

Weight _125_ lbs
_57_ kgs

VITAL SIGNS
Blood pressure _110/70_
Pulse rate _78_
Respiration rate _16_

CASE _Special needs–pregnancy_

1. Under Care of Physician
   Yes [X]   No [ ]
   Condition: _Pregnancy_

2. Hospitalized within the last 5 years
   Yes [ ]   No [X]
   Reason: _____

3. Has or had the following conditions
   Pregnant
   _____

4. Current medications
   Multivitamins
   _____
   _____

5. Smokes or uses tobacco products
   Yes [X]   No [ ]

6. Is pregnant
   Yes [X]   No [ ]   N/A [ ]

MEDICAL HISTORY:
The client reports to be in good health and has a noncontributory history. She is three months pregnant and went to see her physician two weeks ago.

DENTAL HISTORY:
She does not remember her last dental visit, but remembers that it was to get a filling in a wisdom tooth. She reports that she brushes as often as she can, but does not use floss.

SOCIAL HISTORY:
The client is single and is working at a local supermarket on varying shifts. She lives with her boyfriend who is an auto mechanic.

CHIEF COMPLAINT:
"My teeth and gums bleed a lot and they are sore."

ADULT CLINICAL EXAMINATION

Current oral hygiene status
Poor oral hygiene.

Supplemental oral examination findings
1. Heavy calculus and stain in all areas.
2. Acute gingivitis
3. Spontaneous bleeding
4. Heavy bacterial plaque all areas
5. Pain on probing – dental hygienist was unable to probe at initial appointment.

Clinically visible carious lesion

Clinically missing tooth

Furcation

"Through and through" furcation

Probe 1: initial probing depth
Probe 2: probing depth 1 month after scaling and root planing

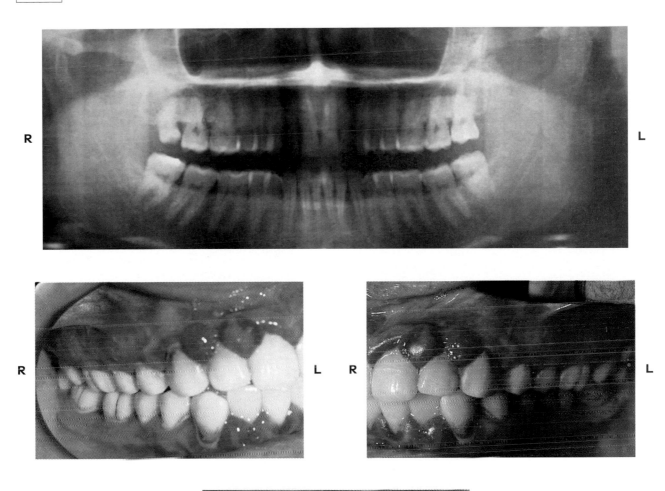

SYNOPSIS
OF PATIENT
HISTORY

Age _____ 68 _____
Sex _____ M _____
Height _____ 5'7" _____

Weight _____ 210 _____ lbs
_____ 95 _____ kgs

CASE _Special needs–visually impaired_

VITAL SIGNS
Blood pressure _____ 130/80 _____
Pulse rate _____ 66 _____
Respiration rate _____ 16 _____

1. Under Care of Physician
   Yes ☒ No ☐
   Condition: _Hypertension_

2. Hospitalized within the last 5 years
   Yes ☐ No ☒
   Reason: _____

3. Has or had the following conditions
   Hypertension, prostate surgery, arthritis,
   retinitis pigmentosa

4. Current medications
   Dyazide, ibuprofen
   _____
   _____

5. Smokes or uses tobacco products
   Yes ☐ No ☒

6. Is pregnant
   Yes ☐ No ☐ N/A ☒

MEDICAL HISTORY:
As a result of retinitis pigmentosa, the client is blind in his left eye and partially sighted in his right eye.

DENTAL HISTORY:
The client receives routine care. He reports brushing twice a day but does not usually floss. He uses a medium toothbrush and a fluoride dentifrice. His teeth are very sensitive to cold and when he brushes.

SOCIAL HISTORY:
The client is retired and divorced. He lives with his daughter and her two teenage sons. He is unable to drive and relies on his daughter for transportation.

CHIEF COMPLAINT:
"My lower right side hurts when I chew something hard."

ADULT CLINICAL EXAMINATION

Current oral hygiene status
Client exhibits good home care.

Supplemental oral examination findings
1. Localized recession on maxillary canines and premolars.
2. Class I mobility #6–11, 23–27.

Clinically visible carious lesion

Clinically missing tooth

△ Furcation

▲ "Through and through" furcation

Probe 1: initial probing depth
Probe 2: probing depth 1 month
 after scaling and root planing

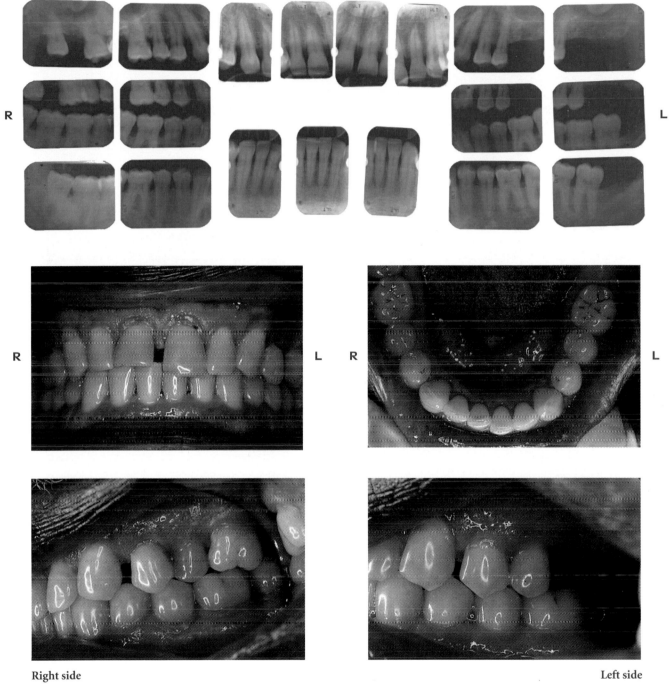

R   L   R   L

Right side   **Left side**

SYNOPSIS OF PATIENT HISTORY

CASE _Geriatric_

Age _86_
Sex _F_
Height _5'0"_

Weight _90_ lbs
_41_ kgs

VITAL SIGNS
Blood pressure _110/70_
Pulse rate _84_
Respiration rate _17_

1. **Under Care of Physician**
   Yes [X]   No [ ]
   Condition: _Squamous cell carcinoma_

2. **Hospitalized within the last 5 years**
   Yes [X]   No [ ]
   Reason: _Surgery to remove right mandible_

3. **Has or had the following conditions**
   Osteoporosis, squamous cell carcinoma

4. **Current medications**
   Aspirin, Nystatin occasionally

5. **Smokes or uses tobacco products**
   Yes [ ]   No [X]

6. **Is pregnant**
   Yes [ ]   No [X]   N/A [ ]

MEDICAL HISTORY:
The client is not currently taking any medications. Two years ago her right mandible was removed and she received 30 radiation treatments and chemotherapy. She has lost 40 lbs. in the last 18 months.

DENTAL HISTORY:
All mandibular teeth and the maxillary molars have been extracted. She has limited opening and severe xerostomia. She had periodontal disease in the past. Note: All radiographs shown were taken prior to the removal of the client's mandibular teeth.

SOCIAL HISTORY:
The client has been a widow for the past 10 years and lives alone in her own home. Stopped smoking 10 years ago. She still uses snuff on occasion.

CHIEF COMPLAINT:
"I need to have my cavities filled."

ADULT CLINICAL EXAMINATION

Current oral hygiene status
Very low plaque score.

Supplemental oral examination findings
1. Limited opening and mandible deviates to the right. Popping sound is evident upon opening.
2. Bilateral tori
3. No bleeding upon probing

Clinically visible carious lesion

Clinically missing tooth

△ Furcation

▲ "Through and through" furcation

Probe 1: initial probing depth
Probe 2: probing depth 1 month after scaling and root planing

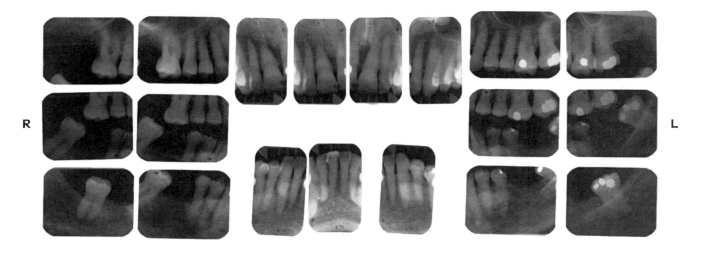

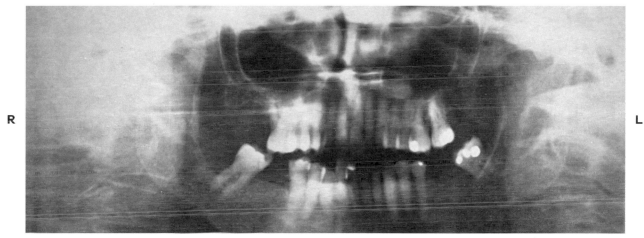

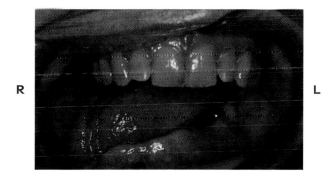

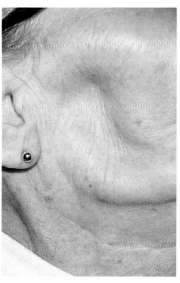

Right side

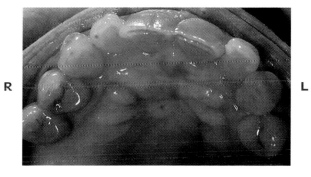

SYNOPSIS OF PATIENT HISTORY

Age __28__
Sex __M__
Height __6'2"__

Weight __170__ lbs
__77__ kgs

VITAL SIGNS
Blood pressure __115/79__
Pulse rate __68__
Respiration rate __24__

CASE _Special needs–Amelogenesis imperfecta_

1. Under Care of Physician
   Yes ☐   No ☒   Condition:_____

2. Hospitalized within the last 5 years
   Yes ☐   No ☒   Reason:_____

3. Has or had the following conditions
   _____
   _____

4. Current medications
   _None_____
   _____
   _____

5. Smokes or uses tobacco products
   Yes ☒   No ☐

6. Is pregnant
   Yes ☐   No ☐   N/A ☒

MEDICAL HISTORY:
The client reports a noncontributory health history, but he is allergic to penicillin.

DENTAL HISTORY:
It has been one year since the client's last dental visit. He reports that his teeth are very sensitive to cold. He brushes twice a day and tries to use floss several times a week.

SOCIAL HISTORY:
The client is married and attends college part-time. He works evenings and weekends in a convenience store. He uses spit tobacco daily.

CHIEF COMPLAINT:
"I want to get my teeth fixed."

ADULT CLINICAL EXAMINATION

	1	2	3	4	5	6	7	8	9	10	11	12	13	14	15	16
Probe 2	6		6		5				4	436			4	444		646
Probe 1	446	7			5		3 3 3	3 4 7				43	4 4	436		646

facial

palatal

	1	2	3	4	5	6	7	8	9	10	11	12	13	14	15	16
Probe 1	556	66	44	445	545	444	444	4	574	454	434	434	5 7		556	
Probe 2	456	66		5	5 5	4 4	4 4	4	46	444	5		5 7		445	

	32	31	30	29	28	27	26	25	24	23	22	21	20	19	18	17
Probe 2	545	655	434	4	333	3	3						4 4 4			
Probe 1	545	745	545	4		3 3	323	323	323	333	323	323	3 4	4 4		3

lingual

facial

	32	31	30	29	28	27	26	25	24	23	22	21	20	19	18	17
Probe 1	546	644	4 4	6							3	4 4	4 5	4		3
Probe 2	5	6 4	4 4	63								4	5			

Current oral hygiene status
Light to moderate bacterial plaque, intrinsic stain on all teeth.

Supplemental oral examination findings
1. Generalized moderate gingivitis.
2. Moderate periodontitis in the UR, UL, and LR.
3. Bleeding at all probing sites.
4. Amelogenesis imperfecta.

🦷 Clinically visible carious lesion

✖ Clinically missing tooth

△ Furcation

▲ "Through and through" furcation

Probe 1: initial probing depth
Probe 2: probing depth 1 month after scaling and root planing

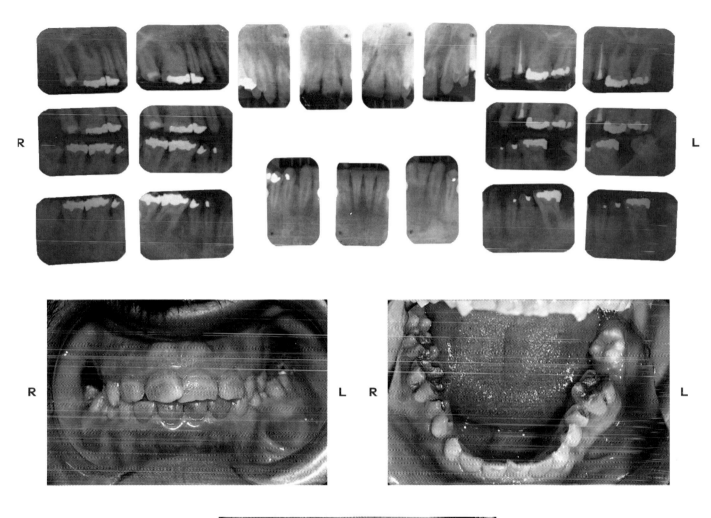

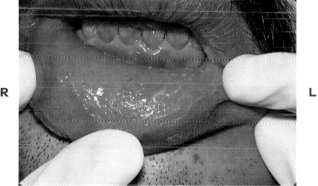

Case F Illustrations on pages I-12–I-13 refer to this case.

212 A bluish area on the facial marginal gingiva of #22 is *MOST* likely which of the following?
A. Subgingival calculus
B. Normal pigmentation
C. Amalgam tattoo
D. Dental caries

213 All of the following should be included in the dental hygiene care plan for this client *EXCEPT* which one?
A. Professional application of fluoride
B. Review toothbrushing with client
C. Review flossing with client
D. Use of disclosing solution to show client areas he is missing

214 Using Angle's classification of malocclusion, the occlusal relationship of the maxillary and mandibular first molars in centric occlusion would be classified as which of the following?
A. Class I
B. Class II Division 1
C. Class II Division 2
D. Class III

215 Which error in technique is represented by the right molar bitewing?
A. Cone cutting
B. Film placed in mouth backwards
C. Incorrect horizontal angulation of x-ray beam
D. Double exposure

216 Which of the following agents can be used to relieve the sensitivity on tooth #5 and 12?
A. Potassium oxalate
B. Benzocaine
C. Chlorhexidine
D. Sodium fluoride
E. A and D

217 Reduction of dentinal hypersensitivity occurs as a result of
A. Parasthesia of the odontoblastic process
B. Formation of crystals that block the dentinal tubules
C. Formation of secondary dentin
D. None of the above

218 Which of the following conditions contributed to the recession on the maxillary canines and premolars on this client?
A. Oral habit
B. Improper use of powered toothbrush
C. Scrub method of toothbrushing
D. Brushing with an abrasive dentrifice

219 Which of the following methods is *BEST* used to instruct this client on toothbrushing techniques?
A. Lecture (conversation) with emphasis on how the correct technique feels in the mouth
B. Pamphlet
C. Interactive video
D. Demonstration

220 All of the following considerations should be implemented when working with a visually impaired individual *EXCEPT* which one?
A. Move hazards out of the way
B. Speak before touching the client
C. Tell the client when you are leaving
D. Hold the client's arm to guide them

221 The broad radiopaque band crossing the neck of tooth #32 represents the image of which of the following?
A. Internal oblique ridge
B. External oblique ridge
C. Artifact due to film bending
D. Wall of mandibular canal

222 A desensitizing agent was applied to tooth #6. This procedure also had been done at the client's last two visits. The client called 6 weeks after his dental hygiene care was completed and reported that tooth #6 was still very sensitive even after the desensitizing agent was applied. Which of the following methods should be considered to alleviate the sensitivity?
A. Apply a dental fluoride varnish
B. Apply a composite resin
C. Extract the tooth
D. Reapply the desensitizing agent

Case G Illustrations on pages I-14–I-15 refer to this case.

223 Referring to the pre-extraction panogram, what is the cause of the radiolucent area in the angle of the mandible, distal to tooth #31?
A. Carcinoma
B. Osteoporosis
C. Sclerotic bone formation
D. Ossifying fibroma

224 The client's xerostomia is so severe that she has problems swallowing food. All of the following should be suggested to her *EXCEPT* which one?
A. Take sips of water before taking a bite of food
B. Eat juicy fruits
C. Use a saliva substitute
D. Take smaller bites

225 This client's severe xerostomia is *MOST* likely caused by which of the following factors?
A. Radiation therapy
B. Chemotherapy
C. Medications
D. Use of chewing gum

226 Which of the following could be recommended to this client as a snack?
A. Ice cream
B. Yogurt
C. Cheese
D. Mints

227 At the time the original lesion was discovered in this client, the clinician could expect to see all of the following *EXCEPT* which one?
   A. Poorly localized bone pain
   B. Painful enlargement of regional lymph nodes
   C. An indurated enlargement
   D. Rough, heterogeneous appearance of the lesion

228 The root morphology of tooth #17 may be described by which of the following terms?
   A. Dilaceration
   B. Flexion
   C. Fusion
   D. Hypercementosis

229 Which of the following factors is most likely the major cause of the client's weight loss?
   A. Poor nutrition
   B. Loss of lower teeth
   C. Xerostomia
   D. Squamous cell carcinoma

230 The cause of the cervical caries in this client is *MOST* likely caused by which of the following conditions?
   A. Xerostomia
   B. Diet
   C. Poor toothbrushing technique
   D. Chemotherapy

231 The radiopaque areas seen on the roots of tooth #20, 21, 27-29 are due to which of the following?
   A. Mandibular tori
   B. Osteoporosis
   C. Carcinoma
   D. Internal oblique ridge

232 What is the appropriate continued care interval for this client?
   A. 1 month
   B. 3 months
   C. 4 months
   D. 6 months

233 All of the following *EXCEPT* which one should be recommended to this client to augment her intake of nutrients.
   A. Puree food in blender
   B. Use liquid nutritional supplements
   C. Drink milkshakes
   D. Drink tomato juice

234 How often should the client perform an oral cancer self-care exam?
   A. Daily
   B. Weekly
   C. Monthly
   D. Every 3 months

235 When instructing this client to perform an oral cancer self-examination, you should encourage her to report all of the following to her dentist immediately *EXCEPT* which one?
   A. Sores that do not heal within 2 weeks
   B. Red or white patches in her mouth
   C. Loss of feeling in the head/neck region
   D. Bad odor in the mouth

Case H Illustrations on pages I-16–I-17 refer to this case.

236 The protuberances on the lingual near the premolars and canines in the mandible are *MOST* likely which of the following?
   A. Exostosis
   B. Tori
   C. Sialoliths
   D. Hyperplasia

237 The dental hygiene care plan for this client should include the use of which of the following?
   A. Sonic/ultrasonic scaler
   B. Airbrasive polisher
   C. Cannula for gingival irrigation
   D. Rubber cup polishing

238 Which of the following *BEST* describes the gingival tissue on the facial of #27?
   A. Acute marginal gingivitis
   B. Chronic marginal gingivitis
   C. Acute papillary gingivitis
   D. Chronic papillary gingivitis

239 The radiolucency associated with the apex of #10 *MOST LIKELY* represents
   A. The image of the anterior palatal foramen
   B. The lateral foci
   C. The greater palatine foramen
   D. A periapical abscess

240 When updating this client's health history, which of the following is the *MOST* important question to ask regarding his epilepsy?
   A. When was your last seizure?
   B. Has your doctor changed your medication?
   C. What type of epilepsy do you have?
   D. Did you take your medication today?

241 The cause of the generalized gingival hyperplasia in this client is *MOST* likely a result of which of the following?
   A. Neglect of his teeth
   B. Client does not use floss
   C. A side-effect of medication
   D. Heavy calculus deposits

242 During the course of dental hygiene care, the client becomes rigid, his eyes roll upward, and he begins to have a seizure. Which of the following is the appropriate course of action?
   A. Try to get the client out of the chair and onto the floor so he does not harm himself
   B. Place a padded tongue blade between his teeth to prevent tongue biting
   C. Call 911 to access the emergency medical system (EMS)
   D. Place the chair in a supine position and if possible turn the client to the side

243 The radiolucent area near the apices of tooth #30 and 31 is *MOST* likely due to which of the following?
   A. Inflammation
   B. Recent extraction
   C. Trauma
   D. Developmental defect

244 Factors present in this client that contribute to gingival enlargement include all of the following *EXCEPT* which one?
A. Mouthbreathing
B. Calculus
C. Smoking
D. Heavy bacterial plaque

245 When comparing the probing depths from the initial visit and those 1 month after scaling and root planing procedures, there does not appear to be much change in the depths. How can this be explained?
A. The calculus was so heavy at the initial probing appointment that readings were probably inaccurate
B. The tissue did not respond as expected to the therapy
C. The side effects of the medication keep the tissue from shrinking
D. A different type of probe was used at the second visit

246 When performing procedures on this client, which of the following actions may precipitate an epileptic attack?
A. Touching particular areas of the client's lip
B. Placing the client in a supine position
C. Flashing the overhead light in the eyes of the client
D. Speaking to the client in a fast manner

247 Which of the following would be the *BEST* approach to planning hard deposit removal on this client?
A. Complete gross scaling during the first appointment
B. Plan anesthesia with each appointment
C. Scale and root plane the anterior teeth during the last appointment
D. Scale and root plane a segment to completion

248 The horizontal radiolucent band in the apical third of the root of tooth #8 represents the image of
A. An artifact
B. A fracture
C. The wall of the nasopalatine canal
D. A bend in the film

249 When selecting a polishing agent to remove the extrinsic stain on this client's teeth, each of the following should be considered *EXCEPT* which one?
A. Tooth sensitivity
B. Type of stain present
C. Number of teeth present
D. Type of restorations present

Case I Illustrations on pages I-18–I-19 refer to this case.

250 The anomaly present on the root of #31 is *BEST* described as which of the following?
A. Dilaceration
B. Fusion
C. Concrescence
D. Taurodont

251 The radiopacity located between the apices of #29 and #30 is *MOST* likely which of the following?
A. Retained primary root tip
B. Supernumerary tooth
C. Hypercementosis
D. Nutrient canal

252 The root and pulp chamber of #20 appears considerably larger than those of the other mandibular premolars. What is the most likely cause of this?
A. Pulp chamber and root anomaly
B. Traumatic occlusion
C. Tooth is rotated
D. Hypercementosis

253 The dental hygiene care plan for this client should include all of the following *EXCEPT* which one?
A. Home use of disclosing tablets
B. Review of toothbrushing techniques
C. Home application of fluoride
D. Oral cancer self-examination

254 Complications from amelogenesis imperfecta include all of the following *EXCEPT* which one?
A. Vulnerability to severe attrition
B. Increased risk for dental caries
C. Increased risk for periodontal disease
D. Increased staining with age

255 Amelogenesis imperfecta is a form of enamel dysplasia resulting from unknown factors. The dentin and pulp of these teeth develop normally, whereas the enamel is easily chipped or worn away.
A. The first sentence is TRUE, the second sentence is FALSE.
B. The first sentence is FALSE, the second sentence is TRUE.
C. Both sentences are FALSE.
D. Both sentences are TRUE.

256 The factor responsible for the localized white lesion in the vestibule and on the buccal mucosa of the lower left lip is *MOST* likely which of the following?
A. Tartar control toothpaste
B. Smokeless tobacco/spit tobacco
C. Lip biting habit
D. Irritation from occlusion

257 Which of the following *BEST* describes the localized lesion on the buccal mucosa on the lip of this client?
A. Corrugated plaquelike
B. Multiple papules
C. Irregular fissured
D. Generalized vesicles

258 The bone loss on the distal of tooth #29 can *BEST* be described by which of the following terms?
A. Vertical
B. Horizontal
C. Intraosseous defect
D. Interdental crater

259 Which of the following bacterial plaque removal devices should *NOT* be recommended to this client?
A. Manual toothbrush
B. End tuft toothbrush
C. Interdental brush
D. Sonic/ultrasonic toothbrush

260 The change in the color of the fixed and attached gingiva in the anterior region is most likely due to which of the following?
A. Tobacco stomatitis
B. Normal pigmentation
C. Medication induced
D. Use of medicated mouthrinses

261 Which of the following dental hygiene services should be provided for this client?
A. Scaling and root planing with hand instruments
B. Use of ultrasonic scaler
C. Rubber cup polishing
D. Airbrasive polishing

Case J Illustrations on pages I-20–I-21 refer to this case.

262 The radiopacity between tooth #24 and 26 is which of the following?
A. Genial tubercle
B. Nutrient canal
C. Mental foramen
D. Exostosis

263 The technique error on the mandibular anterior periapical films can *BEST* be corrected by doing which of the following?
A. Placing the film as far from the teeth as practical to ensure it is parallel to the long axis of the tooth
B. Placing the film as close to the teeth as practical to ensure it is parallel to the long axis of the tooth
C. Direct the central ray of the x-ray beam to a negative 30 degree vertical angle
D. Direct the central ray of the x-ray beam parallel to the long axis of the tooth

264 The radiolucent area in the lower mesial corner of the mandibular premolar film is due to which of the following?
A. Nutrient canal
B. Film crease
C. Mandibular fracture
D. Artifact of film processing

265 What is the proper premedication for this client?
A. Amoxicillin 3.0 g orally 1 hour before procedure
B. Clindamycin 600 mg orally 1 hour before procedure
C. Clindamycin 500 mg orally 1 hour before a procedure and 250 mg 6 hours after initial dose
D. Amoxicillin 500 mg orally 1 hour before a procedure and 250 mg 6 hours after initial dose

266 Which of the following motivational appeals would be *MOST* successful in helping this client to improve his self-care?
A. Reward system
B. Enhance appearance
C. Save money
D. Reduce tooth decay

267 Which of the following could be suggested to this client to help him remove interproximal bacterial plaque?
A. Waxed dental floss
B. Floss fingers
C. Interdental brush
D. End tuft toothbrush

268 The enlargement on the hard palate extending from the lingual of tooth #7 to tooth #10 is due to which of the following?
A. Palatine rugae
B. Palatine fovea
C. Canine eminence
D. Incisive papilla

269 After you speak with the client's caretaker, she reports that he is not brushing and becomes angry when she tries to help him. Which of the following should be suggested to her?
A. Punish him when he does not brush
B. Get a powered toothbrush
C. Buy him a new toothbrush
D. Continue to try to help him brush

270 You are working on the lingual of tooth #9 and you cannot focus the overhead light to provide reflection on the area. What is the *BEST* solution?
A. Lean your head to see
B. Have the client raise his chin
C. Use direct vision
D. Change your operator position

271 While you are instrumenting on this client, you notice that he has trouble keeping his mouth open. Which of the following should be used to alleviate this situation?
A. Local anesthesia
B. Bite block
C. Ask his sister to help you
D. Put more pressure on his lower teeth

272 Which of the following home care methods could be recommended to improve this client's periodontal condition?
A. Brushing with a sodium fluoride gel
B. Rinsing with over-the-counter mouthrinse
C. Using sodium fluoride mouthrinse
D. Brushing with chlorhexidine once a day

273 Which of the following home care products and methods could be recommended to help this client manage his dental caries activity?
A. Brush with an alcohol-free mouthrinse
B. Rinse with fluoridated mouthrinse
C. Brush with prescription fluoride gel
D. Rinse with antiplaque rinse

274 Which of the following restorative materials is *MOST* appropriate for a temporary restoration on tooth #14 on this client?
A. Zinc oxide-eugenol
B. Zinc phosphate cement
C. Composite
D. Glass ionomer cement

275 Which of the following describes the technique error on the mandibular anterior periapical film?
A. Elongation
B. Cone cutting
C. Film placed backward
D. Foreshortening

Case K Illustrations on pages I-22–I-23 refer to this case.

276 Which of the following describes this client's occlusal classification on the right molar side?
A. Underjet
B. Overbite
C. Overjet
D. Crossbite

277 What is the radiopaque band evident in the mandible on both the right and left sides?
A. Styloid process
B. Hyoid bone
C. Wall of the mandibular canal
D. Calcification of facial artery

278 What type of occlusion is present in the anterior area as viewed looking directly onto the teeth of the client?
A. Overbite
B. Overjet
C. Crossbite
D. Underjet

279 The white area on the facial of tooth #3 is *MOST* likely which of the following?
A. Calculus
B. Decalcification
C. Fluorosis
D. Trauma

280 The cause of the white area on the facial of tooth #3 is *MOST* likely due to which of the following factors?
A. Poor brushing habits
B. Ingestion of systemic fluoride
C. Topical application of stannous fluoride
D. Weak tooth structure

281 The client will have orthodontic appliances placed on his teeth soon after these photographs are taken. Which of the following would you recommend to him as an adjunct to his home care after his braces are placed?
A. Interdental brush
B. Floss threader
C. Wooden wedges
D. Water irrigating device

282 Which of the following will be a motivator to help this client improve his home plaque removal routine?
A. Rewards
B. Improvement of appearance
C. Saving money
D. Reducing pain

283 At a subsequent appointment, you placed a dental sealant on tooth #30. After the client rinsed, the sealant came out. Which of the following factors was *MOST* likely the cause of the failure of the sealant placement?
A. Moisture contamination
B. Dated etching solution
C. Insufficient rinsing time after the resin hardens
D. Omission of a post-application fluoride treatment

284 The purpose of using this type of radiograph before making decisions on orthodontic treatment is to detect which one of the following?
A. Dental caries
B. Calculus
C. Vertical bone height
D. Presence/absence of permanent teeth

285 During football season, the client would benefit from a mouth protector because it would
A. Prevent the dislocation or fracture of the maxillary anterior teeth
B. Minimize lacerations by holding the soft tissues away from the teeth
C. Decrease shock to the TMJ and mandibular condyle which would prevent concussions
D. All of the above

286 What is the appropriate continued care interval for this client after the placement of his orthodontic appliances?
A. 1 month
B. 3 months
C. 6 months
D. 9 months

287 You have been asked to obtain alginate impressions on this client and he tells you that he gags easily. Which of the following will help to reduce the client's gagging sensation?
A. Ask the client to concentrate on breathing through his nose
B. Ask the client to rinse with an antimicrobial rinse
C. Spray the client's throat with a topical anesthetic
D. Place the client in the Trendelenburg position

288 After you obtain the client's alginate impressions, you put them in the lab and it is several hours before you are able to pour them up. Which of the following will *MOST* likely occur to the impressions?
A. Solation
B. Gelation
C. Syneresis
D. Imbibition

289 When examining this client's teeth, you notice that the dental sealant on tooth #14 is partially lost. Which of the following should be recommended to this client?
A. No treatment should be rendered at this time
B. Re-etch tooth surface and reapply dental sealant
C. Remove remainder of dental sealant and replace
D. Replace with a restorative material

290 The client asks many questions about the dental sealant placement procedure. Which of the following functions is accomplished by the etching procedure?
A. Produces micropores in the enamel surface
B. Increases the surface tension
C. Produces a hard, lustrous surface
D. Exposes the more porous dentin

291 The facial surfaces of the posterior teeth show white spot demineralization. Which of the following forms of fluoride will *MOST* likely be recommended?
A. Systemic tablets
B. Daily mouthrinses
C. Daily gel in a tray
D. Professionally applied fluoride

Case L Illustrations on pages I-24–I-25 refer to this case.

292 The density of panogram #1 could be improved by
  A. Increasing the kilovoltage
  B. Decreasing the milliamperage
  C. Increasing time in the fixer during processing
  D. Decreasing exposure time

293 The anterior teeth on panogram #1 appear abnormally small. This appearance represents which of the following errors?
  A. Client placed too far back in machine
  B. Client placed too far forward in machine
  C. Client movement
  D. Client head tipped to the right side

294 The white lesions evident on the right and left lateral border of this client's tongue are *MOST* likely which of the following?
  A. Oral candidiasis
  B. Lichen planus
  C. Hairy leukoplakia
  D. Herpetic lesions

295 When the client returned for the 1 month post scaling and root planing appointment, there was no noticeable decrease in the periodontal pocket depths. Which of the following is probably the reason that there was not an improvement?
  A. HIV periodontitis does not always respond to conventional therapy
  B. The client did not follow home care instructions
  C. Her CD4 T lymphocyte count had decreased and her disease had progressed
  D. The client had to change medications

296 Which one of the following is recommended to remove the heavy stain and deposits on the lingual of the mandibular anterior teeth?
  A. Ultrasonic scaler
  B. Air-abrasive polisher
  C. Gracey 1/2 curet
  D. Sickle scaler

297 The client reports that the condition present "around the cheek side of her last tooth" (#17) just happened in the last six weeks. What caused this localized destruction?
  A. Immunocompromised state of the client
  B. Complications from linear gingival erythema
  C. Complications from NUG
  D. Complications from necrotizing ulcerative periodontitis

298 The client is taking Diflucan for which of the following conditions?
  A. Oral candidiasis
  B. Herpetic lesions
  C. Pneumonia
  D. Low CD4 T lymphocyte count

299 Which of the following is a side effect that the dental hygienist should be watching for in a client who has been on Bactrim (co-trimoxozol) therapy for an extended period of time?
  A. Candidiasis
  B. Hairy leukoplakia
  C. Enlarged salivary glands
  D. Enlarged lymph nodes

300 Which of the following should be recommended to this client as part of her immediate self-care therapy?
  A. Povidone-iodine rinses/irrigation
  B. 0.12% chlorhexidine rinses/irrigation
  C. Tetracycline therapy
  D. Anesthetic rinses

301 The gingival condition on the facial of tooth #17 can *BEST* be described by which of the following terms?
  A. Linear gingival erythema
  B. HIV-periodontitis
  C. Necrotizing ulcerative gingivitis
  D. Necrotizing ulcerative periodontitis

302 What method of bacterial plaque removal would be *BEST* for the mandibular anterior teeth on this client?
  A. Interdental brush
  B. Interdental stimulators
  C. Waxed dental floss
  D. Unwaxed dental floss
  E. Polytetrafluoroethylene dental floss

303 At the second scaling appointment for this client, the dental hygienist notices a lesion consisting of multiple clear, fluid-filled vesicles clustered on the vermilion border of the mandibular lip. Which of the following procedures should be followed?
  A. Continue with the appointment as planned
  B. Reschedule the client's appointment
  C. Have the client rinse with chlorhexidine before proceeding
  D. Put a lubricant on the lesion and continue as planned

304 The round to ovoid radiopacities present in the right and left of the first panogram represent which of the following?
  A. Artifact
  B. Processing error
  C. Image of client's earrings
  D. Client napkin chain

305 After the initial periodontal debridement therapy on the mandibular anterior region of this client, which of the following complications could occur?
  A. Delayed healing
  B. Excessive bleeding
  C. Increased tooth mobility
  D. Bacterial endocarditis

Case M Illustrations on pages I-26–I-27 refer to this case.

306 This client lives in the desert Southwest and her water supply is nonfluoridated. What is the optimal amount of fluoride that would be appropriate for the municipal water supply in this area?
A. 0.6 ppm F
B. 1.0 ppm F
C. 2.0 ppm F
D. 2.5 ppm F

307 At the 6-month continued care appointment, the client's mother reports that she had their drinking water tested and the fluoride concentration level is 0.2 ppm. Which of the following fluoride supplement dosage levels would be prescribed for this preschool-age child?
A. 0.25 mg F
B. 0.5 mg F
C. 0.75 mg F
D. 1.0 mg F

308 What is the narrow radiolucent line that extends vertically between tooth #E and F on the maxillary anterior radiograph?
A. Nutrient canal
B. Incisive foramen
C. Bend in the film
D. Median palatine suture

309 The blunted root tips on tooth #O and P visible on the mandibular anterior radiograph are due to which of the following?
A. Improper film placement
B. Physiologic root resorption
C. Root fracture
D. Pathologic process

310 The cause of this child's rampant dental caries is due to all of the following factors *EXCEPT* which one?
A. Nonfluoridated water
B. Poor oral hygiene
C. Diet high in sucrose
D. Soft enamel

311 What term would *BEST* describe the anterior occlusion on this child?
A. Overjet
B. Overbite
C. Open bite
D. Underjet

312 Which of the following should be recommended to this child's parent?
A. Immediate placement of dental sealants on the premolars and molars
B. Placement of dental sealants on the first permanent molar as soon as it erupts
C. Dietary counseling for caries control with parent
D. B and C

313 What is the lethal level of fluoride consumption for a child this age?
A. 0.25 to 0.75 g F
B. 0.5 to 1.0 g F
C. 4 to 5 g F
D. 6 to 10 g F

314 The treatment for acute fluoride toxicity is all of the following *EXCEPT* which one?
A. Induce vomiting
B. Administer milk
C. Monitor respiration
D. Start CPR

315 The child's mother asks you what she should look for if the child is experiencing a "bad reaction" to the fluoride. Which of the following is the *MOST* common initial adverse reaction to fluoride toxicity?
A. Nausea
B. Diarrhea
C. Abdominal cramping
D. Respiratory distress

Case N Illustrations on pages I-28–I-29 refer to this case.

316 This child lives in a rural area in an upper northeastern state. His family's drinking water supply is well water that does not contain the appropriate amount of fluoride. What is the recommended fluoride level for a person living in this climate?
A. 0.6 ppm F
B. 1.0 ppm F
C. 1.2 ppm F
D. 2.0 ppm F

317 The *MOST* likely cause of the rampant dental caries in this child is due to which of the following?
A. Early childhood caries
B. Bubble gum
C. Poor home care
D. Genetic predisposition

318 The hard palate and part of the soft palate of this child have a whitish appearance, the palatal vault is unusually deep and the anterior teeth are slightly protruded. What is the *MOST* likely cause for these features?
A. Thumbsucking habit
B. Mouthbreathing
C. Tongue thrusting
D. Nocturnal bruxism

319 The lesion in the apical of the maxillary primary left central incisor is painful upon palpation and thick yellowish exudate is produced. Which of the following is the *MOST* accurate diagnosis of this lesion?
A. Periapical abscess
B. Periodontal abscess
C. Periapical cyst
D. Periapical granuloma
E. Pericoronitis

320 When talking to the mother about toothbrushing procedures, what should you tell her about the appropriate amount of fluoride dentrifice to use for this child?
A. Pea-size amount of toothpaste
B. Cover entire head of toothbrush
C. Do not use toothpaste
D. ½ inch strip of toothpaste

321 Because this child is only 2½ years old, which of the following can be an effective strategy to manage her care?
A. Use age-appropriate terms
B. Control through restraints
C. Provide quick, efficient treatment
D. Ask the parent to stay in the reception area

322 Which of the following dental indices is an effective measure of the dental caries activity of this child?
A. GI (gingival index)
B. PI (plaque index)
C. Deft (decayed, exfoliated, filled teeth index)
D. OHI-S (oral hygiene index—simplified)

323 When talking to this child's mother, she tells you that she had problems taking the bottle away from her child. All of the following liquids could have contributed to the child's condition *EXCEPT* which one?
A. Diluted milk
B. Nonfluoridated water
C. Organic baby formula
D. Unsweetened apple juice

Case O Illustrations on pages I-30–I-31 refer to this case.

324 Etiologic factors leading to periodontal abscess include all of the following *EXCEPT*:
A. Impaction of foreign objects in the sulcus
B. Incomplete scaling and root planing
C. Intrabony pockets
D. Traumatic occlusion

325 Which of the following terms *BEST* describes the tissue to the lingual of tooth #3 in the photograph?
A. Cyanotic
B. Bulbous
C. Blunted
D. Fibrotic

326 Based on the client data given, what is the appropriate continued care interval for this client?
A. 1 month
B. 3 months
C. 4 months
D. 6 months

327 The crescent-shaped radiolucent area to the distal of #13 is *MOST* likely due to which of the following?
A. Intraradicular cyst
B. Inflamed sinus
C. Recent extraction site
D. Bony defect

328 Teeth #23 and 24 are rotated in which direction? (Refer to the photo labeled "Mandibular.")
A. Mesial
B. Distal
C. Facial
D. Lingual

329 The wearing away of the tooth surfaces on the facial surfaces of the client's maxillary teeth can *BEST* be described as which of the following?
A. Abrasion
B. Attrition
C. Bruxism
D. Periodontal surgery

330 When removing soft deposits from this client's teeth, which of the following methods should be used?
A. Airbrasive polisher
B. Rubber cup
C. Toothbrush
D. Ultrasonic scaler

331 What precautions should be taken when working with this client?
A. Premedication is required
B. Ultrasonic devices should not be used
C. Fluorides should not be administered
D. Vital signs should be taken at each visit

332 During the course of the appointment with this client, she begins to perspire profusely and reports that she is feeling weak and her heart seems to be racing. What is the *MOST* likely cause of this reaction?
A. Diabetic coma
B. Insulin reaction
C. Anxiety
D. Hyperglycemia

333 What action should be taken with the client as she is experiencing the symptoms described in question #332?
A. Administer CPR
B. Give client sugar source
C. Lower back of dental chair and elevate feet
D. Force fluids

334 Xerostomia is commonly exhibited in clients with diabetes mellitus. The xerostomia exhibited occurs from the loss of extracellular fluids due to increased urination.
A. Both statements are *TRUE*.
B. Both statements are *FALSE*.
C. The first statement is *TRUE*, the second statement is *FALSE*.
D. The first statement is *FALSE*, the second statement is *TRUE*.

335 Diseases or conditions that could affect this client due to her diabetes include all of the following *EXCEPT*
A. Polydipsia, polyuria, polyphagia
B. Cyanosis of nailbeds
C. Blindness
D. Coronary heart disease
E. Amputation of extremities

336 The periodontal assessment has revealed that this client has furcation involvement on several teeth. On tooth #19, the furcation invasion allows the probe to extend more than 1 millimeter horizontally but not completely through the furcation. Which of the following is the correct furcation classification?
A. Class I furcation
B. Class II furcation
C. Class III furcation
D. Class IV furcation

337 When planning educational interventions for this client, which of the following measures is *MOST* appropriate to assess this client's periodontal status?
A. Plaque Index
B. Gingival Index
C. Calculus Index
D. DMFS

Answers and Rationales

Section One

1. (D) Diphtheria is not a disease primarily of animals that can be transmitted to man.
   - (A) Tularemia is a zoonotic disease.
   - (B) Brucellosis is a zoonotic disease.
   - (C) Anthrax is a zoonotic disease.
   - (E) Toxoplasmosis is a zoonotic disease.

2. (C) Acute fluoride poisoning should be treated by inducing vomiting in the victim.
   - (A) The victim may drink milk but only after vomiting has been induced.
   - (B, D) Incorrect answer

3. (C) Administration of oxygen is contraindicated in hyperventilation. This patient should be rebreathing air with decreased oxygen content in order to improve symptoms.
   - (A) and (B) Persons with asthma or myocardial infarction should receive oxygen.

4. (B) Photoelectric effect occurs when an inner shell electron is ejected and low level energy is generated when an outer shell electron shifts to an inner vacancy.
   - (A) Compton effect results from an incident electron ejecting an outer shell electron.
   - (C) Thompson scattering occurs when an incident electron passes near an outer shell electron causing vibration and ionization.
   - (D) Coherent scattering is another name for Thompson scattering.

5. (B) Bell's palsy involves paralysis in muscles after bone formation is completed.
   - (A) FAS involves multiple malformations and malocclusions.
   - (C) Cretinism causes malformation in eye spacing and jaw structure.
   - (D) Down syndrome causes a craniofacial malformation with malocclusions.
   - (E) Bilateral cleft lip and palate create major developmental malformations of the palate and alveolar bone that can cause malocclusion.

6. (E) The Water's projection is used to image the maxillary sinuses.
   - (A) The cephalometric projection is better used for orthodontic and facial reconstruction purposes.
   - (B) The lateral oblique mandible projection images the mandible from the canine posteriorly to the body and ramus.
   - (C) The posterior-anterior projection is better used to image changes in the cranial bones.
   - (D) The transcranial projection is better used to image the temporal mandibular joint.

7. (A) Reclining the chair will often abort a near syncopal episode and should be the first thing done for this woman.
   - (B) This should be done once the woman is reclined.
   - (C) This is not indicated unless you have reason to believe that the woman is hypoglycemic.
   - (D) Office staff may be alerted but the chair should be reclined first.

8. (B) While the woman is reclined, the airway may become blocked so this is the first thing to be done.
   - (A) This should not be done.
   - (C) The woman will benefit by remaining in the chair where the head will be lower than the legs, thus increasing blood flow to the brain.
   - (D) If there is any suspicion that the woman is suffering a major respiratory or cardiac event, the EMS should be activated. Based on the situation described, the most likely diagnosis in this woman is syncope due to psychogenic factors.

9. (D) "Fruity" breath odor is associated with diabetic emergency (hyperglycemia).
   - (A, B, C) May be seen in syncope

10. (A) After a syncopal episode, vital signs return to normal.
    - (B) The woman should stay in a reclined position for several minutes to avoid a recurrence of this event.
    - (C) This woman should not feel tired after she recovers. Post-seizure patients may feel sleepy.

11. (A) Once vital signs are normal and the woman feels well, she may go home.
    - (B) No need for this unless the woman does not recover fully or there are other signs or symptoms that make you feel it was more serious than just a syncopal episode.
    - (C) Same as (B)

12. (C) This one-way valve is located between the right atrium and the right ventricle.
    - (A) The AV valve has three flaps.
    - (B) The bicuspid valve is also called the mitral valve.
    - (D) The bicuspid valve is located between these two heart chambers.

13. (A) Therapeutic diagnosis involves use of a medication to see if the suspected condition resolves.
    - (B) Clinical diagnosis is made based upon the clinical picture.
    - (C) Laboratory diagnosis is based upon laboratory tests.
    - (D) Differential diagnosis may involve multiple factors.
    - (E) Historical diagnosis involves several components related to the history of the lesion.

14. (E) Low blood sugar is not a sign or symptom of congestive heart failure (CHF).
    - (A) Shortness of breath occurs with CHF.
    - (B) Cough is a common symptom with CHF.
    - (C) Swelling, especially of the lower extremities, is associated with CHF.
    - (D) Prominent jugular veins may be see in a person with CHF.

15. (D) Growth is delayed in many areas, including the teeth and jaws.
    (A) Autism is a behavioral disorder and does not affect dental development.
    (B) Multiple sclerosis is a neuromuscular disorder of adults and doesn't affect dental development.
    (C) Hyperthyroidism causes accelerated dental development.
    (E) Spina bifida has no effect on dental development.

16. (C) Tissues that have a higher metabolic rate and greater proliferation rate are more radiosensitive. Blood cells are the most radiosensitive on this list.
    (A) Tissues that have a lower metabolic rate and lesser proliferation rate are more radioresistant. Enamel is the most radioresistant on this list.
    (B) Tissues that have a higher metabolic rate and greater proliferation rate are more radiosensitive. Although the lens of the eye is relatively radiosensitive, it is not the most radiosensitive on this list.
    (D) Tissues that have a higher metabolic rate and greater proliferation rate are more radiosensitive. Although the thyroid gland is relatively radiosensitive, it is not the most radiosensitive on this list.

17. (B) This muscle flexes the pronated forearm.
    (A) This muscle flexes the head.
    (C) This muscle extends the head and bends it laterally.
    (D) This muscle extends the head and can bend and rotate it toward the same side as the contracting muscle.

18. (B) Emotional stress is a risk factor associated with necrotizing ulcerative gingivitis (NUG).
    (A) Leukemia is a systemic disease risk factor associated with periodontitis.
    (C) Age is not a risk factor for NUG.
    (D) Tobacco use is a risk factor associated with periodontitis.
    (E) Infrequent dental visits are associated with higher risk for periodontitis.

19. (A) Multinucleated giant cells are most commonly seen in the peripheral giant cell granuloma.
    (B) Numerous inflammatory cells are present in the peripheral giant cell granuloma.
    (C) Enamel and cementum are not components of the peripheral giant cell granuloma.
    (D) The histology of the peripheral giant cell granuloma does not show necrosis of all cells.
    (E) Osteoblasts are bone-forming cells.

20. (C) These two forms account for most of the carbon dioxide in the blood.
    (A) About 10% of the total blood carbon dioxide is dissolved in plasma.
    (B) About 20% of the total blood carbon dioxide is carried attached to an amino acid in hemoglobin.
    (D) Carboxyhemoglobin is an abnormal form of hemoglobin in which the reduced heme is combined with carbon monoxide.

21. (C) This is correct for an adult.
    (A) This is correct for an infant.
    (B) This is correct for a child.
    (D) This is incorrect.

22. (C) Immunity by vaccination results from the host's immune system actively responding to an artificially induced infection.
    (A) Naturally, active immunity would result from actual infection with a pathogen.
    (B) Naturally, passive immunity would result from the passage of antibodies from mother to baby.
    (D) Artificially, passive immunity would result from injection of an immune serum.

23. (C) Normal respiratory rate for a child
    (A) and (B) are incorrect

24. (C) She is progressing to respiratory distress from an immediate allergic reaction.
    (A) This is not a mild reaction nor is it delayed.
    (B) Anaphylactic reaction does not have a mild form.
    (D) Although she is having a skin reaction she is not experiencing hyperventilation.

25. (B) If the child's condition continues to deteriorate, cardiovascular collapse may result.
    (A, C, D) Incorrect answer

26. (C) Naturally occurring radionuclides in the soil and radiation from cosmic energy make up over 80% of the population exposure to ionizing radiation.
    (A) Consumer and industrial products account for a small percentage of the 18% radiation exposure to the population from artificial sources.
    (B) Healing arts, including dental X rays account for 11% of the total population exposure to ionizing radiation.
    (D) Production of nuclear energy accounts for a small percentage of the 18% radiation exposure to the population from artificial sources.

27. (C) A radicular cyst is most commonly associated with a carious tooth.
    (A) A fistula signifies periapical pathosis but is not always present with PAP.
    (B) A dentigerous cyst is most likely associated with an unerupted tooth.
    (D) A radicular cyst is not commonly seen with a supernumerary tooth, unless the tooth is erupted with a carious lesion.
    (E) Impacted third molars are most likely to have a dentigerous cyst surrounding the crown of the unerupted tooth.

28. (D) Four to five modular pieces in the coccygeal are fused and in the adult; this segment may be fused with the sacrum.
    (A) There are seven cervical vertebrae. None of them are fused.
    (B) There are twelve thoracic vertebrae. None of them are fused.
    (C) There are five lumbar vertebrae. None of them are fused.

29. (C) Pedunculated describes a lesion that is stem-like.
    (A) Sessile describes a lesion that is flat at the base.
    (B) A papule is a small elevated lesion that is above the surface of normal surrounding tissue.
    (D) A bulla is an elevated lesion that looks like a blister.
    (E) Lobulated describes a lesion that is fused to make one.

30. (A) Calculus is always overlaid with bacterial plaque in humans and bacterial plaque causes periodontal infection; therefore, its role in harboring pathogens is the primary reason for its removal in periodontal debridement.
    (B) Calculus is primarily a bacterial irritant. See A.
    (C) Plaque and calculus can degenerate cementum in the periodontal pocket; however, this is not the primary reason for its removal in periodontal debridement. See A.
    (D) Subgingival calculus is found coronal to the junctional epithelium in the periodontal pocket; bacteria from the plaque enter the junctional epithelium but calculus does not.

31. (E) A cytokine is a factor produced by cells of the immune system that affect other cells. It is not a bacterial product.
    (A) Capsules are bacterial virulence factors that resist host defenses by impairing phagocytosis.
    (B) Endotoxin is a bacterial virulence factor produced by gram-negative cells.
    (C) Kinase is an enzyme produced by bacteria that aids in virulence.
    (D) Exotoxin is a bacterial virulence factor produced by gram-positive cells.

32. (E) Weight-bearing joints such as hips and knees of adults are affected.
    (A, B, D) Osteoarthritis doesn't affect children.
    (C) Osteoarthritis primarily affects large joints, not small ones.

33. (A) This is correct.
    (B) Heart failure may cause cardiogenic shock.
    (C) Psychologic disorder may cause neurogenic shock.
    (D) Allergic reaction may result in anaphylactic shock.

34. (D) A cannula is a needle-like irrigation tip, and raises safety concerns for home use.
    (A) Mouthrinsing twice daily is safe as long as the antimicrobial agent raises no safety concerns.
    (B) A standard jet tip can be used safely for self-care with proper instruction.
    (C) A subgingival (or marginal) irrigation tip can be used safely at home with proper instruction.

35. (A) Also known as blood pressure cuff.
    (B) Used to listen to the rush of the blood through the artery that is compressed by the cuff
    (C) Name for the sounds heard as the blood flows through the artery that is compressed by the cuff

36. (D) Spironolactone would be an example of a potassium-sparing diuretic that has a major effect on the distal convoluted tubule.
    (A) Carbonic anhydrase inhibitors affect the proximal tubules.
    (B) Loop diuretics affect the thick segments of ascending limbs.
    (C) Thiazides affect the distal convoluted tubules.

37. (A) IgG is the most numerous and acts to neutralize bacterial toxins by enhancing phagocytosis.
    (B) IgM is produced first and activates complement but it is not the most numerous.
    (C) IgE responds in allergic reactions.
    (D) IgD triggers B cell response and is not the most numerous.
    (E) IgA is found in exocrine secretions (e.g., tears, saliva).

38. (E) The airway is hyperreactive, not hyporeactive.
    (A) Bronchospasms lead to airway obstruction.
    (B) Bronchospasms are caused by overreaction to various stimuli.
    (C) Inflammation can be produced by irritation and also contributes to airway obstruction.
    (D) Hypersecretion of mucous glands is an overreaction to stimuli.

39. (C) Repeated radiation exposure may lead to unrepaired effects that accumulate in the tissues.
    (A) Organs are considered critical based on their function, rate of maturity, and inherent sensitivity of cell type.
    (B) Somatic effect refers to the injury occurring in the person being irradiated.
    (D) Genetic effect refers to the exposure of reproductive tissue that results in injury occurring in future generations.
    (E) The latent period refers to the time between exposure and the development of a radiation-induced effect.

40. (A) Human chorionic gonadotropin (hCG) is secreted by trophoblast cells during the first trimester of pregnancy.
    (B) Luteinizing hormone (LH) is secreted from the anterior pituitary.
    (C) As follicles grow, the granulosa cells secrete an increasing amount of estradiol (the principal estrogen).
    (D) Progesterone levels in the blood are negligible before ovulation but rise rapidly to reach a peak during the luteal phase at approximately one week after ovulation.

41. (C) That point on the target where x-radiation is produced by the interaction of accelerating electrons and the target material atoms is called the focal spot.
    (A) The target is embedded in a copper stem.
    (B) This response is incorrect.
    (D) The focusing cup surrounds the tungsten filament on the cathode side of the vacuum tube.
    (E) The tungsten filament produces the electrons when heated.

42. (A) Renal surgery is not a treatment for leukemia.
    (B) Irradiation is used to destroy malignant cells.
    (C) This combination approach destroys malignant cells, injects normal cells, and reduces chances of infection.
    (D) Interferon therapy is a new treatment that has been shown to be effective.
    (E) Bone marrow transplants replace abnormal cells with normal cells.

43. (A) Digoxin (Lanoxin) is often used to treat congestive heart failure (CHF). Swelling of the ankles, shortness of breath, and cough are some signs and symptoms of CHF.
    (B) Stroke is not a heart condition and the symptoms are not consistent with stroke.
    (C) No symptoms indicating angina
    (D) No symptoms indicating myocardial infarction

44. (B) Diuretics are helpful in CHF clients to control fluid retention and edema.
    (A) Keeps heart rate low and not usually used in CHF
    (C) Not used to control water retention
    (D) Used in high blood pressure and sometimes in CHF, but it is not a diuretic

45. (C) CHF client will experience shortness of breath when reclined.
    (A) This may be a side effect of the shortness of breath.
    (B) Ankle edema will decrease upon reclining or elevating the legs.
    (D) See C.

46. (E) The age, gender, and race of the patient plus the fact that the associated teeth are vital are most contributory to the diagnosis of the cementoma.
    (A) Internal resorption can only be seen radiographically.
    (B) The odontoma is evaluated radiographically.
    (C) Unerupted supernumerary teeth are diagnosed from a radiograph.
    (D) Impacted third molars are seen radiographically.

47. (C) With normal gingival contour, average probing depth in moderate periodontitis is 5 to 6 mm with 4 to 5 mm attachment loss and radiographic evidence of bone loss.
    (A) Attachment loss and bone loss do not occur in gingivitis.
    (B) With normal gingival contour, average probing depth in early periodontitis is 3 to 4 mm.
    (D) With normal gingival contour, average probing depth in advanced periodontitis is 7 mm or greater.
    (E) Periodontal pockets do not occur in necrotizing ulcerative periodontitis because soft tissue necrosis is so rapid that it coincides or precedes bone loss, sometimes exposing bone.

48. (D) A nosocomial infection is acquired as a result of a hospital stay.
    (A) A focal infection is localized in one area and spreads elsewhere.
    (B) A subclinical infection occurs when no symptoms are recognized.
    (C) A primary infection is an original infection.
    (E) An opportunistic infection occurs when an organism that does not usually cause disease becomes pathogenic.

49. (B) Acidosis is the term used because the pH is to the acid side of normal.
    (A) A rise in blood pH above 7.45 is known as alkalosis.
    (C) The Bohr effect explains the affinity of hemoglobin for oxygen; it is decreased when pH is lowered.
    (D) This reflex is stimulated by pulmonary stretch receptors.

50. (A) Bremsstrahlung radiation, also called "breaking" radiation is produced when the slowing down process results in a transference of the electron's kinetic energy into x-ray energy.
    (B) Characteristic radiation, also called "discrete" radiation results from the restabilization that occurs in the target material atom, after an orbiting electron is dislodged.
    (C) Discrete radiation is also called "characteristic" radiation and occurs when outer shell electrons move to fill voids left by the ejection of electrons from the inner shells of the target material atoms.
    (D) Particulate is a type of ionizing radiation.

51. (A) Hairy leukoplakia is a condition most often associated with HIV or AIDS.
    (B) White hairy tongue is a variant of normal.
    (C) Fissured tongue is considered a variant of normal.
    (D) Geographic tongue is considered a variant of normal.
    (E) Migratory glossitis is another name for geographic tongue.

52. (C) The medial rectus is innervated by III and rotates the eye toward the midline.
    (A) This muscle is innervated by the occulomotor nerve and rotates the eye upward and toward the midline.
    (B) This muscle is innervated by III and rotates the eye downward and toward the midline.
    (D) This muscle is innervated by VI and rotates the eye away from the midline.

53. (D) External tooth resorption begins in the periodontal ligament.
    (A) Dental caries will not cause external tooth resorption.
    (B) Salivary gland dysfunction has nothing to do with external tooth resorption.
    (C) Medications do not cause external tooth resorption.
    (E) Chemical rinses do not cause external tooth resorption.

54. (B) The characteristic historical, radiographic, and clinical features define the diagnosis for periapical cemental dysplasia.
    (A) The cementoblastoma is a true odontogenic tumor. It is most commonly seen in young adults, involves mandibular posterior teeth, and pain is a clinical characteristic.
    (C) Median mandibular cyst is a rare lesion thought to be odontogenic in origin. There is no race, age, or gender predilection.
    (D) The traumatic bone cyst has no race, gender, or age predilection.
    (E) Odontomas are odontogenic tumors composed of mature tooth structures.

55. (D) Because of his hyperactivity and propensity to injuries, you need to minimize his risk and assure his safety.
    (A) Radiographs may be difficult to obtain, especially a complete set; an exam is more important.
    (B) This could be a consideration, but is not your first priority.
    (C) This is the role of the physician or educational psychologist.
    (E) Toothbrushing is more realistic than flossing.

56. (E) If they had a higher incidence then their primary diagnosis would be mental retardation instead of ADHD.
    (A) The incidence is higher in males, although partially because of more aggressive behavior.
    (B) ADHD can affect any CNS function.
    (C) ADHD most often causes problems with reading, writing, and math.
    (D) Because it is labeled an attention deficit disorder, concentration and memory are problems.

57. (B) No oral manifestations are directly related to the condition.
    (A) Early gingivitis may be present but is related to poor oral hygiene.
    (C) Most medications for this disorder do not cause gingival overgrowth.
    (D) There are no related risk factors for rampant dental caries unless the impaired impulse control leads to constant binging on cariogenic foods or beverages.
    (E) Oral reflexes are more apt to be hyperactive than hypoactive.

58. (C) National laws state that parents have a right to seek free public education for a child with an identified disability.
    (A) Attending school in the local community is an example of mainstreaming.
    (B) ADHD qualifies him for special education services.
    (D) All public buildings must be accessible to people with disabilities.
    (E) ADHD is an example of educational labeling for purposes of acquiring services.

59. (A) There is no evidence that the parents have abused him.
    (B) Because he is prone to accidents and hasn't seen a dentist, he should be checked for oral injuries.
    (C) Dental hygienists should be providing anticipatory guidance to parents about injury-preventive behaviors.
    (D) More information is needed about the causes and types of oral injuries before counseling is attempted.
    (E) This information is needed for counseling and to assure his safety during dental hygiene appointments.

60. (E) A child with ADHD cannot physically remain motionless for that long.
    (A) Placing the instruments out of his reach is to assure his safety and the integrity of your infection control procedures.
    (B) Introducing him to the operatory gradually will reduce his fear and curiosity.
    (C) Desensitization is important to minimize oral reflexes or startle reflexes.
    (D) Short breaks every few minutes will provide some structure but will also accommodate his hyperactivity disorder.

61. (D) Professional oral irrigation is of little value because antimicrobial agents have low substantivity in a periodontal pocket due to presence of serum, proteins, and gingival crevicular fluid.
    (A) Professional oral irrigation is not routinely recommended in nonsurgical periodontal therapy. See D.
    (B) The main effects on periodontal pathogens and tissue are from mechanical debridement rather than irrigation.
    (C) See D.

62. (D) A lymphocyte is an agranular leukocyte (white blood cell).
    (A) A basophil is a granular leukocyte.
    (B) A thrombocyte is a platelet. It is not a white blood cell.
    (C) An erythrocyte is a red blood cell.
    (E) A platelet is not a white blood cell.

63. (B) Resting pressure and the lower number in the blood pressure reading.
    (A) Incorrect answer.
    (C) This is called the systolic pressure.
    (D) Incorrect answer.

64. (D) The filter functions to remove low energy, nonpenetrating wavelengths from the beam.
    (A) This response is incorrect.
    (B) The collimator or diaphragm controls the shape and/or shape of the beam.
    (C) The copper stem functions to absorb heat energy during x-ray production.

65. (A) *Candida albicans* causes a fungal infection that responds to antifungal therapy.
    (B) A bacterial infection would not respond to antifungal treatment.
    (C) A nutritional deficiency will respond to dietary changes that increase the missing dietary nutrients.
    (D) Cold weather alone can cause simple dryness but not necessarily a fungal infection.
    (E) A denture can cause cracked commissures but not necessarily a fungal infection.

66. (B) Arthritis is permanent damage resulting from Lyme disease.
    (A) Scarlet fever is a disease from infection with Group A streptococci.
    (C) Jaundice is a symptom of infection with the Hepatitis B virus.
    (D) Emphysema is a disease of the lungs unrelated to tuberculosis.
    (E) Giardiasis is the name of a prolonged diarrheal disease caused by the protozoa *Giardia lamblia*.

67. (A) Fever is a systemic sign of inflammation.
    (B) Pain is a local sign of inflammation.
    (C) Swelling is a local sign of inflammation.
    (D) Erythema is a local sign of inflammation.
    (E) Edema is a local sign of inflammation.

68. (B) It can be divided into two main parts, the palpebral and orbital portions.
    (A) This muscle surrounds the mouth.
    (C) This muscle depresses the brow.
    (D) This muscle pulls the eyebrow medially and is responsible for the vertical folds beneath the brows at the root of the nose.

69. (B) Neutrophils are highly phagocytic and are active in the initial stages of infection.
    (A) Eosinophils are not phagocytic.
    (C) Basophils are not phagocytic.
    (D) Lymphocytes are not phagocytic.
    (E) Erythrocytes are not phagocytic.

70. (E) The longer the PID, the less divergent the x-ray beam, which decreases the client's radiation exposure. Rectangular PIDs expose the client to less radiation than circular PIDs.
    (A) Closed ended, pointed PIDs increase the client's radiation exposure and should not be used.
    (B, C) The shorter the PID, the more divergent the x-ray beam, which increases the client's radiation exposure.
    (D) The longer the PID, the less divergent the x-ray beam, which decreases the client's radiation exposure. However, circular PIDs expose the client to more radiation than rectangular PIDs.

71. (A) Correct answer
    (B) Produced in the pancreas and involved in glucose utilization
    (C) Oxygen is not produced in the body.

72. (D) Cyanosis and clubbing of the fingers are signs of congenital heart disease.
    (A) Stroke is manifested as paralysis, not cyanosis.
    (B) Hypertensive disease causes increased blood pressure, not clubbing of the fingers.
    (C) Clubbing of the fingers is not a usual symptom of AIDS.
    (E) Cerebral palsy is a neuromuscular disorder that results from brain damage.

73. (B) Obese and pregnant clients should receive chest thrusts in the case of complete airway obstruction.
    (A) Abdominal thrusts are not used in late pregnancy.
    (C) Not indicated
    (D) This will be of no value if the airway is obstructed.

74. (A) This is the correct procedure.
    (B) This will increase pressure of the uterus on the aorta and inferior vena cava, which will decrease cardiac output.
    (C) This should not be done because it would decrease blood flow to the brain.

75. (A) The cricoid cartilage is signet-ring shaped and is attached by membranes to the upper part of the trachea.
    (B) The arytenoid cartilages are shaped like pyramids and are located on the back of the larynx.
    (C) The corniculate cartilages are two tiny cones, one placed on the apex of each arytenoid cartilage.
    (D) The cuneiform cartilages are two tiny rods placed in the mucous membrane folds and join the arytenoids to the epiglottis.

76. (C) The cuff should be 20% greater than the diameter of the upper arm.
    (A) This is the correct client position for taking the blood pressure.
    (B) This is the correct position for the stethoscope.
    (D) This may result in too low of a blood pressure reading.

77. (B) Mast cells are associated with hypersensitivity reactions of an anaphylactic type.
    (A) Neutrophils are associated with inflammatory response to irritation.
    (C) Lymphocytes include T cells that are indirectly associated with cellular immunity and B cells that are associated with humoral immunity.
    (D) Macrophages are directly associated with cell-mediated immunity.
    (E) Plasma cells produce immunoglobulins and antibodies; they are not involved in anaphylactic reactions.

78. (C) Tetracycline fibers have been shown to be effective in reducing periodontal pathogens, inflammations, and probing depths in sites that have not responded to initial therapy.
    (A) Periodontal debridement/root planing is more effective in treatment of periodontitis than tetracycline fiber therapy alone.
    (B) Periodontal debridement/root planing alone is effective in initial therapy; tetracycline fibers may not offer a significant advantage.
    (D) Local delivery of tetracycline fibers is not employed during periodontal flap surgery.

79. (A) The skin is the organ that can most tolerate low rates of blood flow.
    (B, C) See answer A.
    (D) The brain is the organ that can least tolerate low rates of blood flow.

80. (D) Allergy is an altered or enhanced immune reaction.
    (A) Side effects occur when a drug acts on a nontarget organ producing undesirable effects.
    (B) Toxic reactions occur when there is an extension of the drug's effect on the target organ.
    (C) Suprainfections occur when an antibiotic disturbs the normal flora and allows an overgrowth of organisms unaffected or resistant to the antibiotic.
    (E) Adverse reactions are undesirable actions of a drug; this includes allergy, but does not specifically imply involvement of the immune system.

81. (B) Damage to macromolecules through production of a toxic environment is called an indirect effect.
    (A) A direct effect involves the transfer of ionizing energy from the X ray to the DNA.
    (C) This response is incorrect.
    (D) This response is incorrect.

82. (A) Alveolar bone loss can occur with or without apical migration of the gingival margin.
    (B) Tooth position in the arch is an etiologic factor for gingival recession.
    (C) Dehiscence is an etiologic factor for gingival recession.
    (D) Faulty toothbrushing is a common etiologic factor for gingival recession.
    (E) Gingival inflammation can be an etiologic factor for gingival recession.

83. (C) Film speed is determined by crystal size. Larger sized crystals result in a faster speed film. However, resolution is enhanced with a smaller crystal size.
    (A) The second part of the statement is incorrect.
    (B) The first part of the statement is correct.
    (D) The first part of the statement is correct, the second part is incorrect.

84. (A) Regenerative techniques in periodontal surgery are most effective in two- and three-walled defects in the alveolar bone.
    (B) One-walled defects are not indicated for regenerative techniques in periodontal surgery; periodontal flap surgery is.
    (C) Gingival hyperplasia is treated by gingivectomy if severe enough to warrant surgery.
    (D) Gingival recession is not an indication for regenerative techniques; the etiology determines treatment.
    (E) Mucogingival surgery is used to treat mucogingival problems.

85. (D) Fixer contamination results in light or clear stains.
    (A) Fluoride contamination results in dark stains.
    (B) Glove powder contamination results in dark stains.
    (C) Static electricity results in dark streaks or smudges of exposed areas on the film.
    (E) Saliva contamination before processing results in dark stains.

86. (D) Chronic liver disease may result from infection with Hepatitis B and D.
    (A) Hepatitis A does not cause chronic liver disease.
    (B) Neither Hepatitis A nor E cause chronic liver disease.
    (C) Hepatitis E does not cause chronic liver disease.
    (E) Hepatitis A does not cause chronic liver disease.

87. (D) Radiopaque structures are not easily penetrated by X rays, and therefore appear light gray to clear on the resultant image.
    (A) The first part of the statement is incorrect.
    (B) The second part of the statement is correct.
    (C) The first part of the statement is incorrect, the second part is correct.

88. (A) Spina bifida has no associated oral manifestations.
    (B) Bulimia causes multiple oral problems from repeated vomiting.
    (C) Sickle cell anemia creates multiple oral problems with loss of bone trabeculations, delayed eruption, and pain.
    (D) Down syndrome is a craniofacial syndrome with multiple oral manifestations.
    (E) Leukemia causes oral problems such as infections and mucositis.

89. (E) Rampant dental caries is not caused by renal insufficiency.
    (A) Mucosal anemia is a reflection of general anemia.
    (B) Herpes is an opportunistic infection from immunosuppression.
    (C) Calculus deposits tend to be increased in end stage renal disease.
    (D) Calcium leaches out of alveolar bone causing a ground-glass appearance.

90. (C) Seizures are not directly associated with end stage renal disease.
    (A) Hypertension is a clinical manifestation of impaired renal function.
    (B) If a patient is heparinized from hemodialysis, then bleeding potential is enhanced while heparin still is in the bloodstream.
    (D) Some physicians recommend antibiotic premedication for the AV shunt in dialysis patients.
    (E) Renal dysfunction impairs clearance of drugs and affects drug metabolism.

91. (D) Gingival overgrowth is a side effect of Nifedipine.
    (A) Water retention does not generally cause gingival enlargement.
    (B) Accumulation of urea can cause a bad taste but not gingival overgrowth.
    (C) Gingival inflammation is not increased in renal insufficiency.
    (E) Uremic bone disease is present but the papillae do not generally appear larger.

92. (B) Viruses transmitted through blood products are a risk for persons on hemodialysis.
    (A) Hepatitis A is not acquired through blood products.
    (C) TB is not acquired through blood products.
    (D) Hemophilia is an inherited disorder, not acquired through blood products.
    (E) HIV can be acquired in this way, but not Hepatitis A.

93. (A) Dental care is best scheduled 24 hours after dialysis when the client is no longer heparinized and the blood has been dialyzed.
    (B) Clients usually are weak and not ready for dental care immediately before dialysis.
    (C) The blood may still be heparinized and the client is too fatigued after dialysis.
    (D) Dental care should not coincide with dialysis.
    (E) Moderate levels of heparin should not be in the system during dental care because of potential bleeding problems.

94. (D) Overexposure results in radiographs that are too dark.
    (A) The lead foil in the back of the film packet absorbs some of the X rays, resulting in an underexposed image. Underexposure results in a light image.
    (B) Cold processing solution temperatures take longer to develop the image. If time was not adjusted to allow cold solutions more time to work, the resultant image is too light.
    (C) Exhausted chemical solutions are less effective, resulting in images that are too light.
    (E) Underdeveloping results in a light image.

95. (C) This is also known as a nonconvulsive seizure.
    (A) This is a tonic-clonic seizure.
    (B) Person experiencing a psychomotor seizure will have loss of awareness and purposeless movements.
    (D) These symptoms are not consistent with those seen in a stroke victim.
96. (E) Latent infections occur when the causative agent remains inactive in the body for a time and then is reactivated to produce symptoms of the disease.
    (A) Resistant refers to the ability of an organism to ward off the host defenses or antibiotics.
    (B) Cytopathic refers to the ability of a virus to cause cells to deteriorate.
    (C) Opportunistic infections occur when an organism that does not usually cause disease becomes pathogenic.
    (D) Oncogenic viruses are those capable of causing tumors.
97. (A) This is involved in muscle control.
    (B) This gyrus is involved with muscle control.
    (C) It is located in the frontal lobe.
    (D) It is involved with muscle control.
98. (D) Intake of calories in bulimia ranges from 3,500 to 20,000.
    (A) Recurrent binging followed by vomiting is a major characteristic of bulimia.
    (B) Dehydration results from frequent vomiting.
    (C) Vomiting is induced to reduce caloric intake from the binging.
    (E) Depression is an integral component to this psychophysiologic condition.
99. (A) These bones compose the middle ear ossicles.
    (B) They are located in the middle ear.
    (C) Vibrations of the tympanic membrane are transmitted through these ossicles to the stapes.
    (D) Only A is true.
100. (B) Digital imaging uses computer based devices and a conventional x-ray unit to produce video radiographic images.
    (A) Arthography uses the injection of contrast medium to image joint dysfunction.
    (C) Magnetic resonance uses radio frequency emitted from tissue and does not use ionizing radiation.
    (D) Nuclear medicine uses injected isotopes to record radiation emitted from tissues.
    (E) Sialography uses injected contrast agents to evaluate ductal and acinar systems.
101. (A) Beta-blocking agents (β-adrenergic agents) prevent the heart rate from going up. It would be very unusual for the heart rate to go over 100 beats/minute which would be tachycardia.
    (B) Blood pressure can still go up; however, beta-blockers are used to help control blood pressure.
    (C) Beta-blocking agents have no impact on body temperature.

102. (E) Autism creates no problems with mucus accumulation or swallowing.
    (A) Bronchial asthma causes hypersecretion of mucous.
    (B) In emphysema, mucus obstructs airways.
    (C) Mucus obstructs airways in cystic fibrosis.
    (D) People with Parkinson disease have difficulty swallowing.
103. (D) Gingival enlargement does not cause tooth mobility.
    (A) Occlusal trauma can cause tooth mobility.
    (B) When inflammation extends into the periodontal ligament from a periodontal infection or a periapical abscess, it can result in tooth mobility.
    (C) Hormonal changes can cause tooth mobility (e.g., pregnancy).
    (E) Diseases of the jaw, such as osteomyelitis, which destroy bone or roots of the teeth can cause tooth mobility.
104. (C) Diet is an exogenous factor.
    (A) Oral pH is an endogenous factor.
    (B) Saliva is an endogenous factor.
    (D) Oxygen concentration is an endogenous factor.
    (E) Oral microbial interactions are an endogenous factor.
105. (D) Partial airway obstruction with poor air exchange should be treated as complete obstruction, and would indicate Heimlich maneuver.
    (A) May worsen the condition.
    (B) This would be appropriate if the air exchange was good.
    (C) Not indicated.
106. (C) A coin placed over a film for 2 to 3 minutes and then processed is evaluated for a coin image. An outline of the coin indicates unsafe darkroom lighting.
    (A) The coin test does not evaluate film density.
    (B) Processing errors are not determined by the coin test.
    (D) Unit output and consistency are not determined by use of the coin test.
107. (A) Internal resorption occurs when something triggers a pulpal reaction from within the tooth.
    (B) When stimuli begin with the periodontal ligament, it is more likely external resorption.
    (C) With rapid orthodontic movement, resorption of the root is most commonly seen.
    (D) PAP does not usually occur with internal resorption.
    (E) Deep carious lesions are more likely associated with a radicular cyst or a periapical granuloma.
108. (D) The most common cause of a mucocele is trauma to a minor salivary duct.
    (A) Tumor formation does not cause a mucocele.
    (B) Inflammation does not cause the mucocele.
    (C) Obstruction in the duct is most commonly associated with the ranula.
    (E) Blockage at the caruncles does not cause a mucocele.

109. (D) A positive tuberculin skin test is a Type IV hypersensitivity reaction.
  (A) A positive tuberculin skin test is not a Type I hypersensitivity reaction.
  (B) A positive tuberculin skin test is not a Type II hypersensitivity reaction.
  (C) A positive tuberculin skin test is not a Type III hypersensitivity reaction.

110. (C) Prostate cancer generally is characterized by slow progression and treatment has an 85.6% 5-year survival rate, if detected early.
  (A) Lung cancer has one of the lowest 5-year survival rates (13.4%).
  (B) 5-year survival rates from breast cancer are improving and approach 84% or higher when the cancer is detected early.
  (D) 5-year survival rates for ovarian cancer still are only 44% due to late detection and ineffective treatment.
  (E) Colorectal cancer's 5-year survival rate is 61%.

111. (A) Lactobacilli not only produce acid but also tolerate low pH values (aciduric).
  (B) *S. mitis* produce hydrogen peroxide.
  (C) *S. sanguis* produce hydrogen peroxide.
  (D) *Streptococcus viridans* strep produce hydrogen peroxide.

112. (C) Accidental white light exposure results in a dark or black image.
  (A) The fixer functions to remove the undeveloped silver halide crystals, thus the entire image is removed when the film is placed in the fixer before developing.
  (B) No exposure results in a clear or blank film.
  (D) Excessive washing may remove the film emulsion, leaving the film blank.

113. (B) Palpation determines the texture when the lesion is felt or examined with fingers.
  (A) A fissure is a groove showing depth.
  (C) Papillary means small projections found in clusters.
  (D) Coalescence occurs when parts fuse to make one.
  (E) A cyst is an abnormal sac lined with epithelium and surrounded by a connective tissue capsule.

114. (E) *Pneumocystis carinii* is an opportunistic infection often found in HIV infected persons, but does not manifest orally.
  (A) Hairy leukoplakia is an oral manifestation of HIV.
  (B) Candidiasis is an oral manifestation of HIV.
  (C) Linear gingival erythema is an oral manifestation of HIV.
  (D) Papillomavirus (wart) is an oral manifestation of HIV.

115. (B) Dynacirc has been found to show the least amount of gingival tissue proliferation.
  (A) Norvasc causes more tissue response than dynacirc.
  (C) Nifedipine is the generic name for Procardia which causes the most proliferation.
  (D) Procardia causes the most gingival tissue proliferation.
  (E) Nitroglycerine is most commonly prescribed for angina.

116. (D) Localized attachment loss of 2 mm or more would indicate advancing disease; therefore, active therapy should be reinstituted.
  (A) Generalized bacterial plaque would require oral self care education.
  (B) Presence of gingival inflammation would indicate an evaluation of etiology. If related to local factors, such as plaque and calculus, periodontal maintenance procedures would be employed for removal of these factors. If generalized without local etiology, a referral for evaluation of systemic disease would be warranted.
  (C) Gingival recession is a common condition after active periodontal therapy (and resultant tissue shrinkage or repositioning). Progressive recession should be addressed based on etiology.
  (E) Gingival bleeding would be considered the same as gingival inflammation because it is a sign of inflammation. See B.

117. (E) Gummas are inflammatory granulomatous lesions with a central zone of necrosis found in the tertiary stage of syphilis.
  (A) Chancres are found in the primary stage.
  (B) Rashes appear in the secondary stage.
  (C) Chancres are found in the primary stage.
  (D) Gummas are found in the tertiary stage.

118. (E) Supernumerary teeth can often be seen in posterior regions.
  (A) Supernumerary teeth are often unerupted and are therefore seen radiographically.
  (B) Supernumerary teeth are hereditary.
  (C) Supernumerary teeth are associated with certain syndromes.
  (D) The mesioden is the most common supernumerary tooth.

119. (B) Infrahyoid muscles extend between the hyoid bone above and the sternum, clavicle, and scapula below.
  (A) The sternohyoid is an infrahyoid muscle.
  (C) All infrahyoid muscles are flat bands.
  (D) The omohyoid has two bellies.
  (E) The muscles of mastication are the masseter, temporalis, and internal and external pterygoids.

120. (B) The target of penicillin's action is the cell wall and *Mycoplasma* does not have a cell wall.
  (A) Penicillin is the drug of choice (doc) for infections with *Actinomyces*.
  (C) Penicillin is the doc for infections with *Bacillus*.
  (D) Penicillin is the doc for infections with *Leptospira*.
  (E) Penicillin is the doc for infections with *Treponema*.

121. (A) Chewing on an edentulous ridge causes frictional keratosis.
  (B) Mouthwashes do not cause frictional keratosis.
  (C) A malignancy does not cause frictional keratosis.
  (D) High fiber diets do not cause frictional keratosis.
  (E) Smoking heavily may cause hyperkeratosis but not frictional keratosis.

122. (B) Adult periodontitis is slowly progressive and is the most common form of periodontitis.
    (A) Localized juvenile periodontitis is an aggressive form of periodontitis that progresses more rapidly than adult periodontitis.
    (C) Linear gingival erythema is a form of gingivitis that may never progress to periodontitis.
    (D) Refractory periodontitis is an aggressive form of periodontitis that progresses more rapidly than adult periodontitis.

123. (A) Due to visual-spatial perceptual problems, the person cannot use a mirror.
    (B) Auditory memory is affected in left CVA.
    (C) Language centers are affected in left CVA.
    (D) Organizational abilities are more affected in left CVA.
    (E) Right CVA cause left hemiplegia, not right hemiplegia.

124. (B) Hyperplastic candidiasis presents as a raised, white nonremovable plaque.
    (A) Pseudomembranous candidiasis presents as a removable soft, creamy, white plaque with red and/or bleeding base.
    (C) Erythematous candidiasis presents as a smooth, flat, red lesion on the dorsum of the tongue.
    (D) Angular cheilitis presents as cracking or redness around the corners of the mouth.

125. (D) Facial nerve VII supplies the muscles of facial expression.
    (A) The olfactory nerve consists of numerous filaments that originate in the olfactory mucosa and pass through the holes in the cribriform plate of the ethmoid bone.
    (B) The occulomotor nerve (III) leaves the middle cranial fossa through the superior orbital fissure.
    (C) The trigeminal nerve (V) arises with a larger sensory and a smaller motor root from the ventral surface of the pons.

126. (D) Macrophages are large mononuclear cells that play a direct role in cell-mediated immunity.
    (A) B cells are lymphocytes that play a direct role in humoral immunity by forming antigen-antibody complexes.
    (B) T cells are lymphocytes that interact with macrophages to aid the response of B cells by preparing antigen; however, their role is more indirect. See C.
    (C) Mast cells are involved in hypersensitivity reactions of the anaphylactic type.
    (E) Neutrophils are the first inflammatory cell to respond after injury.

127. (E) The mental foramen usually appears radiographically near the apex of the mandibular second premolar. It should be distinguished from periapical pathology by an intact lamina dura around the premolar.
    (A) The incisive foramen would appear on the maxilla.
    (B) The infraorbital foramen would appear on the maxilla.
    (C) The lingual foramen would appear near the mandibular anterior teeth.
    (D) The mandibular foramen would appear on an extraoral film, at the beginning of the mandibular canal on the ramus of the mandible.

128. (E) A man with spinal injury at the T6 level is fairly independent and shouldn't experience any problems with wheelchair transfers.
    (A) A C3 injury makes the person totally dependent on a respirator that may be too cumbersome to move and he will need extra support in the chair for stability.
    (B) A person on a respirator may be too cumbersome to move.
    (C) This client may have impaired respiration, be weak, have muscle wasting, and feel unstable in the chair.
    (D) This person may be too heavy to move and the stress and exertion can precipitate a heart attack.

129. (A) This condition occurs from paralysis and results in a rapid increase in blood pressure and low pulse.
    (B) Autonomic hyperreflexia does not occur in hypothyroidism.
    (C) Autonomic hyperreflexia does not occur in hyperthyroidism.
    (D) This condition is not associated with cardiac arrhythmias.
    (E) Autonomic hyperreflexia does not occur in bronchial asthma.

130. (D) PAP can be associated with a cyst, abscess, or periapical granuloma.
    (A) PAP does not apply to a cyst alone.
    (B) PAP does not apply to a periapical granuloma alone.
    (C) PAP does not apply to an abscess alone.
    (E) PAP does not apply to the periapical granuloma and abscess only.

131. (E) Muscular dystrophy causes problems in dental development, but not enamel dysplasia.
    (A) Enamel dysplasia is sometimes caused by the same agent (such as a virus) that caused the brain damage.
    (B) Enamel dysplasia has been shown to occur at the same time as the cause of the cerebral palsy.
    (C) Causes of the congenital heart disease can also cause enamel dysplasia.
    (D) Sickled cells interfere with enamel formation.

132. (E) Attachment loss is the amount of periodontal support lost due to previous destruction by periodontitis; therefore, it is the single most important criterion for determining extent or severity of periodontitis.
    (A) Tooth mortality can be caused by several factors besides loss of periodontal support (e.g., mobility, hormonal changes).
    (B) Probing depth is affected by position of the gingival margin which may be enlarged coronally or receded apically; therefore, attachment loss measured from the cementoenamel junction as a static reference point is a more accurate criterion for determining extent of periodontal destruction.
    (C) Radiographs have limitations such as their inability to show facial and lingual bone loss or defects, effects of technique and angulation on accuracy of bone level, two-dimensional representation of a three-dimensional anatomy, and inability to assess soft tissue changes.
    (D) Furcation involvement most commonly occurs in advanced periodontitis; therefore, it is not the most important criterion for determining other stages of periodontal destruction in periodontitis; it also only occurs on multi-rooted teeth.

133. (C) Retrocuspid papilla, also referred to as Hirschfeld's papilla, is a small elevated nodule located on the lingual aspect of the mandibular canines.
    (A) Stenson's papilla is located on the buccal mucosa near the parotid gland.
    (B) The incisive papilla is located between the maxillary central incisors on the lingual aspect.
    (C) Papillae are not found on the floor of the mouth.
    (E) Circumvallate papillae are found on the posterior of the dorsal of the tongue.

134. (C) Rheumatic heart disease has no associated oral manifestations.
    (A) Chronic use of alcohol causes dehydration and xerostomia.
    (B) Xerostomia is a side effect of diuretic drug therapies.
    (D) Radiation therapy can damage salivary glands.
    (E) Parotid gland enlargement and decreased salivary flow from hyperglycemia are seen in uncontrolled diabetics.

135. (C) *S. milleri* primarily colonize gingival crevices.
    (A) *S. salivarius* primarily colonize oral soft tissues.
    (B) *S. mitior* primarily colonize nonkeratinized oral tissues.
    (C) *S. mutans* primarily colonize oral hard surfaces.
    (D) *A. naeslundi* primarily colonize the tongue and saliva of children.

136. (E) Cervical abrasion is not usually an oral finding in Down syndrome.
    (A) The small nasomaxillary complex creates a Class III type malocclusion.
    (B) Tooth shape and size are abnormal, and crowded or rotated teeth are common.
    (C) They are highly susceptible to periodontal infections, partly because of connective tissue abnormalities and generalized impaired immune response.
    (D) Tooth eruption may be delayed up to 18 months.

137. (E) Filiform papillae elongate in black hairy tongue.
    (A) Fungiform papillae are mushroom shaped and do not elongate in black hairy tongue.
    (B) Retrocuspid papillae are not on the tongue.
    (C) Foliate papillae are on the lateral borders of the posterior tongue and have nothing to do with black hairy tongue.
    (D) Circumvallate papillae or on the posterior dorsal of the tongue and do not elongate in black hairy tongue.

138. (D) The BANA enzymatic test can be used at chairside to identify three known periodontal pathogens; it does not have to be sent to a laboratory for results.
    (A) DNA probe test must be sent to a laboratory for results.
    (B) Culturing requires laboratory testing for results.
    (C) ELISA immunoassay tests must be sent to a laboratory for results.

139. (A) The trigeminal nerve has three divisions.
    (B) This statement is true.
    (C) This statement is true.
    (D) This statement is true.

140. (D) Cestodes are tapeworms.
    (A, B) Nematodes are roundworms.
    (C, D) Trematodes are flukes.

141. (E) Calcified pulp can only be seen radiographically.
    (A) Supragingival calculus is seen clinically.
    (B) Torus palatinus is diagnosed clinically.
    (C) An erupted mesiodens is a supernumerary tooth between the maxillary centrals and it is diagnosed clinically.
    (D) Retrocuspid papilla is a soft-tissue elevated nodule that is not seen radiographically.

142. (B) Aspirin is recommended therapy for rheumatoid arthritis.
    (A) Aspirin will potentiate bleeding problems.
    (C) Aspirin and certain other antiinflammatory agents contribute to asthmatic symptoms.
    (D) Bleeding problems can be enhanced by aspirin.
    (E) Aspirin irritates the gastric mucosa and can cause bleeding.

143. (A) *S. sanguis* primarily colonize the tongue.
    (B) *S. mutans* primarily colonize oral hard surfaces.
    (C) *S. milleri* primarily colonize gingival crevices.
    (D) *S. mitior* primarily colonize nonkeratinized oral tissues.
    (E) *S. salivarius* primarily colonize oral soft tissues.

144. (E) Interferon has not been found in saliva.
    (A) Salivary flow washes bacteria from the oral cavity.
    (B) Secretory IgA in the saliva inhibits microbial attachment.
    (C) Lysozyme is an enzyme capable of lysing bacterial cell walls.
    (D) Glycoproteins cause bacteria to aggregate and inhibit adherence.

145. (D) Inflammation is the first line of defense to injury.
   (A) Immunity is the second reaction to injury.
   (B) Infection occurs when the body's defenses are not enough to prevent microorganisms from causing disease.
   (C) Hyperplasia is an increase in cells.
   (E) Hypoplasia is the incomplete development of tissues.
146. (A) Fibrin consists of insoluble protein fibers.
   (B) Fluid squeezed from the clot as it retracts is called serum (plasma without fibrinogen).
   (C) Bradykinin stimulates vasodilation.
   (D) Prostaglandins stimulate vasoconstriction.
147. (A) Death in Duchenne MD may occur in adolescence.
   (B) Cerebral palsy is a nonprogressive insult to the brain.
   (C) Autism is a behavior and communication disorder that does not result in early death.
   (D) Schizophrenia is a type of mental illness, not necessarily progressive.
   (E) This seizure disorder can be controlled and is not fatal in most cases.
148. (A) Scalloping around the root commonly describes the radiolucency observed in traumatic bone cysts.
   (B) Stafne bone cysts usually have an oval or elliptical shaped radiolucency in the posterior mandible, inferior to the mandibular canal and not involving teeth.
   (C) Odontogenic keratocysts are radiolucent, diffuse, and often destructive of surrounding structures.
   (D) Primordial cysts develop in place of a third molar or distal to a third molar.
   (E) The ameloblastoma is most commonly found in the mandibular third molar region.
149. (A) Multiple sclerosis is an autoimmune disease of the central nervous system.
   (B) von Willebrand disease is a congenital disorder of the blood clotting mechanism.
   (C) Sickle cell anemia is a defect of hemoglobin.
   (D) Ischemic heart disease is a progressive disease caused by accumulation of atherosclerotic plaques.
   (E) Cystic fibrosis is an inherited disorder of the exocrine glands.
150. (D) Assuring an open airway is a major indication for emergency assistance.
   (A) Rigidity of muscles is a characteristic of this condition, not an emergency.
   (B) Inability to close the eyelids is a result of the condition, but not an emergency.
   (C) Seizures are not associated with this condition.
   (E) Angina is not associated with myasthenia gravis.

Section Two

Case A Answers and Rationales

151. (B) Multiple cardiac complications, including valvular damage, are common in persons who have systemic lupus erythematosus (SLE). Consultation with the client's physician before treatment is required to establish any need for antibiotic pretreatment.
 (A) A medical consultation is not required for arthritis.
 (C) Raynaud's phenomena is a condition exhibited in some individuals who have systemic lupus. There is an abnormal degree of spasm of the blood vessels of the extremities, especially in response to cold temperatures. It is not life-threatening and does not require consultation with the physician.
 (D) Periodontal inflammation by itself does not require a medical consultation.

152. (C) This is the recommended standard regimen for persons at risk for bacterial endocarditis who do not have an allergy to penicillin according to the American Heart Association.
 (A) This is not the AHA recommended dosage.
 (B) This is not the AHA recommended dosage.
 (D) Correct answer is C.

153. (B) Mouthwashes containing alcohol cause further drying of the tissues and could increase his risk for developing carious lesions.
 (A) Fluoridated mouthwashes do not prevent oral fungal infections.
 (C) Fluoridated mouthwashes do not produce an antimicrobial effect.
 (D) Alcohol addiction is not a concern with alcohol-free fluoridated mouthwashes.

154. (C) Although all of the factors mentioned will complicate scaling and root planing, the numerous areas of rampant decay and decalcification will cause the greatest problem. Because many of these areas are located at the gingival margin, complete instrumentation in these areas will be difficult, even with local anesthesia.
 (A) Inadequate oral hygiene will not complicate scaling and root planing procedures.
 (B) Root sensitivity could possibly be a problem, but it is not listed on the client's history.
 (D) Excessive bleeding could possibly be a problem, but the numerous areas of dental caries will be more of a problem.

155. (A) Xerostomia is a common side effect of many medications. In this case, prednisone is known to cause xerostomia. All medications should be investigated before treatment to see if there are any factors that would effect dental/dental hygiene care.
 (B) Xerostomia is not a complication of lupus.
 (C) Xerostomia is not a complication of high blood pressure.
 (D) Xerostomia is not a complication of tobacco use.

156. (A) Heavy interproximal calculus will appear radiographically as an opaque artifact on the proximal surfaces of the teeth.
 (B) Dental caries will appear as a radiolucent area, not radiopaque.
 (C) Enamel pearls would appear more distinctly.
 (D) Exostosis usually appears on the root surfaces of teeth, not interproximal areas.

157. (D) Type IV periodontal class is defined by the American Association of Periodontology as further progression of periodontitis with severe, generalized destruction of the periodontal structures with increased tooth mobility, furcation involvement, and pocket depths 7 mm or greater.
 (A) Type I is defined as gingival disease characterized clinically by changes in color, gingival form, position, surface appearance, and presence of bleeding and/or exudate. This case has advanced beyond this definition.
 (B) Type II is early periodontitis in which the inflammation has progressed into deeper periodontal structures and alveolar bone crest, with slight bone loss. There is usually a slight loss of connective tissue attachment and alveolar bone. This case has advanced beyond this definition.
 (C) Type III is moderate periodontitis, which is an advanced stage with increased destruction of the periodontal structures and noticeable loss of bone support, possibly accompanied by an increase in tooth mobility. There may be furcation involvement in multirooted teeth. This case has advanced beyond this definition.
 (E) Type V is refractory periodontitis. This includes patients with multiple disease sites that continue to demonstrate attachment loss after appropriate therapy; also includes those patients with recurrent disease at single or multiple sites. Until treatment is rendered on this patient, this classification cannot be considered.

158. (D) Because this client has severe arthritis, he probably has trouble using a manual toothbrush. Most of the powered toothbrushes and powered interdental cleaners have large handles that make them easier to use for persons who have limited manual dexterity.
 (A) The small handles on most toothbrushes can be difficult for clients who have trouble grasping small items.
 (B) Many clients with severe arthritis in their hands have difficulty using dental floss.
 (C) Interdental stimulators are small and difficult to use for clients who have arthritis.

159. (B) The sonic/ultrasonic cleaner is contraindicated for areas of decalcification. The other devices listed are not used to remove calculus.
 (A) A rubber cup is used to remove stain, not calculus.
 (C) The airbrasive polisher is used to remove stain, not calculus.
 (D) Water irrigation devices are not designed to remove calculus.

160. (D) Because bleeding upon probing is a sign of disease, the absence of bleeding upon probing along with a decrease in pocket depth would show as an overall decrease in the periodontal disease process.
  - (A) Tissue shrinkage was probably the result in the decrease of the disease process.
  - (B) Better home care techniques probably also resulted in the decrease in the disease process.
  - (C) This would cause an increase in the disease process.

161. (A) The mental foramen is located between the mandibular premolars and appears radiographically as a radiolucent area near the apices of these teeth.
  - (B) This radiolucent area also appears at the tip of #20 and looks just like the area around #29, leading one to conclude that this is not an abscess.
  - (C) Exostosis appears around the roots of teeth and is radiopaque, not radiolucent.
  - (D) This area also appears at the tip of #20 and looks just like the area around #29, leading one to conclude that this is not a cyst.

162. (C) The lateral frenum is located in the buccal vestibule and attaches the lips to the alveolar ridge. If these attachments affix too high on the alveolar gingiva, they can cause excessive recession on the facial surfaces of the teeth in that area.
  - (A) Improper toothbrushing usually affects more than one tooth in the arch.
  - (B) Calculus is present but is not the primary cause of recession.
  - (D) Improper flossing will not cause labial recession.

163. (C) A single application of acidulated phosphate fluoride is more effective than the four applications of sodium fluoride and is more easily tolerated by the client.
  - (A) Sodium fluoride gel requires four applications and is time consuming for the client.
  - (B) Stannous fluoride may be astringent and cause burning of the oral tissues.
  - (D) Sodium fluoride rinse has a lower fluoride content than the gel.

164. (C) This is the description of Class II mobility.
  - (A) This is Class I mobility.
  - (B) Does not correctly describe any class of mobility.
  - (D) This describes Class III mobility.

165. (D) The #2 Nabers probe has curved noncalibrated working ends specifically designed for examination of furcations. This probe is ideal for detecting mesial and distal furcations on maxillary teeth, because adjacent teeth make access difficult or impossible for straight probes.
  - (A) This type of probe is not preferred to detect furcation involvement.
  - (B) This type of probe is not preferred to detect furcation involvement.
  - (C) This type of probe is not preferred to detect furcation involvement.

Case B Answers and Rationales

166. (E) The first four items listed are complications from Sjögren syndrome due to the severe xerostomia that usually accompanies this disorder. However, the salivary gland is not affected.
  - (A) Fissured tongue is a complication from Sjögren syndrome.
  - (B) Intraoral yeast infections are a complication of Sjögren syndrome.
  - (C) Burning mucosa is a complication of Sjögren syndrome.
  - (D) An increase in dental caries is a complication from Sjögren syndrome due to xerostomia.

167. (C) Xerostomia is one of the main symptoms of Sjögren syndrome and is also a common side effect of the drug Prozac.
  - (A) Xerostomia is not a side effect of Librax.
  - (B) Xerostomia is not a side effect of Premarin.
  - (D) Xerostomia is not a side effect of Zantac.

168. (B) This client should definitely receive fluoride therapy due to her history of extensive dental work and xerostomia. Neutral sodium fluoride is the choice because acidulated phosphate fluoride can etch or scratch porcelain surfaces and stannous fluoride may be astringent and cause burning of the oral tissues.
  - (A) Acidulated phosphate fluoride can etch or scratch porcelain surfaces.
  - (C) Stannous fluoride may be astringent and cause burning of the oral tissues.
  - (D) Fluoride should be used on any client who has had extensive dental work.

169. (A) Because this client has had extensive dental work and has severe xerostomia, she should be encouraged to use a topical fluoride gel daily.
  - (B) There is no reason for this client to use chlorhexidine mouthwash.
  - (C) Fluoridated toothpaste is good, but topical fluoride gel will provide more fluoride.
  - (D) There is no therapeutic value to flavored mouthrinses.

170. (D) Festooned gingiva is an enlargement of the marginal gingiva with the formation of a lifesaver-like gingival prominence. Often, the total gingiva is very narrow, with associated apparent recession which is demonstrated very well in this photograph.
  - (A) Cratering of the gingival margin refers to interdental necrosis with ulceration of the papillae, which produces a crater-like defect.
  - (B) Clefting involves a localized recession which is usually V-shaped, apostrophe-shaped, or formed in a slit-like indention and may extend several millimeters toward the mucogingival junction or even to or through the junction.
  - (C) Recession is the exposure of root surface that results from the apical migration of the junctional epithelium.

171. (D) Fungiform papillae are projections that are mushroom-shaped, red, and scattered among the filiform papillae on the dorsal surface of the tongue and contain taste buds responsible for sensing sweet, sour, and salty stimuli.
  (A) These are located in a V formation on the posterior section of the dorsal surface of the tongue and contain taste buds for sensing bitter stimuli.
  (B) The filiform papillae are whitish, hair-like projections that cover the dorsal surface of the tongue.
  (C) Foliate papillae are projections found on the posterior lateral borders of the tongue and contain taste buds responsible for sensing sour and acidic stimuli.

172. (D) Frequent use of air on this client is not necessary and may cause her more discomfort because her tissues are already dry.
  (A) Frequent breaks will make the client more comfortable, because she has problems with TMJ.
  (B) Exercising her jaw frequently will relieve tension on her TMJ.
  (C) Frequent sips of water will help alleviate the discomfort with the client's xerostomia.

173. (A) Although all of these practices will benefit this client, she has a past history of melanoma and should be instructed in oral cancer self-examination techniques.
  (B) Home fluoride is important, but does not have the highest priority for this client.
  (C) The client already reports flossing 2 to 3 times per day.
  (D) Saliva substitutes are important, but not as important as oral cancer self-exam.

174. (B) Due to the client's history of Sjögren syndrome, xerostomia, past history of extensive dental work, and high risk for dental caries, a 3-month continued care interval would be the most appropriate.
  (A) 2 months is probably too frequent for this client because she has good oral hygiene habits.
  (C) 4 months is too long for this client.
  (D) 6 months is definitely too long for this client.

175. (C) Composite restorations appear radiographically as very defined areas of radiolucency.
  (A) Amalgam is not usually used on anterior teeth and the photos of this client do not reveal amalgam restorations on the anterior teeth.
  (B) The photos of this client do not reveal gold restorations on the anterior teeth.
  (D) Dental caries will appear as a radiopacity.

176. (A) The Gracey 1/2 is an area-specific curet designed to scale and root plane anterior teeth.
  (B) The Gracey 11/12 is an area-specific curet designed to be used on the mesial surfaces of posterior teeth.
  (C) The Gracey 13/14 is an area-specific curet designed to be used on the distal surfaces of posterior teeth.
  (D) The Columbia 13/14 is a universal curet designed for the mesial and distal surfaces of posterior teeth.

177. (B) Polishing does abrade the tooth surface and removes tooth substance. As much as 4 microns may be removed in 30 seconds with pumice paste. This lost tooth substance is not replaced and may become significant after repeated polishing. This surface layer also contains the highest concentration of fluoride.
  (A) This answer is true.
  (C) This answer is true.
  (D) This answer is true.

178. (C) Use of rotary instruments or air abrasive extrinsic stain removal techniques produces contaminated aerosols that contaminate the operatory. Additionally, spatter from the rotating polishing cup or brushes can also be hazardous to the clinician.
  (A) Heat generated during extrinsic stain removal is a hazard to the client, not the clinician.
  (B) Removal of surface fluoride affects the client, not the clinician.
  (D) Use of highly abrasive polishing agents affects the client, not the clinician.

Case C Answers and Rationales

179. (B) The shape of the radiolucency is that of a recently extracted tooth. The bone has not yet regenerated at that site.
  (A) No tooth is present at this site.
  (C) There is no reason to suspect that this area is a carcinoma.
  (D) There is no reason to suspect that this area is a radicular cyst.

180. (D) Antibiotics decrease the effectiveness of oral contraceptives; urticaria is a skin reaction that can be observed when someone has an allergy to a substance such as an antibiotic.
  (A) Correct answer—see D.
  (B) Ampicillin does not cause bruising.
  (C) Correct answer—Urticaria is a vascular reaction of the skin characterized by the eruption of pale, evanescent wheals, which are associated with severe itching.

181. (B) Plastic instruments do not scratch or mar the titanium surface or oxide layer on dental implants. These are the instruments of choice. All the other choices will scratch the implant making it more plaque-retentive and could also alter the titanium oxide coating, which changes the biocompatibility that titanium has with bone.
  (A) Metal instruments may scratch the implants.
  (C) The metal tip on the ultrasonic scaler may scratch the implants.
  (D) Coarse polishing paste may scratch the implants.

182. (C) The implants should be probed only if there are signs of fluid perculation inflammation or occlusal trauma around the implant. When necessary, a plastic probe should be used to probe the implants so that they are not scratched.
  (A) The implants should be probed only when disease is suspected.
  (B) Metal instruments may scratch the dental implant.
  (D) The Nabers probe is designed to probe furcation areas.

183. (B) All of the other choices will not scratch the dental implant and are safe to use. A stainless steel coated wire interproximal brush can scratch the implant. A plastic coated wire interproximal brush is available and can be safely used around the dental implant.
   - (A) Powered toothbrushes could be recommended to this client.
   - (C) Superfloss could be recommended to this client.
   - (D) An end-tuft toothbrush could be recommended to this client.

184. (A) Metal is not recommended for use on dental implants because it can damage the surface of the implant materials.
   - (B) Wood is acceptable for use on dental implants.
   - (C) Nylon is acceptable for use on dental implants.
   - (D) Plastic is acceptable for use on dental implants.

185. (B) This is an endosteal screw type dental implant. Endosteal implants are placed within the bone.
   - (A) Subperiosteal implants are made of a custom-fabricated metal framework that rests over the bone of the mandible or maxilla. This is not the type represented here.
   - (C) Transosteal implants consist of a metal plate that is placed in the lower border of the mandible and has pins extending toward the occlusal surface. This is not the type represented here.
   - (D) The correct answer is provided as choice B.

Case D Answers and Rationales

186. (B) Although blood pressure in the range exhibited by this client is elevated, it is not considered to be a medical emergency. Because the client is taking blood pressure medication, he should be questioned on whether he has been taking his medication and when he last visited his physician.
   - (A) This client's blood pressure is elevated and should be checked more frequently than at a 6-month interval.
   - (C, D) Blood pressure exhibited by this client is not considered to be a medical emergency.

187. (A) Monopril is from the drug class angiotension-converting enzyme (ACR) inhibitor and is used to control elevated blood pressure by dilating the arterial and venous vessels.
   - (B) Zocor is from the class of cholesterol lowering agents.
   - (C) Tavist-D is used for the client's sinus problems.

188. (D) Loss of the vermillion border is commonly seen in fair skinned persons who spend a great deal of time in the sun. This client has recently been treated for basal cell carcinoma and spends much of his time in the sun playing golf.
   - (A) The indistinct vermillion border is not part of the normal aging process.
   - (B) Surgery to correct the cleft lip causes a scar, not the indistinct vermillion border.
   - (C) The client does not report a history of herpetic lesions and it would not cause loss of the vermillion border.

189. (C) It appears that a periapical film packet or some other object came into contact with this film during the developing process.
   - (A) Improper developing technique would affect the entire film, not just one spot.
   - (B) Film exposed to light would be completely dark.
   - (D) This artifact does not appear to be a fingerprint.

190. (B) This dark area is present at a previous extraction site and there is a large restoration just posterior to the area. The radiograph also indicates a small radiopacity in this area, so it is most likely an amalgam tattoo.
   - (A) This area could be a melanoma, but is most likely an amalgam tattoo.
   - (C) There is no reason to suspect that this area is Kaposi sarcoma.
   - (D) This area is not representative of a hematoma.

191. (C) Because this client has several open interdental spaces, bridgework, and furcation involvement in several teeth, the interproximal brush is designed to help the client clean these areas more efficiently.
   - (A) Floss is probably not as effective as the interproximal brush for this client.
   - (B) The interdental stimulator is helpful, but the interproximal brush will work better for this client.
   - (D) The floss aid would be difficult to use on this client.

192. (B) Denture stomatitis frequently occurs on the mucosa of denture-bearing tissues as is the case with this client and is associated with constant irritation to the tissues.
   - (A) *Candida albicans* will produce multiple or diffuse white lesions that appear variably thick, patchy and do not rub off with lateral pressure.
   - (C) This describes an infectious disease of the mouth characterized by swollen, spongy gums, ulcers, and loose teeth.
   - (D) These lesions consist of vesicles that rapidly rupture forming painful ulcers. When appearing on the gingiva, they are often diffusely enlarged, erythematous, and ulcerated.

193. (C) Because this client has very light stain and bacterial plaque on the teeth, selective polishing with a soft toothbrush should be an adequate method. Devices that cause aerosolization such as the airbrasive polisher and oral irrigation should not be used due to the client's cleft palate and related sinus problems.
   - (A) Devices that cause aerosolization should not be used due to the client's cleft palate and related sinus problems.
   - (B) Use of the rubber cup is not necessary on this client.
   - (D) An irrigating device will cause aerosolization and could cause the client problems with his sinus condition.

194. (C) Although A and B are good general recommendations, the client's problem with angular cheilosis is dryness of the lips as exhibited in the photos at the middle left and bottom right on page I–8.
    (A) Staying out of the sun is a good recommendation for this client, but does not affect his angular cheilosis.
    (B) Client should use sunblock because he has a history of basal cell carcinoma, but the sunblock will not affect the angular cheilosis.
    (D) Rinsing with chlorhexidine has no effect on the angular cheilosis.

195. (A) As is indicated on the radiographs and in the photograph at the middle right on page I–8, and due to client's history of frequent sinus infections, the dental hygienist should be especially cautious when spraying water or air into his mouth so that it is not forced through the palatal opening into the sinus cavity.
    (B) Speech difficulties of the client will not affect treatment.
    (C) Tooth sensitivity should not be a primary concern in planning care for this client.
    (D) The client's sinus infections do not pose a problem with care planning.

196. (B) Because this area has involvement with the furca, the Gracey 13/14 curet will adapt well to the distal surface of the mesial root.
    (A) The Gracey 11/12 curet is designed to be used on mesial surfaces of posterior teeth.
    (C) The Columbia 13/14 is a universal curet and could work in this area, but is not the preferred instrument.
    (D) The Gracey 4R/4L is a universal curet designed to remove heavy calculus and is not the preferred instrument for this area.

197. (A) Because this client has porcelain and composite restorations, sodium fluoride is preferred as it does not cause etching of the restorations.
    (B) Acidulated phosphate fluoride could cause etching of the porcelain and composite restorations.
    (C) Stannous fluoride may be astringent and cause burning of the tissues.
    (D) This contains a lower amount of available fluoride than choice A.

198. (D) Polishing dental appliances on the dental lathe is not recommended because undue pressure may be put on the appliance and it may break. Also, because the denture is not sterilized and contains bacteria from the client's mouth, it should not be introduced to the polishing wheel.
    (A) This is an acceptable method for cleaning the partial denture.
    (B) This is an acceptable method for cleaning the partial denture.
    (C) This is an acceptable method for cleaning the partial denture.

Case E Answers and Rationales

199. (D) Use of tetracycline to control this client's acute gingival infection is contraindicated as it may cause discoloration of the permanent teeth in the child. The effect occurs during mineralization of the primary teeth beginning at about 4 months gestation and the permanent teeth near and after birth.
    (A) This antibiotic is acceptable for this client.
    (B) This antibiotic is acceptable for this client.
    (C) Penicillin is acceptable for use with this client.

200. (B) Treatment during the second trimester is the best time to perform elective dental restorative procedures when the client is past the stage of morning sickness and the fetus is not as susceptible to injuries.
    (A) During the first trimester, the embryo is highly susceptible to injuries and malformations.
    (C) Treatment during the third trimester is not advisable as the client may be generally uncomfortable and prolonged chair time could create a supine hypotensive syndrome.
    (D) This answer is incorrect.

201. (B) Tooth buds develop between the fourth and fifth week. Initial mineralization occurs from the ninth to the twelfth week.
    (A) This is not the time when teeth begin to develop in the fetus.
    (C) This is not the time when teeth begin to develop in the fetus.
    (D) This is not the time when teeth begin to develop in the fetus.

202. (D) Although her pregnancy may have triggered the severe response of her gingival tissues, the presence of heavy supra- and subgingival deposits confirm the client report that she has not received dental care for quite some time, which would lead to the conclusion of acute/chronic gingivitis. Furthermore there is no loss of interdental papilla and acute pain, which usually accompanies ANUG.
    (A) The pregnancy may have triggered the severity of the response, but is not the primary cause of the condition.
    (B) There is no loss of interdental papilla and acute pain, which usually accompanies ANUG.
    (C) The bone loss is horizontal and consistent throughout the mouth. The bone loss does not indicate acute periodontitis.

203. (D) The other three choices are rich in calcium; cucumbers are not.
    (A) Yogurt is a good source of calcium.
    (B) Salmon with bones is an excellent source of calcium.
    (C) Fresh spinach is a good source of calcium.

204. (A) From other information given in this case, it is evident that this client is truly concerned about the health of her unborn child and could be motivated to improve her own health as it affects that of her child.
    (B) This method could work, but is probably not the most effective.
    (C) This method is probably not as effective as choice A.
    (D) The client does not report pain.

205. (C) It is possible that this woman's pregnancy MAY have contributed to her present condition. However, use of tobacco and neglect of the mouth are factors that adversely affect the oral condition of all persons, directly.
    (A) Tobacco use adversely affects the oral condition of all persons.
    (B) Not using dental floss contributes to inflamed gingival tissues.
    (D) Neglect of dental care contributed to this client's oral condition.
206. (C) Use of chlorhexidine gluconate has been shown to reduce the amount of bacteria present and promote healing of gingival tissues.
    (A) Fluoridated mouthrinses will not affect healing of the gingival tissues.
    (B) This will have no effect on the healing process.
    (D) Mouthwash is indicated for this client.
207. (C) You do not want to introduce drugs for a pregnant client unless it is absolutely necessary. Resolving the inflammation and making the client's mouth more comfortable is more important than obtaining initial periodontal probing measurements.
    (A) The client has not sought dental treatment for some time. You do not want to make it so unpleasant that she will not return for additional care.
    (B) You do not want to introduce drugs for a pregnant client unless it is absolutely necessary.
    (D) You do not want to introduce drugs for a pregnant client unless it is absolutely necessary.
208. (D) The first three choices as well as stillbirth and infant mortality are possible adverse effects on the fetus by the woman who smokes during pregnancy; mental retardation is not associated with smoking.
    (A) Low birth weight can occur as a result of the pregnant woman's smoking habit.
    (B) Premature birth can occur as a result of the pregnant woman's smoking habit.
    (C) Miscarriage is possible in pregnant women who use tobacco.
209. (C) The bright red color denotes an acute inflammatory condition in which there is increased capillary dilation in the area. The condition also is diffuse because it extends farther than just the papilla and marginal gingiva and into the attached gingiva.
    (A) The gingivitis extends beyond the marginal gingiva.
    (B) The gingivitis extends beyond the marginal gingiva and is bright red, which indicates the acute phase.
    (D) The chronic stage does not exhibit the bright red color.
210. (B) Bulbous papilla fills the gingival embrasure but is no longer pyramid shaped. It is swollen and rounded rather than having a sharp peak.
    (A) The papilla no longer fills the gingival embrasure and loses its pyramid shape.
    (C) Cratering of the gingival margin refers to interdental necrosis with ulceration of the papilla which produces a crater-like defect.
    (D) This term refers to the life-saver shaped enlargements of the gingival margin.

211. (D) Gingival tissues that remain inflamed at the evaluation appointment should be reevaluated for the presence of deposits and removed.
    (A) Gingival bleeding and edema indicate that treatment is necessary.
    (B) Probing should be done, but should be followed by removal of the residual deposit.
    (C) Radiographs should be avoided on pregnant women if possible.

Case F Answers and Rationales

212. (B) Melanin is the pigment that gives color to the skin, eyes, hair, mucosa, and gingiva. It is hereditary and developmental and is most commonly observed in a variety of forms in dark-skinned individuals.
    (A) The tissue does not look cyanotic as it would if subgingival calculus were present.
    (C) There are no amalgam restorations present in this client's mouth.
    (D) The area of discussion is on the gingiva. Dental caries occurs only on tooth surfaces.
213. (D) Use of disclosing solution should not be used as an educational tool because the client is visually impaired. It should only be used to gather information for the clinician.
    (A) Fluoride is indicated because the client has areas of recession and sensitivity.
    (B, C) Reviewing home care is acceptable in planning care for this client.
214. (A) In Class I malocclusion, the molar relationship is such that the mesiobuccal cusp of the maxillary permanent first molar occludes with the buccal groove of the mandibular permanent first molar. Additionally, one or more of the following may be present: the anterior teeth may have crowded alignment; abnormal buccolingual tooth position may be present; or the presence of premature occlusal contacts.
    (B) In this type of malocclusion, the buccal groove of the mandibular first permanent molar is distal to the mesiobuccal cusp of the maxillary first permanent molar by at least the width of a premolar. The mandible is retruded and all maxillary incisors are protruded. This is not true with this client.
    (C) In a Class II Division 2 malocclusion, the buccal groove of the mandibular first permanent molar is distal to the mesiobuccal cusp of the maxillary first permanent molar by at least the width of a premolar. The mandible is retruded and one or more maxillary incisors are retruded. This is not true with this client.
    (D) In a Class III occlusal relationship, the buccal groove of the mandibular first permanent molar is mesial to the mesiobuccal cusp of the maxillary first permanent molar by at least the width of a premolar. This is not true with this client.

215. (C) Use of incorrect angulation results in overlap of images of proximal tooth surfaces.
   (A) Cone cutting would be exhibited as an opaque semicircle near one of the corners of the film.
   (B) A grid effect would be present on the film as the result of the lead insert.
   (D) Double exposure would result in overlapping images on the film.

216. (E) Clinical trials of these two agents have found that they are effective in reducing dentinal hypersensitivity.
   (A) This answer is partially correct. Potassium oxalate is effective in reducing dentin hypersensitivity.
   (B) Benzocaine is used as a topical anesthetic.
   (C) Chlorhexidine is used as an anti-plaque and anti-gingivitis agent.
   (D) Sodium fluoride reacts with potassium oxalate.

217. (B) Potassium oxalate and sodium fluoride react with the calcium within the dentinal tubule to form either calcium oxalate crystals or calcium fluoride crystals, which occlude the dentinal tubule.
   (A) This does not occur.
   (C) This is not true.
   (D) Correct answer is B.

218. (C) Recession and abrasion in the canine and premolar regions is usually a result of an improper vigorous toothbrushing technique.
   (A) Oral habits do not cause recession.
   (B) This client does not report using a powered toothbrush. Movement of the powered toothbrushes are designed to prevent abrasion and recession.
   (D) Use of an abrasive dentifrice alone does not cause recession.

219. (A) The other methods listed are inappropriate for a severely visually impaired person.
   (B, C) Inappropriate method for a severely visually impaired person.
   (D) Inappropriate method for a severely visually impaired person, although if used, the demonstration should emphasize how the correct brushing technique feels in the mouth.

220. (D) It is usually easier for the client if they can rest their hand on your arm so you can guide them. The guide gives verbal notice of approaching changes, such as steps or other obstacles. Always ask the client how they prefer to be escorted, so they can let you know what works best for them.
   (A) Hazards should be moved, especially for the visually impaired person.
   (B) Speaking before touching the client will prevent him from being startled.
   (C) Informing the client of your location puts them at ease.

221. (B) Anatomically the external oblique ridge is imaged as a radiopacity that crosses the necks of the molar teeth. Its location is superior to the internal oblique ridge.
   (A) The internal oblique ridge is inferior to the external oblique ridge.
   (C) This is not an artifact, but an anatomical image.
   (D) This radiolucent band is not in the proper location to be the wall of the mandibular canal.

222. (B) If dentinal hypersensitivity persists after several applications of a desensitizing agent in an area that has severe erosion, application of a composite resin should be considered. This will cause a more permanent sealing of the dentinal tubules and decrease dentinal hypersensitivity.
   (A) This may not be effective because a desensitizing agent has already been used several times without positive results.
   (C) This choice is too radical for the symptoms.
   (D) This has already been done several times without positive results.

Case G Answers and Rationales

223. (A) Invasion of bone by malignant neoplastic lesions produces heterogeneous radiolucency with poorly delineated margins. The impression of bone destruction is indicated by areas of ragged cortical erosion and pocket radiolucency often described as a motheaten appearance.
   (B) Osteoporosis appears as a generalized radiolucency.
   (C) Sclerotic bone formation appears as a radiopacity.
   (D) An ossifying fibroma appears as a mixed radiolucent/radiopaque area in the region of the mandibular premolars and premolars.

224. (D) It is not the amount of food put into her mouth, but the fact that she lacks saliva, which moistens food and is the beginning of the digestive process.
   (A) This is an acceptable suggestion to the client.
   (B) This is an acceptable suggestion to this client.
   (C) This is an acceptable suggestion to this client.

225. (A) One oral complication following radiation therapy to the jaws and accompanying salivary glands is severe xerostomia. This condition is progressive and persistent during radiotherapy, and the salivary tissue damage is irreversible in most cases.
   (B) The client has not been on chemotherapy for several years.
   (C) The client reports that she is not taking any medications.
   (D) It would be very difficult for this client to chew gum. If she did, it would stimulate saliva production, not inhibit it.

226. (B) Yogurt provides a large amount of calcium and protein and can be purchased in low-sugar form. The other snacks are either cariogenic or difficult for this client to eat because she does not have lower teeth.
   (A) Ice cream is cariogenic and therefore not a good choice for this client.
   (C) Cheese would be difficult for the client to eat because she has no mandibular teeth.
   (D) Mints are cariogenic and therefore not a good choice for this client.

227. (B) If the regional lymph nodes are involved, it is usually an indication of metastasis of the lesion. However, the nodes will not be painful.
   (A) This symptom would be expected.
   (C) This symptom would be expected.
   (D) This symptom would be expected.

228. (B) Flexion, a sharp bend or curvature of a root, is similar to dilacerations; however, it affects only the root portion of the tooth.
  (A) Dilaceration is a distortion of the root and the crown from their normal vertical position. It is most commonly caused by trauma to or pressure on the developing tooth.
  (C) Fusion is the formation of a single tooth from the union of two adjacent tooth buds. That is not what has occurred with this tooth.
  (D) Hypercementosis is the excessive formation of cementum around the root of a tooth after the tooth has erupted, which is not what has occurred with this tooth.

229. (A) Although the client has lost her ability to chew whole foods, she should be counselled on her diet and nutritional requirements. She should be encouraged to take vitamin and nutritional supplements that will help her to maintain her strength and not lose any additional weight.
  (B) Although she has lost her lower teeth, she can still consume nutritional foods.
  (C) Xerostomia is not a cause of weight loss.
  (D) The carcinoma did not cause the weight loss.

230. (A) Although several of the choices can contribute to cervical caries, the client's severe xerostomia is most likely responsible for her decay. The relative absence of the lubricating saliva deprives the teeth of a primary defense against carious decalcification.
  (B) Diet may be a contributing factor, but the xerostomia is a more serious complication.
  (C) Poor brushing may be a contributing factor, but the xerostomia is a more serious complication.
  (D) Chemotherapy in itself is not a cause of cervical caries.

231. (A) The supplemental findings for this client indicated that she had bilateral mandibular tori. They appear radiographically as radiopaque areas superimposed on the roots of the mandibular teeth which are close to the tori.
  (B) Osteoporosis appears as a radiolucency.
  (C) Carcinoma may appear as an ill-defined radiolucent area.
  (D) The internal oblique ridge is located in the mandibular posterior.

232. (B) The client's severe xerostomia places her in a high-risk category for dental caries and she should probably be seen at least every 3 months.
  (A) This is too frequent for this client.
  (C) This interval is too long for a client with severe xerostomia and cervical caries.
  (D) This interval is too long for a client with severe xerostomia and cervical caries.

233. (D) Most commercial tomato juices are high in salt content and acid, both of which are irritating to xerostomic oral tissues.
  (A) This would help the client's intake of nutrients.
  (B) This would help the client's intake of nutrients.
  (C) This would help the client's intake of nutrients.

234. (B) This client's history of oral cancer necessitates frequent self-examination.
  (A) It is not necessary to perform this examination daily.
  (C) This is too long for a client with a history of oral cancer.
  (D) This is too long for a client with a history of oral cancer.

235. (D) The other three choices are all signs of oral cancer. A bad odor is not necessarily an indication of a precancerous condition and can usually be related to a sinus infection, respiratory infection, or poor oral hygiene.
  (A) This is a sign of oral cancer.
  (B) This is a sign of oral cancer.
  (C) This is a sign of oral cancer.

Case H Answers and Rationales

236. (B) Mandibular tori are a common observation among adults and appear as bony, hard prominent areas on the lingual alveolar process in the canine region. They usually appear bilaterally.
  (A) Exostosis is a bony growth projecting from the surface of the bone. Although this is a bony growth, when it occurs bilaterally on the lingual of mandibular teeth it is more properly called tori.
  (C) These are calcifications in the salivary gland and would also appear radiographically as a radiopacity. They would not be this large nor appear bilaterally as do the protuberances in these photos.
  (D) Hyperplasia occurs as an increase in the size of the tissue. The increase in size in this case is related to bone mass, not gingival tissues.

237. (A) For the comfort of both the client and clinician, initial removal of heavy deposits is best accomplished with a sonic/ultrasonic scaler.
  (B) If the sonic/ultrasonic scaler were used, it also would remove much of the stain, eliminating the need to use the airbrasive polisher.
  (C) Gingival irrigation is usually not indicated on a client with acute gingivitis.
  (D) If the sonic/ultrasonic scaler were used, it would also remove much of the stain, eliminating the need to use the rubber cup for polishing.

238. (A) The gingivitis in this area is bright red and bleeds easily upon probing, an indication of the acute state of gingivitis. It appears as a ring near the gingival margin and does not confine itself to just the papilla.
  (B) The gingivitis is marginal, but in the chronic phase, the tissue is more cyanotic and does not appear bright red as it does in these photos.
  (C) The gingivitis is not confined to just the papillae.
  (D) The gingivitis is not confined to the papillae and is not cyanotic, which indicates the chronic phase of gingivitis.

239. (D) Radiographically, a periapical abscess is a radiolucency associated with the apex of a tooth. The normal lamina dura and periapical space is lost.
    (A) The anterior palatal foramen is a round to ovoid radiolucency in the midline of the maxilla. The image is not associated with a tooth.
    (B) The lateral foci presents as an ill-defined radiolucency in the region of the lateral incisor, but is not tooth associated. As a result, the periodontal ligament and lamina dura would be evident.
    (C) The greater palatine foramen appears as a round to ovoid radiolucency in the maxillary anterior.

240. (D) Although knowledge of the rest of this information is helpful, the clinician should confirm that the client has taken his medication as prescribed before coming for his appointment.
    (A) This is an important question, but not as important as question D.
    (B) This question should be asked, but question D is more important.
    (C) This is not the most important question to ask.

241. (C) Phenytoin sodium is the generic name of a drug used to control seizures. Some common brand names for this drug include Dilantin, Dilantin Kapseals, Diphenylan, Dilantin Infatabs. One common side effect of this drug is gingival overgrowth.
    (A) Dental neglect does not cause gingival hyperplasia.
    (B) Use of floss does not cause gingival hyperplasia.
    (D) Calculus deposits do not cause gingival hyperplasia.

242. (D) It is best to leave the client alone and move things out of the client's way. If possible, you should turn the client on his side to minimize aspiration of secretions. Never force or place anything in the person's mouth as this may cause breakage of the teeth.
    (A) It is best to leave the client alone and move things out of the way.
    (B) Attempting to place an object in the client's mouth could result in injury to the client or the fingers of the person offering assistance.
    (C) It is not necessary to call for emergency help unless status epilepticus occurs and the seizure lasts longer than 5 minutes.

243. (A) Inflammatory result to pulp pathology may be manifested as a radiolucency associated with the apex of a nonvital tooth.
    (B) No extraction has taken place in this area.
    (C) This is not the result of trauma.
    (D) This is a pathological condition, not a developmental defect.

244. (C) Factors that contribute to the severity of gingival overgrowth include mouthbreathing, overhanging or defective restorations, large carious lesions, dental calculus, bacterial plaque, and other factors that retain plaque.
    (A) Mouthbreathing can contribute to gingival enlargement.
    (B) Heavy calculus can contribute to gingival enlargement.
    (D) Heavy plaque can contribute to gingival enlargement.

245. (A) When the calculus is extremely heavy as it is with this client, it is not possible to get accurate probe readings until the deposits have been removed.
    (B) Bleeding points are a more accurate determination of tissue response than probing depths in a client with heavy calculus deposits.
    (C) The medication causes the hyperplasia, but A is a better explanation for the lack of change in the depths.
    (D) All probes use millimeters as the standard of measurement, so even if the markings are different, recording of the depths should be fairly consistent. However, variations in probe thickness and pressure exerted by the clinician can result in some variation in measurements.

246. (C) For some individuals, certain situations or stimuli can increase the likelihood of having a seizure. Some of these include stress, limited sleep, improper diet, or flickering lights and sound. Some sources of flickering lights include television, video games, or shadow and light outdoors.
    (A) This does not precipitate an epileptic attack.
    (B) This does not precipitate an epileptic attack.
    (D) This does not precipitate an epileptic attack.

247. (D) Scaling and root planing a segment of the mouth to completion allows that area the most benefit, because all deposits are removed and root planing is performed. Gross scaling may leave some areas of subgingival deposit that could possibly cause a periodontal abscess or be more difficult to remove at the next visit after tissue shrinkage occurs.
    (A) Gross scaling may leave some areas of subgingival deposit that could possibly cause a periodontal abscess.
    (B) Local anesthesia may or may not be indicated for this client. The client should be consulted.
    (C) There is no reason to do this.

248. (B) The adjacent tooth was lost due to a bicycle accident. It is most likely that this accident also caused a fracture of the root of tooth #8.
    (A) This is not an artifact.
    (C) The nasopalatine canal does not appear in this area.
    (D) A bend in the film would not appear in the middle of a film.

249. (C) Tooth sensitivity, type of stain, and restorations present must be considered when selecting a polishing agent to remove the stain on this client's teeth. The number of teeth present is not a consideration.
    (A) Tooth sensitivity should be considered.
    (B) Type of stain should be considered.
    (D) Type of restorations present should be considered.

Case I Answers and Rationales

250. (D) A taurodont is a tooth in which the pulp chamber is elongated, enlarged, and extends deeply into the region of the roots. The teeth appear normal in all aspects clinically, but radiographs reveal the abnormally large pulp chamber and the more apical location of the furcation.
   (A) This is a severe distortion of a crown or root caused by trauma during tooth formation. It is usually manifested as a severely angulated root.
   (B) This is the formation of a single tooth from the union of two adjacent tooth buds. The two buds are united through the enamel, dentin, and occasionally the pulp.
   (C) Concrescence is the fusion of two teeth at the root through the cementum only. The teeth involved originally were separated but later joined from excessive cementum deposition.

251. (A) Due to the defined shape and location of this radiopacity, it is most likely the root tip of a primary tooth.
   (B) The image of a supernumerary tooth would show a radiodensity similar to enamel within the image.
   (C) Hypercementosis is an excess of cementum deposited on the root of a tooth. This area is not on the root of the tooth.
   (D) Nutrient canals appear as a radiolucency.

252. (C) After looking at the photograph of the mandibular teeth and the incline of the occlusal plane of this tooth, it is obvious that this tooth is rotated 90 degrees from its intended position.
   (A) The pulp chamber and root are normal.
   (B) Traumatic occlusion does not cause tooth rotation.
   (D) Hypercementosis would appear as a radiopaque area at the apex of the tooth.

253. (A) Use of disclosing tablets or solution is contraindicated for this client due to the loss of enamel and exposure of large areas of dentin on many teeth. Because the dentin is more absorbent, it could pick up some of the color from the disclosing solution, further staining the teeth.
   (B) This should be included in the dental hygiene care plan.
   (C) This should be included in the dental hygiene care plan.
   (D) This should be included in the dental hygiene care plan.

254. (C) Because this is an hereditary condition that affects the enamel of the teeth, there is no reason to believe that this would cause an increased risk for periodontal disease.
   (A) This is a complication from amelogenesis imperfecta.
   (B) This is a complication from amelogenesis imperfecta.
   (D) This is a complication from amelogenesis imperfecta.

255. (B) The first statement is false. Amelogenesis imperfecta results from hereditary factors. The second statement is true.
   (A, C, D) Incorrect answer—see rationale for B.

256. (B) The client's daily use of smokeless tobacco/spit tobacco is the factor most likely causing this lesion. Regular use of spit tobacco can cause homogeneous leukoplakia of the oral mucosa.
   (A) Tartar control toothpastes may cause generalized sloughing of the oral mucosa, not a localized lesion like the one in the photograph.
   (C) Lip biting would produce a scarred appearance.
   (D) There is no basis to suspect that irritation from occlusion caused this lesion.

257. (A) The surface of this lesion has a corrugated (wrinkled) surface with a plaque-like appearance, that is slightly raised with a broad, flat top and a "pasted on" appearance.
   (B) Papules are palpable, circumscribed, solid elevations in skin and less than 0.5 cm in diameter, which does not adequately describe this lesion.
   (C) A fissured surface has a deeply cracked appearance rather than the wrinkled appearance of this lesion.
   (D) Vesicles are circumscribed elevations of skin that are less than 0.5 cm in diameter, containing serum, which gives the lesion a clear or translucent, slightly white appearance; this does not describe the lesion in this photograph.

258. (B) A similar rate of bone loss for adjacent teeth in the dentition results in an even decline in the level of the alveolar bone crest and is termed horizontal bone loss.
   (A) Vertical bone loss is a reduction in height of crestal bone that is irregular and is more commonly localized than generalized.
   (C) This type of defect is seen with advanced periodontitis and usually involves tooth mobility and furcation involvement occurring in localized areas.
   (D) This term is usually used to describe the irreversible tissue loss seen in necrotizing ulcerative gingivitis and necrotizing ulcerative periodontitis.

259. (D) The combination of the vibrations from the ultrasonic/sonic brush strokes and the pressure usually applied by client could cause flaking of the remaining fragile enamel.
   (A) A manual toothbrush can be recommended to this client.
   (B) An end tuft toothbrush can be recommended to this client.
   (C) An interdental brush can be recommended to this client.

260. (B) This tissue change is most likely due to normal pigmentation. He is not taking any medications and does not report using a medicated mouthrinse. Because he uses only spit tobacco, tobacco stomatitis would not be a valid reason for the tissue color.
   (A) Tobacco stomatitis would be white, not brown.
   (C) The client is not taking any medications so this answer cannot be correct.
   (D) Medicated mouthrinses will not cause darkening of the gingival tissues.

261. (A) *Hand* scaling and root planing would be necessary to protect the fragile enamel.
   (B) The ultrasonic scaler could cause flaking of the fragile enamel.
   (C) Rubber cup polishing could cause loss of the remaining fragile enamel.
   (D) The air-abrasive polisher could cause loss or flaking of remaining fragile enamel.

Case J Answers and Rationales

262. (A) The genial tubercle is located in the midline of the mandible and appears radiographically as a radiopaque area to the apical of tooth #24 and #25.
   (B) The nutrient canal is not located between the mandibular anterior teeth.
   (C) The mental foramen is located between the mandibular first and second premolars.
   (D) Exostosis appears as a radiopacity around the apices of teeth.

263. (A) The film was not parallel to the long axis of the tooth or the central ray was not projected perpendicular to the film plane.
   (B) This is the cause of the error.
   (C) This has nothing to do with the error on this film.
   (D) This has nothing to do with the error on this film.

264. (B) Bending of the film prior to exposure will result in a dark line in the processed image.
   (A) A nutrient canal would run in a horizontal direction.
   (C) There is no reason to suspect a fracture.
   (D) This is not an artifact of film processing.

265. (B) This is the American Heart Association recommended regimen for prevention of bacterial endocarditis for persons who are allergic to penicillin/amoxicillin.
   (A) Amoxicillin is a form of penicillin. The client is allergic to penicillin.
   (C) This is not the correct dosage of Clindamycin.
   (D) Amoxicillin is a form of penicillin. The client is allergic to penicillin.

266. (A) This client will most likely be motivated by some type of reward system. Because he is a big Elvis fan, perhaps some small reward, like pictures of his hero, could be given to encourage him to improve his home care.
   (B) This could motivate the client, but answer A is a more likely choice.
   (C) This client is cared for by his sister and it is unlikely that saving money would be a motivator.
   (D) This will not work as well as answer A for this client.

267. (B) Floss fingers are very easy to use and do not require as much manual dexterity as the other methods mentioned.
   (A) This requires a higher level of manual dexterity than choice B.
   (C) His interproximal spaces are small. This would not be a good choice.
   (D) This would not be effective in removing interproximal plaque on this client.

268. (A) The palatine rugae are transverse ridges of fibrous tissue extending across the anterior portion of the hard palate.
   (B) The palatine fovea is not located in this area but in the center of the palate near the soft palate.
   (C) The canine eminence is not located in this area but on the facial of the maxillary canines.
   (D) The incisive papilla is located anteriorly to the palatine rugae.

269. (B) Because this client has limited dexterity and takes pride in doing things for himself, perhaps the use of a powered toothbrush may solve both of these problems. Powered brushes are easy to use and well suited to persons who have limited dexterity.
   (A) Punishment would not be a good motivator for this client.
   (C) This could work, but answer B would probably work better.
   (D) This is not currently working and something else should be tried.

270. (B) Leaning your head to see or trying to use direct vision will not work. Asking the client to raise his chin will allow you to more correctly use indirect vision in this area.
   (A) This will not be effective and only cause neck strain.
   (C) It is not possible to use direct vision effectively in this area.
   (D) This will not be effective.

271. (D) The bite block is useful for individuals who have trouble keeping their mouth open. Use of local anesthesia is not indicated for this client and will not help him keep his mouth open.
   (A) There is no reason to use local anesthesia on this client.
   (B) Placing more pressure on the client's mandibular teeth will not cause him to keep his mouth open.
   (C) This would not be a good choice.

272. (D) Chlorhexidine is proven to be effective in destroying bacteria and reducing gingivitis and is safe and effective for use in clients with special needs.
   (A) Sodium fluoride gels will have no effect on the client's periodontal condition.
   (B) Over-the-counter mouthrinses are ineffective in treating periodontal conditions.
   (C) Sodium fluoride mouthrinse will have no effect on the client's periodontal condition.
   (D) Chlorhexidine is proven to be effective in destroying bacteria and reducing gingivitis and is safe and effective for use in clients with special needs.

273. (C) Many clients with Down syndrome have difficulty in "swishing and emptying." Many times they swallow instead of expectorating, which could cause stomach upset or fluoxide toxicity from the ingestion of fluoride.
 (A) This will have no effect on dental caries activity.
 (B) Many patients with Down syndrome have difficulty in rinsing and end up swallowing, which could cause stomach upset or fluoride toxicity with the use of this product.
 (D) Antiplaque rinses have no effect on dental caries activity.
274. (A) Due to the sedative property characteristic of zinc oxide-eugenol, the sensitivity this client feels in tooth #14 can be alleviated.
 (B) This is not used for a temporary restoration.
 (C) This is not used for a temporary restoration.
 (D) This is not used for a temporary restoration.
275. (D) The film was not parallel to the long axis of the tooth, or central ray was not projected perpendicular to the film plane.
 (A) Incorrect—elongation would have caused the roots to appear longer.
 (B) Incorrect—cone cutting would have produced an opaque semicircle near the corner of the film.
 (C) Incorrect—placing the film backwards would have produced a grid-like appearance on the film.

Case K Answers and Rationales

276. (D) The maxillary molar is positioned lingual to its normal position.
 (A) Underjet occurs when the maxillary incisors are lingual to the mandibular incisors.
 (B) Overbite is the vertical distance by which the maxillary incisors overlap the mandibular incisors.
 (C) Overjet occurs when the maxillary incisors are labial to the mandibular incisors.
277. (C) The wall of the mandibular canal appears as a radiopaque band because the central ray of the beam is directed tangential to the curved surface.
 (A) The image of the styloid process is a radiopaque projection from the base of the cranium posterior to the mandible.
 (B) The hyoid bone is the radiopaque structure below the inferior border of the mandible.
 (D) The facial artery crosses the inferior border of the mandible in the region of the apices of the molar/premolar teeth.
278. (A) In a normal overbite, the incisal edges of the maxillary teeth are within the incisal third of the facial surfaces of the mandibular teeth. In this case, the incisal edges of the mandibular teeth are in contact with the maxillary lingual gingival tissue and it is considered very severe overbite.
 (B) Overjet occurs when the maxillary incisors are labial to the mandibular incisors.
 (C) Crossbite occurs when the mandibular teeth are lingual or facial to the normal position.
 (D) Underjet occurs when the maxillary incisors are lingual to the mandibular incisors.

279. (B) Areas of decalcification appear as dull chalky white areas. When exposed to direct light they show loss of translucency of the enamel.
 (A) This answer is incorrect because the white area is within the tooth surface, not on the surface.
 (C) Because this area appears on an isolated tooth, it is probably not fluorosis; fluorosis is more generalized.
 (D) Trauma would not cause this type of white area.
280. (A) Decalcification occurs in areas where bacterial plaque collects and the client finds it difficult to clean.
 (B) This does not cause decalcification.
 (C) This does not cause decalcification.
 (D) This is not a cause of decalcification.
281. (C) Wooden wedges can remove interproximal plaque and clean around the orthodontic brackets. Additionally they help prevent gingivitis by reducing the amount of interproximal plaque.
 (A) This could be used by the client, but would be more difficult to use than some of the other choices.
 (B) This method would be difficult for a 10-year-old child.
 (D) This could be used but would be difficult for a 10-year-old child.
282. (A) At this age the client will respond more readily to a reward than his concern about saving money or improving his appearance. He has not experienced pain with his mouth so that will not be a good motivator either. Because he is a sports fan, appealing to his spirit of winning may be more successful.
 (B) A client of this age may be concerned by appearances, but A is a better motivator.
 (C) This would not be a motivator for a 10-year-old child.
 (D) The client has no pain associated with his mouth.
283. (A) Saliva or water contamination of the etched surface before a sealant is placed is the number one cause of sealant failure.
 (B) There is no shelf life for phosphoric acid; therefore, this answer is incorrect.
 (C) Rinsing the dental sealant after it has undergone polymerization does not affect its retention.
 (D) Placement of fluoride before the sealant is placed can prevent the mechanical bond that is needed for retention of the sealant. Omission of post fluoride does not affect retention either. To prevent recurrent caries around the sealant, the tooth should receive topical fluoride therapy to help remineralize all the etched areas on the occlusal surface that were not covered with a sealant.
284. (D) This type of film is ideal for showing the presence/absence of permanent teeth as well as supernumerary teeth and other areas of concern that cannot be observed in the mouth.
 (A) Small dental caries cannot be detected using this type of film.
 (B) Calculus cannot be detected using this type of film.
 (C) Because of the angulation of the x-ray beam used to make this film, vertical bone height cannot be readily evaluated.

285. (D) All are benefits of wearing a mouth protector.
    (A) This is one benefit of wearing a mouth protector.
    (B) This is one benefit of wearing a mouth protector.
    (C) This is one benefit of wearing a mouth protector.

286. (C) Because the client will be visiting the orthodontist at least monthly, it will not be necessary to treat him any more than every 6 months. If there are contraindications to this, the orthodontist will make additional recommendations.
    (A) The orthodontist will probably check him monthly so there is no reason for him to be treated on a continued care basis.
    (B) This is too frequent because he will be seeing his orthodontist monthly.
    (D) This is too long for this client to go between continued care visits because he has appliances on his teeth and will need to receive regular in-office fluoride treatments.

287. (A) Instructing the client to concentrate on breathing through the nose rather than the mouth is an effective approach to prevent gagging.
    (B) Rinsing with an antimicrobial rinse does not prevent gagging.
    (C) Topical anesthetics should not be used routinely to obtain impressions.
    (D) In this position, the client is supine with the heart higher than the head on a surface inclined downward about 45°.

288. (C) Shrinkage occurs when alginate impressions are exposed to air, as water in the impression is lost through evaporation. This is called syneresis.
    (A) Solation is the process of transforming a colloid gel into a sol or solution. This process occurs with agar hydrocolloid impression material.
    (B) Gelation is the process when a colloid from a sol transforms into a gel. This occurs while the alginate is in the mouth. However, after it is removed, if it is not poured up soon after the impression was made, the alginate will dry out and shrink.
    (D) Imbibition occurs when an alginate impression is stored in water and absorbs additional water, causing it to expand.

289. (B) Partial loss of the dental sealant necessitates re-etching of the tooth surface before reapplication of the sealant material.
    (A) Partial loss of a dental sealant requires treatment.
    (C) There is no reason to remove the remainder of the dental sealant before replacing it.
    (D) A restorative material is not indicated.

290. (A) Phosphoric acid is used to etch the enamel surface to create surface irregularities and increase the adherence of the dental sealant.
    (B) Etching reduces the surface tension.
    (C) This is incorrect as etching produces a rough surface.
    (D) Incorrect—dentin is not exposed by the etching process.

291. (B) Topical application of fluorides is more effective than systemic fluoride therapy in preventing dental caries in this client. Additionally, mouthrinses are indicated in patients whose oral healthcare is complicated by plaque-retentive appliances.
    (A) Systemic tablets are not indicated if this child lives in a fluoridated area.
    (C) Fluoride gel for at-home use is not indicated for a child who does not have dental caries.
    (D) Although fluoride will probably be applied, the client should also use a daily fluoride rinse.

Case L Answers and Rationales

292. (A) Increasing the kilovoltage results in an increase in film density.
    (B) Decreasing the milliamperage would make the film lighter.
    (C) Increasing the time in the fixer would make the film lighter.
    (D) Decreasing the exposure time would make the film lighter.

293. (B) The closer the object is to the film, the smaller its image.
    (A) The anterior teeth would be elongated if the client was placed too far back in the machine.
    (C) Client movement would cause the image to be blurred.
    (D) Tipping the client's head to the side would result in a film with the teeth foreshortened on one side and elongated on the other.

294. (C) Oral hairy leukoplakia is a white lesion found predominately on the lateral margins of the tongue. Virtually all persons who exhibit hairy leukoplakia are HIV+. The surface may be smooth, corrugated or markedly folded.
    (A) Oral candidiasis will produce multiple or diffuse white lesions that appear variable thick, patchy and do not rub off with lateral pressure.
    (B) Lichen planus is characterized by the chronic occurrence of multiple lesions affecting the skin, mucous membranes, or both. It is usually seen in middle aged persons and may or may not be symptomatic.
    (D) Herpetic lesions consist of vesicles that rapidly rupture forming painful ulcers.

295. (A) Necrotizing ulcerative periodontitis and necrotizing ulcerative gingivitis do not always respond well to traditional therapy due to the patient's compromised immune system.
    (B) It is unlikely that this is the reason for the lack of pocket reduction.
    (C) This should not directly influence pocket depth.
    (D) This would not have an effect on the pocket depths.

296. (C) Devices that produce aerosols are contraindicated on HIV+ or AIDS individuals unless an assistant is available to use high speed suctioning. The Gracey 1/2 curet is designed to be used on anterior teeth and can be used to root plane the root surfaces of these teeth.
    (A) Use of an ultrasonic scaler is contraindicated unless an assistant is available to use high speed suctioning.
    (B) Use of the air abrasive polishing system is ineffective for deposit removal.
    (D) Sickle scalers are designed for supragingival calculus removal and are not effective instruments for root planing.

297. (D) Severe soft tissue necrosis and rapid destruction of the periodontal attachment and bone is one of the most distinguishing features of necrotizing ulcerative periodontitis. Frequently NUP affects several localized areas independently, resulting in islands of severely involved periodontium surrounded by relatively normal tissue.
    (A) Her immunocompromised state did not cause the destruction, but because of it her body was not able to fight the infection.
    (B) This destruction is not limited to the gingiva.
    (C) The client does not have NUG.

298. (A) Diflucan (fluconazol) is an antifungal drug that is used to treat oropharyngeal candidiasis and chronic mucocutaneous candidiasis. It is frequently given to HIV+ individuals who are taking multiple medications and is used as a preventive measure.
    (B) Herpetic lesions are caused by a virus and are not affected by an antifungal drug.
    (C) Pneumonia can be caused from either a virus or bacteria and is not affected by an antifungal drug.
    (D) CD4+ count is not affected by an antifungal drug.

299. (A) Bactrim is the brand name for trimethoprim and sulfamethoxazol which act by interfering with bacterial biosynthesis. However, the drug is not selective in the types of bacteria that are destroyed providing ideal conditions for the overgrowth of yeast and fungi.
    (B) Hairy leukoplakia occurs in persons who are HIV+/AIDS but is not a result of drug therapy.
    (C) This is not a common side effect of this drug.
    (D) This is not a common side effect of this drug.

300. (A) In cases where necrotizing lesions and areas of bone sequestration are present, povidone-iodine rinses and irrigation have been shown to be effective; chlorhexidine has a high alcohol content and is not well tolerated by persons with open lesions.
    (B) This should not be recommended as it has a high alcohol content.
    (C) This is not an appropriate recommendation.
    (D) This should not be recommended as it is ineffective in helping this area to heal.

301. (D) This classification includes the criteria for HIV-periodontitis plus the presence of exposed bone, ulceration/necrosis of the attached gingiva, or complaints of severe, deep "bone pain."
    (A) This is incorrect because this condition is not confined to just the gingiva.
    (B) This answer is only partially correct in that it is HIV-periodontitis, but D is a more complete description.
    (C) This is incorrect because this condition is not confined to just the gingiva.

302. (A) The interdental brush will be helpful in eliminating bacterial plaque from the mandibular anterior teeth. Because there are large spaces and pocketing between the teeth, the interdental brush can remove bacterial plaque as well as stimulate the gingival tissue.
    (B) These could be used, but the interdental brush would be a better choice.
    (C) This would not be effective.
    (D) This would not be effective.
    (E) This would not be effective.

303. (B) Clients with active herpetic lesions on the lips, tongue, or oral mucosa should be rescheduled. In the active state, herpetic lesions can be spread to other areas on the client.
    (A) The appointment should not continue as planned.
    (C) Chlorhexidine will not have any effect on the lesions.
    (D) This is not an acceptable choice.

304. (C) Jewelry not removed before exposure are imaged on the film.
    (A) This can be better described than just as an artifact.
    (B) A processing error would not cause these ovoid radiopacities.
    (D) This does not resemble a napkin chain.

305. (A) This client's immune system is compromised and she smokes cigarettes. Both of these factors affect the inflammatory response and healing response in the gingival tissues.
    (B) Excessive bleeding should not occur after treatment.
    (C) If there is any change in tooth mobility, it should be that the tooth is less mobile.
    (D) This client does not report conditions that would predispose her to bacterial endocarditis.

Case M Answers and Rationales

306. (A) In warmer climates, people consume more water than in colder climates; therefore, the concentration of fluoride in the water should be adjusted downward to 0.6 ppm. (1.0 ppm fluoride, is the overall recommended concentration in drinking water in a temperate climate.)
    (B) This is incorrect for someone living in a hot climate where people consume more liquids than those who live in colder climates.
    (C) This level is too high and could possibly cause fluorosis.
    (D) This level is too high and could possibly cause fluorosis.

307. (B) Due to the child's age and the current fluoride concentration in his drinking water, this is the dosage recommended by the American Academy of Pediatric Dentistry.
    (A) This level is too low to produce the desired dosage level.
    (C) This level is too high.
    (D) This level is too high.

308. (D) The median palatine suture appears as a narrow radiolucent band running superiorly from the crest of the alveolar ridge between the central incisors.
    (A) The nutrient canal is not located in this area.
    (B) The incisive foramen is a small circular radiolucent area between the maxillary central incisors.
    (C) This is not a bend in the film.

309. (B) Physiologic root resorption is the response of the primary tooth to the erupting tooth.
    (A) The film is placed properly.
    (C) There is no fracture line on the root of the teeth.
    (D) This is a normal process, not a pathologic one.

310. (D) This is a term erroneously used by some people to explain decay in the teeth.
    (A) Nonfluoridated water contributes to rampant caries.
    (B) Poor oral hygiene contributes to rampant caries.
    (C) A diet high in sucrose contributes to rampant caries.

311. (C) Open bite occurs when there is a lack of occlusal or incisal contract between certain maxillary and mandibular teeth because either or both have failed to reach the line of occlusion. The teeth cannot be brought together, and a space remains as a result of the arching of the line of occlusion.
    (A) Overjet refers to the horizontal distance between the labioincisal surfaces of the mandibular incisors and the linguoincisal surfaces of the maxillary incisors.
    (B) Overbite is the vertical distance by which the maxillary incisors overlap the mandibular incisors.
    (D) Underjet refers to the horizontal distance between the labioincisal surfaces of the maxillary incisors and the linguoincisal surfaces of the mandibular incisors.

312. (D) Sealants are indicated on 1st permanent molars as soon as they are fully erupted. Deep pit and fissures on molars are highly susceptible to occlusal caries. Because the child has a history of rampant caries, sealants should be applied. Additionally, rampant caries has been associated with diets high in sugar consumption.
    (A) These teeth require a restoration, not a dental sealant.
    (B) This answer is partially correct.
    (C) This answer is partially correct.

313. (B) This is the lethal level for a child.
    (A) This is the lethal level of fluoride for an infant.
    (C) This is the lethal level of fluoride for the average adult.
    (D) This choice is incorrect.

314. (D) Cardiopulmonary resuscitation is not the treatment of choice because the heart and breathing are not usually affected initially by fluoride overdose.
    (A) This is an acceptable treatment for fluoride toxicity.
    (B) This is an acceptable treatment for fluoride toxicity.
    (C) This is an acceptable treatment for fluoride toxicity.

315. (A) Nausea is the MOST common initial adverse reaction to fluoride toxicity. Additional reactions include vomiting, hypersalivation, abdominal pain, and diarrhea.
    (B) This can be a reaction, but is not the most common.
    (C) This can be a reaction, but is not the most common.
    (D) This can be a reaction, but is not the most common.

Case N Answers and Rationales

316. (C) The fluoride level should be 1.2 ppm because this is a colder climate and people do not usually consume as much water as they would in a warmer area.
    (A) This level is too low to produce the desired results.
    (B) This level is too low to produce the desired results.
    (D) This level is too high and could cause fluorosis.

317. (A) The appearance of these carious primary teeth is characteristic of early childhood caries/nursing bottle syndrome.
    (B) Use of bubble gum usually causes interproximal caries.
    (C) Poor home care contributed to this problem, but is not the primary cause.
    (D) This answer is incorrect.

318. (A) The pressure of the thumb against the palate and maxillary teeth during early childhood can cause anterior open bite and overjet, labial flare of the maxillary anterior teeth, and a high palatal vault.
    (B) Mouthbreathing can cause gingival hyperplasia, not white lesions on the palate.
    (C) Tongue thrusting would contribute to protrusion of the anterior teeth, not lesions on the palate.
    (D) Bruxism would affect tooth structure, not soft tissues.

319. (A) Due to the purulence and pain involved, this is a periapical abscess, an acute, localized bacterial infection. Given the clinical and radiographic information, the periapical abscess is the BEST diagnosis of this problem.
    (B) A periodontal abscess generally develops from accumulation of exudate or impaction of food within a prominent periodontal defect. No periodontal defect is present at this site.
    (C) A periapical cyst occurs in association with the root of a nonvital tooth. Most are asymptomatic and are discovered on radiographic examination, which does not fit the symptoms with this case.
    (D) A periapical granuloma is a localized mass of chronic granulation tissue that forms at the opening of a pulp canal, generally at the apex of a nonvital tooth root. This is a chronic process and most cases are completely asymptomatic, which does not describe the client's symptoms in this case.
    (E) Pericoronitis is a condition that produces rapid onset of pain associated with a partially erupted tooth.

320. (A) Children aged 6 and under need to be supervised when using toothpaste because they may consume an unnecessary amount of fluoride and develop fluorosis or fluoride toxicity.
    (B) This is too much and could be swallowed by the child.
    (C) A fluoridated toothpaste should be used.
    (D) This is too much and could be swallowed by the child.

321. (A) To manage a child successfully, a common ground for communication must be established. Using words and phrases that the child can understand will improve the child's trust in the clinician.
    (B) Restraints should be reserved as a last resort for client management.
    (C) Quick and efficient care is only successful if you first receive the client's cooperation. Effective communication skills are necessary for this to occur.
    (D) This may or may not be effective.
322. (C) The deft is used to determine the dental caries experience in primary teeth.
    (A) The Gingival Index (GI) is used to assess the severity of gingivitis based on color, consistency, and bleeding on probing, not caries activity.
    (B) The Plaque Index (PI) assesses the thickness of plaque at the gingival area, not caries.
    (D) The Oral Hygiene Index-Simplified (OHI-S) is used to assess oral cleanliness by estimating the tooth surface covered with debris and/or calculus. It is not used to measure dental caries.
323. (B) If a child consumes sugary (natural or refined) or acidic liquids at bedtime, then it can cause dental caries when allowed to remain in the child's mouth.
    (A) Diluted milk contains lactic acid which can contribute to dental caries when allowed to rest in the child's mouth.
    (C) Organic baby formula can cause dental caries when allowed to remain in the child's mouth.
    (D) Unsweetened apple juice contains acids that can contribute to dental caries when allowed to remain in the child's mouth.

Case O Answers and Rationales

324. (D) The other three choices can be responsible for the formation of periodontal abscesses. Traumatic occlusion alone does not usually cause a periodontal abscess.
    (A) This can be responsible for the formation of periodontal abscesses.
    (B) This can be responsible for the formation of periodontal abscesses.
    (C) This can be responsible for the formation of periodontal abscesses.
325. (A) Cyanotic tissue has a bluish tinge caused by excess concentration of reduced hemoglobin in the blood.
    (B) Bulbous gingiva fills the gingival embrasure but is no longer pyramid shaped. It is swollen and rounded rather than having a sharp peak and covers part of the facial or lingual surface of the tooth.
    (C) The gingiva no longer fills the gingival embrasure and loses its pyramid shape, but the gingiva is not swollen.
    (D) The surface texture appears firm, but has heavier stippling.

326. (B) Because this client has had periodontal surgery in the past and currently has draining fistulas, it would be best to observe her on a more frequent basis to monitor home care and the condition of the recurring fistulas. Additionally, because this client is an insulin-dependent diabetic, delayed healing and periodontal involvement are common complications.
    (A) This is too frequent.
    (C) This is too long for a person with periodontal problem and abscesses.
    (D) This is too long for a periodontally involved client.
327. (C) Due to the shape and location of this radiolucency, it is probably the site of a recently extracted tooth.
    (A) An intraradicular cyst usually appears as a round to ovoid radiolucency.
    (B) The sinus is located superior to the extraction site.
    (D) A radiolucency is present in place of a missing tooth and the client has a history of tooth extractions.
328. (A) The central axis of the tooth has rotated toward the midline thus the tooth is rotated to the mesial.
    (B) This choice is incorrect.
    (C) This choice is incorrect.
    (D) This choice is incorrect.
329. (A) Abrasion is defined as the mechanical wearing away of tooth substance by forces other than mastication. The most common cause is an abrasive dentifrice applied with vigorous horizontal toothbrushing.
    (B) Attrition is the wearing away of a tooth as a result of tooth-to-tooth contact.
    (C) Bruxism is the stress induced behavior of grinding the teeth together.
    (D) Periodontal surgery would affect the gingiva and bone structure not the surface of the tooth.
330. (C) Selective toothbrushing with a soft toothbrush is indicated for this client due to the many areas of exposed cementum and because there is very little stain on the teeth.
    (A) There is no reason to use the air-abrasive polisher on this client.
    (B) A prophy cup is not necessary to remove soft deposits.
    (D) An ultrasonic scaler is not used to remove soft deposits from the teeth.
331. (B) Ultrasonic devices should not be used on or near clients with cardiac pacemakers because they may interfere with the proper functioning of the pacemaker.
    (A) Premedication is not required for a client with a pacemaker.
    (C) There is no reason to refrain from using fluoride on this client.
    (D) The client's vital signs are within normal levels and there is no reason to reassess at each appointment.

332. (B) If the client has failed to eat in her normal pattern, but continues to take her regular insulin injection, an insulin reaction may occur. This is a result of too much insulin in the blood and too little glucose.
    (A) Signs of a diabetic coma include dry, flushed skin and a weak pulse and there may be a fruity odor to the breath. These are not the signs exhibited by this client.
    (C) This client has had extensive dental treatment and it is unlikely that anxiety is the problem.
    (D) Hyperglycemia is another name for diabetic coma. See rationale for A.
333. (B) Client should be given a source of sugar such as orange juice, sweet drinks or hard candy.
    (A) CPR is not indicated on a person who is breathing and has a pulse.
    (C) This is an inappropriate action for this client.
    (D) This is an inappropriate action for this client.
334. (A) The second sentence in the question supports the first sentence.
    (B) This answer is incorrect as both statements are true.
    (C) This answer is incorrect as both statements are true.
    (D) This answer is incorrect as both statements are true.
335. (B) Bluish discoloration of the nailbed is an early sign of cyanosis resulting from inadequate blood oxygenation or peripheral circulation. All of the other conditions listed above are diseases or conditions that can affect persons with diabetes.
    (A) These conditions could affect the person with diabetes.
    (C) This can be a complication of diabetes.
    (D) This is a complication of diabetes.
    (E) This is a complication of diabetes.

336. (B) Class II furcation invasion occurs when the bone loss allows the probe to extend more than a millimeter horizontally into the furcation. However, there is still some bone intact between the roots and the probe will not pass completely through to the opposite furcation.
    (A) Class I furcation involvement exhibits slight bone loss in the furca. The Nabors probe does not penetrate between the roots of the teeth and the radiographic evidence of furcation involvement usually is not found.
    (C) Class III furcation involvement occurs when the interradicular bone is absent but the entrance(s) to the furcation are covered by gingival tissue. Involvement cannot be visualized clinically, but appears as a distinct area of radiolucency on radiographs.
    (D) In Class IV furcation involvement, the interradicular bone is destroyed and the gingiva has receded apically exposing the opening(s) to the furcation. It can be visualized clinically and on radiographs.
337. (B) The Gingival Index (GI) measures gingival inflammation including bleeding, rather than the amount of deposit, calculus or dental caries history.
    (A) Plaque Index assesses amount of bacterial plaque not periodontal status.
    (C) This index measures calculus not periodontal status.
    (D) This index measures dental caries history not periodontal status.

Index

Page numbers in *italics* denote figures; those followed by "t" denote tables.

Frontal lobe of brain, 88
Frontal plane, 58-59
Frontal sinus, 68, *70*
Fructose, 360, 365t
Fructose intolerance, 366
FSH. *See* Follicle-stimulating hormone
5-FU. *See* Fluorouracil
Fulcrums, 538
Full-mouth radiographic survey, 167, *169*
Full-time employment, 696
Full-wave rectification, 151
Fungal infections
  central nervous system, 278
  drug therapy for, 343-344
  respiratory, 271
  of skin, hair, and nails, 268
Fungi, 246, 255-256
Fungicide, 292
Fungiform papillae, 40, 127, *127*
Furcation areas, 129, 462
  classes I to IV, 542
  probe examination of, 542
Furosemide, 345t
Fusing, 429
Fusion, 229
Fusobacterium, 284, 285, 290t
Future trends
  in community oral health planning and
      practice, 664-665
  in National Board Dental Hygiene Examina-
      tion, 10
  in state and regional clinical examinations,
      17-18

*Gage and Pickett: Mosby's 1997 Dental Drug
    Reference,* 325
Galactose, 360, 365t
Galactosemia, 366
Gallbladder, *108,* 109
  lipid intake and disease of, 373
Galvanic corrosion, 408
Gamma rays, 150, 191
Gantrisin. *See* Sulfisoxazole
Gap junctions, 21
Garamycin. *See* Gentamicin
Gas exchange, 106t, 106-107
Gastric artery, 100
Gastrocnemius muscle, 84t
Gastroduodenal artery, 100
Gastroepiploic artery, 100
Gastrointestinal agents, 349
Gastrointestinal system, 107-111, *108*
  infections of, 271-274, 272t
Gauze strips for bacterial plaque control, 504
GCF. *See* Gingival crevicular fluid
Gemination, 229
General anesthetics, 334-335
  interaction with adrenergic drugs, 330
Generators for x-ray machines, 151
Generic names of drugs, 324
Genetic factors
  dental caries and, 632
  periodontal disease and, 455

Genetic recombination, 253
Genetics, microbial, 253
Genitalia, 116-118
  female, 117-118
  male, 116-117
Gentamicin, 343
Genu, *89*
Geographic barriers to oral healthcare, 567
Geographic tongue, 231
Geopen. *See* Carbenicillin
Germ cells, 34
German measles, 269, 290t
Germicide, 292
Gestures, 709
"Ghost-teeth," 230
GI. *See* Gingival Index
Giardia lamblia, 256
Gigantism, pituitary, 113
Gingiva, 449-452, *450*
  amalgam tattoo of, 230
  appearance of, 50
  attached, 450
      measuring amount of, 542-543, *543*
  cancer of, 214
  clinical features of, 452
  definition of, 449
  histology of, 49, 50, 450-452, *451*
  interdental, 450
  interproximal, 130
  marginal (free), 449-450
  melanin pigmentation of, 230
  probe examination of, 540
  recession (atrophy) of, 468-469
Gingival bleeding, 460-461
  prevalence of, 632
  on probing, 543
Gingival Bleeding Index, 461
Gingival crevicular fluid (GCF), 463
Gingival curettage, 473, 474, 545
Gingival fibers, 47, 451, *451*
Gingival fibromatosis, 205-206
Gingival groove, 449-450, *450*
Gingival hyperplasia, 468
  in leukemia, 592, *592*
  phenytoin-induced, 574, 574-575
Gingival Index (GI), 461, 635t
Gingival margin, 449
Gingival pocket, 534, *534,* 535, 541
Gingival sulcus, 450, *450*
  depth of, 461
  microbial proliferation in, 279
Gingival tissue packs, 421
Gingival wall of pocket, 534-535
Gingivectomy, 474
Gingivitis, 285-286, 456, 464-466
  acute necrotizing ulcerative, 207, 285, 455,
      464-465
  associated with hormonal changes, 465
  classification of, 464
  desquamative changes, 465-466
  drug-induced overgrowth, 455, 465
  epidemiology of, 632-633
  indices of, 461, 635t

Gingivitis—cont'd
  linear gingival erythema (HIV), 285, 465
  microbiology of, 284, 284t, 285
  nutrition and, 388
  scorbutic, 465
  stages I to IV, 456-457
Gingivitis index, 460
Glabella, *68*
Gland(s), 25, 64
  adrenal, *112,* 115-116
  Brunner's, 107
  bulbourethral (Cowper's), 116
  endocrine, 25, 64, *112,* 112-116
  exocrine, 25, 64
  mammary, 117
  pancreas, *108, 109, 112,* 115
  parathyroid, *112,* 114-115
  parotid, 107, *108*
  pituitary, *112,* 113t, 113-114
  prostate, 116
  salivary, 128
  sublingual, 107, *108*
  submandibular, 107, *108*
  thyroid, 35, *112,* 114
Glandular fever, 210
Glans penis, 116
Glass ceramics, 430
Glass envelope of x-ray unit, 152
Glass ionomers, 420-421, *422,* 422-423, *424,*
      431, 431t
Glaucoma, 575
Glenoid cavity, 73
Glenoid fossa, 68
Glial cells, 32
Gliding, 65
Glipizide, 348
Globulomaxillary cysts, 216
Glomerular filtration rate, 111
Glomerulonephritis, 289t
Glossitis. *See also* Tongue
  benign migratory, 231
  diet and, 398
  gonococcal, 275, *275*
  Hunter's, 220
  Moeller's, 220
  nutrition and, 388
Glossopalatine arch, *127,* 128
Glossopharyngeal nerve (IX), *90,* 92
Glottis, 104, *104*
Glove powder artifacts on films, 163
Gloves, 294-295, 300
Glucagon, 115, 362
Glucocorticoids, 116, 347
Glucose, 360, 361, 365t, 383
Glucosuria, 115
Glucotrol. *See* Glipizide
Glue sniffing, 350
Glutaraldehyde, 311
Gluteal nerve, 83t
Gluteus maximus muscle, 83t
Gluteus medius muscle, 83t
Gluteus minimus muscle, 83t
Glyburide, 348

Oral histology—cont'd
 oral mucosa, 38-40, *39*
 periodontal ligament, *47*, 47-49, *48*
 pulp tissue, 42-43
 tissues of tooth, 40-46, *41*, *44*
 tooth development, 36-38, *36-38*
Oral hygiene indices, 636t-637t
Oral hypoglycemic agents, 348
Oral irrigation, 472, 507-508
Oral sulfonylureas, 115
Oral surgery, dietary modifications for, 396-397
Orban-type explorer, 544
Orbicularis oculi muscle, 77t
Orbicularis oris muscle, 77t
Orbit, *66*
Orbital fissure, *68*, *71*
Ordinal scale, 654
Organization of book, 18
Orinase. *See* Tolbutamide
Oropharynx, 104
Orthodontics, 47
 bands, 508
 brackets, 508
 cements for, 421
 dietary modifications for, 397
 wires, 508
Orthopnea, 105
Orudis KT. *See* Ketoprofen
OSHA. *See* Occupational Safety and Health Administration
Osler-Vasquez disease, 221
Osmosis, 63
Osmotic pressure, 63
Osseous resective surgery, 474
Ossicles, auditory, 94
Ossification, 64
 endochondral, 29, 64
 intramembranous, 64
Ossifying fibroma, *192*
Osteitis
 condensing, *185*
 deformans (hyperplastica), 226
Osteoarthritis, 580t
Osteoblasts, 29, 64
 nutrient effects on, 383
Osteoclasts, 28, 29
 nutrient effects on, 383
Osteocytes, 28, 29
Osteogenic sarcoma, *189*
Osteoma, 204
Osteomalacia, 227
Osteons, 28
Osteoporosis, 226-227
Otitis externa, 267
Otitis media, 289t, 576t
Otosclerosis, 576t
Outer enamel epithelium (OEE), 36, *37*
Ovarian artery, 101
Ovarian veins, 102
Ovaries, *112*, 117
Overbite, 139, *140*
 excessive, 141

Overdeveloped films, 162
Overdoses, 737-738
Overhang removal
 definition of, 545
 rationale for, 546
Overjet, 139, *140*
 excessive, 141
Overtime, 697
Oxacillin, 341
Oxazepam, 336
β-Oxidation, 372
Oxidation-reduction reactions, 252
Oxidative phosphorylation, 361
Oxidizing agents, 471-472
Oxycodone, 339
Oxygen
 in blood, 95, 106
 diffusion from capillary to tissue, *106*
 effect on composition of oral flora, 280
 intake during pregnancy, 732
 in respiration, 106t, 106-107
Oxygen administration, 727, 733. *See also* Emergencies, medical
Oxygenating agents, 471
Oxyhemoglobin, 95, 106
Oxytalan fibers, 27
Oxytocin, 114

P waves, 97
Pacemakers, 588
Pacinian corpuscles, 94
Packaging instruments, 307
Paget's disease, 226
Paid absences, 699
Pain, 337
 dentinal hypersensitivity, 42, 518-519
 management of, 337t, 337-339
 stimuli for, 519
Paint sniffing, 350
Paint-on systems for fluoride application, 512-513
Paired true-false items on test, 7-8
Palate, 128
 cancer of, 214
 cleft, 35, 577, *577*, 602t
 development of, 35
 hard, *71*, 128
 papillary hyperplasia of, 202
 "pipe smoker's," 212
 pleomorphic adenoma involving, 215
 soft, 128
 during swallowing, 107
Palatine bones, 71
Palatine foramen, *71*
Palatine fovea, *127*, 128
Palatine process, 70, *71*
Palatine raphe, *127*, 128
Palatine tonsils, 98, *127*, 129
Palm grasp, 538
Palmar, defined, 59
Palmar vein, 101
Palmaris longus muscle, 80t
Pancreas, *108*, 109, *112*, 115

Pancreatic duct, 109
Pancreatic enzymes, 110, 360t
Pancreaticoduodenal artery, 100
Pancreatitis, 373
Pandemic, defined, 627
Panoramic radiography, 173-175, *174*
 anatomy on, *181*
 artifacts on, *182*
 for localization, 176-177
 technical errors in, 175
Pantothenic acid, 375t
Papilla(e)
 circumvallate, 40, 127, *127*
 dental, 37, *37*
 filiform, 40, 127, *127*
 foliate, 40, 127, *127*
 fungiform, 40, 127, *127*
 incisive, 128
 interdental, 450
 lingual, 40
 parotid, 127
Papilloma, 40, 201
Papillomatosis, palatal, 202
Papillon-Lefévre syndrome, 455
Parainfluenza, 291t
Paralleling technique, 166, *166*
Parameter, defined, 654
"Parameters of Practice," 758
Parametric statistical procedures, 655, 656
Parasitism, 253, 279
Parasympathetic nervous system, 32, 82, 93
Parasympatholytics, 329
Parasympathomimetics, 327-329, *328*
Parathion, 328
Parathyroid glands, *112*, 114-115
 hyperparathyroidism, 226
Parathyroid hormone (PTH), 114-115
Parenteral drug administration, 326
Parietal artery, 101
Parietal bone, *67-70*, *68*
Parietal lobe of brain, 88
Parietal veins, 101
Parkinson disease, 579-580, 603t
Parkinsonism, 346
Parotid glands, 107, *108*
 pleomorphic adenoma involving, 215
Parotid papilla, 127
Parotitis, 290t
Pars distalis, 113
Pars intermedia, 114
Pars tuberalis, 114
Particulate radiation, 149
Partnership, legal, 769
Part-time employment, 696
Passive behavior, 709
Patella, *66*, 74
Patent ductus arteriosus, 587
Paternalism, 765
Pathocil. *See* Dicloxacillin
Pathogen, 258
Pathology, oral, 200-245
 abnormalities of teeth, 228-230
 acquired immunodeficiency syndrome, 224